C000071662

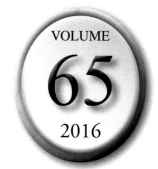

VOLUME
65
2016

INSTRUCTIONAL COURSE LECTURES

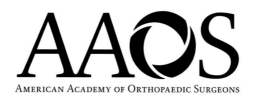

AMERICAN ACADEMY OF ORTHOPAEDIC SURGEONS

VOLUME

65

2016

INSTRUCTIONAL COURSE LECTURES

Edited by

Thomas (Quin)Throckmorton, MD
Associate Professor
Department of Orthopaedic Surgery
University of Tennessee-Campbell Clinic
Memphis, Tennessee

Tad L. Gerlinger, MD
Assistant Professor
Midwest Orthopaedics at Rush
Rush University Medical Center
Chicago, Illinois

Published 2016 by the
American Academy
of Orthopaedic Surgeons
9400 West Higgins Road
Rosemont, IL 60018

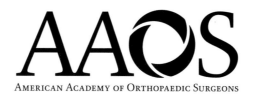

AMERICAN ACADEMY OF ORTHOPAEDIC SURGEONS

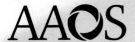

AAOS
AMERICAN ACADEMY OF ORTHOPAEDIC SURGEONS

American Academy of Orthopaedic Surgeons Board of Directors, 2015-2016

David D. Teuscher, MD
President

Gerald R. Williams Jr, MD
First Vice President

William J. Maloney, MD
Second Vice President

Frederick M. Azar, MD
Treasurer

Frederick M. Azar, MD
Past President

Lisa K. Cannada, MD

Howard R. Epps, MD

Daniel C. Farber, MD

Daniel K. Guy, MD

Lawrence S. Halperin, MD

David A. Halsey, MD

David J. Mansfield, MD

Raj D. Rao, MD

Brian G. Smith, MD

Ken Sowards, MBA

Jennifer M. Weiss, MD

Karen L. Hackett, FACHE, CAE (*Ex-officio*)

Staff

Ellen C. Moore, *Chief Education Officer*

Hans Koelsch, PhD, *Director, Department of Publications*

Lisa Claxton Moore, *Senior Manager, Book Program*

Kathleen Anderson, *Senior Editor*

Michelle Wild, *Associate Senior Editor*

Courtney Dunker, *Editorial Production Manager*

Abram Fassler, *Publishing Systems Manager*

Suzanne O'Reilly, *Graphic Designer*

Susan Morritz Baim, *Production Coordinator*

Karen Danca, *Permissions Coordinator*

Charlie Baldwin, *Digital and Print Production Specialist*

Hollie Muir, *Digital and Print Production Specialist*

Emily Nickel, *Page Production Assistant*

Rachel Winokur, *Editorial Coordinator*

Genevieve Charet, *Editorial Coordinator*

Sylvia Orellana, *Publications Assistant*

Instructional Course Lectures, Volume 65

The material presented in the *Instructional Course Lectures, Volume 65* has been made available by the American Academy of Orthopaedic Surgeons for educational purposes only. This material is not intended to present the only, or necessarily best, methods or procedures for the medical situations discussed, but rather is intended to represent an approach, view, statement, or opinion of the author(s) or producer(s), which may be helpful to others who face similar situations.

Some drugs or medical devices demonstrated in Academy courses or described in Academy print or electronic publications have not been cleared by the Food and Drug Administration (FDA) or have been cleared for specific uses only. The FDA has stated that it is the responsibility of the physician to determine the FDA clearance status of each drug or device he or she wishes to use in clinical practice.

Furthermore, any statements about commercial products are solely the opinion(s) of the author(s) and do not represent an Academy endorsement or evaluation of these products. These statements may not be used in advertising or for any commercial purpose.

All rights reserved. No part of this publication may be reproduced, stored in a retrieval system, or transmitted, in any form, or by any means, electronic, mechanical, photocopying, recording, or otherwise, without prior written permission from the publisher.

Published 2016 by the
American Academy of Orthopaedic Surgeons
9400 West Higgins Road
Rosemont, IL 60018

Copyright 2016
by the American Academy of Orthopaedic Surgeons

ISBN: 978-1-62552-435-5

ISSN: 0065-6895

Printed in the USA

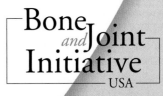

Acknowledgments

Editorial Board
Instructional Course Lectures, Volume 65
Thomas (Quin) Throckmorton, MD
Editor

Tad L. Gerlinger, MD
Assistant Editor

Section Editors
Paul J. Duwelius, MD
Adult Reconstruction: Hip

Thomas J. Errico, MD
Spine

Martin Joseph Herman, MD
Pediatrics

Kerwyn Jones, MD
Practice Management

Paul J. Juliano, MD
Foot and Ankle

Mark D. Lazarus, MD
Shoulder and Elbow

Adolph V. Lombardi Jr, MD
Adult Reconstruction: Knee

Bradley J. Nelson, MD
Sports Medicine and Arthroscopy

John T. Ruth, MD
Trauma

Editorial Board Members
Jonathan E. Buzzell, MD
J. Chris Coetzee, MD
Meghan N. Imrie, MD
Madhav A. Karunakar, MD
Ira H. Kirschenbaum, MD
Patrick M. Osborn, MD
Judith Siegel, MD
Lewis Evan Zionts, MD

Explore the full portfolio of AAOS educational programs and publications across the orthopaedic spectrum for every stage of an orthopaedic surgeon's career, at www.aaos.org/store. The AAOS, in partnership with Jones & Bartlett Learning, also offers a comprehensive collection of educational and training resources for emergency medical providers, from first responders to critical care transport paramedics. Learn more at www.aaos.org/ems.

Contributors

Jeffrey S. Abrams, MD
Clinical Professor, Department of Orthopaedics, Seton Hall University, Orange, New Jersey, Attending Surgeon, Department of Surgery, University Medical Center of Princeton, Princeton, New Jersey

Joshua Abzug, MD
Assistant Professor, Director of Pediatric Orthopaedics, Director of University of Maryland Brachial Plexus Clinic, Deputy Surgeon-in-Chief of Maryland Children's Hospital, Department of Orthopaedics, University of Maryland Medical System, Baltimore, Maryland

Samuel B. Adams Jr, MD
Assistant Professor, Department of Orthopaedic Surgery, Duke University, Durham, North Carolina

Thomas C. Alexander Jr, MD
Orthopaedic Surgeon, Steadman Hawkins Clinic of the Carolinas, Greenville Health System, Greenville, South Carolina

Annunziato Amendola, MD
Professor of Orthopaedic Surgery, Kim and John Callaghan Endowed Chair, Director of Sports Medicine, Department of Orthopaedics and Rehabilitation, University of Iowa Hospitals and Clinics, Iowa City, Iowa

Paul A. Anderson, MD
Professor, Department of Orthopedic Surgery and Rehabilitation, University of Wisconsin, Madison, Wisconsin

Michael Archdeacon, MD
Professor and Chairman, Department of Orthopaedic Surgery, University of Cincinnati, College of Medicine, Cincinnati, Ohio

George S. Athwal, MD, FRCSC
Associate Professor, Roth/McFarlane Hand and Upper Limb Center, The University of Western Ontario, London, Ontario, Canada

Matthew S. Austin, MD
Associate Professor of Orthopaedic Surgery, Rothman Institute, Thomas Jefferson University Hospital, Philadelphia, Pennsylvania

Sameer Badarudeen, MD, MPH
Fellow, Department of Orthopaedic Surgery, University of Louisville, Louisville, Kentucky

Donald S. Bae, MD
Associate Professor of Orthopaedic Surgery, Department of Orthopaedic Surgery, Boston Children's Hospital/Harvard Medical School, Boston, Massachusetts

John W. Barrington, MD
Orthopaedic Surgeon, Joint Replacement Center of Texas, Plano Orthopaedics and Sports Medicine Center, Plano, Texas

Carl J. Basamania, MD
Orthopaedic Surgeon, The Polyclinic, Seattle, Washington

William R. Beach, MD
Orthopaedic Surgeon, Tuckahoe Orthopaedics, Richmond, Virginia

Paul E. Beaulé, MD, FRCSC
Professor of Surgery, Department of Orthopedic Surgery, University of Ottawa, Ottawa, Ontario, Canada

Keith R. Berend, MD
Vice President, Joint Implant Surgeons, New Albany, Ohio

Michael E. Berend, MD
Midwest Center for Joint Replacement, Indianapolis, Indiana

Richard A. Berger, MD
Assistant Professor, Department of Arthroplasty, Rush University Medical Center, Chicago, Illinois

Jack M. Bert, MD
Physician, Minnesota Bone and Joint Specialists, Adjunct Clinical Professor, University of Minnesota School of Medicine, Woodbury, Minnesota

Alan H. Beyer, MD
Executive Medical Director, Hoag Orthopedic Institute, Irvine, California

Mohit Bhandari, MD, PhD, FRCSC
Professor and Academic Chair, Department of Surgery, Division of Orthopaedic Surgery, McMaster University, Hamilton, Ontario, Canada

Jesse Bible, MD, MHS
Orthopaedic Spine Fellow, Department of Orthopaedics, University of Pittsburgh Medical Center, Pittsburgh, Pennsylvania

Eric M. Bluman, MD, PhD
Assistant Professor, Department of Orthopaedic Surgery, Harvard Medical School, Boston, Massachusetts

Jared Bookman, BA
Medical Student, NYU School of Medicine, New York, New York

Joseph Bosco, MD
Vice Chair of Clinical Affairs, Department of Orthopaedic Surgery, NYU Hospital for Joint Diseases, New York, New York

Christina L. Boulton, MD
Assistant Professor, Division of Orthopaedic Traumatology, R. Adams Cowley Shock Trauma Center, University of Maryland School of Medicine, Baltimore, Maryland

Daniel Bouton, MD
Resident, Department of Orthopedic Surgery, Akron General Medical Center, Akron, Ohio

Kevin J. Bozic, MD, MDA
Professor and Chair, Department of Surgery and Perioperative Care, Dell Medical School at the University of Texas at Austin, Austin, Texas

Jonathan P. Braman, MD
Associate Professor, Department of Orthopaedic Surgery, University of Minnesota, Minneapolis, Minnesota

Brian Brighton, MD, MPH
Pediatric Orthopaedic Surgeon, Department of Orthopaedic Surgery, Carolinas HealthCare System/Levine Children's Hospital, Charlotte, North Carolina

Darrel S. Brodke, MD
Professor and Vice Chair, Department of Orthopaedics, University of Utah, Salt Lake City, Utah

Stephen S. Burkhart, MD
Orthopaedic Surgeon, The San Antonio Orthopaedic Group, San Antonio, Texas

Jeffrey Cherian, DO
Orthopedic Research Fellow, Rubin Institute for Advanced Orthopedics, Sinai Hospital of Baltimore, Baltimore, Maryland

Emilie V. Cheung, MD
Associate Professor, Department of Orthopedic Surgery, Stanford University, Redwood City, California

Kenneth Chin, MD
Orthopaedic Resident, Department of Orthopaedics, University of Maryland, Baltimore, Maryland

Christopher P. Chiodo, MD
Foot and Ankle Division Chief, Department of Orthopedic Surgery, Brigham and Women's Hospital/Harvard Medical School, Boston, Massachusetts

Theodore J. Choma, MD
Professor and Vice Chairman, Department of Orthopaedic Surgery, University of Missouri, Columbia, Missouri

John Clohisy, MD
Daniel C. and Betty B. Viehmann Distinguished Professor of Orthopaedic Surgery, Department of Orthopaedic Surgery, Washington University School of Medicine, St. Louis, Missouri

Edward V. Craig, MD, MPH
Attending Surgeon, Hospital for Special Surgery, New York, New York

Michael B. Cross, MD
Assistant Attending Orthopaedic Surgeon, Department of Adult Reconstruction and Joint Replacement, Hospital for Special Surgery, New York, New York

Alan H. Daniels, MD
Assistant Professor, Department of Orthopedics, Brown University, Providence, Rhode Island

David Dare, MD
Orthopaedic Surgery Resident, Department of Academic Training, Hospital for Special Surgery, New York, New York

Roberto Diaz, MD
Orthopaedic Surgery Fellow, Department of Orthopaedic Surgery, Stanford University, Redwood City, California

David M. Dines, MD
Senior Attending, Sports Medicine and Shoulder Service, Hospital for Special Surgery, New York, New York

Joshua S. Dines, MD
Orthopedic Surgeon, Sports Medicine and Shoulder Service, Hospital for Special Surgery, New York, New York

James P. Doran, MD
Adult Reconstruction Research Fellow, Department of Orthopaedic Surgery, NYU Langone Medical Center, Hospital for Joint Diseases, New York, New York

Lawrence D. Dorr, MD
Professor of Clinical, Department of Orthopaedic Surgery, Keck School of Medicine of University of Southern California, Los Angeles, California

Naven Duggal, MD
Department of Orthopaedic Surgery, Syracuse Orthopedic Specialists, Syracuse, New York

Mark E. Easley, MD
Associate Professor, Department of Orthopaedic Surgery, Duke University, Durham, North Carolina

Craig P. Eberson, MD
Chief, Division of Pediatric Orthopaedics, Associate Professor, Department of Orthopaedics, Alpert Medical School at Brown University, Providence, Rhode Island

Emmanuel Edusei, BS
Research Assistant, Department of Orthopaedic Surgery, NYU Hospital for Joint Diseases, New York, New York

T. Bradley Edwards, MD
Attending Shoulder Surgeon, Fondren Orthopedic Group, Texas Orthopedic Hospital, Houston, Texas

Randa Elmallah, MD
Orthopedic Research Fellow, Rubin Institute for Advanced Orthopedics, Sinai Hospital of Baltimore, Baltimore, Maryland

Mouhanad M. El-Othmani, MD
Post-Doctorate Research Fellow, Department of Orthopedic Surgery, Southern Illinois University School of Medicine, Springfield, Illinois

Larry D. Field, MD
Physician, Department of Orthopaedics, Mississippi Sports Medicine and Orthopaedic Center, Jackson, Mississippi

Mark A. Frankle, MD
Chief of Shoulder and Elbow Surgery, Department of Shoulder and Elbow Surgery, Florida Orthopaedic Institute, Tampa, Florida

Leesa M. Galatz, MD
Professor of Orthopaedic Surgery, Department of Orthopaedic Surgery, Washington University School of Medicine, St. Louis, Missouri

Kevin L. Garvin, MD
Professor and Chair, Department of Orthopaedic Surgery and Rehabilitation, University of Nebraska Medical Center, Omaha, Nebraska

C. David Geier Jr, MD
Medical Director, East Cooper Sports Medicine, Sport Medicine Specialists of Charleston, East Cooper Medical Center, Mount Pleasant, South Carolina

Mohit Gilotra, MD
Assistant Professor, Department of Orthopaedic Surgery, University of Maryland, Baltimore, Maryland

Michael Ginnetti, BSc
Medical Student, Division of Orthopaedics and Rehabilitation, Southern Illinois University School of Medicine, Springfield, Illinois

Nicholas J. Giori, MD, PhD
Associate Professor, Department of Orthopedic Surgery, Stanford University, Stanford, California

Tyson Gofton, PhD
Guelph, Ontario, Canada

Wade T. Gofton, BScH, MD, MEd, FRCSC
Physician, Associate Professor, Department of Surgery, Division of Orthopedic Surgery, University of Ottawa, Ottawa, Ontario, Canada

Tyler A. Gonzalez, MD, MBA
Orthopaedic Surgery Resident, Department of Orthopaedic Surgery, Brigham and Women's Hospital, Boston, Massachusetts

A. Seth Greenwald, DPhil (Oxon)
Director, Orthopaedic Research Laboratories, Cleveland, Ohio

Gordon I. Groh, MD
Orthopedic Surgeon, Blue Ridge Bone & Joint, Asheville, North Carolina

Christopher E. Gross, MD
Assistant Professor, Department of Orthopaedic Surgery, Medical University of South Carolina, Charleston, South Carolina

Kenneth Gundle, MD
Resident Orthopaedic Surgeon, Department of Orthopaedics and Sports Medicine, University of Washington, Seattle, Washington

William Hamilton, MD
Anderson Orthopaedic Research Institute, Alexandria, Virginia

Alicia Harrison, MD
Assistant Professor, Department of Orthopaedic Surgery, University of Minnesota, Minneapolis, Minnesota

Robert A. Hart, MD
Professor, Department of Orthopaedics and Rehabilitation, Oregon Health & Science University, Portland, Oregon

Richard J. Hawkins, MD
Orthopaedic Surgeon, Steadman Hawkins Clinic of the Carolinas, Greenville Health System, Greenville, South Carolina

Brandon J. Hayes, MD
Clinical Foot and Ankle Fellow, Department of Orthopaedic Surgery, Harvard School of Medicine, Boston, Massachusetts

William L. Healy, MD
Kaplan Joint Center, Newton Wellesley Hospital, Massachusetts General Hospital, Boston, Massachusetts

Martin Herman, MD
Orthopaedic Surgeon, Department of Orthopedic Surgery and Pediatrics, Drexel University College of Medicine, Philadelphia, Pennsylvania

Kirby D. Hitt, MD
Head of Adult Reconstruction and Joint Replacement, Baylor Scott and White Healthcare
Assistant Professor, Texas A&M University, Temple, Texas

Christine Ann Ho, MD
Associate Professor, Department of Orthopaedics, University of Texas Southwestern Medical School, Texas Scottish Rite Hospital for Children–Children's Healthcare, Dallas, Texas

Bernard D. Horn, MD
Assistant Professor, Clinical Orthopaedic Surgery, Department of Orthopaedic Surgery, Perelman School of Medicine University, Philadelphia, Pennsylvania

Patrick Horrigan, MD
Resident Physician, Department of Orthopaedic Surgery, University of Minnesota, Minneapolis, Minnesota

Jason M. Hurst, MD
Senior Associate, Joint Implant Surgeons, New Albany, Ohio

Richard Iorio, MD
Chief of Adult Reconstruction, Department of Orthopaedic Surgery, NYU Langone Medical Center, Hospital for Joint Diseases, New York, New York

David S. Jevsevar, MD, MBA
Chair, Department of Orthopaedics, Dartmouth-Hitchcock Medical Center, Lebanon, New Hampshire

Clifford B. Jones, MD, FACS
Chief, Centers for Orthopaedic Trauma and Bone Health, The CORE Institute, Banner University of Arizona, Musculoskeletal Health Institute, Phoenix, Arizona

Jonathan R.M. Kaplan, MD
Orthopaedic Surgery Foot and Ankle Fellow, Institute for Foot & Ankle Reconstruction, Mercy Medical Center, Baltimore, Maryland

John W. Karl, MD, MPH
Resident, Department of Orthopaedic Surgery,
Columbia University Medical Center, New York,
New York

W. Ben Kibler, MD
Medical Director, Shoulder Center of Kentucky,
Lexington Clinic, Lexington, Kentucky

Paul R. Kim, MD, FRCSC
Associate Professor, Division of Orthopaedics,
University of Ottawa, Ottawa, Ontario, Canada

Karl Koenig, MD, MS
Division Leader, Arthroplasty, Department of
Orthopaedics, Dartmouth-Hitchcock Medical
Center, Lebanon, New Hampshire

Stephen A. Kottmeier, MD
Clinical Professor of Orthopedic Surgery, Director
of Orthopedic Trauma, Department of Orthopedic
Surgery, State University of New York Health
Science Center at Stony Brook, Stony Brook, New
York

Scott H. Kozin, MD
Chief of Staff, Shriners Hospital for Children,
Philadelphia, Pennsylvania

John E. Kuhn, MD
Kenneth D. Schermerhorn Professor of
Orthopaedics and Rehabilitation, Department of
Orthopaedic Surgery, Vanderbilt University Medical
School, Nashville, Tennessee

Alexander Kurdi, BSc
Medical Student, Southern Illinois University School
of Medicine, Springfield, Illinois

J.M. Lane, MD
Professor of Orthopaedic Surgery, Department of
Orthopaedics, Weill Cornell Medical College, New
York, New York

Carlos J. Lavernia, MD
Director, The Center for Advanced Orthopedics,
Chief of Orthopedics, Larkin Hospital, Larkin
Community Hospital, South Miami, Florida

Joon Y. Lee, MD
Associate Professor, Department of Orthopaedics,
University of Pittsburgh Medical Center, Pittsburgh,
Pennsylvania

J. Martin Leland III, MD
Orthopaedic Sports Surgeon and Medical Director
of Sports Medicine, Division of Orthopaedic
Surgery, University Hospitals Geauga Medical
Center, Cleveland, Ohio

Brett Levine, MD, MS
Residency Program Director and Assistant Professor,
Department of Orthopedics, Rush University
Medical Center, Chicago, Illinois

William N. Levine, MD
Frank E. Stinchfield Professor and Chairman,
Department of Orthopedic Surgery, New York
Presbyterian/Columbia University Medical Center,
New York, New York

Courtland Lewis, MD
Physician in Chief, Hartford Healthcare Bone &
Joint Institute, Hartford, Connecticut

Moe R. Lim, MD
Associate Professor, Department of Orthopaedics,
University of North Carolina–Chapel Hill, Chapel
Hill, North Carolina

Adolph V. Lombardi Jr, MD, FACS
President, Joint Implant Surgeons, New Albany,
Ohio

Adam J. Lorenzetti, MD
Orthopaedic Surgeon, Department of Shoulder
and Elbow Surgery, Florida Orthopaedic Institute,
Tampa, Florida

Dean G. Lorich, MD
Associate Director, Orthopaedic Trauma Service,
Hospital for Special Surgery, New York, New York

Arthur L. Malkani, MD
Professor, Chief of Adult Reconstruction,
Department of Orthopaedic Surgery, University of
Louisville, Louisville, Kentucky

Dean K. Matsuda, MD
Director, Hip Arthroscopy, Department of
Orthopedics, DISC Sports and Spine Centers,
Marina del Rey, California

Robert A. McGuire, MD
Professor, Department of Orthopaedics, University
of Mississippi Medical Center, Jackson, Mississippi

Louis F. McIntyre, MD
Louis F. McIntyre, MD, PC, White Plains, New York

Mark A. Mighell, MD
Shoulder and Elbow Surgeon, Florida Orthopaedic Institute, Tampa, Florida

William M. Mihalko, MD, PhD
Professor and J.R. Hyde Chair of Excellence in Biomedical Engineering, Department of Orthopaedic Surgery and Biomedical Engineering, Campbell Clinic, University of Tennessee, Memphis, Tennessee

Hassan R. Mir, MD, MBA
Associate Professor of Orthopaedic Trauma, Department of Orthopaedics and Rehabilitation, Vanderbilt University, Nashville, Tennessee

Nicholas G. Mohtadi, MD, MSc, FRCSC
Clinical Professor, Sports Medicine Centre, University of Calgary, Calgary, Alberta, Canada

Michael A. Mont, MD
Director, Rubin Institute for Advanced Orthopedics, Sinai Hospital of Baltimore, Baltimore, Maryland

Brent J. Morris, MD
Orthopedic Surgeon, Lexington Clinic, Lexington, Kentucky

Michael J. Morris, MD
Senior Associate, Joint Implant Surgeons, New Albany, Ohio

Mark S. Myerson, MD
Medical Director, Institute for Foot & Ankle Reconstruction, Mercy Medical Center, Baltimore, Maryland

Peggy L. Naas, MD, MBA
Chief Medical Officer, Healthcare Performance Improvement, Virginia Beach, Virginia

Caleb Netting, MD
Resident, Department of Orthopaedic Surgery, University of Ottawa, Ottawa, Ontario, Canada

Mai Nguyen, MD
Resident Physician, Department of Orthopaedics and Rehabilitation, University of Iowa Hospitals and Clinics, Iowa City, Iowa

James A. Nunley, MD
Goldner Jones Professor of Orthopaedic Surgery, Director of Foot and Ankle Surgery, Duke University, Durham, North Carolina

Ryan M. Nunley, MD
Associate Professor, Department of Orthopaedic Surgery, Washington University, St. Louis, Missouri

Michael J. O'Brien, MD
Assistant Professor, Department of Orthopaedics, Tulane University School of Medicine, New Orleans, Louisiana

Alex Pagé, MD, FRCSC
Arthroplasty Fellow, Department of Orthopaedics, University of Ottawa, Ottawa, Ontario, Canada

Gurpal S. Pannu, MD
Orthopaedic Surgery Resident, Department of Orthopaedic Surgery, Drexel University College of Medicine, Philadelphia, Pennsylvania

Steven R. Papp, MD, MSc, FRCSC
Orthopaedic Surgeon, Assistant Professor, Department of Orthopaedic Surgery, University of Ottawa, Ottawa, Ontario, Canada

Brian S. Parsley, MD
Clinical Associate Professor, Barnhart Department of Orthopaedic Surgery, Baylor College of Medicine, Houston, Texas

Javad Parvizi, MD, FRCS
Professor of Orthopedic Surgery, Joint Replacement Program, Rothman Institute, Philadelphia, Pennsylvania

Vincent D. Pellegrini Jr, MD
John A. Siegling Professor and Chair, Department of Orthopaedics, Medical University of South Carolina, Charleston, South Carolina

Marc J. Philippon, MD
The Steadman Clinic, The Steadman Philippon Research Institute, Vail, Colorado

Mark A. Piasio, MD, MBA
Medical Director, Department of Quality Management and Provider Strategy, Highmark, Pittsburgh, Pennsylvania

Matthew Provencher, MD
Chief, Sports Medicine Service, Massachusetts
General Hospital, Boston, Massachusetts

Peter Pyrko, MD, PhD
Arthroplasty Fellow, Joint Replacement Program,
Rothman Institute, Philadelphia, Pennsylvania

Glenn Rechtine, MD
Spine Surgeon, Department of Spine/Orthopaedics/
Surgery, Charles George VA Medical Center,
Asheville, North Carolina

Eric T. Ricchetti, MD
Staff, Department of Orthopaedic Surgery,
Cleveland Clinic, Cleveland, Ohio

Jeffrey A. Rihn, MD
Associate Professor, Department of Orthopaedic
Surgery, Thomas Jefferson University, The Rothman
Institute, Philadelphia, Pennsylvania

Todd F. Ritzman, MD
Director of Education, Department of Orthopedic
Surgery, Akron Children's Hospital, Akron, Ohio

Aaron G. Rosenberg, MD
Professor of Surgery, Department of Orthopedic
Surgery, Rush University Medical Center, Chicago,
Illinois

Elliot Row, MD
Orthopaedic Surgery Resident-PGY4, Department
of Orthopaedic Surgery and Department of Trauma,
Stony Brook University Hospital, Stony Brook, New
York

George V. Russell Jr, MD, MBA
Professor and Chairman, Department of
Orthopaedics, University of Mississippi Medical
Center, Jackson, Mississippi

Richard K.N. Ryu, MD
Senior Surgeon, The Ryu Hurvitz Orthopedic
Clinic, Santa Barbara, California

Ranjan Sachdev, MD, MBA, CHC
Sachdev Orthopaedics, Easton, Pennsylvania

Marc R. Safran, MD
Professor, Department of Orthopaedic Surgery,
Stanford University, Redwood City, California

Jamal K. Saleh, BSc
Second Year Medical Student, San Francisco,
California

Jasmine Saleh, MD
Intramural Research Training Award Fellow,
National Institutes of Health, Bethesda, Maryland

**Khaled J. Saleh, BSc, MD, MSc, FRCSC,
MHCM**
Professor and Chair of the Department of
Orthopaedic Surgery, Director of Clinical and
Translational Research, Southern Illinois University
School of Medicine, Springfield, Illinois

Charles Saltzman, MD
Professor and Chair, Department of Orthopaedics,
University of Utah, Salt Lake City, Utah

Thomas G. Sampson, MD
Medical Director of Post Street Surgery Center,
Orthopaedic Consultant at the Veterans
Administration Hospital, San Francisco, California

Joaquin Sanchez-Sotelo, MD, PhD
Consultant and Professor of Orthopedics,
Department of Orthopedic Surgery, Mayo Clinic,
Rochester, Minnesota

Sheila Sanders, RN, BSN, DNC
Nurse Clinician, Department of Orthopaedics, Rush
University Medical Center, Chicago, Illinois

Felix H. Savoie III, MD
Professor and Vice Chairman, Department of
Orthopaedics, Tulane University School of
Medicine, New Orleans, Louisiana

Giles R. Scuderi, MD
Vice President, Orthopaedic Service Line, North
Shore LIJ Health System, New York, New York

Peter K. Sculco, MD
Adult Reconstruction Fellow, Department of
Orthopedic Surgery, Mayo Clinic, Rochester,
Minnesota

Kevin G. Shea, MD
Department of Orthopedic Surgery, St. Lukes
Health System, Boise, Idaho

Rafael J. Sierra, MD
Professor, Department of Orthopedic Surgery, Mayo
Clinic, Rochester, Minnesota

Lance Silverman, MD
Orthopaedic Surgeon, Silverman Ankle & Foot, Edina, Minnesota

Peter Simon, PhD
Staff Scientist, Phillip Spiegel Orthopaedic Research Laboratory, Foundation for Orthopaedic Research and Education, Tampa, Florida

James Slover, MD, MS
Assistant Professor, Department of Orthopaedic Surgery, NYU Langone Medical Center, Hospital for Joint Diseases, New York, New York

Jeremy T. Smith, MD
Associate Orthopaedic Surgeon, Department of Orthopaedics, Brigham and Women's Hospital, Boston, Massachusetts

Michael Solomon, MBChB, FRACS (Ortho)
Doctor, Department of Orthopaedics, Prince of Wales Hospital, Sydney, New South Wales, Australia

John W. Sperling, MD, MBA
Consultant, Department of Orthopedics, Professor of Orthopedic Surgery, Mayo Clinic College of Medicine, Department of Orthopedic Surgery, Mayo Clinic, Rochester, Minnesota

Jeffrey B. Stambough, MD
Resident, Orthopaedic Surgery, Department of Orthopaedic Surgery, Washington University, St. Louis, Missouri

Scott P. Steinmann, MD
Consultant, Department of Orthopedic Surgery, Mayo Clinic, Rochester, Minnesota

Geoffey P. Stone, MD
Orthopaedic Surgeon, Department of Shoulder and Elbow Surgery, Florida Orthopaedic Institute, Tampa, Florida

Alexandra Styhl, BA
Clinical Research Intern, Intermountain Orthopedics, St. Luke's, Boise, Idaho

Tanishq Suryavanshi
Student, Department of Health Sciences, McMaster University Faculty of Health Sciences, Hamilton, Ontario, Canada

Benjamin W. Szerlip, DO
Shoulder and Elbow Fellow, Fondren Orthopedic Group, Texas Orthopedic Hospital, Houston, Texas

Robert Z. Tashjian, MD
Associate Professor, Department of Orthopaedics, University of Utah School of Medicine, Salt Lake City, Utah

Collin Tebo, BA
Medical Student, Department of Orthopaedic Surgery, Hospital for Special Surgery, New York, New York

John M. Tokish, MD
Orthopaedic Surgeon, Steadman Hawkins Clinic of the Carolinas, Greenville Health System, Greenville, South Carolina

Paul Tornetta III, MD
Director, Orthopaedic Trauma, Department of Orthopaedic Surgery, Boston Medical Center, Boston, Massachusetts

Tony H. Tzeng, BS
Research Fellow, Department of Orthopedic Surgery, Southern Illinois University School of Medicine, Springfield, Illinois

Ekaterina Urch, MD
Orthopaedic Surgery Resident, Department of Orthopaedic Surgery, Hospital for Special Surgery, New York, New York

Roger P. van Riet, MD, PhD
Orthopedic Surgeon, Department of Orthopedic Surgery, AZ Monica, Antwerp, Belgium

Jesus M. Villa, MD
Research Fellow, The Center for Advanced Orthopedics at Larkin Hospital, Arthritis Surgery Research Foundation, South Miami, Florida

Benjamin Voss, BS
Southern Illinois University School of Medicine, Springfield, Illinois

J. Tracy Watson, MD
Professor of Orthopaedic Surgery, Chief of Orthopaedic Trauma Service, Saint Louis University School of Medicine, St. Louis, Missouri

Stuart L. Weinstein, MD
Ignacio V. Ponseti Chair and Professor, Department of Orthopaedic Surgery, University of Iowa, Iowa City, Iowa

Jessica Jane Wingfield, MD
Resident, Department of Orthopedic Surgery, University of Texas Southwestern, Dallas, Texas

Brian R. Wolf, MD, MS
Congdon Professor, Vice Chairman and Head Team Physician, Department of Orthopaedics and Rehabilitation, University of Iowa, Iowa City, Iowa

Erik Wright, BS
Medical Student, Department of Orthopedics, Southern Illinois School of Medicine, Springfield, Illinois

Stephen Yu, MD
Adult Reconstruction Research Fellow, Department of Orthopaedic Surgery, NYU Hospital for Joint Diseases, New York, New York

Stephen J. Zabinski, MD
Director of the Division of Orthopedic Surgery, Shore Orthopedic University Associates, Shore Medical Center, Somers Point, New Jersey

Joseph D. Zuckerman, MD
Chairman, Department of Orthopaedic Surgery, NYU Langone Medical Center, Hospital for Joint Diseases, New York, New York

Preface

As a trainee and young surgeon, the Instructional Course Lectures (ICLs) presented at the American Academy of Orthopaedic Surgeons (AAOS) Annual Meeting were the epitome of orthopaedic education. With leaders in our field volunteering to share their research, experience, and insight, the ICLs represented a unique forum for learning tried-and-true methods to improve patient care and outcomes. This volume of ICLs continues that tradition, with 52 chapters on topics that were presented at the 2015 Annual Meeting held in Las Vegas, NV. Coming after landmark changes in the healthcare system, such as the Affordable Care Act and ICD-10, this volume includes topics in traditional subspecialties but also includes a section relevant to important healthcare policy shifts. It is my hope that these additional chapters on the practice of orthopaedics will be useful to members regardless of their age, subspecialty, or practice type.

The list of individuals who have made this undertaking possible is extensive: the contributing authors, the specialty Instructional Course committees, the Central Instructional Courses Committee, and the AAOS editorial staff. The authors generously volunteered their time and effort to share their expertise. The specialty Instructional Course committee chairs and members functioned as section editors and editorial board members for this volume and provided valuable content editing in this era of increased subspecialization. I am honored to have served on the Central Instructional Courses Committee with terrific people, such as Robert Hart, 2013 chair; Craig J. Della Valle, 2014 chair; Tad L. Gerlinger, 2016 chair; and Jay Parvizi, 2017 chair. The previous chairs, Mark Pagnano and Paul Tornetta, also were instrumental in laying the groundwork for the ICL program. Many thanks to Fred Azar (2014 AAOS President) and Bill Mihalko (2015 Central Program Committee Chair); I could not have asked for better partners or friends.

Additional thanks to the AAOS staff, including Kathie Niesen, April Holmes, Scottie Rangel, Nicole Williams, and Domenic Picardo. My sincerest gratitude as well to Michelle Wild, Lisa Claxton Moore, Kathleen Anderson, Rachel Winokur, and Katie Hovany, all of whom work with a large group of volunteer authors to achieve an organized and well-written textbook and a useful video supplement. Without their dedication, responsiveness, and persistence, this volume would not be possible. A final round of thanks is due to my family; you are my rock and my greatest happiness. To my wife, Alyssa, who somehow tolerates my absences and maintains a busy surgical practice of her own, and to my children, Charlie and Porter, for their unwavering support and affection.

The ICL series is constantly evolving. Orthopaedic education is rapidly changing and it is the goal of the Central Instructional Courses Committee to change with it. The Committee recognizes that the AAOS membership increasingly values interaction as part of its educational experience. The debut and unprecedented success of the "case-based ICLs" is evidence of this trend, and the Committee is working to expand the number and breadth of those courses at future Annual Meetings. The value of multimedia also is an area of emphasis for the Central Instructional Courses Committee. The ICLs that focus on technical skills represent an effort to provide AAOS members with step-by-step video demonstrations of surgical techniques that range from simple to complex. The Committee's emphasis on the practice of orthopaedics is reflected in the expanded career development course offerings. With these and other innovations, it is intended that the ICLs will be a staple of orthopaedic education well into the future.

Thomas (Quin) Throckmorton, MD
Memphis, Tennessee

Table of Contents

Section 3: Adult Reconstruction: Hip and Knee

Section 7: Sports Medicine

Section 8: Orthopaedic Medicine

Section 9: The Practice of Orthopaedics

Video Abstracts

Chapter 1 Surgical Exposure Trends and Controversies in Extremity Fracture Care

Video: Kottmeier SA, Row E, Watson JT, Jones CB: *Posteromedial Tibial Plateau Fixation in the Prone Position: Applications of the Lobenhoffer Approach*. Stony Brook, NY, 2015. (21 min)

This video demonstrates posterior ankle approach strategies for the treatment of high-energy fractures. The goals of treatment are to preserve motion, strength, stability, and painless function; restore articular congruity, articular alignment, and limb axis; and preserve regional blood supply and the soft-tissue envelope. The pathoanatomy of posterior pilon fractures versus posterior malleolus fractures is discussed, and a classification scheme is illustrated. Indications for fixation of posterior malleolus fractures are discussed. The differences between syndesmotic screw fixation alone and syndesmotic screw fixation with posterior malleolus fixation are outlined. The protocol of staged (initial posterior pilon fixation) strategies is described. Anterior soft-tissue concerns are addressed with case discussions. The posterolateral approach to the malleolus is demonstrated. Techniques for reduction are listed. A posteromedial approach, which may be appropriate for posterior malleolus fractures with medial extension, is then described. Patients in whom simultaneous approaches may be necessary are described.

Video: Row E, Kottmeier SA, Burns C, Tornetta P III, Lorich D: *Posterior Ankle Approach Strategies (For Fracture Fixation)*. Stony Brook, NY, 2015. (13 min)

This video demonstrates a critical assessment of radiographic and clinical outcomes for the management of complex articular fragments of the proximal tibia. It also demonstrates several aspects worthy of re-evaluation and potential modification, including a refined understanding of fracture pathoanatomy and classification, surgical access (surgical exposure) and timing, preferential fixation constructs, and implant design modifications.

Chapter 5 Arthroscopic Rotator Cuff Repair: Indication and Technique

Video: O'Brien MJ: *Fiber Tape Rotator Cuff Repair*. New Orleans, LA, 2015. (2 min)

This video demonstrates a double-row rotator cuff repair in a 45-year-old, right hand dominant, male firefighter. A full-thickness supraspinatus tear is seen arthroscopically, and a microfracture has been performed on the greater tuberosity to facilitate healing. The medial-row anchor is placed just beyond the articular cartilage margin and contains fiber tape and No. 2 suture. A percutaneous suture passer is used for retrograde suture passing. The suture is placed in a mattress pattern. The fiber tape is passed medially and between the mattress sutures. The mattress sutures are tied first, which reduces the supraspinatus tendon over the anchor to the greater tuberosity bone. The fiber tape is brought over the top of the mattress sutures, tensioned appropriately, and secured to the tuberosity with a knotless lateral anchor. This provides excellent tension-free compression of the tendon to the underlying bone.

Chapter 8 Biomechanics of Reverse Shoulder Arthroplasty: Current Concepts

Video: Frankle MA: *Indications for Reverse Total Shoulder Arthroplasty*. Temple Terrace, FL, 2015. (10 min)

Reverse total shoulder arthroplasty (RSA) was developed as a salvage procedure, but it is currently used for the primary treatment of a number of shoulder conditions. RSA can be used to treat conditions that disrupt the Matsen center line; this concept is illustrated and discussed. Restoration of the rotation point of the humeral head back toward the center line after RSA is illustrated. The surgical technique begins with a standard humeral head cut. Then, the glenoid surface is prepared, the glenosphere baseplate is implanted, and the glenosphere is applied and fixed to the baseplate. The humeral component is placed, and the joint is reduced to ensure that adequate tension has been restored to the shoulder. The next case demonstrates the use of RSA for the treatment of eccentric osteoarthritis and glenoid bone loss. The possible need to alter the version of the baseplate and the "spine line" is discussed and illustrated. Bone graft can be applied for additional support. A technique is demonstrated for the treatment of considerable bone loss, and the baseplate is implanted over a humeral head bone graft. Another case demonstrates the use of RSA for the treatment of an acute proximal humerus fracture. Problems with hemiarthroplasty are discussed. Repair of the tuberosities after implantation of the prosthesis proceeds according to the Black and Tan technique, which was described by Dr. Jonathan C. Levy. The technique begins with the placement of tag sutures and removal of the humeral head. Sutures and fiber tape, both of which will secure the greater tuberosity, are placed. The glenosphere is placed, and the humerus is reamed. Holes for the sutures are drilled in the humerus, and a cement restrictor is placed. The humeral implant is inserted after cement and morcellized bone graft are placed, and the polyethylene liner is positioned and impacted into the implant. The shoulder is reduced, and the sutures reduce the tuberosities. All sutures and the fiber tape are fixed, and the shoulder is taken through a range of motion.

Chapter 11 Reverse Shoulder Arthroplasty for Trauma: When, Where, and How

Video: Szerlip BW, Morris BJ, Edwards TB: *Reverse Shoulder Arthroplasty for Trauma: When, Where, and How.* Houston, TX, 2015. (9 min)

Reverse shoulder arthroplasty has become increasingly popular for the treatment of complex shoulder injuries, including proximal humerus fractures and fixed glenohumeral dislocation, in the elderly population. The early to midterm results of reverse shoulder arthroplasty for the treatment of proximal humerus fractures are promising compared with the results of unconstrained humeral head replacement, and patients may have more predictable improvement with less dependence on bone healing and rehabilitation. However, long-term follow-up is needed, and surgeons must be familiar with various complications that are specific to reverse shoulder arthroplasty. To achieve optimal patient outcomes for the management of traumatic shoulder injuries, surgeons must have a comprehensive understanding of the current implant options, indications, and surgical techniques for reverse shoulder arthroplasty.

Chapter 12 All Things Clavicle: From Acromioclavicular to Sternoclavicular and All Points in Between

Video: Kibler WB: *AC Joint Reconstruction.* Lexington, KY, 2015. (10 min)

A biomechanically-based surgical treatment approach for high-grade acromioclavicular (AC) joint injuries is necessary to restore the clavicle's key role as a mobile strut for scapular and arm motion, the AC joint's role as the unifying link in the screw axis mechanism that governs normal scapulohumeral rhythm, and the three-dimensional nature of the normal kinematics of the clavicle and scapula that facilitate arm function. This video demonstrates execution of a surgical technique; a modification of that surgical technique proposed by Mazzocca, which includes allograft reconstruction of both the conoid and trapezoid ligaments through anatomically positioned clavicle drill holes; the use of graft tails to reconstruct the superior AC ligament via a novel docking technique; and anatomic repair of the native anterior and posterior AC ligaments. Favorable functional outcomes have been achieved with anatomic coracoclavicular ligament reconstruction and repair/reconstruction of the AC ligaments.

Chapter 15 Preventing Leg Length Discrepancy and Instability After Total Hip Arthroplasty

Video: Lavernia CJ: *The Importance of the Posterior Superior Iliac Spines When Assessing Leg Length.* Coral Gables, FL, 2015. (12 sec)

In this video, a patient is viewed from behind while he is standing on a set of blocks that are used to level the pelvis. The patient's pelvic tilt changes as he steps onto the blocks.

Video: Lavernia CJ: *An Inexpensive Method to Assess Length.* Coral Gables, FL, 2015. (22 sec)

This video demonstrates a very simple and cheap technique to assess leg length discrepancy. Plywood of different thicknesses can be stacked. These can be 1- or 0.5-cm thick. The patient's pelvis is levelled by stacking the plywood pieces and observing the position of the patient's posterior superior iliac spines.

Video: Lavernia CJ: *Placement of the Tool Beneath the Patient*. Coral Gables, FL, 2015. (23 sec)

This video demonstrates placement of plywood pieces under the patient's leg and having him walk in situ to assess how comfortable he feels. A set of plywood pieces is too high for the patient; however, this can only be seen when viewing the patient from behind and observing the position of his posterior superior iliac spines.

Video: Lavernia CJ: *Where is the Problem*? Coral Gables, FL, 2015. (20 sec)

This video demonstrates the importance of assessing leg length in a seated position to determine the location at which the discrepancy actually occurs. A patient with a tibial fracture will have normal femurs if compared side-by-side in a sitting position with the femurs directly under the shoulders.

Video: Lavernia CJ: *Preoperative Planning*. Coral Gables, FL, 2015. (19 sec)

This video demonstrates the importance of preoperative planning with the use of digital or acetate templates on a standard or digital radiograph. Hip replacement surgery should always include preoperative planning to determine exactly what offset and size of stem should be used.

Chapter 16 The Difficult Primary Total Knee Arthroplasty

Video: Hitt KD: *Varus Preoperative Examination*. Temple, TX, 2015. (17 sec)

A preoperative examination that is performed under anesthesia can help the surgeon direct his focus on appropriate soft-tissue balancing and release techniques. This video demonstrates a fixed varus deformity in extension that appears to correct in flexion.

Video: Hitt KD: *Varus Approach and Osteophyte Removal*. Temple, TX, 2015. (1 min)

A varus approach to the knee begins with the surgeon's preferred approach, whether it be medial parapatellar, midvastus, or subvastus, and release of the anteromedial capsule to the midcoronal plane on the medial side. An examination in extension reveals the amount of correction of the fixed varus deformity that is appreciated. If the knee is not corrected in extension, osteophytes can be removed from the medial femoral condyle and the tibial plateau. Release of the deep medial collateral ligament that extends posteromedially to include the semimembranosus can be performed, especially in patients who have associated fixed flexion contracture. A repeat examination reveals correction of the fixed deformity, and subsequent bony preparation can be undertaken.

Video: Hitt KD: *Varus Balancing*. Temple, TX, 2015. (36 sec)

This video demonstrates residual lateral laxity with contracture on the medial side. This can be addressed by downsizing the tibial tray, lateralizing the tray, and removing uncapped bone medially. This decompresses the tight medial structures and helps facilitate balancing in extension.

Video: Hitt KD: *Varus Micropuncture*. Temple, TX, 2015. (22 sec)

Laminar spreaders are used to tension the medial and lateral soft tissues if lateral opening is seen compared with the medial side. A micropuncture technique with a 20-gauge needle is performed to help facilitate balancing in extension on the medial side.

Video: Hitt KD: *Valgus Preoperative Examination*. Temple, TX, 2015. (30 sec)

An intraoperative assessment for correctable or fixed deformities can help determine the amount of release required. In this video, the left knee examination reveals a fixed deformity in extension that corrects in flexion, whereas the right knee examination reveals a passively correctable deformity.

Video: Hitt KD: *Valgus Approach*. Temple, TX, 2015. (1 min)

Overrelease of the medial structures should be avoided in a valgus approach to the knee. Medial release should be taken to the midcoronal plane. The anterolateral capsule can be released off the tibia behind the fat pad. The release extends laterally to help facilitate lateralization of the patella and correction of the contracted lateral capsule.

Video: Hitt KD: *Valgus Micropuncture*. Temple, TX, 2015. (2 min)

This video demonstrates the anatomic landmarks used for placement of the femoral component with appropriate rotation in a valgus knee. This is achieved using a combination of the posterior condylar axis, the transcondylar axis, and the Whiteside line. Internal rotation, which can occur in a deficient lateral femoral condyle, is thus avoided. In managing a valgus knee, underresection of the tibial plateau is encouraged because of attenuation of the medial structures. This prevents the need for larger-than-normal polyethylene inserts. In all total knee replacements, any posterior condylar bone that extends beyond the limits of the femoral implant should be removed to facilitate extension. Any residual tightness in extension can be addressed by tensioning the medial and lateral soft-tissue structures, using a micropuncture technique with a 20-gauge needle on the affected structures, and confirming appropriate balancing. In flexion, the micropuncture technique can be performed on posterolateral structures to help facilitate flexion balance.

Chapter 20 Role of Fresh Osteochondral Allografts for Large Talar Osteochondral Lesions

Video Excerpt: Easley ME: Osteochondral lesions of the talus. *J Am Acad Orthop Surg* 2010;18(10):616-630. (6 min)

This video demonstrates both autologous chondrocyte implantation and osteochondral allografting for the treatment of osteochondral lesions of the talus. These techniques fill the defect with near-normal hyaline cartilage. Lesions that involve a substantial portion of the talus or the talar shoulder are difficult to treat with osteochondral allografting or autologous chondrocyte implantation and are best managed with structural allograft reconstruction. Moreover, structural allograft reconstruction may be a reasonable alternative to ankle arthrodesis if osteochondral allografting or autologous chondrocyte implantation have failed. The challenge in structural allograft reconstruction often is obtaining an appropriate talar allograft.

Chapter 27 The Difficult Supracondylar Humerus Fracture: Flexion-Type Injuries

Video: Koerner J, Sabharwal S: *Percutaneous Pinning of Supracondylar Humerus Fractures*. Philadelphia, PA, 2013. (11 min)

Pediatric supracondylar humerus fractures are common injuries. Treatment begins with an evaluation to assess the patient's overlying skin for open fractures, bruising, or puckering, all of which may indicate more severe trauma and possible difficulty in achieving an adequate closed reduction. A thorough neurovascular examination must be documented, radiographs must be obtained, and splinting should be performed. Determining if surgical treatment is required and the timing of surgery is based on radiographs and the physical examination. Use of the proper surgical equipment, setup, and patient positioning are crucial for successful treatment. The reduction is followed by percutaneous pinning and casting. This video demonstrates the physical examination, the operating room setup, patient positioning, and postoperative care. The technique for reduction as well as pin placement and configuration are detailed. Common pitfalls and complications, such as vascular compromise, neurologic injury, and loss of reduction as well as techniques to avoid these, are covered. Difficult cases, with pearls for successful treatment, also are presented.

Chapter 31 Arthroscopic Management of Anterior, Posterior, and Multidirectional Shoulder Instabilities

Video: Field LD: *Arthroscopic Management of Shoulder Instabilities: Anterior, Posterior, and Multidirectional.* Jackson, MS, 2015. (12 min)

This video demonstrates an example of anterior shoulder instability, with reconstruction, remplissage, and repair of a bony Bankart fragment; an example of posterior instability; and examples of multidirectional instability. First, a Hill-Sachs lesion is repaired with remplissage before bony Bankart repair. It is important that remplissage be performed before Bankart repair to allow access to the posterior humeral head defect. Next, a large, bony Bankart lesion is débrided and repaired with anchors that are placed in the glenoid neck; the suture limbs are passed medially through the fracture fragment to allow for labral ligamentous tissue reapproximation and retensioning. The next case is a 24-year-old athlete who has a history of posterior instability. After 4 months of nonsurgical treatment and no improvement, the posterior labrum is arthroscopically repaired to provide good reapproximation of the labrum, complete coverage of the articular cartilage defect, and supplemental capsular plication. Two patients who have multidirectional instability are next demonstrated. In the first patient, suture capsulorrhaphy is accomplished with the use of a retrograde suture retriever that is passed through the inferior capsule to create a horizontal mattress suture construct pattern. The second patient with multidirectional instability has substantial capsular laxity. A probe demonstrates the lack of labral pathology and the underdeveloped labral tissue that is often present in patients who have multidirectional instability. This lack of tissue can make capsular fixation difficult, and creates a need for suture anchors. The finished capsulorrhaphy is demonstrated through the anterior portal camera.

Chapter 32 Hip Arthroscopy: Tales From the Crypt

Video: Philippon MJ: *Hip Arthroscopy With Bone Augmentation*. Vail, CO, 2015. (1 min)

This video demonstrates a patient who had proximal femoral bone loss that was reconstructed with a fresh-frozen femoral head allograft. Three bone fragments were fixed with four screws and contoured with the use of an arthroscopic burr to cover a surface area of 3 cm × 2 cm.

Trauma

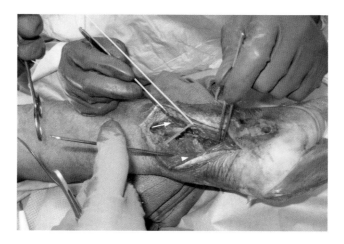

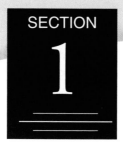

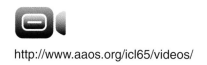
http://www.aaos.org/icl65/videos/

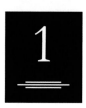

Surgical Exposure Trends and Controversies in Extremity Fracture Care

Stephen A. Kottmeier, MD
Elliot Row, MD
Paul Tornetta III, MD
Clifford B. Jones, MD, FACS
Dean G. Lorich, MD
J. Tracy Watson, MD

Abstract

Surgical exposures for the management of extremity fractures continue to evolve. Strategies to achieve satisfactory articular reconstitution require surgeons to have an appreciation and understanding of various conventional and contemporary surgical approaches. The recent literature has witnessed a surge in studies on surgical approaches for the fixation of extremity fractures. This increased interest in surgical exposures resulted from not only a desire to enhance outcomes and minimize complications but also a recognition of the inadequacies of traditionally accepted surgical exposures. Contemporary exposures may be modifications or combinations of existing exposures. All surgical exposures require proper surgical execution and familiarity with regional anatomic structures. Exposures, whether conventional or contemporary, must provide sufficient access for reduction and implant insertion. Proper exposure selection can greatly enhance a surgeon's ability to achieve acceptable reduction and adequate fixation. Unique characteristics of both the patient and his or her fracture pathoanatomy may dictate the surgical approach. Patient positioning, imaging access, and concomitant comorbidities (medical, systemic trauma, and regional extremity related) also must be considered. Minimally invasive methods of reduction and fixation are attractive and have merit; however, adherence to them while failing to achieve satisfactory reduction and fixation will not generate a desirable outcome. Surgeons should be aware of several site-specific anatomic regions in which evolving surgical exposures and strategies for extremity fracture management have had favorable outcomes.

Instr Course Lect 2016;65:3–24.

Skeletal reconstruction requires not only the proper selection of surgical tools and implants but also the means by which to introduce them within the surgical site. Patient positioning, adequate imaging, and the atraumatic insertion of devices (including the proper trajectory of implants during the course of insertion) must be considered. For example, the lesion in a medial condyle fracture of the distal femur (**Figure 1, A**) does not violate the lateral column or osseous cortical integrity. Ideally, a medial condyle fracture of the distal femur should be managed only with a medial approach and medially applied implant. In this example, the treating surgeon was familiar only, or primarily, with the application of lateral implants via lateral exposures (**Figure 1, B**). Malreduction and biomechanically ineffective and undesirable fixation, which resulted in a sustained state of articular and metadiaphyseal malreduction, were the

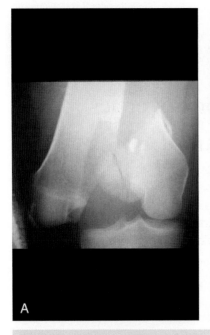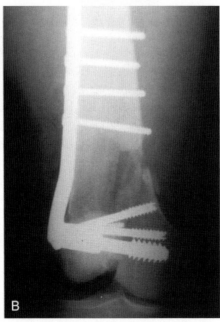

Figure 1 AP radiographs demonstrate a medial monocondylar distal fracture of a right femur (**A**) that should have been managed with medial exposure and medially applied fixation, but was instead managed with lateral exposure and laterally applied fixation (**B**).

outcomes of the procedure. A proper understanding of morphologic characteristics of this fracture pattern would have directed the surgeon to a better means for fracture access, which would have yielded a more desirable reduction and enhanced biomechanical stability. As implants continue to evolve, the surgical exposures required for their efficacy also must evolve.

Proximal Humerus Fractures

Displaced proximal humerus fractures continue to present surgeons with therapeutic challenges. Surgical management of proximal humerus fractures must provide satisfactory reduction and fixation to allow for early shoulder range of motion and, thus, restoration of function. Although locking screw fixation and fixed angle interfaces with site-specific plate contouring are appealing, the results of these techniques have been less than universally successful and predictable. Techniques to insert implants with design modifications continue to evolve in an effort to improve their performance. The

restoration of medial column support is important to ensure maintenance of reduction.[1,2] Methods to minimize regional devascularization while introducing fixation constructs of sufficient integrity continue to be refined. Surgeons are able to favorably enhance the mechanical and biologic environment by modifying several variables that are within their control. The importance of adequate surgical access, and, accordingly, proper approach selection has a substantial effect on outcomes.

Deltopectoral Approach

The deltopectoral approach is the standard surgical approach for the management of proximal humerus fractures. Limitations and liabilities inherent to the deltopectoral approach have been increasingly recognized. The anterior position of the deltopectoral approach does not provide surgeons with direct access to the plating zone nor does it provide easy access to the greater tuberosity fracture components. Substantial muscle retraction and manipulation are required to overcome these deficiencies. In addition, implant and drill trajectory may be compromised with the deltopectoral approach, which may predispose the patient to anterior plate placement and result in a mechanically compromised fixation. Partial detachment of the deltoid insertion inferiorly may be required to allow for proper lateral plate positioning. Because it has been reported that the anterior deltoid has a functional and anatomic intolerance to partial detachment of its insertion,[3] plate contouring and redesign have been suggested to allow for anterior plate placement inferiorly. Dissatisfaction with the deltopectoral approach has prompted several investigators to develop, modify, and pursue alternatives.

Dr. Tornetta or an immediate family member has received royalties from Smith & Nephew. Dr. Jones or an immediate family member serves as a board member, owner, officer, or committee member of the Orthopaedic Trauma Association. Dr. Watson or an immediate family member has received royalties from Biomet and Smith & Nephew; is a member of a speakers' bureau or has made paid presentations on behalf of Biomet, Ellipse Technologies, and Smith & Nephew; serves as a paid consultant to Biomet, Bioventus, and Smith & Nephew; serves as an unpaid consultant to Accelalox, Acumed, and Ellipse Technologies; has received nonincome support (such as equipment or services), commercially derived honoraria, or other non-research–related funding (such as paid travel) from Biomet; and serves as a board member, owner, officer, or committee member of the Orthopaedic Trauma Association. None of the following authors or any immediate family member has received anything of value from or has stock or stock options held in a commercial company or institution related directly or indirectly to the subject of this chapter: Dr. Kottmeier, Dr. Row, and Dr. Lorich.

Transdeltoid Approaches

Transdeltoid approaches were created to adhere to the tenets of less invasive fracture fixation. These approaches, regardless of incision orientation, are established within the avascular raphe between the anterior and middle deltoid. Compared with the deltopectoral approach, transdeltoid approaches are more remote from the critical anterior blood supply of the osteoarticular segment of the proximal humerus. Direct access to the underlying plating zone is provided by transdeltoid approaches. This 3-cm hypovascular region of the plating zone between the greater and lesser tuberosities resides between the anterior and posterior penetrating vessels of the humeral head. Unlike the deltopectoral approach, transdeltoid approaches, which provide a direct approach to the plate application site, facilitate mobilization and reduction of fracture components.[4] Fracture planes reside immediately beneath the developed interval, and the typically posteriorly retracted greater tuberosity can be readily retrieved. In addition, the deltoid presents less hindrance with implant trajectory and insertion with transdeltoid approaches. Transdeltoid approaches, regardless of incision orientation, allow for endosteal substitution and arthroplasty options if fixation is problematic.[5,6]

The widespread acceptance of transdeltoid approaches may be limited by the perception of axillary nerve vulnerability. However, a potential attribute of transdeltoid approaches is the identification and protection of the axillary nerve if it is within the proximity of displaced fractures, an attribute that is not provided with the deltopectoral approach. Regardless of incision orientations for transdeltoid splitting approaches, the anterior branch of the axillary nerve is identified and palpated on the deltoid undersurface to its emergence from the quadrilateral space posteriorly. Distal extension of the split deltoid is pursued with caution. The anterior branch of the axillary nerve is identified within the zone of the split deltoid and can be predictably found approximately 6 cm distal to the anterior acromion.[7] As it traverses the surgical field, the axillary nerve is mobilized only enough to allow for positioning of the plate underneath it. A proximal window is established superior to the axillary nerve through which the locking plate and proximal locking screws are introduced. An inferior window is developed below the axillary nerve for fixation of screws within the lower limits of the plate.

Several studies have demonstrated the absence of any clinically apparent neurologic deficits to the axillary nerve with the transdeltoid splitting approach.[8-11] Gavaskar et al[12] reported transient electrophysiologic changes with the transdeltoid splitting approach; however, these changes did not result in any detrimental clinical sequelae. Axillary nerve vulnerability is a concern with any revision surgery or attempt at implant extraction with secondary procedures; however, Robinson et al[13] did not report any deleterious outcomes with such efforts. The authors suggested limited dissection in the proximity of the axillary nerve, which again was readily identified and easily protected.

The patient is placed in either the beach-chair or semisupine position with the image intensifier positioned on the opposite side of the surgical table. Rotation of the image intensifier allows for satisfactory AP and modified axial imaging. The entire upper extremity as well as the anterior and posterior hemithorax are prepped and draped within the surgical field to allow for limb manipulation.

The Edinburg shoulder strap incision described by Robinson and Page[9,14] creates a distally based elliptical flap with its apex centered over the acromion (**Figure 2, A**). The Edinburg shoulder strap incision is cosmetically appealing and made within the relaxed skin tension lines. If necessary for problematic fracture-dislocation variants, the Edinburg shoulder strap incision accommodates a deltopectoral exposure within the anterior portion of the incision. The Edinburgh shoulder strap incision does not allow for distal extension to address fractures with substantial diaphyseal concerns. In such cases the linear anterolateral incision described by Gardner et al[10] may be preferable (**Figure 2, B**). In addition, a standard anterolateral approach to the humeral shaft also may be used (**Figure 2, C**). Dissection and plate fixation within the deltoid insertion distally addresses diaphyseal concerns. Robinson and Murray[15] reported no clinical detachment or dysfunction to the deltoid with this more extensile approach. With any of the incisions, detachment of the origin of the deltoid may be pursued as necessary (**Figure 3, A**) but demands meticulous subsequent transosseous suture closure to limit catastrophic detachment (**Figure 3, B**).

After the surgical incision is complete, deep dissection within the subcutaneous tissues overlying the deltoid fascia is performed. The fat stripe within the avascular raphae between the anterior and middle deltoids is identified (**Figure 4, A**). The deltoid is then incised in line with its fibers, beginning proximally and extending distally, for no more than 3 cm. Blunt

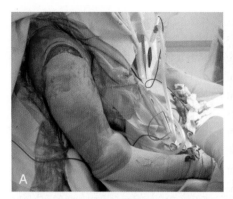
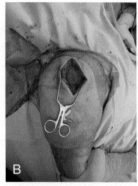
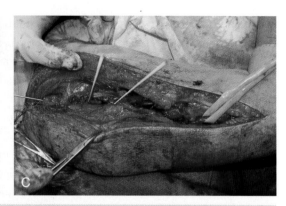

Figure 2 Intraoperative photographs show potential exposures for the treatment of a displaced proximal humerus fracture with the use of a transdeltoid splitting approach. **A,** The Edinburg shoulder strap incision creates a distally based elliptical flap (deltoid splitting). **B,** The linear anterolateral incision is made within the raphe between the anterior and middle deltoids (deltoid splitting). **C,** The extensile anterolateral approach (deltoid splitting), in which the radial nerve is identified distally and protected within a Penrose drain. (Panel B is reproduced from Kottmeier SA, Jones CB, Tornetta P III, Russell TA: Locked and minimally invasive plating: A paradigm shift? Metadiaphyseal site-specific concerns and controversies. *Instr Course Lect* 2013;62:41-59.)

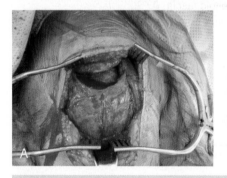
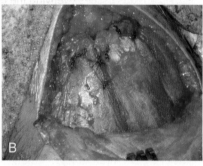

Figure 3 Intraoperative photographs of an Edinburg shoulder strap incision show proximal deltoid detachment (**A**) and meticulous deltoid transosseous suture reattachment (**B**).

dissection is pursued only within the proximity of the palpated nerve on the undersurface of the deltoid. The nerve may be readily identified and palpated with the surgeon's index finger directed distally and laterally. The axillary nerve is predictably found and palpated as a cordlike structure within the loose connective tissue between the deltoid and the humerus. In a cadaver model study, Gardner et al[7] reported that the axillary nerve was "distinct and predictably found" in all the cadaver models. In this study, no nerve branches other than the main anterior axillary trunk traversed the deltoid raphe. The authors reported

that the distance from the superior edge of the axillary nerve to the lateral prominence of the greater tuberosity was approximately 35.5 mm, and the distance from the superior edge of the axillary nerve to the undersurface of the acromion was approximately 63.3 mm. If a displaced fracture is present, the greater tuberosity may be an unreliable landmark for axillary nerve identification. The axillary nerve is protected within adjacent connective tissue using a sling (**Figure 4, B**). Circumferential dissection of the axillary nerve is discouraged.

Care should be taken to avoid any tension on the axillary nerve as the

plate is positioned beneath it. Similarly, the area above and below the axillary nerve should be protected during screw insertion. Fracture surfaces are cleared of debris, and interposed soft tissues are mobilized with the insertion of nonabsorbable sutures within the tuberosities. Because of the proximity of fracture components to the incision, deep dissection anteriorly and posteriorly beneath the deltoid is typically not required and is discouraged. Controversy exists with regard to the relative contributions of osseous and articular blood supply, both anteriorly and posteriorly. A study by Hettrich et al[16] challenged the consensus that arterial blood supply to the humeral head is provided primarily anteriorly. Using a gadolinium-enhanced MRI cadaver perfusion model study, the authors attempted to objectively quantify the relative contribution of blood flow from the anterior and posterior humeral circumflex arteries to the humeral head. A greater percentage of blood flow was provided to the humeral head from the posterior humeral circumflex artery compared with the anterior humeral circumflex artery. Accordingly, sub-deltoid dissection and the positioning of retractors and reduction aids anteriorly and posteriorly should be limited to that required to attain a satisfactory reduction and fixation.

Proximal Tibia Fractures

Contemporary classifications of tibial plateau fractures have increasingly adopted the notion of quadrants and columns, which has provided surgeons with a better understanding of plausible circumferential access to the proximal tibia. Conventional two-dimensional classifications are limited with regard to the characterization of posterior shearing or coronal plane fractures that involve the retrotibial proximal articular surface. Such classifications endorse only medial and lateral fixation and limit the notion of posterior access and fixation. Luo et al[17] described a three-column, CT-based classification for complex multiplanar tibial plateau fractures (**Figure 5**). The authors reported that an enhanced and correct CT-based morphologic classification of a multiplanar tibial plateau fracture is achieved only after the application of a previously applied distracting transarticular external fixator. Using axial CT analysis, the authors divided the tibial plateau into three regions (lateral, medial, and posterior columns). To conform to the three-column fracture assignment, at least one independent articular fragment was identified within each of the three columns. The merits of three-dimensional CT reconstruction analysis in combination with the axial CT-assigned classification also were reported. Because of an increased recognition of the limitations of surgical approaches and implant design, the medial column of metadiaphyseal, medial

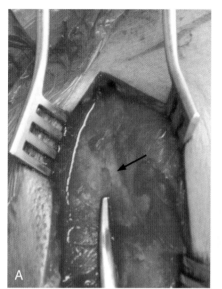
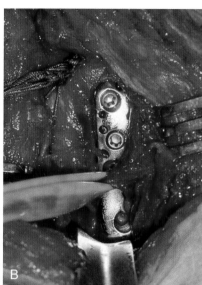

Figure 4   Intraoperative photographs show deep dissection within the subcutaneous tissues overlying the deltoid fascia. **A,** Subcutaneous flaps are developed, and the fat stripe (arrow) within the raphe between the anterior and middle deltoid is identified. **B,** The axillary nerve is bluntly dissected and protected within a Penrose drain. Two windows are established: one above the nerve, through which the plate is inserted and proximally secured, and another inferiorly, through which the shaft of the plate is secured. (Panel B is reproduced from Kottmeier SA, Jones CB, Tornetta P III, Russell TA: Locked and minimally invasive plating: A paradigm shift? Metadiaphyseal site-specific concerns and controversies. *Instr Course Lect* 2013;62:41-59.)

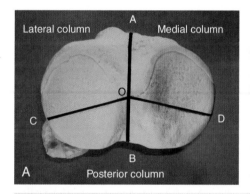
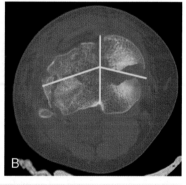

Figure 5   Bone model (**A**) and axial CT scan (**B**) demonstrate the three-column classification of proximal tibial plateau fractures described by Luo et al.[17] The three columns are separated by three connecting lines (OA, OC, and OD). Point O is the center of the knee (midpoint of two tibial spines). Point A represents the anterior tibial tuberosity. Point C is the most anterior point of the fibular head. Point D is the posteromedial ridge of the proximal tibia. Point B is the posterior sulcus of the tibial plateau, which intersects the posterior column into the medial and lateral parts.

monocondylar, and bicondylar fractures has received recent attention. A continuously improving comprehension of regional pathoanatomy and fracture morphology also has contributed to this increased interest.

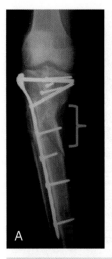
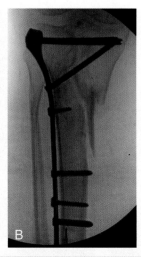
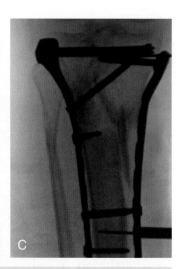

Figure 6 **A,** AP radiograph of a fixed angle (locking) interface device that was used to stabilize a highly comminuted (bracketed area) metadiaphyseal fracture of the proximal tibia demonstrates substantial medial column compromise with subsequent implant failure. **B,** AP fluoroscopic image shows locking plate fixation of a proximal tibia fracture with medial column comminution. **C,** AP fluoroscopic image shows adjuvant medial column plating with subcutaneous insertion and proximal unicortical fixation. (Panel A is reproduced from Kottmeier SA, Jones CB, Tornetta P III, Russell TA: Locked and minimally invasive plating: A paradigm shift? Metadiaphyseal site-specific concerns and controversies. *Instr Course Lect* 2013;62:41-59.)

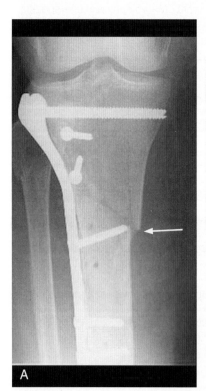
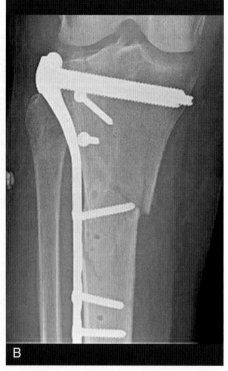

Figure 7 AP radiographs demonstrate that locking plate fixation of a proximal tibia fracture without medial column reduction (arrow; **A**) will result in varus drift (**B**).

Metadiaphyseal Fractures

Metadiaphyseal fractures of the proximal tibia are uniquely challenging because of the tenuous soft-tissue envelope and, often, short and comminuted proximal fragment. Because of these concerns, laterally applied fixed-angle devices that are compatible with minimally invasive insertion techniques are particularly attractive for use in proximal tibia fractures. Surgical priorities include reestablishing limb axis, articular congruity, and joint function. Laterally applied fixed-angle devices, which are intended to resist varus collapse, are not without limitations. There is growing concern for a seemingly overdependence on the angle stable screw interface for the sustained and sufficient management of varus forces (**Figure 6, A**). Occasionally, adjuvant medial column support may be beneficial and desirable (**Figure 6, B** and **C**). Whether it is acceptable to use a single laterally applied locking plate or augment the construct with adjuvant medial plating is an important question that surgeons should answer.

Watson et al[18] stressed the need for surgeons to ascertain the integrity of the medial osseous column of the proximal tibia as well as its reduction parameters. The authors suggested that a lateral locking plate will be sufficient and not result in subsequent varus collapse only if certain criteria, such as medial column reduction (**Figure 7**), medial cortical opposition, and a medial condylar component of sufficient size, are met. In the absence of medial column reduction or in the presence of medial comminution, adjunctive medial plating should be considered.

A distraction CT scan taken after transarticular external fixation determines the size and location of the medial

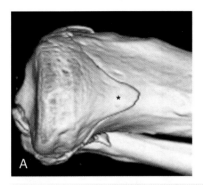
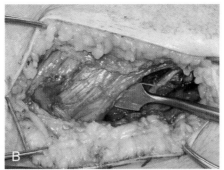
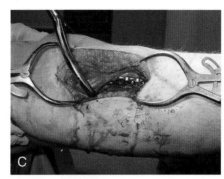

Figure 8   Images show the treatment strategy for a displaced bicondylar tibial plateau fracture. **A,** Lateral three-dimensional CT reconstruction of a medial condyle helps localize the inferior apex of the fracture (asterisk). **B,** Intraoperative photograph shows the posteromedial approach with the pes tendons elevated, which allows for exposure and reduction of the fracture apex. **C,** The plate is applied posteromedially over the identified fracture apex, which provides antiglide support.

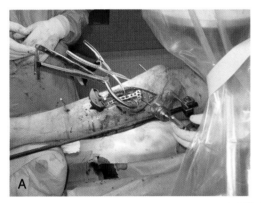
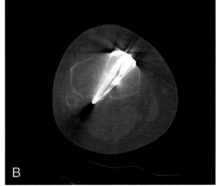
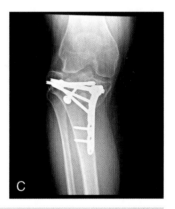

Figure 9   Images demonstrate incorrect plate placement for the fixation of a medial tibial plateau fracture. **A,** Intraoperative photograph shows the anteromedial application of a plate. **B,** Axial CT scan demonstrates that the plate is ineffectually positioned to address the fracture. **C,** AP radiograph demonstrates improper positioning of the anteromedial plate, which rendered the plate incapable of withstanding an applied axial load.

condyle fracture and helps suggest the fixation strategy. Three-dimensional CT reconstructions better orient surgeons to the site of apical discontinuity, which facilitates the strategic placement of antiglide devices at the apex inferiorly (**Figure 8, A**). Three-dimensional CT reconstructions can identify the preferred location for surgical access and incision placement. Implant application and positioning that is less than ideal will likely lead to construct failure and medial column collapse. Apical application of the plate enhances construct rigidity. Deviation from apical application of the plate can lead to construct

failure. For some fracture variants, medial, rather than posteromedial or posterior, application of a plate will result in less favorable construct integrity and, ultimately, failure. A false sense of security may be provided with medially based precontoured periarticular plates that are designed to fit the anteromedial tibial face (**Figure 9, A**). A plate applied anteromedially, which is intended to address a posteromedial variant, will not provide apical fixation and commonly results in varus collapse (**Figure 9, B and C**). These not infrequent fracture variants must be recognized, and surgical exposures and fixation strategies

must be patterned for their optimal management.

Medial surgical approaches for the management of metadiaphyseal fractures of the proximal tibia include a direct medial approach to the anteromedial surface either through or underneath the pes anserinus tendons (**Figure 8, B and C**). Alternative medial column approaches include a posteromedial approach at the pes-medial gastrocnemius interval and the direct posterior approach. The skin incision should be made to allow access to the apex of the medial condyle and is predetermined with the use of

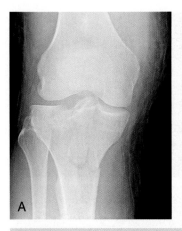 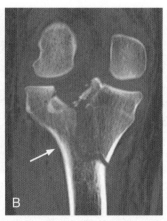 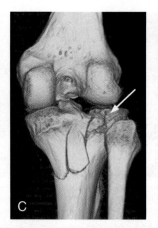 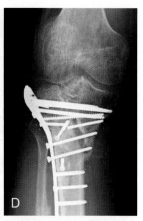

Figure 10 Images show how imaging can be used to differentiate isolated medial tibial plateau fractures from a bicondylar tibial plateau fracture variant. **A,** AP radiograph of a medial proximal (right) tibia fracture (Moore type I) demonstrates widening of the proximal tibia laterally with respect to the overlying lateral femoral condyle, which may be misinterpreted as a lateral plateau fracture. **B,** Coronal CT scan demonstrates the absence of any cortical compromise laterally (arrow), which is consistent with a medial condyle fracture. **C,** Posterior three-dimensional CT reconstruction demonstrates articular extension within the lateral compartment (arrow), which also is consistent with a medial condyle fracture. **D,** AP radiograph demonstrates a medial monocondylar proximal tibia fracture that was inaccurately classified and improperly managed with a laterally based device.

three-dimensional reconstructive CT images. Methods for medial column plate augmentation have been described and incorporate minimally invasive techniques. The capture area for locking screws is dependent on plate design. Variable angle locking screws may offer some latitude to increase the capture area required; however, it may be limited and insufficient. Unicortical screws usually are sufficient within the initially fixated medial construct, which limits the potential for conflicting insertion of implants (gridlock) with subsequent lateral column plating.

Medial Monocondylar Fractures

Isolated posteromedial split fractures of the tibial plateau (Moore type I) represent a fracture-dislocation with concerning osseous and soft-tissue injury[19,20] (**Figure 10, A**). These patterns may be mistakenly interpreted as a lateral tibial plateau fracture. Careful scrutiny of imaging studies, particularly CT scans, will identify an intact cortical column

laterally (**Figure 10, B**). An obliquely or coronally oriented isolated fragment that involves a substantial portion of the posteromedial condyle also is demonstrated (**Figure 10, C**). These lesions are frequently associated with potentially encroaching central articular depression of the lateral condyle. The use of a laterally based approach with primarily lateral fixation likely will result in inadequate reduction and undesirable and insufficient fixation (**Figure 10, D**).

Isolated posteromedial split fractures of the tibial plateau are preferentially managed with a posteromedial (Loebenhoeffer) approach and the patient placed in the prone position.[21-23] The involved extremity is elevated on bolsters to facilitate imaging. Both the patient and the surgical table are rotated to enhance accurate lateral imaging. The surgeon is positioned on the opposite side of the radiolucent table. Either a linear or curvilinear (within or just superior to the retropopliteal crease) incision is made with well-developed skin flaps (**Figure 11, A**). Elevation of the

medial margin of the medial gastrocnemius is begun within the midportion of the wound and is extended proximally to its origin. The pes tendons and their attachments may be maintained or divided as necessary. The popliteal vessels are neither formally encountered nor mobilized. Next, the popliteus is mobilized with subperiosteal elevation along its medial margin that extends laterally. Retractors are positioned on the lateral tibial osseous margin and gentle retraction is used to limit the risk of venous thrombosis and neurovascular injury. The posteromedial fracture is mobilized to allow for extraction of interposed hematoma soft tissue and osteochondral debris. Mobilization of the posteromedial fracture is facilitated by placing the patient's knee in a position of flexion. The inferior apex of the retrocondylar medial fracture serves as an indirect reduction aid and a means for effective fixation with the use of antiglide techniques (**Figure 11, B**). Placing the patient's knee in extension facilitates reduction (**Figure 11, C**).

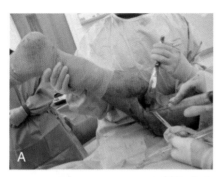
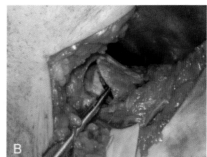
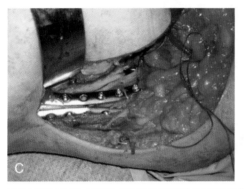
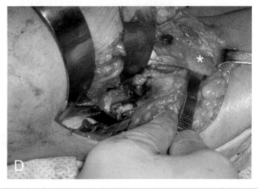
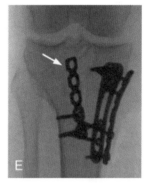

Figure 11   Images show the management of a medial monocondylar proximal tibia fracture. **A,** Intraoperative photograph shows the posteromedial (Loebenhoffer) approach over a left knee with the patient placed in the prone position and the surgeon standing on the opposite side of the surgical table. Intraoperative photographs show that knee flexion allows for mobilization of the fracture (**B**), and knee extension aids in fracture reduction and subsequent plate application (**C**). **D,** Intraoperative photograph shows that the origin of the medial gastrocnemius (asterisk) is identified and can be sectioned to enhance exposure, which allows access to the posterolateral aspect of the proximal tibia. **E,** AP radiograph demonstrates final implant insertion. The arrow indicates a laterally positioned plate that was introduced via the posteromedial approach.

Occasionally, fracture patterns may extend laterally within the subchondral region of the lateral femoral condyle. This lateral extension occurs in the absence of any lateral cortical compromise. Accurate reduction may necessitate extraction or reduction of these lateral osteochondral components, which require a more extensile version of the posteromedial (Loebenhoeffer) approach. In such circumstances, the medial gastrocnemius tendon is sectioned proximally to enhance exposure, reduction, and subsequent fixation[24] (**Figure 11, D**). Sectioning of the gastrocnemius tendon should be performed inferior to its origin to limit compromise to its arterial supply. Fixation constructs may be extended laterally with the posteromedial

(Loebenhoeffer) approach to allow for reduction and fixation of the lateral extensions of these primarily medial fractures (**Figure 11, E**). The gastrocnemius origin is subsequently repaired, and the soft tissues are closed in layers. Some studies have encouraged immobilization in a position of flexion to limit wound healing concerns; however, this has been associated with some sustained extension deficits.

Bicondylar Fractures

The frequent presence of a coronally oriented posteromedial fragment has been increasingly appreciated in bicondylar fracture patterns (**Figure 12, A**). These fragments have been described in 60% to 75% of Orthopaedic Trauma

Association C-type bicondylar tibial plateau fractures.[25,26] Coronally oriented posteromedial fragments typically encompass as much as 25% of the entire knee joint surface. If unrecognized or inadequately reduced and fixated, articular incongruity and limb malalignment with compromised clinical outcomes may result.[27] Contemporary laterally applied locking plates may not provide sufficient fixation or engage these posteromedial variants[28] (**Figure 12, B** and **C**); however, these factors depend on the type of implant and operator insertion. Both the plate design and the location of application may influence posteromedial fragment capture.

To provide an adequate and preserved reduction, the surgeon may

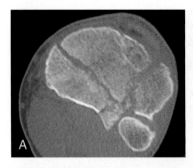
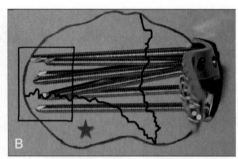
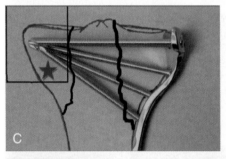
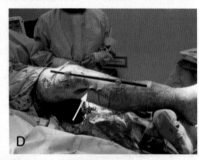

Figure 12 Images show the management of a bicondylar tibial plateau fracture with a coronally oriented posteromedial component. **A,** Axial CT scan demonstrates a proximal tibial plateau fracture with a coronally oriented posteromedial component. **B** and **C,** Sketches with implants show the design characteristics of contemporary locking plates, which may not effectively engage coronally oriented posteromedial proximal tibia fractures. The location of the fragments is shown by the stars. **D,** Intraoperative photograph shows dual plate fixation using a medial approach over the left knee with the patient placed in the supine position. The arrow indicates the required, sometimes compromising trajectory of the implant insertion devices (drills, depth gauges, screws). (Reproduced from Kottmeier SA, Jones CB, Tornetta P III, Russell TA: Locked and minimally invasive plating: A paradigm shift? Metadiaphyseal site-specific concerns and controversies. *Instr Course Lect* 2013;62:41-59.)

perform dual plate fixation, which uses both anterolateral and posteromedial approaches.[29-31] Dual plate fixation is commonly performed with simultaneous surgical access strategies and the patient placed in the supine position. Weil et al[32] described the importance of proper patient and limb positioning. Adequate reduction and fixation of the posteromedial fragment with the patient placed in the supine position may be complicated by knee extension that is required for reduction as well as the limited exposure and conflicts with screw and drill trajectory (**Figure 12, D**). Typically, medial condyle reduction is performed first because the medial

condyle is often less comminuted than its lateral counterpart and serves as a foundation on which to build the lateral articular and lateral column components. If the patient is placed in the supine position, the knee tends to drift into varus, which complicates both reduction and the maintenance of reduction during fixation. In this situation, valgus and extension are commonly required to provide effective reduction. Although overcome with some effort, these deforming forces are increasingly problematic as fracture complexity increases. Patients who have systemic comorbidities may require dual plate reduction in the supine position.

Alternatively, the surgeon may use a staged strategy, which provides fixation of the medial column with the patient placed in the prone position, to initiate the reconstructive effort (**Figure 13, A** through **D**). Reduction and stabilization of the medial column is followed by repositioning of the patient supine and re-preparation of the limb (same setting) for lateral column and articular surface fixation (**Figure 13, E** through **H**). Prone positioning of the patient and the posteromedial (Loebenhoffer) approach that was previously discussed allow for excellent and efficient reduction maneuvers and easy implant insertion (drill and screw trajectory). Implants introduced for reduction of the medial condyle must not compete with implants introduced for the subsequent fixation of the lateral condyle. In addition to the inconveniences of patient and limb re-preparation, the staged strategy does not allow for simultaneous reduction of the medial and lateral condylar components. Further, the staged strategy mandates accurate and anatomic reduction of the medial condyle before subsequent fixation of the lateral condyle. Luo et al[17] described patient preparation and positioning in a floating position that allowed for simultaneous anterior and posterior access; however, this approach may include both the attributes and liabilities of supine- (simultaneous) and prone- (followed by supine) staged approaches.

Watson et al[33] described a staged treatment strategy for the management of complex three-column tibial plateau fracture-dislocations. The authors reported a displaced vertical shear fracture of the posterior column with lateral and medial column fractures. These three-column fracture-dislocations typically had substantial posterior

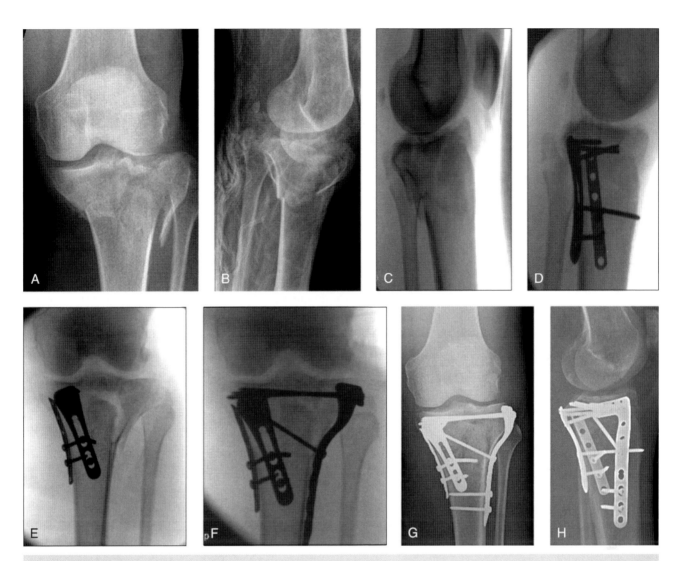

Figure 13   Images demonstrate staged fixation of a bicondylar tibial plateau fracture with a coronally oriented posteromedial component. AP (**A**) and lateral (**B**) radiographs demonstrate a high-energy bicondylar proximal left tibia fracture with inferior subsidence of both condyles. Lateral fluoroscopic images show that the patient was initially placed in the prone position (**C**), and the medial column was reduced and stabilized only (**D**). AP fluoroscopic images show that after reconstitution of the medial column foundation, the patient was repositioned supine (**E**), and the lateral column and articular surface were then addressed (**F**). Postoperative AP (**G**) and lateral (**H**) radiographs demonstrate final fixation.

column compromise with resultant knee subluxation. The authors concluded that such complex three-column injuries were rare and unique compared with more common posteromedial condylar components found in bicondylar fractures. Further, the authors cautioned that unfamiliarity with and, accordingly, the absence of the recognition of these fracture patterns would likely result in an ineffective treatment strategy. Prompt recognition and

stabilization of the posterior column component with the patient placed in the prone position was encouraged to initially restore limb length, alignment, and stability, as well as to resolve subluxation. This was performed in combination with the application of a transarticular external fixator to allow the soft tissues to recover. Definitive fixation of the remaining components was performed in delayed fashion. A postoperative CT scan was obtained in

the interim to better strategize fixation of and access to the lateral and medial columns.

Distal Tibia Fractures

Early fracture classifications that described plateau and pilon injuries largely emphasized a coronal mindset with an emphasis on medial and lateral fracture site involvement and surgical access. Accordingly, indications and strategies for fixation were based on this mindset.

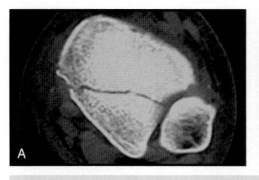 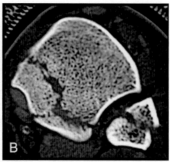

Figure 14   Axial CT scans demonstrate type I (**A**) and type II (**B**) posterior malleolus fractures described by Haraguchi et al.[34]

Contemporary fracture classifications have challenged earlier classifications by adopting the notion of quadrants and columns. Contemporary classifications have generated a heightened interest in and placed emphasis on circumferential access as well as staged and simultaneous fixation strategies. These evolving approaches help address the limitations of previously adopted exposures as well as the occasional incompatibility of implants and their designs.

Posterior Malleolus Fractures

Fractures that involve the posterior malleolus of the ankle warrant, and are increasingly receiving, attention. The preferred treatment for posterior malleolus ankle fracture variants is controversial and evolving. Inadequate or improper assessment of posterior malleolus ankle fractures may result in posterior ankle instability and altered ankle reaction forces that contribute to arthrosis. The terms and definitions for posterior malleolus ankle fractures, including what truly defines and constitutes a posterior malleolus fracture and a posterior pilon fracture, remain vague. The term "posterior pilon" has been used to designate a lesion that results from a lesser energy mechanism of injury rather than a higher energy mechanism of injury. Efforts to characterize

posterior pilon fractures group them between rotational ankle fractures and conventional high-energy pilon fractures.

Early fracture classifications distinguished posterior malleolus fractures that involved the posterolateral corner of the distal tibia (Volkmann fragment) from those that involved the entire posterior or posteromedial tibial plafond. Posterior malleolus fractures that involve the posterolateral corner result from avulsion forces imparted by the intact posteroinferior tibiofibular ligament and from applied rotational forces. Posterior malleolus fractures that involve the entire posterior malleolus result secondary to axial loading and posterior shearing forces. These lesions commonly exit the medial tibial cortex with or without articular impaction, and the medial malleolus may be fractured and displaced in isolation or in combination.

Haraguchi et al[34] conducted a CT study to better discern the unique and common anatomic presentations of posterior malleolus fractures. The authors distinguished three types of posterior malleolus fractures: type I, posterolateral-oblique (**Figure 14, A**); type II, transverse medial-extension (**Figure 14, B**); and type III, small-shell. Type I posterior malleolus

fractures typically involve the posterolateral corner of the tibial plafond in the form of a large triangular fragment that exits dorsally before the medial malleolus. Type II posterior malleolus fractures are typically transverse with medial extension that is characterized by a fracture line that extends from the fibular notch of the tibia to the medial malleolus. Type II fractures that extend to the anterior portion of the medial malleolus may frequently have two fragments (posterolateral and posteromedial). The authors reported that the mean fragment area comprised approximately 12% of the cross-sectional area of the tibial plafond in type I posterior malleolus fractures and approximately 30% of the cross-sectional area of the tibial plafond in type II posterior malleolus fractures. The authors also reported that type II posterior malleolus fractures often had two fragments, some of which involved the entire medial malleolus. The authors reported that these posterior malleolus two-part fracture variants were not infrequent and demanded identification to ensure proper surgical access, reduction, and fixation.

The major fracture lines in type I and type II posterior malleolus fractures are not always consistent. The degree of comminution and obliquity of the fracture fragment depends on both the magnitude and the direction of applied force. Assessment of posterior malleolus fractures on conventional radiographs alone may prove inaccurate; therefore, CT is required to determine the exact size, location, and orientation of the fracture fragments. Proper identification and scrutiny of type I and type II posterior malleolus fracture variants may dictate surgical access strategies.

Uncertainty exists with regard to the potential negative influence of posterior malleolus fractures on subsequent ankle performance. Some studies have attempted to assess the role of the posterior malleolus in stabilization of the ankle.[35,36] Other studies have attempted to assess the contact area dimensions of the posterior malleolus and, accordingly, its potential influence on ankle dynamics and the evolution of arthrosis. Contact stress aberrations have been intuitively implicated in the origin of arthrosis. In a cadaver model study, Fitzpatrick et al[37] performed a kinematic and contact stress analysis of posterior malleolus fractures. The authors did not report talar subluxation or increases in contact stresses in any of the simulated posterior malleolus fractures; however, the authors reported an abnormal redistribution of forces to regions of the ankle that were unaccustomed to such forces, which suggested that anatomic fixation did not fully restore the stress patterns. In a cadaver model study, Hartford et al[38] reported corresponding decreases in the tibiotalar contact area with increasingly larger fracture fragments; however, the integrity of the deltoid ligament did not appear to influence the contact area.

The origin of arthrosis has been described in clinical scenarios but remains uncertain. Clinical studies have suggested that posterior malleolus injuries are associated with a higher incidence of posttraumatic arthrosis compared with bimalleolar fractures variants.[39-41] Chondral damage sustained at the time of injury and residual joint instability are potential sources of arthrosis. The clinical and biomechanical evidence that dictates the proper surgical indications for the management of posterior malleolus fractures is elusive and without scientific validity.

Historically, fibular stabilization has been advocated to indirectly reduce and stabilize posterior malleolus fractures, which renders fixation unnecessary. An intact posteroinferior tibiofibular ligament, by way of ligamentotaxis, may help address smaller fractures; however, it is unlikely that larger posterolateral fractures, particularly those with an associated posteromedial (dual) fracture configuration, will be restored within acceptable parameters with such efforts. Fixation with the use of anterior-to-posterior percutaneous techniques may be considered for fracture patterns with no or minimal displacement. Such fixation constructs may be inadequate for more displaced or unstable lesions and may result in construct failure as well as disastrous functional and clinical outcomes.

Conventional medial or lateral surgical approaches to the distal posterior tibial articular surface may not provide sufficient access or allow for easy implant insertion. In addition, regions with marginal impaction are difficult to address with medial or lateral surgical approaches. Central regions of articular impaction also are difficult to access with medial or lateral surgical approaches, and a sustained position of malreduction may precipitate arthrosis. Several surgical approaches, including posteromedial and posterolateral approaches as well as dual access via both simultaneously, have been described for posterior malleolus fragment reduction and fixation. The often highly variable fracture configurations of posterior malleolus fractures require surgeons to select an ideal approach or a combination of several approaches.[42]

In a multicenter study, Tornetta et al[43] described the indications and results for 72 patients with posterior malleolus

fractures who were treated with surgical fixation. The cohort included patients who had bimalleolar and trimalleolar fractures but specifically excluded patients who had pilon fracture variants. Indications included displaced fracture patterns that involved more than 30% of the joint surface or had posterior ankle instability. The authors emphasized the advantages of the posterolateral approach, which provided access to both the lateral and posterior malleoli, as well as direct and sufficient exposure, which allowed for accurate reduction and rigid plate fixation. The authors reported a slightly higher rate of noninfected healing complications compared with standard lateral and medial malleolar approaches.

Bois and Dust[44] described a posteromedial surgical approach for the management of posterior malleolus fractures that had associated posterior ankle fracture-dislocations. A large posterior malleolus fragment was identified in each of the 17 patients. All but two patients underwent surgical fixation with the use of the posteromedial approach; the two remaining patients were managed with a dual posteromedial and posterolateral approach. The authors reported excellent visualization of the entire posterior malleolar surface with the posteromedial approach, which was initiated within the tendon sheath of the tibialis posterior tendon. The authors advocated for a dual posteromedial and posterolateral approach because it allowed for enhanced access and preferential implant site application, if required. The authors encouraged careful preoperative scrutiny of CT scans to determine fracture configuration (medial versus lateral).

Several caveats are worthy of consideration in performing retromalleolar

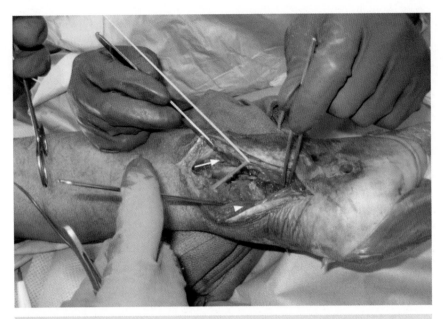

Figure 15 Intraoperative photograph shows the posterolateral approach to a right ankle, which includes lateral positioning of the ankle and a linear posterolateral skin incision. The peroneal tendons are mobilized laterally (arrow), the sural nerve is positioned within the vessel loop, the flexor hallucis longus muscle is mobilized medially (arrowhead), and the retromalleolar surface is exposed.

fixation. Surgeons should avoid the introduction of excessively long implants (screws) posteriorly because anterior implant-related prominence and discomfort may result. This may be recognized only after the patient is returned to the supine position. Surgeons who pursue fibular fixation first, with the application and positioning of implants that may conflict with satisfactory fluoroscopic imaging second, may potentially compromise the assessment of posterior malleolus fracture reduction and implant orientation.

Access to both the lateral and posterior malleoli is provided with the posterolateral approach. The patient is placed in either the lateral (**Figure 15**) or, preferably, the prone position. Bolsters are positioned to allow for passive flexion of both the knee and ankle during surgical reduction. A longitudinal incision is made between the posterior border of the fibula and the

lateral border of the Achilles tendon. Superficial dissection is carried down to the interval between the peroneal and Achilles tendons. The sural nerve is then encountered and is protected throughout the course of dissection. Next, the overlying fascia of the flexor hallucis longus muscle is identified and incised, and the muscle is elevated from the interosseous membrane and lateral tibia. Next, the muscle is retracted medially to expose the distal aspect of the posterior tibia as well as the posterior and medial margins of the fibula. The longitudinally positioned peroneal artery is protected, and its transverse perforators are ligated and divided as necessary. Dissection is maintained superficial to the ankle capsule to prevent the potential disruption of the posterior syndesmotic ligaments. Subperiosteal elevation of the retromalleolar fragment is performed superiorly to identify its apical spike. The superior spike is an

excellent confirmation of accurate anatomic reduction; however, assessment of the fracture margins both medially and laterally is required to further confirm the adequacy of reduction. Because posterior malleolus fractures more often present with lateral displacement than medial displacement, a medial soft-tissue hinge is provided and aids in reduction. Occasionally, incarcerated fragments or more complex fracture variants (type II with medial extension) may demand a medial approach or a dual posteromedial and posterolateral approach.

The fracture is sufficiently mobilized to allow for evacuation of the interposed soft tissues, hematoma, and early callus as well as any displaced osteochondral fragments that may compromise reduction. Marginal impaction is reduced under direct visualization and lateral fluoroscopic guidance. Passive dorsiflexion of the ankle helps restore length and further facilitates fracture reduction; however, ball-spike pushers, reduction clamps, and other directly applied reduction aids may be required if passive dorsiflexion of the ankle is insufficient. Excessive passive dorsiflexion of the ankle may result in posterior translation of the talus; an anteriorly directed force is required to counteract this reduction complication. Infrequently, a femoral distractor may be required to facilitate reduction. Distal pin insertion should be performed within the talar body rather than the calcaneus to provide collinear distraction (**Figure 16**).

Although some studies have advocated for screw insertion only to secure the posterior malleolus, other studies have advocated for antiglide plate application, which may aid in fracture reduction and in the sustained maintenance

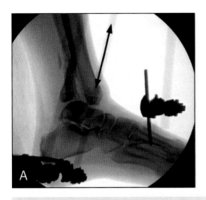
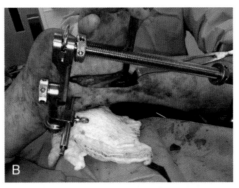
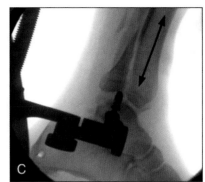

Figure 16   Images show reduction of a posterior fracture-dislocation of the ankle. **A,** Lateral fluoroscopic image shows that transarticular distraction with a calcaneal pin does not provide a collinear force, which results in subluxation. **B,** Intraoperative photograph shows the application of a femoral distractor with the inclusion of a talar body pin. **C,** Lateral fluoroscopic image shows the resolution of subluxation. The double-sided arrow in panels A and C represent the preferred distraction forces imparted by the applied distractor.

of construct integrity[43,45] (**Figure 17**). A true lateral view of the ankle under fluoroscopic guidance is required to confirm satisfactory reduction of the articular fragment and concentric reduction of the ankle joint. Fixation of the fibula can be performed via the same incision, either medial or lateral to the mobilized peroneal tendons; however, the tendon sheath should be maintained inferiorly within the proximity of the distal fibula to ensure the presence of tendon stability within the retrofibular groove. The proximity of posteriorly applied retrofibular implants to the adjacent peroneal tendons must be considered to minimize implant-related discomfort.

Fixation of medial malleolus fractures via a standard medial approach is easily achieved with the patient placed in the lateral position as well as with free draping of the limb and external rotation. Fixation is more complicated with the patient placed in the prone position, but is certainly feasible; however, any anteromedial marginal impaction must be anticipated and addressed preoperatively because it may complicate the procedure with the patient placed in the prone position. The inclusion of a simultaneous posteromedial approach

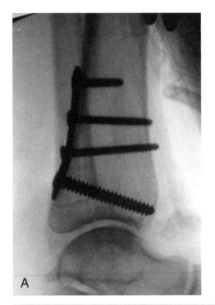
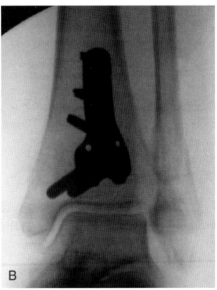

Figure 17   Lateral (**A**) and AP (**B**) fluoroscopic images show retromalleolar fixation of an ankle with the use of antiglide fixation.

may be beneficial and, occasionally, is essential. Ideally, a dual approach should be anticipated preoperatively to allow for preferential placement of the patient in the prone position.

The patient is placed in either the supine or prone position on a radiolucent table. If the patient is placed in the supine position, figure-of-4 positioning of the ipsilateral hip facilitates access to the medial aspect of the ankle. The skin incision follows the posteromedial

border of the distal tibia and medial malleolus in continuity with the tibialis posterior tendon. The incision is extended proximally to the level required to gain sufficient access to the most superior portion of the fracture. Full-thickness skin flaps are developed. Next, the flexor retinaculum overlying the tibialis posterior tendon sheath is identified, and the saphenous vein and nerve are protected within the anterior soft tissues. The tibialis posterior

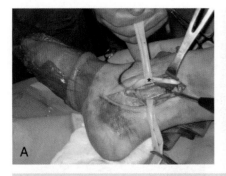 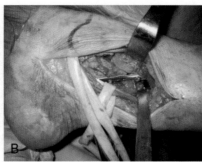

Figure 18 Intraoperative photographs show the posteromedial approach for fixation of a medial malleolar fracture of a right ankle. **A,** The posterior tibialis is mobilized anteriorly with the use of a Penrose drain (asterisk), and the flexor digitorum longus is retracted posteriorly. The fracture, which enters the retromalleolar groove, is mobilized with an elevator. **B,** An antiglide plate is applied to the retromalleolar surface at the superior apex of the fracture.

tendon sheath is incised throughout the entire length of the surgical incision. The flexor digitorum longus is retracted posteriorly to protect the neurovascular bundle, and the posterior tibialis is mobilized and retracted anteriorly (**Figure 18, A**). Alternatively, both tendons may be directed anteriorly and provisionally secured within the medial malleolus with an overlying pin, which enhances access to the fracture and allows for insertion of implants. The fracture site is identified within the floor of the tendon sheath. Dissection is continued both laterally and medially to allow for adequate exposure of the fracture margins. Components of both the posterior and medial malleolus fractures may be sufficiently mobilized to allow for joint inspection and articular reconstitution. In a manner similar to that previously discussed for the posterolateral approach, reduction forceps and pointed ball-spike pushers as well as undercontoured antiglide plates are used to facilitate reduction. The cortical osseous margins at the apex and medial lateral extents of the fracture must be simultaneously assessed and reduced to ensure adequate anatomic reduction (**Figure 18, B**). The posterior tibial

tendon is mobilized posteriorly from its position of anterior displacement as necessary to facilitate the introduction of medial malleolar implants. Next, fibular fixation is performed with either a direct lateral or posterolateral approach to the ankle. An incongruous reduction of the posterior malleolus will result in any of the aforementioned scenarios if fibular malreduction occurs before posterior malleolar fixation. Care should be taken in the placement of posteromedial implants to prevent posterior tendon irritation and resultant injury. Similar to lateral peroneal tendon sheath closure, a secure closure of the posterior tibial tendon sheath is required to avoid postsurgical tendon instability.

In some patients, a dual incision approach that includes a simultaneous posterolateral approach may be required. As previously mentioned, a dual approach should be determined preoperatively with the careful scrutiny of CT scans to allow for placement of the patient in the required prone position (**Figure 19**). An accurate assessment of regional marginal impaction, incarcerated fragments, and fracture configuration complexities will help determine if a dual approach is necessary.

Pilon Fractures

High-energy pilon fractures present a surgical challenge because of the often compromised and vulnerable soft tissues. The principles of delayed treatment and temporary transarticular spanning external fixation have provided surgeons with a successful strategy to resolve these concerns. The goals of surgical intervention include restoration of axial alignment, anatomic articular reconstruction, and the introduction of early range of motion. Surgical access should not introduce additional compromise to the osseous and soft-tissue vascular supply. Although minimally invasive approaches are attractive, they are primarily suited to manage fracture patterns with minimal or easily managed articular involvement. Surgical exposure selection requires surgeons to have an accurate understanding of the fracture pathoanatomy and regional soft-tissue anatomy.

Conventional pilon exposures include the anteromedial, direct anterior, and anterolateral approaches as well as versions and modifications of these approaches. Recently, the role of posterior approaches, including their attributes and limitations, has been investigated. Several studies explored the role of the posterolateral approach for the management of fracture patterns that were receptive to it.[46-48] Because the posterolateral approach does not require extensive surgical flaps or undermining dissection, the studies hypothesized that abundant and robust regional soft tissues would result in fewer wound healing complications. Although the results of several studies supported this hypothesis,[46-48] Bhattacharyya et al[49] reported a 33% infection and wound healing complication rate.

The posterolateral approach provides excellent visualization of the posterior aspect of the tibia, the posterior malleolus fragments, and the posterolateral aspect of the fibula; however, it provides only limited visualization of the anterior articular surface. Fracture patterns with moderate or extensive anterior comminution require a staged approach. Ketz and Sanders[46] reported frustration with accurate reduction of the posterior malleolus fragment in high-energy pilon fractures that were managed with standard anterior midline approaches. The authors advocated the posterolateral approach with posterior malleolus plating in certain patients (**Figure 20**). A postoperative CT scan was obtained to critically assess the adequacy of posterior reduction and fixation. Next, a staged anterior fixation was performed in a delayed fashion as soft-tissue recovery allowed. The authors determined that this protocol, with initial anatomic restoration posteriorly, enhanced subsequent articular reduction in select fracture patterns. This technique demonstrated improvement over approaches that used anterior incisions only with indirect posterior reduction. The authors reported that if the posterior fragment was anatomically reduced and stable, the fracture would then be converted (upgraded) to a simpler Orthopaedic Trauma Association 43B pilon fracture pattern. These authors reported both improved articular reductions and superior functional outcomes with this technique. Similarly, Assal et al[50] acknowledged the advantages of initial posterior column reconstruction; however, the authors used a posteromedial exposure and reported enhanced access to the entire retromalleolar surface. Staged approaches were performed both in a delayed fashion and in the same setting. Screws introduced posteriorly during

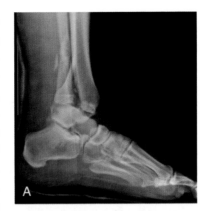
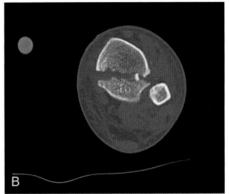
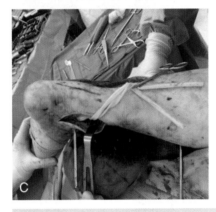
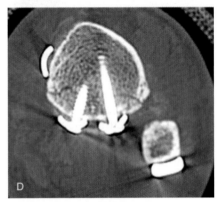

Figure 19 Images show the dual (posteromedial and posterolateral) approach for fixation of a posteriorly dislocated ankle with incarcerated fragments. **A,** Lateral radiograph demonstrates a posterior left ankle dislocation. **B,** Axial CT scan demonstrates several concerns, including incarcerated fragments, fracture orientation, and possible limitations for lateral access. **C,** Intraoperative photograph shows that these difficulties were anticipated and the patient was placed in the prone position for dual access. **D,** Axial CT demonstrates reduction and fixation with a dual plate construct.

the initial stage were unicortical only to limit conflict with subsequent anterior reconstruction in the supine positon.

Posteromedial access for the management of pilon fractures may be useful in several unique situations. Dunbar et al[51] described a subset of pilon fractures with an oblique extension to the diaphysis, which poses a specific and additional treatment dilemma (**Figure 21, A** through **C**). The authors encountered difficulties in reduction of these pilon fracture variants at the time of delayed definitive fixation. The authors reported the insertion, often posteromedially, of an antiglide plate via a

small proximal incision that was remote from the zone of injury (**Figure 21, D**). Length, rotation, and alignment were reestablished with this fragment, which often was in continuity with either a substantial articular anterolateral or posterolateral fragment. These steps were performed in the very early or immediate phases of treatment and followed by additional delayed articular reduction as soft-tissue recovery allowed. This approach converts a more complex articular Orthopaedic Trauma Association 43C pilon fracture pattern to a simpler Orthopaedic Trauma Association 43B pilon fracture pattern, or upgrades

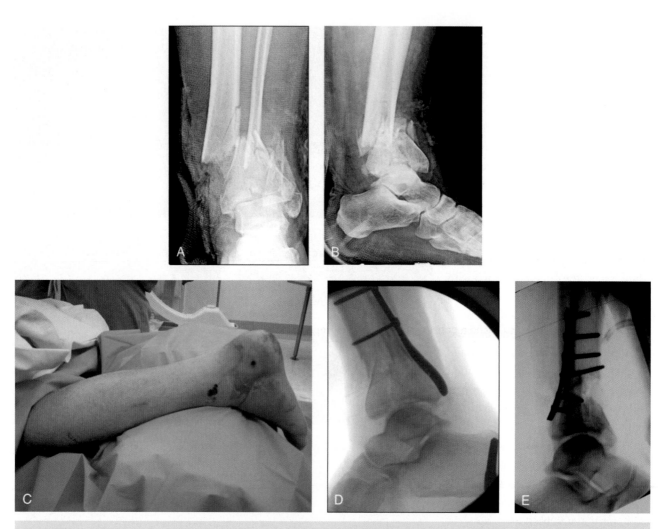

Figure 20 Images show the staged posterolateral approach with posterior malleolar plating for the fixation of a tibial pilon fracture. AP (**A**) and lateral (**B**) radiographs demonstrate a complex unstable tibial pilon fracture. **C,** Intraoperative photograph shows that the patient was placed in the prone position for initial staged posterior column reconstitution. **D,** Lateral fluoroscopic image shows that a template was established posteriorly, upon which anterior reconstruction was subsequently performed using a staged supine anterior approach. **E,** Lateral fluoroscopic image shows the posterior application of a device that is limited to unicortical fixation to prevent conflict with subsequent anteriorly introduced implants.

the fracture. Eastman et al[52] advocated a posteromedial incision if suspicion of entrapped structures exists in otherwise conventional articular reconstruction of pilon fractures. The authors identified interposition of the tibialis posterior tendon and, on occasion, the posterior tibial neurovascular bundle. Careful scrutiny of CT scans before surgery was encouraged to identify interposition of the tibialis posterior tendon and the posterior tibial neurovascular bundle

and to determine the option for remedy during surgical fixation.

Summary

As new implants and the means for surgically introducing them continue to evolve, surgeons must consider the attributes and limitations not only of the devices but also the options for surgical access. Contemporary strategies for satisfactory skeletal reconstruction mandate surgeons have an understanding

of various desirable and preferential exposures. The proper exposure can greatly enhance acceptable reduction and adequate fixation; however, a balance must be attained between an effective approach for reduction and the preservation of soft tissues and subsequent osseous viability. Vulnerable regional anatomic structures must be respected. In the management of complex high-energy osteoarticular injuries, more surgeries (staged) and

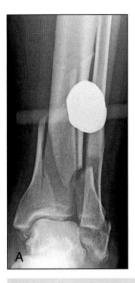
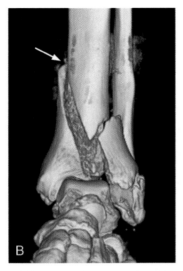
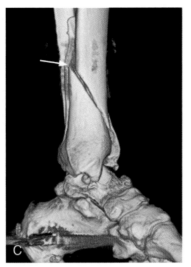
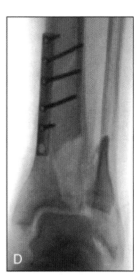

Figure 21   Images show the posteromedial approach (upgrading) for fixation of a pilon fracture variant. AP radiograph (**A**) and AP (**B**) and lateral (**C**) three-dimensional CT reconstructions demonstrate a pilon fracture variant with oblique diaphyseal extension and a considerable articular component (arrow in panels B and C). **D,** AP radiograph demonstrates limited dissection and insertion of a plate remote from the compromised soft tissues, which restored length acutely.

more incisions (strategically placed), if properly executed, may be less perilous to the soft tissues. Unique characteristics of both the patient and his or her fracture pathoanatomy may dictate the surgical approach. Seemingly minor details must be considered, including patient positioning, imaging access, and urinary catheterization. Patient systemic and regional comorbidities, both medical and trauma related, must be accurately assessed. Inadequacies in both implant design and surgical exposures must continue to be reassessed. Surgeons who adopt new surgical techniques must critically assess the literature to determine if studies include evidence-based medicine or nothing more than junk science. In addition, surgeons must reflect on not only the collective experience of other surgeons but also their own personal experience.

References

1. Gardner MJ, Weil Y, Barker JU, Kelly BT, Helfet DL, Lorich DG: The importance of medial support in locked plating of proximal humerus fractures. *J Orthop Trauma* 2007;21(3):185-191.

2. Little MT, Berkes MB, Schottel PC, et al: The impact of preoperative coronal plane deformity on proximal humerus fixation with endosteal augmentation. *J Orthop Trauma* 2014;28(6):338-347.

3. Morgan SJ, Furry K, Parekh AA, Agudelo JF, Smith WR: The deltoid muscle: An anatomic description of the deltoid insertion to the proximal humerus. *J Orthop Trauma* 2006;20(1):19-21.

4. Gardner MJ, Voos JE, Wanich T, Helfet DL, Lorich DG: Vascular implications of minimally invasive plating of proximal humerus fractures. *J Orthop Trauma* 2006;20(9):602-607.

5. Gardner MJ, Boraiah S, Helfet DL, Lorich DG: Indirect medial reduction and strut support of proximal humerus fractures using an endosteal implant. *J Orthop Trauma* 2008;22(3):195-200.

6. Hettrich CM, Neviaser A, Beamer BS, Paul O, Helfet DL, Lorich DG: Locked plating of the proximal humerus using an endosteal implant. *J Orthop Trauma* 2012;26(4):212-215.

7. Gardner MJ, Griffith MH, Dines JS, Briggs SM, Weiland AJ, Lorich DG: The extended anterolateral acromial approach allows minimally invasive access to the proximal humerus. *Clin Orthop Relat Res* 2005;434:123-129.

8. Khan LA, Robinson CM, Will E, Whittaker R: Assessment of axillary nerve function and functional outcome after fixation of complex proximal humeral fractures using the extended deltoid-splitting approach. *Injury* 2009;40(2):181-185.

9. Robinson CM, Page RS: Severely impacted valgus proximal humeral fractures: Results of operative treatment. *J Bone Joint Surg Am* 2003;85(9):1647-1655.

10. Gardner MJ, Boraiah S, Helfet DL, Lorich DG: The anterolateral acromial approach for fractures of the proximal humerus. *J Orthop Trauma* 2008;22(2):132-137.

11. Laflamme GY, Rouleau DM, Berry GK, Beaumont PH, Reindl R, Harvey EJ: Percutaneous humeral plating of fractures of the proximal humerus: Results of a prospective multicenter clinical trial. *J Orthop Trauma* 2008;22(3):153-158.

12. Gavaskar AS, Chowdary N, Abraham S: Complex proximal humerus fractures treated with locked plating utilizing an extended deltoid split approach with a shoulder strap incision. *J Orthop Trauma* 2013;27(2):73-76.

13. Robinson CM, Khan L, Akhtar A, Whittaker R: The extended deltoid-splitting approach to the proximal humerus. *J Orthop Trauma* 2007;21(9):657-662.

14. Robinson CM, Page RS. Severely impacted valgus proximal humeral fractures. *J Bone Joint Surg Am* 2004;86(suppl 1):143-155.

15. Robinson CM, Murray IR: The extended deltoid-splitting approach to the proximal humerus: Variations and extensions. *J Bone Joint Surg Br* 2011;93(3):387-392.

16. Hettrich CM, Boraiah S, Dyke JP, Neviaser A, Helfet DL, Lorich DG: Quantitative assessment of the vascularity of the proximal part of the humerus. *J Bone Joint Surg Am* 2010;92(4):943-948.

17. Luo CF, Sun H, Zhang B, Zeng BF: Three-column fixation for complex tibial plateau fractures. *J Orthop Trauma* 2010;24(11):683-692.

18. Watson JT, Karges D Jackman J: Lateral locking plates for the treatment of bicondylar tibial plateau fractures: A treatment protocol, indications, and results. Presented at the Annual Meeting of the Orthopaedic Trauma Association, Boston, MA, October 17-20, 2007.

19. Moore TM: Fracture—dislocation of the knee. *Clin Orthop Relat Res* 1981;156:128-140.

20. De Boeck H, Opdecam P: Posteromedial tibial plateau fractures: Operative treatment by posterior approach. *Clin Orthop Relat Res* 1995;320:125-128.

21. Fakler JK, Ryzewicz M, Hartshorn C, Morgan SJ, Stahel PF, Smith WR: Optimizing the management of Moore type I postero-medial split fracture dislocations of the tibial head: Description of the Lobenhoffer approach. *J Orthop Trauma* 2007;21(5):330-336.

22. Galla M, Lobenhoffer P: The direct, dorsal approach to the treatment of unstable tibial posteromedial fracture-dislocations. *Unfallchirurg* 2003;106(3):241-247.

23. Lobenhoffer P, Gerich T, Bertram T, Lattermann C, Pohlemann T, Tscheme H: Particular posteromedial and posterolateral approaches for the treatment of tibial head fractures. *Unfallchirurg* 1997;100(12):957-967.

24. Bhattacharyya T, McCarty LP III, Harris MB, et al: The posterior shearing tibial plateau fracture: Treatment and results via a posterior approach. *J Orthop Trauma* 2005;19(5):305-310.

25. Barei DP, O'Mara TJ, Taitsman LA, Dunbar RP, Nork SE: Frequency and fracture morphology of the posteromedial fragment in bicondylar tibial plateau fracture patterns. *J Orthop Trauma* 2008;22(3):176-182.

26. Higgins TF, Kemper D, Klatt J: Incidence and morphology of the posteromedial fragment in bicondylar tibial plateau fractures. *J Orthop Trauma* 2009;23(1):45-51.

27. Weaver M, Strom AC, Smith RM, Harris MB, Lhowe D, Vrahas MS: Fracture pattern and fixation type related to loss of reduction in bicondylar tibial plateau fractures. Presented at the Annual Meeting of the Orthopaedic Trauma Association, San Diego, CA, October 17-10, 2009.

28. Yoo BJ, Beingessner DM, Barei DP: Stabilization of the posteromedial fragment in bicondylar tibial plateau fractures: A mechanical comparison of locking and nonlocking single and dual plating methods. *J Trauma* 2010;69(1):148-155.

29. Barei DP, Nork SE, Mills WJ, Henley MB, Benirschke SK: Complications associated with internal fixation of high-energy bicondylar tibial plateau fractures utilizing a two-incision technique. *J Orthop Trauma* 2004;18(10):649-657.

30. Bendayan J, Noblin JD, Freeland AE: Posteromedial second incision to reduce and stabilize a displaced posterior fragment that can occur in Schatzker type V bicondylar tibial plateau fractures. *Orthopedics* 1996;19(10):903-904.

31. Georgiadis GM: Combined anterior and posterior approaches for complex tibial plateau fractures. *J Bone Joint Surg Br* 1994;76(2):285-289.

32. Weil YA, Gardner MJ, Boraiah S, Helfet DL, Lorich DG: Posteromedial supine approach for reduction and fixation of medial and bicondylar tibial plateau fractures. *J Orthop Trauma* 2008;22(5):357-362.

33. Watson JT, Boudreau JA, Karges D, Kuldjanov D: Paper No. 084. Staged treatment for complex 3 column tibial plateau fracture dislocations. AAOS 2014 Annual Meeting Proceedings. Rosemont, IL, American Academy of Orthopaedic Surgeons, 2014.

34. Haraguchi N, Haruyama H, Toga H, Kato F: Pathoanatomy of posterior malleolar fractures of the ankle. *J Bone Joint Surg Am* 2006;88(5):1085-1092.

35. Harper MC: Posterior instability of the talus: An anatomic evaluation. *Foot Ankle* 1989;10(1):36-39.

36. Raasch WG, Larkin JJ, Draganich LF: Assessment of the posterior malleolus as a restraint to posterior subluxation of the ankle. *J Bone Joint Surg Am* 1992;74(8):1201-1206.

37. Fitzpatrick DC, Otto JK, McKinley TO, Marsh JL, Brown TD: Kinematic and contact stress analysis of posterior malleolus fractures of the ankle. *J Orthop Trauma* 2004;18(5):271-278.

38. Hartford JM, Gorczyca JT, McNamara JL, Mayor MB: Tibiotalar contact area: Contribution of posterior malleolus and deltoid ligament. *Clin Orthop Relat Res* 1995;320:182-187.

39. Broos PL, Bisschop AP: Operative treatment of ankle fractures in adults: Correlation between types of fracture and final results. *Injury* 1991;22(5):403-406.

40. Jaskulka RA, Ittner G, Schedl R: Fractures of the posterior tibial margin: Their role in the prognosis of malleolar fractures. *J Trauma* 1989;29(11):1565-1570.

41. McDaniel WJ, Wilson FC: Trimalleolar fractures of the ankle: An end result study. *Clin Orthop Relat Res* 1977;122:37-45.

42. Amorosa LF, Brown GD, Greisberg J: A surgical approach to posterior pilon fractures. *J Orthop Trauma* 2010;24(3):188-193.

43. Tornetta P III, Ricci W, Nork S, Collinge C, Steen B: The posterolateral approach to the tibia for displaced posterior malleolar injuries. *J Orthop Trauma* 2011;25(2):123-126.

44. Bois AJ, Dust W: Posterior fracture dislocation of the ankle: Technique and clinical experience using a posteromedial surgical approach. *J Orthop Trauma* 2008;22(9):629-636.

45. Amorosa LF, Chen L, Greisberg JA: New surgical approach to posterior pilon fractures. *Techniques in Foot & Ankle Surgery* 2009;8(2):60-64.

46. Ketz J, Sanders R: Staged posterior tibial plating for the treatment of Orthopaedic Trauma Association 43C2 and 43C3 tibial pilon fractures. *J Orthop Trauma* 2012;26(6):341-347.

47. Konrath GA, Hopkins G II: Posterolateral approach for tibial pilon fractures: A report of two cases. *J Orthop Trauma* 1999;13(8):586-589.

48. Sheerin DV, Turen CH, Nascone JW: Reconstruction of distal tibia fractures using a posterolateral approach and a blade plate. *J Orthop Trauma* 2006;20(4):247-252.

49. Bhattacharyya T, Crichlow R, Gobezie R, Kim E, Vrahas MS: Complications associated with the posterolateral approach for pilon fractures. *J Orthop Trauma* 2006;20(2):104-107.

50. Assal M, Ray A, Fasel JH, Stern R: A modified posteromedial approach combined with extensile anterior for the treatment of complex tibial pilon fractures (AO/OTA 43-C). *J Orthop Trauma* 2014;28(6):e138-e145.

51. Dunbar RP, Barei DP, Kubiak EN, Nork SE, Henley MB: Early limited internal fixation of diaphyseal extensions in select pilon fractures: Upgrading AO/OTA type C fractures to AO/OTA type B. *J Orthop Trauma* 2008;22(6):426-429.

52. Eastman JG, Firoozabadi R, Benirschke SK, Barei DP, Dunbar RP: Entrapped posteromedial structures in pilon fractures. *J Orthop Trauma* 2014;28(9):528-533.

Video References

Kottmeier SA, Row E, Watson JT, Jones CB: Video. *Posteromedial Tibial Plateau Fixation in the Prone Position: Applications of the Lobenhoffer Approach.* Stony Brook, NY, 2015.

Row E, Kottmeier SA, Burns C, Tornetta P III, Lorich DG: Video. *Posterior Ankle Approach Strategies (For Fracture Fixation).* Stony Brook, NY, 2015.

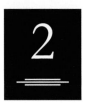

Lower Extremity Fracture Reduction: Tips, Tricks, and Techniques So That You Leave the Operating Room Satisfied

Hassan R. Mir, MD, MBA
Christina L. Boulton, MD
George V. Russell Jr, MD, MBA
Michael Archdeacon, MD

Abstract

It can be challenging for surgeons to obtain proper alignment and to create stable constructs for the maintenance of many lower extremity fractures until union is achieved. Whether lower extremity fractures are treated with plates and screws or intramedullary nails, there are numerous pearls that may help surgeons deal with these difficult injuries. Various intraoperative techniques can be used for lower extremity fracture reduction and stabilization. The use of several reduction tools, tips, and tricks may facilitate the care of lower extremity fractures and, subsequently, improve patient outcomes.

Instr Course Lect 2016;65:25–40.

Proximal Femur Fractures

Fractures of the proximal femur can be very difficult to reduce and stabilize because of the regional anatomy and the associated deforming forces. The prevention of varus malalignment is paramount. The successful union of fractures in this anatomic region is often compromised as a result of the tenuous blood supply in the subtrochanteric and femoral neck and head regions. Various strategies to obtain reduction of proximal femur fracture variants and, ultimately, to achieve successful union with function restoration are available.

Surgical Table Selection and Patient Positioning

A fracture table and a radiolucent flat-top table are the most common surgical table choices for proximal femur fracture fixation. Both tables require the patient to be placed in either the supine or lateral position. A fracture table assists in length restoration via a traction pin or boot traction; however, excessive traction can frequently accentuate proximal femoral flexion and abduction. In cases in which the authors of this chapter use a fracture table, they allow the table to

Dr. Mir or an immediate family member serves as a paid consultant to or is an employee of Acumed and Smith & Nephew; has stock or stock options held in Core Orthopaedics; and serves as a board member, owner, officer, or committee member of the American Academy of Orthopaedic Surgeons Council on Advocacy, the American Academy of Orthopaedic Surgeons Diversity Advisory Board, the Foundation for Orthopaedic Trauma Nominating and Membership Committees, and the Orthopaedic Trauma Association Public Relations Committee. Dr. Boulton or an immediate family member serves as an unpaid consultant to Advanced Orthopaedic Systems. Dr. Russell or an immediate family member is a member of a speakers' bureau or has made paid presentations on behalf of Acumed and AO North America; serves as a paid consultant to or is an employee of Acumed; has received research or institutional support from the Major Extremity Trauma Research Consortium and Synthes; has stock or stock options held in Zimmer; and serves as a board member, owner, officer, or committee member of the American Academy of Orthopaedic Surgeons, the American Academy of Orthopaedic Surgeons Board of Councilors, and the Orthopaedic Trauma Association Research Committee. Dr. Archdeacon or an immediate family member serves as a paid consultant to or is an employee of Stryker, and serves as a board member, owner, officer, or committee member of the Ohio Orthopaedic Society and the Orthopaedic Trauma Association.

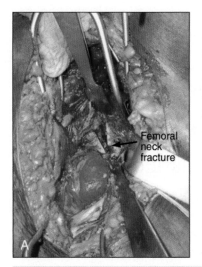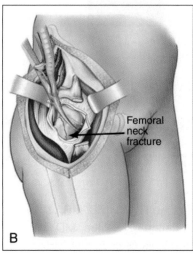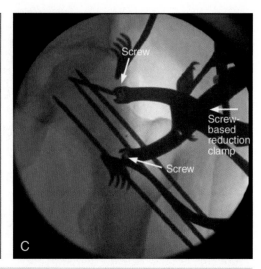

Figure 1   Images demonstrate open reduction of a femoral neck fracture. **A,** Intraoperative photograph shows an open anterior Smith-Petersen approach. **B,** Illustration shows pointed reduction clamp application. **C,** Intraoperative AP fluoroscopic image demonstrates screw-based reduction clamp application.

support the limb and to provide some hip flexion. The authors obtain provisional clamp reduction and then apply more distraction to regain length. Deformity as a result of excessive traction is less problematic for closed reduction of most intertrochanteric and femoral neck fractures. For open reduction of femoral neck fractures, a radiolucent flat-top table with the patient positioned supine and with the hip flexed allows for an anterior hip approach.

The lateral decubitus position on a radiolucent flat-top table is advantageous for most subtrochanteric and intertrochanteric fractures because it neutralizes the gravitational forces that act on the femur in the major plane of motion during hip flexion and extension, facilitates reduction and exposure as adipose tissue falls away from the plane of surgical dissection, and is easily compatible with intraoperative image intensification.[1] AP radiographs of the proximal femur require slight overrotation to account for hip anteversion. True lateral radiographs of the proximal femur require correct rotation to fully

appreciate the collinear nature of the femoral neck and shaft.

Fracture Reduction

Reduction of proximal femur fractures can be accomplished with percutaneous techniques, minimally invasive techniques, or open reduction. Regardless of the technique, it is critical for the surgeon to minimize soft-tissue stripping to preserve the tenuous blood supply of the subtrochanteric and femoral neck and head regions. Because of the cantilever nature of the proximal femur, fractures of the subtrochanteric, intertrochanteric, and femoral neck regions have a tendency toward varus malalignment. To control the proximal neck segment and prevent varus malalignment, a percutaneous Schanz pin or a spiked-ball pusher, which correct flexion, adduction, and rotation, can be used. If these maneuvers prove inadequate, standard reduction or Verbrugge bone clamps can facilitate the stabilization of subtrochanteric segments.[2] Occasionally, femoral neck fractures can be reduced with a fracture table, which

applies moderate traction and internal rotation with medialization of the shaft. It is imperative that anatomic reduction of the femoral neck be performed in younger patients to reduce the risk of nonunion or osteonecrosis.

If anatomic reduction cannot be obtained with percutaneous or minimally invasive techniques, then open reduction is necessary. A Smith-Petersen approach with the use of pointed reduction clamps or screw-based reduction clamps allows for open reduction of femoral neck fractures (**Figure 1**). For open reduction of intertrochanteric and subtrochanteric fractures, one of the authors of this chapter (M.A.) prefers a direct lateral approach with the patient placed in the lateral decubitus position because it elevates the vastus lateralis.[1] Frequently, the trochanteric segment can be easily reduced with clamps or reduction plates[3] (**Figure 2**). Other adjuvant techniques include the placement of bumps under the leg to correct coronal plane deformity, the use of cerclage wires and cables for spiral and oblique components, and the use of universal

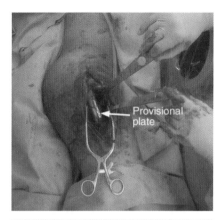

Figure 2 Intraoperative photograph shows provisional plate reduction of a subtrochanteric fracture of the femur with the patient placed in the lateral position.

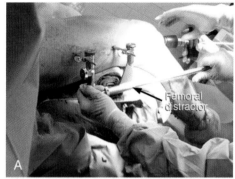

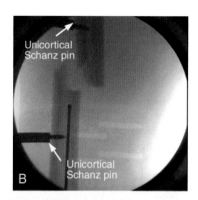

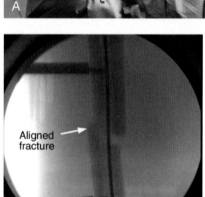

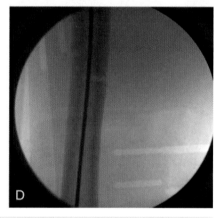

Figure 3 Intraoperative photograph (**A**) and intraoperative AP fluoroscopic images (**B** through **D**) demonstrate the use of a percutaneous femoral distractor with unicortical Schanz pins to attain anatomic alignment of the femoral shaft for the passage of a guidewire before reaming is begun. This case example shows retrograde femoral nailing; however, the concept is the same for antegrade femoral nailing.

or femoral distractors to control multiplane deformities (**Figure 3**).

Fracture Stabilization

After reduction has been obtained, internal fixation is performed with the use of several implants that are specific to each fracture variant. For femoral neck fractures, cannulated screws, which can be placed percutaneously, must be positioned along the central inferior neck and more superiorly along the anterior and posterior neck in an inverted triangle pattern. Alternatively, a sliding hip screw and side plate, with or without an antirotation screw, can be used to stabilize the femoral neck.[4] An antiglide plate can be placed on the medial femoral neck of more vertically oriented femoral neck fractures to supplement other forms of fixation (**Figure 4**).

For intertrochanteric and subtrochanteric fractures, either a cephalomedullary nail or a fixed-angle plate construct can be used.[5] If the reduction is not anatomic and the medial buttress is not restored, the authors of this chapter prefer to use a nail device, which serves as a bridging device. If a

nail is used, care must be taken to prevent lateralization of the reamer, which will result in an oval entry portal and predispose the fracture to varus malreduction. Medialization of the reamer, which forces the reamer medially, can be assisted with the use of a cannulated entry portal sleeve or the finger hole of a surgical instrument. This helps create a circular entry portal that maintains anatomic alignment during nail insertion (**Figure 5**).

One of the authors of this chapter (M.A.) prefers to use a plate for fixation of anatomic reductions because it serves as a neutralization device or a tension band. A fixed-angle plate is ideally suited to the anatomy of the proximal

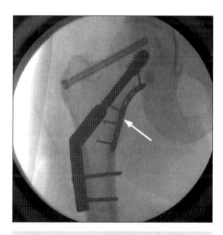

Figure 4 Intraoperative AP fluoroscopic image demonstrates the use of an antiglide plate (arrow) to supplement a dynamic hip screw and an antirotation screw for fixation of a vertically oriented femoral neck fracture.

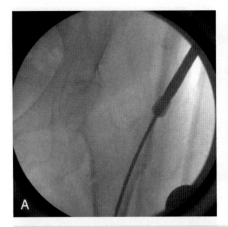
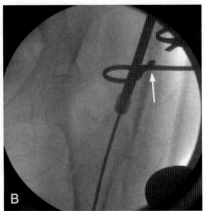

Figure 5   A, Intraoperative AP fluoroscopic image demonstrates a reamer path that is too lateral. **B,** Intraoperative AP fluoroscopic image demonstrates medialization of a reamer with the finger hole of a surgical instrument (arrow) to create a circular trochanteric entry portal that maintains anatomic alignment during nail insertion.

femur. Fixed-angle implants include a 95° fixed-angle blade plate, a condylar screw and side plate, and proximal femoral locking plates. Recent literature has reported very poor results for unstable proximal femur fractures that are fixed with proximal femoral locking plates;[6] however, one of the authors of this chapter (M.A.) has reported very good results with proximal femoral locking plates for the fixation of anatomic reductions that have had the medial buttress restored.[1] If the medial buttress is intact, the laterally based plate serves as a tension band or neutralization device. Regardless of the technique chosen for reduction and stabilization of proximal femur fractures, it is critical for surgeons to consider the technical factors of proximal femur fracture fixation, such as preservation of blood supply, anatomic reduction with the prevention of varus malalignment, and appropriate implant choice and application, to achieve good outcomes.

Femoral and Tibial Shaft Fractures

Femoral and tibial shaft fractures are commonly treated with intramedullary nails. Intramedullary nailing techniques are included in every surgical resident's education and are frequently utilized by many surgeons. There are many ways to perform intramedullary nailing of femoral and tibial shaft fractures; however, there are a few tips that can help ensure that intramedullary nailing is safe and effective.

Femoral Shaft Fractures
Surgical Table Selection and Patient Positioning
Femoral shaft fractures can be treated on a fracture table or a radiolucent flat-top table. A fracture table is useful if surgical assistants are not available because it can help the surgeon obtain and maintain fracture reduction. A fracture table also allows the surgeon to easily obtain lateral fluoroscopic images of the proximal femur. Despite the advantages of a fracture table, patient positioning may be a challenge and the surgeon has a limited ability to address associated injuries.

A radiolucent flat-top table is a popular choice for the treatment of femoral shaft fractures because it allows for easier patient positioning and allows the surgical team to address associated injuries; however, the ease of patient positioning is offset by the challenge of obtaining and maintaining fracture reduction. A radiolucent flat-top table may come with traction setups, or traction can be improvised to gain axial length. Positioning pillows can be used for coronal and sagittal plane adjustments. Surgical assistants are required more often if femoral fractures are stabilized on a radiolucent flat-top table. It may be difficult for the surgeon to obtain lateral fluoroscopic images of the proximal femur and femoral neck with the use of a radiolucent flat-top table, which can be problematic during the placement of cephalomedullary nails.

Patients who have femoral shaft fractures are routinely placed in the supine or lateral position. The lateral position is not used frequently and not usually used on a fracture table. The lateral position allows for easy access to the piriformis fossa; however, this advantage has been mitigated by the use of trochanteric entry portals. Lateral patient positioning can be done on a radiolucent flat-top table; however, it may be difficult for the surgeon to obtain lateral fluoroscopic images of the proximal femur.

The supine position is the primary patient position used for femoral nailing and can be done on both a fracture table and a radiolucent flat-top table. The supine position makes the procedure easier for the entire surgical team. Supine positioning of the patient on a flat-top table allows the surgical team to address associated injuries. If a flat-top table is used, a bump can be placed under the ipsilateral hip to allow for easier access to the entry portal.

Entry Portals and Fracture Reduction

The creation of the entry portal is a critical step in fracture reduction. A piriformis entry portal is the traditional entry portal to the proximal femur. A piriformis entry portal is especially beneficial for proximal shaft fractures because it allows for nailing along the anatomic axis of the femur and because it negates deforming forces with the use of an off-axis nail. Because it is difficult to localize the bony insertion site for a piriformis entry portal, many surgeons instead use trochanteric entry portals.

It is easier to localize the bony insertion site for a trochanteric entry portal because many patients have a palpable greater trochanter. The use of a straight nail with a trochanteric entry portal should be avoided. When selecting the entrance angle, the surgeon must account for the proximal bend in the trochanteric-specific nail. The starting point for trochanteric-specific nails is easy to locate; however, because trochanteric-specific nails are curved and are inserted into a trochanteric entry portal that is not linear with the anatomic axis of the femur, their use for proximal femoral shaft fractures is difficult and prone to malreduction unless the surgeon gives careful attention to technique.

Retrograde femoral nailing continues to gain popularity because it is easy to localize the entry portal. It also is easy to position the patient and to locate the starting point for the nail. A disadvantage of retrograde femoral nailing is that the starting point for the nail violates the articular cartilage of the distal femur; however, this has not been reported to have lasting detrimental effects.[7]

Reduction maneuvers for femoral shaft fractures largely depend on the

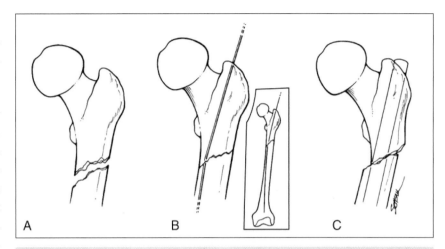

Figure 6   Illustration shows common femoral shaft fracture fixation errors to avoid. **A,** A proximal femoral shaft fracture is shown. **B,** A trochanteric entry portal has been created, but the entrance angle into the proximal femur is too medially oriented despite guidewire termination in the center of the distal femur (inset). **C,** Malalignment has occurred after eccentric reaming and the insertion of a straight nail through the trochanteric entry portal.

surgical table and patient position selected; however, the surgical team should have various aides to assist with fracture reduction. Positioning pillows are helpful for provisional fracture reduction. Hooks, clamps, Schanz pins, spiked-ball pushers, reduction wrenches, and crutches are some tools that are useful for fracture reduction. After reduction has been obtained, it is critical that the surgeon give close attention to the position of the guidewire. The entrance angle of the guidewire into the distal segment can be as critical as the entrance angle of the guidewire into the proximal segment. The surgeon should verify that the guidewire is positioned in the middle of the femoral canal with the use of AP and lateral fluoroscopic imaging. This is especially important for shaft fractures that border the femoral metaphysis. Malpositioned guidewires can lead to eccentric reaming and the placement of a rigid rod along an eccentric path, which can cause malalignment (**Figure 6**).

Tibial Shaft Fractures

Intramedullary nailing of tibial shaft fractures is commonly performed on a standard surgical table with the use of a radiolucent triangle to aid access to the proximal tibia. If intramedullary nailing is performed with the knee in extension, positioning pillows are helpful for provisional fracture alignment. The use of a flat-top table may make it difficult for the surgeon to reach over the end of the table to access the patient. Reduction techniques for tibial shaft fractures are similar to the reduction techniques described for femoral shaft fractures; however, distractors and external fixators are more commonly used in femoral shaft fractures to gain length across the fracture zone. Open fractures are more common with tibial shaft fractures and offer the surgeon the opportunity to reduce the fracture under direct visualization with the use of clamps and plates with unicortical screws (**Figure 7**). The plates can be left in place or, if stable nailing has been accomplished, can be removed.

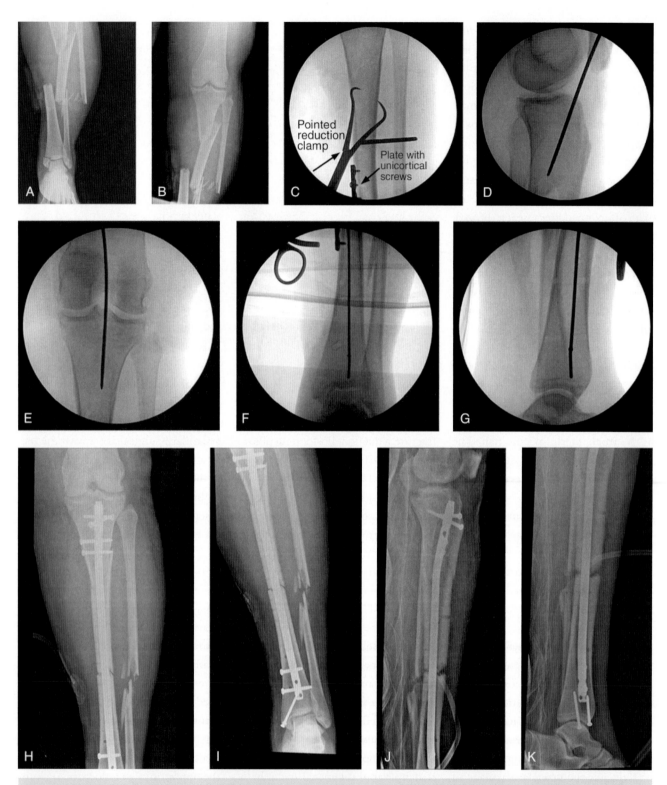

Figure 7 Images of the leg of a patient who was involved in a motorcycle crash. Preoperative AP radiographs (**A** and **B**) demonstrate that the patient sustained a type IIIB open tibial shaft fracture and a fibular shaft fracture. **C,** Intraoperative AP fluoroscopic image demonstrates fracture reduction through the open tibia fracture. Note the plate that was used to hold the distal portion of the intercalary segment in reduction. Intraoperative AP (**D** and **G**) and lateral (**E** and **F**) fluoroscopic images demonstrate guidewire and pin placement in the proximal and distal segments of the tibia. Note the positioning of the guidewire along the anatomic axis of the tibia. Postoperative AP (**H** and **I**) and lateral (**J** and **K**) radiographs demonstrate final reduction and fixation.

© 2016 AAOS Instructional Course Lectures, Volume 65

Although various entry portals for tibial nails can be used to negate the deforming forces about the proximal tibia, the standard entry portal is just medial to the lateral tibial eminence and, ideally, parallel to the anterior tibial cortex.[8] This positioning of the entry portal is in line with the anatomic axis of the tibia. The entrance angle of the guidewire into the distal segment must be carefully executed, and the surgeon should verify that the guidewire is positioned in the center of the distal segment with the use of AP and lateral fluoroscopic imaging. Failure to position the guidewire in the center of the distal segment will lead to malalignment.

Periarticular Knee Fractures

Many of the fracture reduction principles and techniques previously discussed can be applied to both the distal femur and the proximal tibia. Anatomic reduction of the articular surface is best achieved via direct reduction; therefore, adequate visualization is paramount. Because of comminution, the restoration of metadiaphyseal length, alignment, and rotation is typically performed via indirect reduction, unless direct reduction is possible.

Patient Positioning

The patient is positioned supine to allow access to the medial and lateral distal femur and the proximal tibia via a variety of surgical approaches.[9,10] A radiolucent triangle or bone foam is typically placed under the knee. Supine positioning of the patient facilitates anatomic and fluoroscopic comparisons between the injured and uninjured limbs for length, alignment, and rotation. Prone positioning of the patient can be used for a direct posterior approach to the proximal tibia.[11]

Distal Femoral Plating

To maintain control of an intra-articular fracture of the distal femur in multiple planes, threaded joystick Kirschner wires (K-wires) are placed into the main condylar fragment. A pointed reduction clamp is very useful for reduction of coronal plane fractures (ie, Hoffa fractures). A periarticular reduction clamp is used for compression of the intercondylar split; however, the surgeon should prevent overcompression if notch comminution is present. Bicortical lag screws are used for fixation of the main intercondylar fracture (**Figure 8**), and unicortical lag screws are used for fixation of coronal plane fractures. Lag screws should be placed so as not to interfere with primary implant placement. Because of the shape of the distal femur, special care must be taken to avoid screw perforation of the intercondylar notch and to avoid prominent medial screw tips.

Metaphyseal comminution of the distal femur may make the restoration of rotation, length, and alignment a challenge. Because it is difficult to assess alignment within the limited frame of the fluoroscope, it may be helpful to obtain a full-length intraoperative radiograph. A universal distractor can be placed to restore length; however, the pins must be placed with caution to avoid rotational malreduction. Percutaneous Schanz pins, spiked-ball pushers, compression devices, and nonlocking screws can be used to manipulate the shaft component. External bumps or the percutaneous placement of a bone hook under the distal fragment can be used to correct apex posterior deformity. Medialization of the articular block, which may result from incorrect positioning of the plate (too posterior or too distal), malreduction (commonly, valgus or external rotation), loss of the metaphyseal flare as a result of comminution (which causes nonlocking screws to lateralize the intact shaft), or a mismatch between the patient's anatomy and the plate contour, is a common concern after distal femoral plating. Deformity can be avoided by reducing the plate to the distal segment and then using locking screws to fix the plate without apposition to the shaft. A blunt-tipped locking screw can be used to medially force the shaft into the correct position over the articular block (**Figure 9**).

Proximal Tibial Plating

Three common difficulties of lateral tibial plateau fractures are inadequate visualization, incomplete joint elevation, and condylar widening. Tagging sutures can be placed during the creation of a lateral submeniscal arthrotomy to allow for retraction and better visualization of the lateral joint surface. A laterally placed femoral distractor allows the knee to be brought into varus, which further improves visualization. Most of the lateral tibial joint depression can be visualized and corrected using a submeniscal arthrotomy in conjunction with the lateral metaphyseal split fracture. To elevate the lateral depressed fragments in cases in which the lateral split is not visible, a lateral split can be created with the use of an osteotome or a medial cortical window can be created with the use of a burr. Articular fragments with minimal subchondral bone can be rafted with the use of mini-fragment screws or threaded K-wires that are cut flush and left in place after reduction. Unicortical small- or mini-fragment reduction plates, which allow for the removal of clamps, may help simplify a complex fracture pattern. Periarticular reduction

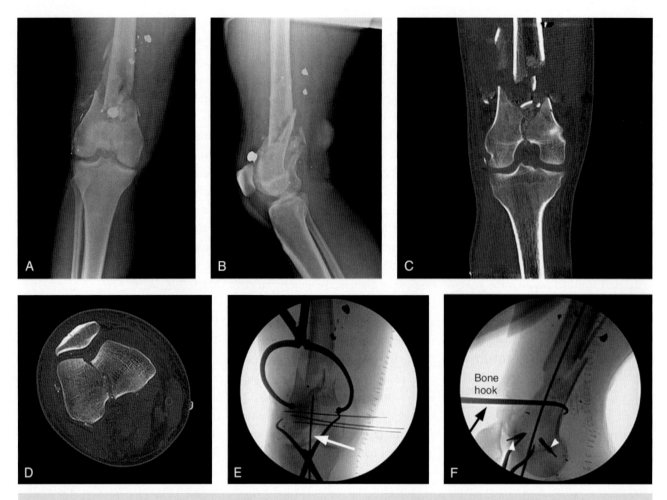

Figure 8 Images demonstrate plating of a distal femur fracture. Preoperative AP (**A**) and lateral (**B**) radiographs and preoperative coronal (**C**) and axial (**D**) CT scans demonstrate an intra-articular fracture of the distal femur. **E**, Intraoperative AP fluoroscopic image demonstrates initial reduction of the intercondylar split with the use of a periarticular reduction clamp, a pointed reduction clamp, and provisional K-wire fixation as well as the placement of a guide pin (arrow) for a retrograde femoral nail. **F**, Intraoperative lateral fluoroscopic image demonstrates the placement of two lag screws (arrowheads) for fixation of the joint, which allows for removal of the larger clamp. Note the placement of the screws around the nail pathway.

clamps can be used to restore condylar width. To avoid cortical perforation in osteoporotic bone, care should be taken to use a foot plate or place a clamp over the plate.

Reduction of displaced medial tibial plateau fractures can sometimes be performed with the use of percutaneous clamps, but often requires a separate medial exposure (**Figure 10**). Although direct visualization of the medial joint surface is rarely required, it can be obtained via a submeniscal arthrotomy and by working around the superficial medial collateral ligament. Although lateral locking plates allow for fixed-angle rafting of both the lateral and medial joints, the typical trajectory of the screws from lateral locking plates provides inadequate support for the separate posteromedial fragment.[12-14] Dual surgical approaches are necessary if the posteromedial fragment cannot be both reduced and stabilized via a single lateral approach. The authors of this chapter prefer to treat most bicondylar fractures with dual plating to provide buttress support for the posteromedial fracture component and to prevent varus collapse (**Figure 11**).

Distal Femoral and Proximal Tibial Nailing

Nail fixation of distal femur and proximal tibia fractures is typically reserved for extra-articular fractures or fractures with simple articular splits that are amenable to indirect reduction and percutaneous fixation before nailing.

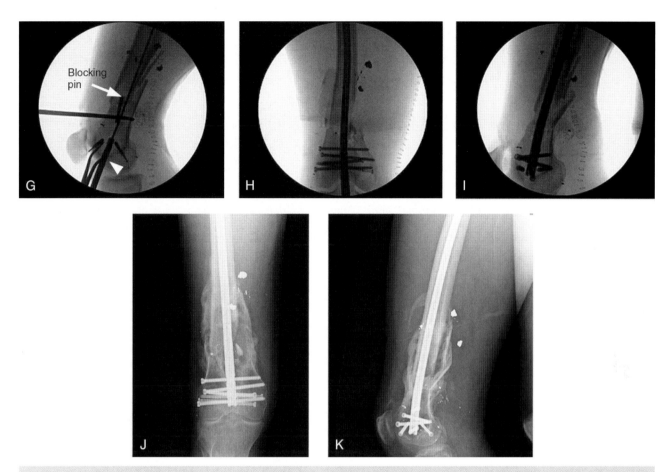

Figure 8 *(continued)*   G, Intraoperative lateral fluoroscopic image demonstrates the use of a bone hook to correct distal fragment extension and the use of an anterior blocking pin to force the reamer (arrowhead) posteriorly through the distal fragment. Postoperative AP (H) and lateral (I) fluoroscopic images and AP (J) and lateral (K) radiographs taken at 3-month follow-up demonstrate alignment of the distal femur fracture.

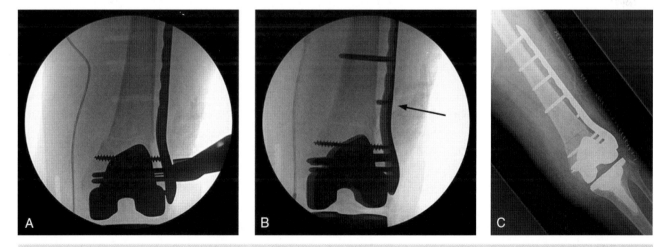

Figure 9   A, AP fluoroscopic image demonstrates medialization of an articular block that will worsen if the shaft is pulled toward the plate laterally. B, AP fluoroscopic image demonstrates correction of alignment with the use of a short, blunt-tipped locking screw (arrow), which is placed distally against the bone to exert a medial force on the shaft, and the use of locking screws, which are placed with the plate slightly proud. C, Postoperative AP radiograph demonstrates anatomic alignment.

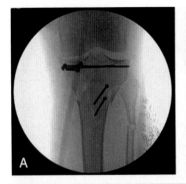
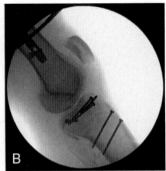
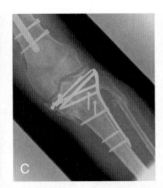
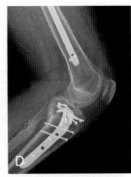

Figure 10   AP (**A**) and lateral (**B**) fluoroscopic images of the leg of a patient who had compartment syndrome demonstrate the percutaneous placement of provisional lag screws to stabilize the tibial tubercle and the medial articular fragments. AP (**C**) and lateral (**D**) radiographs demonstrate delayed definitive fixation with the use of a lateral locking plate.

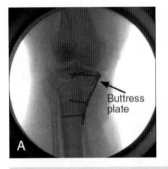
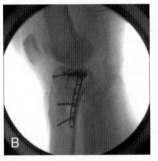
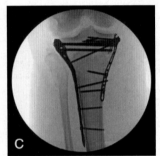
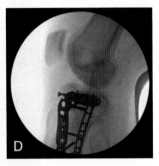

Figure 11   Fluoroscopic images demonstrate staged dual plating of a bicondylar tibial plateau fracture. AP (**A**) and lateral (**B**) views show that medial fixation was initially performed. AP (**C**) and lateral (**D**) views show that lateral fixation was performed at a later date.

Modern nails offer multiple multiplanar interlocking screw options and many offer fixed-angle screws. It is paramount that the surgeon locates the correct nail starting point and uses the correct nail trajectory. Suprapatellar nailing of proximal tibia fractures with the leg in the semiextended position decreases proximal fragment displacement. The placement of unicortical reduction plates is helpful for provisional fixation.

Blocking screws, which can be placed anywhere with adequate bone stock, can be used to maintain or facilitate reduction.[15,16] Blocking screws should be placed more than 1 cm from the fracture line to the minimize risk of fracture propagation. Commonly, blocking screws are placed before

reaming to help prevent an anticipated deformity during nail insertion. Alternatively, blocking screws can be placed around a well-positioned nail to limit postoperative toggle of an osteoporotic metaphyseal segment (**Figure 12**).

Ankle Fractures
Surgical Approaches

A direct lateral approach for reduction and fixation of ankle fractures should be familiar to most surgeons. A posterolateral approach along the posterior border of the fibula, performed anterior to the peroneal tendons or in the interval between the peroneal tendons and flexor hallucis longus, can be used for fixation of the fibula and the posterior malleolus, respectively. To

attain adequate visualization with this approach, the patient should be placed in the prone or floppy lateral position. The medial ankle can be approached through a variety of incisions; however, one of the authors of this chapter (H.R.M.) prefers to use a straight vertical incision because it can be easily extended.

Reduction and Fixation

For simple fibula fracture patterns, reduction is performed via direct clamp application. Indirect reduction techniques, such as the use of a push screw with a lamina spreader or the placement of a pin from the distal segment into the talus (which first requires medial stability and fixation), can be used to regain

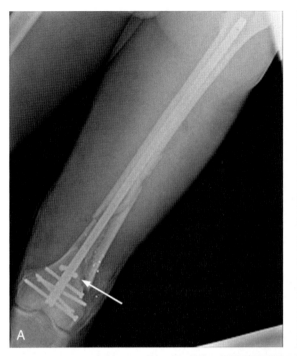

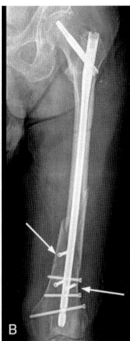

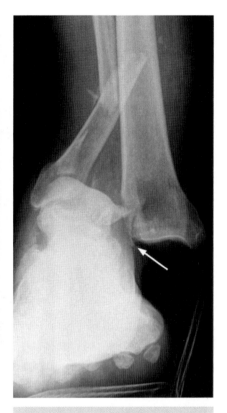

Figure 12   AP radiographs demonstrate the placement of blocking screws (arrows) adjacent to a retrograde (**A**) and an antegrade (**B**) nail in the distal femur to prevent the toggle of a metaphyseal or short distal segment.

Figure 13   AP radiograph demonstrates a log-splitter ankle fracture-dislocation as well as a tibial plafond fracture (arrow) and dramatic syndesmotic displacement.

length and alignment in comminuted fractures. The fixation of oblique and spiral fibula fractures is accomplished with the use of a lag screw and a neutralization plate. Additional constructs that can be used for the fixation of fibular fractures include posterior antiglide plates, bridge plates for comminuted fractures, and intramedullary implants for axially stable fractures.

The fixation of medial malleolus fractures can be accomplished with the use of partially threaded cancellous screws; however, bicortical lag screws are biomechanically superior, and, in some cases, may be beneficial.[17] Buttress plates can be used for vertical fracture patterns, and a mini-fragment T-plate can be used for fracture variants that have separate anterior and posterior collicular fragments.

Fractures of the posterior malleolus are fixed to restore articular congruity

and the stability of the syndesmotic complex.[18] Direct reduction, with the use of provisional K-wires, or indirect reduction, with the use of a buttress plate or percutaneous clamps, can be performed. Typically, fixation is accomplished with a buttress plate that is placed posteriorly or with lag screws that are placed from either the front or back of the ankle. To ensure accurate reduction of the syndesmosis, the surgeon should obtain contralateral radiographs.[19] A wide periarticular clamp, rather than a pointed reduction clamp, should be used to avoid unnecessary pressure on the soft tissues. Open reduction may be helpful; however, it is imperative that the surgeon work through the torn ligament and not detach the intact side. One of the authors of this chapter (H.R.M.) prefers to use 3.5-mm screws for fixation of three cortices; however, there is a

substantial ongoing debate on the number of screws, the size of the screws, and the number of cortices that should be used, and the use of nonabsorbable, heavy suture implants. High-energy ankle fracture-dislocations that combine rotational and axial forces may involve the tibial plafond[20] (**Figure 13**). Anterolateral fragments can be directly reduced via a limited anterolateral approach and secured with lag screws or a buttress plate.

Pilon Fractures
Surgical Approaches

Anteromedial and anterolateral approaches can be used for reduction and fixation of the distal tibia; however, one of the authors of this chapter (H.R.M.)

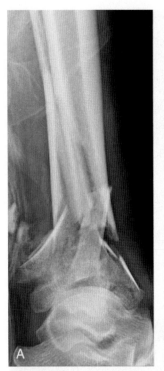
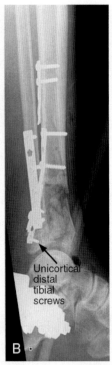
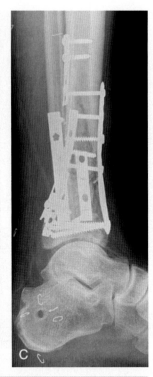

Figure 14 Lateral radiographs demonstrate staged fixation of a posterior pilon fracture (**A**). Initial fixation was performed on the date of injury and included the placement of a spanning external fixator and posterior plating (**B**). Placement of the final fixation construct was performed at a later date in a staged manner (**C**).

prefers a direct approach between the tibialis anterior and extensor hallucis longus. The posterolateral approach previously discussed with respect to reduction and fixation of ankle fractures is often useful. The posteromedial side can be approached by retracting all structures medial to and including the flexor hallucis longus, which protects the neurovascular bundle, or can be approached through the posterior tibialis tendon sheath. The keys to all of these approaches are meticulous soft-tissue technique and protection of the neurovascular structures. A limited medial approach with a 3-cm incision centered over the medial distal tibia allows for the use of minimally invasive percutaneous plate osteosynthesis. Similarly, a limited anterolateral approach with a 3-cm incision in line with the fourth

ray and centered over the ankle joint allows for the use of the minimally invasive percutaneous plate osteosynthesis technique; however, the surgeon should exercise caution because anterior neurovascular bundle entrapment may occur proximally.

Reduction and Fixation

A universal distractor is an invaluable tool that can be used to gain fracture length and direct intra-articular visualization. One of the authors of this chapter (H.R.M.) prefers to place a pin in the talar neck to create the appropriate force vector. It is helpful for the surgeon to think of the pilon as four areas that need to be stabilized: lateral (fibula), posterior (Volkmann), anterior (Chaput), and medial (malleolus/plafond). The goals are to achieve anatomic joint reduction and

fixation and to build stable metaphyseal columns. In some cases, it may be difficult to start with the articular reduction and then connect the articular block to the shaft; therefore, it may be helpful to first fix simple metaphyseal fractures to build a column and then reconstruct the articular segments.

Early fixation of the fibula and posterior malleolus in combination with external fixation followed by staged anterior fixation may be useful[21] (**Figure 14**). For most cases, one of the authors of this chapter (H.R.M.) applies a simple spanning external fixator and obtains a CT scan initially and then performs all definitive fixation in a staged manner; this technique, described by Liporace and Yoon[22] allows for the surgical planning of incisions and fixation. Depending on the particular fracture pattern, combinations of locking and nonlocking small-fragment implants may be indicated. Mini-fragment implants can help address individual fragments or act as brim plates. Useful adjuncts to address osteochondral-impacted fragments include bioabsorbable pins and bone graft substitute to fill the cancellous metaphyseal void. Long, bicortical, medial malleolar screws can be used for medial column support if surface implants pose a risk (ie, open fracture with medial wound). Some simple pilon fractures are amenable to intramedullary nail fixation with lag screws at the plafond level. In select cases, fibular fixation can be performed with a plate or an intramedullary implant.

Calcaneal Fractures
Surgical Approaches

Although an extensile lateral approach, which uses an L-shaped incision and a full-thickness skin flap, can be used

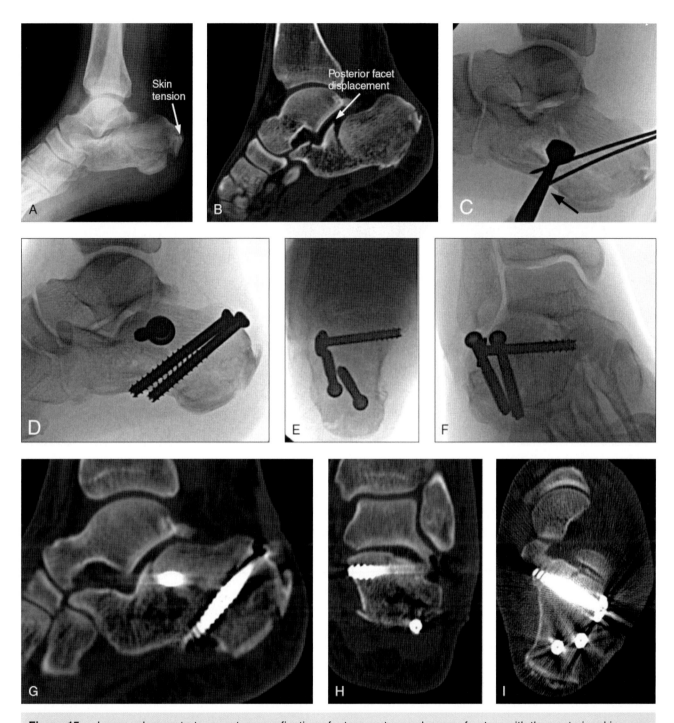

Figure 15   Images demonstrate percutaneous fixation of a tongue-type calcaneus fracture with the posterior skin under tension. Preoperative lateral radiograph (**A**) and sagittal CT scan (**B**) demonstrate a tongue-type fracture of the calcaneus. **C,** Lateral fluoroscopic image demonstrates percutaneous reduction with the use of an elevator (arrow) and the placement of guide pins for cannulated screws. Postoperative lateral (**D**), axial (**E**), and mortise (**F**) fluoroscopic images and sagittal (**G**), coronal (**H**), and axial (**I**) CT scans demonstrate reduction and fixation.

for reduction and fixation of calcaneal fractures, there is a risk for injury to the peroneal tendons and the sural nerve and also a concern for wound corner necrosis. A medial approach, which is occasionally used for sustentacular fractures, also can be used for medial reduction and fixation of open calcaneus fractures.[23] The sinus tarsi approach is minimally invasive and provides good visualization of the subtalar joint;[24] however, this approach may be

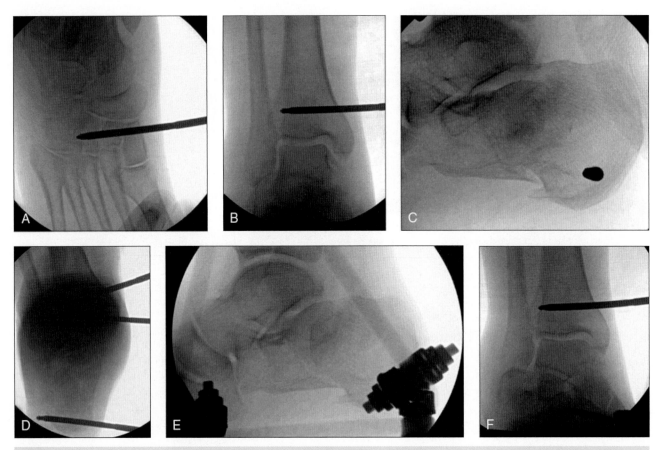

Figure 16 Fluoroscopic images demonstrate medial spanning external fixation of a calcaneal fracture. AP (**A**), mortise (**B**), and lateral (**C**) views demonstrate the placement of Schanz pins into the cuneiforms (**A**), distal tibia (**B**), and calcaneal tuberosity (**C**). Axial (**D**), lateral (**E**), and mortise (**F**) views demonstrate the restoration of bony- and soft-tissue alignment and length, which allows staged definitive internal fixation to be performed at a later date after edema has subsided.

difficult if tuberosity comminution or complex fracture patterns are present or if patients have long delays to surgery. Percutaneous approaches can be used for tongue-type fracture patterns or for some patients who have simple joint-depression type fracture patterns and are at risk for wound complications (**Figure 15**).

Reduction and Fixation

The goal of reduction and fixation is to secure the posterior facet, tuberosity, anterior process, and medial sustentacular fragment. To restore anatomic alignment of the injured extremity, the surgeon should obtain imaging of the contralateral side for comparison. A mortise radiograph of the ankle provides adequate visualization of the subtalar joint and allows the surgeon to judge posterior facet reduction. A heel-leg angle axial radiograph helps the surgeon restore alignment and avoid varus alignment. Fixation of the posterior facet is commonly performed with lag screws, and the remaining fixation is performed with a lateral perimeter plate that has options for locking screws.[25] The surgeon has the option to leave the metaphyseal void, which is usually present below the posterior facet, unfilled or to fill it with allograft chips or bone substitute. Staged fixation with external fixation or percutaneous pinning to maintain soft-tissue length is gaining popularity (**Figure 16**).

Summary

The surgical hurdles that accompany many lower extremity fractures can be overcome with good preoperative planning. To improve patient outcomes, surgeons must understand the advantages and disadvantages of various patient positions, surgical approaches, fracture reduction methods, and fixation constructs. Surgeons can use several reduction tips, tricks, and techniques as guides for the management of unique patient and fracture scenarios.

References

1. Connelly CL, Archdeacon MT: The lateral decubitus approach for complex proximal femur fractures: anatomic reduction and locking plate neutralization: A technical trick. *J Orthop Trauma* 2012;26(4):252-257.

2. Afsari A, Liporace F, Lindvall E, Infante A Jr, Sagi HC, Haidukewych GJ: Clamp-assisted reduction of high subtrochanteric fractures of the femur: Surgical technique. *J Bone Joint Surg Am* 2010;92(suppl 1 pt 2):217-225.

3. Archdeacon MT, Wyrick JD: Reduction plating for provisional fracture fixation. *J Orthop Trauma* 2006;20(3):206-211.

4. Thein R, Herman A, Kedem P, Chechik A, Shazar N: Osteosynthesis of unstable intracapsular femoral neck fracture by dynamic locking plate or screw fixation: Early results. *J Orthop Trauma* 2014;28(2):70-76.

5. French BG, Tornetta P III: Use of an interlocked cephalomedullary nail for subtrochanteric fracture stabilization. *Clin Orthop Relat Res* 1998;348:95-100.

6. Johnson B, Stevenson J, Chamma R, et al: Short-term follow-up of pertrochanteric fractures treated using the proximal femoral locking plate. *J Orthop Trauma* 2014;28(5):283-287.

7. Ostrum RF, Agarwal A, Lakatos R, Poka A: Prospective comparison of retrograde and antegrade femoral intramedullary nailing. *J Orthop Trauma* 2000;14(7):496-501.

8. Tornetta P III, Riina J, Geller J, Purban W: Intraarticular anatomic risks of tibial nailing. *J Orthop Trauma* 1999;13(4):247-251.

9. Kregor PJ: Distal femur fractures with complex articular involvement: Management by articular exposure and submuscular fixation. *Orthop Clin North Am* 2002;33(1):153-175, ix.

10. Starr AJ, Jones AL, Reinert CM: The "swashbuckler": A modified anterior approach for fractures of the distal femur. *J Orthop Trauma* 1999;13(2):138-140.

11. Yu GR, Xia J, Zhou JQ, Yang YF: Low-energy fracture of posterolateral tibial plateau: Treatment by a posterolateral prone approach. *J Trauma Acute Care Surg* 2012;72(5):1416-1423.

12. Weaver MJ, Harris MB, Strom AC, et al: Fracture pattern and fixation type related to loss of reduction in bicondylar tibial plateau fractures. *Injury* 2012;43(6):864-869.

13. Weil YA, Gardner MJ, Boraiah S, Helfet DL, Lorich DG: Posteromedial supine approach for reduction and fixation of medial and bicondylar tibial plateau fractures. *J Orthop Trauma* 2008;22(5):357-362.

14. Yoo BJ, Beingessner DM, Barei DP: Stabilization of the posteromedial fragment in bicondylar tibial plateau fractures: A mechanical comparison of locking and nonlocking single and dual plating methods. *J Trauma* 2010;69(1):148-155.

15. Krettek C, Miclau T, Schandelmaier P, Stephan C, Möhlmann U, Tscherne H: The mechanical effect of blocking screws ("Poller screws") in stabilizing tibia fractures with short proximal or distal fragments after insertion of small-diameter intramedullary nails. *J Orthop Trauma* 1999;13(8):550-553.

16. Seyhan M, Cakmak S, Donmez F, Gereli A: Blocking screws for the treatment of distal femur fractures. *Orthopedics* 2013;36(7):e936-e941.

17. Ricci WM, Tornetta P, Borrelli J Jr: Lag screw fixation of medial malleolar fractures: A biomechanical, radiographic, and clinical comparison of unicortical partially threaded lag screws and bicortical fully threaded lag screws. *J Orthop Trauma* 2012;26(10):602-606.

18. Gardner MJ, Brodsky A, Briggs SM, Nielson JH, Lorich DG: Fixation of posterior malleolar fractures provides greater syndesmotic stability. *Clin Orthop Relat Res* 2006;447:165-171.

19. Sagi HC, Shah AR, Sanders RW: The functional consequence of syndesmotic joint malreduction at a minimum 2-year follow-up. *J Orthop Trauma* 2012;26(7):439-443.

20. Bible JE, Sivasubramaniam PG, Jahangir AA, Evans JM, Mir HR: High-energy transsyndesmotic ankle fracture dislocation—the "Logsplitter" injury. *J Orthop Trauma* 2014;28(4):200-204.

21. Ketz J, Sanders R: Staged posterior tibial plating for the treatment of Orthopaedic Trauma Association 43C2 and 43C3 tibial pilon fractures. *J Orthop Trauma* 2012;26(6):341-347.

22. Liporace FA, Yoon RS: Decisions and staging leading to definitive open management of pilon fractures: Where have we come from and where are we now? *J Orthop Trauma* 2012;26(8):488-498.

23. Beltran MJ, Collinge CA: Outcomes of high-grade open calcaneus fractures managed with open reduction via the medial wound and percutaneous screw fixation. *J Orthop Trauma* 2012;26(11):662-670.

24. Femino JE, Vaseenon T, Levin DA, Yian EH: Modification of the sinus tarsi approach for open reduction and plate fixation of intra-articular calcaneus fractures: The limits of proximal extension based upon the vascular anatomy of the lateral calcaneal artery. *Iowa Orthop J* 2010;30:161-167.

25. Swanson SA, Clare MP, Sanders RW: Management of intra-articular fractures of the calcaneus. *Foot Ankle Clin* 2008;13(4):659-678.

Fractures and Dislocations About the Elbow and Their Adverse Sequelae: Contemporary Perspectives

Patrick Horrigan, MD

Jonathan P. Braman, MD

Alicia Harrison, MD

Abstract

Fractures and dislocations of the elbow can result in adverse outcomes. The elbow is a unique joint that allows for great mobility but is predisposed to instability, either simple or complex, in traumatic settings. Even simple elbow instability, in which no fracture is present, may be associated with tremendous soft-tissue injury. Surgical treatment is often required for complex instability in which various fractures are present. The treatment goals for fixation of elbow fractures and dislocations include stable fracture fixation, a stable concentrically reduced joint, and early range of motion. Continued pain, stiffness, and instability as well as heterotopic ossification are common sequelae of elbow fractures and dislocations.

Instr Course Lect 2016;65:41–52.

Background

The elbow is the second most commonly dislocated major joint in adults, with a dislocation incidence ranging from 2.9 to 6 per 100,000 persons.[1-3] Dislocations of the elbow are either simple or complex. Simple elbow dislocations do not have accompanying fractures. Complex elbow dislocations have an associated fracture that may involve the coronoid, radial head, and/or proximal ulna. A recent epidemiologic study suggested a male preponderance for elbow dislocation, with a fall being the cause of dislocation in most patients.[2] An estimated 90% of elbow dislocations involve posterior displacement of the forearm relative to the humerus. Adverse outcomes may occur in the treatment of elbow fractures and dislocations; therefore, a good working knowledge of elbow anatomy is essential to achieve anatomic fracture fixation, concentric reduction, and early range of motion. An understanding of both bony and soft-tissue anatomy is crucial for the management of elbow dislocations. It is important for surgeons to understand the components of elbow anatomy that contribute to stability as well as how to manage simple and complex elbow instability and the common sequelae of each treatment.

Anatomy and Biomechanics of the Elbow

The elbow is composed of the articular components of the distal humerus and the proximal radius and ulna as well as the surrounding ligamentous and capsular attachments. The elbow has both the ability of rotating motion via the proximal radioulnar and radiocapitellar

Dr. Braman or an immediate family member has received royalties from Sawbones/Pacific Research Laboratories; has received nonincome support (such as equipment or services), commercially derived honoraria, or other non-research–related funding (such as paid travel) from Stryker; and serves as a board member, owner, officer, or committee member of the American Academy of Orthopaedic Surgeons, the American Orthopaedic Association, and the American Shoulder and Elbow Surgeons. Dr. Harrison or an immediate family member serves as a board member, owner, officer, or committee member of the American College of Surgeons and the Minnesota Orthopaedic Society. Neither Dr. Horrigan nor any immediate family member has received anything of value from or has stock or stock options held in a commercial company or institution related directly or indirectly to the subject of this chapter.

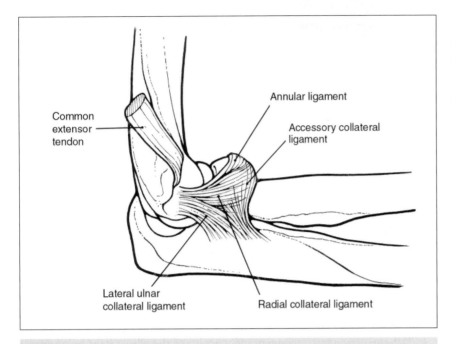

Common extensor tendon

Annular ligament

Accessory collateral ligament

Lateral ulnar collateral ligament

Radial collateral ligament

Figure 1   Illustration shows the anatomy of the lateral ligamentous complex of the elbow. Lateral ulnar collateral ligament = radial ulnohumeral ligament. (Reproduced from Yadao MA, Savoie FH III, Field LD: Posterolateral rotatory instability of the elbow. *Instr Course Lect* 2004;53:607-614.)

joints through pronation and supination as well as hinge-like motion via the ulnohumeral joint through flexion and extension. A biomechanical understanding of the bony and soft-tissue components that contribute to elbow stability can help guide the treatment of both simple and complex elbow instability.

The articular surface of the distal humerus consists of the trochlea and the capitellum. The highly irregular features of these bony surfaces that are congruent with the proximal radius and ulna provide inherent osseous stability to the elbow.[4] The radial head is a secondary stabilizer of the elbow. It articulates with the capitellum and the lesser sigmoid notch of the ulna and, therefore, is almost completely covered with articular cartilage. With the forearm in neutral rotation, the lateral aspect of the radial head is the only area without hyaline cartilage, which makes it a common

location for implant placement in the setting of a fracture. The proximal ulna includes both the greater sigmoid notch and the lesser sigmoid notch. The greater sigmoid notch is the region of primary articulation between the ulna and the humerus and articulates with the apex of the trochlea. The lesser notch articulates with the radial head as part of the proximal radioulnar joint. The coronoid process, which is a component of the greater sigmoid notch, plays a key role in elbow stability. Osseous stability is enhanced in elbow flexion if the coronoid process engages in the coronoid fossa of the distal humerus.

Surgeons also should have a thorough understanding of the ligamentous stabilizers of the elbow, including the lateral collateral ligament (LCL) complex and the medial collateral ligament (MCL). The MCL is composed of the anterior bundle, the posterior bundle, and the transverse ligament. The

anterior bundle originates from the medial epicondyle and inserts on the sublime tubercle of the coronoid. The anterior bundle of the MCL is important in preventing valgus and posteromedial rotatory instability. The LCL complex includes the lateral ulnar collateral ligament (LUCL), the radial collateral ligament, the annular ligament, and the accessory collateral ligament (**Figure 1**). This lateral ligamentous complex originates at the inferior surface of the lateral humeral epicondyle. By way of its insertion just distal to the annular ligament on the crista supinatoris of the ulna, the LUCL is important in preventing varus and posterolateral rotatory instability.

The elbow is inherently stable as a result of the articular congruence of the ulna and humerus as well as capsular and ligamentous contributions. Instability can lead to marked loss of function and may jeopardize functional independence. A thorough understanding of the biomechanics of elbow instability provides surgeons with the scientific basis for treatment.[5]

The specific anatomic structures already mentioned are classified as either primary or secondary stabilizers. The primary stabilizers are the ulnohumeral joint, the anterior bundle of the MCL, and the LUCL. These structures are termed primary stabilizers because disruption of any one is believed to render the elbow unstable.[6] The ulnohumeral joint plays a primary role in elbow stabilization throughout flexion and extension. An et al[7] evaluated the role of the ulnohumeral joint by performing serial excisions of the olecranon, which demonstrated that the ulnohumeral joint significantly contributes to stability with valgus stress. The coronoid process also has been identified as an important stabilizer to varus stress. Hull et al[8] reported that only transverse cuts that removed more than 50% of the coronoid process resulted in a significant decrease in resistance to varus stress, which was accentuated in extension. Closkey et al[9] reported a significant increase in displacement during axial loading only if more than 50% of the coronoid was removed.

Schneeberger et al[10] reported on the contribution of both the radial head and the coronoid process to posterolateral rotatory instability. The authors reported that it was important to either reconstruct or replace the radial head in the setting of posterolateral rotatory instability. If a fracture consisted of less than 30% of the coronoid and had intact collateral ligaments, a concurrent radial head fracture produced instability at three separate flexion angles. In this situation, ulnohumeral stability was restored by restoring only the radial head. Fractures of the radial head and fractures that consisted of 50% or more of the coronoid process created instability that could not be restored with only radial head replacement.

Jeon et al[11] reported that approximately 60% of the coronoid and approximately 40% of the radial head contribute to total articular surface. In addition, the authors reported that coronoid fractures that comprised up to 40% of the total articular surface were stable in the presence of an intact radial head and no ligament ruptures. As more studies on elbow stability are published, surgeons' understanding of bony contributions to elbow stability is becoming more sophisticated.

Simple Elbow Dislocation

Dislocation of the elbow without an associated fracture is considered a simple dislocation; however, major soft-tissue injuries may be associated with simple elbow dislocations. Associated injuries occur in 10% to 15% of patients who have elbow dislocations and include ipsilateral humerus, distal radius, ulnar, and carpal bone fractures as well as soft-tissue sprains and disruptions, such as Essex-Lopresti lesions.[12] Most elbow dislocations occur during sporting activities, especially in patients younger than 30 years, and most elbow dislocations result after a fall onto an outstretched hand.[3]

The mechanism and order of soft-tissue disruption in simple elbow dislocations are controversial. O'Driscoll et al[13,14] introduced the concept of posterolateral rotatory instability and suggested that the LCL ruptures first in axial compression and forced elbow flexion. LCL rupture is followed by anterior and posterior capsular disruption and, finally, MCL rupture. A different study suggested that ligament disruption may begin medially.[15] In a recent video analysis of in vivo elbow dislocations, Schreiber et al[16] reported that a substantial valgus deformity of the elbow was present in most elbow dislocations regardless of forearm position. The authors suggested that rupture of the anterior bundle of the MCL may be necessary before dislocation occurs.

Patient History and Examination

Regardless of the mechanism and order of ligament disruption, patients with acute elbow dislocations usually have easily identifiable soft-tissue swelling and deformity about the elbow. A neurovascular examination should be performed before and after reduction, and the ipsilateral wrist and shoulder should be assessed for concomitant injury.

Reduction should be performed with procedural sedation (with or without local anesthetic) and the use of gentle traction, anterior manipulation of the proximal ulna, and elbow flexion. Any mechanical blocks to forearm rotation should be noted, and the arc of motion should be recorded. Postreduction radiographs should be obtained in two planes to evaluate concentric reduction of the joint. Widening of the joint space may suggest instability or the presence of osteochondral fragments in the joint space.[12]

Nonsurgical Treatment

The inherent bony stability and congruity of the elbow joint help protect ruptured ligamentous structures in simple elbow dislocations. For this reason, nonsurgical treatment may be used to manage most simple elbow dislocations that remain stable through postreduction arc of motion.[12,17-20] Maripuri et al[21] performed a retrospective review that compared above-elbow plaster cast immobilization with simple sling immobilization for the treatment of simple elbow dislocations. The authors reported that, at a minimum follow-up of 2 years, patients who were treated with a simple sling had significantly better Mayo Elbow Performance Index scores, better Quick Disabilities of the Arm, Shoulder and Hand questionnaire scores, and a faster return to work compared with patients who were treated with plaster casting.

In general, early radiographic follow-up is recommended within 1 week of injury and reduction to ensure concentric reduction of the elbow in the early postinjury period. Several studies have reported that, if joint congruity is maintained, early range of motion predictably decreases the likelihood of elbow stiffness and loss of extension.[22-24] Motion may be increased as tolerated in patients who demonstrate elbow stability past 60° of extension. If instability occurs past 60° of extension, an extension-blocking hinged elbow brace can be applied and set to 5° less than the point of instability and may be increased by up to 20° per week to regain motion.[5]

Surgical Treatment

Although MCL disruption is present in simple elbow dislocations, surgical treatment is rarely indicated.[12] In a randomized controlled trial that compared surgical versus nonsurgical treatment, Josefsson et al[25] reported that surgery did not produce better results than cast immobilization followed by active range of motion. In this study, surgery involved both medial and lateral longitudinal incisions as well as exploration and repair of the respective ruptured ligamentous complexes. Results were measured via range of motion at follow-up and the number of patient complaints with regard to treatment, neither of which were significantly in favor of one treatment method.

Data that specifically pertain to the surgical treatment of simple elbow dislocations are sparse. In recent decades, attention was paid to repair of both the medial and lateral ligamentous complexes.[25] This was followed by a focus on the medial ligamentous complex, which was believed to be most important to elbow stability.[12] Current data extrapolated from studies on complex elbow dislocations focus on repair of only the LCL.

Micic et al[26] reported on a series of 18 male and 2 female patients who underwent surgery for the treatment of instability after simple elbow dislocation.

Instability was defined as an elbow dislocation that required an extension block splint set at more than 45° of flexion to maintain reduction. The authors addressed the LCL first and the MCL second. The authors reported that the LCL was disrupted in 80% of dislocations, and that 55% of the dislocations involved MCL ruptures. The authors defined intraoperative stability as a lack of anterior subluxation of the humerus in full extension. The authors reported that elbow stabilization with suture anchors may aid in early functional range of motion. In a study of 17 patients who had elbow dislocations and either no fracture or only capsuloligamentous avulsion fractures, Duckworth et al[27] reported that eight patients underwent LCL repair, seven patients underwent LCL and MCL repair, and two patients required hinged external fixator application after ligamentous repair.

A small case series suggested that simple medial elbow dislocations may warrant special surgical attention given their predisposition to instability.[28] The LCL and extensor tendon origin were disrupted in the four patients who were treated. Therefore, surgeons should have a heightened awareness for the potential for surgical intervention in patients who have medial instability.

Complications

Substantial ligamentous and capsular injuries often accompany simple elbow dislocations, and the injury—despite favorable outcomes—may not be entirely benign. In an epidemiologic review of 110 dislocations in a well-defined patient population, 56% of patients reported subjective stiffness after injury, and 62% of patients reported residual pain.[3] Eight percent of patients reported subjective instability, and 8% of patients

(all but one patient being different from those who reported subjective instability) reported objective instability.

Objective measures of complications after simple elbow dislocation are better established in the literature.[22,29] Loss of elbow extension is the most commonly reported complication, with mean losses ranging from 10° to 15°.[12,22] It has been suggested that postinjury immobilization for more than 3 weeks leads to a greater loss of motion without any advantage of stability.[24] Greater loss of extension may be seen in patients who are managed surgically, and may be the result of a greater degree of soft-tissue disruption.[26,27] The treatment of posttraumatic elbow stiffness relies on the identification of its cause, whether from involvement of the articular surfaces (intrinsic) or the surrounding soft tissues (extrinsic). Most elbow stiffness results from a combination of intrinsic and extrinsic causes.[30,31] Nonsurgical options for the management of posttraumatic stiffness include progressive static bracing or dynamic bracing as well as splinting and examination under anesthesia.[30] Flexion less than 130° and extension less than 30° are common surgical indications; however, surgery may be pursued outside these range-of-motion parameters depending on the patient's functional demands. Surgery may be performed via several surgical approaches and techniques, with the use of either arthroscopic or open procedures.[32-36] Although early postoperative initiation of motion is encouraged, Lindenhovius et al[37] reported no benefit of continuous passive motion of the elbow after open contracture release for the treatment of elbow stiffness.

Heterotopic ossification (HO) is relatively common after simple elbow dislocations; however, questions exist on its role in painful and stiff range of motion. HO is reported in approximately 3% of simple elbow dislocations, and surgical excision is rarely required.[38] Some forms of HO are asymptomatic calcifications of ligamentous avulsion injuries. Risk factors for HO include the amount of soft-tissue trauma, associated central nervous system injury, and aggressive passive manipulation of the injured elbow.[39] The use of indomethacin for prophylaxis against HO in elbow dislocations should follow treatment principles similar to those for total hip arthroplasty.[40]

Several studies have reported subtle instability after simple elbow dislocations.[1-3] Posterolateral rotatory instability, which renders the elbow most unstable in extension and forearm supination, is the most common type of subtle instability reported.[13] Treatment algorithms for chronic elbow instability after simple elbow dislocation are similar to those for acute injuries because identification of the source and the type of instability guides decision making. For chronic posterolateral rotatory instability, ligamentous reconstruction with the use of autograft (palmaris longus, plantaris, or gracilis) or allograft has produced more reproducible outcomes than repair of only local tissue.[41] Instability also may be attributed to disruption of the radioulnar interosseous membrane with or without concomitant distal or proximal radioulnar joint disruption (Essex-Lopresti variants).

Neurovascular injury is a rare but important complication of simple elbow dislocations. Neurapraxia of the ulnar nerve most commonly occurs after simple elbow dislocations but typically resolves after reduction. Brachial artery disruption has been reported in anterior dislocations and other injuries.

Complex Elbow Dislocations
Elbow Dislocation With Radial Head Fracture
Diagnosis and Classification
Elbow dislocations accompanied by an isolated radial head fracture are a relatively common fracture-dislocation pattern. A common mechanism of injury often includes a fall onto an outstretched arm. Many radial head fractures are quite small and are often first recognized on postreduction radiographs. A typical patient examination may include early loss of motion despite intra-articular injection of anesthetic. Because plain radiographs may not clearly define these fractures, a CT scan may be obtained to define the degree of fracture displacement and comminution. CT also will allow the surgeon to rule out any other associated fractures or bony injuries.

Most surgeons use the Broberg and Morrey[42] modification or the Mason[43] system to classify the size and displacement of radial head fracture fragments. Type I fractures are nondisplaced or displaced less than 2 mm. Type II fractures are displaced more than 2 mm and involve more than 30% of the articular surface. Type III fractures are comminuted. Type IV fractures are a radial head fracture with an associated elbow dislocation.

Treatment
The management of elbow dislocations with an associated radial head fracture is predicated on achieving a stable joint with functional range of motion. Certain patient factors, such as preinjury function, medical comorbidities, and postinjury expectations, play a role in treatment decision making. Nonsurgical treatment is recommended for type I injuries (nondisplaced or displaced

<2 mm) with a stable elbow. If the reduced elbow is stable and no blocks to motion exist, the patient may be treated similar to a patient who has a simple elbow dislocation, encouraging early motion after a brief period of immobilization. If the elbow is unstable, the patient should be treated surgically to address ligamentous stabilization and fracture fixation. Unstable type I injuries are unusual, and most type I injuries can be treated nonsurgically. In a study of 54 patients with type I injuries who were treated nonsurgically, Shulman et al[44] reported that no patients experienced a complication.

Less agreement exists on the recommended treatment for type II radial head fractures. Surgical fixation is advised for type II injuries with elbow instability or if patient factors, such as the examination, expectations, or activities, dictate. Studies have reported good results for type II injuries that are managed either nonsurgically[45,46] or surgically.[47,48] Type III radial head fractures are most often treated surgically. The surgical treatment options for type III fractures include radial head arthroplasty or open reduction and internal fixation (ORIF). Type IV fractures are discussed later.

Complications
Multiple studies report higher complication rates if ORIF is selected for the management of a fracture pattern that involves three or more fragments.[47-51] For this reason, many surgeons favor radial head replacement for the management of a multifragmented radial head fracture (Type III). In a study of 45 patients who underwent treatment for multifragmented radial head fractures, Chen et al[51] reported a 47.9% complication rate for patients who underwent

ORIF compared with a 13.6% complication rate for those who underwent radial head arthroplasty.

Although elbow fracture-dislocations that involve an isolated noncomminuted radial head fracture are able to be treated with good outcomes, adverse sequelae can and do occur, particularly in fractures with more comminution or displacement. The most common complication is stiffness that sometimes requires capsular release. Other adverse sequelae, which are similar for all of the complex patterns discussed in this chapter, include posttraumatic arthritis, HO, neuropathy, infection, malunion, and nonunion.

Higher overall complication rates have been reported in patients who have radial head fractures with additional bony injuries or instability (type IV). Pike et al[52] compared the results of ORIF for the treatment of simple radial head fractures with the results of ORIF for the treatment of radial head fractures with instability or other fracture patterns. The overall complication rates were high for both groups (13% for simple patterns versus 25% for complex patterns). Disabling stiffness was seen in both groups and required capsular release in 3% of the simple patterns and 20% of the complex patterns. Capsular release was more likely if three or more radial head fragments were present.

The Terrible Triad
Diagnosis and Classification
Elbow dislocations accompanied by radial head and coronoid fractures are called the terrible triad because the literature has repeatedly documented poor outcomes for this injury pattern. Ring et al[53] reported an unsatisfactory outcome in 7 of 11 patients who had

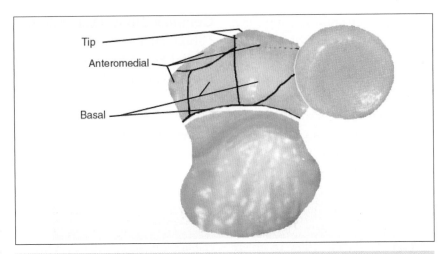

Figure 2   Illustration shows the proposed classification system for coronoid fractures described by O'Driscoll et al.[57] This classification system, which is based on anatomic location, with subtypes classified according to the severity of coronoid involvement, and considers the mechanism of injury as well as the associated fractures and soft-tissue injuries, dictates the surgical approach and treatment. (Reproduced from O'Driscoll SW, Jupiter JB, Cohen MS, Ring D, McKee MD: Difficult elbow fractures: Pearls and pitfalls. *Instr Course Lect* 2003;52:113-134.)

a terrible triad injury. A better understanding of elbow anatomy and the stabilizers of the elbow has led to improved techniques for the management of terrible triad injuries. Current studies have outlined an algorithm that has led to improved outcomes.[54,55]

A classification scheme for terrible triad injuries does not exist; however, classification schemes exist for the separate components of the terrible triad. The radial head classification system was previously discussed. Regan and Morrey[56] classified coronoid fractures based on the height of the coronoid fracture fragment. Type I fractures consist of an avulsion of the tip of the coronoid process, type II fractures consist of a fracture that involves at least 50% of the coronoid process, and type III fractures consist of a fracture that involves more than 50% of the coronoid. All three types of coronoid fractures are subclassified based on the absence (A) or presence (B) of dislocation.

O'Driscoll et al[57] proposed a classification scheme in which the fracture pattern is based on the surrounding anatomy (**Figure 2**). This system divides the coronoid process into the tip (type I), the anteromedial facet (type II), and the base (type III). Coronoid tip fractures (type I) are subclassified based on whether the fragments are less than or greater than 2 mm. Fractures of the anteromedial facet (type II) are subclassified into three subtypes. Subtype 1 fractures do not involve the coronoid tip and extend from medial to the tip to just anterior to the sublime tubercle. Subtype 2 fractures are subtype 1 fractures that involve the coronoid tip. Subtype 3 fractures involve the anteromedial rim of the coronoid and the sublime tubercle. Basal coronoid fractures (type III) consist of a fracture through the body of the coronoid process that involves at least 50% of the coronoid height. Basal fractures are subclassified into subtype 1 fractures, which involve

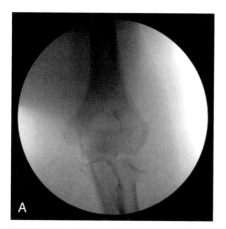

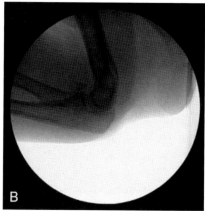

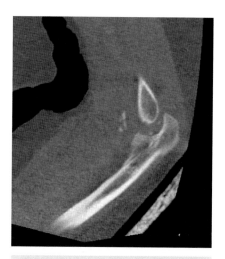

Figure 3   AP (**A**) and lateral (**B**) elbow radiographs of a terrible triad injury demonstrate a radial head fracture and coronoid fracture after closed reduction.

Figure 4   Sagittal CT scan of the same elbow shown in Figure 3 demonstrates comminution of the coronoid and intra-articular fragments.

only the coronoid process, and subtype 2 fractures, which include a coronoid body fracture as well as an olecranon fracture.

Prereduction and postreduction radiographs should be obtained (**Figure 3**). A postreduction CT scan is essential to define the precise fracture lines, which are important in surgical planning for terrible triad injuries (**Figure 4**). Many surgeons find three-dimensional CT reconstruction helpful in surgical planning.

Treatment

Most terrible triad injuries require surgery. The indications for nonsurgical treatment include CT documentation of a minimally displaced radial head fracture without mechanical block, a coronoid fracture that involves only the tip, and concentric reduction after relocation. The elbow must be stable enough to allow for early range of motion. Good results have been reported if these principles are applied.[58] Many surgeons use a static splint with the elbow positioned in neutral pronosupination for 7 to 10 days, after which time active motion is initiated and radiographic

documentation of concentric joint reduction is confirmed (**Figure 5**).

Complications

The most common complications of terrible triad injuries are residual instability, malunion, nonunion, stiffness, HO, infection, and ulnar neuropathy.[54,59-61] In a systematic literature review of 312 patients who underwent surgical management for terrible triad injuries, Chen et al[61] reported that 70 patients (22.4%) had complications that required revision surgery because of problems related to stiffness, hardware failure, instability, or ulnar neuropathy.

Residual instability is one of the biggest challenges in the treatment of terrible triad injuries. Residual instability may be caused by concomitant ligamentous injuries as well as the technical challenges inherent to fixation of the coronoid, which is often fragmented. Terada et al[62] reported that chronic elbow instability was more common in terrible triad patterns that involved smaller fractures of the coronoid process; however, Beingessner et al[63] reported that, with regard to elbow

stability, collateral ligament repair was more important than fixation in type I coronoid fractures. Furthermore, in a recent study of 14 patients who had terrible triad injuries with type I or type II coronoid fractures, Papatheodorou et al[64] reported successful outcomes without coronoid fixation if radial head replacement or fixation and reconstruction of the LUCL complex restored intraoperative elbow stability.

Postoperative elbow stiffness is a common and challenging complication of terrible triad elbow injuries. Because of this common complication, early range of motion is necessary, and stability should be confirmed intraoperatively to ensure that early motion will be possible. Static progressive splinting is initiated for patients who have early signs of stiffness. If stiffness is recalcitrant to therapy and splinting, patients may be treated with either open or arthroscopic capsular release.

HO is a common complication of terrible triad injuries; however, it does not usually require surgical treatment. In a systematic review of 312 patients

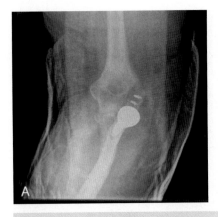
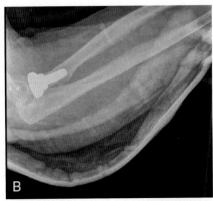

Figure 5 AP (**A**) and lateral (**B**) elbow radiographs demonstrate concentric elbow reduction after radial head replacement, repair of the lateral ligamentous complex, and suture fixation of the coronoid fracture.

who underwent surgical management for terrible triad injuries, Chen et al[61] reported that HO developed in 12.5% of the patients. Shukla et al[65] reported that multiple reduction attempts was a risk factor for HO; however, time to surgery and other factors were not reported to influence the risk of HO. Open capsular excision may improve function for patients in whom HO develops and is clinically significant. In a study of 46 patients who underwent open capsular excision, Ring et al[66] reported a mean flexion arc of almost 100° at mean follow-up of 48 months.

Hardware failure requires revision surgery and, in many patients, is the result of radial neck fracture fixation failure. Ring et al[48] reported a risk for both early and late fixation failure as well as poor results in patients who had comminuted radial head or neck fractures. The sequelae of hardware fixation and the fracture pattern itself may lead to another complication of terrible triad injuries: posttraumatic arthritis. Chondral damage at the time of the injury, residual articular incongruity, or instability can contribute to the development of arthrosis. The treatment options for arthrosis include débridement or osteophyte excision, biologic resurfacing, radial head excision or arthroplasty, and total elbow arthroplasty.

Fortunately, infection is not the most common complication of terrible triad injuries; however, it may be devastating if it occurs. Superficial infections may be managed with irrigation and débridement. Deep infections often require hardware removal, local antibiotic treatment, and an extended course of organism-specific intravenous antibiotics.

The Monteggia Lesion
Diagnosis and Classification
Bado[67] described an injury pattern that involves an ulnar fracture with an associated radiocapitellar dislocation as a Monteggia lesion, which he classified into four types. Type I injuries involve an anterior radial head dislocation and a diaphyseal ulnar fracture with anterior angulation. Type II injuries involve a posterior or posterolateral radial head dislocation and a diaphyseal ulnar fracture with posterior angulation. Type III injuries involve a lateral or anterolateral radial head dislocation with a metaphyseal ulnar fracture. Type IV injuries involve an anterior radial head dislocation with a fracture of the proximal third of the radius and the ulna at the same level.

Jupiter et al[68] subclassified type II Monteggia lesions because the specific anatomic features unique to this pattern are important for appropriate treatment. The type II subclassification includes: type IIA, a fracture at the level of the greater sigmoid notch; type IIB, an ulnar fracture distal to the coronoid at the metaphyseal-diaphyseal junction; type IIC, a diaphyseal ulnar fracture; and type IID, comminuted fractures that involve multiple regions.

Plain orthogonal radiographs often are adequate to recognize the presence of a Monteggia lesion; however, CT is frequently necessary to identify the extent of the fracture and the position of all the fracture fragments.

Treatment
Skeletally mature patients who have Monteggia fractures require surgical management to anatomically reduce the ulnar fracture with the use of rigid fixation, ensure concentric joint reduction, and allow for early postoperative range of motion. Closed reduction attempts are unsuccessful in many patients. Comminution of the ulnar fracture shortens the ulna, which prevents stable reduction of the radial head. In such cases, multiple reduction attempts should be avoided because such efforts have been reported to increase the risk of HO.[65] Surgical treatment involves ORIF of the ulna, which may require variable plating systems and, possibly, bone graft as well as the management of any potential radial head fracture with either fixation or arthroplasty. The techniques for surgical management of Monteggia fractures have been well described in the literature.[69]

Complications

Monteggia fractures may be challenging to treat and can result in various complications, relatively poor outcomes, and a high rate of revision surgery. Complications include malreduction or malunion (with associated persistent radial head subluxation), nonunion, neurologic injury, and HO. In a multicenter study of 67 adults who had Monteggia fractures that were treated with ORIF, Reynders et al[70] reported that, at a 1- to 14-year follow-up, the overall complication rate was 43%, with fair or poor results noted in 46.3% of patients. The authors reported that, overall, the fair or poor results were associated with type II and type IV Monteggia lesions. In a study of 47 patients who sustained a Monteggia fracture, Konrad et al[71] reported that, at a mean follow-up of 8.4 years, 26% of patients required revision surgery within 1 year of the initial surgery. The authors reported that type II Monteggia fractures, with more frequent radial head and coronoid fractures, were predictive of a poorer long-term functional outcome. Many surgeons obtain anatomic ulnar reduction and concentric radiocapitellar reduction as well as ensure rigid fracture fixation to allow for safe early postoperative motion. Attention to these principles may help avoid some of the more common pitfalls of Monteggia fractures.

Anteromedial Coronoid Fracture With Varus Posteromedial Instability

An anteromedial coronoid fracture that is accompanied by elbow instability without a radial head fracture is an injury pattern that has received attention only relatively recently. This fracture pattern is less common, is less well understood and studied, and may initially be misdiagnosed. If the coronoid fracture and/or elbow instability goes unnoticed, the patient is at risk for elbow arthrosis secondary to subluxation or instability. An injury or postreduction CT scan can help identify the coronoid fracture and define the injury pattern.

Relatively limited literature exists to guide the treatment of anteromedial coronoid fractures with varus posteromedial instability. A small group of studies have provided surgeons with an understanding of the injury and the mechanical forces involved.[72-74] As awareness of this injury pattern improved, additional studies that suggested guidelines for the management of anteromedial coronoid fractures with varus posteromedial instability have been published.[75,76] Doornberg and Ring[77] documented the outcomes of a series of 18 patients who had anteromedial coronoid fractures, 15 of whom underwent surgical treatment and three of whom were treated nonsurgically. At a mean follow-up of 26 months, six patients had persistent varus subluxation of the elbow, which was the result of loss of fracture fixation in two patients and the fracture not being treated initially in the remaining four patients. The six patients with persistent varus subluxation of the elbow had arthrosis and fair or poor results. The remaining 12 patients were reported to have good or excellent results.

Summary

Simple and complex elbow instability can have lasting effects on a patient's function. Stable fracture fixation, a stable concentrically reduced joint, and early range of motion are the goals of treatment. If surgical treatment is necessary, the surgeon should ensure anatomic reduction of the proximal ulna, appropriately address coronoid fractures, securely fix or replace the radial head, and ensure restoration of lateral ligamentous stability. Intraoperative stability should be confirmed so early range of motion can be initiated. Adherence to these principles decreases the likelihood of an adverse outcome, such as stiffness, recurrent instability, or posttraumatic arthritis. Surgeons who have an improved understanding of elbow anatomy and instability as well as updated treatment algorithms may further improve the outcomes of patients who have simple or complex elbow fractures and dislocations.

References

1. Linscheid RL, Wheeler DK: Elbow dislocations. *JAMA* 1965;194(11):1171-1176.

2. Stoneback JW, Owens BD, Sykes J, Athwal GS, Pointer L, Wolf JM: Incidence of elbow dislocations in the United States population. *J Bone Joint Surg Am* 2012;94(3):240-245.

3. Anakwe RE, Middleton SD, Jenkins PJ, McQueen MM, Court-Brown CM: Patient-reported outcomes after simple dislocation of the elbow. *J Bone Joint Surg Am* 2011;93(13):1220-1226.

4. Bryce CD, Armstrong AD: Anatomy and biomechanics of the elbow. *Orthop Clin North Am* 2008;39(2):141-154, v.

5. Morrey BF, Sanchez-Sotelo J: *The Elbow and Its Disorders*. Philadelphia, PA, Saunders Elsevier, 2009, pp 11-39.

6. O'Driscoll SW, Jupiter JB, King GJ, Hotchkiss RN, Morrey BF: The unstable elbow. *Instr Course Lect* 2001;50:89-102.

7. An KN, Morrey BF, Chao EY: The effect of partial removal of proximal ulna on elbow constraint. *Clin Orthop Relat Res* 1986;209:270-279.

8. Hull JR, Owen JR, Fern SE, Wayne JS, Boardman ND III: Role of the coronoid process in varus osteoarticular stability of the elbow. *J Shoulder Elbow Surg* 2005;14(4):441-446.

9. Closkey RF, Goode JR, Kirschen-baum D, Cody RP: The role of the coronoid process in elbow stability: A biomechanical analysis of axial loading. *J Bone Joint Surg Am* 2000;82(12):1749-1753.

10. Schneeberger AG, Sadowski MM, Jacob HA: Coronoid process and radial head as posterolateral rotatory stabilizers of the elbow. *J Bone Joint Surg Am* 2004;86(5):975-982.

11. Jeon IH, Sanchez-Sotelo J, Zhao K, An KN, Morrey BM: The contribution of the coronoid and radial head to the stability of the elbow. *J Bone Joint Surg Br* 2012;94(1):86-92.

12. Cohen MS, Hastings H II: Acute elbow dislocation: Evaluation and management. *J Am Acad Orthop Surg* 1998;6(1):15-23.

13. O'Driscoll SW, Bell DF, Morrey BF: Posterolateral rotatory instability of the elbow. *J Bone Joint Surg Am* 1991;73(3):440-446.

14. O'Driscoll SW, Morrey BF, Korinek S, An KN: Elbow subluxation and dislocation. A spectrum of instability. *Clin Orthop Relat Res* 1992;280:186-197.

15. Rhyou IH, Kim YS: New mechanism of the posterior elbow dislocation. *Knee Surg Sports Traumatol Arthrosc* 2012;20(12):2535-2541.

16. Schreiber JJ, Warren RF, Hotchkiss RN, Daluiski A: An online video investigation into the mechanism of elbow dislocation. *J Hand Surg Am* 2013;38(3):488-494.

17. Sheps DM, Hildebrand KA, Boorman RS: Simple dislocations of the elbow: Evaluation and treatment. *Hand Clin* 2004;20(4):389-404.

18. Rafai M, Largab A, Cohen D, Trafeh M: Pure posterior luxation of the elbow in adults: Immobilization or early mobilization: A randomized prospective study of 50 cases. *Chir Main* 1999;18(4):272-278.

19. Ross G, McDevitt ER, Chronister R, Ove PN: Treatment of simple elbow dislocation using an immediate motion protocol. *Am J Sports Med* 1999;27(3):308-311.

20. Hildebrand KA, Patterson SD, King GJ: Acute elbow dislocations: Simple and complex. *Orthop Clin North Am* 1999;30(1):63-79.

21. Maripuri SN, Debnath UK, Rao P, Mohanty K: Simple elbow dislocation among adults: A comparative study of two different methods of treatment. *Injury* 2007;38(11):1254-1258.

22. Mehlhoff TL, Noble PC, Bennett JB, Tullos HS: Simple dislocation of the elbow in the adult: Results after closed treatment. *J Bone Joint Surg Am* 1988;70(2):244-249.

23. Protzman RR: Dislocation of the elbow joint. *J Bone Joint Surg Am* 1978;60(4):539-541.

24. Schippinger G, Seibert FJ, Steinböck J, Kucharczyk M: Management of simple elbow dislocations: Does the period of immobilization affect the eventual results? *Langenbecks Arch Surg* 1999;384(3):294-297.

25. Josefsson PO, Gentz CF, Johnell O, Wendeberg B: Surgical versus non-surgical treatment of ligamentous injuries following dislocation of the elbow joint: A prospective randomized study. *J Bone Joint Surg Am* 1987;69(4):605-608.

26. Micic I, Kim SY, Park IH, Kim PT, Jeon IH: Surgical management of unstable elbow dislocation without intra-articular fracture. *Int Orthop* 2009;33(4):1141-1147.

27. Duckworth AD, Ring D, Kulijdian A, McKee MD: Unstable elbow dislocations. *J Shoulder Elbow Surg* 2008;17(2):281-286.

28. Jockel CR, Katolik LI, Zelouf DS: Simple medial elbow dislocations: A rare injury at risk for early instability. *J Hand Surg Am* 2013;38(9):1768-1773.

29. Martin BD, Johansen JA, Edwards SG: Complications related to simple dislocations of the elbow. *Hand Clin* 2008;24(1):9-25.

30. Charalambous CP, Morrey BF: Post-traumatic elbow stiffness. *J Bone Joint Surg Am* 2012;94(15):1428-1437.

31. Everding NG, Maschke SD, Hoyen HA, Evans PJ: Prevention and treatment of elbow stiffness: A 5-year update. *J Hand Surg Am* 2013;38(12):2496-2507.

32. Ayadi D, Etienne P, Burny F, Schuind F: Results of open arthrolysis for elbow stiffness: A series of 22 cases. *Acta Orthop Belg* 2011;77(4):453-457.

33. Lindenhovius AL, Doornberg JN, Ring D, Jupiter JB: Health status after open elbow contracture release. *J Bone Joint Surg Am* 2010;92(12):2187-2195.

34. Tosun B, Gundes H, Buluc L, Sarlak AY: The use of combined lateral and medial releases in the treatment of post-traumatic contracture of the elbow. *Int Orthop* 2007;31(5):635-638.

35. Gundlach U, Eygendaal D: Surgical treatment of posttraumatic stiffness of the elbow: 2-year outcome in 21 patients after a column procedure. *Acta Orthop* 2008;79(1):74-77.

36. Park MJ, Chang MJ, Lee YB, Kang HJ: Surgical release for posttraumatic loss of elbow flexion. *J Bone Joint Surg Am* 2010;92(16):2692-2699.

37. Lindenhovius AL, van de Luijt-gaarden K, Ring D, Jupiter J: Open elbow contracture release: Postoperative management with and without continuous passive motion. *J Hand Surg Am* 2009;34(5):858-865.

38. Thompson HC III, Garcia A: Myositis ossificans: Aftermath of elbow injuries. *Clin Orthop Relat Res* 1967;50:129-134.

39. Summerfield SL, DiGiovanni C, Weiss AP: Heterotopic ossification of the elbow. *J Shoulder Elbow Surg* 1997;6(3):321-332.

40. Schmidt SA, Kjaersgaard-Andersen P, Pedersen NW, Kristensen SS, Pedersen P, Nielsen JB: The use of indomethacin to prevent the formation of heterotopic bone after total hip replacement: A randomized, double-blind clinical trial. *J Bone Joint Surg Am* 1988;70(6):834-838.

41. Murthi AM, Keener JD, Armstrong AD, Getz CL: The recurrent unstable elbow: Diagnosis and treatment. *J Bone Joint Surg Am* 2010;92(8):1794-1804.

42. Broberg MA, Morrey BF: Results of treatment of fracture-dislocations of the elbow. *Clin Orthop Relat Res* 1987;216:109-119.

43. Mason ML: Some observations on fractures of the head of the radius with a review of one hundred cases. *Br J Surg* 1954;42(172):123-132.

44. Shulman BS, Lee JH, Liporace FA, Egol KA: Minimally displaced radial head/neck fractures (Mason type-I,

OTA types 21A2.2 and 21B2.1): Are we "over treating" our patients? *J Orthop Trauma* 2015;29(2):e31-e35.

45. Herbertsson P, Josefsson PO, Hasserius R, Karlsson C, Besjakov J, Karlsson M: Uncomplicated Mason type-II and III fractures of the radial head and neck in adults: A long-term follow-up study. *J Bone Joint Surg Am* 2004;86(3):569-574.

46. Akesson T, Herbertsson P, Josefsson PO, Hasserius R, Besjakov J, Karlsson MK: Primary nonoperative treatment of moderately displaced two-part fractures of the radial head. *J Bone Joint Surg Am* 2006;88(9):1909-1914.

47. King GJ, Evans DC, Kellam JF: Open reduction and internal fixation of radial head fractures. *J Orthop Trauma* 1991;5(1):21-28.

48. Ring D, Quintero J, Jupiter JB: Open reduction and internal fixation of fractures of the radial head. *J Bone Joint Surg Am* 2002;84(10):1811-1815.

49. Lindenhovius AL, Felsch Q, Doornberg JN, Ring D, Kloen P: Open reduction and internal fixation compared with excision for unstable displaced fractures of the radial head. *J Hand Surg Am* 2007;32(5):630-636.

50. Pike JM, Athwal GS, Faber KJ, King GJ: Radial head fractures—an update. *J Hand Surg Am* 2009;34(3):557-565.

51. Chen X, Wang SC, Cao LH, Yang GQ, Li M, Su JC: Comparison between radial head replacement and open reduction and internal fixation in clinical treatment of unstable, multi-fragmented radial head fractures. *Int Orthop* 2011;35(7):1071-1076.

52. Pike JM, Grewal R, Athwal GS, Faber KJ, King GJ: Open reduction and internal fixation of radial head fractures: Do outcomes differ between simple and complex injuries? *Clin Orthop Relat Res* 2014;472(7):2120-2127.

53. Ring D, Jupiter JB, Zilberfarb J: Posterior dislocation of the elbow with fractures of the radial head and coronoid. *J Bone Joint Surg Am* 2002;84(4):547-551.

54. Pugh DM, Wild LM, Schemitsch EH, King GJ, McKee MD: Standard surgical protocol to treat elbow dislocations with radial head and

coronoid fractures. *J Bone Joint Surg Am* 2004;86(6):1122-1130.

55. Mathew PK, Athwal GS, King GJ: Terrible triad injury of the elbow: Current concepts. *J Am Acad Orthop Surg* 2009;17(3):137-151.

56. Regan W, Morrey B: Fractures of the coronoid process of the ulna. *J Bone Joint Surg Am* 1989;71(9):1348-1354.

57. O'Driscoll SW, Jupiter JB, Cohen MS, Ring D, McKee MD: Difficult elbow fractures: Pearls and pitfalls. *Instr Course Lect* 2003;52:113-134.

58. Chan K, MacDermid JC, Faber KJ, King GJ, Athwal GS: Can we treat select terrible triad injuries nonoperatively? *Clin Orthop Relat Res* 2014;472(7):2092-2099.

59. Pugh DM, McKee MD: The "terrible triad" of the elbow. *Tech Hand Up Extrem Surg* 2002;6(1):21-29.

60. Ring D: Fractures of the coronoid process of the ulna. *J Hand Surg Am* 2006;31(10):1679-1689.

61. Chen HW, Liu GD, Wu LJ: Complications of treating terrible triad injury of the elbow: A systematic review. *PLoS One* 2014;9(5):e97476.

62. Terada N, Yamada H, Seki T, Urabe T, Takayama S: The importance of reducing small fractures of the coronoid process in the treatment of unstable elbow dislocation. *J Shoulder Elbow Surg* 2000;9(4):344-346.

63. Beingessner DM, Stacpoole RA, Dunning CE, Johnson JA, King GJ: The effect of suture fixation of type I coronoid fractures on the kinematics and stability of the elbow with and without medial collateral ligament repair. *J Shoulder Elbow Surg* 2007;16(2):213-217.

64. Papatheodorou LK, Rubright JH, Heim KA, Weiser RW, Sotereanos DG: Terrible triad injuries of the elbow: Does the coronoid always need to be fixed? *Clin Orthop Relat Res* 2014;472(7):2084-2091.

65. Shukla DR, Pillai G, McAnany S, Hausman M, Parsons BO: Heterotopic ossification formation after fracture-dislocations of the elbow. *J Shoulder Elbow Surg* 2015;24(3):333-338.

66. Ring D, Adey L, Zurakowski D, Jupiter JB: Elbow capsulectomy for posttraumatic elbow stiffness. *J Hand Surg Am* 2006;31(8):1264-1271.

67. Bado JL: The Monteggia lesion. *Clin Orthop Relat Res* 1967;50:71-86.

68. Jupiter JB, Leibovic SJ, Ribbans W, Wilk RM: The posterior Monteggia lesion. *J Orthop Trauma* 1991;5(4):395-402.

69. Athwal GS, Ramsey ML, Steinmann SP, Wolf JM: Fractures and dislocations of the elbow: A return to the basics. *Instr Course Lect* 2011;60:199-214.

70. Reynders P, De Groote W, Rondia J, Govaerts K, Stoffelen D, Broos PL: Monteggia lesions in adults. A multicenter Bota study. *Acta Orthop Belg* 1996;62(suppl 1):78-83.

71. Konrad GG, Kundel K, Kreuz PC, Oberst M, Sudkamp NP: Monteggia fractures in adults: Long-term results and prognostic factors. *J Bone Joint Surg Br* 2007;89(3):354-360.

72. Pollock JW, Brownhill J, Ferreira L, McDonald CP, Johnson J, King G: The effect of anteromedial facet fractures of the coronoid and lateral collateral ligament injury on elbow stability and kinematics. *J Bone Joint Surg Am* 2009;91(6):1448-1458.

73. Doornberg JN, de Jong IM, Lindenhovius AL, Ring D: The anteromedial facet of the coronoid process of the ulna. *J Shoulder Elbow Surg* 2007;16(5):667-670.

74. Sanchez-Sotelo J, O'Driscoll SW, Morrey BF: Anteromedial fracture of the coronoid process of the ulna. *J Shoulder Elbow Surg* 2006;15(5):e5-e8.

75. Rhyou IH, Kim KC, Lee JH, Kim SY: Strategic approach to O'Driscoll type 2 anteromedial coronoid facet fracture. *J Shoulder Elbow Surg* 2014;23(7):924-932.

76. Park SM, Lee JS, Jung JY, Kim JY, Song KS: How should anteromedial coronoid facet fracture be managed? A surgical strategy based on O'Driscoll classification and ligament injury. *J Shoulder Elbow Surg* 2015;24(1):74-82.

77. Doornberg JN, Ring DC: Fracture of the anteromedial facet of the coronoid process. *J Bone Joint Surg Am* 2006;88(10):2216-2224.

Shoulder and Elbow

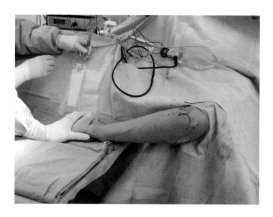

The Unstable Elbow: Current Concepts in Diagnosis and Treatment

Robert Z. Tashjian, MD
Brian R. Wolf, MD, MS
Roger P. van Riet, MD, PhD
Scott P. Steinmann, MD

Abstract

Elbow instability is common and may occur after a variety of injuries, including falls or direct blows. Instability can be classified as either acute or chronic. Acute instability is classified as simple (without fracture) or complex (with associated fracture). Chronic instability is classified as a chronically dislocated or recurrently unstable elbow. Recurrent instability commonly presents as isolated medial or lateral collateral ligament insufficiency. A chronically dislocated elbow is often more complex, involving both osseous and ligamentous injuries. The treatment of simple dislocations typically involves closed reduction and nonsurgical management. Chronic recurrent lateral and medial collateral ligament insufficiencies have very different clinical characteristics, but definitive treatment frequently involves ligament reconstruction. Complex instability usually requires surgery, which includes open reduction and internal fixation of coronoid and olecranon fractures, repair or replacement of radial head fractures, and lateral collateral ligament repair. Medial collateral ligament repair and/or external fixation are rarely required to restore stability. It is important for surgeons to understand current concepts in the diagnosis and management of acute and chronic elbow instability as well as the preferred surgical treatments and techniques for the management of these injuries.

Instr Course Lect 2016;65:55–82.

The incidence of acute simple elbow dislocations is 6 per 100,000 per year. Patients who have acute simple elbow dislocations are typically young, with a median age of 30 years and a peak incidence between 10 and 20 years.[1,2] Approximately one-half of elbow dislocations are simple dislocations without an associated fracture.[3,4] Posterolateral dislocation is the most common direction for an elbow dislocation. The lateral collateral ligament (LCL) first tears from its humeral origin followed by anterior capsular tearing and, finally, medial collateral ligament (MCL) tearing; however, the MCL occasionally remains intact, especially in the setting of an associated fracture.[5-8] Complex dislocations are associated with fractures, including fractures of the radial head, the coronoid process, the olecranon,

Dr. Tashjian or an immediate family member serves as a paid consultant to Mitek and Tornier. Dr. Wolf or an immediate family member serves as a paid consultant to CONMED Linvatec; has received research or institutional support from the Orthopaedic Research and Education Foundation; and has received nonincome support (such as equipment or services), commercially derived honoraria, or other non-research–related funding (such as paid travel) from Arthrex. Dr. van Riet or an immediate family member is a member of a speakers' bureau or has made paid presentations on behalf of Acumed; serves as a paid consultant to Acumed; and serves as a board member, owner, officer, or committee member of the Belgian Elbow and Shoulder Society. Dr. Steinmann or an immediate family member has received royalties from Arthrex, Biomet, and Innovative Medical Device Sourcing; serves as a paid consultant to Acumed, Arthrex, Articulinx, Biomet, and Elsevier; and serves as a board member, owner, officer, or committee member of the American Shoulder and Elbow Surgeons and the American Society for Surgery of the Hand.

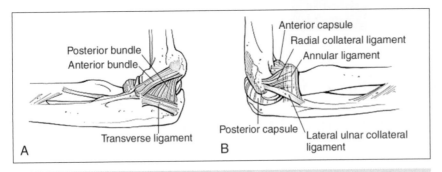

Figure 1   Illustrations show the structure of the medial collateral ligament complex (**A**) and the lateral collateral ligament complex (**B**). (Reproduced from Tashjian RZ, Katarincic JA: Complex elbow instability. *J Am Acad Orthop Surg* 2006;14[5]:278-286.)

Table 1
Lateral and Medial Collateral Ligaments of the Elbow

Ligament	Origin	Insertion
Lateral collateral ligament complex		
Radial collateral ligament	Lateral epicondyle (humerus)	Annular ligament
Lateral ulnar collateral ligament	Lateral epicondyle (humerus)	Supinator crest (ulna)
Annular ligament	Anterior margin of the lesser sigmoid notch (ulna)	Supinator crest (ulna)
Medial collateral ligament complex		
Anterior band	Anteroinferior aspect of medial epicondyle	Sublime tubercle (coronoid)
Posterior band	Posteroinferior aspect of medial epicondyle	Olecranon
Transverse band	Coronoid	Olecranon

and the distal humerus. Compared with simple dislocations, a greater risk of recurrent instability and arthritis occurs with complex dislocations.[9,10] Complex dislocation patterns include transolecranon fracture-dislocations, posterior Monteggia fracture-dislocations, terrible triad injuries, and varus posteromedial rotatory instability (PMRI) that is associated with anteromedial coronoid facet fractures.

Chronic elbow instability often includes MCL and LCL insufficiency, which typically results from a dislocation with insufficient LCL healing and

lead to posterolateral rotatory instability (PLRI).[11] Other etiologies of PLRI include LCL insufficiency in the setting of cubitus varus deformity and iatrogenic LCL injury after lateral surgical approaches.[12] MCL insufficiency often is a chronic attritional process that occurs in overhead throwing athletes and results in pain and limited sport-related function. Most patients often report pain during high-level overhead activities but no symptoms of instability during lower levels of activity.

It is important for orthopaedic surgeons to understand the current

techniques for the diagnosis and treatment of the most common forms of acute (simple and complex) and chronic (MCL or LCL insufficiency) instability. Surgeons should understand the anatomy and biomechanics associated with elbow instability as well as the clinical scenarios and treatment algorithms for each diagnosis.

Anatomy and Biomechanics

The radius, the ulna, and the humerus articulate at the elbow to form three joints: the radiohumeral, ulnohumeral, and proximal radiohumeral joints. The elbow is one of the most congruent joints of the human body. The capsule, the LCL complex, and the extensor tendons on the lateral side as well as the MCL complex and the flexor-pronator group on the medial side further stabilize the elbow (**Figure 1, A** and **B**).

The LCL complex consists of the radial collateral ligament (RCL), the lateral ulnar collateral ligament (LUCL), and the annular ligament. The RCL and LUCL share their origins on the lateral epicondyle and are not individually identifiable at this level[13] (**Table 1**). The MCL complex also is divided into three distinct structures: the anterior, posterior, and transverse bands. The anterior and posterior bands originate from the medial epicondyle. The anterior band inserts on the sublime tubercle on the ulna and is the primary stabilizing structure of the MCL complex for valgus stability[14] (**Table 1**).

The articulation and its surrounding soft tissues, including the capsule, ligaments, and muscles, determine elbow stability. The contribution of the articulation and its surrounding soft tissues depends on the position of the elbow and the direction of stress placed on the elbow. The MCL is the primary stabilizer to valgus stress, and the radial head is a secondary stabilizer to valgus stress.[15] The bony articulation is the most important structure that resists varus stress, with less influence from the anterior capsule and the RCL.[16] The LUCL resists external rotation stresses to the elbow; however, sectioning of the LUCL alone does not induce a clear PLRI pattern, which requires both the RCL and the LUCL to be injured.[13-18] Resection of the radial head or the coronoid increases the magnitude of PLRI.[19] Muscles also play a role in maintaining elbow stability. Contraction of the extensor muscles decreases laxity in LCL-deficient elbows, and, conversely, sectioning of the muscles decreases stability.[17,20] The stabilizing effect of the muscles is greater on the medial side, with the flexor carpi ulnaris (FCU) as the main stabilizer.[21]

Simple Dislocations

Most simple elbow dislocations occur after a fall onto an outstretched hand. Some patients may immediately relocate the arm via muscle contraction or by forcefully moving the elbow. The clinical examination of an acutely dislocated elbow is limited, but the dislocation will be readily apparent via an inspection of the elbow. The elbow will be swollen and painful to touch. A thorough neurovascular examination should be performed initially.

Plain radiographs, including AP and lateral views of the elbow, are sufficient to diagnose an acute elbow dislocation. Radiographs will show the dislocated joint and any displaced fragments. Prereduction advanced imaging, such as CT, is not indicated. Radiographs should be repeated after the reduction maneuver is performed because sometimes fractures become visible only

after the elbow is reduced. CT may be ordered if associated bony lesions are suspected. MRI will reveal the extent of the soft-tissue injury but rarely changes the treatment plan.

Although a dislocated elbow often can be reduced with the patient under limited sedation, occasionally reduction may need to be performed with the patient under general anesthesia. After reduction, the elbow is reexamined by moving the elbow from flexion to extension with the forearm in neutral rotation. Typically, the elbow will be stable in flexion and become increasingly unstable with extension.

Nonsurgical Management

Some controversy exists regarding the nonsurgical treatment of simple elbow dislocations. Historically, up to 3 weeks of immobilization has been recommended; however, studies have reported that functional treatment with immediate mobilization in a brace or a sling for comfort is safe with regard to redislocation rates and may lead to improved functional results.[22,23] If radiographic signs of subluxation persist, an exercise program may help to further stabilize the elbow.[24] Although long-term results report some degenerative changes and persistent medial instability in approximately 50% of patients who are treated with nonsurgical measures, no recurrent ulnohumeral dislocations have been reported.[25] Rarely, persistent chronic instability may develop, which is typically caused by a failure of the LCL to heal.

In general, after reduction, the elbow can be splinted temporarily for pain control. One week after injury, patients should be reexamined and radiographs should be obtained to confirm a reduced ulnohumeral joint. After a

reduced ulnohumeral joint is confirmed, patients may use the affected arm with a dynamic elbow brace as tolerated for the next 4 to 6 weeks. If signs of residual instability are present at the terminal 30° of extension, an extension block may be used progressively, allowing increased extension in increments of 30° every 2 weeks, starting with a 60° extension block. Surgical repair of the LCL should be considered for patients who have instability at more than 30° of extension.

Surgical Management

In general, compared with closed reduction and nonsurgical treatment, no data suggest that acute surgery yields better outcomes for simple dislocations.[8] Surgery may be indicated if the elbow remains grossly unstable after closed reduction, especially if instability remains at more than 30° to 45° of terminal extension. Acute lateral ligament repair, which can be performed either open or arthroscopically, without a medial repair typically stabilizes the elbow.[26] It is not uncommon for patients to have an avulsion of the common extensor tendon mass.[8] The LCL is most commonly avulsed from the humerus.[8] Depending on the surgeon's preference, the LCL can be reattached at the isometric point on the lateral epicondyle with the use of either bone tunnels or a bone anchor.

LCL Injuries of the Elbow and Chronic PLRI

PLRI occurs when the radial head and the ulna rotate externally off the distal humerus, which leads to posterior displacement and subluxation of the radial head relative to the capitellum. The radius and the ulna move as a unit because the proximal radioulnar joint remains intact. O'Driscoll et al[27] first

Table 2
Clinical Tests for Posterolateral Rotatory Instability

Test	Execution	Positive Test
Pivot shift apprehension test[29]	Flexion/extension of the elbow with valgus stress, hypersupination, and axial load	Apprehension
Pivot shift instability test[29]	Flexion/extension of the elbow with valgus stress, hypersupination, and axial load	Ranging from subluxation dimple in soft spot to full dislocation of the elbow
Posterolateral drawer test[29]	Elbow at 90° of flexion, external rotation of the forearm as a unit while palpating the radiohumeral joint	Palpable posterior subluxation of the radial head
Tabletop test[29]	Press-up maneuver with the forearm supinated from extension to flexion. The examiner supports the radial head, and the test is repeated.	Pain and apprehension with the elbow at 40° of flexion; decreased pain when examiner supports radial head.
Chair sign[30]	Push up from a chair. Elbow at 90° of flexion, forearms supinated, and arms abducted to greater than shoulder width	Apprehension or inability to fully extend the elbow
Push-up test[30]	Push up from the floor. Elbow at 90° of flexion, forearms supinated, and arms abducted to greater than shoulder width	Apprehension or inability to fully extend the elbow

described PLRI in 1991. Although the overall incidence of PLRI is relatively uncommon, PLRI is the most common form of chronic recurrent elbow instability. Instability typically results from an elbow dislocation in which the LCL complex fails to heal.[11] Some patients may have a history of one or more simple dislocations; others may not have a documented dislocation but may have had a relatively minor trauma that led to persistent and symptomatic subluxation of the elbow.[27] Instead of a preceding traumatic event, patients may have a history of multiple cortisone injections and secondary LCL insufficiency. Long-standing cubitus varus deformity may result in chronic LCL attenuation and instability.[28] Finally, PLRI may occur after surgery on the lateral side of the elbow (eg, after a release for lateral epicondylitis with an iatrogenic injury).[12] Patients report lateral elbow

pain, clicking, mechanical symptoms, and instability of the proximal radius, all of which are aggravated by activities that create an axial load on the externally rotated forearm in extension (eg, pushing up from a chair).

The diagnosis of PLRI is predominantly clinical. Varus laxity may be present in patients who have complete LCL ruptures. Several specific clinical tests for PLRI have been described[29,30] (**Table 2**). Although the pivot shift test is sensitive, its specificity is low in patients who are awake; the specificity of the pivot shift test is improved if the patient is anesthetized. The posterolateral drawer test is more specific than the pivot shift test because patients will have less apprehension if the test is performed when they are awake.[31] The tabletop test, the chair sign, and the push-up test all are useful and sensitive tests to help confirm instability.[29,32]

Radiographs and CT scans may reveal indirect signs of ligamentous injury, such as calcification of the ligament, subluxation of the joint, or an impression fracture on the posterior aspect of the capitellum. Coonrad et al[33] described the drop sign, which includes widening of the ulnohumeral joint more than 4 mm as seen on a lateral radiograph, as suggestive of PLRI. In most patients, radiographs and CT scans will be negative. An MRI may help visualize a ruptured LCL in patients who have chronic PLRI.[30] Cartilage lesions, which are common and may have a negative effect on the outcome of treatment, also may be detected via MRI.

Nonsurgical Management
Nonsurgical management of PLRI is limited. Bracing and activity modification may be attempted; however, because the elbow is commonly placed in a position at risk for instability during activities of daily living, instability is difficult to avoid. Anconeus and extensor strengthening may help limit mild PLRI. In general, surgical treatment is typically required to stabilize the joint.

Surgical Management
Various surgical options are available to treat patients who have chronic PLRI. Primary repair of the chronically ruptured LCL complex has been described with variable results. Repair is the first line of treatment for ligament injuries that have occurred within 6 weeks; however, surgeons should be ready to perform a reconstruction if necessary. Although more chronic injuries have been treated with repair alone, the outcomes have been varied. In a study of 34 patients who underwent primary repair for the treatment of PLRI, Daluiski et al[34] reported no difference in

outcomes between patients treated early and those treated in a delayed fashion. No patients in the delayed treatment group (>30 days) required further treatment. In a study that compared the results of direct repair and ligament reconstruction, Sanchez-Sotelo et al[35] reported better results and improved Mayo Elbow Performance Scores (MEPSs) in patients who underwent reconstruction compared with those who underwent ligament repair. Ligament reconstruction with the use of a tissue graft is the preferred technique for most patients who have chronic injuries, with reliable results and restoration of stability reported in 85% to 90% of patients.[35-37]

Various surgical techniques are available for LUCL reconstruction. Distal graft fixation options include a two-tunnel technique and a single-tunnel technique. The single-tunnel technique is fixed with an interference screw, a cortical button, or suture anchors. Proximal fixation options include a three-tunnel technique and a single-tunnel docking technique. Various grafts, including allograft and autograft, are available, and many tendons, including the palmaris, plantaris, Achilles, semitendinosus, and gracilis, have sufficient strength to reconstruct the LCL complex.[38]

One of the authors of this chapter (R.P.vR.) adapted an arthroscopic technique for treatment of PLRI that was described by Savoie et al[26] to treat patients with stage 1 and stage 2 PLRI (ie, stress pivot shift radiographs under anesthesia that show radiohumeral subluxation or a perched ulnohumeral joint on the coronoid). The technique consists of imbrication of the LCL from the lateral epicondyle to the soft-spot portal and then the supinator crest with

the use of a No. 2 polydioxanone suture. The suture is then doubled, and the tails are passed subcutaneously back to the soft-spot portal and tied. An LCL reconstruction is preferred in patients who have stage 3 PLRI (ie, ulnohumeral dislocation under the stress pivot shift test). LCL reconstruction also is a reasonable treatment for patients who have stage 1 and stage 2 PLRI; however, one of the authors of this chapter (R.P.vR.) prefers an arthroscopic technique for plication (**Figure 2**).

The open technique for lateral ligament reconstruction uses an incision that is centered over the lateral epicondyle. The Kocher interval is identified between the anconeus and the extensor carpi ulnaris. Among the various graft choices, one of the authors of this chapter (R.P.vR.) prefers to use an extensor hallucis longus allograft that is approximately 20 cm. In addition, cortical bone button fixation of both the ulna (intramedullary) and the humerus (posterior cortex) is the preferred fixation technique of one of the authors of this chapter (R.P.vR.). A single tunnel in the ulna (4.5 mm) and a single tunnel in the humerus (6.0 mm) are used. The elbow is fully reduced and held with the forearm in pronation as the graft is tightened in 30° of flexion. The LUCL has been shown to be lax in extension and tighten in flexion; therefore, the graft should be tensioned in approximately 30° of flexion to allow the reconstruction to tighten further when the elbow is flexed.[39]

The results of LCL reconstruction are very good in 80% to 90% of patients.[35-37,40] In a study of 33 patients who underwent ligament reconstruction, Sanchez-Sotelo et al[35] reported that elbow stability was restored in all but five patients. The mean MEPS was 85 at a

mean follow-up of 6 years. Better results were seen in patients who had posttraumatic etiology and in patients who had subjective instability compared with patients who had only pain. In a study of 18 patients who underwent ligament reconstruction with the use of a triceps graft, Olsen and Søjbjerg[40] reported no recurrent subluxations at a mean follow-up of 44 months. Seventeen patients were satisfied with their outcome, and only one patient was considered to have failed surgery. In a study of six patients who underwent reconstruction and four patients who underwent LCL repair, Lee and Teo[37] reported that no patients had residual instability, and 80% of the results were considered good or excellent. The authors reported that patients who underwent reconstruction fared better than patients who underwent LCL repair. In a study of eight patients who underwent LCL reconstruction with the use of a graft and the proximal docking technique, Jones et al[36] reported that, at a mean follow-up of 7.1 years, 75% of patients had resolution of elbow instability, and 25% of patients reported occasional elbow instability. The authors reported that the mean MEPS was 87.5, and all patients were satisfied with their outcomes.

MCL Injuries of the Elbow

Injuries to the MCL of the elbow have increased considerably during the past decade, which is likely related to more adolescents participating in year-round sports, especially baseball.[41] Baseball players and javelin throwers are especially at risk for MCL injuries because their sports place tremendous amounts of valgus stress on the elbow. Baseball players who participate in their sport for more than 8 months per year have a 500% increased risk for MCL injuries

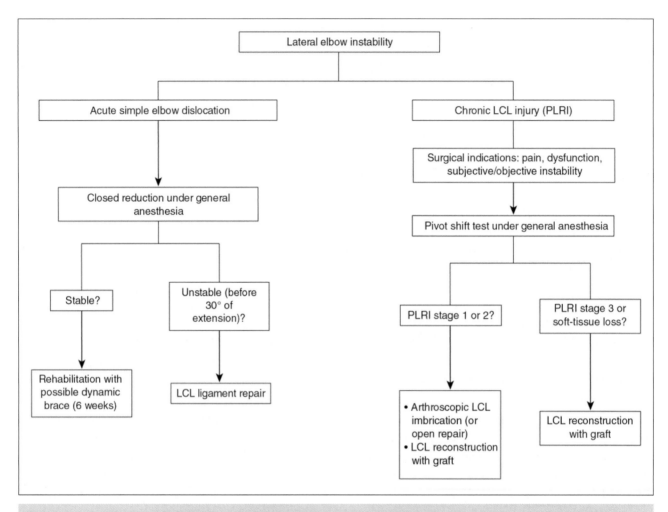

Figure 2 Algorithm for the management of acute simple elbow dislocations and chronic lateral collateral ligament (LCL) injuries. PLRI = posterolateral rotatory instability.

that require surgery.[42] For adolescent baseball players, more than 100 innings pitched per year and high pitch counts during games also have been reported to be risk factors for MCL injuries that require surgery. Fatigue also is a substantial risk factor for the development of an MCL injury in a thrower, regardless of his or her age. It is estimated that one-third of professional baseball pitchers have undergone surgery for an MCL injury. MCL injuries also are seen in gymnasts, wrestlers, and football players.

History and Evaluation

MCL injuries can be characterized by an acute pop in the elbow with substantial pain and an abrupt loss of normal velocity and control or by the gradual onset of vague medial elbow pain, loss of control, and reduced velocity. Historically, an acute pop in the elbow with substantial pain and an abrupt loss of normal velocity and control was believed to correlate with an acute rupture of the MCL, whereas the gradual onset of vague medial elbow pain, loss of control, and reduced velocity represented chronic attritional damage to the MCL. The patient usually notes pain during the late cocking phase and the early acceleration phase of throwing motion.

A physical examination of the elbow may reveal swelling over the medial elbow at the level of the epicondyle, especially in the acute setting. Tenderness may be elicited over the ulnar collateral ligament (UCL), which sits deep to the FCU and the flexor pronator mass. Several provocative tests can be performed to evaluate the MCL. All tests place a valgus stress on the MCL and will elicit pain over the ligament if the MCL is injured. These tests include the milking maneuver,[43] in which the patient is seated and the shoulder is abducted to 90° with valgus stress placed on the elbow. Another frequently used test is the moving valgus stress test,[44] which can be performed with the patient in either the seated or supine position and the arm abducted in the throwing position. The supine position allows the examination table to stabilize the arm and scapula while the surgeon applies valgus loads in varying degrees of shoulder abduction and varying angles of elbow flexion (**Figure 3**). Pain is elicited in the shear angle from 70° to 120° of flexion. Patients will report sharp medial elbow pain in this arc of motion and will have limited pain outside this arc of motion.

Imaging for a suspected MCL injury begins with AP and lateral radiographs of the elbow. The radiographs should be carefully scrutinized for calcification or bony prominence off the sublime tubercle of the ulna or off the distal aspect of the medial epicondyle. Chronic MCL injuries may demonstrate spurring of the medial olecranon and olecranon fossa and, possibly, loose bodies. Stress injuries of the medial epicondyle and the olecranon also may be seen on radiographs. Direct imaging of the MCL is best accomplished with MRI or MRI combined with an arthrogram. Arthrogram MRI may allow for better visualization of partial MCL injuries and avulsions, either proximally or distally. The distal peel-off of the MCL from the sublime tubercle will demonstrate a T sign, in which dye leaks over the ulna and under the partial avulsion of the MCL. Ultrasound is becoming a more frequently used diagnostic modality for MCL injuries and is beneficial because dynamic imaging can be performed while stressing the elbow.

Classification

MCL injuries can be classified with MRI to assess damage to the ligament. Grade I injuries are partial injuries, in which fluid is seen along the ligament or edema is seen within the ligament but without fiber tearing. Grade II injuries

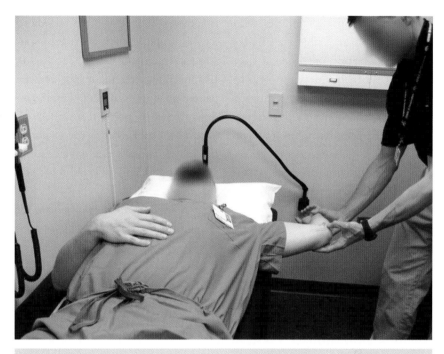

Figure 3   Clinical photograph shows the moving valgus stress test, which is performed with the patient placed in the supine position.

also are partial injuries with some fiber tearing but without complete disruption. A wide range of grade II injuries exist, from low grade, in which a minimal percentage of fibers are torn, to high grade, in which a higher percentage of the ligament thickness is damaged. Grade III injuries are complete injuries across all ligament fibers (**Figure 4**).

Nonsurgical Management

Several options exist for the treatment of MCL injuries. Nonsurgical treatment is recommended for MCL injuries in patients who are nonthrowers. Most nonthrowing patients will have good outcomes with a period of activity modification, possible bracing, physical therapy, and rest. A hinged brace may be used for 4 to 6 weeks to provide stability and comfort; occasionally, bracing may be used for a patient who is a position player if the patient attempts a return to active play. Most patients who

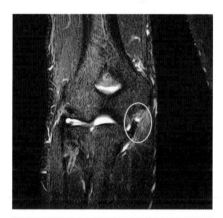

Figure 4   Sagittal T2-weighted MRI of the elbow demonstrates a complete medial collateral ligament tear (circle).

are not throwers also will have good outcomes with nonsurgical treatment. Historically, baseball players have not successfully returned to a high level of throwing reliably if MCL injuries were treated nonsurgically; however, most historical studies did not differentiate between patients who had partial tears and patients who had complete tears.[45]

Throwers with partial injuries who are treated nonsurgically have a better likelihood of good outcomes if they are withheld from throwing for 6 to 12 weeks. Physical therapy is performed to correct any motion abnormalities of the shoulder and to strengthen the arm, the shoulder, the core, and the lower extremities. Pitching mechanics can be examined and corrected during the time that the elbow is allowed to rest and heal.[46]

In recent years, new adjunctive treatments have been used to supplement the healing of MCL injuries, especially partial tears. Under ultrasonography, platelet-rich plasma may be injected into and around a damaged MCL. In a study on the use of platelet-rich plasma for the treatment of partial tears, Podesta et al[47] described a rehabilitation and return-to-throwing algorithm, which included only gentle range of motion for the first 2 weeks after the injection(s). Strengthening of the upper extremity is started approximately 3 weeks after the injection(s), and some valgus stretch is instituted 5 to 6 weeks after the injection(s). Strengthening is increased gradually, and a throwing program is initiated 8 to 10 weeks after injection(s) if the patient is symptom free. Return to play is allowed 12 to 14 weeks after the injection(s). The authors reported that 88% of athletes (30 of 34) who used this algorithm successfully returned to play.[47]

Surgical Management

The surgical indications for MCL injuries include failure of nonsurgical treatment, full-thickness and high-grade partial tears in patients who are high-level throwers, and a desire to return to a throwing or elbow-stressing sport. The discussion on surgery in patients who are throwing athletes often is complex because it often takes 2 to 3 months to determine if a trial of nonsurgical treatment will be successful. If nonsurgical treatment fails and the patient undergoes surgery, then the ultimate return to sport is further delayed. Careful consideration of the extent of the injury, the physical examination, and an individual patient's goals and situation is critical.

Primarily, there are two options for the surgical treatment of MCL injuries: direct repair or graft placement and fixation. Direct repair of the MCL is solely applicable to avulsion injuries. A recent study reported high success rates in patients who underwent suture anchor repair of MCL avulsion injuries off the sublime tubercle or the medial epicondyle.[48] It is important to note that all patients in this study were athletes younger than 20 years. The authors directly repaired the avulsion injuries by placing a single, double-loaded suture anchor in the medial epicondyle or at the sublime tubercle, depending on the site of avulsion. An accelerated rehabilitation program of approximately 4 months allowed for earlier return to sport than that typically seen in patients who undergo complete ligament reconstruction.

Several techniques can be used for graft placement and fixation,[49] including the figure-of-8 Jobe technique and the modified Jobe technique; the American Sports Medicine Institute technique; and the use of interference screws, suture anchors, and suture buttons in various combinations.[50] One of the authors of this chapter (B.R.W.) prefers to use the docking technique described by Dodson and Altchek.[51]

Concomitant pathology, which is present in a substantial percentage of patients who undergo surgery for the treatment of MCL injuries, necessitates elbow arthroscopy.[52] The indications for elbow arthroscopy at the time of reconstructive surgery are guided by both the physical examination and imaging studies. If spurring is seen posteromedially on imaging studies and the clinical examination is consistent with posteromedial impingement, then elbow arthroscopy is performed to débride the superior medial olecranon and the medial olecranon. Patients who are throwers may have concomitant articular cartilage injury, loose bodies, and synovitis, all of which can be addressed with arthroscopy. Arthroscopy is typically performed in the same setting but before elbow repair or reconstruction.

MCL reconstruction can be performed with the patient placed in either the supine or prone position. One of the authors of this chapter (B.R.W.) prefers to perform MCL reconstruction with the patient placed in the prone position. Prone positioning places the elbow in a varus position and optimizes visualization for both the surgeon and the assistant during the procedure. In addition, the prone position is a more customary position for elbow arthroscopy, which is often performed before MCL reconstruction. For reconstruction, the shoulder is internally rotated, and the forearm is supported on a padded Mayo stand (**Figure 5**). If reconstruction is performed with the patient placed in the supine position, a hand table attachment is used while the shoulder is abducted and externally rotated.

The most common graft source for MCL reconstruction is autologous ipsilateral or contralateral palmaris longus tendon tissue. The ipsilateral or contralateral gracilis hamstring tendon also may be used. Palmaris harvest is performed by making a 1-cm incision on the distal flexion crease of the wrist (**Figure 6**). It is helpful to mark the tendon on the patient as he or she demonstrates the tendon; this should be done in the preoperative area. Although performed less frequently, allograft also may be used for reconstruction. Savoie et al[53] reported a 94% success rate for MCL reconstruction with the use of a hamstring allograft.

The surgical approach for reconstruction uses an 8- to 12-cm incision that extends from 4 to 5 cm proximal to 5 to 7 cm distal to the medial epicondyle (**Figure 7, A**). The medial antebrachial nerve should be identified and protected as the deep fascia is approached. Approximately 40% of patients with MCL injuries who require surgery will have associated ulnar nerve symptoms. The ulnar nerve should be addressed with subcutaneous transposition during MCL reconstruction if the patient had ulnar dysesthesias with throwing, had a grossly positive Tinel test during the physical examination, has a subluxating ulnar nerve, or has an ulnar nerve that is perching on the medial epicondyle. Given the proximity of the MCL to the ulnar nerve, the MCL is exposed via a muscle-splitting approach through the FCU raphe with the use of blunt dissection and blunt retractors. The native injured ligament is split longitudinally (**Figure 7, B**), which allows for assessment of the ligament injury and, more importantly, clear identification of the joint line.

Using a 2.5- to 3.5-mm burr or drill, a transosseous tunnel is made below the sublime tubercle of the ulna approximately 15 mm distal to the joint line. Holes are created anterior and posterior to the tubercle and connected beneath the bone bridge with the use of curets (**Figure 7, C**). Commercial sets are

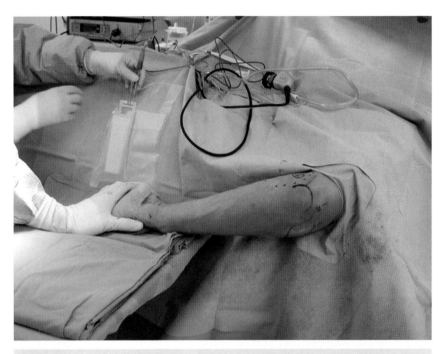

Figure 5   Intraoperative photograph shows a patient placed in the prone position for medial collateral ligament reconstruction.

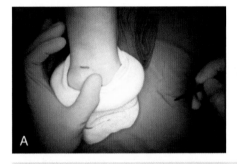
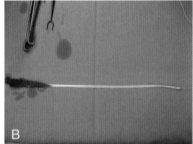

Figure 6   Intraoperative photographs show a graft procedure for medial collateral ligament reconstruction. A 1-cm incision is made at the distal flexion crease of the wrist over the palmaris longus (**A**) to obtain a palmaris longus graft (**B**).

available to assist with tunnel drilling. Care must be taken to maintain a stout bone bridge. Using a 4- to 5-mm burr or drill, a humeral tunnel is made at the anterior medial epicondyle (**Figure 7, D**). Ideally, the tunnel should be started slightly lateral to the midline of the inferior surface of the medial epicondyle and angled 30° posterior in the sagittal plane and 15° lateral in the coronal plane[54] to maximize possible tunnel length. The humeral tunnel should be

15 to 20 mm in depth. Using a pencil-tip burr or a 1.8-mm drill, two exit tunnels for sutures are then made from the superior epicondyle connecting into the humeral tunnel.

The prepared end of the tendon graft is then passed through the ulna (**Figure 7, E**). The prepared end of the tendon graft with sutures is pulled up into the humeral tunnel, with sutures exiting one of the superior holes. The elbow is placed at 60° and in varus.

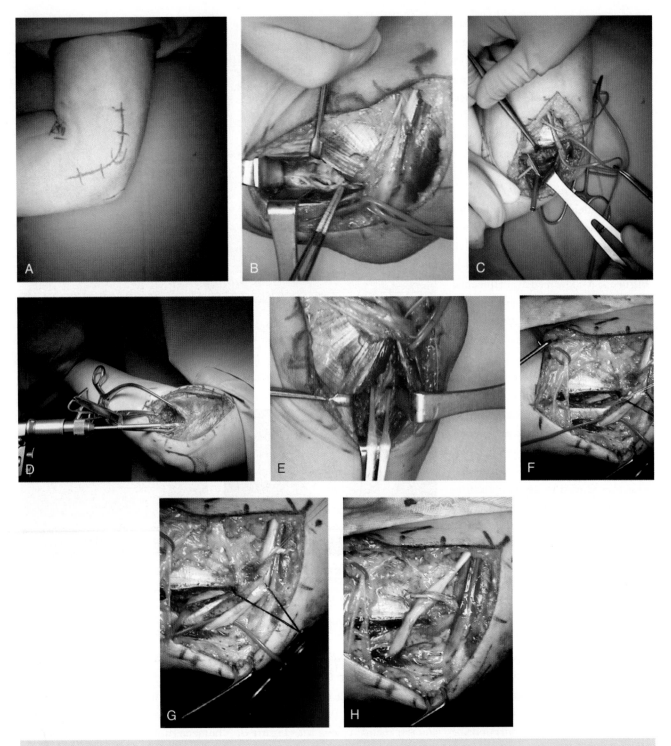

Figure 7 Intraoperative photographs show the surgical approach for medial collateral ligament reconstruction. **A,** The incision is centered over the medial epicondyle. **B,** A muscle-splitting approach through the flexor carpi ulnaris raphe is used to expose the medial collateral ligament. **C,** A guide is placed to create the ulnar tunnels in a converging manner anterior and posterior to the sublime tubercle. **D,** A 4.5-mm drill is used to create the humeral tunnel on the medial epicondyle. **E,** The graft is passed through the ulnar tunnels. **F,** One limb of the graft is docked into the humeral tunnels, and the second limb of the graft is cut to the appropriate length and prepared with locking sutures. **G,** The sutures are tied proximally over the bone bridge on the superior epicondyle to complete the graft construct. **H,** Subcutaneous ulnar nerve transposition uses a strip of the medial intermuscular septum as a sling to loosely stabilize the nerve and prevent subluxation back into the cubital tunnel.

The second limb of the graft is drawn proximally and measured so that at least 10 to 15 mm of graft will enter the humeral tunnel. The second limb of the graft is prepared with suture similar to the first limb, and the graft is cut to the appropriate length (**Figure 7, F**). The native MCL is repaired with a running size 0 permanent stitch. The second limb of the graft is drawn up into the humeral tunnel, with sutures exiting the other superior suture hole. The graft is then docked, and tension is checked; both limbs of the graft should be tight. The forearm is supinated, and the elbow is held in 45° to 60° of flexion with varus stress as the suture limbs are tied together proximally over the epicondyle (**Figure 7, G**).

The fascia of the FCU split is closed. If necessary, the ulnar nerve is transposed with the use of a strip of the medial intermuscular septum, which acts as a fascial sling to prevent the nerve from subluxating back into the groove (**Figure 7, H**). Postoperatively, the patient's elbow is placed in a hinged elbow brace, which allows motion from 45° to 90°. Full motion is gradually restored during a 6-week period. Strengthening of the shoulder, arm, and forearm—while avoiding valgus stress—begins 6 to 8 weeks after surgery. A throwing program is started 14 to 18 weeks after surgery. Throwers are typically ready for position play 6 to 7 months after surgery. A return to mound pitching typically occurs 9 to 12 months after surgery.

Outcomes

In general, MCL reconstruction outcomes are quite good. Cain et al[55] reported an 84% return-to-play rate in 1,281 athletes who underwent reconstruction with the American Sports Medicine Institute technique. Dodson et al[56] reported a 90% return-to-play rate at the same or at a higher level for patients who underwent reconstruction with the docking technique. Using the Kerlan-Jobe Orthopaedic Clinic score, Jones et al[57] reported excellent outcomes in 93% of athletes aged 15 to 18 years who underwent reconstruction. Savoie et al[53] reported an 88% return-to-play rate at the same or at a higher level and good or excellent outcomes in 93% of patients who underwent reconstruction with the use of tissue allografts.

Watson et al[58] summarized the results of 1,368 patients who underwent MCL reconstruction in 14 clinical studies. The authors reported an overall 79% return-to-play rate and an overall 18.6% complication rate after reconstruction. Among contemporary techniques, complications were lower in patients who underwent reconstruction with the modified docking technique (4.3%) compared with patients who underwent reconstruction with the modified Jobe (19.1%) and interference screw (10%) techniques. The most common complication after reconstruction was ulnar neuropathy, which occurred at a rate of 12.9%. In a prior systematic review, Vitale and Ahmad[52] reported more ulnar nerve complications in patients who underwent an obligatory ulnar nerve transposition compared with those who only underwent ulnar nerve transposition if they had preoperative symptoms or ulnar nerve instability at the time of surgery. The authors also reported that patients who underwent reconstruction with the use of a muscle-splitting approach had fewer complications and better outcomes compared with patients who underwent reconstruction with detachment of the flexor-pronator mass.

Overall, MCL injuries are becoming more common in throwing athletes. A careful examination and advanced imaging studies are important to diagnose MCL injuries. Nonsurgical treatment options can be attempted in patients who are nonthrowers and in athletes who have partial tears. Surgical repair or reconstruction can be performed in patients who fail nonsurgical treatment or have complete ligament injuries.

Fracture-Dislocations

Olecranon fractures account for approximately 10% of all upper extremity fractures in adults. Approximately 85% of olecranon fractures are simple displaced transverse fractures.[59] Olecranon fractures with an associated dislocation are infrequently reported in the literature. Olecranon fracture-dislocations are categorized as either transolecranon fracture-dislocations or posterior Monteggia fracture-dislocations. The mechanism of injury, at-risk patient population, structural injury pattern, repair technique, postoperative rehabilitation recommendations, and functional outcomes are unique to each fracture pattern. Surgeons should understand the differences between these two injury patterns to optimize treatment and final clinical outcomes.

Transolecranon Fracture-Dislocations

Transolecranon fracture-dislocations are comminuted fractures of the proximal ulna that result in subluxation or dislocation of the radial head anteriorly on the distal humerus (**Figure 8**). Transolecranon fracture-dislocations typically result from a high-energy injury to the dorsum of the forearm and often occur in young patients who have good bone quality. The injury pattern

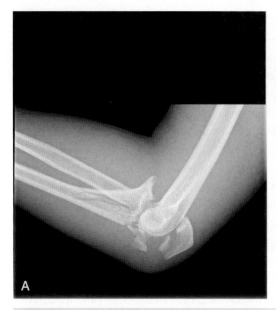
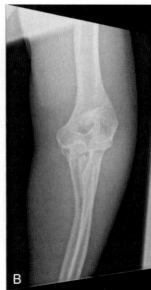

Figure 8 Lateral (**A**) and AP (**B**) radiographs of the elbow demonstrate a transolecranon fracture-dislocation.

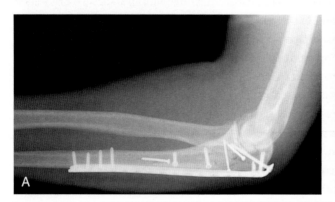
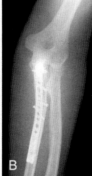

Figure 9 Lateral (**A**) and AP (**B**) radiographs of the elbow demonstrate a transolecranon fracture-dislocation that was surgically repaired with multiple small interfragmentary screws and a long dorsal 3.5-mm contoured olecranon plate.

of a highly comminuted transolecranon fracture includes a proximal radioulnar joint that is not injured and radial and ulnar shafts that translate anteriorly on the distal humerus in the same direction. The lack of disruption of the proximal radioulnar joint is a key difference between transolecranon fracture-dislocations and posterior Monteggia fracture-dislocations.[60] The distal humerus is driven into the olecranon fracture, which results in subluxation.

Radial and neck fractures are uncommon; however, if a coronoid fracture occurs, it is typically a large, basal injury.[61] Compared with posterior Monteggia fracture-dislocations, in which the LCL is injured in approximately two-thirds of patients, the MCL and LCL are typically uninjured in transolecranon fracture-dislocations.[60,61] Restoration of the trochlear notch with stable fixation in patients who have transolecranon fracture-dislocations

typically leads to very good outcomes and low levels of posttraumatic arthritis as long as the contour of the notch is restored independent of comminution[60] (**Figure 9**).

In general, transolecranon fracture-dislocations require surgical repair. The key to repair is restoration of the trochlear notch with stable fixation using a dorsally applied 3.5-mm reconstruction or compression plate. Higher failure rates have been reported if a tension band device or a one-third tubular plate is used.[60,62,63] If stable fixation is achieved, aggressive postoperative physical therapy can be performed with limited protection because there is no reliance on soft-tissue ligament healing.

Medial and lateral surgical windows are not typically required for the surgical treatment of transolecranon fracture-dislocations. A direct posterior approach allows access to the dorsal aspect of the olecranon and the ulnar shaft, the location at which most of the procedure is performed. Typically, the fracture can be reduced in a distal to proximal direction, sequentially repairing each fragment back to the more distal segment. Each fragment is temporarily reduced with the use of Kirschner wires, followed by screw fixation with the use of independent screws. If the coronoid process is fractured, reduction is facilitated by reducing the coronoid process inside the joint by working distal to proximal through the olecranon fracture. Long dorsal plate fixation is required after anatomic reduction of all articular segments to restore the trochlear notch. Because medial and lateral plating do not allow for adequate resistance to tensile forces, a 3.5-mm precontoured olecranon plate with locking screws in the proximal olecranon fragment and at least three screws in the distal ulnar fragment are used. Common errors include malreduction of the trochlear notch, which results from comminution and inadequate fixation of the coronoid. If accessory medial plating of the coronoid is required, the Taylor-Scham (take-down of the ulnar head of the FCU, which leaves a stump on the humerus for repair) or the FCU-splitting approach can be used for placement of a small 2.0- or 2.4-mm T- or L-shaped plate.[64] Because the ligamentous structures are typically intact in transolecranon fracture-dislocations, no ligament repair or reattachment is required. After bony stability has been achieved and the trochlear notch is re-created, elbow stability should be restored.

A long arm splint with the elbow positioned at 90° and in neutral rotation is used for 1 week postoperatively. If stable fixation is achieved, the authors of this chapter allow full passive and active-assisted range of motion of the elbow but limit active extension starting at 1 week postoperatively. A sling may still be used to protect the elbow between physical therapy sessions for another 2 to 3 weeks. The sling should be discontinued at 3 weeks postoperatively. Resistive strengthening of the elbow as well as continued stretching may be initiated at 3 months postoperatively if signs of radiographic union are present. Return to all activities and contact sports is allowed at 5 months postoperatively.

Posterior Monteggia Fracture-Dislocations

Fractures of the ulna accompanied by a dislocation of the proximal radioulnar joint are known as Monteggia fracture-dislocations. The traditional classification of Monteggia

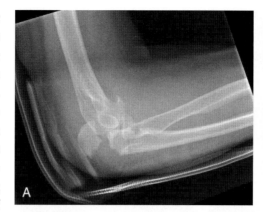
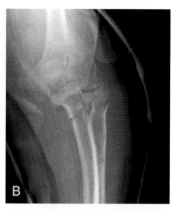

Figure 10   Lateral (**A**) and AP (**B**) radiographs of the elbow demonstrate a posterior Monteggia fracture-dislocation.

fracture-dislocations is based on the direction of radial head dislocation (anterior, lateral, or posterior). Posterior Monteggia fracture-dislocations are the most common injury pattern in adults and are classified as a Bado type II injury.[65] Bado type II injury patterns include a proximal radioulnar joint that is disrupted, with a radial head that dislocates posteriorly and the apex of a proximal ulna fracture that is directed anteriorly. Jupiter et al[66] further classified Bado type II injuries based on the location of the ulnar fracture: type IIa fractures involve the distal olecranon and coronoid process; type IIb fractures occur at the metaphyseal-diaphyseal junction; type IIc fractures are diaphyseal; and type IId fractures extend along the proximal third to proximal half of the ulna. These injuries typically occur in older patients, and osteoporosis often is present, which may compromise stable internal fixation.[61] A low-energy fall onto an outstretched arm is the most common mechanism of injury. A comminuted fracture of the olecranon, which is commonly associated with fractures of the coronoid process (frequently) and the radial head (almost always), typically occurs in patients who sustain a posterior Monteggia

fracture-dislocation (**Figure 10**). Associated LCL complex injuries occur in as many as two-thirds of patients who have a posterior Monteggia fracture-dislocation, and associated ulnohumeral instability may occur as well.[67,68]

The surgical treatment of posterior Monteggia fracture-dislocations typically involves treating all of the pathologic structures, including anatomic axial alignment of the ulnar fracture (primary goal), repair or replacement of radial head and coronoid fractures, and repair of the injured LCL complex (**Figure 11**). Ulnar fractures should be treated with a dorsally applied reconstruction or compression plate. Because of the increased risk for complications, including proximal radioulnar synostosis, ulnar malunion, PLRI, and fixation failure that results from osteoporotic bone, the overall results of patients who are treated for posterior Monteggia fracture-dislocations are slightly worse compared with the results of patients who are treated for transolecranon fracture-dislocations.[67] Associated radial head and coronoid fractures negatively affect the surgical outcomes of patients who have posterior Monteggia fracture-dislocations.[67,69] Because of less stable fixation that is associated with

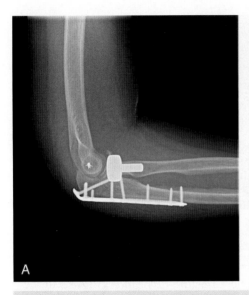
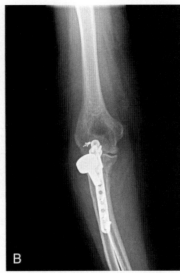

Figure 11 Lateral (**A**) and AP (**B**) radiographs of the elbow demonstrate a posterior Monteggia fracture-dislocation that was surgically repaired with a contoured 3.5-mm dorsally applied olecranon plate, suture fixation of a small type I coronoid fracture, radial head arthroplasty, and lateral collateral ligament repair.

osteoporosis and the protection that is required for a repaired LCL complex, the postoperative rehabilitation for patients who undergo treatment for posterior Monteggia fracture-dislocations must be more cautious compared with the postoperative rehabilitation for patients who undergo treatment for transolecranon fracture-dislocations. Despite these limitations, reasonable outcomes can still be achieved with a structured rehabilitation program.

The treatment for posterior Monteggia fracture-dislocations essentially follows the principles of fixation for terrible triad injuries (discussed later) rather than that for simple olecranon fractures. In most patients, a posterior Monteggia fracture-dislocation can be considered a terrible triad injury plus an olecranon fracture. The principles of fixation for posterior Monteggia fracture-dislocations include open reduction and internal fixation (ORIF) rather than arthroplasty of associated radial head fractures, ORIF of

coronoid fractures, repair of the LCL complex, and fixation of the olecranon fracture. Typically, the radial head fracture is first approached via a Kocher, a Kaplan, or an extensor digitorum communis (EDC)-splitting approach. If a type I coronoid fracture is present, suture fixation is performed using drill holes through the dorsal aspect of the ulna. If larger coronoid fractures are present, a separate medial approach is performed using the Taylor-Scham or the FCU-splitting approach as well as an ulnar nerve transposition.[64] Medial-sided fixation of substantially displaced coronoid fractures includes screw or plate fixation. If coronoid fixation is required, olecranon fracture fixation should be performed first to provide a stable base for repair of the coronoid. Olecranon fracture fixation should be performed with a dorsally applied 3.5-mm compression or reconstruction plate with at least three screw holes located distal to the fracture site. To complete the procedure, LCL repair should

be anatomically performed at the isometric point of the lateral epicondyle with the use of either suture anchors or drill holes.

A long arm splint with the elbow positioned at 90° and in neutral rotation is used for 1 week postoperatively. If stable fixation is achieved, the authors of this chapter allow full passive range of motion of the elbow but limit extension to 30° short of full starting at 1 week postoperatively. A sling may be used to protect the elbow between physical therapy sessions. At 6 weeks postoperatively, sling use is discontinued, and the authors of this chapter allow 5- to 10-lb lifting and continued active and passive stretching in all planes with no triceps protection. Isometric strengthening also is allowed at 6 weeks postoperatively. Progressive resistive strengthening of the elbow as well as continued stretching is initiated at 3 months postoperatively if signs of radiographic union are present. Return to all activities and contact sports is allowed at 5 months postoperatively.

Terrible Triad Injuries

Terrible triad injuries are classified as complex dislocations with associated radial head and coronoid fractures. Hotchkiss[70] originally named the injury pattern the "terrible triad" because of the historically poor results seen in the treatment of patients who had these injuries. Common problems associated with nonsurgical and historical surgical techniques (radial head excision with no treatment of the LCL or the coronoid) include persistent instability, stiffness, and early arthritis.[71] Ring et al[71] reported that 7 of 11 patients who were treated nonsurgically or with historical surgical treatments had unsatisfactory results.

As surgeons' understanding of terrible triad injuries increased, an algorithmic approach, which includes fixation or replacement of the radial head; fixation of the coronoid fracture; repair of the LCL complex; and possible repair of the MCL complex with or without placement of an external fixator in patients who have persistent instability after treatment of the radial head, the coronoid, and the LCL, was developed.[72] Reasonable outcomes can be achieved with the use of this algorithmic approach, as shown by Pugh et al[72] in a study that reported a mean postoperative flexion arc of 112° and good or excellent results in 77% of patients. Despite these improvements, complications, such as persistent instability, heterotopic bone formation, stiffness, infection, ulnar neuropathy, nonunion, and malunion, are still common, and revision surgery is required in as many as 28% of patients.[73] Several issues regarding the treatment of terrible triad injuries, including the potential for nonsurgical management in isolated patients, the need for repair in patients who have very small coronoid tip fractures, methods to approximate radial head size during arthroplasty, and static versus dynamic external fixation, are still evolving.

Pathophysiology

Most terrible triad injuries are the result of either a low-energy fall from a standing position in patients who have poorer bone quality or high-energy elbow trauma in young patients who have good bone quality. A posteriorly directed force on the elbow that results from a fall, which levers the ulna out of the trochlea, is typically the mechanism of injury.[70] An axial load on the supinated forearm creates a valgus

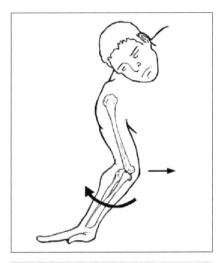

Figure 12   Illustration shows that the combination of an axial load with supinating (curved arrow) and valgus (straight arrow) forces may result in a terrible triad injury. (Reproduced from Wyrick JD, Dailey SK, Gunzenhaeuser JM, Casstevens EC: Management of complex elbow dislocations: A mechanistic approach. *J Am Acad Orthop Surg* 2015;23[5]:297-306.)

and posterolateral rotatory moment, which results in failure of the lateral ligaments first, then the anterior capsule, and then, potentially, the medial ligaments[27] (**Figure 12**). As the elbow dislocates, the radial head and the coronoid process frequently can fracture. Terrible triad injuries must be differentiated from anteromedial facet fractures of the coronoid (discussed later), which also occur with a dislocation of the elbow but are secondary to a varus, posteromedially directed force with the elbow in flexion[74] (**Figure 13**).

Fractures of the radial head are classified based on articular involvement and the extent of comminution. The radial head is an important secondary stabilizer of the elbow that provides approximately 30% of valgus stability.[15,75] The radial head also is a primary restraint to PLRI.[19] In a biomechanical study, Schneeberger et al[19] reported that

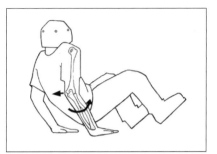

Figure 13   Illustration shows that the combination of an axial load with pronating (curved arrow) and varus (straight arrow) forces may result in an anteromedial facet fracture of the coronoid. (Reproduced from Wyrick JD, Dailey SK, Gunzenhaeuser JM, Casstevens EC: Management of complex elbow dislocations: A mechanistic approach. *J Am Acad Orthop Surg* 2015;23[5]:297-306.)

isolated radial head excision in cadaver models with intact ligaments led to increased rotatory laxity. The authors reported that radial head excision and excision of 30% of a coronoid fracture in cadaver models with intact ligaments resulted in ulnohumeral subluxation rather than just posterolateral rotatory laxity.[19] In this scenario, radial head replacement corrected subluxation; however, posterolateral rotatory displacement still existed, and coronoid fixation was required to stabilize the elbow.[19] Consequently, restoration of both the radial head and the coronoid was required to restore stability in cadaver models that had substantial (>30%) fractures. It has been clinically shown that radial head excision without ligament repair in patients who have terrible triad injuries results in a high risk for recurrent instability; therefore, it is not recommended.[71] Based on these data, complete restoration of the radial head with either repair or replacement is required to restore elbow stability in patients who have terrible triad injuries. In general, even small articular fragments of the radial head should be repaired because they can provide a substantial amount of stabilizing function to the arm in supination. If repair is not possible, then replacement should be strongly considered because excision may lead to poor outcomes.

Because the coronoid provides the elbow with a substantial amount of stabilizing function, even small fractures may lead to substantial instability. Biomechanically, the coronoid process provides the elbow with increasing resistance to posterior subluxation as the elbow is extended past a flexion angle of 30°.[76] The coronoid process also provides axial, posteromedial, and posterolateral elbow stability. Small coronoid fractures (<10% of the total coronoid height) have been reported to have little effect on elbow stability.[77] Larger coronoid fractures have a progressively larger influence on elbow stability.[78] Coronoid process fractures are typically simple, transverse, and small in patients who have a terrible triad injury,[79] with a mean height of 35% of the total coronoid height; therefore, based on biomechanical data on the restoration of joint stability, most coronoid process fractures should be repaired.[80] Coronoid fragments always have some anterior capsule attached, which may be useful for suture repair of the fracture.

Evaluation

The skin should be examined for open wounds and abrasions. Medial ecchymosis may suggest a more severe medial-sided injury. A complete neurovascular examination of the upper extremity and an assessment of the distal radioulnar joint should be performed. Tenderness and instability of the distal radioulnar joint in a dorsal to palmar

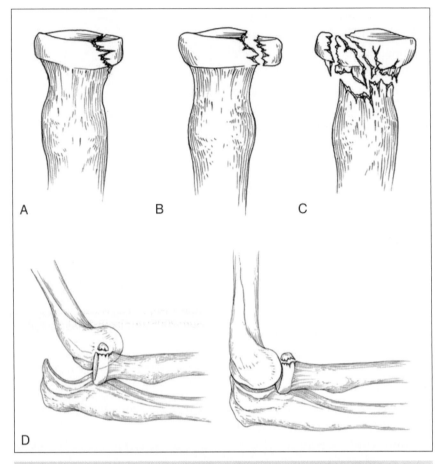

Figure 14 Illustration shows the Mason classification of radial head fractures. **A,** Type I, nondisplaced. **B,** Type II, displaced partial articular fracture. **C,** Type III, comminuted fracture. **D,** A type IV injury indicates an associated ipsilateral ulnohumeral dislocation. (Reproduced from Mathew PK, Athwal GS, King GJ: Terrible triad injury of the elbow: Current concepts. *J Am Acad Orthop Surg* 2009;17[3]:137-151.)

direction may suggest a longitudinal (Essex-Lopresti) injury.

Typical imaging studies include AP and lateral radiographs of the elbow before and after reduction. Radiographs should be scrutinized for fractures of the proximal ulna and radius as well as the distal humerus, including the capitellum and the trochlea. PA and lateral wrist and forearm radiographs should be obtained to rule out an injury to the distal radioulnar joint. Advanced imaging, specifically CT with three-dimensional reconstructions and digital subtraction of the humerus, is

routinely obtained to further classify the proximal radius and coronoid fractures. Digital subtraction allows for easy classification of coronoid fractures based on the classification system described by O'Driscoll et al.[81]

Classification systems have been developed for the individual parts of terrible triad injuries, specifically radial head and coronoid process fractures. The Mason classification (**Figure 14**), which was modified by Hotchkiss,[82] categorizes radial head fractures into three types.[83] Type I radial head injuries are nondisplaced or mildly displaced partial articular fractures that have less than 2 mm of displacement and no mechanical block. Type I radial head injuries are uncommon in patients who have terrible triad injuries. Type II radial head injuries are partial articular fractures that have more than 2 mm of displacement and may be reparable. Type III radial head injuries are comminuted fractures and typically require excision or replacement. Type II and type III radial head injuries are common in patients who have terrible triad injuries, and treatment requires repair or replacement. Excision of the entire radial head is contraindicated for the reasons previously discussed.

The classification system described by O'Driscoll et al[81] categorizes coronoid fractures based on the region of the coronoid fracture. The classification splits the coronoid into different regions: the tip, the anteromedial facet, and the base (**Figure 15**; **Table 3**). Tip fractures, which are the most commonly seen injuries in patients who have terrible triad injuries, are subdivided into those that are greater than or less than 2 mm. Anteromedial facet injuries are subdivided into subtype 1 (in isolation), subtype 2 (anteromedial facet plus the tip), and subtype 3 (anteromedial facet extending into the sublime tubercle) fractures. Anteromedial facet injuries are typically seen in patients who have varus PMRI but not in patients who have terrible triad injuries. Coronoid base injuries are fractures through the body of the coronoid that involve at least 50% of the total coronoid height. Coronoid base injuries are less common in patients who have terrible triad injuries and are more commonly associated with a concomitant olecranon fracture or posterior Monteggia or transolecranon fracture-dislocations.

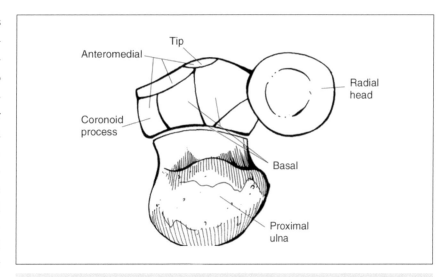

Figure 15   Illustration shows the O'Driscoll coronoid fracture classification system, including tip, anteromedial facet, and basal fractures. (Reproduced from Tashjian RZ, Katarincic JA: Complex elbow instability. *J Am Acad Orthop Surg* 2006;14[5]:278-286.)

Table 3
O'Driscoll Coronoid Fracture Classification

Fracture	Subtype	Description
Tip	1	≤2 mm of coronoid height
	2	>2 mm of coronoid height
Anteromedial	1	Anteromedial rim
	2	Anteromedial rim and tip
	3	Anteromedial rim and sublime tubercle (± tip)
Basal	1	Coronoid body and base
	2	Transolecranon basal coronoid fracture

Reproduced from Tashjian RZ, Katarincic JA: Complex elbow instability. *J Am Acad Orthop Surg* 2006;14(5):278-286.

Treatment

In general, most patients who have terrible triad injuries require surgical treatment. Recently, nonsurgical management has been considered for certain isolated patients. Chan et al[84] evaluated 12 patients who underwent nonsurgical treatment for a terrible triad injury. Nonsurgical treatment was indicated in these patients if they had a concentric joint reduction, a radial head fracture that did not cause a mechanical block to rotation, a small type 1 or type 2 Regan-Morrey coronoid fracture, and a stable arc of motion to a minimum of 30° of extension within the first 10 days after injury. At a minimum 12-month follow-up, 11 of 12 patients were stable and had healed fractures, with 134° of flexion and 6° of extension as well as a mean MEPS of 94. One patient required surgery for the treatment of early instability. In general, patients who, after reduction, have congruent ulnohumeral and radiohumeral articulations, have nondisplaced radial head or neck

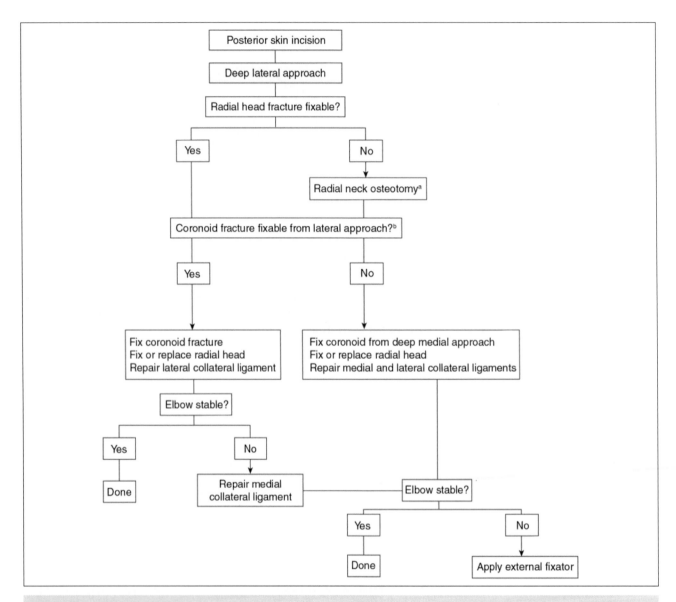

Figure 16   Algorithm for the surgical management of terrible triad injuries.
[a]In preparation for radial head replacement. If fragment size is less than 25% of the radial head, then fragment excision may be considered.
[b]Type I coronoid fractures may not require repair.
(Reproduced from Mathew PK, Athwal GS, King GJ: Terrible triad injury of the elbow: Current concepts. *J Am Acad Orthop Surg* 2009;17[3]:137-151.)

fractures, and remain stable through a full range of elbow flexion/extension motion in neutral rotation are the best candidates for nonsurgical treatment. Nonsurgical treatment should include a short period of immobilization (1 week) followed by progression in range of motion. Serial radiographs should be obtained at short intervals

to confirm fracture healing and maintenance of a stable reduction.

If surgery is required, a systematic approach, which includes fixation of substantial (>10%) coronoid fracture fragments, repair or replacement of substantial radial head fractures, and LCL repair, should be applied. If stability is not attained after treatment of

the coronoid fracture, radial head fracture, and LCL injury, other procedures (MCL/flexor pronator repair, dynamic or static external fixation) can be performed (**Figure 16**).

A lateral incision (with an additional medial approach if required) and a posterior incision are the two primary incisions used to repair terrible triad injuries. The advantages of a posterior incision are the ability to access the medial and lateral sides of the joint, a more cosmetic incision, and limited risk for cutaneous nerve injury. The primary disadvantage of a posterior incision is that large cutaneous flaps are developed, which may lead to hematoma or seroma formation. The deep lateral approach to the elbow is made through the lateral extensor muscles, either through the Kocher interval (between the extensor carpi ulnaris and the anconeus) or through an EDC split. Distal extension of an EDC split may injure the posterior interosseous nerve, and distal extension of the Kocher interval may injure the LCL. If the Kocher interval is used, the Kaplan interval (extensor carpi radialis longus and the common extensor) may be used as well to gain additional access to the anterior joint and the coronoid process (**Figure 17**).

Based on biomechanical data, most coronoid fractures should be fixed, with the possible exclusion of very small fragments (<10% of the total coronoid height).[77] Most coronoid fractures can be repaired with a suture grasping technique, in which No. 2 high-strength suture is passed at the coronoid fragment bone/soft-tissue interface and then passed through bone tunnels in the base of the fracture on the ulna and tied over the posterior aspect of the proximal ulna. Lasso suture repair has been reported to be more stable intraoperatively, both before and after LUCL repair, compared with suture anchor or screw fixation.[85] Compared with lasso suture repair, screw fixation is associated with a higher rate of implant failure, and anchor fixation is associated with a higher rate of nonunion.[85] Basal or anteromedial facet fractures (discussed later) are less commonly associated with classic

terrible triad injuries (posterolateral dislocation).[79] Larger coronoid fractures typically require fixation via a medial approach with the use of a plate or screws.[86] Access to the medial coronoid is attained between the two heads of the FCU or by detaching the ulnar head of the FCU (Taylor-Scham approach).[64,83] Fixation is performed with either 2.0- or 2.4-mm T- or L-shaped plates or precontoured coronoid plates.

The options for surgical management of radial head fractures in patients who have terrible triad injuries include fragment excision, ORIF, or radial head arthroplasty. Fragment excision is a reasonable treatment option for patients who have small, nonreparable fragments (<25% to 30%) that do not articulate with the lesser sigmoid notch if stability of the elbow is achieved after coronoid and LCL repair. The anterolateral head, which is typically injured in patients who have fracture-dislocations, is critical for stability; therefore, care must be taken during excision because even a small amount of bone loss may lead to instability. A rotational osteotomy may be considered in patients who have small irreparable fragments only if persistent instability exists with extension in supination and if most of the remaining head is intact. If stability is not restored, then arthroplasty should be performed unless repair is feasible.

Fixation of the proximal radius should be considered in patients who have radial neck fractures with limited neck comminution and an intact head or in patients who have partial articular fractures with a maximum of two free fragments that are not comminuted. Plate fixation is useful for radial neck fractures, and plates should be placed in the safe zone, which is the area at which the radius does not articulate

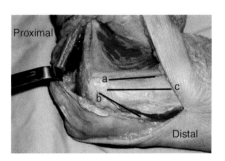

Figure 17 Lateral intraoperative photograph of a right elbow shows the relative location of the Kaplan interval (line a), the Kocher interval (line b), and the extensor digitorum communis split (line c). (Adapted from Cheung EV, Steinmann SP: Surgical approaches to the elbow. *J Am Acad Orthop Surg* 2009;17[5]:325-333.)

with the proximal radioulnar joint. The plate should be placed directly lateral with the arm in neutral rotation. Stiffness is a common problem after plating and often requires hardware removal. Crossed-screw fixation, which is another technique for radial neck fixation, may limit stiffness seen with plate fixation.

Radial head arthroplasty is indicated for patients who have comminuted Mason type III fractures, surgical neck fractures with substantial neck comminution, and partial radial head fractures with several fragments that do not allow for fixation. Overstuffing should be avoided because it will substantially limit elbow range of motion, specifically flexion, as well as result in pain and capitellar erosion. The diameter of the implant should be slightly undersized using the minimum, rather than the maximum, diameter of the head. The lesser sigmoid notch is an unreliable landmark for determining the implant diameter.[87] The best guide for radial head height involves matching the proximal articular surface of the radial head arthroplasty with the lateral edge of the coronoid at its junction with the lesser sigmoid notch. Doornberg et al[88] reported that the radial head is, on average, 0.9 mm more proximal than the lateral edge of the coronoid process. Severe overlengthening (>6 mm) is apparent on radiographs in patients who have medial ulnohumeral joint incongruity.[89] To avoid overlengthening, the articular surface should be even with the lateral edge of the coronoid.

The LCL complex must be repaired after fixation of the coronoid and either fixation or arthroplasty of the radial head. LCL complex repair should be performed with the use of either bone tunnels or suture anchors. The LUCL must be repaired to its isometric point on the humerus, which is located approximately at the center of the capitellum. In an in vivo MRI kinematic study of a normal elbow joint, Moritomo et al[39] reported that the isometric point of the LCL was approximately 2 mm proximal to the center of the capitellum.

After LCL repair and radial head and coronoid fixation, the elbow should be brought through a full range of flexion and extension in neutral rotation under fluoroscopy. If the ulnohumeral joint is persistently unstable (dislocating in extension), further treatment is required. If instability persists, then the MCL as well as the flexors and pronators should be repaired. If instability still persists, then static or dynamic external fixation should be used. Other alternatives for persistent instability include crossed-pin fixation of the joint. Dynamic fixators are an effective treatment to restore motion and function in patients who have persistent instability after surgical treatment for complex instability.[90,91] Several studies have reported a high rate of complications

(37%) after dynamic fixation.[90-92] Complications associated with hinge fixation include infection, radial nerve injury, recurrent instability, broken pins, and nonunion.[90-92] Dynamic fixators may drive the elbow into further instability if applied without exactly identifying the isometric point of the LCL. Ring et al[92] reported lower complication rates in patients who underwent crossed-pin fixation of the elbow for the treatment of persistent instability compared with patients who underwent hinged fixation for the treatment of similar symptoms. Static fixators may be a reasonable compromise between hinged fixation and crossed-pin fixation for surgeons who are uncomfortable with placing pins across the joint.

Slight persistent ulnohumeral widening (the drop sign) that is seen on lateral radiographs should be monitored postoperatively because residual widening often results from incompetent forearm flexors, which should be treated with active flexor exercises and the avoidance of varus stress.[24] Subluxation typically resolves within 1 to 2 weeks, and very low rates of persistent instability exist despite initial ulnohumeral joint widening.[24,93] Postoperative rehabilitation for terrible triad injuries is similar to that for posterior Monteggia fracture-dislocations.

Outcomes

Several authors have reported excellent outcomes for patients with terrible triad injuries who were treated with the standardized fixation protocol previously discussed[72,85,94] (**Figure 18**). In a study of 36 patients who underwent either radial head ORIF or replacement, coronoid repair, and LCL repair for the treatment of a terrible triad injury, Pugh et al[72] reported that the mean arc

of flexion-extension was 112° and the mean arc of forearm rotation was 136° at a mean of follow-up of 34 months. The mean MEPS was 88. Eight patients underwent revision surgery for the treatment of complications, including synostosis (two patients), recurrent instability (one patient), elbow stiffness (four patients), and infection (one patient).[72] In a study of 35 patients with terrible triad injuries who underwent treatment with a systemic protocol, Lindenhovius et al[94] reported that stability and strength were restored independent of time to treatment (within 2 weeks of injury [acute] or after 3 weeks of injury [subacute]). The authors reported that the mean arc of flexion was 119° in the acute group and 100° in the subacute group. MEPSs were similar in the acute (90) and subacute groups (87).[94] Garrigues et al[85] reported similar results, with a mean flexion arc of 115° and a mean MEPS of 90. The authors reported that patients who underwent suture repair of the coronoid had fewer complications and better stability compared with patients who underwent either suture anchor fixation or ORIF of coronoid fractures.

Postoperative complications occur in approximately 20% to 25% of patients.[72,85,94,95] Recurrent instability is not common in patients who undergo treatment with the use of the standardized fixation protocol previously discussed. Historically, instability was common after surgical treatment that did not adhere to these principles. Stiffness is common, and approximately 10% of patients require a release. Heterotopic ossification, which often is present with stiffness, occurs in approximately 10% of patients. Infection is very uncommon but occurs in approximately one-half of patients if an external fixator is used;

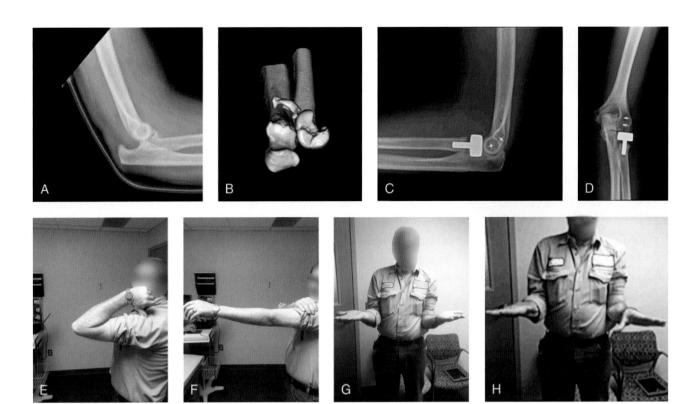

Figure 18   Images of a patient who had a terrible triad injury with a comminuted radial head fracture and a coronoid tip fracture who was treated with radial head arthroplasty, suture fixation of the coronoid fracture, and lateral collateral ligament repair. **A,** Preoperative lateral elbow radiograph demonstrates a subluxed ulnohumeral joint with a comminuted radial head and a coronoid tip fracture. **B,** Preoperative three-dimensional CT reconstruction of the elbow demonstrates an O'Driscoll type I coronoid tip fracture and a Mason type III radial head fracture. Postoperative lateral (**C**) and AP (**D**) elbow radiographs demonstrate final fixation. Clinical photographs taken 6 months postoperatively show flexion (**E**), extension (**F**), supination (**G**), and pronation (**H**).

therefore, surgeons should avoid the use of a fixator. Some arthritis is common (70%), but it is typically not clinically important. Ulnar neuritis, which also is a common postoperative complication, affects approximately 10% of patients.

Anteromedial Facet Fractures of the Coronoid Process (Varus PMRI)

The coronoid process plays a critical role in maintaining stability of the elbow joint. Historically, fractures of the coronoid process were defined by their overall size based on the classification system described by Regan and Morrey.[96] Several recent classification systems have been created to define fractures of the coronoid process by their location and their associated injury patterns.[81,97] O'Driscoll et al[81] created the coronoid fracture classification system previously discussed. Type II fractures, which involve the anteromedial facet, include three subtypes. Subtype 1 fractures involve the rim. Subtype 2 fractures involve the rim and tip. Subtype 3 fractures involve the rim and sublime tubercle. Adams et al[97] classified coronoid fractures based on CT scans. The authors reported that oblique anteromedial fractures, which are equivalent to O'Driscoll type II fractures, accounted for 17% of coronoid process injuries. The authors also reported on a newly described oblique anterolateral fracture pattern, which accounted for 7% of coronoid process injuries and did not often require surgical fixation. Conversely, anteromedial facet fractures often require surgical treatment to avoid the development of early rapid arthritis.[81] Aggressive surgical fixation for most coronoid process injuries has been supported biomechanically and suggested clinically;[86,98] however, recent studies have recognized that not all anteromedial facet fractures require surgical repair.[99,100]

Pathophysiology

Varus PMRI of the elbow results from a fall backward onto both hands, in which there was axial loading of the arm

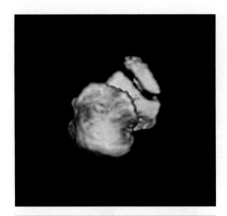

Figure 19 Three-dimensional CT reconstruction of an elbow with the humerus and radius subtracted. The ulna is rotated to evaluate the articular surface, which confirms an O'Driscoll type II subtype 2 anteromedial facet fracture of the coronoid.

with pronating and varus forces. Varus PMRI will result in a rupture of the LCL complex, and the trochlea will fracture the anteromedial facet of the coronoid. Doornberg et al[101] reported that 58% of the anteromedial facet is unsupported by the proximal ulna, which places it at risk for fracture in the mechanism of injury already mentioned. The radial head is typically preserved without injury.[99,100] The MCL also can be damaged in this injury pattern.[99,100] Rhyou et al[100] reported concomitant repair of the MCL in 3 of 18 patients. Park et al[99] reported MCL injury in 6 of 11 patients, 3 of whom required surgical repair because of residual instability after LCL repair and coronoid fracture fixation. The treatment strategy for anteromedial facet fractures of the coronoid process potentially includes nonsurgical treatment, LCL repair only, anteromedial facet repair only, or both LCL repair and anteromedial facet repair. The surgical indications for anteromedial facet fractures of the coronoid process continue to evolve as clinical information on their outcomes becomes available.

Evaluation

The initial clinical and radiographic evaluation for patients who have coronoid process injuries is similar to that for patients who have a terrible triad injury. The history should query patients on the dislocation as well as the position of the hands and arms at the time of the injury. Radiographs must be carefully reviewed because anteromedial facet injuries often may be very subtle. The medial joint space often is narrowed or incongruent on AP radiographs. The fracture may be difficult to see on lateral radiographs; however, Sanchez-Sotelo et al[74] described a double-crescent sign in the setting of a depressed fracture. Three-dimensional CT reconstructions with the radius and humerus subtracted are critical to evaluate coronoid process injuries. The ulna can be rotated to view the articular surface from proximal to distal, which allows for classification of the injury based on the O'Driscoll classification system (**Figure 19**). The fracture should be evaluated for displacement as well as the subtype classification. Varus stress radiographs also may be obtained to evaluate for medial joint space collapse and lateral joint space widening.

On physical examination, the patient should be placed in the supine position and brought through a full range of elbow flexion and extension to offload the LCL. The patient should be queried about symptoms of instability or grinding, both of which are indications for surgical repair.

Treatment

Because this injury pattern has been recognized only in the past 10 years and it is, overall, much less common than other forms of complex elbow instability, studies on the outcomes of clinical care for patients who underwent treatment for coronoid process injuries are limited. Because of these limited data, the indications for nonsurgical and surgical treatment of coronoid process injuries are still evolving. Initially, all injuries were believed to require surgical fixation of both the LCL and the anteromedial facet fracture.[86] As knowledge of coronoid process injuries improved, the treatment algorithm, which is based on fracture pattern, size, and location; stress radiographs; and clinical symptoms, has been refined.[99,100]

All patients should initially be treated with closed reduction and splinting, after which the elbow should be reexamined. Varus stress radiographs with the forearm placed in pronation should be obtained in the setting of an anteromedial facet fracture that has minimal displacement with no static collapse of the medial ulnohumeral joint space seen on AP radiographs. If no medial collapse of the ulnohumeral joint space, no lateral gapping, and a firm end point are seen, the patient can be considered for nonsurgical treatment. Passive elbow flexion and extension should be evaluated with the patient placed in the supine position. If no crepitus or feelings of instability exist and stress radiographs are negative, nonsurgical treatment can be considered. If nonsurgical treatment is selected, flexion and extension exercises with the patient in the supine position as well as passive supination and pronation with the elbow positioned in 90° of elbow flexion should begin 1 week after injury. A sling should be worn for 6 weeks to protect the elbow between physical therapy sessions. Radiographs should be obtained every week for the first 3 weeks as well as 6 weeks after injury to confirm maintenance of alignment and no collapse. Six weeks after injury, the sling should be discontinued, and progression stretching may be performed, with strengthening initiated 3 months after injury. Patients may return to activities as tolerated 4 to 5 months after injury.

Surgery is recommended if substantial displacement with subluxation is seen on radiographs or if positive varus stress or clinical symptoms of grinding or instability with supine overhead elbow flexion and extension are apparent. Surgery may include LCL repair only, anteromedial facet repair only, or both. In a study of 11 patients who had isolated anteromedial facet fractures, Park et al[99] treated patients who had O'Driscoll type II subtype 1 fractures with LCL repair only and patients who had O'Driscoll type II subtype 2 and subtype 3 fractures with LCL repair and buttress plating.[99] Rhyou et al[100] recommended treatment based on fracture fragment size (articular height as defined by Pollock et al[98]). If the fragment was smaller than or equal to 5 mm, the authors did not repair the fracture.[100] If the fragment was larger than 6 mm and not comminuted, the authors repaired the facture via a medial approach.[98,100] If varus stress testing under fluoroscopy with the forearm positioned in pronation revealed a firm end point with a congruent medial ulnohumeral joint, the authors did not repair the LCL.[100] If loss of congruency occurred, the authors repaired the LCL.[100] This treatment algorithm allowed some patients who had very small fractures and a stable elbow to undergo nonsurgical treatment. Nonsurgical treatment can be considered for slightly larger fragments if no grinding or instability exists during overhead flexion and extension with the patient placed in the supine position.

A variety of medial approaches may be used to surgically repair coronoid process fractures. Surgical techniques include an over-the-top approach, which uses a 50:50 flexor-pronator split anterior to the ulnar nerve; a through-the-bed approach to the ulnar nerve, which splits the two heads of the FCU; and a slightly posterior approach, with takedown of the ulnar head of the FCU (the Taylor-Scham approach).[64,83] Only a very small number of fractures, many of which can be treated nonsurgically, can be repaired via the over-the-top approach with the use of suture fixation; therefore, the over-the-top approach is uncommonly used. The mainstays of fixation include the FCU-splitting and the Taylor-Scham approaches. Many surgeons prefer the FCU-splitting approach; however, the incidence of ulnar neuropathy is approximately 10% in patients who undergo surgical treatment with this exposure.[86,99] Working through the FCU often requires extensive dissection of the ulnar nerve and may place a substantial amount of traction on the nerve. Although the Taylor-Scham approach may require take-down of the FCU, the entire FCU and the transposed ulnar nerve can be elevated anteriorly to eliminate all traction during fixation.

Internal fixation can be achieved using suture, screws, or a buttress plate. Small 2.0- or 2.4-mm T- or L-shaped plates can be used as a buttress. If the fracture is small, suture fixation passed through dorsal drill holes may be a reasonable alternative. Extensive knowledge of joint anatomy is required to prevent intra-articular penetration or penetration of the lesser sigmoid notch if screw fixation is performed, either alone or through a plate. In general, screw trajectory should be distal

and dorsal, and preoperative planning should be performed to prevent joint penetration. The UCL often is attached to the fracture fragment in an O'Driscoll type II subtype 3 fracture and is still attached to the sublime tubercle in O'Driscoll type II subtype 1 or subtype 2 fractures; therefore, it should be protected. Dissection of the FCU muscle off the proximal ulna in a distal to proximal direction during exposure will prevent inadvertent injury to the anterior band of the UCL. LCL repair should be performed in a fashion similar to that for a terrible triad injury, to the lateral epicondylar isometric point with the use of bone tunnels or suture anchors. Postoperative rehabilitation is similar to that for terrible triad injuries.

Outcomes

Overall, limited data exist on the outcomes for patients who undergo surgical treatment for anteromedial facet fractures in the setting of varus PMRI (**Figure 20**). Doornberg and Ring[86] reported on a series of 18 patients who had anteromedial facet fractures, 15 of whom were treated surgically, and three of whom were treated nonsurgically. The coronoid was fixed with a plate in nine patients, a screw in one patient, and sutures in one patient. The coronoid was not repaired in the remaining seven patients. At mean follow-up of 26 months, the authors reported that six patients had malalignment of the fracture and varus subluxation, which was caused by a lack of fixation in four patients and a loss of fixation in two patients. All six of the patients with malalignment and varus subluxation had fair or poor results. The remaining 12 patients had good or excellent outcomes. There was a 17% incidence of ulnar neuropathy in patients who

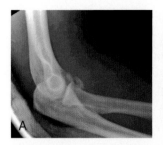 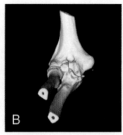 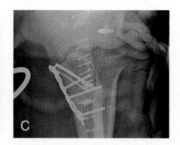 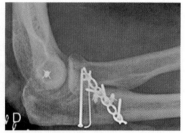

Figure 20   Images show an anteromedial facet fracture of the coronoid that was treated with open reduction and internal fixation. **A,** Preoperative lateral radiograph demonstrates a displaced O'Driscoll type II anteromedial facet fracture of the coronoid. **B,** Preoperative three-dimensional CT reconstruction demonstrates a displaced and comminuted anteromedial facet fracture. Postoperative AP (**C**) and lateral (**D**) radiographs taken after open reduction and internal fixation via a medial approach with the use of a buttress plate and screw fixation and lateral collateral ligament repair with the use of a suture anchor.

underwent repair via the FCU-splitting approach. The three patients who were treated nonsurgically had maintenance of alignment of the fracture and had excellent results based on the rating system described by Broberg and Morrey.[9] The authors recommended that surgical fixation of anteromedial facet fractures be performed to prevent malalignment, except in patients who have very small fractures with no subluxation and no radiocapitellar joint opening with varus stress.

In a study of 18 patients who had coronoid fractures, Rhyou et al[100] repaired only fractures that were larger than 5 mm in size (articular height as defined by Pollock et al[98]) and repaired the LCL only if an incongruent medial ulnohumeral joint was present during varus stress in pronation as seen under fluoroscopy.[98,100] The authors reported 2 patients who had O'Driscoll type II subtype 1 fractures, 14 patients who had O'Driscoll type II subtype 2 fractures, and 2 patients who had O'Driscoll type II subtype 3 fractures. Seven patients were treated with ORIF only, four patients were treated with LCL repair only, six patients were treated with LCL repair and ORIF, and one patient was managed nonsurgically.

ORIF included the use of cannulated screws in two patients, Kirschner wires with tension-band wiring in seven patients, and a buttress plate in two patients. The UCL was repaired in three patients. The mean MEPS was 98 (range, 85 to 100) at a mean follow-up of 37 months. There was no difference in outcomes between the subtypes. The authors provided a treatment algorithm that defined the size of the small fractures with no subluxation that were previously described by Doornberg and Ring.[86] Park et al[99] reviewed 11 patients with isolated anteromedial facet fractures who were treated with ORIF. The authors treated patients who had O'Driscoll type II subtype 1 fractures with LCL repair only and patients who had O'Driscoll type II subtype 2 and subtype 3 fractures with LCL repair and ORIF. Three patients required MCL repair. At a mean follow-up of 31 months, the mean range of motion was 128°, and the mean MEPS was 89. Ten patients had good or excellent results. Two of the 11 patients complained of postoperative ulnar neuropathic symptoms, one of whom already had ulnar neuropathic symptoms at the time of surgery. The patient who had preoperative ulnar neuropathic symptoms

underwent ulnar nerve exploration at the time of surgery, and the nerve was anteriorly transposed in the subcutaneous area. This patient fully recovered by 3 months postoperatively. The patient who had new-onset ulnar neuritis still had mild numbness in the ulnar nerve distribution 25 months postoperatively. All 11 patients in the study were treated with the FCU-splitting approach.

Overall, the surgical repair of varus PMRI can lead to excellent outcomes. Surgical repair typically consists of LCL repair with ORIF of the fracture. Small fractures (<6 mm in height) may be considered for nonsurgical management. Similarly, the LCL often does not require repair if the elbow is stable to varus stress in pronation as seen under fluoroscopy. Larger fractures also may be considered for nonsurgical management if minimal displacement, no static subluxation, a negative varus stress test, and no sensation of instability or grinding with supine overhead flexion and extension are present after injury. If surgery is required, a medial approach with buttress plate fixation will typically lead to reasonable outcomes. The FCU-splitting approach has a 10% to 15% incidence of postoperative ulnar neuropathy; therefore, an alternate approach, including the Taylor-Scham approach, which limits traction on the nerve, should be considered if exposure is difficult with an FCU-splitting approach.

Summary

Elbow instability varies from isolated soft-tissue injuries to combined soft-tissue and bony injuries. Simple dislocations can be easily treated nonsurgically with limited long-term sequelae and only rarely require surgical repair for the treatment of persistent instability. PLRI usually results from failure of the LCL to heal after a dislocation, and surgical treatment often is required to restore stability, with most patients requiring graft reconstruction. Arthroscopic techniques for the treatment of PLRI are promising and may be an option for patients who have more limited instability. MCL injuries are becoming more common, especially in young patients who are throwers, and attempts should be made to curb excessive throwing. Rehabilitation remains the mainstay of initial treatment for most injuries. If rehabilitation fails, reconstruction with a graft helps most patients return to play at a similar level but requires more than 1 year for recovery.

Fracture-dislocations include transolecranon fracture-dislocations, posterior Monteggia fracture-dislocations, terrible triad injuries, and anteromedial facet fractures of the coronoid with associated varus PMRI. Long, stable, dorsally applied plate fixation of the olecranon is required to achieve optimal results in patients who have posterior Monteggia and transolecranon fracture-dislocations. Outcomes for patients who have posterior Monteggia and transolecranon fracture-dislocations are typically very good;

however, because of the lack of good bone quality, radial head and smaller coronoid fractures, and ligamentous injuries, all of which are typically seen in patients who have posterior Monteggia fracture-dislocations, outcomes are more predictable in patients who have transolecranon fracture-dislocations. Appropriate recognition of these injury patterns is essential to provide effective treatment and maximize outcomes. Excellent outcomes can be attained in patients who have terrible triad injuries with the use of an algorithmic approach to repair or replace radial head fractures, repair substantial coronoid fractures, and repair the LCL. Anteromedial facet fractures of the coronoid associated with PMRI often require fixation and LCL repair; however, certain patients may be treated with isolated fracture fixation, ligament repair, or nonsurgical management based on the fracture size and pattern and elbow stability. Restoration of function and range of motion with a stable elbow can be attained in patients who have terrible triad injuries and anteromedial facet fractures if a systematic treatment approach is used.

References

1. Josefsson PO, Nilsson BE: Incidence of elbow dislocation. *Acta Orthop Scand* 1986;57(6):537-538.

2. Hobgood ER, Khan SO, Field LD: Acute dislocations of the adult elbow. *Hand Clin* 2008;24(1):1-7.

3. Conn J Jr, Wade PA: Injuries of the elbow: A ten year review. *J Trauma* 1961;1(3):248-268.

4. Josefsson PO, Johnell O, Gentz CF: Long-term sequelae of simple dislocation of the elbow. *J Bone Joint Surg Am* 1984;66(6):927-930.

5. Neviaser JS, Wickstrom JK: Dislocation of the elbow: A retrospective study of 115 patients. *South Med J* 1977;70(2):172-173.

6. O'Driscoll SW, Morrey BF, Korinek S, et al: Elbow subluxation and dislocation: A spectrum of instability. *Clin Orthop Relat Res* 1992;280:186-197.

7. Josefsson PO, Gentz CF, Johnell O, Wendeberg B: Surgical versus non-surgical treatment of ligamentous injuries following dislocation of the elbow joint: A prospective randomized study. *J Bone Joint Surg Am* 1987;69(4):605-608.

8. McKee MD, Schemitsch EH, Sala MJ, O'Driscoll SW: The pathoanatomy of lateral ligamentous disruption in complex elbow instability. *J Shoulder Elbow Surg* 2003;12(4):391-396.

9. Broberg MA, Morrey BF: Results of treatment of fracture-dislocations of the elbow. *Clin Orthop Relat Res* 1987;216:109-119.

10. Josefsson PO, Gentz CF, Johnell O, Wendeberg B: Dislocations of the elbow and intraarticular fractures. *Clin Orthop Relat Res* 1989;246:126-130.

11. Steinmann, SP, O'Driscoll SW: Elbow instability. *Curr Orthop* 2002;16(5):341-348.

12. Kalainov DM, Cohen MS: Posterolateral rotatory instability of the elbow in association with lateral epicondylitis: A report of three cases. *J Bone Joint Surg Am* 2005;87(5):1120-1125.

13. Dunning CE, Zarzour ZD, Patterson SD, Johnson JA, King GJ: Ligamentous stabilizers against posterolateral rotatory instability of the elbow. *J Bone Joint Surg Am* 2001;83(12):1823-1828.

14. Morrey BF: Anatomy of the elbow joint, in Morrey BF, ed: *The Elbow and Its Disorders*, ed 3. Philadelphia, PA, WB Saunders, 2000, pp 13-42.

15. Morrey BF, Tanaka S, An KN: Valgus stability of the elbow: A definition of primary and secondary constraints. *Clin Orthop Relat Res* 1991;265:187-195.

16. Morrey BF, An KN: Articular and ligamentous contributions to the stability of the elbow joint. *Am J Sports Med* 1983;11(5):315-319.

17. McAdams TR, Masters GW, Srivastava S: The effect of arthroscopic sectioning of the lateral ligament complex of the elbow on posterolateral

rotary stability. *J Shoulder Elbow Surg* 2005;14(3):298-301.

18. Olsen BS, Søjbjerg JO, Nielsen KK, Vaesel MT, Dalstra M, Sneppen O: Posterolateral elbow joint instability: The basic kinematics. *J Shoulder Elbow Surg* 1998;7(1):19-29.

19. Schneeberger AG, Sadowski MM, Jacob HA: Coronoid process and radial head as posterolateral rotatory stabilizers of the elbow. *J Bone Joint Surg Am* 2004;86(5):975-982.

20. Dunning CE, Zarzour ZD, Patterson SD, Johnson JA, King GJ: Muscle forces and pronation stabilize the lateral ligament deficient elbow. *Clin Orthop Relat Res* 2001;388:118-124.

21. Park MC, Ahmad CS: Dynamic contributions of the flexor-pronator mass to elbow valgus stability. *J Bone Joint Surg Am* 2004;86(10):2268-2274.

22. Rafai M, Largab A, Cohen D, Trafeh M: Pure posterior luxation of the elbow in adults: Immobilization or early mobilization: A randomized prospective study of 50 cases. *Chir Main* 1999;18(4):272-278.

23. Maripuri SN, Debnath UK, Rao P, Mohanty K: Simple elbow dislocation among adults: A comparative study of two different methods of treatment. *Injury* 2007;38(11):1254-1258.

24. Duckworth AD, Kulijdian A, McKee MD, Ring D: Residual subluxation of the elbow after dislocation or fracture-dislocation: Treatment with active elbow exercises and avoidance of varus stress. *J Shoulder Elbow Surg* 2008;17(2):276-280.

25. Eygendaal D, Verdegaal SH, Obermann WR, van Vugt AB, Pöll RG, Rozing PM: Posterolateral dislocation of the elbow joint: Relationship to medial instability. *J Bone Joint Surg Am* 2000;82(4):555-560.

26. Savoie FH III, O'Brien MJ, Field LD, Gurley DJ: Arthroscopic and open radial ulnohumeral ligament reconstruction for posterolateral rotatory instability of the elbow. *Clin Sports Med* 2010;29(4):611-618.

27. O'Driscoll SW, Bell DF, Morrey BF: Posterolateral rotatory instability of the elbow. *J Bone Joint Surg Am* 1991;73(3):440-446.

28. O'Driscoll SW, Spinner RJ, McKee MD, et al: Tardy posterolateral rotatory instability of the elbow due to cubitus varus. *J Bone Joint Surg Am* 2001;83(9):1358-1369.

29. Regan W, Lapner PC: Prospective evaluation of two diagnostic apprehension signs for posterolateral instability of the elbow. *J Shoulder Elbow Surg* 2006;15(3):344-346.

30. Potter HG, Weiland AJ, Schatz JA, Paletta GA, Hotchkiss RN: Posterolateral rotatory instability of the elbow: Usefulness of MR imaging in diagnosis. *Radiology* 1997;204(1):185-189.

31. O'Driscoll SW: Classification and evaluation of recurrent instability of the elbow. *Clin Orthop Relat Res* 2000;370:34-43.

32. Arvind CH, Hargreaves DG: Table top relocation test—New clinical test for posterolateral rotatory instability of the elbow. *J Shoulder Elbow Surg* 2006;15(4):500-501.

33. Coonrad RW, Roush TF, Major NM, Basamania CJ: The drop sign, a radiographic warning sign of elbow instability. *J Shoulder Elbow Surg* 2005;14(3):312-317.

34. Daluiski A, Schrumpf MA, Schreiber JJ, Nguyen JT, Hotchkiss RN: Direct repair for managing acute and chronic lateral ulnar collateral ligament disruptions. *J Hand Surg Am* 2014;39(6):1125-1129.

35. Sanchez-Sotelo J, Morrey BF, O'Driscoll SW: Ligamentous repair and reconstruction for posterolateral rotatory instability of the elbow. *J Bone Joint Surg Br* 2005;87(1):54-61.

36. Jones KJ, Dodson CC, Osbahr DC, et al: The docking technique for lateral ulnar collateral ligament reconstruction: Surgical technique and clinical outcomes. *J Shoulder Elbow Surg* 2012;21(3):389-395.

37. Lee BP, Teo LH: Surgical reconstruction for posterolateral rotatory instability of the elbow. *J Shoulder Elbow Surg* 2003;12(5):476-479.

38. Baumfeld JA, van Riet RP, Zobitz ME, Eygendaal D, An KN, Steinmann SP: Triceps tendon properties and its potential as an

autograft. *J Shoulder Elbow Surg* 2010;19(5):697-699.

39. Moritomo H, Murase T, Arimitsu S, Oka K, Yoshikawa H, Sugamoto K: The in vivo isometric point of the lateral ligament of the elbow. *J Bone Joint Surg Am* 2007;89(9):2011-2017.

40. Olsen BS, Søjbjerg JO: The treatment of recurrent posterolateral instability of the elbow. *J Bone Joint Surg Br* 2003;85(3):342-346.

41. Fleisig GS, Andrews JR: Prevention of elbow injuries in youth baseball pitchers. *Sports Health* 2012;4(5):419-424.

42. Olsen SJ II, Fleisig GS, Dun S, Loftice J, Andrews JR: Risk factors for shoulder and elbow injuries in adolescent baseball pitchers. *Am J Sports Med* 2006;34(6):905-912.

43. Bruce JR, Andrews JR: Ulnar collateral ligament injuries in the throwing athlete. *J Am Acad Orthop Surg* 2014;22(5):315-325.

44. O'Driscoll SW, Lawton RL, Smith AM: The "moving valgus stress test" for medial collateral ligament tears of the elbow. *Am J Sports Med* 2005;33(2):231-239.

45. Rettig AC, Sherrill C, Snead DS, Mendler JC, Mieling P: Nonoperative treatment of ulnar collateral ligament injuries in throwing athletes. *Am J Sports Med* 2001;29(1):15-17.

46. Wilk KE, Macrina LC, Cain EL, Dugas JR, Andrews JR: Rehabilitation of the overhead athlete's elbow. *Sports Health* 2012;4(5):404-414.

47. Podesta L, Crow SA, Volkmer D, Bert T, Yocum LA: Treatment of partial ulnar collateral ligament tears in the elbow with platelet-rich plasma. *Am J Sports Med* 2013;41(7):1689-1694.

48. Savoie FH III, Trenhaile SW, Roberts J, Field LD, Ramsey JR: Primary repair of ulnar collateral ligament injuries of the elbow in young athletes: A case series of injuries to the proximal and distal ends of the ligament. *Am J Sports Med* 2008;36(6):1066-1072.

49. Jones KJ, Osbahr DC, Schrumpf MA, Dines JS, Altchek DW: Ulnar collateral ligament reconstruction in throwing athletes: A review of current concepts. AAOS exhibit selection. *J Bone Joint Surg Am* 2012;94(8):e49.

50. Andrews JR, Jost PW, Cain EL: The ulnar collateral ligament procedure revisited: The procedure we use. *Sports Health* 2012;4(5):438-441.

51. Dodson CC, Altchek DW: Ulnar collateral ligament reconstruction revisited: The procedure I use and why. *Sports Health* 2012;4(5):433-437.

52. Vitale MA, Ahmad CS: The outcome of elbow ulnar collateral ligament reconstruction in overhead athletes: A systematic review. *Am J Sports Med* 2008;36(6):1193-1205.

53. Savoie FH III, Morgan C, Yaste J, Hurt J, Field L: Medial ulnar collateral ligament reconstruction using hamstring allograft in overhead throwing athletes. *J Bone Joint Surg Am* 2013;95(12):1062-1066.

54. Byram IR, Khanna K, Gardner TR, Ahmad CS: Characterizing bone tunnel placement in medial ulnar collateral ligament reconstruction using patient-specific 3-dimensional computed tomography modeling. *Am J Sports Med* 2013;41(4):894-902.

55. Cain EL Jr, Andrews JR, Dugas JR, et al: Outcome of ulnar collateral ligament reconstruction of the elbow in 1281 athletes: Results in 743 athletes with minimum 2-year follow-up. *Am J Sports Med* 2010;38(12):2426-2434.

56. Dodson CC, Thomas A, Dines JS, et a: Medial ulnar collateral ligament reconstruction of the elbow in throwing athletes. *Am J Sports Med* 2006;34(12):1926-1932.

57. Jones KJ, Dines JS, Rebolledo BJ, et al: Operative management of ulnar collateral ligament insufficiency in adolescent athletes. *Am J Sports Med* 2014;42(1):117-121.

58. Watson JN, McQueen P, Hutchinson MR: A systematic review of ulnar collateral ligament reconstruction techniques. *Am J Sports Med* 2014;42(10):2510-2516.

59. Baecher N, Edwards S: Olecranon fractures. *J Hand Surg Am* 2013;38(3):593-604.

60. Ring D, Jupiter JB, Sanders RW, Mast J, Simpson NS: Transolecranon fracture-dislocation of the elbow. *J Orthop Trauma* 1997;11(8):545-550.

61. Ring D, Jupiter JB, Simpson NS: Monteggia fractures in adults. *J Bone Joint Surg Am* 1998;80(12):1733-1744.

62. Mortazavi SM, Asadollahi S, Tahririan MA: Functional outcome following treatment of transolecranon fracture-dislocation of the elbow. *Injury* 2006;37(3):284-288.

63. Mouhsine E, Akiki A, Castagna A, et al: Transolecranon anterior fracture dislocation. *J Shoulder Elbow Surg* 2007;16(3):352-357.

64. Taylor TK, Scham SM: A posteromedial approach to the proximal end of the ulna for the internal fixation of olecranon fractures. *J Trauma* 1969;9(7):594-602.

65. Bado JL: The Monteggia lesion. *Clin Orthop Relat Res* 1967;50:71-86.

66. Jupiter JB, Leibovic SJ, Ribbans W, Wilk RM: The posterior Monteggia lesion. *J Orthop Trauma* 1991;5(4):395-402.

67. Ring D: Monteggia fractures. *Orthop Clin North Am* 2013;44(1):59-66.

68. Strauss EJ, Tejwani NC, Preston CF, Egol KA: The posterior Monteggia lesion with associated ulnohumeral instability. *J Bone Joint Surg Br* 2006;88(1):84-89.

69. Konrad GG, Kundel K, Kreuz PC, Oberst M, Sudkamp NP: Monteggia fractures in adults: Long-term results and prognostic factors. *J Bone Joint Surg Br* 2007;89(3):354-360.

70. Hotchkiss RN: Fractures and dislocations of the elbow, in Rockwood CA Jr, Green DP, Bucholz RW, Heckman JD, eds: *Rockwood and Green's Fractures in Adults*, ed 4. Philadelphia, PA, Lippincott-Raven, 1996, vol 1, pp 929-1024.

71. Ring D, Jupiter JB, Zilberfarb J: Posterior dislocation of the elbow with fractures of the radial head and coronoid. *J Bone Joint Surg Am* 2002;84(4):547-551.

72. Pugh DM, Wild LM, Schemitsch EH, King GJ, McKee MD: Standard surgical protocol to treat elbow dislocations with radial head and coronoid fractures. *J Bone Joint Surg Am* 2004;86(6):1122-1130.

73. Bohn K, Ipaktchi K, Livermore M, Cao J, Banegas R: Current treatment concepts for "terrible triad" injuries of the elbow. *Orthopedics* 2014;37(12):831-837.

74. Sanchez-Sotelo J, O'Driscoll SW, Morrey BF: Medial oblique compression fracture of the coronoid process of the ulna. *J Shoulder Elbow Surg* 2005;14(1):60-64.

75. Hotchkiss RN, Weiland AJ: Valgus stability of the elbow. *J Orthop Res* 1987;5(3):372-377.

76. Mezera K, Hotchkiss RN: Fractures and dislocations of the elbow, in Rockwood CA Jr, Green DP, Bucholz RW, Heckman JD, eds: *Rockwood and Green's Fractures in Adults*, ed 5. Philadelphia, PA, Lippincott-Raven, 2001, pp 921-952.

77. Beingessner DM, Stacpoole RA, Dunning CE, Johnson JA, King GJ: The effect of suture fixation of type I coronoid fractures on the kinematics and stability of the elbow with and without medial collateral ligament repair. *J Shoulder Elbow Surg* 2007;16(2):213-217.

78. Mathew PK, Athwal GS, King GJ: Terrible triad injury of the elbow: Current concepts. *J Am Acad Orthop Surg* 2009;17(3):137-151.

79. Doornberg JN, Ring D: Coronoid fracture patterns. *J Hand Surg Am* 2006;31(1):45-52.

80. Doornberg JN, van Duijn J, Ring D: Coronoid fracture height in terrible-triad injuries. *J Hand Surg Am* 2006;31(5):794-797.

81. O'Driscoll SW, Jupiter JB, Cohen MS, Ring D, McKee MD: Difficult elbow fractures: Pearls and pitfalls. *Instr Course Lect* 2003;52:113-134.

82. Hotchkiss RN: Displaced fractures of the radial head: Internal fixation or excision? *J Am Acad Orthop Surg* 1997;5(1):1-10.

83. Ring D, Doornberg JN: Fracture of the anteromedial facet of the coronoid process: Surgical technique. *J Bone Joint Surg Am* 2007; 89(suppl 2 pt 2):267-283.

84. Chan K, MacDermid JC, Faber KJ, King GJ, Athwal GS: Can we treat select terrible triad injuries

nonoperatively? *Clin Orthop Relat Res* 2014;472(7):2092-2099.

85. Garrigues GE, Wray WH III, Lindenhovius AL, Ring DC, Ruch DS: Fixation of the coronoid process in elbow fracture-dislocations. *J Bone Joint Surg Am* 2011;93(20):1873-1881.

86. Doornberg JN, Ring DC: Fracture of the anteromedial facet of the coronoid process. *J Bone Joint Surg Am* 2006;88(10):2216-2224.

87. Alolabi B, Studer A, Gray A, et al: Selecting the diameter of a radial head implant: An assessment of local landmarks. *J Shoulder Elbow Surg* 2013;22(10):1395-1399.

88. Doornberg JN, Linzel DS, Zurakowski D, Ring D: Reference points for radial head prosthesis size. *J Hand Surg Am* 2006;31(1):53-57.

89. Frank SG, Grewal R, Johnson J, Faber KJ, King GJ, Athwal GS: Determination of correct implant size in radial head arthroplasty to avoid overlengthening. *J Bone Joint Surg Am* 2009;91(7):1738-1746.

90. Iordens GI, Den Hartog D, Van Lieshout EM, et al: Good functional recovery of complex elbow dislocations treated with hinged external fixation: A multicenter prospective study. *Clin Orthop Relat Res* 2015;473(4):1451-1461.

91. McKee MD, Bowden SH, King GJ, et al: Management of recurrent, complex instability of the elbow with a hinged external fixator. *J Bone Joint Surg Br* 1998;80(6):1031-1036.

92. Ring D, Bruinsma WE, Jupiter JB: Complications of hinged external fixation compared with cross-pinning of the elbow for acute and subacute instability. *Clin Orthop Relat Res* 2014;472(7):2044-2048.

93. Rhyou IH, Lim KS, Kim KC, Lee JH, Ahn KB, Moon SC: Drop sign of the elbow joint after surgical stabilization of an unstable simple posterolateral dislocation: Natural course and contributing factors. *J Shoulder Elbow Surg* 2015;24(7):1081-1089.

94. Lindenhovius AL, Jupiter JB, Ring D: Comparison of acute versus subacute treatment of terrible triad injuries of the elbow. *J Hand Surg Am* 2008;33(6):920-926.

95. Egol KA, Immerman I, Paksima N, Tejwani N, Koval KJ: Fracture-dislocation of the elbow functional outcome following treatment with a standardized protocol. *Bull NYU Hosp Jt Dis* 2007;65(4):263-270.

96. Regan W, Morrey B: Fractures of the coronoid process of the ulna. *J Bone Joint Surg Am* 1989;71(9):1348-1354.

97. Adams JE, Sanchez-Sotelo J, Kallina CF IV, Morrey BF, Steinmann SP: Fractures of the coronoid: Morphology based upon computer tomography scanning. *J Shoulder Elbow Surg* 2012;21(6):782-788.

98. Pollock JW, Brownhill J, Ferreira L, McDonald CP, Johnson J, King G: The effect of anteromedial facet fractures of the coronoid and lateral collateral ligament injury on elbow stability and kinematics. *J Bone Joint Surg Am* 2009;91(6):1448-1458.

99. Park SM, Lee JS, Jung JY, Kim JY, Song KS: How should anteromedial coronoid facet fracture be managed? A surgical strategy based on O'Driscoll classification and ligament injury. *J Shoulder Elbow Surg* 2015;24(1):74-82.

100. Rhyou IH, Kim KC, Lee JH, Kim SY: Strategic approach to O'Driscoll type 2 anteromedial coronoid facet fracture. *J Shoulder Elbow Surg* 2014;23(7):924-932.

101. Doornberg JN, de Jong IM, Lindenhovius AL, Ring D: The anteromedial facet of the coronoid process of the ulna. *J Shoulder Elbow Surg* 2007;16(5):667-670.

© 2016 AAOS Instructional Course Lectures, Volume 65

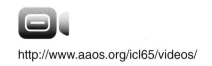

http://www.aaos.org/icl65/videos/

Arthroscopic Rotator Cuff Repair: Indication and Technique

Mohit Gilotra, MD

Michael J. O'Brien, MD

Felix H. Savoie III, MD

Abstract

Shoulder arthroscopy and rotator cuff repair techniques are frequently used by most practicing orthopaedic surgeons. A thorough patient history and physical examination can often confirm the presence of a rotator cuff tear, and imaging can be used to evaluate the extent of the injury. The indication for rotator cuff repair is a painful shoulder refractory to nonsurgical management. Arthroscopic techniques, including capsular and coracohumeral ligament releases to decrease tension on the repair, facilitate successful rotator cuff repair. Biomechanically, a double-row transosseous-equivalent rotator cuff repair provides excellent results for medium-size rotator cuff tears. Larger, retracted rotator cuff tears may be better repaired with oblique convergence sutures and a medial single-row rotator cuff repair. The biology of healing, the preservation of blood supply, and the trephination of the bony healing bed are essential parts of all rotator cuff repair procedures. Protection of the rotator cuff repair with an abduction sling for 4 to 8 weeks postoperatively and the delay of active motion until early healing has occurred will improve outcomes.

Instr Course Lect 2016;65:83–92.

Shoulder pain from a rotator cuff tear is one of the most common reasons patients present to an outpatient physician. Over five million doctor visits between 1998 and 2004 were attributed to rotator cuff symptoms.[1] Most full-thickness rotator cuff tears present in patients older than 55 years.[2,3] McMahon et al[4] reported that the frequency of symptomatic full-thickness rotator cuff tears in senior athletes older than 60 years was 21.3%; however, the authors noted a larger distribution of shoulders with partial-thickness rotator cuff tears and tendinosis. The incidence of symptomatic rotator cuff tears is expected to increase as the population ages.

The economic effects of the treatment for rotator cuff tears are substantial because of the high cost of diagnostic imaging, outpatient visits, injections, and physical therapy. Yeranosian et al[5] reported that preoperative charges associated with rotator cuff

Dr. O'Brien or an immediate family member serves as a paid consultant to or is an employee of Smith & Nephew; has received research or institutional support from DePuy and Mitek; has received nonincome support (such as equipment or services), commercially derived honoraria, or other non-research–related funding (such as paid travel) from DePuy, Mitek, and Smith & Nephew; and serves as a board member, owner, officer, or committee member of the Arthroscopy Association of North America and the Association of American Medical Colleges. Dr. Savoie or an immediate family member is a member of a speakers' bureau or has made paid presentations on behalf of Mitek and Smith & Nephew; serves as an unpaid consultant to Biomet, Exactech, Mitek, Rotation Medical, and Smith & Nephew; has received research or institutional support from Mitek; and serves as a board member, owner, officer, or committee member of the American Shoulder and Elbow Surgeons and the Arthroscopy Association of North America. Neither Dr. Gilotra nor any immediate family member has received anything of value from or has stock or stock options held in a commercial company or institution related directly or indirectly to the subject of this chapter.

repair, not including the charges associated with the actual surgical procedure, averaged more than $1,500 per patient. Conversely, surgical repair in a select patient population may actually result in cost savings. In a recent study, Mather et al[6] used a Markov decision model to explore the societal and economic value of rotator cuff repair. Direct and indirect costs and savings were estimated based on national survey data, patient-reported outcomes, and Medicare reimbursements. The authors estimated that lifetime societal savings for rotator cuff repair was higher than $70,000 for younger patients and was still cost effective for patients of all ages.[6]

Successful surgical management of a symptomatic rotator cuff tear is dependent on appropriate preoperative patient evaluation and preparation, intraoperative capsular and ligament releases, biomechanically sound rotator cuff repair techniques, attention to the biology of healing, and postoperative protection of the rotator cuff repair.

Patient Evaluation

Patient history focuses on patient age, the presence or absence of trauma, medical comorbidities such as diabetes or smoking, and previous rotator cuff treatment. Traumatic or acute rotator cuff tears, especially in younger patients, are often symptomatic and are more likely to require surgical intervention than their atraumatic counterparts.

Symptoms

The two hallmarks of a rotator cuff tear are pain with overhead activities and pain at night. Weakness is often present as well. Symptomatic rotator cuff tears affect daily activities and occupation-specific tasks. Pain associated with weakness may indicate a larger rotator cuff tear; however, symptoms of weakness are better corroborated with rotator cuff tests.

Physical Examination

The physical examination begins with an inspection of the patient's posture. Patients who have shoulder pain will often sit hunched forward with the scapula protracted. In the setting of a long-standing rotator cuff tear, there may be visible atrophy of the supraspinatus and/or infraspinatus muscles. Palpation allows the examiner to confirm or rule out other possible sources of pain. The acromioclavicular joint and the biceps tendon are easy landmarks to palpate. Palpation of the biceps tendon at the subpectoral location isolates biceps tenosynovitis from other diagnoses that present with anterior shoulder pain. If possible, palpation of the defect in the rotator cuff with the use of the techniques described by Codman[7] and Wolf and Agrawal[8] can help determine if a rotator cuff tear is the source of pain.

In a painful shoulder, it is helpful to determine passive range of motion as well as active range of motion with and without pain. Passive range of motion should be full, but it is often difficult to assess if a patient's shoulder is too painful. The inferior glide test can help discern the presence of adhesive capsulitis (**Figure 1**). During the first 10° to 30° of abduction, the humerus should slightly glide inferiorly. In the setting of adhesive capsulitis and a tight rotator interval, the humerus will not glide. The examiner should cradle the patient's forearm with one arm and push down on the patient's humerus with the other arm while forcing the proximal humerus inferiorly. This test will elicit pain only during early adhesive capsulitis.

Rotator Cuff Tests

Provocative tests can help isolate a full-thickness or partial-thickness supraspinatus tear. The Whipple test, performed with the patient's scapula retracted (**Figure 2**), is specific for partial- or full-thickness supraspinatus tears.[9] Supraspinatus isolation testing, performed with the patient's arm outstretched in the plane of the scapula with the thumb up and then down, will be positive only if a full-thickness supraspinatus tear is present. Weakness or buckling (giving way) during provocative testing indicates a positive test. A negative supraspinatus isolation test and a positive Whipple test is indicative of a partial-thickness supraspinatus tear; however, if both tests are positive, then a full-thickness supraspinatus tear likely exists.[10]

The upper (transverse portion) infraspinatus is tested in 90° of abduction and 45° to 90° of external rotation against resistance, and the lower (oblique portion) infraspinatus is tested in neutral adduction against resistance in external rotation.[11] Tests for the subscapularis include the belly-press, lift-off, and bear-hug tests.[12] The belly-press test and the bear-hug test performed at 45° of shoulder flexion are used to isolate the upper subscapularis.[13] The lift-off test is more difficult to perform, especially if the patient lacks internal rotation.

Tests for impingement are categorized as anterior, lateral, or coracoid and are strictly anatomically based. Anterior impingement is diagnosed with the Neer and Hawkins tests. For the Neer test, the examiner elevates the patient's shoulder in the scapular plane, which abuts the enthesophyte on the underside of the anterolateral acromion against the top of the rotator

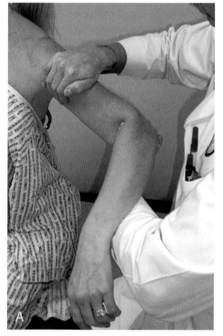
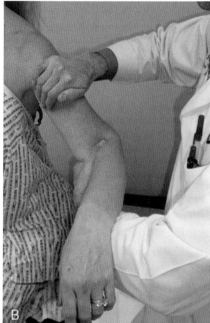
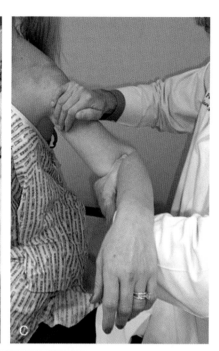

Figure 1   Clinical photographs demonstrate the inferior glide test. **A,** The patient's arm is positioned in abduction. **B,** The examiner places a slight inferior axial load on the patient's arm. **C,** The examiner gently displaces the proximal humerus inferiorly. A positive inferior glide test will elicit pain. (Copyright Felix H. Savoie III, MD, New Orleans, LA.)

cuff. A Neer sign is present if pain is elicited in 90° to 120° of flexion. For the Hawkins test, the examiner rotates the patient's abducted shoulder from external rotation into internal rotation, which abuts the supraspinatus against the coracoacromial arch. Pain indicates a positive Hawkins sign. Pain with 100° to 120° of passive abduction is indicative of lateral impingement. To confirm a diagnosis of coracoid impingement, the examiner applies a slight anterior force to the humeral head with the patient's arm abducted 45° to 60° and rotates the lessor tuberosity against the coracoid while feeling for crepitus.[14,15]

Imaging

Imaging studies help confirm a diagnosis that is suspected based on the patient's history and physical examination. Although the rotator cuff itself is not visualized on radiographs, there are some key findings that may assist in the diagnosis of a rotator cuff tear. Cortical thickening and subcortical sclerosis of the greater tuberosity may correspond with rotator cuff disease, but has not been substantiated.[16] Acromial slope morphology is best visualized on a supraspinatus outlet radiograph[17] (**Figure 3**). The lateral acromial angle, the acromial index, and the critical shoulder angle, all of which may predict degenerative rotator cuff tears, are more easily measured on a true AP (ie, Grashey view) radiograph.[18] A decreased acromiohumeral distance with pseudoarticulation between the humerus and the acromion is a sign of a massive rotator cuff tear.

Advanced imaging can help the surgeon further evaluate the rotator cuff and classify the tear pattern. MRI and ultrasonography are the most common advanced imaging modalities. Ultrasonography is less expensive than MRI, is useful in the setting of an implant,

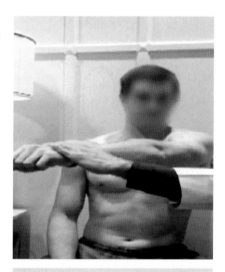

Figure 2   Clinical photograph demonstrates the Whipple test. The patient holds his arm in front of the opposite shoulder with the palm facing down and resists a downward force applied by the examiner. A positive Whipple test will elicit weakness. (Copyright Felix H. Savoie III, MD, New Orleans, LA.)

and allows for evaluation of the shoulder in dynamic positions.[19] MRI is less

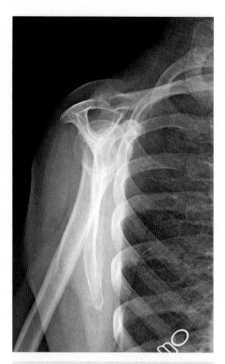

Figure 3 Supraspinatus outlet radiograph demonstrates acromial slope morphology. (Copyright Felix H. Savoie III, MD, New Orleans, LA.)

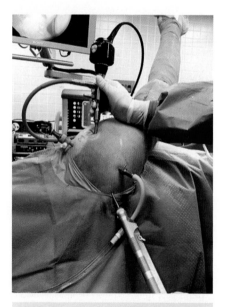

Figure 4 Intraoperative photograph shows a patient placed in the lateral decubitus position, which helps the surgeon view the rotator cuff from the lateral portal. (Copyright Felix H. Savoie III, MD, New Orleans, LA.)

operator dependent than ultrasonography, better defines complex tear patterns as well as the degree of atrophy and fatty infiltration, and is able to identify concurrent intra-articular pathology.[20]

Surgical Technique

Surgery begins with an examination under anesthesia. The range of motion of the surgical limb should be documented and compared with the contralateral side. Shoulder arthroscopy can be performed in the beach-chair or lateral decubitus position. The beach-chair position reduces the risk of brachial plexus strain and neurovascular stretch from traction and is easy to convert to an open approach, if necessary.[21] The lateral decubitus position is faster to set up than the beach-chair position, provides an improved intra-articular view with humeral traction, and decreases the risk of ischemic neurologic events[22] (**Figure 4**).

Regardless of the patient position selected, arthroscopic visualization, which can be obtained with either an arthroscopic pump or gravity tubing, is necessary. If a patient's capillary blood pressure is consistently higher than the arthroscopic pump pressure, excess bleeding, which impairs arthroscopic visualization, may occur. Therefore, the surgeon should attempt to maintain the patient's systolic blood pressure below 90 mm Hg and the arthroscopic pump or gravity pressure at or above 60 mm Hg. Limiting outflow from multiple portals also can help minimize bleeding.[23]

Classification and Treatment by Rotator Cuff Tear Size
Partial-Thickness Rotator Cuff Tears
Partial-thickness rotator cuff tears are classified as bursal-sided or articular-sided based on the location and depth of the tear. Although less common, bursal-sided rotator cuff tears are more likely to progress to full-thickness rotator cuff tears. Bursal-sided rotator cuff tears tend to occur in younger patients secondary to trauma.[24] In a study on the preservation of the articular-sided tendon during bursal-sided rotator cuff repair, Koh et al[25] reported good clinical results, with 88% of patients healed based on postoperative MRI. Cordasco et al[26] reported a 38% failure rate for patients with grade 2B (3- to 6-mm-deep) bursal-sided rotator cuff tears who were treated with débridement alone. If the depth of a bursal-sided rotator cuff tear is more than 3 mm, then a repair with an acromioplasty to treat any extrinsic pathology is recommended.[26] To repair a bursal-sided rotator cuff tear, the surgeon places an anchor into the lateral aspect of the greater tuberosity and then retrieves the sutures through the more medial aspect of the torn tendon; this creates a lateral single-row repair.

Partial-thickness articular-sided tendon avulsion rotator cuff tears are much more common than partial-thickness bursal-sided rotator cuff tears. The articular side has a greater modulus of elasticity, decreased vascularity, and higher eccentric forces than the bursal side.[27] The classification of partial-thickness articular-side tendon avulsion rotator cuff tears is based on both depth grade and delamination distance. The amount of depth and delamination that warrants a repair or a débridement alone is controversial.

Arthroscopic rotator cuff repair is attempted for symptomatic rotator cuff tears that extend to more than 50% of the rotator cuff footprint or to an articular tear depth of more than 5 mm. Rotator cuff tears that fit these criteria can be treated with a transtendinous rotator cuff repair (**Figure 5**) or with complete detachment and a full-thickness rotator cuff repair.[28] A transtendinous rotator cuff repair is most easily performed with the dual spinal-needle technique and suture shuttling. The rotator cuff tear is débrided, and the exposed greater tuberosity is abraded. An 18-gauge spinal needle is placed lateral to the acromion, through the rotator cuff, and medial and posterior to the extent of the rotator cuff tear. A monofilament suture, which is used as a shuttle, is then passed through the spinal needle and into the joint and retrieved through the anterior cannula. A second spinal needle is placed through the anteriormost lateral aspect of the intact supraspinatus tendon and into the joint. A second monofilament suture is then passed through the second needle and retrieved through the anterior cannula. The two sutures are then used to pass a more permanent stitch, which is retrieved through the subacromial bursa and tied down, thereby completing the repair. Placement of the sutures too medial in the rotator cuff may result in shoulder stiffness and may place the repair site under excessive tension, which increases the risk of rotator cuff repair failure. In a review of 50 patients who had transtendinous rotator cuff repairs, Duralde et al[29] reported a 98% patient satisfaction rate, with significant improvement in American Shoulder and Elbow Surgeons scores, excluding workers' compensation patients. In a recent systematic review, Strauss et al[30] reported that both in situ transtendinous repair and complete detachment and transtendinous repair techniques led to favorable outcomes, especially if

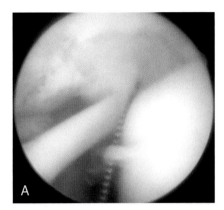
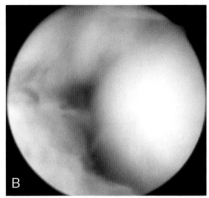

Figure 5   Arthroscopic images demonstrate a transtendinous repair of a partial-thickness articular-sided rotator cuff tear. **A,** A suture is passed through the tear. **B,** The suture is tied to reduce the tear. (Copyright Felix H. Savoie III, MD, New Orleans, LA.)

the rotator cuff tear extended to more than 50% of the rotator cuff footprint.

Rotator cuff repairs after complete detachment are performed with a standard single- or double-row technique and seem to decrease the risk of early stiffness; however, takedown of some intact enthesis may increase the risk of rotator cuff repair failure. In a study of the outcomes of partial-thickness articular-sided rotator cuff repair techniques, Shin[31] randomized patients into an arthroscopic rotator cuff repair with transtendinous technique group and an arthroscopic rotator cuff repair after complete takedown group. The author reported that although both groups did well, recovery and initial pain relief was better, especially in the first 3 months after surgery, for patients in the complete takedown group. There were no re-tears in the transtendinous technique group, but there were two repair failures in the complete takedown group.[31]

Medium and Large Full-Thickness Rotator Cuff Tears

The terms "medium" and "large" are relative descriptors of full-thickness rotator cuff tears. According to Bassett and Cofield,[32] rotator cuff tear size is based on the amount of uncovered tuberosity, in which 2 to 3 cm is considered a medium rotator cuff tear, and 3 to 5 cm is considered a large rotator cuff tear. In general, a one-tendon tear is considered medium, and a tear that includes two or more tendons is considered large. Regardless of the rotator cuff tear size, the goal of surgery is pain relief and the restoration of function without tendon failure. The technical goal of surgery is to attain a tension-free rotator cuff repair that covers the greater tuberosity. The incidence of rotator cuff re-tear varies from 11% to 94% based on the series, surgical technique used, and radiologic mode of interpretation.[33-35] In a cohort study of 1,000 patients who had rotator cuff repairs, Le et al[36] reported that risk factors for failure included patient age, size of the rotator cuff tear, fatty infiltration, and chronicity. Although rotator cuff repair integrity may not be an important factor for pain relief, recent literature suggests that it does help with shoulder function, especially in younger and active patients.[37,38]

To effectively plan a rotator cuff repair, it is important that the surgeon

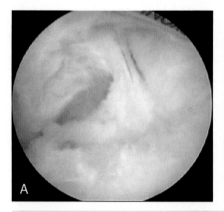
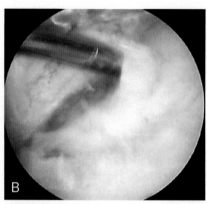

Figure 6 Arthroscopic images demonstrate an anterior interval slide for repair of a large rotator cuff tear. **A,** The coracohumeral ligament is identified from the lateral portal. **B,** The coracohumeral ligament is released with an incision. A 4.5-mm full-radius resector is used as a probe. (Copyright Felix H. Savoie III, MD, New Orleans, LA.)

determine the shape of the rotator cuff tear with the use of preoperative imaging and arthroscopy. Most rotator cuff tears are classified as crescent-shaped, U-shaped, L-shaped, or massive contracted.[39] Crescent-shaped rotator cuff tears are larger from anterior to posterior than from lateral to medial. Crescent-shaped rotator cuff tears are mobile and are able to be reduced to the greater tuberosity without much tension. U-shaped rotator cuff tears have a greater extension medially toward the glenoid rim, but do not have substantial lateral mobility of either the anterior or posterior limb. True U-shaped rotator cuff tears are relatively rare and may require a side-to-side repair. The more commonly occurring L-shaped and reverse L-shaped rotator cuff tears have a medial extension similar to a U-shaped rotator cuff tear, but either the anterior or posterior limb of an L-shaped rotator cuff tear is more mobile than those of a U-shaped rotator cuff tear. The mobile limb is reduced with an oblique side-to-side repair before tendon-to-bone repair.

Not all rotator cuff tear patterns are the same; the treatment of a U- or L-shaped rotator cuff tear without margin convergence increases tensile stress and increases the risk of rotator cuff repair failure.[23] To attain a secure rotator cuff repair, the first step is to release any adhesions between the torn, retraced tendon and the surrounding tissue. The capsule beneath the rotator cuff tear can be released to facilitate easier mobilization. If loss of motion occurs on examination under anesthesia, the inferior capsule may also be released to allow for inferior displacement of the humeral head on the glenoid and to decrease tension on the repair.

Occasionally, a capsular release will not provide enough mobilization for larger chronic rotator cuff tears; therefore, interval slides can be used to improve the ease of the rotator cuff repair. To perform an anterior interval slide, the surgeon releases the supraspinatus tendon from the rotator cuff interval and incises the contracted coracohumeral ligament[40] (**Figure 6**). In a study of more than 40 patients who had rotator cuff repairs with the use of an anterior interval slide, Tauro[41] reported that all patients had improved American Shoulder and Elbow Surgeons scores at 2-year follow-up; however, rotator cuff integrity was not evaluated. If an anterior interval slide does not provide enough mobilization, then a posterior interval slide can be used. A posterior interval slide is useful if a partial rotator cuff repair is being considered because it separates the supraspinatus tendon from the infraspinatus tendon. While viewing the scapular spine through the lateral portal, the surgeon places traction stitches into the infraspinatus tendon and the supraspinatus tendon and pulls them posteriorly and anteriorly, respectively. The surgeon then uses arthroscopic scissors to separate the two muscle tendon units by cutting toward the scapular spine, taking care to avoid injury to the infraspinatus branch of the suprascapular nerve. In a study on the usefulness of the posterior interval slide for patients who had large to massive rotator cuff tears, Kim et al[42] reported that patients who were treated with a posterior interval slide in addition to a complete rotator cuff repair did not have better outcomes at 2-year follow-up than patients who were treated with a partial rotator cuff repair and margin convergence alone.

Arthroscopic rotator cuff repair is commonly performed with the use of either a single or double row of suture anchors. Traditionally, a double-row arthroscopic rotator cuff repair consists of two separate rows of anchors that alternate from medial to lateral. The strength of an arthroscopic rotator cuff repair is dependent on the number of sutures that cross the repair rather than the number of rows used.[43] The double-row transosseous-equivalent rotator cuff repair (**Figure 7**) has recently come into favor because some biomechanical studies have reported that it increases the footprint contact

© 2016 AAOS Instructional Course Lectures, Volume 65

force area, increases load to failure, and minimizes gap formation.[44-46] Clinically, patients who have a double-row transosseous-equivalent rotator cuff repair or a double-row rotator cuff repair have a decreased re-tear rate compared with patients who have a single-row rotator cuff repair;[47-49] however, most studies have not demonstrated a difference in subjective and objective outcomes scores between these techniques.

Massive and Irreparable Rotator Cuff Tears

Technically, almost all rotator cuff tears are repairable; however, chronicity, muscle atrophy, and extensive fatty infiltration are contraindications for rotator cuff repair. If the supraspinatus tendon is completely atrophied, then a partial rotator cuff repair may be indicated to provide some pain relief and to balance the shoulder or improve the rotator cuff force couple. If the supraspinatus tendon is irreparable, then a partial repair of the subscapularis or infraspinatus tendon may be indicated, even in the presence of a superior defect, to maintain a stable fulcrum for the deltoid. In a study of 24 patients who underwent partial rotator cuff repair for irreparable large or massive rotator cuff tears, Mori et al[50] reported that the re-tear rate was higher than 40%. In a retrospective review of 1,128 consecutive patients who had arthroscopic rotator cuff repairs, Iagulli et al[51] identified 97 patients who had massive rotator cuff tears. The authors reported that complete rotator cuff repair was achieved in 52 patients, whereas partial rotator cuff repair was only possible in 45 patients. Both groups of patients showed significant improvement in postoperative University of California-Los Angeles shoulder scores, and there was no

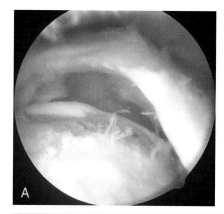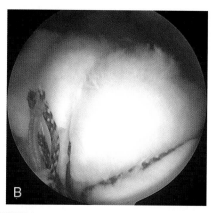

Figure 7   Arthroscopic images demonstrate a double-row transosseous-equivalent rotator cuff repair. **A,** A medium-size rotator cuff tear is identified from the lateral portal. **B,** After sutures from the medial row are passed through the rotator cuff, the repair is completed by tacking the sutures down to the lateral anchors. (Copyright Felix H. Savoie III, MD, New Orleans, LA.)

significant difference in postoperative outcomes between the two groups.[51] Rotator cuff débridement, with or without biceps tenotomy, is a final arthroscopic treatment option for massive rotator cuff tears. Although there are some short-term improvements in pain relief for patients who have rotator cuff débridement with biceps tenotomy, the long-term functional results are not predictable.[52]

The keys to a satisfactory massive rotator cuff repair are capsular and ligament releases and oblique convergence sutures. The first step for repair of a massive, retracted rotator cuff tear is to release the capsule, the coracohumeral ligament, and any adhesions above or below the rotator cuff muscle tendon unit that may prevent it from sliding back to its insertion. After the tendon is completely mobilized, the repair begins with the placement of an oblique convergence suture between the midportion of the supraspinatus tendon and the subscapularis tendon; this requires the use of a retrograde retriever, which is placed through either a Neviaser portal or a posteromedial accessory portal. The placement of a second or third

oblique convergence suture may be helpful. After the supraspinatus tendon is reduced back to the greater tuberosity, a standard single- or double-row rotator cuff repair can be performed.

Postoperative Rehabilitation

A progressive rehabilitation plan and patient compliance are paramount for rotator cuff healing and a satisfactory outcome. For the first 6 weeks postoperatively, the rotator cuff repair is protected with a pillow abduction device sling and only pain-free passive motion is allowed. Formal physical therapy, which includes supine passive flexion and external rotation, is initiated 1 month postoperatively to promote motion and some strengthening. All active motion should return by 3 months postoperatively. Early improvement of motion may be a sign of poor patient compliance. Patients are usually able to return to unrestricted activity within 4 to 8 months.[53] In a study to determine when rotator cuff re-tears commonly occur during the postoperative period, Ahmad et al[54] reported that poor patient compliance was highest in the second 6 weeks postoperatively and was a significant prognostic factor for rotator cuff re-tear.

Postoperative rehabilitation for any tendon repair has traditionally consisted of early passive motion because it both protects the repair and prevents stiffness; however, this has recently changed for rotator cuff repairs. In a randomized controlled trial of 124 patients who had small and medium full-thickness rotator cuff tears, Keener et al[55] reported no difference in outcomes or rotator cuff integrity for patients who were allowed early passive motion compared with patients who were immobilized. Similar results were reported in a prospective study by Cuff et al.[56] Two recent meta-analyses reported higher rotator cuff re-tear rates for patients who were allowed early passive motion, but also noted that these patients had slightly improved forward flexion.[57,58] Ultimately, there may be a slight advantage for patients with small and medium rotator cuff tears who are allowed early passive motion, but the risk of rotator cuff repair failure increases with larger rotator cuff tears.

Summary

Arthroscopic rotator cuff repair is now indicated for rotator cuff tears of all sizes. A thorough patient history and a focused physical examination can help in proper patient selection. The technique the surgeon selects for arthroscopic rotator cuff repair is dependent on rotator cuff tear size, morphology, and patient biology. Good outcomes are contingent on all the aforementioned factors.

References

1. Department of Research & Scientific Affairs, American Academy of Orthopaedic Surgeons: Physician visits for musculoskeletal symptoms and complaints. Rosemont, IL, American Academy of Orthopaedic Surgeons, updated November 2013. Available at: www.aaos.org/research/stats/patientstats.asp. Accessed June 4, 2015.

2. Dwyer T, Razmjou H, Holtby R: Full-thickness rotator cuff tears in patients younger than 55 years: Clinical outcome of arthroscopic repair in comparison with older patients. *Knee Surg Sports Traumatol Arthrosc* 2015;23(2):508-513.

3. Tokish JM: The mature athlete's shoulder. *Sports Health* 2014;6(1):31-35.

4. McMahon PJ, Prasad A, Francis KA: What is the prevalence of senior-athlete rotator cuff injuries and are they associated with pain and dysfunction? *Clin Orthop Relat Res* 2014;472(8):2427-2432.

5. Yeranosian MG, Terrell RD, Wang JC, McAllister DR, Petrigliano FA: The costs associated with the evaluation of rotator cuff tears before surgical repair. *J Shoulder Elbow Surg* 2013;22(12):1662-1666.

6. Mather RC III, Koenig L, Acevedo D, et al: The societal and economic value of rotator cuff repair. *J Bone Joint Surg Am* 2013;95(22):1993-2000.

7. Codman EA: *The Shoulder: Rupture of the Supraspinatus Tendon and Other Lesions in or About the Subacromial Bursa.* Boston, MA, Thomas Todd, 1934, pp 123-177.

8. Wolf EM, Agrawal V: Transdeltoid palpation (the rent test) in the diagnosis of rotator cuff tears. *J Shoulder Elbow Surg* 2001;10(5):470-473.

9. Savoie FH III, Field LD, Atchinson S: Anterior superior instability with rotator cuff tearing: SLAC lesion. *Orthop Clin North Am* 2001;32(3):457-461, ix.

10. Holtby R, Razmjou H: Validity of the supraspinatus test as a single clinical test in diagnosing patients with rotator cuff pathology. *J Orthop Sports Phys Ther* 2004;34(4):194-200.

11. Hughes PC, Green RA, Taylor NF: Isolation of infraspinatus in clinical test positions. *J Sci Med Sport* 2014;17(3):256-260.

12. Pennock AT, Pennington WW, Torry MR, et al: The influence of arm and shoulder position on the bear-hug, belly-press, and lift-off tests: An electromyographic study. *Am J Sports Med* 2011;39(11):2338-2346.

13. Chao S, Thomas S, Yucha D, Kelly JD IV, Driban J, Swanik K: An electromyographic assessment of the "bear hug": An examination for the evaluation of the subscapularis muscle. *Arthroscopy* 2008;24(11):1265-1270.

14. Osti L, Soldati F, Del Buono A, Massari L: Subcoracoid impingement and subscapularis tendon: Is there any truth? *Muscles Ligaments Tendons J* 2013;3(2):101-105.

15. Dines DM, Warren RF, Inglis AE, Pavlov H: The coracoid impingement syndrome. *J Bone Joint Surg Br* 1990;72(2):314-316.

16. Huang LF, Rubin DA, Britton CA: Greater tuberosity changes as revealed by radiography: Lack of clinical usefulness in patients with rotator cuff disease. *AJR Am J Roentgenol* 1999;172(5):1381-1388.

17. Bigliani LU, Ticker JB, Flatow EL, Soslowsky LJ, Mow VC: The relationship of acromial architecture to rotator cuff disease. *Clin Sports Med* 1991;10(4):823-838.

18. Moor BK, Wieser K, Slankamenac K, Gerber C, Bouaicha S: Relationship of individual scapular anatomy and degenerative rotator cuff tears. *J Shoulder Elbow Surg* 2014;23(4):536-541.

19. Teefey SA, Hasan SA, Middleton WD, Patel M, Wright RW, Yamaguchi K: Ultrasonography of the rotator cuff: A comparison of ultrasonographic and arthroscopic findings in one hundred consecutive cases. *J Bone Joint Surg Am* 2000;82(4):498-504.

20. Teefey SA, Rubin DA, Middleton WD, Hildebolt CF, Leibold RA, Yamaguchi K: Detection and quantification of rotator cuff tears: Comparison of ultrasonographic, magnetic resonance imaging, and arthroscopic findings in seventy-one consecutive cases. *J Bone Joint Surg Am* 2004;86(4):708-716.

21. Skyhar MJ, Altchek DW, Warren RF, Wickiewicz TL, O'Brien SJ: Shoulder arthroscopy with the patient in the beach-chair position. *Arthroscopy* 1988;4(4):256-259.

© 2016 AAOS Instructional Course Lectures, Volume 65

22. Murphy GS, Szokol JW, Marymont JH, et al: Cerebral oxygen desaturation events assessed by near-infrared spectroscopy during shoulder arthroscopy in the beach chair and lateral decubitus positions. *Anesth Analg* 2010;111(2):496-505.

23. Burkhart SS, Lo IK: Arthroscopic rotator cuff repair. *J Am Acad Orthop Surg* 2006;14(6):333-346.

24. Oh JH, Oh CH, Kim SH, Kim JH, Yoon JP, Jung JH: Clinical features of partial anterior bursal-sided supraspinatus tendon (PABST) lesions. *J Shoulder Elbow Surg* 2012;21(3):295-303.

25. Koh KH, Shon MS, Lim TK, Yoo JC: Clinical and magnetic resonance imaging results of arthroscopic full-layer repair of bursal-side partial-thickness rotator cuff tears. *Am J Sports Med* 2011;39(8):1660-1667.

26. Cordasco FA, Backer M, Craig EV, Klein D, Warren RF: The partial-thickness rotator cuff tear: Is acromioplasty without repair sufficient? *Am J Sports Med* 2002;30(2):257-260.

27. Itoi E, Berglund LJ, Grabowski JJ, et al: Tensile properties of the supraspinatus tendon. *J Orthop Res* 1995;13(4):578-584.

28. Wolff AB, Sethi P, Sutton KM, Covey AS, Magit DP, Medvecky M: Partial-thickness rotator cuff tears. *J Am Acad Orthop Surg* 2006;14(13):715-725.

29. Duralde XA, McClelland WB Jr: The clinical results of arthroscopic transtendinous repair of grade III partial articular-sided supraspinatus tendon tears. *Arthroscopy* 2012;28(2):160-168.

30. Strauss EJ, Salata MJ, Kercher J, et al: Multimedia article: The arthroscopic management of partial-thickness rotator cuff tears. A systematic review of the literature. *Arthroscopy* 2011;27(4):568-580.

31. Shin SJ: A comparison of 2 repair techniques for partial-thickness articular-sided rotator cuff tears. *Arthroscopy* 2012;28(1):25-33.

32. Bassett RW, Cofield RH: Acute tears of the rotator cuff: The timing of surgical repair. *Clin Orthop Relat Res* 1983;175:18-24.

33. Harryman DT II, Mack LA, Wang KY, Jackins SE, Richardson ML, Matsen FA III: Repairs of the rotator cuff: Correlation of functional results with integrity of the cuff. *J Bone Joint Surg Am* 1991;73(7):982-989.

34. Galatz LM, Ball CM, Teefey SA, Middleton WD, Yamaguchi K: The outcome and repair integrity of completely arthroscopically repaired large and massive rotator cuff tears. *J Bone Joint Surg Am* 2004;86(2):219-224.

35. Gerber C, Fuchs B, Hodler J: The results of repair of massive tears of the rotator cuff. *J Bone Joint Surg Am* 2000;82(4):505-515.

36. Le BT, Wu XL, Lam PH, Murrell GA: Factors predicting rotator cuff retears: An analysis of 1000 consecutive rotator cuff repairs. *Am J Sports Med* 2014;42(5):1134-1142.

37. Kim HM, Caldwell JM, Buza JA, et al: Factors affecting satisfaction and shoulder function in patients with a recurrent rotator cuff tear. *J Bone Joint Surg Am* 2014;96(2):106-112.

38. Namdari S, Donegan RP, Chamberlain AM, Galatz LM, Yamaguchi K, Keener JD: Factors affecting outcome after structural failure of repaired rotator cuff tears. *J Bone Joint Surg Am* 2014;96(2):99-105.

39. Davidson J, Burkhart SS: The geometric classification of rotator cuff tears: A system linking tear pattern to treatment and prognosis. *Arthroscopy* 2010;26(3):417-424.

40. Tauro JC: Arthroscopic "interval slide" in the repair of large rotator cuff tears. *Arthroscopy* 1999;15(5):527-530.

41. Tauro JC: Arthroscopic repair of large rotator cuff tears using the interval slide technique. *Arthroscopy* 2004;20(1):13-21.

42. Kim SJ, Kim SH, Lee SK, Seo JW, Chun YM: Arthroscopic repair of massive contracted rotator cuff tears: Aggressive release with anterior and posterior interval slides do not improve cuff healing and integrity. *J Bone Joint Surg Am* 2013;95(16):1482-1488.

43. Jost PW, Khair MM, Chen DX, Wright TM, Kelly AM, Rodeo SA: Suture number determines strength of rotator cuff repair. *J Bone Joint Surg Am* 2012;94(14):e100.

44. Park MC, ElAttrache NS, Tibone JE, Ahmad CS, Jun BJ, Lee TQ: Part I: Footprint contact characteristics for a transosseous-equivalent rotator cuff repair technique compared with a double-row repair technique. *J Shoulder Elbow Surg* 2007;16(4):461-468.

45. Park MC, Pirolo JM, Park CJ, Tibone JE, McGarry MH, Lee TQ: The effect of abduction and rotation on footprint contact for single-row, double-row, and modified double-row rotator cuff repair techniques. *Am J Sports Med* 2009;37(8):1599-1608.

46. Mazzocca AD, Bollier MJ, Ciminiello AM, et al: Biomechanical evaluation of arthroscopic rotator cuff repairs over time. *Arthroscopy* 2010;26(5):592-599.

47. McCormick F, Gupta A, Bruce B, et al: Single-row, double-row, and transosseous equivalent techniques for isolated supraspinatus tendon tears with minimal atrophy: A retrospective comparative outcome and radiographic analysis at minimum 2-year follow-up. *Int J Shoulder Surg* 2014;8(1):15-20.

48. Millett PJ, Warth RJ, Dornan GJ, Lee JT, Spiegl UJ: Clinical and structural outcomes after arthroscopic single-row versus double-row rotator cuff repair: A systematic review and meta-analysis of level I randomized clinical trials. *J Shoulder Elbow Surg* 2014;23(4):586-597.

49. Mascarenhas R, Chalmers PN, Sayegh ET, et al: Is double-row rotator cuff repair clinically superior to single-row rotator cuff repair: A systematic review of overlapping meta-analyses. *Arthroscopy* 2014;30(9):1156-1165.

50. Mori D, Funakoshi N, Yamashita F: Arthroscopic surgery of irreparable large or massive rotator cuff tears with low-grade fatty degeneration of the infraspinatus: Patch autograft procedure versus partial repair procedure. *Arthroscopy* 2013;29(12):1911-1921.

51. Iagulli ND, Field LD, Hobgood ER, Ramsey JR, Savoie FH III: Comparison of partial versus complete arthroscopic repair of massive rotator cuff tears. *Am J Sports Med* 2012;40(5):1022-1026.

52. Klinger HM, Spahn G, Baums MH, Steckel H: Arthroscopic debridement of irreparable massive rotator cuff tears—a comparison of debridement alone and combined procedure with biceps tenotomy. *Acta Chir Belg* 2005;105(3):297-301.

53. Iannotti JP, Deutsch A, Green A, et al: Time to failure after rotator cuff repair: A prospective imaging study. *J Bone Joint Surg Am* 2013;95(11):965-971.

54. Ahmad S, Haber M, Bokor DJ: The influence of intraoperative factors and postoperative rehabilitation compliance on the integrity of the rotator cuff after arthroscopic repair. *J Shoulder Elbow Surg* 2015;24(2):229-235.

55. Keener JD, Galatz LM, Stobbs-Cucchi G, Patton R, Yamaguchi K: Rehabilitation following arthroscopic rotator cuff repair: A prospective randomized trial of immobilization compared with early motion. *J Bone Joint Surg Am* 2014;96(1):11-19.

56. Cuff DJ, Pupello DR: Prospective randomized study of arthroscopic rotator cuff repair using an early versus delayed postoperative physical therapy protocol. *J Shoulder Elbow Surg* 2012;21(11):1450-1455.

57. Chang KV, Hung CY, Han DS, Chen WS, Wang TG, Chien KL: Early versus delayed passive range of motion exercise for arthroscopic rotator cuff repair: A meta-analysis of randomized controlled trials. *Am J Sports Med* 2015;43(5):1265-1273.

58. Kluczynski MA, Nayyar S, Marzo JM, Bisson LJ: Early versus delayed passive range of motion after rotator cuff repair: A systematic review and meta-analysis. *Am J Sports Med* 2015;43(8):2057-2063.

Video Reference

O'Brien MJ: Video. *Fiber Tape Rotator Cuff Repair.* New Orleans, LA, 2015.

Challenges and Controversies in Treating Massive Rotator Cuff Tears

Stephen S. Burkhart, MD
Eric T. Ricchetti, MD
William N. Levine, MD
Leesa M. Galatz, MD

Abstract

Massive rotator cuff tears present several challenges for orthopaedic surgeons. Many rotator cuff tears can be repaired; however, some chronic rotator cuff tears require advanced reconstructive techniques. Repair, if possible, is the optimal treatment for rotator cuff tears. In general, muscle transfers are an option for patients younger than 60 years who do not have pseudoparalysis. Arthroplasty is an option for older patients who have concomitant arthritis and for patients who have pseudoparalysis. Biologic augmentation in the setting of rotator cuff tears continues to evolve, and the application of biologic products should be guided by sound evidence and cost-benefit considerations.

Instr Course Lect 2016;65:93–108.

Massive rotator cuff tears are clinically challenging for orthopaedic surgeons. Most rotator cuff tears reflect the natural degeneration of the tendon over time. In addition, as rotator cuff tears progress, the muscle tissue, which is designed to bear load, concomitantly undergoes degeneration, which is reflected as fat accumulation, collagen accumulation, and loss of plasticity. These changes compromise reparability and affect healing. Large and massive rotator cuff tears are difficult to repair, and there is a positive correlation between tear size and recurrence after repair. Repair is desirable in most patients, but other options, such as muscle transfers and reverse shoulder arthroplasty, are appropriate in certain clinical scenarios. Orthopaedic surgeons should be aware of the various treatment options, expert recommendations, and the latest science to appropriately treat patients who have massive rotator cuff tears.

Tricks for Repairing Massive Rotator Cuff Tears

Massive rotator cuff tears typically involve two or more tendons[1] and are larger than 5 cm in diameter.[2] Almost all massive rotator cuff tears can be fully repaired with the use of proper techniques. In a study of 126 massive rotator cuff tears that were evaluated at a mean follow-up of 8.2 years, Denard et al[3] reported that 85% of the tears were completely repaired, and 15% were partially repaired. To achieve a high rate of complete repair in massive rotator cuff tears, interval slides[4,5] were required in 43% of the cases. Therefore, a thorough knowledge of advanced arthroscopic techniques is necessary to achieve successful repair

Dr. Burkhart or an immediate family member has received royalties from Arthrex, and serves as a paid consultant to or is an employee of Arthrex. Dr. Ricchetti or an immediate family member has received research or institutional support from DePuy. Dr. Levine or an immediate family member serves as an unpaid consultant to Zimmer, and serves as a board member, owner, officer, or committee member of the American Board of Orthopaedic Surgery and the American Orthopaedic Association. Dr. Galatz or an immediate family member serves as a board member, owner, officer, or committee member of the American Academy of Orthopaedic Surgeons and the American Shoulder and Elbow Surgeons.

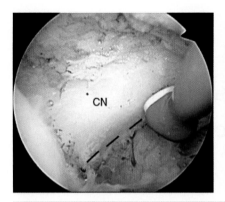
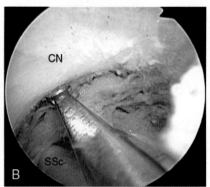
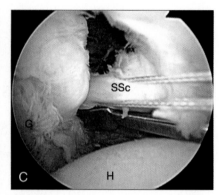

Figure 1   Arthroscopic images show a three-sided release of a retracted, adhesed subscapularis tendon tear in a right shoulder viewed from a posterior portal with the use of a 70° arthroscope. **A,** The posterolateral coracoid is skeletonized to the level of the coracoid neck (CN) (dashed lines) and the coracoid base with the use of electrocautery. **B,** A 30° elevator is introduced from an anterosuperolateral working portal, and adhesions between the superior subscapularis tendon (SSc) and the coracoid neck (CN) are released. The elevator is inserted only to the base of its blade, which is enough to release the adhesions to the coracoid. **C,** A 15° elevator is introduced from an anterosuperolateral portal and frees the subscapularis tendon (SSc) from adhesions between its posterior border and the glenoid (G). H = humerus. (Reproduced with permission from Burkhart SS, Lo IKY, Brady PC, Denard PJ: Subscapularis tendon tears, in *The Cowboy's Companion: A Trail Guide for the Arthroscopic Shoulder Surgeon*. Philadelphia, PA, Lippincott, Williams & Wilkins, 2012, pp 101-128.)

of massive rotator cuff tears. Even with pseudoparalysis, 90% of patients regain overhead elevation after arthroscopic rotator cuff repair.[3] Most massive rotator cuff tears are fully repairable and demonstrate substantial improvement after arthroscopic repair.

In general, most massive rotator cuff tears involve portions of the subscapularis, supraspinatus, and infraspinatus tendons; the biceps tendon is usually subluxated if the subscapularis is torn. The surgeon should approach such a tear in two stages: the subscapularis/biceps tendon component should be addressed first, after which the supraspinatus and infraspinatus should be repaired. Identification of the comma sign in association with subscapularis tears is critical because the junction of the comma tissue with the superolateral subscapularis should be repaired at the superomedial corner of the lesser tuberosity to restore normal anatomy.[6] The comma tissue, which is composed of the confluence of the superior glenohumeral ligament complex and the

coracohumeral ligament, is visible as a curved, thickened area at the upper subscapularis.[6] Furthermore, coracoplasty should be performed if the subcoracoid space is less than 7 mm.[7] Prior to repair of the subscapularis, a biceps tenotomy or tenodesis should be performed at the discretion of the surgeon. If the subscapularis is adhesed and retracted, a three-sided release will typically provide adequate excursion for repair without the need to specifically expose the neurovascular structures[8,9] (**Figure 1**). If the subscapularis tendon will not quite reach the lesser tuberosity bone bed, the bone bed may be medialized 5 to 7 mm without adversely affecting function.[10] The authors of this chapter prefer to preserve the comma tissue, even if releases are performed, because the subscapularis repair will reduce tension on the supraspinatus repair via the bridging effect of the comma between these two tendons. An anatomic repair is optimal, and every attempt should be made to restore the native position of the repaired tissue.

After the subscapularis, biceps, and coracoid have been addressed, the surgeon should proceed with the second phase of the procedure: repair of the supraspinatus and infraspinatus. Recognition of the tear pattern is essential because the tear pattern is the repair pattern, and proper recognition will allow the surgeon to repair the tear under minimal tension.[11] Combinations of margin convergence[12] and tendon-to-bone fixation should be used as indicated.

Massive retracted tears that lack adequate excursion to allow repair back to the greater tuberosity will require releases to gain excursion. Release of the capsule below the tendon and above the superior glenoid will usually yield less than 1 cm of lateral excursion, and other releases are usually necessary. In general, for contracted massive rotator cuff tears, the authors of this chapter use a modified double-interval slide technique, which consists of an anterior interval slide in continuity (release of the rotator interval tissue) plus a posterior interval slide.[4,5] The anterior interval slide will usually yield approximately 2 cm of additional lateral excursion of the cuff, and the posterior interval slide will typically provide 4 to 5 cm of additional lateral excursion. The individual flaps should then be repaired to bone with suture anchors, most often with a single-row technique, although, occasionally, a double-row repair may be possible. After fixation of the two tendon flaps to bone, the split between them should be closed with side-to-side sutures. If tendon quality is poor, the authors of this chapter reinforce the repair with the use of high-strength surgical tape that is placed as an inverted mattress stitch and secured laterally with anchors designed for fixation of the rotator cuff and placement of the greater tuberosity in a load-sharing rip-stop construct.[13] If the anterior flap still will not reach the greater tuberosity after a modified double-interval slide, the authors of this chapter have found that it is best to repair the infraspinatus (to balance the force couple with the subscapularis) and then advance the supraspinatus as much as possible as well as perform a side-to-side repair of the supraspinatus to the infraspinatus, which leaves a residual defect but achieves a substantial partial repair.

In dissection of the muscle-tendon units, it is helpful to expose the scapular spine by following the acromial arc posteromedially and removing the surrounding fat pad until the keel-shaped scapular spine is visible. This landmark will help identify the raphe between the supraspinatus and infraspinatus. The cut for the posterior interval slide should be made at the raphe while pulling laterally on the supraspinatus and infraspinatus tendons with the traction sutures to avoid damage to

the suprascapular nerve at the base of the scapular spine (**Figure 2**). Another helpful tip for adequate dissection of the rotator cuff is to excise any bursal leaders that may be present in the posterior or lateral gutters. Bursal leaders are fibrous bands that extend from the rotator cuff and insert into the internal deltoid fascia (rather than inserting into the greater tuberosity as do tendons). These bursal leaders must be excised and not used in the repair because they are not rotator cuff tissue.

The load-sharing rip-stop construct can dramatically increase the strength of a repair if tendon tissue is deficient (**Figure 3**). The inverted mattress high-strength surgical tape serves both as a rip-stop for the simple sutures from the medial anchors as well as a load-sharing element to the lateral anchors. The interlocking of the high-strength surgical tape with simple sutures is advantageous over a single row of high-strength surgical tape or a standard single-row suture anchor repair because it provides a rip-stop effect to prevent suture cut-out, load-sharing between rows, and an interlocking and self-reinforcing construct. Massive rotator cuff tears are almost always repairable if the surgeon recognizes the tear pattern and applies the appropriate biomechanical principles to maximize tendon excursion and optimize the strength of the repair construct.

Augmentation in Rotator Cuff Repair

Despite improvements in knowledge of rotator cuff pathology and advances in surgical treatment, healing after rotator cuff repair remains a substantial clinical challenge, particularly for large or massive rotator cuff tears. Failure rates after the repair of large to massive

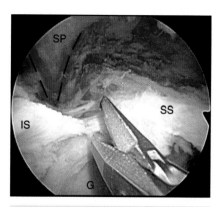

Figure 2   Arthroscopic image of a right shoulder viewed from a posterolateral portal shows a posterior interval slide that is performed with the use of arthroscopic scissors. G = glenoid, IS = infraspinatus tendon, SS = supraspinatus tendon, SP = scapular spine (dashed line). (Reproduced with permission from Burkhart SS, Lo IKY, Brady PC, Denard PJ: Large and massive rotator cuff tears, in *The Cowboy's Companion: A Trail Guide for the Arthroscopic Shoulder Surgeon.* Philadelphia, PA, Lippincott, Williams & Wilkins, 2012, pp 129-164.)

rotator cuff tears are between 25% and 94%,[14-21] depending on factors such as patient age, tear size and chronicity, muscle atrophy and fatty infiltration, tendon quality, repair technique, and postoperative rehabilitation. Therefore, additional strategies are necessary to augment the rotator cuff repair site by improving the mechanical integrity of the repair and/or the biologic healing environment. Preclinical and clinical studies on tissue-engineering therapies for rotator cuff repair augmentation have included the use of scaffold devices, platelet-rich plasma (PRP), specific growth factors, cell seeding, stem cells, and a combination of these treatments. The following techniques are currently available for clinical use to augment healing after rotator cuff repair.

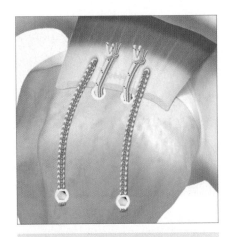

Figure 3 Illustration shows the load-sharing rip-stop construct for maximizing fixation strength in a deficient tendon. The inverted-mattress high-strength surgical tape acts as a rip-stop for the simple sutures from the suture anchors and also shares the load through its lateral fixation anchors. (Reproduced with permission from Burkhart SS, Lo IKY, Brady PC, Denard PJ: Managing poor tissue and bone quality in arthroscopic rotator cuff repair, in *The Cowboy's Companion: A Trail Guide for the Arthroscopic Shoulder Surgeon.* Philadelphia, PA, Lippincott, Williams & Wilkins, 2012, pp 180-196.)

Scaffold Devices

Scaffold devices derived from human and nonhuman mammalian extracellular matrix (ECM) and/or synthetic polymers are currently marketed for rotator cuff repair in humans. ECM scaffolds derived from nonhuman sources and synthetic scaffolds have been approved through the FDA's 510(k) regulatory process as medical devices that are considered a nonsignificant risk product for use in humans.[22] Nonhuman-derived ECM scaffolds have specifically been cleared as augmentation devices for rotator cuff tears that are repaired by suture or suture anchors. Conversely, human-derived ECM scaffolds are classified as human tissue for transplantation and do not require FDA clearance.[23,24]

Scaffolds have both potential mechanical and biologic benefits as augmentation devices in rotator cuff repair, with the ideal graft mechanically off-loading the repair site in the early postoperative healing phase when failure commonly occurs[25,26] and biologically improving the rate and quality of tendon healing. ECM devices, in particular, are believed to provide a chemically and structurally instructive environment for host cells and new tissue formation via their natural composition, three-dimensional structure, and degradation by-products.[27,28] Synthetic scaffolds may not provide such a biologic effect during healing; however, their ability to maintain durable mechanical properties over time may mechanically stabilize the repair construct until host tissue healing occurs.

Although the material properties of each scaffold are important in its ability to augment the mechanical properties of a rotator cuff repair, the characteristics of the augmented repair construct as a whole are equally or more important. Factors such as a scaffold's geometry and suture-retention properties as well as the surgical technique of graft application (including the number, type, and location of fixation sutures and pretensioning of the scaffold at the time of repair) all affect the mechanical performance of the device in situ.[22,29]

The indications for the clinical use of scaffolds as augmentation devices in rotator cuff repair have not been well defined. The most common indication has been in situations in which the failure rate after repair is high, including primary repair of chronic, large to massive rotator cuff tears; primary repair in the presence of other potential negative risk factors for healing (eg, tobacco use, diabetes); and revision surgery repairs. Although FDA-approved only as augmentation devices, scaffolds also have been used as interpositional grafts in irreparable rotator cuff tears or tears that are only partially repairable. There is a relatively even split in published clinical studies that report outcomes of scaffolds that are applied as augmentation devices and used as interpositional grafts in rotator cuff repair[30-46] (**Tables 1** and **2**). The conclusions drawn from these studies are limited because of small sample sizes, short-term follow-up, and no control or comparative groups. Almost all published studies are level IV case series, with most studies reporting improvements in pain, function, and clinical outcome scores from the preoperative state.[30-46] Variability exists across these studies in the type of graft applied, the type of rotator cuff tears treated, and the method of surgical application (open versus arthroscopic or augmentation versus interposition). In addition, radiographic healing rates vary across the studies, which may relate in part to a lack of criteria to define the quality of healing at the repair site, including what constitutes healed native tendon tissue in the presence of a graft.

Currently, only two randomized clinical trials that evaluated scaffold devices have been published.[31,47] One study investigated the use of non–cross-linked porcine small intestine submucosa (Restore Orthobiologic Implant, DePuy) for the augmentation of open rotator cuff repair of chronic tendon tears and reported a severe, sterile, postoperative inflammatory reaction in 3 of 15 patients who received the graft.[47] This reaction was noted at a similar rate in other clinical series that used the device.[48,49] Because of this finding and the lack of clinical benefit of the graft, the American Academy of Orthopaedic Surgeons does not currently recommend the use of Restore Orthobiologic Implant to treat rotator cuff tears in humans.[50] More recently, a prospective randomized clinical trial that investigated the use of non–cross-linked human dermis (GraftJacket, Wright Medical Technology) for the augmentation of arthroscopic repair of chronic two-tendon tears reported significantly better American Shoulder and Elbow Surgeons Subjective Shoulder Scale and Constant assessment scores as well as significantly improved healing rates compared with nonaugmented repairs (85% versus 40%, respectively;[31] **Table 1**). Some methodologic inconsistencies with regard to the number of anchors used per group and the use of PRP in certain patients were present in this study; however, the study suggests the potential benefit of augmentation in rotator cuff repair and the need for further investigation of scaffold devices.

Studies have reported on the clinical use of synthetic scaffolds in rotator cuff repair[34-37,44] (**Tables 1** and **2**); however, a recent retrospective study reported significantly better outcome scores and lower retear rates in open repairs of massive posterosuperior tears that were augmented with a polypropylene mesh synthetic scaffold (Repol Angimesh, Angiologica B.M. S.r.l.) compared with those augmented with a bovine-derived pericardium ECM patch (Tutopatch, Tutogen Medical GmbH) or nonaugmented repairs (17%, 51%, and 41% retear rates, respectively;[34] **Table 1**).

Further prospective, comparative studies are necessary to better define the indications, surgical application, safety, mechanism of action, and

efficacy of ECM and synthetic scaffold devices. Peer-reviewed clinical data do not exist for many of the scaffold devices currently available to surgeons. The unique physical, chemical, and/or biologic characteristics of a device as well as how and when the device is used play critical roles in its effectiveness for rotator cuff repair. Currently, because of the paucity of clinical evidence, the American Academy of Orthopaedic Surgeons cannot recommend for or against the use of soft-tissue allografts or other xenografts to treat patients who have rotator cuff tears.[50]

PRP and Growth Factors

Substantial clinical interest in the use of PRP for rotator cuff repair has increased in recent years. PRP is a readily available clinical source of growth factors known to play a role in tendon healing, including platelet-derived growth factor, vascular endothelial growth factor, transforming growth factor-β1, fibroblast growth factor, endothelial growth factor, human growth factor, and insulin-like growth factor-1.[51-53] The ability to concentrate these growth factors in one source has the potential to improve the biologic healing environment and, thus, the quality and rate of healing after rotator cuff repair. However, variability exists in the composition and preparation of different PRP formulations.[51,54] In addition, substantial differences in the PRP preparation produced from a given system have been reported to occur across and within individuals,[55] and patients also may fail to concentrate platelets with one preparation system but be successful with another.[56] This wide variability in PRP preparations and patient response likely affects the biologic effect on tissue healing.

In contrast to the clinical literature on the use of scaffold devices in rotator cuff repair, numerous high-level prospective clinical studies have been published in recent years on the use of PRP for augmentation of rotator cuff repair.[57-70] Most of these well-designed studies have reported no significant difference in clinical outcomes and retear rates after arthroscopic rotator cuff repair with or without PRP, including a meta-analysis of recent randomized clinical trials.[57,60,61,63,65-70] A small number of studies have reported significant differences in retear rates at short-term follow-up but no significant difference in clinical outcomes.[58,59,62,64] Therefore, insufficient evidence currently exists to support the use of PRP in the augmentation of rotator cuff repairs. It is challenging to draw definitive conclusions from the existing clinical data on PRP because of variability across studies in the choice and the application method for PRP preparation, rotator cuff tear size and repair technique, and the postoperative rehabilitation protocol. Numerous questions on the optimal timing, dosing, mode of application, and formulation of PRP in rotator cuff repair have the potential to be investigated and may help define a clinical benefit and indications for use.

Stem Cells

Stem cells also may potentially enhance the biologic healing of rotator cuff repair; however, investigation of their use has been mostly limited to preclinical studies. In a recent case-controlled study, Hernigou et al[71] reported on the use of mesenchymal stem cells (MSCs) in the arthroscopic single-row repair of medium-sized supraspinatus tears. Forty-five patients who underwent repair with injection of their own iliac

Table 1

Results of Scaffold Devices in Rotator Cuff Repair Augmentation

Device (Material)	Author(s) (Year)	Level of Evidence	Tear Size (Sample Size)	Scaffold Application Technique	Mean Follow-up in Months	MRI (US) Failure Rate	Mean Scores[a]	Outcomes
GraftJacket, Wright Medical Technology (human dermis)	Burkhead et al[32] (2007)	Level IV (case series)	Massive tears (n = 17)	Open, augmentation	14	3 (12)	**UCLA** Pre: 9.06 Post: 26.12	No adverse events reported; scores, strength, and ROM improved; 14 of 17 patients satisfied with outcome; recurrent tears were smaller than preoperative size.
	Barber et al[31] (2012)	Level II (prospective RCT)	Chronic, two-tendon tears >3 cm (NA: n = 20; A: n = 22)	Arthroscopic, augmentation	12–38	NA: 9 (15) A: 3 (20)	**UCLA** NA: 28.3 A: 28.2 **Constant** NA: 85.3 A: 91.9 **ASES** NA: 94.8 A: 98.9	No adverse events reported; A group had significantly better Constant and ASES scores and a significantly better healing rate according to MRI arthrograms compared with NA group.
Biomerix RCR Patch, Biomerix (polycarbonate polyurethane)	Encalada-Diaz et al[35] (2011)	Level IV (case series)	Open, small or medium tears, mean size = 2 cm (n = 10)	Open, augmentation	12	1 (10)	**ASES** Pre: 44 Post: 73.3 **UCLA** Post: 29.2 **Simple Shoulder** Pre: 3.6 Post: 7.7	Smaller tears (single tendon tears of supraspinatus or infraspinatus); no adverse events reported; scores, pain, and ROM improved.
Acellular human dermal matrix (human dermis)	Rotini et al[38] (2011)	Level IV (case series)	Large or massive tears (n = 5)	Arthroscopic (n = 2) or open (n = 3), augmentation	12–18	2 (5)	**Constant** Pre: 64 Post: 88	No adverse events reported; healed repairs showed graft incorporation into native tissue on MRI.

A = augmented, ASES = American Shoulder and Elbow Surgeons Subjective Shoulder Scale, Constant = Constant assessment score, DASH = Disabilities of the Arm, Shoulder and Hand questionnaire, FLEX-SF = Flexilevel Scale of Shoulder Function, HD = human dermis, NA = nonaugmented, Pre = preoperative, Post = postoperative, RA = Repol Angimesh, RCR = rotator cuff repair, RCT = randomized controlled trial, ROM = range of motion, Simple Shoulder = Simple Shoulder Test, TP = Tutopatch, UCLA = University of California–Los Angeles Shoulder Rating Scale, US = ultrasound.

[a]American Shoulder and Elbow Surgens Subjective Shoulder Scale score is measured out of 100 points; Constant assessment score is measured out of 100 points; Flexilevel Scale of Shoulder Function is measured out of 100 points; Simple Shoulder Test is measured out of 12 points; University of California–Los Angeles Shoulder Rating Scale score is measured out of 35 points.

Table 1 (continued)
Results of Scaffold Devices in Rotator Cuff Repair Augmentation

Device (Material)	Author(s) (Year)	Level of Evidence	Tear Size (Sample Size)	Scaffold Application Technique	Mean Follow-up in Months	MRI (US) Failure Rate	Mean Scores[a]	Outcomes
Allopatch HD, MTF Sports Medicine (human dermis)	Agrawal[30] (2012)	Level IV (case series)	Large and massive or recurrent tears (n = 14)	Arthroscopic, augmentation	14–19	2 (14)	**FLEX-SF** Pre: 53.7 Post: 79.7 **Constant** Pre: 49.7 Post: 81.1	No adverse events reported; scores, pain, strength, and ROM improved; recurrent tears were smaller than preoperative size.
SportMesh, Biomet (polyurethane urea)	Petriccioli et al[36] (2013)	Level IV (case series)	Subscapularis tears: two-thirds to complete tendon (n = 10)	Open, augmentation	12–34	1 (10)	**Constant** Pre: 47 Post: 69	No adverse events reported; scores, pain, and strength improved; 6 excellent, 2 good, and 2 fair results per DASH.
Zimmer Collagen Repair Patch, Zimmer (porcine dermis)	Cho et al[33] (2014)	Level IV (case series)	Massive tears (n = 5)	Mini-open, augmentation	14–27	1 (5)	**UCLA** Pre: 15.4 Post: 31.2 **ASES** Pre: 39.4 Post: 86.4	No adverse events reported; scores and pain improved; 1 partial retear.
Tutopatch,Tutogen Medical GmbH (bovine-derived pericardium); Repol Angimesh, Angiologica B.M. S.r.l. (polypropylene)	Ciampi et al[34] (2014)	Level III (retrospective comparative study)	Massive posterosuperior tears (NA: n = 51; TP: n = 49; RA: n = 52)	Open, augmentation	36	NA: 21 (51) TP: 25 (49) RA: 9 (52)	**UCLA** NA: 14.88 TP: 14.69 RA: 24.61	No adverse events reported; the RA group had significantly better UCLA scores, strength, and ROM at 36 months; the retear rate was significantly lower in the RA group.
X-Repair, Synthasome (poly-L-lactide)	Proctor[37] (2014)	Level IV (case series)	Large or massive tears (n = 18)	Arthroscopic, augmentation	35–47	4 (18)	**ASES** Pre: 26 Post: 70	No adverse events reported; mean ASES score for intact repairs = 82.

A = augmented, ASES = American Shoulder and Elbow Surgeons Subjective Shoulder Scale, Constant = Constant assessment score, DASH = Disabilities of the Arm, Shoulder and Hand questionnaire, FLEX-SF = Flexilevel Scale of Shoulder Function, HD = human dermis, NA = nonaugmented, Pre = preoperative, Post = postoperative, RA = Repol Angimesh, RCR = rotator cuff repair, RCT = randomized controlled trial, ROM = range of motion, Simple Shoulder = Simple Shoulder Test, TP = Tutopatch, UCLA = University of California–Los Angeles Shoulder Rating Scale, US = ultrasound.

[a] American Shoulder and Elbow Surgeons Subjective Shoulder Scale score is measured out of 100 points; Constant assessment score is measured out of 100 points; Flexilevel Scale of Shoulder Function is measured out of 100 points; Simple Shoulder Test is measured out of 12 points; University of California–Los Angeles Shoulder Rating Scale score is measured out of 35 points.

Table 2

Results of Scaffold Devices in Rotator Cuff Repair Interposition

Device (Material)	Authors (Year)[a]	Tear Size (Sample Size)	Scaffold Application Technique	Mean Follow-up	MRI (US) Failure Rate	Mean Scores[b]	Outcomes
GraftJacket, Wright Medical Technology (human dermis)	Dopirak et al[41] (2007); Bond et al[40] (2008)	Massive irreparable tears (n = 16)	Arthroscopic, interposition	12–38 months	3 (16)	**UCLA** Pre: 18.4 Post: 30.4 **Constant** Pre: 53.8 Post: 84	No adverse events reported; scores, pain, strength, and ROM improved; 15 of 16 patients satisfied with outcome; 13 patients had full incorporation of graft into native tissue on MRI.
	Wong et al[46] (2010) (update from Bond et al[40] [2008])	Massive irreparable tears (n = 45)	Arthroscopic, interposition	24–68 months	NR	**UCLA** Pre: 18.4 Post: 27.5 **WORC** Post: 75.2 **ASES** Post: 84.1	Deep wound infection developed in 1 (immunocompromised) patient, which required arthroscopic irrigation as well as débridement and antibiotics; 1 long-term neuropraxia occurred and resolved at 1 year; surgical time noted to be consistently less than 3 hours.
	Gupta et al[42] (2012)	Massive irreparable tears (n = 24)	Mini-open, interposition	29–42 months	5 (19)	**SF-12** Pre: 48.8 Post: 56.8 **ASES** Pre: 66.6 Post: 88.7	No adverse events reported; scores, pain, strength, and ROM improved; all patients satisfied with outcome; no complete retears, only partial retears.
Zimmer Collagen Repair Patch, Zimmer (porcine dermis)	Soler et al[45] (2007)	Massive tears (n = 4)	Open, interposition	3–6 months	4 (4)	NR	Older patient population (71–82 years); graft disruption occurred between 3 and 6 months after surgery in all patients; inflammatory reaction seen in all patients, with graft disintegration and tissue necrosis observed at revision surgery.

ASES = American Shoulder and Elbow Surgeons Subjective Shoulder Scale, Constant = Constant assessment score, LARS = ligament advanced reinforcement system, NR = not reported, Pre = preoperative, Post = postoperative, ROM = range of motion, SF-12 = Medical Outcomes Study 12-Item Short Form, Oxford = Oxford Shoulder Scale, UCLA = University of California–Los Angeles Shoulder Rating Scale, US = ultrasound, WORC = Western Ontario Rotator Cuff Index.

[a]All studies are Level IV (case series).

[b]American Shoulder and Elbow Surgeons Subjective Shoulder Scale score is measured out of 100 points; Constant assessment score is measured out of 100 points; Medical Outcomes Study 12-Item Short Form is measured out of 100 points; Oxford Shoulder Scale is measured out of 60 points; University of California–Los Angeles Shoulder Rating Scale score is measured out of 35 points; Western Ontario Rotator Cuff Index is measured out of 100 points.

Table 2 (continued)
Results of Scaffold Devices in Rotator Cuff Repair Interposition

Device (Material)	Authors (Year)[a]	Tear Size (Sample Size)	Scaffold Application Technique	Mean Follow-up	MRI (US) Failure Rate	Mean Scores[b]	Outcomes
	Badhe et al[39] (2008)	Large or massive tears (n = 10)	Open, interposition	3–5 years	2 (10)	**Constant** Pre: 41 Post: 62	No adverse events reported; scores, pain, ROM, and abduction power improved; 9 of 10 patients satisfied with outcome.
Conexa, Tornier (porcine dermis)	Gupta et al[43] (2013)	Massive irreparable tears (n = 27)	Mini-open, interposition	24–40 months	6 (22)	**SF-12** Pre: 48.4 Post: 56.6 **ASES** Pre: 62.7 Post: 91.8	No adverse events reported; scores, pain, strength, and ROM improved; all but 1 patient satisfied with outcome; 1 complete retear and 5 partial retears.
LARS graft (polyester terephthalate)	Petrie and Ismaiel[44] (2013)	Massive irreparable tears (n = 31)	Open, interposition	24–72 months	NR	**Oxford** Pre: 46.7 Post: 30.6	No adverse events reported; graft not always secured medially to retracted tear stump; lower Oxford score was better; scores and pain improved; 2 revisions with graft failure noted, but other patients were not imaged postoperatively for healing.

ASES = American Shoulder and Elbow Surgeons Subjective Shoulder Scale, Constant = Constant assessment score, LARS = ligament advanced reinforcement system, NR = not reported, Pre = preoperative, Post = postoperative, ROM = range of motion, SF-12 = Medical Outcomes Study 12-Item Short Form, Oxford = Oxford Shoulder Scale, UCLA = University of California—Los Angeles Shoulder Rating Scale, US = ultrasound, WORC = Western Ontario Rotator Cuff Index.

[a]All studies are Level IV (case series).

[b]American Shoulder and Elbow Surgeons Subjective Shoulder Scale score is measured out of 100 points; Constant assessment score is measured out of 100 points; Medical Outcomes Study 12-Item Short Form is measured out of 100 points; Oxford Shoulder Scale is measured out of 60 points; University of California—Los Angeles Shoulder Rating Scale score is measured out of 35 points; Western Ontario Rotator Cuff Index is measured out of 100 points.

crest bone marrow-derived MSCs were compared with 45 patients who underwent repair alone, including MRI evaluation at 3 months, 6 months, 1 year, 2 years, and a minimum 10-year follow-up. MSCs were injected after repair into both the repaired tendon and the bone at the repair footprint. Healing rates at 6 months postoperatively were significantly higher in the MSC group compared with the control group (100% versus 67%, respectively), and the durability of the repair was significantly higher in the MSC group compared with the control group at a minimum 10-year follow-up (87% versus 44% intact repairs, respectively).

Conclusions

Several augmentation strategies are clinically available for use in rotator cuff repair; however, limited clinical evidence exists to demonstrate their efficacy in improving healing rates as well as patient functional outcomes and their appropriate surgical indications. The effectiveness of a particular augmentation product depends on the manner in which it is applied, formulated, and delivered, and it may be possible that certain products are efficacious for particular patient populations and/or surgical indications but not for others. Further investigation on the mechanism of action, safety, surgical application, and appropriate indications of these devices is necessary to optimize their use. Combination therapies also may hold promise.

Tendon Transfers

Decision making in the setting of massive rotator cuff tears often is convoluted. Healing is a major topic of discussion, research, and investigation; although healing is considered

important, the literature reports that some patients have good outcomes after a rotator cuff repair in the absence of anatomic healing.[16,72,73] Most clinicians agree that some patients do not have good outcomes after rotator cuff repair for several reasons, including stiffness or loss of balance between posterior and anterior force vectors, which allows for loss of containment within the coracoacromial arch and relative instability. Younger patients tolerate this very poorly because many of these patients have high activity expectations and notice a loss of strength in both work and recreational activities. A reverse shoulder replacement is an established option for the treatment of massive, irreparable tears; patients who are not indicated for reverse shoulder replacement should be considered as appropriate candidates for a muscle transfer procedure. Historically, latissimus dorsi transfers have been the transfer of choice for the treatment of massive rotator cuff tears.[74-77] More recently, transfer of the lower trapezius has been used and offers some advantages.[78] Long-term outcomes are forthcoming because lower trapezius transfer is a relatively new procedure.

Indications for Muscle Transfer

Relative Indications

Most patients who are indicated for muscle transfers are younger than 60 years. Although there is no specific age delineation, patients indicated for a reverse shoulder replacement should be at least 65 years old. Chronologic age should not be the only determinant because some patients may be good candidates based on physiologic age and activity considerations. In general, patients who are still of working age have activity demands that make

reverse shoulder replacement less desirable. Importantly, a muscle transfer will not restore enough strength to maintain a manual labor job that requires frequent heavy lifting; therefore, activity requirements should be considered preoperatively. Patient compliance also is a factor because the rehabilitation is a long process, and it generally takes a full year to reach maximal medical improvement after a muscle transfer.

Range of motion also is an important consideration. Experts vary in opinion, but, in general, most agree that a muscle transfer is more effective at restoring external rotation power and augmenting overhead elevation by alleviating pain. Therefore, careful consideration should be given to patients who have true pseudoparalysis because they may be better served with arthroplasty. In the opinion of the authors of this chapter, a patient should be able to reach 90° of elevation to be a candidate for a muscle transfer.

Absolute Indications

Absolute indications include a painful posterosuperior rotator cuff tear that involves the supraspinatus only or both the supraspinatus and the infraspinatus and that is not repairable and not responsive to nonsurgical treatment, such as injections and physical therapy. The reparability of a tear is based on MRI or ultrasound findings of massive size with retraction and muscle degeneration, such as atrophy and fatty degeneration. A transfer can be performed in the primary setting, but failure of a previous attempt at repair is very common. The deltoid muscle should be intact and functioning because loss of deltoid function is a bad prognosticator of outcome. An intact subscapularis is important for a satisfactory outcome. Advanced arthritic changes are a contraindication for a muscle transfer; however, a muscle transfer can be performed in patients who have mild, early arthritic changes.

Latissimus Dorsi Transfer

Transfer of the latissimus dorsi tendon is usually performed with the patient placed in the lateral decubitus position. The tendon is harvested from the posterior approach, and a second incision is made over the lateral shoulder to secure the tendon to the greater tuberosity. Previous sutures and anchors should be removed to provide a surface for tendon healing that is as clean as possible. Some techniques describe harvest of the latissimus dorsi tendon alone, whereas others describe harvest of the latissimus dorsi and the teres major together.[79] The insertion sites of these muscles vary; most have a separate insertion for each muscle, whereas some have a confluent insertion that is composed of both muscles and tendons. The theoretic advantage of harvesting both is increased strength; however, this has not been demonstrated definitively. The disadvantage of harvesting both is that the teres major has a shorter excursion and can tether the transfer.

Outcomes for muscle transfer procedures may be difficult to interpret. In general, studies report a 60% to 80% satisfaction rate.[74,76,77,80,81] Constant assessment scores are rarely higher than 75. The techniques, patient characteristics, and indications for surgery vary greatly; however, surgeons agree that results are better in patients who have an intact subscapularis, and that an intact and functioning teres minor also positively affects the final results.

Trapezius Transfer

A lower trapezius transfer was originally described to treat brachial plexus injuries, particularly those of the upper trunk.[82,83] The original technique has been modified and used to treat massive rotator cuff tears. The trapezius transfer offers the advantage of firing in phase with the rotator cuff, and patients can be easily taught to recruit this muscle in shoulder elevation. The disadvantage of trapezius transfer is that the excursion of the tendon-muscle unit is limited, so a bridge graft is necessary to attach the lower trapezius to the greater tuberosity.

The procedure is performed with the patient placed in the lateral decubitus position. The lower trapezius is harvested via an incision adjacent to the medial border of the scapula. The raphe between the lower and middle trapezius is identified to preserve the middle and upper trapezius because they are necessary to maintain normal shoulder kinematics. The authors of this chapter use an Achilles tendon allograft to bridge the gap to the greater tuberosity. The plane superficial to the infraspinatus and deep to the deltoid is developed to facilitate the transfer. The distal end of the graft is attached to the greater tuberosity with the use of anchors. On occasion in a revision surgery, the greater tuberosity may have poor bone stock because of previous anchor placement. In this situation, the authors of this chapter pass the sutures through the humeral head from anterior to posterior with the use of a Beath needle and tie the sutures over a button.

Arthroplasty for Rotator Cuff Tears

Massive rotator cuff tears with arthritis, cuff tear arthropathy, and failed massive irreparable rotator cuff repairs remain challenging diagnoses in shoulder surgery. Arthroplasty treatment options include hemiarthroplasty (stemmed or resurfacing), anatomic total shoulder arthroplasty (if the rotator cuff is considered repairable—although this is rare), and reverse total shoulder arthroplasty (RTSA). Selection of the appropriate arthroplasty option involves a thorough understanding of the patient's age, the patient's activity level, the physical examination, and the technical aspects and complications related to each specific arthroplasty option.

Patient Characteristics

A patient's age and activity level play a substantial role in selection of the appropriate arthroplasty option. Patients who are younger than 50 years are typically best treated with anatomic arthroplasty options. Although these recommendations are a guideline, exceptions may always occur. In general, if a patient has forward elevation greater than 90°, results will be excellent; this was demonstrated in a study by Goldberg et al[84] that reported excellent results in 14 of 16 patients who were treated with hemiarthroplasty. Long-term concerns for complications of RTSA make hemiarthroplasty an attractive option for younger patients; however, this is counterbalanced by the high failure rate of hemiarthroplasty, with ongoing reports of pain and failure to improve active function if preoperative range of motion is less than 90° (especially in patients who have true pseudoparalysis).

To determine the best surgical option, the surgeon also must consider the patient's activity level. Very few data currently exist to guide surgeons; however, a shoulder activity level scale has been developed to determine shoulder activity norms based on patient age and sex.[85,86] For example, rotator cuff disease and instability are associated with higher activity levels compared with osteoarthritis. Although these data exist, they have not been incorporated in the current literature.

Physical Examination

A thorough physical examination is critical to selection of the appropriate shoulder arthroplasty option. Prior surgical procedures also will influence selection. As previously discussed, the preservation of active forward elevation is a key determinant of outcomes.[84] In addition, subscapularis and teres minor function should be carefully evaluated because the failure of either muscle has been reported to lead to poorer results if hemiarthroplasty is performed.[87,88]

Resurfacing/ Hemiarthroplasty

Resurfacing arthroplasty is attractive because of its bone-preserving potential. Although resurfacing arthroplasty has always been lauded as an advantageous procedure, few studies currently exist to support this claim. Boileau et al[89] reported poorer results in patients who underwent revision of failed arthroplasty to RTSA. A recent study reported good results for hemiarthroplasty at a short-term follow-up (mean, 38 months), with 19 of 24 patients satisfied or very satisfied.[87] This study reported that the preoperative assessment of teres minor function had a direct correlation with postoperative patient satisfaction, external rotation strength, and function. Patients with severe preoperative subscapularis dysfunction (n = 3) had poorer outcomes than those with intact or partially intact tendons. Technical pearls of the study included placing the resurfacing arthroplasty in more valgus alignment to cover the humeral surface. With

longer follow-up, however, Levy and Copeland[90] reported that stemless resurfacing arthroplasty results were much poorer in patients who had cuff tear arthropathy compared with those who had osteoarthritis. The adjusted Constant assessment scores of patients who had cuff tear arthropathy were 61.3%, and those of patients who had osteoarthritis were 93.7%. In a study of 33 shoulders in 33 patients who underwent stemmed hemiarthroplasty for the treatment of cuff tear arthropathy, Sanchez-Sotelo et al[91] reported that, at a mean 5-year follow-up (range, 2 to 11 years), satisfactory outcomes were achieved in only 67% of the patients, with persistent pain, decreased functional improvement, and anterosuperior instability being the most common complications reported.[91]

Reverse Total Shoulder Replacement

Reverse shoulder replacement has dramatically changed the treatment options and potential outcomes for patients who have cuff tear arthropathy. As previously mentioned, the use of hemiarthroplasty and resurfacing arthroplasty led to variable outcomes, especially for pain relief and functional gains. Conversely, RTSA leads to fairly predictable pain relief and improved active range of motion. The classic indications for RTSA include stage IV and stage V Hamada disease; however, the indications have expanded substantially in the past decade.[92]

Patients younger than 65 years who undergo RTSA must be advised that the results may be quite good, but that the complication rate is higher compared with older patients. In a cohort study of 46 shoulders in 41 patients who underwent RTSA, Ek et al[93] reported

significantly improved pain scores, forward elevation, and strength at a 5- to 15-year follow-up; however, at least one or more complications occurred in 15 shoulders (37.5%), and six failures required conversion to hemiarthroplasty. In addition, 10 shoulders (25%) required partial or total component exchange, conversion to hemiarthroplasty, or removal. In a study of 60 shoulders in 60 patients who underwent RTSA, Frankle et al[94] reported that, at a minimum follow-up of 2 years, 57 of 60 patients were satisfied with the procedure; however, 17% of patients had at least one complication. In addition, eight patients had failed procedures (12%), five of whom required revision to another RTSA (one patient had two revisions) and two of whom required conversion to hemiarthroplasty.[94]

Hemiarthroplasty Versus RTSA

Several recent studies have compared hemiarthroplasty with RTSA, and concluded that RTSA is typically favored over hemiarthroplasty. In a study of the New Zealand Joint Registry that compared 102 hemiarthroplasty procedures with 102 RTSA procedures, Young et al[95] reported that patients who underwent RTSA had improved outcome scores that were maintained 5 years after surgery. The authors reported no difference in shoulders that required revision surgery during the study period (nine hemiarthroplasty and five RTSA). Similarly, in a study of 20 hemiarthroplasty and 36 RTSA procedures, Leung et al[96] reported that the results of RTSA were superior with respect to Shoulder Pain and Disability Index scores and active forward elevation. Cost-effectiveness studies have become increasingly important because they demonstrate that the costs of intervention are worth the value they provide for patients. Several recent studies have reported that, despite the high costs, RTSA is cost effective compared with hemiarthroplasty.[97,98]

Summary

Many advanced surgical techniques can facilitate the sound repair of massive rotator cuff tears, and, historically, many of these techniques result in good outcomes. Muscle transfer is an option for patients who have an irreparable rotator cuff tear and is often used in patients younger than 60 years, especially in the revision setting. Early results of muscle transfers are promising, and new muscle transfers have expanded the list of treatment options. Since its inception, reverse shoulder arthroplasty has been a reliable treatment option for patients with rotator cuff tears who did not previously have a satisfactory treatment option. Research in tendon biology is advancing rapidly. The introduction of new methodologies to treat degenerated tendon and muscle will likely occur in the next several years.

References

1. Gerber C, Fuchs B, Hodler J: The results of repair of massive tears of the rotator cuff. *J Bone Joint Surg Am* 2000;82(4):505-515.

2. Cofield RH, Parvizi J, Hoffmeyer PJ, Lanzer WL, Ilstrup DM, Rowland CM: Surgical repair of chronic rotator cuff tears: A prospective long-term study. *J Bone Joint Surg Am* 2001;83(1):71-77.

3. Denard PJ, Jiwani AZ, Lädermann A, Burkhart SS: Long-term outcome of arthroscopic massive rotator cuff repair: The importance of double-row fixation. *Arthroscopy* 2012;28(7):909-915.

4. Lo IK, Burkhart SS: Arthroscopic repair of massive, contracted, immobile rotator cuff tears using single and double interval slides: Technique and preliminary results. *Arthroscopy* 2004;20(1):22-33.

5. Lo IK, Burkhart SS: The interval slide in continuity: A method of mobilizing the anterosuperior rotator cuff without disrupting the tear margins. *Arthroscopy* 2004;20(4):435-441.

6. Lo IK, Burkhart SS: The comma sign: An arthroscopic guide to the torn subscapularis tendon. *Arthroscopy* 2003;19(3):334-337.

7. Lo IK, Parten PM, Burkhart SS: Combined subcoracoid and subacromial impingement in association with anterosuperior rotator cuff tears: An arthroscopic approach. *Arthroscopy* 2003;19(10):1068-1078.

8. Richards DP, Burkhart SS, Lo IK: Subscapularis tears: Arthroscopic repair techniques. *Orthop Clin North Am* 2003;34(4):485-498.

9. Burkhart SS, Lo IKY, Brady PC, Denard PJ: *The Cowboy's Companion: A Trail Guide for the Arthroscopic Shoulder Surgeon*. Philadelphia, PA, Lippincott, Williams & Wilkins, 2012.

10. Denard PJ, Burkhart SS: Medialization of the subscapularis footprint does not affect functional outcome of arthroscopic repair. *Arthroscopy* 2012;28(11):1608-1614.

11. Davidson J, Burkhart SS: The geometric classification of rotator cuff tears: A system linking tear pattern to treatment and prognosis. *Arthroscopy* 2010;26(3):417-424.

12. Burkhart SS, Athanasiou KA, Wirth MA: Margin convergence: A method of reducing strain in massive rotator cuff tears. *Arthroscopy* 1996;12(3):335-338.

13. Burkhart SS, Denard PJ, Konicek J, Hanypsiak BT: Biomechanical validation of load-sharing rip-stop fixation for the repair of tissue-deficient rotator cuff tears. *Am J Sports Med* 2014;42(2):457-462.

14. Tashjian RZ, Hollins AM, Kim HM, et al: Factors affecting healing rates after arthroscopic double-row rotator cuff repair. *Am J Sports Med* 2010;38(12):2435-2442.

15. Toussaint B, Schnaser E, Bosley J, Lefebvre Y, Gobezie R: Early structural and functional outcomes for arthroscopic double-row transosseous-equivalent rotator cuff repair. *Am J Sports Med* 2011;39(6):1217-1225.

16. Galatz LM, Ball CM, Teefey SA, Middleton WD, Yamaguchi K: The outcome and repair integrity of completely arthroscopically repaired large and massive rotator cuff tears. *J Bone Joint Surg Am* 2004;86(2):219-224.

17. Harryman DT II, Mack LA, Wang KY, Jackins SE, Richardson ML, Matsen FA III: Repairs of the rotator cuff: Correlation of functional results with integrity of the cuff. *J Bone Joint Surg Am* 1991;73(7):982-989.

18. Zumstein MA, Jost B, Hempel J, Hodler J, Gerber C: The clinical and structural long-term results of open repair of massive tears of the rotator cuff. *J Bone Joint Surg Am* 2008;90(11):2423-2431.

19. Bishop J, Klepps S, Lo IK, Bird J, Gladstone JN, Flatow EL: Cuff integrity after arthroscopic versus open rotator cuff repair: A prospective study. *J Shoulder Elbow Surg* 2006;15(3):290-299.

20. Boileau P, Brassart N, Watkinson DJ, Carles M, Hatzidakis AM, Krishnan SG: Arthroscopic repair of full-thickness tears of the supraspinatus: Does the tendon really heal? *J Bone Joint Surg Am* 2005;87(6):1229-1240.

21. Duquin TR, Buyea C, Bisson LJ: Which method of rotator cuff repair leads to the highest rate of structural healing? A systematic review. *Am J Sports Med* 2010;38(4):835-841.

22. Derwin KA, Kovacevic D, Kim MS, Ricchetti ET: Biologic augmentation of rotator cuff healing, in Nicholson GP, ed: *Orthopaedic Knowledge Update: Shoulder and Elbow*, ed 4. Rosemont, IL, American Academy of Orthopaedic Surgeons, 2013, pp 31-44.

23. Derwin KA, Badylak SF, Steinmann SP, Iannotti JP: Extracellular matrix scaffold devices for rotator cuff repair. *J Shoulder Elbow Surg* 2010;19(3):467-476.

24. Ricchetti ET, Aurora A, Iannotti JP, Derwin KA: Scaffold devices for rotator cuff repair. *J Shoulder Elbow Surg* 2012;21(2):251-265.

25. Iannotti JP, Deutsch A, Green A, et al: Time to failure after rotator cuff repair: A prospective imaging study. *J Bone Joint Surg Am* 2013;95(11):965-971.

26. McCarron JA, Derwin KA, Bey MJ, et al: Failure with continuity in rotator cuff repair "healing." *Am J Sports Med* 2013;41(1):134-141.

27. Badylak SF, Freytes DO, Gilbert TW: Extracellular matrix as a biological scaffold material: Structure and function. *Acta Biomater* 2009;5(1):1-13.

28. Reing JE, Zhang L, Myers-Irvin J, et al: Degradation products of extracellular matrix affect cell migration and proliferation. *Tissue Eng Part A* 2009;15(3):605-614.

29. Sahoo S, Greeson CB, McCarron JA, et al: Effect of pretension and suture needle type on mechanical properties of acellular human dermis patches for rotator cuff repair. *J Shoulder Elbow Surg* 2012;21(10):1413-1421.

30. Agrawal V: Healing rates for challenging rotator cuff tears utilizing an acellular human dermal reinforcement graft. *Int J Shoulder Surg* 2012;6(2):36-44.

31. Barber FA, Burns JP, Deutsch A, Labbé MR, Litchfield RB: A prospective, randomized evaluation of acellular human dermal matrix augmentation for arthroscopic rotator cuff repair. *Arthroscopy* 2012;28(1):8-15.

32. Burkhead WZ, Schiffern SC, Krishnan SG: Use of GraftJacket as an augmentation for massive rotator cuff tears. *Seminars in Arthroplasty* 2007;18(1):11-18.

33. Cho CH, Lee SM, Lee YK, Shin HK: Mini-open suture bridge repair with porcine dermal patch augmentation for massive rotator cuff tear: Surgical technique and preliminary results. *Clin Orthop Surg* 2014;6(3):329-335.

34. Ciampi P, Scotti C, Nonis A, et al: The benefit of synthetic versus biological patch augmentation in the repair of posterosuperior massive rotator cuff tears: A 3-year follow-up study. *Am J Sports Med* 2014;42(5):1169-1175.

35. Encalada-Diaz I, Cole BJ, Macgillivray JD, et al: Rotator cuff repair augmentation using a novel polycarbonate polyurethane patch: Preliminary results at 12 months' follow-up. *J Shoulder Elbow Surg* 2011;20(5):788-794.

36. Petriccioli D, Bertone C, Marchi G, Mujahed I: Open repair of isolated traumatic subscapularis tendon tears with a synthetic soft tissue reinforcement. *Musculoskelet Surg* 2013; 97(suppl 1):63-68.

37. Proctor CS: Long-term successful arthroscopic repair of large and massive rotator cuff tears with a functional and degradable reinforcement device. *J Shoulder Elbow Surg* 2014;23(10):1508-1513.

38. Rotini R, Marinelli A, Guerra E, et al: Human dermal matrix scaffold augmentation for large and massive rotator cuff repairs: Preliminary clinical and MRI results at 1-year follow-up. *Musculoskelet Surg* 2011;95(suppl 1): S13-S23.

39. Badhe SP, Lawrence TM, Smith FD, Lunn PG: An assessment of porcine dermal xenograft as an augmentation graft in the treatment of extensive rotator cuff tears. *J Shoulder Elbow Surg* 2008;17(1, suppl):35S-39S.

40. Bond JL, Dopirak RM, Higgins J, Burns J, Snyder SJ: Arthroscopic replacement of massive, irreparable rotator cuff tears using a GraftJacket allograft: Technique and preliminary results. *Arthroscopy* 2008;24(4): 403.e1-409.e8.

41. Dopirak R, Bond JL, Snyder SJ: Arthroscopic total rotator cuff replacement with an acellular human dermal allograft matrix. *Int J Shoulder Surg* 2007;1(1):7-15.

42. Gupta AK, Hug K, Berkoff DJ, et al: Dermal tissue allograft for the repair of massive irreparable rotator cuff tears. *Am J Sports Med* 2012;40(1):141-147.

43. Gupta AK, Hug K, Boggess B, Gavigan M, Toth AP: Massive or 2-tendon rotator cuff tears in active patients with minimal glenohumeral arthritis: Clinical and radiographic outcomes of reconstruction using dermal tissue matrix xenograft. *Am J Sports Med* 2013;41(4):872-879.

44. Petrie MJ, Ismaiel AH: Treatment of massive rotator-cuff tears with a polyester ligament (LARS) patch. *Acta Orthop Belg* 2013;79(6):620-625.

45. Soler JA, Gidwani S, Curtis MJ: Early complications from the use of porcine dermal collagen implants (Permacol) as bridging constructs in the repair of massive rotator cuff tears: A report of 4 cases. *Acta Orthop Belg* 2007;73(4):432-436.

46. Wong I, Burns J, Snyder S: Arthroscopic GraftJacket repair of rotator cuff tears. *J Shoulder Elbow Surg* 2010;19(2, suppl):104-109.

47. Iannotti JP, Codsi MJ, Kwon YW, Derwin K, Ciccone J, Brems JJ: Porcine small intestine submucosa augmentation of surgical repair of chronic two-tendon rotator cuff tears: A randomized, controlled trial. *J Bone Joint Surg Am* 2006;88(6):1238-1244.

48. Malcarney HL, Bonar F, Murrell GA: Early inflammatory reaction after rotator cuff repair with a porcine small intestine submucosal implant: A report of 4 cases. *Am J Sports Med* 2005;33(6):907-911.

49. Walton JR, Bowman NK, Khatib Y, Linklater J, Murrell GA: Restore orthobiologic implant: Not recommended for augmentation of rotator cuff repairs. *J Bone Joint Surg Am* 2007;89(4):786-791.

50. Pedowitz RA, Yamaguchi K, Ahmad CS, et al: Optimizing the management of rotator cuff problems. *J Am Acad Orthop Surg* 2011;19(6):368-379.

51. Hall MP, Band PA, Meislin RJ, Jazrawi LM, Cardone DA: Platelet-rich plasma: Current concepts and application in sports medicine. *J Am Acad Orthop Surg* 2009;17(10):602-608.

52. Kobayashi M, Itoi E, Minagawa H, et al: Expression of growth factors in the early phase of supraspinatus tendon healing in rabbits. *J Shoulder Elbow Surg* 2006;15(3):371-377.

53. Thomopoulos S, Hattersley G, Rosen V, et al: The localized expression of extracellular matrix components in healing tendon insertion sites: An in situ hybridization study. *J Orthop Res* 2002;20(3):454-463.

54. Castillo TN, Pouliot MA, Kim HJ, Dragoo JL: Comparison of growth factor and platelet concentration from commercial platelet-rich plasma separation systems. *Am J Sports Med* 2011;39(2):266-271.

55. Mazzocca AD, McCarthy MB, Chowaniec DM, et al: Platelet-rich plasma differs according to preparation method and human variability. *J Bone Joint Surg Am* 2012;94(4):308-316.

56. Boswell SG, Cole BJ, Sundman EA, Karas V, Fortier LA: Platelet-rich plasma: A milieu of bioactive factors. *Arthroscopy* 2012;28(3):429-439.

57. Antuña S, Barco R, Martínez Diez JM, Sánchez Márquez JM: Platelet-rich fibrin in arthroscopic repair of massive rotator cuff tears: A prospective randomized pilot clinical trial. *Acta Orthop Belg* 2013;79(1):25-30.

58. Barber FA, Hrnack SA, Snyder SJ, Hapa O: Rotator cuff repair healing influenced by platelet-rich plasma construct augmentation. *Arthroscopy* 2011;27(8):1029-1035.

59. Bergeson AG, Tashjian RZ, Greis PE, Crim J, Stoddard GJ, Burks RT: Effects of platelet-rich fibrin matrix on repair integrity of at-risk rotator cuff tears. *Am J Sports Med* 2012;40(2):286-293.

60. Castricini R, Longo UG, De Benedetto M, et al: Platelet-rich plasma augmentation for arthroscopic rotator cuff repair: A randomized controlled trial. *Am J Sports Med* 2011;39(2):258-265.

61. Charousset C, Zaoui A, Bellaïche L, Piterman M: Does autologous leukocyte-platelet-rich plasma improve tendon healing in arthroscopic repair of large or massive rotator cuff tears? *Arthroscopy* 2014;30(4):428-435.

62. Gumina S, Campagna V, Ferrazza G, et al: Use of platelet-leukocyte membrane in arthroscopic repair of large rotator cuff tears: A prospective randomized study. *J Bone Joint Surg Am* 2012;94(15):1345-1352.

63. Jo CH, Kim JE, Yoon KS, et al: Does platelet-rich plasma accelerate recovery after rotator cuff repair? A prospective cohort study. *Am J Sports Med* 2011;39(10):2082-2090.

64. Jo CH, Shin JS, Lee YG, et al: Platelet-rich plasma for arthroscopic repair of large to massive rotator cuff tears: A randomized, single-blind, parallel-group trial. *Am J Sports Med* 2013;41(10):2240-2248.

65. Malavolta EA, Gracitelli ME, Ferreira Neto AA, Assunção JH, Bordalo-Rodrigues M, de Camargo OP: Platelet-rich plasma in rotator cuff repair: A prospective randomized study. *Am J Sports Med* 2014;42(10):2446-2454.

66. Randelli P, Arrigoni P, Ragone V, Aliprandi A, Cabitza P: Platelet rich plasma in arthroscopic rotator cuff repair: A prospective RCT study, 2-year follow-up. *J Shoulder Elbow Surg* 2011;20(4):518-528.

67. Rodeo SA, Delos D, Williams RJ, Adler RS, Pearle A, Warren RF: The effect of platelet-rich fibrin matrix on rotator cuff tendon healing: A prospective, randomized clinical study. *Am J Sports Med* 2012;40(6):1234-1241.

68. Ruiz-Moneo P, Molano-Muñoz J, Prieto E, Algorta J: Plasma rich in growth factors in arthroscopic rotator cuff repair: A randomized, double-blind, controlled clinical trial. *Arthroscopy* 2013;29(1):2-9.

69. Weber SC, Kauffman JI, Parise C, Weber SJ, Katz SD: Platelet-rich fibrin matrix in the management of arthroscopic repair of the rotator cuff: A prospective, randomized, double-blinded study. *Am J Sports Med* 2013;41(2):263-270.

70. Zhao JG, Zhao L, Jiang YX, Wang ZL, Wang J, Zhang P: Platelet-rich plasma in arthroscopic rotator cuff repair: A meta-analysis of randomized controlled trials. *Arthroscopy* 2015;31(1):125-135.

71. Hernigou P, Flouzat Lachaniette CH, Delambre J, et al: Biologic augmentation of rotator cuff repair with mesenchymal stem cells during arthroscopy improves healing and prevents further tears: A case-controlled study. *Int Orthop* 2014;38(9):1811-1818.

72. Charousset C, Bellaïche L, Kalra K, Petrover D: Arthroscopic repair of full-thickness rotator cuff tears: Is there tendon healing in patients aged 65 years or older? *Arthroscopy* 2010;26(3):302-309.

73. Gulotta LV, Nho SJ, Dodson CC, et al: Prospective evaluation of arthroscopic rotator cuff repairs at 5 years: Part I—functional outcomes and radiographic healing rates. *J Shoulder Elbow Surg* 2011;20(6):934-940.

74. Gerber C, Rahm SA, Catanzaro S, Farshad M, Moor BK: Latissimus dorsi tendon transfer for treatment of irreparable posterosuperior rotator cuff tears: Long-term results at a minimum follow-up of ten years. *J Bone Joint Surg Am* 2013;95(21):1920-1926.

75. Oh JH, Tilan J, Chen YJ, Chung KC, McGarry MH, Lee TQ: Biomechanical effect of latissimus dorsi tendon transfer for irreparable massive cuff tear. *J Shoulder Elbow Surg* 2013;22(2):150-157.

76. Henseler JF, Nagels J, Nelissen RG, de Groot JH: Does the latissimus dorsi tendon transfer for massive rotator cuff tears remain active postoperatively and restore active external rotation? *J Shoulder Elbow Surg* 2014;23(4):553-560.

77. Nové-Josserand L, Costa P, Liotard JP, Safar JF, Walch G, Zilber S: Results of latissimus dorsi tendon transfer for irreparable cuff tears. *Orthop Traumatol Surg Res* 2009;95(2):108-113.

78. Omid R, Lee B: Tendon transfers for irreparable rotator cuff tears. *J Am Acad Orthop Surg* 2013;21(8):492-501.

79. Wang AA, Strauch RJ, Flatow EL, Bigliani LU, Rosenwasser MP: The teres major muscle: An anatomic study of its use as a tendon transfer. *J Shoulder Elbow Surg* 1999;8(4):334-338.

80. Birmingham PM, Neviaser RJ: Outcome of latissimus dorsi transfer as a salvage procedure for failed rotator cuff repair with loss of elevation. *J Shoulder Elbow Surg* 2008;17(6):871-874.

81. Gerber C, Wirth SH, Farshad M: Treatment options for massive rotator cuff tears. *J Shoulder Elbow Surg* 2011;20(2, suppl):S20-S29.

82. Elhassan B: Lower trapezius transfer for shoulder external rotation in patients with paralytic shoulder. *J Hand Surg Am* 2014;39(3):556-562.

83. Elhassan B, Bishop AT, Hartzler RU, Shin AY, Spinner RJ: Tendon transfer options about the shoulder in patients with brachial plexus injury. *J Bone Joint Surg Am* 2012;94(15):1391-1398.

84. Goldberg SS, Bell JE, Kim HJ, Bak SF, Levine WN, Bigliani LU: Hemiarthroplasty for the rotator cuff-deficient shoulder. *J Bone Joint Surg Am* 2008;90(3):554-559.

85. Brophy RH, Lin K, Smith MV: The role of activity level in orthopaedics: An important prognostic and outcome variable. *J Am Acad Orthop Surg* 2014;22(7):430-436.

86. Hepper CT, Smith MV, Steger-May K, Brophy RH: Normative data of shoulder activity level by age and sex. *Am J Sports Med* 2013;41(5):1146-1151.

87. Pape G, Bruckner T, Loew M, Zeifang F: Treatment of severe cuff tear arthropathy with the humeral head resurfacing arthroplasty: Two-year minimum follow-up. *J Shoulder Elbow Surg* 2013;22(1):e1-e7.

88. Simovitch RW, Helmy N, Zumstein MA, Gerber C: Impact of fatty infiltration of the teres minor muscle on the outcome of reverse total shoulder arthroplasty. *J Bone Joint Surg Am* 2007;89(5):934-939.

89. Boileau P, Watkinson D, Hatzidakis AM, Hovorka I: Neer Award 2005: The Grammont reverse shoulder prosthesis. Results in cuff tear arthritis, fracture sequelae, and revision arthroplasty. *J Shoulder Elbow Surg* 2006;15(5):527-540.

90. Levy O, Copeland SA: Cementless surface replacement arthroplasty of the shoulder: 5- to 10-year results with the Copeland mark-2 prosthesis. *J Bone Joint Surg Br* 2001;83(2):213-221.

91. Sanchez-Sotelo J, Cofield RH, Rowland CM: Shoulder hemiarthroplasty for glenohumeral arthritis associated with severe rotator cuff deficiency. *J Bone Joint Surg Am* 2001;83(12):1814-1822.

92. Hamada K, Fukuda H, Mikasa M, Kobayashi Y: Roentgenographic findings in massive rotator cuff tears: A long-term observation. *Clin Orthop Relat Res* 1990;254:92-96.

93. Ek ET, Neukom L, Catanzaro S, Gerber C: Reverse total shoulder arthroplasty for massive irreparable rotator cuff tears in patients younger than 65 years old: Results after five to fifteen years. *J Shoulder Elbow Surg* 2013;22(9):1199-1208.

94. Frankle M, Levy JC, Pupello D, et al: The reverse shoulder prosthesis for glenohumeral arthritis associated with severe rotator cuff deficiency: A minimum two-year follow-up study of sixty patients surgical technique. *J Bone Joint Surg Am* 2006; 88(suppl 1 pt 2):178-190.

95. Young SW, Zhu M, Walker CG, Poon PC: Comparison of functional outcomes of reverse shoulder arthroplasty with those of hemiarthroplasty in the treatment of cuff-tear arthropathy: A matched-pair analysis. *J Bone Joint Surg Am* 2013;95(10):910-915.

96. Leung B, Horodyski M, Struk AM, Wright TW: Functional outcome of hemiarthroplasty compared with reverse total shoulder arthroplasty in the treatment of rotator cuff tear arthropathy. *J Shoulder Elbow Surg* 2012;21(3):319-323.

97. Coe MP, Greiwe RM, Joshi R, et al: The cost-effectiveness of reverse total shoulder arthroplasty compared with hemiarthroplasty for rotator cuff tear arthropathy. *J Shoulder Elbow Surg* 2012;21(10):1278-1288.

98. Renfree KJ, Hattrup SJ, Chang YH: Cost utility analysis of reverse total shoulder arthroplasty. *J Shoulder Elbow Surg* 2013;22(12):1656-1661.

Shoulder Arthroplasty: Key Steps to Improve Outcomes and Minimize Complications

Emilie V. Cheung, MD
Roberto Diaz, MD
George S. Athwal, MD, FRCSC
Joaquin Sanchez-Sotelo, MD, PhD
John W. Sperling, MD, MBA

Abstract

Advances in shoulder replacement surgery have allowed for the successful treatment of various shoulder conditions. As the elderly population increases and the surgical indications for shoulder replacement surgery continue to expand, the number of shoulder replacements performed annually will continue to increase. Accordingly, the number of complications also will be expected to increase. Successful shoulder replacement outcomes require surgeons to have a thorough understanding of the surgical indications, surgical technique, and potential complications of the procedure. By reviewing the key aspects of shoulder replacement surgery and focusing on the surgical technique and common complications for both anatomic and reverse total shoulder arthroplasty, surgeons can help improve outcomes and minimize complications.

Instr Course Lect 2016;65:109–126.

Advances in shoulder replacement surgery have enabled orthopaedic surgeons to successfully treat various shoulder conditions by alleviating pain and restoring function. As the elderly population increases, the number of shoulder

replacement surgeries performed annually continues to increase. Between 2000 and 2008, the number of shoulder arthroplasties performed annually in the United States increased 2.5-fold and coincided with an 11% increase in the elderly population.[1] As shoulder replacement surgeries increase, the number of complications related to shoulder replacement surgery also is expected to increase. Shoulder replacement surgery is a technically demanding procedure and successful outcomes are dependent on several factors, including proper patient selection, surgical technique, and rehabilitation. Surgeons who have a thorough understanding of the surgical indications, the surgical technique, and the potential complications that may arise before, during, and after shoulder replacement surgery can help improve outcomes and minimize complications.

Surgical Technique

Successful outcomes in shoulder replacement surgery are highly dependent

Dr. Athwal or an immediate family member has received royalties from Imascap; serves as a paid consultant to or is an employee of DePuy, Smith & Nephew, and Tornier; and has received research or institutional support from DePuy, Exactech, Smith & Nephew, Tornier, and Zimmer. Dr. Sanchez-Sotelo or an immediate family member has received royalties from Stryker; has received research or institutional support from Biomet, Stryker, DePuy, and Zimmer; and serves as a board member, owner, officer, or committee member of the American Academy of Orthopaedic Surgeons International Committee and the American Shoulder and Elbow Surgeons. Dr. Sperling or an immediate family member has received royalties from Biomet and DJ Orthopaedics, and serves as a paid consultant to or is an employee of Tornier. Dr. Cheung or an immediate family member serves as a paid consultant to or is an employee of Exactech, and serves as a board member, owner, officer, or committee member of the American Academy of Orthopaedic Surgeons. Neither Dr. Diaz nor any immediate family member has received anything of value from or has stock or stock options held in a commercial company or institution related directly or indirectly to the subject of this chapter.

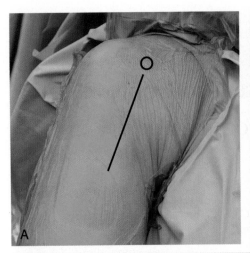

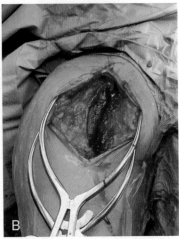

Figure 1   Intraoperative photographs show the planned incision (solid line) for the deltopectoral approach (**A**) and the deltopectoral interval with the cephalic vein shifted laterally (**B**). The circle in panel **A** represents the Mohrenheim fossa.

on surgical exposure. Adequate exposure facilitates humeral and glenoid preparation and allows for proper component placement. A general anesthetic with or without regional anesthesia is administered. The patient is placed in the beach-chair position at a 30° to 45° incline, and an arm-holder device may be used to facilitate intraoperative positioning. The patient's body and head are properly secured, and all bony prominences are adequately padded. The contralateral arm is placed on a well-padded arm holder. It is important to ensure that the surgical limb can be adducted and hyperextended to facilitate the preparation of the humerus intraoperatively. Routine surgical antibiotic prophylaxis is administered.

The deltopectoral approach is the most commonly used surgical approach for shoulder replacement surgery. The surgical incision begins inferior to the coracoid process, but may be extended proximally to improve visualization, and extends along the deltopectoral interval toward the center of the humerus (**Figure 1, A**). A small triangle of fat known as the Mohrenheim fossa, located at the proximal aspect of the incision, helps in identification of the deltopectoral interval. The cephalic vein is identified within the deltopectoral interval and is protected and retracted laterally or medially, depending on surgeon preference (**Figure 1, B**). The subdeltoid and subacromial spaces are then developed bluntly, and any adhesions are released, taking care not to injure the axillary nerve, which lies underneath the deltoid. A standard deltoid retractor is placed around the humeral head, which assists in retracting the deltoid muscle laterally. To increase exposure, the superior third of the pectoralis major tendon insertion on the humerus may be released. The clavipectoral fascia is incised along the lateral border of the conjoined tendon. The plane under the conjoined tendon is then developed bluntly, and retractors are carefully placed underneath the conjoined tendon. The anterior circumflex humeral artery and its venae

comitantes are cauterized because they lie inferior to the subscapularis muscle. The long head of the biceps can be palpated along the intertubercular groove and its sheath is incised. The tendon is dissected proximally along the rotator interval with curved dissecting scissors and is released near its origin. The authors of this chapter routinely perform a biceps tenodesis to the pectoralis major tendon. The subscapularis tendon, which frequently is covered by a thickened bursa that must be excised, is then identified.

Subscapularis Release

Subscapularis release techniques include subscapularis tenotomy, subscapularis peel, and lesser tuberosity osteotomy. Advocates for lesser tuberosity osteotomy report improved biomechanical strength and function when compared with subscapularis tenotomy;[2-7] however, lesser tuberosity osteotomy is a more technically demanding procedure and patients may be at risk for intraoperative fractures and nonunion.[8] Other biomechanical studies have failed to show a significant difference between subscapularis tenotomy and lesser tuberosity osteotomy with respect to improved biomechanical strength.[3,9] In a randomized prospective trial, Lapner et al[10] reported no statistically significant differences between subscapularis peel and lesser tuberosity osteotomy. Caplan et al[11] reported good functional results after performing subscapularis tenotomy in 45 shoulders.

The authors of this chapter prefer to use subscapularis tenotomy for subscapularis release. With the use of a scalpel, the rotator interval is incised, and the subscapularis is released along its insertion on the lesser tuberosity. The arm is placed in approximately 30° of external rotation to prevent injury to the axillary nerve, which lies at the inferior border of the subscapularis. A Darrach retractor may be placed deep to the conjoint tendon and anteroinferior to the subscapularis to isolate the subscapularis and protect the axillary nerve. The subscapularis and the anterior capsule are incised in a full-thickness fashion. The subscapularis is tagged with sutures for later repair and to prevent medial retraction into the chest during subsequent humeral and glenoid preparation. The circumplex vessels are isolated and cauterized or suture ligated to prevent continued bleeding during and after surgery. The inferior capsule is then released directly from the bone. With the arm in external rotation, flexion, and adduction, the release is continued to the 5-o'clock position on a right shoulder or the 7-o'clock position on a left shoulder around the peripheral osteophyte.

Humeral Head Exposure

Humeral head dislocation is performed through gentle adduction, extension, and external rotation of the humerus. Adequate exposure requires a complete release of the inferior capsule, which improves visualization of the humeral head and facilitates osteophyte removal. The degree of osteophyte formation will vary for each patient and is dependent on the type of disease and its severity. Failure to completely remove posterior osteophytes may limit glenoid exposure. Care should be taken to identify the supraspinatus and infraspinatus insertions at the greater tuberosity to prevent injury to the rotator cuff during humeral head resection. After proper visualization of the rotator cuff is achieved, humeral head resection can proceed. Humeral head resection may

be performed freehand or with the assistance of cutting jigs (**Figure 2**). If a freehand cut is performed, then the saw blade is directed along the anatomic neck of the humerus just above the rotator cuff insertion. Alternatively, depending on the instrument system and surgeon's preference, a cutting jig may be used.

Glenoid Exposure

Glenoid exposure is the most challenging aspect of shoulder replacement surgery. Several key steps are necessary for adequate glenoid exposure and to ensure proper glenoid component placement. A paralytic agent may be administered by an anesthesiologist to assist with exposure in challenging cases. One of the key aspects for adequate glenoid exposure is the ability of the surgeon to retract the humerus posteriorly using a posterior glenoid retractor. Various retractors exist, but the authors of this chapter most commonly use a Fukuda retractor or a Bankart retractor. Excessive force on the posterior glenoid retractor should be avoided because it can cause fracture to the proximal humerus and injury to the axillary nerve. Inadequate glenoid exposure may be caused by a lack of deltoid mobilization, inadequate humeral head resection, inadequate osteophyte removal, and insufficient capsular release. Correcting one of the following problems can help prevent inadequate glenoid exposure.

Lack of Deltoid Mobilization
Deltoid mobilization may be limited by incomplete release of subdeltoid adhesions or inadequate dissection near its clavicular origin. Placing the arm in slight abduction can relax the deltoid and facilitate glenoid exposure.

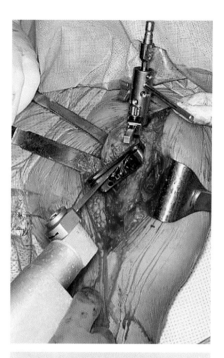

Figure 2   Intraoperative photograph shows resection of the humeral head with a cutting jig.

Inadequate Humeral Head Resection
The supraspinatus insertion can be used as a reference to assess the adequacy of humeral head resection. If a ridge exists between the lateral aspect of the humeral head and the rotator cuff, then additional humeral head resection should be performed. This also is an important step because inadequate humeral head resection will result in a proud humeral component that may cause irritation to the articular portion of the supraspinatus tendon in an anatomic total shoulder replacement. Extreme care should be taken to avoid inadvertently cutting the rotator cuff.

Inadequate Osteophyte Removal
As previously mentioned, inadequate osteophyte removal may limit glenoid exposure. Circumferential removal of osteophytes may help decrease the volume of the proximal humerus and allow for more access to the glenoid.

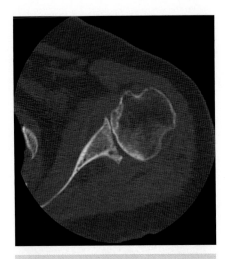

Figure 3 Preoperative CT scan of the shoulder demonstrates mild posterior glenoid wear.

Osteophytes can be removed with an osteotome and a rongeur.

Insufficient Capsular Release

Contracture of the posterior capsule may limit posterior translation of the proximal humerus. If the proximal humerus cannot be adequately displaced posteriorly, then additional posterior capsular release should be performed. Care should be taken to avoid aggressive posterior capsular release in patients who have a history of posterior instability because it may lead to instability.

Retractor Placement

After the humerus is adequately mobilized posteriorly, a Fukuda retractor or a two-pronged retractor is placed along the posterior aspect of the glenoid. Proper retractor placement is important for glenoid visualization and to protect the axillary nerve. A Darrach retractor may be placed along the inferior glenoid to protect the axillary nerve and to increase exposure to the inferior glenoid. The labrum is then carefully released from the inferior glenoid.

Labrum Resection

The glenoid labrum is completely excised to fully visualize the entire bony glenoid face. Proper glenoid visualization is important for understanding the morphology of the glenoid. Adequate glenoid exposure allows better assessment of wear patterns and appropriate sizing and placement of glenoid components. To achieve optimal exposure during surgery and optimal postoperative range of motion, capsular release along the glenoid also is necessary. The interior surface of the subscapularis is released with blunt dissection just prior to the placement of an anterior glenoid retractor. The capsular release is continued inferiorly to release the soft tissue along the inferior scapular pillar at the triceps origin. A forked inferior glenoid retractor may help provide adequate soft-tissue tension and help peel away the capsular adhesions along the inferior scapular pillar.

Primary Total Shoulder Arthroplasty

Indications

Total shoulder arthroplasty (TSA) is the treatment of choice for patients who have end-stage glenohumeral arthritis with a competent rotator cuff. The primary goals of TSA are pain relief and function restoration. The indications for TSA continue to expand and younger patients are now being considered candidates; however, the ideal candidate for TSA is typically older than 50 years and has severe glenohumeral arthritis that is refractory to conservative management. The indications for TSA include primary osteoarthritis, rheumatoid arthritis, humeral head osteonecrosis, and posttraumatic arthritis. To prevent early glenoid component failure, a competent rotator cuff or a rotator cuff tear that is amendable to intraoperative repair is required.[12]

Preoperative Evaluation

The physical examination of the shoulder should focus on the integrity of the rotator cuff muscles and the range of motion of the shoulder. Limited range of motion translates to a more difficult surgical exposure and the need for additional soft-tissue releases. Typically, a lack of external rotation is seen in the setting of hypertropic osteophytes and obliterated glenohumeral joint space. In this situation, it is necessary for the surgeon to perform a generous humeral release to disarticulate the shoulder for proper implant preparation. In addition, the subscapularis may need to be released along its articular surface in order to provide adequate excursion for later reattachment.

Imaging

Radiographs of the shoulder, including AP, Grashey, and axillary views, should be obtained. The authors of this chapter routinely obtain CT scans of the surgical shoulder to evaluate for glenoid version, glenoid wear, and osteophyte formation (**Figure 3**). If there is any concern for the integrity of the rotator cuff, clinically or radiographically, then an MRI or a CT arthrogram should be obtained.

Surgical Technique

The deltopectoral approach is the preferred approach and is performed as previously described. After adequate exposure of the proximal humerus is attained, the rotator cuff is examined. If the rotator cuff is compromised and not amendable to repair at the time of TSA, then an alternative procedure, such as hemiarthroplasty or reverse total shoulder arthroplasty (RTSA), should be performed.[13]

The humeral head is cut just slightly above the location of the rotator cuff insertion, taking care not to injure the tendons. Sequential reaming of the humeral canal is performed and is followed by broaching to the appropriate sized stem (**Figure 4**). It is important to note that the humeral canal, not the entry point, dictates the stem position. Most modern shoulder replacement systems allow the humeral head to be offset to restore the patient's anatomy. The humeral head can be set to 30° of retroversion or to the patient's native retroversion value with a freehand cut.

Glenoid exposure is performed as previously described. The center of the glenoid face is identified for placement of a central guidewire (**Figure 5**). Based on preoperative imaging, the glenoid is reamed to normalize the glenoid version and to create a smooth glenoid surface for placement of the glenoid component (**Figure 6**). Both the glenoid version and the glenoid wear pattern should be scrutinized on preoperative imaging. If glenoid bone stock is sufficient, then posterior glenoid wear may be corrected by preferentially reaming the anterior glenoid. If glenoid bone stock is deficient, then bone grafting or the use of an augmented glenoid component may be required. The glenoid component is appropriately sized such that the prosthesis is fully supported, with surface area contact along the entire backside of the glenoid component. Drill holes for a keeled or pegged component are created (**Figure 7**). To prevent rocking, which may lead to early glenoid component failure, it is imperative that the trial glenoid component be fully seated on

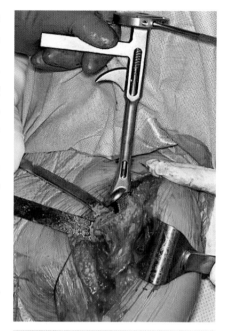

Figure 4   Intraoperative photograph shows broaching of the humeral stem with a version rod that is set to 30° of retroversion.

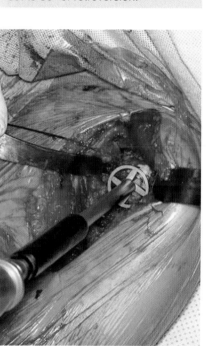

Figure 6   Intraoperative photograph shows glenoid reaming.

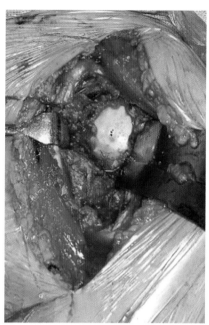

Figure 5   Intraoperative photograph shows the center of the glenoid face.

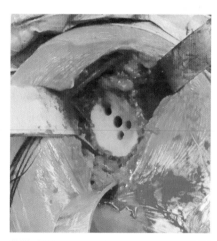

Figure 7   Intraoperative photograph shows the glenoid with drill holes for a pegged glenoid component.

the glenoid. After the drill holes have been thoroughly irrigated and dried, the final glenoid component is inserted

with careful cementing technique. The cement is allowed to cure, and the posterior glenoid retractor is removed, taking care not to damage the glenoid component.

The arm is repositioned in adduction, extension, and external rotation for

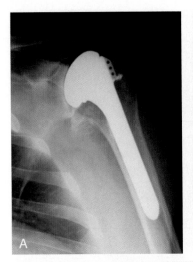 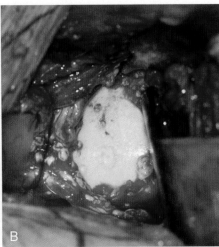 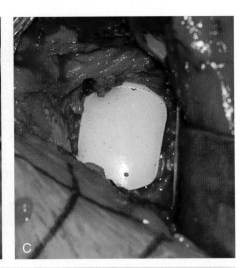

Figure 8 **A,** AP radiograph of the shoulder of a patient who had shoulder pain after hemiarthroplasty demonstrates glenoid erosion. **B,** Intraoperative photograph of the shoulder of the same patient shows glenoid erosion. **C,** Intraoperative photograph shows placement of a glenoid component.

the insertion of a cemented or press-fit humeral stem. A trial humeral head is used for head sizing and to determine the offset for maximum coverage of the proximal humerus. Component trialing is performed so that the humeral head is able to be translated 50% posteriorly, superiorly, and inferiorly. After placing the final implants, a meticulous tension-free subscapularis repair is performed. Transosseous sutures may be placed through the lesser tuberosity before stem insertion to strengthen the subscapularis repair.

Complications

Incidence

Complications after anatomic TSA are not uncommon. In a literature review of 4,010 shoulder prostheses, 66% of which were TSAs and 33% of which were humeral hemiarthroplasties, Gonzalez et al[14] reported a complication rate of 22.6% and a reoperation rate of 11.2%. Complications included painful glenoid erosion of the unresurfaced glenoid in the presence of a humeral hemiarthroplasty (20.6%), glenoid

loosening (14.3%), humeral loosening (6%), instability (4.6%), secondary rotator cuff tear (2.7%), neurologic lesion (1.8%), and infection (1.1%).[14] Management of TSA complications with revision surgery presents several challenges. It is extremely difficult to address glenoid bone loss and instability in the setting of a deficient rotator cuff or capsule or to remove fully textured or cemented stems. The diagnosis of infection may be difficult, particularly for low-virulent pathogens such as *Propionibacterium acnes*. Increased awareness of infection, the availability of reverse implants, improved glenoid components, and the liberal use of bone graft may help in the management of these complications.

Glenoid Problems

Glenoid erosion should be suspected in any patient who has been treated with hemiarthroplasty and reports progressive shoulder pain (**Figure 8, A** and **B**). Risk factors for glenoid erosion include preexisting cartilage injury, overstuffing of implants, and, possibly, overuse.

Serial radiographs may reveal progressive bone loss. A CT scan can help quantify the degree of bone loss and help evaluate fatty atrophy of the rotator cuff musculature, which may indirectly indicate a chronic rotator cuff tear. In the setting of a painful anatomic TSA, a CT arthrogram may be performed to determine if glenoid component loosening is present. Treatment of glenoid erosion in patients who have a competent rotator cuff consists of conversion to TSA via implantation of a glenoid component and exchange of the humeral head (**Figure 8, C**). Predictable pain relief can be achieved, but range of motion oftentimes is decreased compared with an uncomplicated primary TSA.

Patients who have glenoid loosening may present with persistent shoulder pain in the setting of a previously well-functioning TSA. Because well-positioned radiographs that demonstrate glenoid loosening are difficult to attain unless they are performed under fluoroscopic guidance, it may be difficult to diagnose glenoid loosening based on radiographs alone. However, radiographs may reveal radiolucent lines and changes in component position (**Figure 9**). A CT arthrogram can help establish the diagnosis by demonstrating contrast leakage behind the glenoid component. A CT arthrogram also assists in evaluating the condition of the rotator cuff by revealing extravasation of contrast dye through a rotator cuff tear. Treatment options for glenoid loosening include glenoid component revision, conversion to hemiarthroplasty, or conversion to RTSA. Glenoid revision provides good pain relief; however, satisfactory fixation of the glenoid component may not be possible. Conversion to hemiarthroplasty, which may be accompanied by bone grafting of glenoid bone defects, if present, is another option; however, pain relief after bone grafting procedures is less predictable. If the graft incorporates into the surrounding bone, then revision to TSA can later be performed if pain is still unsatisfactory.[15] Revision to RTSA provides excellent pain relief and predictable component fixation; however, the complications associated with RTSA and revision surgery should be discussed with the patient. Glenoid fixation may still be difficult to achieve in the revision setting, and range of motion usually is decreased compared with range of motion after RTSA for other indications.

Instability and Rotator Cuff Failure
Most patients who have shoulder instability after anatomic TSA have a combination of soft-tissue imbalance and component malposition.[16,17] Instability can occur in any direction: anteriorly, posteriorly, inferiorly, or superiorly. Anterior instability is most commonly a result of anterior capsule and subscapularis insufficiency.

Increased glenoid component anteversion, possibly related to anterior glenoid bone loss, may also contribute to anterior instability. Similarly, posterior instability may result from injury to or deficiency of the posterior capsule or the rotator cuff. Excessive component retroversion may also contribute to posterior instability. Inferior instability may result from a weak deltoid or from shortening of the humerus, which may occur in the setting of a proximal humerus fracture. Instability after TSA most commonly occurs in the superior direction. A deficient rotator cuff is the most common reason for superior instability. Rotator cuff failure leads to proximal migration of the humeral head during attempted forward elevation.

Treatment options for instability include component revision, soft-tissue reconstruction, and rotator cuff repair; however, these options are associated with a high rate of failure, particularly in patients who have posttraumatic arthritis.[17] Therefore, patients who demonstrate rotator cuff insufficiency or instability are best treated with revision to RTSA.[18] Every attempt should be made to prevent instability while performing primary TSA. To help prevent excessive anteversion or retroversion during component placement, preoperative images should be scrutinized for glenoid bone loss. Proper soft-tissue tension is established by selecting an appropriately sized humeral head and by performing capsular releases or plication, if necessary. To prevent postoperative failure, a meticulous repair of the subscapularis tendon should be performed and a structured postoperative physical therapy program that protects the subscapularis repair should be initiated.

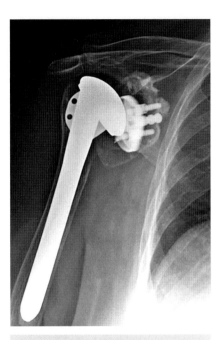

Figure 9 AP radiograph of the shoulder demonstrates lucency behind the glenoid component, which suggests glenoid component loosening.

Periprosthetic Fractures
The incidence of periprosthetic fractures after TSA is approximately 1% to 2%.[19-21] Although periprosthetic fractures are a rare complication, they can cause substantial disability to the patient and may be difficult to treat. Periprosthetic fractures may occur intraoperatively or postoperatively. Risk factors for periprosthetic fractures include advanced age, rheumatoid arthritis, osteopenia or osteoporosis, and inadequate surgical exposure.[19] Periprosthetic fractures may result from trauma, excessive torsional forces secondary to poor surgical exposure, excessive endosteal reaming, insertion of an oversized broach or stem, or attempted removal of a well-fixed stem during revision surgery. Periprosthetic fractures are classified into three different types: fractures that involve the greater tuberosity, fractures around

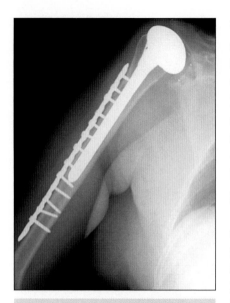

Figure 10 AP radiograph of the shoulder demonstrates plate fixation of a humeral shaft fracture.

the stem, and fractures distal to the stem.[19] Periprosthetic fractures around the stem are subclassified as fractures with a well-fixed stem, fractures with a loose stem, or fractures with substantial bone loss.

Treatment options for greater tuberosity fractures that are identified at the time of surgery include suture fixation and intraoperative conversion to RTSA. If adequate fixation cannot be achieved with suture fixation, or if there is a concern for the development of a nonunion, then conversion to RTSA is the preferred treatment. Fractures that are associated with a well-fixed stem can generally be treated with plate fixation (**Figure 10**); however, conversion to a long-stemmed prosthesis may also be considered. Fractures that are associated with a loose stem are best treated with revision to a long-stemmed humeral prosthesis. A plate or strut may be used to augment the fixation. If there is severe humeral bone loss, then an allograft-prosthetic composite or an endoprosthesis may

be considered. Fractures that occur distal to a well-fixed humeral stem can be treated in a manner similar to that used for nonperiprosthetic fractures. Fractures with satisfactory alignment can be treated conservatively; however, if substantial displacement exists, or if the patient cannot tolerate functional bracing, plate fixation should be performed.

Every attempt should be made to minimize the risk of intraoperative periprosthetic fractures. Preoperative images should be used to measure the humeral canal size for appropriate selection of broaches and final stem sizes. Adequate exposure should be attained to help minimize the forces placed on the humeral shaft that may result in a fracture. Forceful impaction of the broach on the humeral stem should be avoided to minimize the risk of a humeral fracture.

Primary RTSA
Indications
The indications for primary RTSA continue to expand, but, in general, include disorders in which a patient has a nonfunctional rotator cuff. Essentially, RTSA offers a solution for many shoulder conditions that are not amendable to treatment with an anatomic total shoulder replacement. Primary RTSA can be used to treat rotator cuff tear arthropathy, posttraumatic arthritis with rotator cuff insufficiency, four-part proximal humerus fractures, malunion, nonunion, fixed glenohumeral dislocations, and substantial glenoid bone deficiency.

Preoperative Evaluation
The evaluation of a patient who is being considered for primary RTSA includes a thorough patient history and

physical examination. Surgeons should place particular attention on the overall functional status of the patient and the functional demands on the involved limb. Patients who are heavy laborers or have increased functional requirements, such as the need for weight-bearing transfers or the permanent use of crutches, may not be ideal candidates for RTSA.

Imaging
Radiographs of the shoulder, including AP and axillary views, should be obtained. A CT scan is routinely obtained to evaluate for glenoid version, glenoid wear, and osteophyte formation (**Figure 3**). The CT scan also helps determine the entry point of the glenoid and the amount of reaming required for glenoid preparation.

Surgical Technique
The deltopectoral approach is performed as previously described. The humeral head is cut slightly above the location of the rotator cuff insertion. In patients who have rotator cuff tear arthropathy, the rotator cuff insertion may be absent. Similar to anatomic TSA, sequential reaming of the humeral canal is performed and is followed by broaching to the appropriate sized stem (**Figure 4**). As with TSA, the humeral canal, not the entry point, dictates the stem position. In general, retroversion is set to 30°. Some surgeons, depending on the design of the implant, prefer a less retroverted prosthesis; however, this has not been precisely quantified in the literature.

The surgeon should ensure that the inferior portion of the glenoid is well visualized. Additional release of the inferior capsule and the triceps insertion may be necessary. Extreme caution

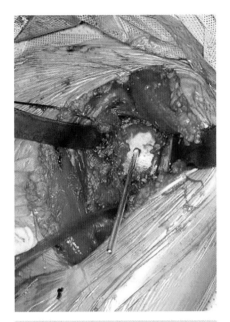

Figure 11 Intraoperative photograph shows placement of a guidewire with 10° of inferior tilt along the central axis of the glenoid.

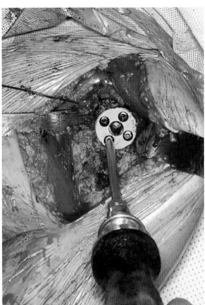

Figure 12 Intraoperative photograph shows insertion of the glenoid baseplate.

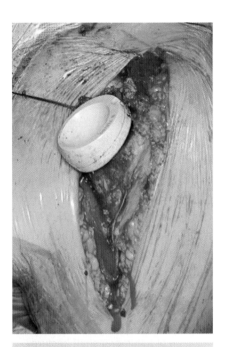

Figure 13 Intraoperative photograph shows placement of the trial glenosphere.

should be exercised during this step to prevent injury to the axillary nerve. The starting point on the glenoid face, which is indicated on the glenosphere size and the implant specifications, is identified. For example, for a given glenosphere size, care should be taken to not place the baseplate too superiorly, or there will be inadequate coverage of the inferior glenoid; this will lead to scapular impingement and eventual contact with the humeral component.[22,23] Care should be taken to avoid superior tilt on the baseplate because it has been associated with early glenoid loosening. Many surgeons believe that placement of the glenosphere with a 10° inferior tilt in relation to the articular surface of the glenoid minimizes the risk of scapular notching. This is extremely useful if shoulders with advanced rotator cuff arthropathy have superior glenoid erosion. Some systems have cannulated reamers that ream along

a central guidewire, which allows the surgeon to more clearly visualize the degree of bony correction (**Figures 5** and **11**). Guided by the preoperative CT scan, minimal reaming of the glenoid is performed. The glenoid baseplate is then inserted with the superior screw directed toward the coracoid base where there tends to be more abundant bone for bicortical fixation. The peripheral screws are directed to gain bicortical fixation (**Figure 12**).

The size of the glenosphere is determined by the size of the patient's glenoid. Many surgeons prefer to offset the glenosphere inferiorly to prevent scapular notching.[22,23] A trial glenosphere is placed, and the stability of the shoulder is tested (**Figures 13** and **14**). The tension of the conjoint tendon is assessed. Because of the altered biomechanics and relative distalization of the humerus in reverse TSA, the conjoint tendon is often supraphysiologic on palpation. To prevent complications,

such as acromial stress fractures and overtensioning of the deltoid, the authors of this chapter favor less tension of the deltoid. Because the exact amount of deltoid tension necessary has yet to be determined in the literature, final deltoid tension is surgeon-dependent and based on surgeon experience.

Complications

Incidence

Complications after RTSA increase with decreased surgeon experience, revision surgery, and increased surgical complexity.[24] Complication rates ranging from 8% to 75% have been reported in the literature[25-29] (**Table 1**). This wide variation is largely a result of the differences in the definition of a complication. In a systematic review of the literature to determine the incidence of adverse events after RTSA, Zumstein et al[30] defined a "problem" as an event not likely to affect a patient's final outcome. Problems included radiographic scapular notching, hematomas, heterotopic ossification, phlebitis, intraoperative dislocations, and intraoperative cement extravasation. The authors defined a "complication" as an event likely to have a negative effect on a patient's final outcome. Complications included fractures, infections, dislocations, nerve palsies, aseptic loosening of humeral or glenoid components, modular stem or polyethylene disassociations, and glenoid screw problems. The authors reported a complication rate of 24% and a problem rate of 44%.[30] Adverse

events most frequently encountered after RTSA include scapular notching, instability, acromial fractures, implant disassembly, and infection.

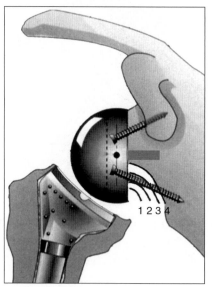

Figure 15 Illustration demonstrates the scapular notching classification described by Sirveaux et al.[25] Grade 1 defects are confined to the pillar. Grade 2 defects extend to the level of the lower screw. Grade 3 defects extend beyond the lower screw. Grade 4 defects extend under the baseplate. (Reproduced with permission from Sirveaux F, Favard L, Oudet D, Huquet D, Walch G, Molé D: Grammont inverted total shoulder arthroplasty in the treatment of glenohumeral osteoarthritis with massive rupture of the cuff: Results of a multicentre study of 80 shoulders. *J Bone Joint Surg Br* 2004;86[3]:388-395.)

Scapular Notching

Scapular notching refers to bone loss that occurs along the inferior portion of the scapular neck, which is caused by mechanical impingement of the humeral prosthesis or humeral bone on the scapular neck. Sirveaux et al[25] developed a system that classified scapular notching into four grades (**Figure 15**). Scapular notching incidence rates ranging from zero to 97% have been reported in the literature[25,26,28,29,31-36] (**Table 2**). Several authors have reported that scapular notching has no effect on functional outcome scores,[22,26,31] whereas other authors have reported a decrease in Constant assessment scores.[25,37] Although the clinical significance of scapular notching is still a subject of debate, it is reasonable to believe that the prevention of bone loss and polyethylene wear may help improve component survivability. A significant risk factor for scapular notching is superior glenoid wear that may occur as a result of rotator cuff tear arthropathy.[22] Preparation of a glenoid that has superior wear may lead to the placement of a glenoid baseplate with superior tilt. This unfavorable glenoid position decreases the clearance of the humeral component during arm adduction, which results in the increased abutment of the humeral component against the scapular neck and, most importantly, leads to early glenoid component failure. To minimize

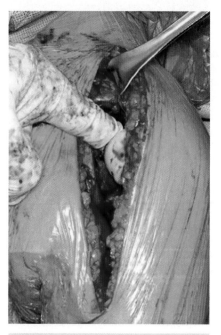

Figure 14 Intraoperative photograph shows reduction using the trial glenosphere to determine deltoid tension.

Table 1
Complication Rates for Reverse Total Shoulder Arthroplasty

Authors (Year)	No. of Shoulders	Mean Follow-up (months)	Complication Rate (%)
Rittmeister and Kerschbaumer[27] (2001)	8	54	75
Sirveaux et al[25] (2004)	80	44	15
Vanhove and Beugnies[28] (2004)	24	31	8
Frankle et al[29] (2005)	60	33	17
Werner et al[26] (2005)	58	38	50

Table 2

Reported Incidence of Scapular Notching

Authors (Year)	No. of Shoulders	Mean Patient Age in Years (Range)	Prosthesis Type[a]	Mean Follow-up in Months (Range)	No. of Shoulders with Scapular Notching
Sirveaux et al[32] (2001)	80	72 (58–86)	Delta III	44.5 (24–101)	50 (65%)
Valenti et al[33] (2001)	22	70 (55–87)	Delta III	84 (60–108)	19 (86%)
Boulahia et al[34] (2002)	16	77 (66–80)	Delta III	35 (24–65)	10 (63%)
De Wilde et al[35] (2003)	13	49 (26–68)	Delta III	36 (5–120)	4 (31%)
Sirveaux et al[25] (2004)	80	72.8 (60–86)	Delta III	44.5 (24–97)	49 (63.6%)
Vanhove and Beugnies[28] (2004)	24	71 (55–85)	Delta III	31 (11–50)	14 (50%)
Boileau et al[31] (2005)	45	NR	Delta III	40 (24–72)	24 (74%)
Frankle et al[29] (2005)	60	71 (34–86)	Reverse Shoulder Prosthesis	33 (24–68)	0
Werner et al[26] (2005)	58	68 (44–84)	Delta III	38 (24–NR)	56 (97%)

NR = not reported.

[a]Prostheses included the Delta III Reverse Shoulder System (DePuy Orthopaedics) and the Reverse Shoulder Prosthesis (Encore Medical).

Adapted with permission from Wierks C, Skolasky RL, Ji JH, McFarland EG: Reverse total shoulder replacement: Intraoperative and early postoperative complications. *Clin Orthop Relat Res* 2009;467(1):225-234.

scapular notching, the authors of this chapter recommend placement of the glenosphere in an inferior rather than superior position and the use of a humeral component with a more vertical angle of inclination.

Nyffeler et al[23] recommended that the glenoid baseplate be placed flush with the inferior glenoid rim because this position results in overhang of the glenosphere beyond the scapular neck, which increases the clearance of the polyethylene component during arm adduction. The use of a larger glenosphere also will increase the component overhang. In addition, a larger glenosphere will lateralize the center of rotation, which increases the clearance of the humeral component from the scapular neck. Lateralization of the center of rotation of the glenosphere also can be accomplished by using glenoid bone graft or an offset glenosphere.[38,39] The use of a humeral component with a smaller angle of inclination, which effectively increases the clearance of the humeral component from the scapular neck, may also minimize scapular notching.

Instability

A semiconstrained ball-in-socket prosthesis that converts the normal shear forces of a native glenohumeral joint into compressive forces created by the deltoid muscle is used for RTSA. This configuration creates a fixed fulcrum of rotation that allows the deltoid to elevate the arm of a patient who has a deficient rotator cuff. Despite the inherent stability of this prosthesis, prosthetic dislocations and instability are common complications after RTSA. Prosthetic dislocation rates ranging from 2.4% to 31% have been reported after RTSA.[26,40-42] The direction of instability after RTSA is most commonly anterior for dislocations that occur with the arm in an adducted, extended, and internally rotated position.[42,43] The risk factors for instability include male sex, a body mass index higher than 30 kg/m^2, revision surgery, and an unsatisfactory subscapularis repair.[44] In a prospective evaluation of 138 RTSAs, Edwards et al[45] reported a dislocation rate of 5.1%. The authors reported that the risk of a postoperative dislocation was significantly higher ($P < 0.012$) for patients who had an irreparable subscapularis compared with patients who underwent subscapularis repair at the time of surgery.

Postoperative instability may be a challenge for both the patient and the surgeon. It is of paramount importance for the surgeon to identify factors that may lead to instability. Factors that contribute to instability can be categorized as patient factors, surgical factors, and implant factors. Patient-related factors include compliance, prior surgery, deltoid dysfunction, and axillary nerve injury. Patients should be screened for dementia and the ability to adhere to postoperative restrictions. Postoperative delirium should be identified and treated because it can be a risk factor for early dislocation. The function of the deltoid also should be carefully assessed. An incompetent deltoid, as a result of muscular atrophy, prior stroke, or axillary nerve injury, can contribute to instability because proper deltoid tensioning will be difficult. An incompetent deltoid also will result in a poor functional outcome. Electromyogram and nerve conduction studies are a useful preoperative tool to evaluate deltoid function.

Surgical factors include bone or soft-tissue impingement, an unsatisfactory subscapularis repair, surgical approach, humeral length, and soft-tissue tensioning. Mechanical impingement, which may cause instability, should be identified intraoperatively. Common areas of impingement include the inferior aspect of the glenoid neck and the area along the posterior glenoid. Impinging structures should be released or excised as required. In revision cases, any heterotopic bone or consolidated scar tissue that is encountered must be adequately and carefully removed. Although the results are controversial, several authors reported that an unsatisfactory subscapularis tendon repair is a risk

factor for instability;[44,45] however, Clark et al[46] reported no significant difference in the complication rates for patients with or without subscapularis repair. Surgical approaches for RTSA include the anterosuperior approach and the deltopectoral approach, which is more common. Several authors have reported a lower dislocation rate if RTSA is performed via an anterosuperior approach;[47,48] however, because this technique uses a transdeltoid approach, there is an increased risk for axillary nerve injury and deltoid weakening. In a study of RTSA stability using a mechanical model, Gutiérrez et al[49] reported that appropriate soft-tissue tension is the most important factor in providing stability. Appropriate soft-tissue tension can be achieved by restoring humeral length.[50] Humeral length is restored through the preservation of as much proximal humeral and glenoid bone as possible. If there is proximal humeral bone loss, then a thicker polyethylene component can be used or a spacer can be added to restore proper humeral length. If there is substantial glenoid bone loss, then the center of rotation can be optimized by increasing the glenosphere offset, using augments to minimize glenoid reaming, or by using bone graft to lateralize the glenosphere. Other implant factors that can increase stability include the use of a deeper humeral socket, the use of a larger size glenosphere, and an increased angle of inclination; however, these factors appear to be less important than proper tensioning of the soft-tissue envelope.

Acromial Fractures
A successful RTSA outcome is dependent on the ability of the deltoid muscle to restore shoulder function.

Increased demands on the deltoid muscle translate to increased forces along the acromion, which may result in acromial fractures. A fracture of the acromion effectively weakens the deltoid and can impair shoulder function. The incidence of acromial fractures after RTSA ranges from 1% to 7%.[51] Although the exact cause of acromial fractures is unknown, overtensioning of the deltoid muscle, osteoporosis, and screw stress risers may be risk factors. Patients who have acromial fractures present with pain along the acromion, which is exacerbated with palpation, or with a decline in shoulder function. The diagnosis of acromial fractures is primarily clinical, but can be made using radiographs or, in some cases, CT scans[52] (**Figure 16**). Levy et al[51] developed a system that classified acromial fractures into three types (**Figure 17**). Treatment of acromial fractures is mainly nonsurgical. Patients are placed in a shoulder immobilizer with an abduction pillow for 6 to 8 weeks. Pain relief after an acromial fracture is usually good; however, forward elevation is typically decreased.[51]

Implant Disassembly
The incidence of implant disassembly after RTSA ranges from 3% to 5%.[30] Implant disassembly typically results from improper intraoperative component linkage. Subtle findings on postoperative radiographs may suggest improper component linkage (**Figure 18**). Prevention is the best form of treatment. To minimize implant disassembly, surgeons should have a thorough understanding of the implants being used and their linking mechanisms. Adequate visualization and the prevention of soft-tissue

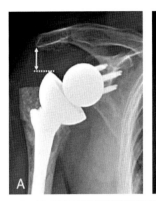
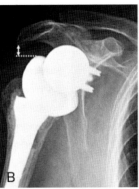
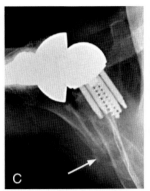
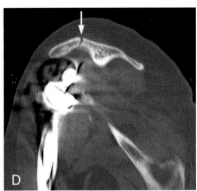

Figure 16   A, Postoperative AP radiograph of the shoulder of a patient taken 7 weeks after reverse total shoulder arthroplasty. **B,** AP radiograph of the shoulder of the same patient taken after she sustained a fall. The radiograph (**B**), taken 12 weeks after reverse total shoulder arthroplasty, demonstrates decreased distance (line with arrowheads) from the lateral acromion to the superior aspect of the humeral component (dotted line) compared with panel **A**, which suggests an acromial fracture. An axillary radiograph (**C**) and coronal CT scan (**D**) both confirm the presence of an acromial fracture (arrows). (Panels A, B, and C reproduced with permission from Levy JC, Blum S: Postoperative acromion base fracture resulting in subsequent instability of reverse shoulder replacement. *J Shoulder Elbow Surg* 2012;21[4]:e14-e18. Panel D courtesy of Jonathan C. Levy, MD, Fort Lauderdale, FL.)

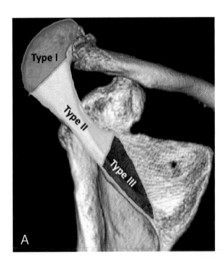
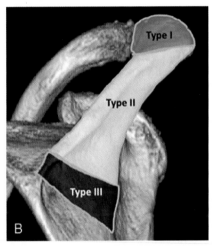
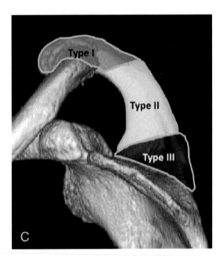

Figure 17   Posterior (A), posterosuperior (B), and superior (C) 3D reconstruction views of the scapula demonstrate the acromial fracture classification described by Levy et al.[51] Type I fractures involve a portion of the anterior and middle deltoid origin. Type II fractures involve at least the entire middle portion of the deltoid origin and sometimes a portion of the posterior deltoid origin. Type III fractures involve the entire middle and posterior deltoid origin. (Reproduced with permission from Levy JC, Anderson C, Samson A: Classification of postoperative acromial fractures following reverse shoulder arthroplasty. *J Bone Joint Surg Am* 2013;95[15]:e104.)

interposition during component placement are crucial. The use of monoblock components also can help prevent implant disassembly.

Periprosthetic Infections
Presentation
TSA infection rates range from zero to 4%.[53,54] RTSA infection rates range from 1% to 10%.[26,43,55,56] The potential risk factors for infection include revision surgery, postoperative hematoma, dead space, and other host-related factors. The most common pathogen isolated in periprosthetic infections is *P acnes*.[57] Higher concentrations of *P acnes* appear to be present in the shoulder region. Levy et al[58] reported the presence of *P acnes* in 41.8% of patients (23 of 55) who had intraoperative cultures taken during primary shoulder replacement surgery. *P acnes* does not typically present with the classic signs of inflammation that are seen with more virulent pathogens, such as erythema, swelling, or fever. The most common presenting symptom of *P acnes* is shoulder pain.

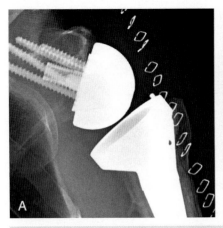
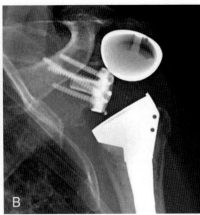

Figure 18   **A,** Immediate postoperative AP radiograph demonstrates improper linkage of the glenosphere and the baseplate. **B,** AP radiograph demonstrates disassembly of the glenosphere and the baseplate.

Patients who report persistent shoulder pain after surgery should be evaluated for a periprosthetic infection. Because of the indolent nature of *P acnes*, symptoms may not develop in some patients until several years after the index procedure.

Diagnosis

The diagnosis of a periprosthetic infection includes a thorough patient history, physical examination, review of serial radiographs, blood work, and joint aspiration. Peripheral blood tests should include a complete blood count with differential, erythrocyte sedimentation rate, and C-reactive protein level; however, several studies have shown that these laboratory markers are frequently within normal limits in patients who have *P acnes* infections.[59,60] Cultures from aspirated joint fluid may also fail to grow pathogens.

A recent study by Frangiamore et al[61] reported that synovial fluid interleukin-6 analysis was more sensitive and specific for the diagnosis of prosthetic joint infection than erythrocyte sedimentation rates and C-reactive protein levels. The authors

measured synovial fluid interleukin-6 levels with the use of a cytokine immunoassay and determined the ideal cutoff value to be 359.3 pg/mL.[61] Synovial fluid interleukin-6 levels were significantly elevated in patients who had *P acnes* infections; therefore, if institutions have the capability to perform such assays, then synovial fluid interleukin-6 analysis may be a good test for the diagnosis of periprosthetic joint infections.[61]

Obtaining intraoperative cultures is currently the preferred method for diagnosis of a periprosthetic infection. Three to five intraoperative cultures should be obtained. Cultures should be held for at least 10 days because *P acnes* has a longer incubation period.[62] Many laboratories discard cultures after 3 to 5 days. To ensure the proper handling of cultures and to increase the accuracy of diagnosis, it is highly recommended that treating physicians be familiar with their institution's microbiology laboratory practices.

Management

Treatment options for periprosthetic shoulder infections include chronic

suppression, irrigation and débridement, single-stage prosthetic reimplantation, two-stage prosthetic reimplantation, arthrodesis, and resection arthroplasty. A treatment algorithm for the management of periprosthetic shoulder infections is presented in **Figure 19**. Acute infections that are diagnosed within 6 weeks of the onset of symptoms can be treated with irrigation, débridement, polyethylene-liner exchange, and parenteral antibiotics. Infections presenting more than 6 weeks after the index procedure may be best treated with a two-stage prosthetic reimplantation as long as the patient can medically tolerate repeated interventions.

Two-stage prosthetic reimplantation is the most common procedure used to treat periprosthetic shoulder infections. In the first stage, the implant is removed, and the surgical site is irrigated and débrided thoroughly. An antibiotic-loaded cement spacer is inserted, and parenteral antibiotics are administered for a minimum of 6 weeks. A cement spacer can be created in the operating room, or the surgeon can use one of the many commercially available antibiotic spacers. Gentamicin-loaded cement is typically used, and, in many cases, tobramycin, cefoxitin, or vancomycin are added based on intraoperative cultures. Stage two, prosthetic reimplantation, is performed after antibiotic therapy is completed and there are no clinical signs of infection (**Figure 20**). Repeat intraoperative cultures are obtained; if cultures are positive, then the patient should be placed on chronic antibiotic suppression therapy.

Some surgeons advocate for open biopsy before implantation, particularly in cases of *P acnes* infection, to ensure that the infection has been eradicated.[63] Single-stage prosthetic reimplantation

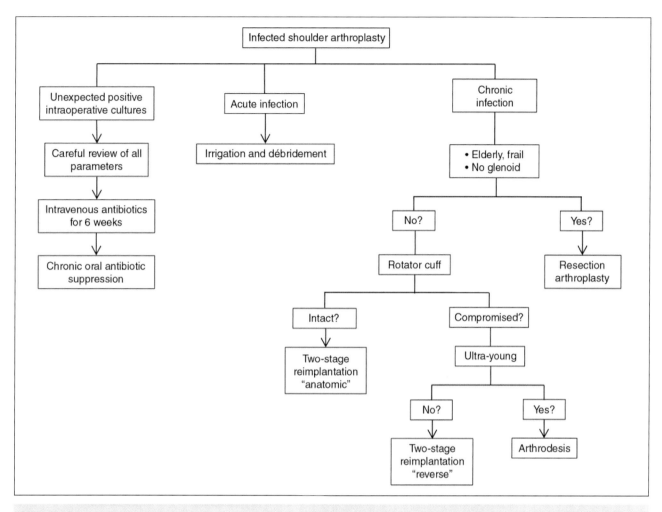

Figure 19   Treatment algorithm for the management of periprosthetic shoulder infections.

has been described in some small series with good results.[64,65] Shoulder arthrodesis or resection arthroplasty may be the best procedure in the rare case that a patient is not a candidate for reimplantation with an anatomic TSA or a RTSA.

Summary

Advances in shoulder arthroplasty have allowed for the successful treatment of various shoulder conditions. Successful shoulder arthroplasty outcomes require surgeons to have a thorough understanding of the surgical indications, surgical technique, and potential complications of the procedure. Surgeons

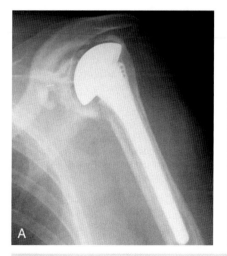
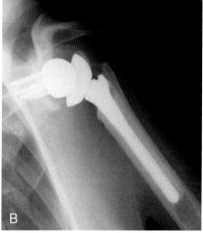

Figure 20   A, Preoperative AP radiograph of the shoulder of a man aged 73 years who had a *Propionibacterium acnes* infection demonstrates moderate glenoid bone loss and a poor rotator cuff. **B,** Postoperative AP radiograph of same patient taken 8 weeks after a two-stage prosthesis reimplantation.

who perform RTSA should be familiar with the potential complications and how to prevent and address them.

References

1. Kim SH, Wise BL, Zhang Y, Szabo RM: Increasing incidence of shoulder arthroplasty in the United States. *J Bone Joint Surg Am* 2011;93(24):2249-2254.

2. Van den Berghe GR, Nguyen B, Patil S, et al: A biomechanical evaluation of three surgical techniques for subscapularis repair. *J Shoulder Elbow Surg* 2008;17(1):156-161.

3. Van Thiel GS, Wang VM, Wang FC, et al: Biomechanical similarities among subscapularis repairs after shoulder arthroplasty. *J Shoulder Elbow Surg* 2010;19(5):657-663.

4. Gerber C, Yian EH, Pfirrmann CA, Zumstein MA, Werner CM: Subscapularis muscle function and structure after total shoulder replacement with lesser tuberosity osteotomy and repair. *J Bone Joint Surg Am* 2005;87(8):1739-1745.

5. Ponce BA, Ahluwalia RS, Mazzocca AD, Gobezie RG, Warner JJ, Millett PJ: Biomechanical and clinical evaluation of a novel lesser tuberosity repair technique in total shoulder arthroplasty. *J Bone Joint Surg Am* 2005;87(suppl 2):1-8.

6. Scalise JJ, Ciccone J, Iannotti JP: Clinical, radiographic, and ultrasonographic comparison of subscapularis tenotomy and lesser tuberosity osteotomy for total shoulder arthroplasty. *J Bone Joint Surg Am* 2010;92(7):1627-1634.

7. Krishnan SG, Stewart DG, Reineck JR, Lin KC, Buzzell JE, Burkhead WZ: Subscapularis repair after shoulder arthroplasty: Biomechanical and clinical validation of a novel technique. *J Shoulder Elbow Surg* 2009;18(2):184-192, discussion 197-198.

8. Budge MD, Nolan EM, Wiater JM: Lesser tuberosity osteotomy versus subscapularis tenotomy: Technique and rationale. *Oper Tech Orthop* 2011;21(1):39-43.

9. Giuseffi SA, Wongtriratanachai P, Omae H, et al: Biomechanical comparison of lesser tuberosity osteotomy versus subscapularis tenotomy in total shoulder arthroplasty. *J Shoulder Elbow Surg* 2012;21(8):1087-1095.

10. Lapner PL, Sabri E, Rakhra K, Bell K, Athwal GS: Comparison of lesser tuberosity osteotomy to subscapularis peel in shoulder arthroplasty: A randomized controlled trial. *J Bone Joint Surg Am* 2012;94(24):2239-2246.

11. Caplan JL, Whitfield B, Neviaser RJ: Subscapularis function after primary tendon to tendon repair in patients after replacement arthroplasty of the shoulder. *J Shoulder Elbow Surg* 2009;18(2):193-198.

12. Barrett WP, Franklin JL, Jackins SE, Wyss CR, Matsen FA III: Total shoulder arthroplasty. *J Bone Joint Surg Am* 1987;69(6):865-872.

13. Simone JP, Streubel PH, Sperling JW, Schleck CD, Cofield RH, Athwal GS: Anatomical total shoulder replacement with rotator cuff repair for osteoarthritis of the shoulder. *Bone Joint J* 2014;96(2):224-228.

14. Gonzalez JF, Alami GB, Baque F, Walch G, Boileau P: Complications of unconstrained shoulder prostheses. *J Shoulder Elbow Surg* 2011;20(4):666-682.

15. Antuna SA, Sperling JW, Cofield RH, Rowland CM: Glenoid revision surgery after total shoulder arthroplasty. *J Shoulder Elbow Surg* 2001;10(3):217-224.

16. Warren RF, Coleman SH, Dines JS: Instability after arthroplasty: The shoulder. *J Arthroplasty* 2002;17(4, suppl 1):28-31.

17. Sanchez-Sotelo J, Sperling JW, Rowland CM, Cofield RH: Instability after shoulder arthroplasty: Results of surgical treatment. *J Bone Joint Surg Am* 2003;85(4):622-631.

18. Abdel MP, Hattrup SJ, Sperling JW, Cofield RH, Kreofsky CR, Sanchez-Sotelo J: Revision of an unstable hemiarthroplasty or anatomical total shoulder replacement using a reverse design prosthesis. *Bone Joint J* 2013;95(5):668-672.

19. Campbell JT, Moore RS, Iannotti JP, Norris TR, Williams GR: Periprosthetic humeral fractures: Mechanisms of fracture and treatment options. *J Shoulder Elbow Surg* 1998;7(4):406-413.

20. Steinmann SP, Cheung EV: Treatment of periprosthetic humerus fractures associated with shoulder arthroplasty. *J Am Acad Orthop Surg* 2008;16(4):199-207.

21. Sewell MD, Kang SN, Al-Hadithy N, et al: Management of periprosthetic fracture of the humerus with severe bone loss and loosening of the humeral component after total shoulder replacement. *J Bone Joint Surg Br* 2012;94(10):1382-1389.

22. Lévigne C, Boileau P, Favard L, et al: Scapular notching in reverse shoulder arthroplasty. *J Shoulder Elbow Surg* 2008;17(6):925-935.

23. Nyffeler RW, Werner CM, Gerber C: Biomechanical relevance of glenoid component positioning in the reverse Delta III total shoulder prosthesis. *J Shoulder Elbow Surg* 2005;14(5):524-528.

24. Kempton LB, Ankerson E, Wiater JM: A complication-based learning curve from 200 reverse shoulder arthroplasties. *Clin Orthop Relat Res* 2011;469(9):2496-2504.

25. Sirveaux F, Favard L, Oudet D, Huquet D, Walch G, Molé D: Grammont inverted total shoulder arthroplasty in the treatment of glenohumeral osteoarthritis with massive rupture of the cuff: Results of a multicentre study of 80 shoulders. *J Bone Joint Surg Br* 2004;86(3):388-395.

26. Werner CM, Steinmann PA, Gilbart M, Gerber C: Treatment of painful pseudoparesis due to irreparable rotator cuff dysfunction with the Delta III reverse-ball-and-socket total shoulder prosthesis. *J Bone Joint Surg Am* 2005;87(7):1476-1486.

27. Rittmeister M, Kerschbaumer F: Grammont reverse total shoulder arthroplasty in patients with rheumatoid arthritis and nonreconstructible rotator cuff lesions. *J Shoulder Elbow Surg* 2001;10(1):17-22.

28. Vanhove B, Beugnies A: Grammont's reverse shoulder prosthesis for rotator cuff arthropathy: A retrospective

study of 32 cases. *Acta Orthop Belg* 2004;70(3):219-225.

29. Frankle M, Siegal S, Pupello D, Saleem A, Mighell M, Vasey M: The Reverse Shoulder Prosthesis for glenohumeral arthritis associated with severe rotator cuff deficiency: A minimum two-year follow-up study of sixty patients. *J Bone Joint Surg Am* 2005;87(8):1697-1705.

30. Zumstein MA, Pinedo M, Old J, Boileau P: Problems, complications, reoperations, and revisions in reverse total shoulder arthroplasty: A systematic review. *J Shoulder Elbow Surg* 2011;20(1):146-157.

31. Boileau P, Watkinson DJ, Hatzidakis AM, Balg F: Grammont reverse prosthesis: Design, rationale, and biomechanics. *J Shoulder Elbow Surg* 2005;14(1, suppl S):147S-161S.

32. Sirveaux F, Favard L, Oudet D, Huguet D, Lautman S: Grammont inverted total shoulder arthroplasty in the treatment of glenohumeral osteoarthritis with massive and non-repairable cuff rupture, in Walch G, Boileau P, Mole D, eds: *2000 Shoulder Prostheses…Two to Ten Year Follow-up.* Montpellier, France, Sauramps Medical, 2001, pp 247-252.

33. Valenti PH, Boutens D, Nerot C: Delta 3 reversed prosthesis for osteoarthritis with massive rotator cuff tear: Long-term results (>5 years), in Walch G, Boileau P, Molé D, eds: *2000 Shoulder Prostheses…Two to Ten Year Follow-up.* Montpellier, France, Sauramps Medical, 2001, pp 253-259.

34. Boulahia A, Edwards TB, Walch G, Baratta RV: Early results of a reverse design prosthesis in the treatment of arthritis of the shoulder in elderly patients with a large rotator cuff tear. *Orthopedics* 2002;25(2):129-133.

35. De Wilde L, Sys G, Julien Y, Van Ovost E, Poffyn B, Trouilloud P: The reversed Delta shoulder prosthesis in reconstruction of the proximal humerus after tumour resection. *Acta Orthop Belg* 2003;69(6):495-500.

36. Wierks C, Skolasky RL, Ji JH, McFarland EG: Reverse total shoulder replacement: Intraoperative and early postoperative complications. *Clin Orthop Relat Res* 2009;467(1):225-234.

37. Simovitch RW, Zumstein MA, Lohri E, Helmy N, Gerber C: Predictors of scapular notching in patients managed with the Delta III reverse total shoulder replacement. *J Bone Joint Surg Am* 2007;89(3):588-600.

38. Athwal GS, MacDermid JC, Reddy KM, Marsh JP, Faber KJ, Drosdowech D: Does bony increased-offset reverse shoulder arthroplasty decrease scapular notching? *J Shoulder Elbow Surg* 2015;24(3):468-473.

39. Boileau P, Moineau G, Roussanne Y, O'Shea K: Bony increased-offset reversed shoulder arthroplasty: Minimizing scapular impingement while maximizing glenoid fixation. *Clin Orthop Relat Res* 2011;469(9):2558-2567.

40. Bufquin T, Hersan A, Hubert L, Massin P: Reverse shoulder arthroplasty for the treatment of three- and four-part fractures of the proximal humerus in the elderly: A prospective review of 43 cases with a short-term follow-up. *J Bone Joint Surg Br* 2007;89(4):516-520.

41. Cazeneuve JF, Cristofari DJ: The reverse shoulder prosthesis in the treatment of fractures of the proximal humerus in the elderly. *J Bone Joint Surg Br* 2010;92(4):535-539.

42. Gerber C, Pennington SD, Nyffeler RW: Reverse total shoulder arthroplasty. *J Am Acad Orthop Surg* 2009;17(5):284-295.

43. Cheung E, Willis M, Walker M, Clark R, Frankle MA: Complications in reverse total shoulder arthroplasty. *J Am Acad Orthop Surg* 2011;19(7):439-449.

44. Chalmers PN, Rahman Z, Romeo AA, Nicholson GP: Early dislocation after reverse total shoulder arthroplasty. *J Shoulder Elbow Surg* 2014;23(5):737-744.

45. Edwards TB, Williams MD, Labriola JE, Elkousy HA, Gartsman GM, O'Connor DP: Subscapularis insufficiency and the risk of shoulder dislocation after reverse shoulder arthroplasty. *J Shoulder Elbow Surg* 2009;18(6):892-896.

46. Clark JC, Ritchie J, Song FS, et al: Complication rates, dislocation, pain, and postoperative range of motion after reverse shoulder arthroplasty in

patients with and without repair of the subscapularis. *J Shoulder Elbow Surg* 2012;21(1):36-41.

47. Affonso J, Nicholson GP, Frankle MA, et al: Complications of the reverse prosthesis: Prevention and treatment. *Instr Course Lect* 2012;61:157-168.

48. Molé D, Wein F, Dézaly C, Valenti P, Sirveaux F: Surgical technique: The anterosuperior approach for reverse shoulder arthroplasty. *Clin Orthop Relat Res* 2011;469(9):2461-2468.

49. Gutiérrez S, Keller TS, Levy JC, Lee WE III, Luo ZP: Hierarchy of stability factors in reverse shoulder arthroplasty. *Clin Orthop Relat Res* 2008;466(3):670-676.

50. Lädermann A, Williams MD, Melis B, Hoffmeyer P, Walch G: Objective evaluation of lengthening in reverse shoulder arthroplasty. *J Shoulder Elbow Surg* 2009;18(4):588-595.

51. Levy JC, Anderson C, Samson A: Classification of postoperative acromial fractures following reverse shoulder arthroplasty. *J Bone Joint Surg Am* 2013;95(15):e104.

52. Levy JC, Blum S: Postoperative acromion base fracture resulting in subsequent instability of reverse shoulder replacement. *J Shoulder Elbow Surg* 2012;21(4):e14-e18.

53. Coste JS, Reig S, Trojani C, Berg M, Walch G, Boileau P: The management of infection in arthroplasty of the shoulder. *J Bone Joint Surg Br* 2004;86(1):65-69.

54. Sperling JW, Kozak TK, Hanssen AD, Cofield RH: Infection after shoulder arthroplasty. *Clin Orthop Relat Res* 2001;382:206-216.

55. Cuff D, Pupello D, Virani N, Levy J, Frankle M: Reverse shoulder arthroplasty for the treatment of rotator cuff deficiency. *J Bone Joint Surg Am* 2008;90(6):1244-1251.

56. Wall B, Nové-Josserand L, O'Connor DP, Edwards TB, Walch G: Reverse total shoulder arthroplasty: A review of results according to etiology. *J Bone Joint Surg Am* 2007;89(7):1476-1485.

57. Horneff JG, Hsu JE, Huffman GR: Propionibacterium acnes infections in shoulder surgery. *Orthop Clin North Am* 2014;45(4):515-521.

58. Levy O, Iyer S, Atoun E, et al: Propionibacterium acnes: An underestimated etiology in the pathogenesis of osteoarthritis? *J Shoulder Elbow Surg* 2013;22(4):505-511.

59. Pottinger P, Butler-Wu S, Neradilek MB, et al: Prognostic factors for bacterial cultures positive for Propionibacterium acnes and other organisms in a large series of revision shoulder arthroplasties performed for stiffness, pain, or loosening. *J Bone Joint Surg Am* 2012;94(22):2075-2083.

60. Zeller V, Ghorbani A, Strady C, Leonard P, Mamoudy P, Desplaces N: Propionibacterium acnes: An agent of prosthetic joint infection and colonization. *J Infect* 2007;55(2):119-124.

61. Frangiamore SJ, Saleh A, Kovak MF, et al: Synovial fluid interleukin-6 as a predictor of periprosthetic shoulder infection. *J Bone Joint Surg Am* 2015;97(1):63-70.

62. Zimmerli W, Trampuz A, Ochsner PE: Prosthetic-joint infections. *N Engl J Med* 2004;351(16):1645-1654.

63. Zhang AL, Feeley BT, Schwartz BS, Chung TT, Ma CB: Management of deep postoperative shoulder infections: Is there a role for open biopsy during staged treatment? *J Shoulder Elbow Surg* 2015;24(1):e15-e20.

64. Klatte TO, Kendoff D, Kamath AF, et al: Single-stage revision for fungal peri-prosthetic joint infection: A single-centre experience. *Bone Joint J* 2014;96(4):492-496.

65. Beekman PD, Katusic D, Berghs BM, Karelse A, De Wilde L: One-stage revision for patients with a chronically infected reverse total shoulder replacement. *J Bone Joint Surg Br* 2010;92(6):817-822.

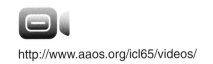

http://www.aaos.org/icl65/videos/

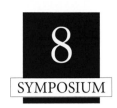

SYMPOSIUM

Biomechanics of Reverse Shoulder Arthroplasty: Current Concepts

Adam J. Lorenzetti, MD

Geoffrey P. Stone, MD

Peter Simon, PhD

Mark A. Frankle, MD

Abstract

The evolution of reverse shoulder arthroplasty has provided surgeons with new solutions for many complex shoulder problems. A primary goal of orthopaedics is the restoration or re-creation of functional anatomy to reduce pain and improve function, which can be accomplished by either repairing injured structures or replacing them as anatomically as possible. If reconstructible tissue is lacking or not available, which is seen in patients who have complex shoulder conditions such as an irreparable rotator cuff–deficient shoulder, cuff tear arthropathy, or severe glenoid bone loss, substantial problems may arise. Historically, hemiarthroplasty or glenoid grafting with total shoulder arthroplasty yielded inconsistent and unsatisfactory results. Underlying pathologies in patients who have an irreparable rotator cuff–deficient shoulder, cuff tear arthropathy, or severe glenoid bone loss can considerably alter the mechanical function of the shoulder and create treatment dilemmas that are difficult to overcome. A better biomechanical understanding of these pathologic adaptations has improved treatment options. In the past three decades, reverse total shoulder arthroplasty was developed to treat these complex shoulder conditions not by specifically re-creating the anatomy but by using the remaining functional tissue to improve shoulder balance. Reverse total shoulder arthroplasty has achieved reliable improvements in both pain and function. Initial implant designs lacked scientific evidence to support the design rationale, and many implants failed because surgeons did not completely understand the forces involved or the pathology being treated. Implant function and clinical results will continue to improve as surgeons' biomechanical understanding of shoulder disease and reverse shoulder arthroplasty implants increases.

Instr Course Lect 2016;65:127–144.

Reverse shoulder arthroplasty (RSA) has revolutionized the treatment of complex shoulder conditions that were previously believed to be irreparable. RSA includes the use of a nonanatomic implant; the pursuit of ideal biomechanics has improved patient outcomes, function, and implant survival. Surgeons should be aware of recent advances in RSA implant designs as well as the rationale and controversies that drive implant development. In addition, it is important for surgeons to understand the influence of current clinical and biomechanical evidence and its effect on improvements in RSA function and outcomes.

A Brief History of RSA

Initially developed as a limited salvage procedure, RSA has become the standard procedure for the treatment of cuff tear arthropathy (CTA); however, it has been increasingly indicated for other complex shoulder conditions, including massive rotator cuff tears,[1] proximal humerus fractures,[2,3] failed arthroplasty,[4,5] osteoarthritis with an intact rotator cuff, and severe glenoid deficiency. In 1983, Neer et al[6] coined the term "cuff tear arthropathy" to describe a condition that involved massive multiple rotator cuff tears and the associated morphologic changes of the glenohumeral joint. CTA results from glenohumeral instability that is caused by a lack of balanced cuff tension, which, in turn, creates unbalanced dynamic forces across the joint. This leads to a spectrum of disease that may be either isolated or combined glenoid- and humeral-sided wear, which is often found in eccentric patterns. The initial solution advocated by Neer et al[6] for the treatment of CTA was hemiarthroplasty; however, this treatment did not specifically address joint instability, and subsequent studies have reported unpredictable and poor results, including inadequate restoration of functional range of motion (ROM).[6-11]

More constrained implants were used in an attempt to correct stability, but these attempts were met with high rates of clinical failure as a result of the implants' inability to withstand forces at the glenosphere-bone junction during shoulder motion.[12-16] A breakthrough occurred in 1985 when Grammont and Baulot[17] developed a semiconstrained reverse prosthesis; the authors' initial design included a cemented humeral and glenoid component; the prosthesis was subsequently modified and, in 1991,

became the Delta III reverse shoulder prosthesis (DePuy).

The initial clinical results of the Delta III reverse shoulder prosthesis were very promising, with substantial decreases in pain and improvements in clinical function reported at 2-year follow-up in early case studies.[17,18] The Delta III reverse shoulder prosthesis design biomechanically overcame the early difficulty of inadequate glenoid fixation by adding locked screw fixation and improving the metallic ingrowth material. The prosthesis design also used theoretic assumptions on shoulder biomechanics to reduce stresses on the glenoid-bone interface, which explain improved glenoid implant survival. Boileau et al[19] hypothesized that a humeral center of rotation (COR) that was located as close as possible to the bone-glenosphere junction would decrease baseplate loosening and the number of failures seen with previous prosthesis designs. The authors reported that enhanced deltoid function, which moved the COR medially to the glenoid surface, theoretically explained the functional improvement that was clinically observed in patients. In addition, enhanced deltoid muscle fiber recruitment allowed for a more efficient deltoid lever arm. The prosthesis design also used a large glenosphere (36 or 42 mm) and a humeral component with a neck-shaft angle of 155° to distalize the humerus and tension the deltoid. The authors theorized that tensioning

the deltoid muscle would result in compression between the humeral socket and the glenosphere, which would subsequently stabilize the prosthetic articulation.

Although the Delta III reverse shoulder prosthesis design helped establish RSA as a viable option for CTA, several problems remained. Mechanical impingement between the medial aspect of the humeral component and the inferior scapula (ie, scapular notching) was reported in 24.5% to 96% of patients in several studies[19,20] and was a concern for long-term implant survival. In addition, clinical results of the Delta III reverse shoulder prosthesis revealed substantial limitations in external rotation because the remaining rotator cuff was no longer appropriately tensioned; several studies considered muscle transfers to restore external rotation.[21-26] Shifting the proximal humerus more medially may result in a loss of cosmesis, with patient complaints of a loss of normal deltoid contour. Finally, because instability is managed via humeral distalization, there is an inherent increased risk of neurapraxia if overlengthening occurs, which may result in a prosthesis that has less inherent stability.[27] Recognition of these drawbacks led to substantial clinical and basic science studies that focused on improving RSA prosthesis designs and surgical techniques.

Biomechanics of a Normal and Diseased Shoulder

A normal shoulder lacks a level of intrinsic stability imparted by the bony morphology that exists in other ball-and-socket joints, such as the hip. Shoulder stability, which can be understood with the concept of concavity-compression, requires an

Dr. Frankle or an immediate family member has received royalties from DJO Surgical; is a member of a speakers' bureau or has made paid presentations on behalf of DJO Surgical; serves as a paid consultant to DJO Surgical; has received research or institutional support from BioMimetic Therapeutics and DJO Surgical; has received nonincome support (such as equipment or services), commercially derived honoraria, or other non-research–related funding (such as paid travel) from DJO Surgical; and serves as a board member, owner, officer, or committee member of the American Academy of Orthopaedic Surgeons and the American Shoulder and Elbow Surgeons. None of the following authors or any immediate family member has received anything of value from or has stock or stock options held in a commercial company or institution related directly or indirectly to the subject of this chapter: Dr. Lorenzetti, Dr. Stone, and Dr. Simon.

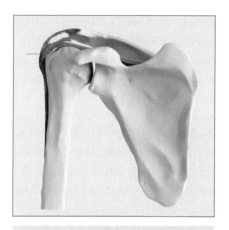

Figure 1 Anatomic illustration of a normal shoulder shows the compressive force of the intact rotator cuff muscles that balances the proximal pull of the deltoid.

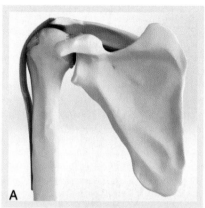

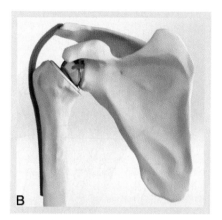

Figure 2 Anatomic illustrations show a diseased shoulder. **A,** A massive rotator cuff tear without glenohumeral osteoarthritis leads to unbalanced proximal pull of the deltoid and instability of the shoulder joint with proximal humeral migration. **B,** Reverse shoulder arthroplasty restores balance by converting the proximal deltoid pull into compression across a stable fulcrum.

adequate amount of compression of the humeral head into the shallow glenoid fossa.[28,29] If the cavity (ie, the glenoid socket) is deeper, less compressive load is required to resist a given displacing force. A normal shoulder requires a functioning rotator cuff that provides a balanced compressive load to maintain stability between the humeral head and the glenoid (**Figure 1**). This allows the shoulder to resist the proximal translational force of the deltoid and allows for smooth shoulder ROM with minimal translation as the rotator cuff dynamically responds to changes in the displacing forces.

In a diseased shoulder that has rotator cuff deficiency, a loss of balanced compressive forces leads to pathologic instability at the glenohumeral joint. A spectrum of pathologic entities with various clinical presentations, from intact rotator cuffs with soft-tissue imbalance that leads to eccentric wear to massive rotator cuff tears with or without arthritis, exists (**Figure 2**). It is essential for surgeons to recognize these different pathologies to determine the proper treatment. The surgeon must

evaluate the articular surface, ligamentous stability, soft-tissue compliance, and periscapular musculature in conjunction with the amount of rotator cuff disease. In addition, anatomic total shoulder arthroplasty (TSA) may lead to poor results in patients who have an untorn rotator cuff and other pathology such as capsular insufficiency, eccentric bone loss, and static or dynamic instability that signal rotator cuff deficiency.

The glenoid center line is another important biomechanical shoulder principle.[30] In a normal glenoid, the center line is perpendicular to the articular surface of the glenoid and directed, in most patients, approximately 10° posterior (retroverted) to the plane of the scapula. The center line acts as a pillar on which the humeral head rests; the coupling of glenohumeral and scapulothoracic motions maintains the center line beneath the humeral head throughout ROM to provide adequate support. In rotator cuff deficiency, unbalanced muscular forces disrupt this relationship and shift the humeral head away from the glenoid center line, which results in eccentric loads across the joint

that may lead to wear; however, glenoid wear patterns in cuff deficiency may consist of no wear or superior, inferior, anterior, posterior, or global wear.[31] Abnormal wear patterns are likely the result of an altered biomechanical environment and often result in eccentric glenoid wear patterns.[6,32,33]

Ideally, the glenoid component should be placed along the glenoid center line to help restore normal shoulder relationships and provide a stable column of bone for implant fixation; however, this placement is not always possible because of glenoid bone deficiency, which compromises glenoid fixation. In patients who have severe or eccentric glenoid wear, stable baseplate fixation can be achieved only by placing the component along the alternative glenoid center line[31] (**Figure 3**). This alternative center line is aimed at the dense bone at which the scapular spine meets the body of the scapula; it is not necessarily perpendicular to the remaining glenoid face. The center line in a rotator cuff–deficient shoulder that has little glenoid wear can provide excellent fixation for the glenoid baseplate

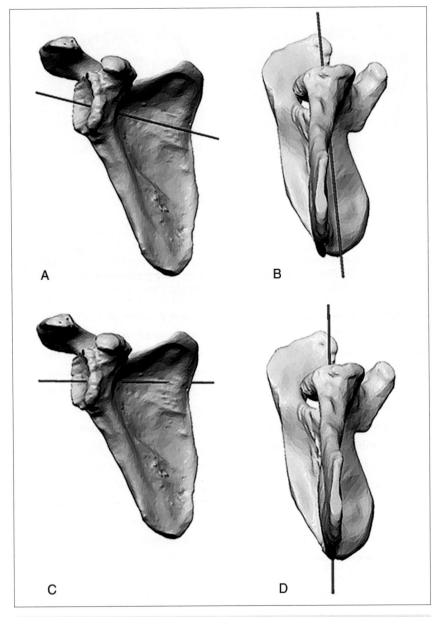

Figure 3 Three-dimensional computer models of a shoulder demonstrate glenoid component placement. Anterior (**A**) and inferior (**B**) views demonstrate ideal glenoid component placement along the glenoid center line (blue line). Anterior (**C**) and inferior (**D**) views demonstrate alternative center line (blue line) glenoid component placement along the scapular spine. (Reproduced with permission from Frankle MA, Teramoto A, Luo ZP, Levy JC, Pupello D: Glenoid morphology in reverse shoulder arthroplasty: Classification and surgical implications. *J Shoulder Elbow Surg* 2009;18[6]:874-885.)

three-dimensional CT reconstructions from 92 patients without bony deformities who underwent RSA. The authors reported that although humeral head size, glenoid width, lateral offset, and moment arm all independently increased linearly, the rate of increase varied. Using their initial data, the authors investigated the effect of prosthetic/patient size mismatch and reported that such a mismatch may have adverse effects on soft-tissue strain and middle deltoid moment arm. This study emphasizes that patient size (as determined by measured morphometric parameters) should be considered in the selection of proper implants to avoid large deviations in nonanatomic reconstructions.[34]

Humeral Fixation

Humeral fixation has changed considerably since RSA was introduced. All humeral components were initially fixed with cement, which provided good results and continues to be frequently used in certain patients.[35] Although cement provides initial stable prosthetic attachment, long-term failure of the cement-bone or cement-prosthetic interface is possible. Humeral loosening, although not considered a major issue in TSA, is more of a concern in RSA. Farvard et al[36] reported that, at a minimum follow-up of 8 years, the humeral loosening rate for patients who underwent anatomic TSA was 1.5%, and the humeral loosening rate for patients who underwent RSA was 3.6%. This significant difference may be caused by the semiconstrained RSA prosthesis design that compensates for loss of rotator cuff stability, which increases the forces placed on the bone implant interface.[36]

Similar to the evolution of total hip arthroplasty, a trend for press-fit RSA humeral stems, which allow

in RSA. Surgeons should know which glenoid wear patterns make the center line unusable so bone loss can be compensated for with adequate fixation along the alternative center line.

To better understand the effect of a patient's size on glenohumeral anatomy, Cabezas et al[34] evaluated 11 anatomic measurements and 7 glenohumeral relationships with the use of preoperative for osseointegration, has emerged. The direct structural connection between living bone and the surface of a load-carrying implant is achieved by applying grit-blasted or porous-coated surface finishes to certain portions of the implant, which allow for bony ingrowth or ongrowth. Optimal bony ingrowth requires stable attachment of the prosthesis to the bone while limiting bone-prosthetic interface micromotion to less than 150 μm and a surface that is conducive to osseous healing.[37] The optimal surface characteristics depend on the type of coating surface finishes used; the material porosity, which is typically 65% to 80% for most orthopaedic applications; and the optimal surface roughness of the coating surface finishes.[38] The advantages of uncemented fixation include faster surgical time, the potential for biologic prosthetic fixation, and the avoidance of cement-related complications. Several recent studies have reported that the results of uncemented humeral fixation are comparable with those of cemented stems;[39,40] however, because limited biomechanical data are available on RSA humeral fixation and because uncemented fixation has its own advantages, the decision of whether to use cement should be made using intraoperative judgment. Although it is the current practice of the authors of this chapter to press fit most primary RSAs, there are still patients in whom the authors commonly cement the humeral stem, including patients in whom normal mechanical support provided by the proximal humerus is absent as a result of bone loss, which has been reported to diminish humeral fixation.[41] In addition, the authors of this chapter have a low threshold for the use of cement in primary procedures for patients

in whom humeral component stability is in question, such as in patients who have severe osteoporosis.

Glenoid Baseplate Fixation

Glenoid fixation universally uses uncemented techniques that compress the baseplate to the glenoid bone stock. Similar to humeral fixation, the goal is to prevent micromotion and allow for osseointegration, which will help decrease glenoid failure rates. Glenoid baseplate fixation is achieved by using the basic AO principles of bone healing: compression and neutralization. Most baseplate designs use a backside coating that encourages bony ingrowth or ongrowth as well as a variable configuration of peripheral screws that provide further stabilization. Stable baseplate fixation can be achieved with either a press-fit peg with peripheral compression screw fixation or a central axis screw. After the baseplate is properly compressed to the glenoid bone, forces can be neutralized with locking screws, which minimize micromotion.[42,43] A study that compared the different methods of baseplate fixation reported that a peg/peripheral screw system provided a compressive force of 200 N, and central screw fixation provided a compressive force of 2,000 N.[44] In addition, a 2.3-fold increase in load to failure was reported between the central screw (629 N) and the central post (269 N).[44] For patients in whom bony ingrowth is critical, such as those who require bone grafting, this increased compressive force provides the most optimal platform for bony ingrowth.

The inability of baseplate fixation to overcome forces at the bone-implant interface before bony ingrowth has been attributed to glenoid baseplate failure.[45] In a central peg design that relies on

peripheral compression, it is imperative for the surgeon to place the peripheral screw into the highest quality glenoid bone stock.[46] This bone stock can be found in the three major columns of scapular bone: the base of the coracoid, the spine of the scapula, and the scapular pillar.[47] However, because of the varied spectrum of glenoid bone deficiency in CTA as well as revision arthroplasty, these typically optimal locations may be compromised, which may lead to inadequate fixation. Glenoid morphology analysis has helped surgeons better understand these anatomic variations and provide better treatment options. In a study of 216 glenoids that required RSA, Frankle et al[31] reported that 62.5% of the glenoids had normal morphology. If a normal glenoid was present, the anatomic center line was used for glenoid baseplate fixation. Abnormal glenoid morphology was reported in 37.5% of the glenoids, with eccentric bone loss posteriorly (17.6%), superiorly (9.3%), anteriorly (4.2%), or globally (6.5%). If abnormal glenoid morphology was encountered, the anatomic center line would not provide optimal glenoid fixation, and the alternative center line was used.

The authors of this chapter use a system that includes a compressive lag screw that has variation in the thread pitch; the central core is 3.2 mm, and the outer thread diameter is 6.5 mm (**Figure 4**). The benefits of substantial initial compression combined with the flexibility to apply compression along the alternative center line if glenoid morphology dictates provides surgeons with an important tool. The baseplate also contains 5.0-mm fixed locking screws. In a study that compared 5.0-mm fixed locking screws with 3.5-mm unlocked compression screws,

Harman et al[42] reported that the 5.0-mm screws had 29% less micromotion. A subsequent clinical study reported that the use of 5.0-mm peripheral locking screws with a central compression screw and a lateralized COR reduced glenoid failure to 0.4%.[48] Another benefit is that intraoperative tactile feedback is provided from the friction between the baseplate and bone (ie, the bite); this is commonly helpful in patients who have alterations in glenoid morphology, who have bone loss, in whom bone grafting is used, and in whom the sufficiency of implant purchase is in question. The use of a glenosphere that contacts the glenoid is another method to improve fixation and baseplate stability, especially during bone grafting. In a study of the effects of implant-bone contact on implant stability, Nigro et al[49] used a virtual computer model to allow the glenosphere underside to contact the glenoid and, thus, increase the composite baseplate-glenoid contact area. The authors reported a decrease in both baseplate stress and micromotion for all seven implant designs tested if the glenosphere was in contact with the glenoid. In addition, a greater reduction in stress and micromotion was reported as the glenosphere size increased.[49]

Glenosphere Design

Because RSA is not meant to replicate normal shoulder anatomy, the proper position and design of the glenosphere is an active area of discussion, debate, and research. Glenoid designs fall into two main categories: glenospheres that place the COR at the glenosphere-bone interface, and, thus, mimic the original Grammont design, and eccentric glenospheres that move the COR away from the glenosphere-bone interface. Eccentric offset designs include lateral offset

designs, which bring the COR closer to the anatomic COR, and inferior offset designs, which further distalize the articulation in an attempt to improve adduction and impingement-free ROM. Several basic science studies have examined the biomechanical forces at the glenoid and impingement-free ROM with these different glenoid designs in an attempt to elucidate optimal glenoid positioning and, thus, improve implant longevity and patient function.[50-56]

The Grammont reverse prosthesis was designed with a humeral component in substantial valgus (155° neck-shaft angle) and a hemisphere with a COR directly at the point of implant fixation (ie, the implant/bony glenoid surface; **Figure 5**). Grammont believed that glenoid baseplate failure in earlier designs was related to the amount of shear stress across the glenoid component, and that simply medializing the glenosphere COR to the glenoid face would dramatically reduce this stress. In Grammont's theory, the valgus humeral component would tension the deltoid by lengthening the humerus and, thus, enhance deltoid recruitment, which would allow for a more efficient deltoid lever arm. These substantial deviations from the normal anatomic positioning of the humerus resulted in complications, including prosthetic abutment of the scapula, alterations in shoulder function, and an abnormal cosmetic appearance. Despite the clinical improvements seen with Grammont's device, several mechanical problems, including a substantial reduction in impingement-free ROM and a substantial alteration in inferior and lateral offset of the proximal humerus, remained. These problems led to numerous biomechanical and clinical studies that attempted to improve the design of RSA prostheses.

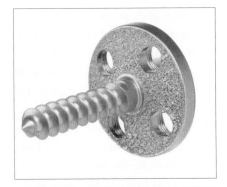

Figure 4   Photograph shows a 6.5-mm central lag screw for DJO's reverse shoulder prosthesis.

Inferior eccentric glenosphere designs were developed specifically to reduce the high rate of impingement between the lateral border of the scapula and the medial humeral socket and subsequent scapular notching,[50] both of which have been reported with traditional Grammont-style prostheses.[57,58] In a study that compared concentric and eccentric glenosphere designs, De Biase et al[59] reported a reduction in the rate of notching with the use of an inferior eccentric design; however, no clinically significant difference was reported between patients with and without notching at 2-year follow-up. Mizuno et al[60] used an inferior eccentric glenosphere and did not report a difference in the rate of notching but did report a decrease in the severity of notching at early follow-up. In a randomized controlled trial, Poon et al[61] did not report a difference in the rate of notching or clinical outcomes if an inferior eccentric glenosphere was used. Gutiérrez et al[51] used a computer model to show that an inferior eccentric glenosphere, if placed inferiorly, will result in an unbalanced force-distribution profile, which may lead to shear forces at the bone-implant interface and early failure. An inferior eccentric glenosphere also places the humerus in a more distal position if the arm is adducted, which may adversely affect deltoid contour, stability, and soft-tissue tensioning.

Lateral (or less medial) eccentric glenospheres shift the COR into a more anatomic position and avoid overdistalization of the humerus but still result in deltoid tensioning. Lateralization offers many benefits, including improved glenohumeral impingement-free adduction and abduction[52-54] and improved stability.[55,56] In addition, lateralization of the humerus lengthens and tensions the remaining intact posterior cuff musculature, which improves external rotation force.[48] The authors of this chapter have found that maintaining the humerus in a more anatomic position facilitates repair of the subscapularis, which may improve stability[62] and internal rotation force. Improvements in implant designs have resolved initial glenoid-sided concerns, and studies have reported greater glenoid fixation, lower rates of mechanical failure, and a decrease in scapular notching.[63,64]

Glenoid Positioning

The effects of glenoid component positioning on implant survival were not appreciated until 2006. An analysis of initial failures of lateral-offset RSAs that were implanted with 3.5-mm unlocked peripheral screws revealed a common radiographic appearance: The glenospheres were superiorly tilted.[65] This was not surprising given that the initial population was composed primarily of patients with CTA who exhibited superior glenoid wear. Initially, major alterations were not made to the glenoid at the time the baseplate was implanted; therefore, the baseplates were often implanted at the native glenoid inclination, which resulted in a

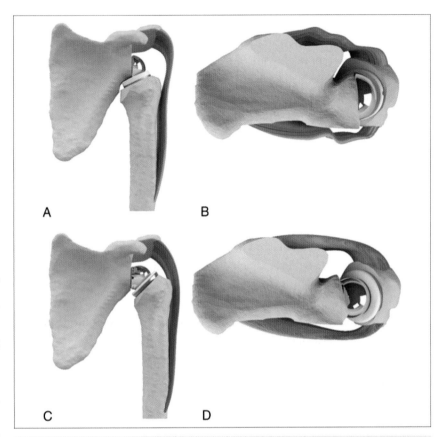

Figure 5   Anatomic illustrations of a shoulder show two reverse shoulder prostheses. Anterior (**A**) and superior (**B**) views show a Grammont-style design with a 155° neck-shaft angle and a medialized center of rotation to the glenoid face with medialization and distalization of the proximal humerus. Anterior (**C**) and superior (**D**) views show a lateral offset design with a more varus neck-shaft angle, which shifts the proximal humerus into a more lateral and anatomic position and, thus, tensions the deltoid and remaining rotator cuff. The acromion and coracoid have been removed for better visualization of the articulating space. (Reproduced from Otto RJ, Nigro PT, Frankle MA: Reverse shoulder arthroplasty for chronic shoulder pathology, in Nicholson GP, ed: *Orthopaedic Knowledge Update: Shoulder and Elbow*, ed 4. Rosemont, IL, American Academy of Orthopaedic Surgeons, 2013, pp 379-396.)

component with superior tilt. Gutierrez et al[66] compared different glenosphere implantation angles (15° of superior tilt, 15° of inferior tilt, and neutral tilt) and reported that inferior tilt of the glenosphere by 15° resulted in the most uniform compressive forces and the least amount of tensile forces and micromotion. This optimum scenario requires either inferior glenoid reaming or, in larger defects, glenoid bone grafting. The effect of baseplate positioning and the distribution of forces across the

baseplate-bone interface continue to be areas of interest.

Gutierrez et al[66] investigated the forces at the baseplate-bone interface for three different glenosphere designs (concentric, lateral eccentric, and inferior eccentric) that were placed in three different positions (superior tilt, neutral, and inferior tilt). In this study, a computer simulation that was based on a previously validated biomechanical study was used to evaluate the forces in the previously mentioned scenarios.

The results showed a predictable pattern of forces at the baseplate-bone junction that corresponded with the type of offset used and the tilt in which the glenoid was placed. The most even distribution of forces was reported with a glenosphere that had a lateralized or concentric COR and was placed in inferior tilt; the most uneven distribution of forces was seen with a glenosphere that had either a concentric or lateral COR and was placed in superior tilt.[66] Interestingly, glenospheres that had inferior offset demonstrated increasingly uneven forces if placed in inferior tilt versus neutral or, even, superior tilt.

Glenohumeral Stability

Loss of glenohumeral stability is central to a pathologic rotator cuff. RSA restores functional stability, and several factors play critical roles in achieving and maintaining stability. Early results of RSA that was performed with the classic Grammont-style prosthesis included dislocation rates up to 30%[67,68] and highlighted the need for further implant design innovation. Several key contributors to postoperative instability include soft-tissue tension, glenosphere diameter, humeral-socket constraint, impingement, and axillary nerve and deltoid function. Gutiérrez et al[55] evaluated the effect of several key factors on stability by systematically changing the variables and examining how much translational force (perpendicular to the prosthesis) was required to dislocate the prosthesis for the different combinations. A hierarchy of importance for stability was established among the factors, with increasing compressive force being the most important factor, followed by humeral socket depth; glenosphere size was the least important factor. Based on these data, Gutiérrez et al[55] reported that the ratio between the diameter of the glenosphere and the radius of the humeral socket (d/R ratio) was a critical determinant of translational stability. Devices with an increased d/R ratio have more inherent stability and are more constrained (ie, for a specific ball size, the deeper the socket, the more stable and resistant it is to dislocation),[69,70] which echoes the concept of concavity-compression described by Matsen and Lippitt;[29] however, a substantial tradeoff in impingement-free ROM occurs as socket depth increases. Gutiérrez et al[71] evaluated this relationship with the use of computer simulation and reported that increasing constraint decreased impingement-free ROM in most patients.

Patient bony anatomy plays an important role in RSA stability. Substantial bone loss, as a result of either overmedialization of the joint in the presence of glenoid bone loss or loss of the deltoid wrapping effect (the compressive effect of the deltoid muscle that results from the path it takes between attachment sites on the humerus, scapula, and clavicle over the tuberosities) in the presence of humeral bone loss, may decrease tension in the shoulder soft-tissue envelope and reduce the compressive force at the joint. Proper prosthetic selection and surgical technique compensate for this bone deficiency by repositioning the humerus and restoring the required tension. Prosthetic design options include various glenosphere offset and sizes, varying humeral neck-shaft angles, and varying humeral insert thickness. Surgical technique options include the level and version of the humeral osteotomy, placement of the humeral socket (inset versus onset), placement of the glenosphere, and the use of glenoid or humeral bone grafting.

A Grammont-style prosthesis with a valgus neck cut tensions the remaining soft tissues by placing the humerus in an inferior position, which effectively lengthens the humerus and, thus, increases the acromial-tuberosity distance. This may increase compression between the ball and socket and provide a stable reduction;[19] however, the vector of pull is no longer in an anatomic plane after the humerus is substantially lengthened. In patients who have glenoid bone loss, a medialized COR may place a distracting force on the humeral component, which increases the risk of dislocation.[19,72] The humerus can be further lengthened and tensioned by using an inferior eccentric glenosphere, a larger glenosphere with inferior overhang, a more valgus humeral neck-shaft angle, and humeral augments; however, increasing humeral length increases the risk of acromial stress fracture, brachial plexopathy, deltoid overtensioning, and loss of motion.

Another method to increase compressive force at the joint involves increasing the glenoid-tuberosity distance by shifting the humerus laterally. This can be achieved by using a lateral eccentric glenosphere, using a more varus humeral component or neck cut, translating the humeral component so the intramedullary stem is lateral to the socket, and insetting the humeral socket. The potential consequences of increasing the glenoid-tuberosity distance include greater component or bony impingement. Using several implant designs as well as several glenosphere and humeral socket sizes, Freilich et al[73] evaluated changes in capsular volume as well as vertical and horizontal humeral shift. The authors reported that the humeral neck-shaft angle was the most important factor that affected intra-articular volume; the diameter and offset of the glenosphere had less of an effect on intra-articular volume. The authors reported that lateralization of the glenosphere followed by the humeral neck-shaft angle were the most important factors that affected lateral humeral displacement. Finally, the authors reported that the humeral neck-shaft angle was the most important factor that affected deltoid length; glenosphere location and humeral offset had less of an effect on deltoid length. It is important for surgeons to remember that stability is a highly complex issue affected by numerous implant- and patient-related factors, and that hardware selection and changes made in implant configuration may have multifactorial effects.[74]

Range of Motion

As previously discussed, RSA designs and techniques that help provide a more stable implant may, in fact, detract from maximal ROM and, thus, overall postoperative function. To achieve the best outcomes, a balance must be attained between stability and consistent and adequate impingement-free ROM. Surgeons can help predict postoperative ROM by altering potential prosthetic design components in space relative to the bony structures of the shoulder—namely the glenoid, the acromion, and the scapular neck—that may be sources of impingement during motion and at rest. With many Grammont-based designs, the medial aspect of the humeral socket often impinges on the inferior scapular pillar, even if the patient's arm is in the resting position at his or her side. This impingement may result in the radiographic appearance of bone erosion along the inferior scapular

neck, which is termed scapular notching, and has been reported to result in inferior scapular wear, osteolysis, and polyethylene wear.[13] Impingement after RSA also may contribute to prosthetic instability, unexplained pain, and long-term prosthetic loosening.

Several studies have suggested placing the glenoid baseplate more inferiorly on the glenoid to avoid an adduction deficit.[75,76] In a study on the effects of several different glenoid positions on glenohumeral ROM, Nyffeler et al[75] reported that inferior glenosphere placement with the glenosphere's inferior edge overhanging the glenoid's inferior edge resulted in a significant improvement in adduction and abduction ROM. Chou et al[50] reported similar results with the use of large-diameter, inferior eccentric glenospheres that created a similar implant overhang. Roche et al[77] distalized the glenoid attachment and the prosthetic design by increasing the glenosphere thickness, which yielded improvements in impingement-free ROM.

To better understand the factors that contribute to scapular notching and determine the hierarchy of factors necessary to avoid an adduction deficit, Gutiérrez et al[78] biomechanically examined the effect of moving the COR further from the glenoid. The authors reported that ROM improvements correlated with increased distances of the COR from the glenoid because it allowed for more clearance of the humeral socket before impingement. Gutiérrez et al[52] expanded on these findings by using a virtual model that simulated 243 prosthetic design and surgical technique combinations to reassess different combinations of prosthetic design and surgical technique factors when moving the humerus from 0° of abduction until

superior impingement on the scapula or acromion occurred. The authors reported that the most important factor for avoiding an adduction deficit was a more varus humeral neck-shaft angle of 130°, followed by an inferior glenosphere position on the glenoid, a 10-mm lateral offset of the COR, inferior tilt of the glenosphere, and a larger glenosphere size. The authors also reported that the most important factor for maximizing abduction impingement-free ROM was the use of a lateralized glenosphere COR, followed by inferior glenoid component placement, inferior glenoid component tilt, the use a humeral implant with a lower neck-shaft angle, and a larger glenosphere. Given that previous studies had examined abduction only, Virani et al[79] used the validated virtual model to examine the effects of 216 prosthetic design and surgical technique combinations on abduction, flexion/extension, and internal/external rotation. The authors reported that the humeral neck-shaft angle had the greatest effect on abduction and flexion/extension, and glenosphere placement on the glenoid had the greatest effect on internal and external rotation. Overall, the authors concluded that a higher lateralization of glenosphere COR offset maximized motion in all planes, inferior glenosphere placement maximized internal and external rotation, a valgus humeral neck-shaft angle maximized motion in abduction, and a varus humeral neck-shaft angle maximized flexion/extension.

Surgeons must understand that maximizing impingement-free ROM is not only important to achieve ultimate ROM but also may play a critical role in the survivability of the implant. Similar to hip arthroplasty, polyethylene wear, which may result in osteolysis and polyethylene disease, is a major consequence of mechanical impingement. RSA patients with scapular notching have been reported to have inferior clinical results, which may lead to bone loss and eventual catastrophic failure of the glenoid component.[57,80,81] To minimize scapular notching, surgeons should make a maximum effort to optimize impingement-free ROM. It also is important for surgeons to be aware of the multifactorial nature of shoulder ROM, and that changes made to improve one plane of motion may have unintended effects in others.

External Rotation Strength

Although the clinical results of the Grammont-style RSA prosthesis have shown improvements in both pain relief and functional recovery, external rotation improvements have been unreliable. Postoperatively, some patients still have weak external rotation and others exhibit a loss in overall external rotation.[20,82-85] This loss can be attributed to both biologic (fatty infiltration, muscle atrophy, etc) and biomechanical factors. Regardless of prosthetic design, a reduction in external force will occur in patients who have complete teres minor and infraspinatus muscle loss as the force generator is completely lost. Depending on the amount of tissue loss, the potential maximum force output from these muscles will predictably decline; however, in patients who have comparable muscle loss, the optimal length-tension of active muscle units has an effect and the biomechanical consequences of medializing the COR to the glenoid negatively alters the length-tension relationship of the remaining rotator cuff muscles.[86] In addition, the cuff-force vector is no longer in an anatomic plane in patients who

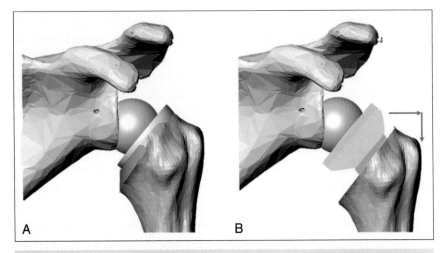

Figure 6 Anatomic illustrations of a shoulder show the consequences of retaining the humeral stem in conversion to a reverse shoulder prosthesis. **A,** Stem removal and replacement allows the stem to be inset, which facilitates a more anatomic position of the humerus. **B,** Stem retention and conversion requires an onset humeral socket, which may lead to increased distalization and lateralization of the humerus (arrows).

have a distalized humerus. This altered anatomy decreases muscular efficiency and explains the resultant loss of external rotation strength. Further, evidence suggests that patients who experience external rotation improvements are more satisfied with their outcomes.[84]

Improvements in external rotation were observed more consistently if surgeons used a prosthesis that had a more lateral COR. In patients who have rotator cuff deficiency, the unstable, proximally migrated humerus prevents the remaining intact rotator cuff muscles from properly functioning. Chacon et al[87] hypothesized that restoring the humerus to a more anatomic position would provide adequate tension to the remaining posterior rotator cuff muscles, which could restore strength and, potentially, more normal function to the remaining muscles. In addition, because restoration of maximal passive ROM is a prerequisite for achieving active external rotation, the authors believed that the use of a prosthetic design that would maximize humeral-glenoid

impingement-free ROM would create the potential for functional recovery of external rotation. Clinical studies have reported that, in a variety of pathologic conditions, restoration of a more anatomic lateral offset of the humerus has led to postoperative increases in external rotation.[48,87-90]

Modularity

As RSA indications continue to expand, the ability of surgeons to revise a well-fixed TSA or hemiarthroplasty is becoming more of a concern. The removal of a well-fixed stemmed prosthesis may result in several inherent intraoperative complications, such as radial nerve palsy, bone loss, humeral fractures, and increased soft-tissue compromise. Many current devices are modular systems that use the same stem for both anatomic and reverse implants (**Figure 6**). Several small studies have supported revision to RSA with stem retention because it avoids neurologic and stem removal complications.[91-93] Wieser et al[94] reported substantially less blood loss and reduced surgical times for patients who underwent RSA with humeral stem retention compared with patients who underwent RSA with stem exchange; however, the authors did support the removal of well-fixed stems in patients in whom substantial stem malposition was encountered.[94]

Although modular revision has many benefits, it also has biomechanical consequences. The ideal position of the humeral stem in an anatomic TSA may not be the same in RSA and is highly debatable. Alterations in the spatial relationship of the humerus to its surrounding structures have a multifactorial effect that may result in unforeseen consequences (**Figure 7**). In a study of 14 patients who underwent revision to RSA for failed hemiarthroplasty, Werner et al[93] reported a mean humeral lengthening of 2.6 cm during conversion to a modular stem. Although the authors did not report any neurologic complications, they discussed the potential risk for excessive lengthening. Deltoid overtensioning may lead to adduction contractures and altered joint kinematics as well as increased glenoid forces, which may increase the risk of early glenoid loosening.

Minimal biomechanical data on modular components are available in the current literature. In a study on the biomechanical effects of onlay RSA humeral tray positioning in a prosthesis with a medialized COR, Berhouet et al[95] reported less superior impingement during abduction, scapular plane elevation, and rotation of the shoulder if the humeral tray was placed laterally or posteriorly. In addition, the authors reported that the subscapularis rotational moment arm increased with posterior offset, and the infraspinatus and teres minor rotational moment

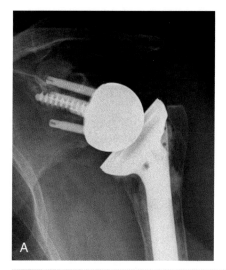
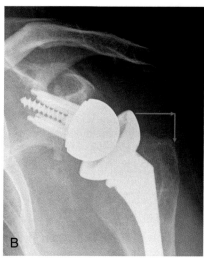

Figure 7   Postoperative AP shoulder radiographs demonstrate conversion to a reverse shoulder prosthesis after stem removal (**A**) and after stem conversion (**B**). Panel B demonstrates an increase in humeral distalization and lateralization (arrows) as well as an increase in glenoid- and acromial-tuberosity distances.

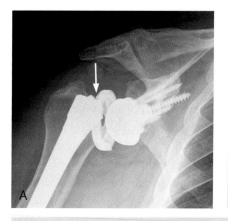
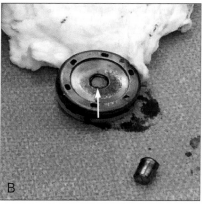

Figure 8   **A,** AP radiograph of a shoulder demonstrates failure at the modular humeral junction (arrow). **B,** Photograph of the explant shows that failure was a result of inadequate proximal bony support and implant fatigue (arrow).

arms increased with anterior offset.[95] This study highlights that an ideal humeral stem position remains elusive in nonanatomic shoulder implants. It also highlights that each onlay position has benefits and drawbacks that may affect outcomes. Compared with a monoblock component, modular systems have an increased risk of failure at the modular component, which is a result of the increased number of component interfaces[96,97] (**Figure 8**). Increased modularity

provides surgeons with options that may be conceptually attractive but remain, at some level, clinically unknown.

Current Clinical Application of Applied Knowledge

The biomechanical aspects of rotator cuff disease have implications on proper treatment. Attempts should be made to repair structures anatomically; however, the key to reduced pain and improved function is neutralizing the

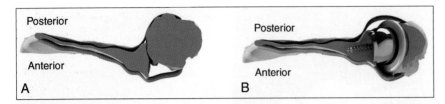

Figure 9 Anatomic illustrations of a shoulder with eccentric osteoarthritis. **A,** The humeral head demonstrates posterior wear and subluxation. **B,** Restoration of a stable fulcrum with reverse shoulder arthroplasty to neutralize the deforming forces.

mechanical deforming forces that lead to the different disease states. The spectrum of rotator cuff disease is varied; an improved understanding of these different disease states has enabled surgeons to use implant technology to provide better treatments than were previously possible.

A subtle form of rotator cuff imbalance is seen in patients who have eccentrically (posterior) worn glenohumeral osteoarthritis with an intact rotator cuff (**Figure 9**). Usually, this group of patients has previously been treated with TSA and various techniques to restore joint alignment, which reestablishes the humerus over the glenoid center line structurally but only addresses eccentricity. Previous treatments typically ignore the dynamic contribution of the rotator cuff and the abnormal forces across the joint that contribute to eccentric wear, which leads to poor long-term survival and inconsistent results.[98] It has been reported at early follow-up that early glenoid loosening develops in patients who have osteoarthritis with eccentric wear patterns and are treated with TSA at twice the rate of those who have concentric wear patterns and are treated with TSA.[99] Improved and consistent clinical results have been recently reported (short to medium follow-up) in patients who underwent RSA for the treatment of glenohumeral osteoarthritis with a biconcave glenoid because RSA corrected the soft-tissue imbalance with a semiconstrained implant.[60,100] The use of a semiconstrained implant (RSA in patients who have an intact rotator cuff is an off-label use in the United States) allows the previously subluxed humeral head to articulate with a fixed fulcrum that has a fixed COR, which neutralizes the deforming posteriorly directed force.

A massive rotator cuff tear without glenohumeral arthritis, in which the humeral head may appear aligned with the glenoid center line on static radiographs, is another form of rotator cuff deficiency. The appearance of the rotator cuff tear on radiographs may make it seem stable; however, during dynamic activity, the cuff is unable to maintain adequate compression and the humerus disassociates from the glenoid as a result of the pull of the deltoid. This may lead to pseudoparalysis and, if the coracoacromial ligament was removed during a previous arthroscopy, the humeral head may escape from the coracoacromial arch. No articular degeneration can be seen because there is no longer contact between the humeral head and the glenoid; however, depending on the degree of instability and the time to presentation, different eccentric wear patterns may develop. RSA is an effective treatment for these injuries because the deltoid will pull the humeral socket into the glenosphere, which will result in compression across a stable fulcrum, and will convert the previous deforming force to an effective lever arm (RSA in patients who have an intact rotator cuff is an off-label use in the United States).[1]

In the most severe form of rotator cuff deficiency (a massive rotator cuff tear with complete loss of static soft-tissue support), the pull of the deltoid is unopposed, which leads to migration of the humeral head into the subacromial space and abutment into the acromion. Patients with this form of rotator cuff deficiency have a humeral head that is statically subluxated proximally, which leads to both eccentric glenohumeral wear and abutment between the greater tuberosity and the acromion (ie, acromial erosion or acetabularization; **Figure 10**). Functional motion requires not only restoration of the force couple of the shoulder but also distalization of the humerus to avoid superior impingement. The restoration of length-tension relationships, joint stability, and a fixed stable fulcrum is vital to restore function in many other shoulder pathologies, including failed arthroplasty, severe glenoid bone loss (**Figure 11**), and four-part proximal humerus fractures (**Figure 12**). A better understanding of these concepts has led to advancements in prosthetic design and, thus, improvements in impingement-free ROM, implant survival, and, ultimately, clinical outcomes.

Summary

The evolution of RSA has been driven by an improved biomechanical understanding of the diseased shoulder and the effects of implant design. Advancements in humeral surface coatings and compressive lag screw baseplate designs have improved cementless component

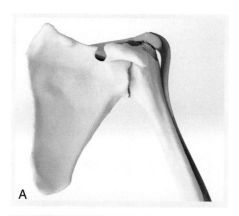
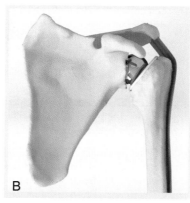

Figure 10 Anatomic illustrations of a shoulder with severe rotator cuff tear arthropathy. **A,** Superior migration of the proximal humerus leads to glenoid wear and a locked fulcrum as a result of increased friction at the joint interface. **B,** Reverse shoulder arthroplasty distalizes the humerus into a more anatomic position to restore the force couple.

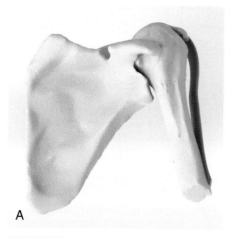
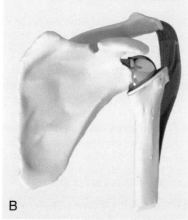

Figure 11 Anatomic illustrations of a shoulder with glenoid bone loss. **A,** Severe superior glenoid bone loss results in an unstable fulcrum and subluxation of the humeral head in the direction of the deficit. **B,** A stable fulcrum is restored with the use of reverse shoulder arthroplasty and the superior placement of a glenoid bone graft behind the baseplate.

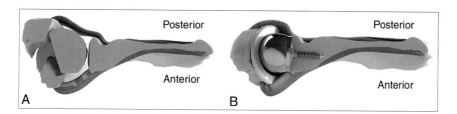

Figure 12 Anatomic illustrations of a shoulder with a four-part proximal humerus fracture. **A,** Displacement occurs as a result of the pull of the posterior cuff on the greater tuberosity and anterior pull of the subscapularis on the lesser tuberosity. **B,** Reapproximation of the tuberosities to a stable cemented implant neutralizes these forces and allows for an optimal healing environment.

fixation via osseointegration. Positioning the COR in a more anatomic position with the use of a lateralized glenosphere, a more varus humeral neck-shaft angle, and an inset humeral socket have reduced the incidence of scapular notching, improved glenohumeral stability, improved impingement free ROM, and improved external rotation by more appropriately tensioning the remaining posterior rotator cuff. The increase in implant options, including advanced modularity, coupled with improved knowledge of complex shoulder conditions have increased the indications for and improved the outcomes of RSA. Because RSA is still a relatively new technology that is rapidly evolving, further biomechanical research and long-term follow-up are necessary to verify the clinical validity of implant designs.

References

1. Mulieri P, Dunning P, Klein S, Pupello D, Frankle M: Reverse shoulder arthroplasty for the treatment of irreparable rotator cuff tear without glenohumeral arthritis. *J Bone Joint Surg Am* 2010;92(15):2544-2556.

2. Cuff DJ, Pupello DR: Comparison of hemiarthroplasty and reverse shoulder arthroplasty for the treatment of proximal humeral fractures in elderly patients. *J Bone Joint Surg Am* 2013;95(22):2050-2055.

3. Sebastiá-Forcada E, Cebrián-Gómez R, Lizaur-Utrilla A, Gil-Guillén V: Reverse shoulder arthroplasty versus hemiarthroplasty for acute proximal humeral fractures: A blinded, randomized, controlled, prospective study. *J Shoulder Elbow Surg* 2014;23(10):1419-1426.

4. Walker M, Willis MP, Brooks JP, Pupello D, Mulieri PJ, Frankle MA: The use of the reverse shoulder arthroplasty for treatment of failed total shoulder arthroplasty. *J Shoulder Elbow Surg* 2012;21(4):514-522.

5. Black EM, Roberts SM, Siegel E, Yannopoulos P, Higgins LD, Warner JJ: Reverse shoulder arthroplasty as salvage for failed prior arthroplasty in patients 65 years of age or younger. *J Shoulder Elbow Surg* 2014;23(7):1036-1042.

6. Neer CS II, Craig EV, Fukuda H: Cuff-tear arthropathy. *J Bone Joint Surg Am* 1983;65(9):1232-1244.

7. Cofield RH: Total shoulder arthroplasty with the Neer prosthesis. *J Bone Joint Surg Am* 1984;66(6):899-906.

8. Field LD, Dines DM, Zabinski SJ, Warren RF: Hemiarthroplasty of the shoulder for rotator cuff arthropathy. *J Shoulder Elbow Surg* 1997;6(1):18-23.

9. Sanchez-Sotelo J, Cofield RH, Rowland CM: Shoulder hemiarthroplasty for glenohumeral arthritis associated with severe rotator cuff deficiency. *J Bone Joint Surg Am* 2001;83(12):1814-1822.

10. Williams GR Jr, Rockwood CA Jr: Hemiarthroplasty in rotator cuff-deficient shoulders. *J Shoulder Elbow Surg* 1996;5(5):362-367.

11. Zuckerman JD, Scott AJ, Gallagher MA: Hemiarthroplasty for cuff tear arthropathy. *J Shoulder Elbow Surg* 2000;9(3):169-172.

12. Bayley J, Kessel L: The Kessel total shoulder replacement, in Bayley J, Kessel L, eds: *Shoulder Surgery*. New York, NY, Springer-Verlag, 1982, pp 160-164.

13. Nyffeler RW, Werner CM, Simmen BR, Gerber C: Analysis of a retrieved Delta III total shoulder prosthesis. *J Bone Joint Surg Br* 2004;86(8):1187-1191.

14. Coughlin MJ, Morris JM, West WF: The semiconstrained total shoulder arthroplasty. *J Bone Joint Surg Am* 1979;61(4):574-581.

15. Laurence M: Replacement arthroplasty of the rotator cuff deficient shoulder. *J Bone Joint Surg Br* 1991;73(6):916-919.

16. Post M, Jablon M: Constrained total shoulder arthroplasty: Long-term follow-up observations. *Clin Orthop Relat Res* 1983;173:109-116.

17. Grammont PM, Baulot E: Delta shoulder prosthesis for rotator cuff rupture. *Orthopedics* 1993;16(1):65-68.

18. Boulahia A, Edwards TB, Walch G, Baratta RV: Early results of a reverse design prosthesis in the treatment of arthritis of the shoulder in elderly patients with a large rotator cuff tear. *Orthopedics* 2002;25(2):129-133.

19. Boileau P, Watkinson DJ, Hatzidakis AM, Balg F: Grammont reverse prosthesis: Design, rationale, and biomechanics. *J Shoulder Elbow Surg* 2005;14(1 suppl S):147S-161S.

20. Werner CM, Steinmann PA, Gilbart M, Gerber C: Treatment of painful pseudoparesis due to irreparable rotator cuff dysfunction with the Delta III reverse-ball-and-socket total shoulder prosthesis. *J Bone Joint Surg Am* 2005;87(7):1476-1486.

21. Warner JJ: Management of massive irreparable rotator cuff tears: The role of tendon transfer. *Instr Course Lect* 2001;50:63-71.

22. Boileau P, Chuinard C, Roussanne Y, Bicknell RT, Rochet N, Trojani C: Reverse shoulder arthroplasty combined with a modified latissimus dorsi and teres major tendon transfer for shoulder pseudoparalysis associated with dropping arm. *Clin Orthop Relat Res* 2008;466(3):584-593.

23. Boileau P, Chuinard C, Roussanne Y, Neyton L, Trojani C: Modified latissimus dorsi and teres major transfer through a single delto-pectoral approach for external rotation deficit of the shoulder: As an isolated procedure or with a reverse arthroplasty. *J Shoulder Elbow Surg* 2007;16(6):671-682.

24. Favre P, Loeb MD, Helmy N, Gerber C: Latissimus dorsi transfer to restore external rotation with reverse shoulder arthroplasty: A biomechanical study. *J Shoulder Elbow Surg* 2008;17(4):650-658.

25. Gerber C, Maquieira G, Espinosa N: Latissimus dorsi transfer for the treatment of irreparable rotator cuff tears. *J Bone Joint Surg Am* 2006;88(1):113-120.

26. Gerber C, Pennington SD, Lingenfelter EJ, Sukthankar A: Reverse Delta-III total shoulder replacement combined with latissimus dorsi transfer: A preliminary report. *J Bone Joint Surg Am* 2007;89(5):940-947.

27. Gagey O, Hue E: Mechanics of the deltoid muscle: A new approach. *Clin Orthop Relat Res* 2000;375:250-257.

28. Lippitt SB, Vanderhooft JE, Harris SL, Sidles JA, Harryman DT II, Matsen FA III: Glenohumeral stability from concavity-compression: A quantitative analysis. *J Shoulder Elbow Surg* 1993;2(1):27-35.

29. Matsen FA III, Lippitt SB: Principles of glenohumeral stability, in **Matsen FA III, Lippitt SB, DeBartolo SE,** eds: *Shoulder Surgery: Principles and Procedures*. Philadelphia, PA, Saunders, 2004, pp 80-90.

30. Matsen FA III, Lippitt SB: Principles of glenoid concavity, in **Matsen FA III, Lippitt SB, DeBartolo SE,** eds: *Shoulder Surgery: Principles and Procedures*. Philadelphia, PA, Saunders, 2004, pp 91-120.

31. Frankle MA, Teramoto A, Luo ZP, Levy JC, Pupello D: Glenoid morphology in reverse shoulder arthroplasty: Classification and surgical implications. *J Shoulder Elbow Surg* 2009;18(6):874-885.

32. Ecklund KJ, Lee TQ, Tibone J, Gupta R: Rotator cuff tear arthropathy. *J Am Acad Orthop Surg* 2007;15(6):340-349.

33. Visotsky JL, Basamania C, Seebauer L, Rockwood CA, Jensen KL: Cuff tear arthropathy: Pathogenesis, classification, and algorithm for treatment. *J Bone Joint Surg Am* 2004;86(suppl 2):35-40.

34. Cabezas AF, Gutiérrez S, Teusink MJ, et al: Kinematic impact of size on the existing glenohumeral joint in patients undergoing reverse shoulder arthroplasty. *Clin Biomech (Bristol, Avon)* 2014;29(6):622-628.

35. Guery J, Favard L, Sirveaux F, Oudet D, Mole D, Walch G: Reverse total shoulder arthroplasty. Survivorship analysis of eighty replacements followed for five to ten years. *J Bone Joint Surg Am* 2006;88(8):1742-1747.

36. Favard L, Katz D, Colmar M, Benkalfate T, Thomazeau H, Emily S: Total shoulder arthroplasty—arthroplasty for glenohumeral arthropathies: Results and complications

after a minimum follow-up of 8 years according to the type of arthroplasty and etiology. *Orthop Traumatol Surg Res* 2012;98(4 suppl):S41-S47.

37. Jasty M, Bragdon C, Burke D, O'Connor D, Lowenstein J, Harris WH: In vivo skeletal responses to porous-surfaced implants subjected to small induced motions. *J Bone Joint Surg Am* 1997;79(5):707-714.

38. Bobyn JD, Toh KK, Hacking SA, Tanzer M, Krygier JJ: Tissue response to porous tantalum acetabular cups: A canine model. *J Arthroplasty* 1999;14(3):347-354.

39. Wiater JM, Moravek JE Jr, Budge MD, Koueiter DM, Marcantonio D, Wiater BP: Clinical and radiographic results of cementless reverse total shoulder arthroplasty: A comparative study with 2 to 5 years of follow-up. *J Shoulder Elbow Surg* 2014;23(8):1208-1214.

40. Bogle A, Budge M, Richman A, Miller RJ, Wiater JM, Voloshin I: Radiographic results of fully uncemented trabecular metal reverse shoulder system at 1 and 2 years' follow-up. *J Shoulder Elbow Surg* 2013;22(4):e20-e25.

41. Gutierrez S, Pupello D, Comiskey C, Frankle M: Stability of reverse shoulder humeral implants in a proximal humeral bone loss model. Presented at the 56th Annual Meeting of the Orthopaedic Research Society, New Orleans, LA, March 6-9, 2010.

42. Harman M, Frankle M, Vasey M, Banks S: Initial glenoid component fixation in "reverse" total shoulder arthroplasty: A biomechanical evaluation. *J Shoulder Elbow Surg* 2005; 14(1 suppl S):162S-167S.

43. Hopkins AR, Hansen UN, Bull AM, Emery R, Amis AA: Fixation of the reversed shoulder prosthesis. *J Shoulder Elbow Surg* 2008;17(6):974-980.

44. Frankle MA, Virani N, Pupello D, Gutierrez S: Rationale and biomechanics of the reversed shoulder prosthesis: The American experience, in Frankle MA, ed: *Rotator Cuff Deficiency of the Shoulder*. New York, NY, Thieme, 2008, pp 76-104.

45. Frankle M, Siegal S, Pupello D, Saleem A, Mighell M, Vasey M: The reverse shoulder prosthesis for glenohumeral arthritis associated

with severe rotator cuff deficiency: A minimum two-year follow-up study of sixty patients. *J Bone Joint Surg Am* 2005;87(8):1697-1705.

46. Chebli C, Huber P, Watling J, Bertelsen A, Bicknell RT, Matsen F III: Factors affecting fixation of the glenoid component of a reverse total shoulder prothesis. *J Shoulder Elbow Surg* 2008;17(2):323-327.

47. Humphrey CS, Kelly JD II, Norris TR: Optimizing glenosphere position and fixation in reverse shoulder arthroplasty, part two: The three-column concept. *J Shoulder Elbow Surg* 2008;17(4):595-601.

48. Cuff D, Pupello D, Virani N, Levy J, Frankle M: Reverse shoulder arthroplasty for the treatment of rotator cuff deficiency. *J Bone Joint Surg Am* 2008;90(6):1244-1251.

49. Nigro PT, Gutiérrez S, Frankle MA: Improving glenoid-side load sharing in a virtual reverse shoulder arthroplasty model. *J Shoulder Elbow Surg* 2013;22(7):954-962.

50. Chou J, Malak SF, Anderson IA, Astley T, Poon PC: Biomechanical evaluation of different designs of glenospheres in the SMR reverse total shoulder prosthesis: Range of motion and risk of scapular notching. *J Shoulder Elbow Surg* 2009;18(3):354-359.

51. Gutiérrez S, Walker M, Willis M, Pupello DR, Frankle MA: Effects of tilt and glenosphere eccentricity on baseplate/bone interface forces in a computational model, validated by a mechanical model, of reverse shoulder arthroplasty. *J Shoulder Elbow Surg* 2011;20(5):732-739.

52. Gutiérrez S, Comiskey CA IV, Luo ZP, Pupello DR, Frankle MA: Range of impingement-free abduction and adduction deficit after reverse shoulder arthroplasty: Hierarchy of surgical and implant-design-related factors. *J Bone Joint Surg Am* 2008;90(12):2606-2615.

53. Gutiérrez S, Levy JC, Frankle MA, et al: Evaluation of abduction range of motion and avoidance of inferior scapular impingement in a reverse shoulder model. *J Shoulder Elbow Surg* 2008;17(4):608-615.

54. Berhouet J, Garaud P, Favard L: Evaluation of the role of glenosphere design and humeral component retroversion in avoiding scapular notching during reverse shoulder arthroplasty. *J Shoulder Elbow Surg* 2014;23(2):151-158.

55. Gutiérrez S, Keller TS, Levy JC, Lee WE III, Luo ZP: Hierarchy of stability factors in reverse shoulder arthroplasty. *Clin Orthop Relat Res* 2008;466(3):670-676.

56. Henninger HB, Barg A, Anderson AE, Bachus KN, Burks RT, Tashjian RZ: Effect of lateral offset center of rotation in reverse total shoulder arthroplasty: A biomechanical study. *J Shoulder Elbow Surg* 2012;21(9):1128-1135.

57. Simovitch RW, Zumstein MA, Lohri E, Helmy N, Gerber C: Predictors of scapular notching in patients managed with the Delta III reverse total shoulder replacement. *J Bone Joint Surg Am* 2007;89(3):588-600.

58. Sirveaux F, Favard L, Oudet D, Huquet D, Walch G, Molé D: Grammont inverted total shoulder arthroplasty in the treatment of glenohumeral osteoarthritis with massive rupture of the cuff: Results of a multicentre study of 80 shoulders. *J Bone Joint Surg Br* 2004;86(3):388-395.

59. De Biase CF, Ziveri G, Delcogliano M, et al: The use of an eccentric glenosphere compared with a concentric glenosphere in reverse total shoulder arthroplasty: Two-year minimum follow-up results. *Int Orthop* 2013;37(10):1949-1955.

60. Mizuno N, Denard PJ, Raiss P, Walch G: Reverse total shoulder arthroplasty for primary glenohumeral osteoarthritis in patients with a biconcave glenoid. *J Bone Joint Surg Am* 2013;95(14):1297-1304.

61. Poon PC, Chou J, Young SW, Astley T: A comparison of concentric and eccentric glenospheres in reverse shoulder arthroplasty: A randomized controlled trial. *J Bone Joint Surg Am* 2014;96(16):e138.

62. Edwards TB, Williams MD, Labriola JE, Elkousy HA, Gartsman GM, O'Connor DP: Subscapularis insufficiency and the risk of shoulder

dislocation after reverse shoulder arthroplasty. *J Shoulder Elbow Surg* 2009;18(6):892-896.

63. Cuff D, Clark R, Pupello D, Frankle M: Reverse shoulder arthroplasty for the treatment of rotator cuff deficiency: A concise follow-up, at a minimum of five years, of a previous report. *J Bone Joint Surg Am* 2012;94(21):1996-2000.

64. Valenti P, Sauzières P, Katz D, Kalouche I, Kilinc AS: Do less medialized reverse shoulder prostheses increase motion and reduce notching? *Clin Orthop Relat Res* 2011;469(9):2550-2557.

65. Frankle MA, Siegal S, Pupello DR, Gutierrez S, Griewe M, Mighell MA: Coronal plane tilt angle affects risk of catastrophic failure in patients treated with a reverse shoulder prosthesis. *J Shoulder Elbow Surg* 2007;16(2):e46.

66. Gutierrez S, Pupello D, Frankle M: Effects of eccentric glenospheres and baseplate tilts on shear stress in reverse shoulder implants. Presented at the 56th Annual Meeting of the Orthopaedic Research Society, New Orleans, LA, March 6-9, 2010.

67. Nové-Josserand L: Prosthetic instability: Clinical presentation (early, late) type of reduction, unique or recurrent, causes, etiologies, treatments, results. Presented at the Nice Shoulder Course 2006: Arthroscopy & Arthroplasty Current Concepts, Nice, France, June 3, 2006.

68. De Wilde LF, Van Ovost E, Uyttendaele D, Verdonk R: Results of an inverted shoulder prosthesis after resection for tumor of the proximal humerus.. *Rev Chir Orthop Reparatrice Appar Mot* 2002;88(4):373-378.

69. Anglin C, Wyss UP, Pichora DR: Shoulder prosthesis subluxation: Theory and experiment. *J Shoulder Elbow Surg* 2000;9(2):104-114.

70. Karduna AR, Williams GR, Williams JL, Iannotti JP: Glenohumeral joint translations before and after total shoulder arthroplasty: A study in cadavera. *J Bone Joint Surg Am* 1997;79(8):1166-1174.

71. Gutiérrez S, Luo ZP, Levy J, Frankle MA: Arc of motion and socket depth in reverse shoulder implants. *Clin Biomech (Bristol, Avon)* 2009;24(6):473-479.

72. Norris TR, Kelly JD, Humphrey CS: Management of glenoid bone defects in revision shoulder arthroplasty: A new application of the reverse total shoulder prosthesis. *Tech Shoulder Elbow Surg* 2007;8(1):37-46

73. Freilich R, Gutiérrez S, Pupello D, Lee W, Frankle M: Analysis of joint volume, humeral displacement and deltoid length changes after reverse shoulder arthroplasty: Hierarchy of surgical and implant-related factors. Presented at the 56th Annual Meeting of the Orthopaedic Research Society, New Orleans, LA, March 6-9, 2010.

74. Tashjian RZ, Burks RT, Zhang Y, Henninger HB: Reverse total shoulder arthroplasty: A biomechanical evaluation of humeral and glenosphere hardware configuration. *J Shoulder Elbow Surg* 2015;24(3):e68-e77.

75. Nyffeler RW, Werner CM, Gerber C: Biomechanical relevance of glenoid component positioning in the reverse Delta III total shoulder prosthesis. *J Shoulder Elbow Surg* 2005;14(5):524-528.

76. Lévigne C, Boileau P, Favard L, et al: Scapular notching in reverse shoulder arthroplasty. *J Shoulder Elbow Surg* 2008;17(6):925-935.

77. Roche C, Flurin PH, Wright T, Crosby LA, Mauldin M, Zuckerman JD: An evaluation of the relationships between reverse shoulder design parameters and range of motion, impingement, and stability. *J Shoulder Elbow Surg* 2009;18(5):734-741.

78. Gutiérrez S, Levy JC, Lee WE III, Keller TS, Maitland ME: Center of rotation affects abduction range of motion of reverse shoulder arthroplasty. *Clin Orthop Relat Res* 2007;458:78-82.

79. Virani NA, Cabezas A, Gutiérrez S, Santoni BG, Otto R, Frankle M: Reverse shoulder arthroplasty components and surgical techniques that restore glenohumeral motion. *J Shoulder Elbow Surg* 2013;22(2):179-187.

80. Delloye C, Joris D, Colette A, Eudier A, Dubuc JE: Mechanical complications of total shoulder inverted prosthesis. *Rev Chir Orthop Reparatrice Appar Mot* 2002;88(4):410-414.

81. Van Seymortier P, Stoffelen D, Fortems Y, Reynders P: The reverse shoulder prosthesis (Delta III) in acute shoulder fractures: Technical considerations with respect to stability. *Acta Orthop Belg* 2006;72(4):474-477.

82. Boileau P, Watkinson D, Hatzidakis AM, Hovorka I: Neer Award 2005: The Grammont reverse shoulder prosthesis. Results in cuff tear arthritis, fracture sequelae, and revision arthroplasty. *J Shoulder Elbow Surg* 2006;15(5):527-540.

83. Wall B, Nové-Josserand L, O'Connor DP, Edwards TB, Walch G: Reverse total shoulder arthroplasty: A review of results according to etiology. *J Bone Joint Surg Am* 2007;89(7):1476-1485.

84. Simovitch RW, Helmy N, Zumstein MA, Gerber C: Impact of fatty infiltration of the teres minor muscle on the outcome of reverse total shoulder arthroplasty. *J Bone Joint Surg Am* 2007;89(5):934-939.

85. Favard L, Lautmann S, Sirveau F, Oudet D, Kerjean Y, Huget D: Hemi arthroplasty versus reverse arthroplasty in the treatment of osteoarthritis with massive rotator cuff tear, in Walch G, Boileau P, Molé D, eds: *2000 Shoulder Prostheses: Two to Ten Year Follow Up.* Paris, France, Sauramps Medical, 2001, pp 261-268.

86. Herrmann S, König C, Heller M, Perka C, Greiner S: Reverse shoulder arthroplasty leads to significant biomechanical changes in the remaining rotator cuff. *J Orthop Surg Res* 2011;6:42.

87. Chacon A, Virani N, Shannon R, Levy JC, Pupello D, Frankle M: Revision arthroplasty with use of a reverse shoulder prosthesis-allograft composite. *J Bone Joint Surg Am* 2009;91(1):119-127.

88. Levy J, Frankle M, Mighell M, Pupello D: The use of the reverse shoulder prosthesis for the treatment of failed hemiarthroplasty for proximal humeral fracture. *J Bone Joint Surg Am* 2007;89(2):292-300.

89. Levy JC, Virani N, Pupello D, Frankle M: Use of the reverse shoulder prosthesis for the treatment of failed hemiarthroplasty in patients with glenohumeral arthritis and rotator

cuff deficiency. *J Bone Joint Surg Br* 2007;89(2):189-195.

90. Frankle M, Levy JC, Pupello D, et al: The reverse shoulder prosthesis for glenohumeral arthritis associated with severe rotator cuff deficiency: A minimum two-year follow-up study of sixty patients surgical technique. *J Bone Joint Surg Am* 2006; 88(suppl 1 pt 2):178-190.

91. Groh GI, Wirth MA: Results of revision from hemiarthroplasty to total shoulder arthroplasty utilizing modular component systems. *J Shoulder Elbow Surg* 2011;20(5):778-782.

92. Castagna A, Delcogliano M, de Caro F, et al: Conversion of shoulder arthroplasty to reverse implants: Clinical and radiological results using a modular system. *Int Orthop* 2013;37(7):1297-1305.

93. Werner BS, Boehm D, Gohlke F: Revision to reverse shoulder arthroplasty with retention of the humeral component. *Acta Orthop* 2013;84(5):473-478.

94. Wieser K, Borbas P, Ek ET, Meyer DC, Gerber C: Conversion of stemmed hemi- or total to reverse total shoulder arthroplasty: Advantages of a modular stem design. *Clin Orthop Relat Res* 2015;473(2):651-660.

95. Berhouet J, Kontaxis A, Gulotta LV, et al: Effects of the humeral tray component positioning for onlay reverse shoulder arthroplasty design: A biomechanical analysis. *J Shoulder Elbow Surg* 2015;24(4):569-577.

96. Cuff D, Levy JC, Gutiérrez S, Frankle MA: Torsional stability of modular and non-modular reverse shoulder humeral components in a proximal humeral bone loss model. *J Shoulder Elbow Surg* 2011;20(4):646-651.

97. Ansari F, Major C, Norris TR, Gunther SB, Ries M, Pruitt L: Unscrewing instability of modular reverse shoulder prosthesis increases propensity for in vivo fracture: A report of two cases. *J Shoulder Elbow Surg* 2014;23(2):e40-e45.

98. Cil A, Sperling JW, Cofield RH: Nonstandard glenoid components for bone deficiencies in shoulder arthroplasty. *J Shoulder Elbow Surg* 2014;23(7):e149-e157.

99. Hussey MM, Hussey MM, Steen BM, et al: The effects of glenoid wear patterns on patients with osteoarthritis in total shoulder arthroplasty: An assessment of outcomes and value. *J Shoulder Elbow Surg* 2015;24(5):682-690.

100. McFarland EG, Huri G, Hyun Y, Garbis NG: Use of the reverse total shoulder arthroplasty (RTSA) for patients with osteoarthritis and glenoid bone loss: An alternative to bone grafting. Presented at the American Shoulder and Elbow Surgeons 2013 Closed Meeting, Las Vegas, NV, October 13-15, 2013.

Video Reference

Frankle MA: Video. *Indications for Reverse Total Shoulder Arthroplasty.* Temple Terrace, FL, 2015.

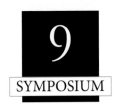

Scapular Notching

David Dare, MD
Joshua S. Dines, MD
Collin Tebo, BA
T. Bradley Edwards, MD
Edward V. Craig, MD, MPH
David M. Dines, MD

Abstract

Developed in 1985, the Grammont-style reverse total shoulder arthroplasty offered a biomechanical advantage for the deltoid muscle as well as predictably reduced pain and improved shoulder function in rotator cuff–deficient shoulders. Despite favorable outcomes, reverse total shoulder arthroplasty is associated with a unique set of complications, one of which is scapular notching. Scapular notching is believed to be a result of mechanical impingement of the humeral component on the lateral scapular pillar. Although it appears that scapular notching progresses with time, its effect on implant survivorship and clinical outcomes is unknown. Factors associated with scapular notching are categorized into several groups, including patient-specific risk factors, surgical approach and technique, and prosthetic design. Surgical strategies to reduce the rate of scapular notching include inferior positioning of the glenosphere, inferior tilting of the glenosphere, and increasing the size of the glenosphere. A lateralized center of rotation and a decreased humeral shaft-neck angle also decrease the incidence of scapular notching. As the indications for reverse total shoulder arthroplasty expand, it is important for orthopaedic surgeons to understand the etiology and incidence, predictive factors, and clinical relevance of scapular notching as well as strategies to avoid it.

Instr Course Lect 2016;65:145–156.

Conventional total shoulder arthroplasty (TSA) reliably decreases pain and improves shoulder function in patients who have glenohumeral arthritis and a functioning rotator cuff. In patients who have a deficient rotator cuff, however, standard unconstrained TSA creates altered glenohumeral kinematics, which results in decreased patient satisfaction and increased complications.[1] Reverse TSA (RTSA) was developed to compensate for an absent or malfunctioning rotator cuff. Initial designs were fraught with complications, including instability,[2] poor active shoulder motion,[2,3] and catastrophic failure of the glenoid;[2] however, modern implants and surgical techniques have contributed to improved postoperative clinical scores, improved patient satisfaction, decreased pain, and increased active motion.[4-6] Although RTSA addresses unique problems, it also is associated with unique complications, which include scapular notching.

Developed in 1985, the Grammont-style RTSA focuses on four key principles, one of which dictates that the center of rotation be medialized and distalized. This principle confers a biomechanical advantage for the deltoid muscle as well as predictably reduces pain and improves shoulder function. The biomechanics of the Grammont-style RTSA also created the potential for scapular notching. In early studies, the incidence of scapular notching ranged from 44% to 100%.[2,7-9]

Factors associated with scapular notching are categorized into several groups, including patient-specific risk factors, surgical approach and technique, and prosthetic design. It is important for orthopaedic surgeons to understand the etiology and incidence, predictive factors, and clinical relevance of scapular notching as well as strategies to avoid it.

Etiology and Classification

Scapular notching is thought to be a result of mechanical impingement of the superomedial lip of the humeral component on the inferior scapular neck when the arm is adducted, which causes an osseous defect via direct contact that is potentially compounded by a biologic response to polyethylene wear debris.[5,10] The osseous defect in the scapular neck typically occurs inferior to the glenosphere, but also may be found anterior or posterior, depending on the implant design and the positioning of the glenosphere and humeral component.[11]

Radiographic evaluation of scapular notching includes true AP and axillary views. A true AP radiograph of the shoulder in the scapular plane allows for direct examination of the scapular neck without overlap from the humeral prosthesis. Axillary radiographs may demonstrate extension of scapular notching anterior and posterior to the scapular neck. Because

scapular notching, in some cases, may be posteroinferior to the location at which the scapular pillar arises, a scapular notch may at times be best visualized on axillary lateral radiographs. It also should be noted that the presence of a bony spur medial to a scapular notch may make the scapular notch appear larger. Although the etiology of these bone spurs or osteophytes is unknown, it is hypothesized that they result from traction of the long head of the triceps.[12]

Sirveaux et al[7] developed a classification system to define the extent of scapular neck erosion (**Figure 1**). Because it may be difficult to accurately assess scapular notching on radiographs, Lévigne et al[13] prefer to regroup Sirveaux grades 1 and 2 into a single group and grades 3 and 4 into another.

Incidence

Scapular notching is usually observed within 1 year postoperatively, with most studies reporting scapular neck osteolysis between 1 and 14 months postoperatively.[2,12] The rate of scapular notching has been reported to range from zero to 96%. In a retrospective review of the postoperative radiographs of 48 patients, Werner et al[5] reported that scapular notching was exceedingly prevalent, with scapular notching evident in 96% of patients. Fifty-four percent of the patients had grade 1 or grade 2 scapular notching, and 46%

of the patients had grade 3 or grade 4 scapular notching. Lévigne et al[13] observed scapular notching in 312 of 461 shoulders (68%). Twenty-two percent of the shoulders had grade 1 scapular notching, 23% of the shoulders had grade 2 scapular notching, 13% of the shoulders had grade 3 scapular notching, and 10% of the shoulders had grade 4 scapular notching. Simovitch et al,[12] Sirveaux et al,[7] and Boileau et al[3] reported scapular notching in 44%, 64%, and 74%, respectively. More recently, Al-Hadithy et al[14] reported scapular notching in 28 of 41 shoulders (68%). Fifty-four percent of the shoulders had grade 1 or grade 2 scapular notching, and 6 patients had grade 3 or grade 4 scapular notching. Roche et al[15] calculated the weighted mean rate of scapular notching for reverse shoulders prostheses with a more medialized center of rotation to be approximately 68%, and reported that notches classified as greater than grade 2 occurred in approximately 21% of patients[3,5,7,8,12,13,16-19] (**Table 1**). Improvements in surgical technique and prosthetic design have substantially decreased the rate of scapular notching in recent years.[20-24] In the past 5 years, Valenti et al,[20] Boileau et al,[21] De Biase et al,[22] Cuff et al,[23] Li et al,[25] and Giuseffi et al[24] reported scapular notching rates of zero, 19%, zero, 9%, 11%, and 6.8%, respectively.

Dr. J.S. Dines or an immediate family member has received royalties from Biomet, and is a member of a speakers' bureau or has made paid presentations on behalf of Arthrex, CONMED Linvatec, and Ossur. Dr. Edwards or an immediate family member has received royalties from Tornier, OrthoHelix Surgical Designs, and Shoulder Options; is a member of a speakers' bureau or has made paid presentations on behalf of Tornier; serves as a paid consultant to Kinamed and Tornier; has received research or institutional support from Tornier; has received nonincome support (such as equipment or services), commercially derived honoraria, or other non-research–related funding (such as paid travel) from Tornier; and serves as a board member, owner, officer, or committee member of the American Shoulder and Elbow Surgeons. Dr. Craig or an immediate family member has received royalties from Biomet; is a member of a speakers' bureau or has made paid presentations on behalf of Biomet; serves as a paid consultant to Biomet; and serves as a board member, owner, officer, or committee member of the American Academy of Orthopaedic Surgeons and the American Shoulder and Elbow Surgeons. Dr. D.M. Dines or an immediate family member has received royalties from Biomet; serves as a paid consultant to Wright Medical Technology; has received nonincome support (such as equipment or services), commercially derived honoraria, or other non-research–related funding (such as paid travel) from Biomet; and serves as a board member, owner, officer, or committee member of the American Shoulder and Elbow Surgeons. Neither of the following authors nor any immediate family member has received anything of value from or has stock or stock options held in a commercial company or institution related directly or indirectly to the subject of this chapter: Dr. Dare and Mr. Tebo.

© 2016 AAOS Instructional Course Lectures, Volume 65

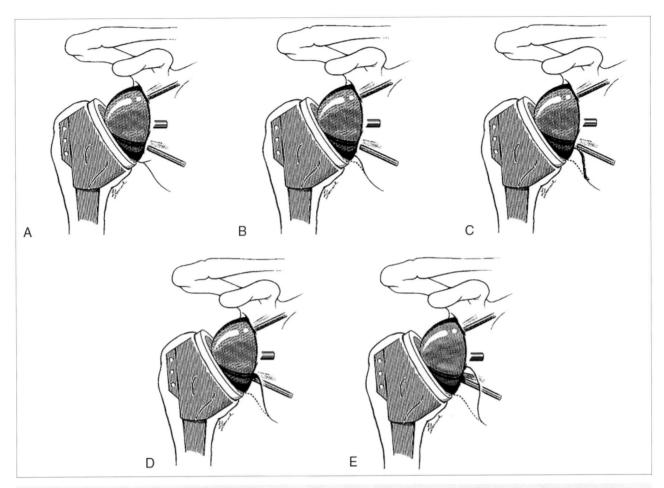

Figure 1   Illustration shows the classification system for scapular notching that was described by Sirveaux et al.[7] **A,** Grade 0 (no notch). **B,** Grade 1 (small notch). **C,** Grade 2 (erosion to the inferior screw). **D,** Grade 3 (erosion over the inferior screw). **E,** Grade 4 (erosion to the central peg). (Reproduced with permission from McFarland EG, Sanguanjit P, Tasaki A, Keyurapan E, Fishman EK, Fayad LM: The reverse shoulder prosthesis: A review of imaging features and complications. *Skeletal Radiol* 2006;35[7]:488-496.)

Radiographic Progression, Implant Survival, and Clinical Relevance

Scapular notching is generally observed within 1 year after RTSA.[2] Whether scapular notching progresses over time is debated. Werner et al[5] and Simovitch et al[12] suggest that scapular notching plateaus with time. Werner et al[5] reported that 79% of patients who had a scapular notch postoperatively did not show evidence of progression on subsequent radiographs over a period of 1 year. The remaining 21% of patients had a scapular notch that increased by a maximum of one grade by 38 months postoperatively. Similarly, Simovitch et al[12] reported that patients who had scapular notching plateaued at 18 months postoperatively, and there was no evidence of progression at 24 months postoperatively. Al-Hadithy et al[14] reported that scapular notches, all of which were visible on radiographs at 12 months, were noted in 28 shoulders (68%), only three of which progressed with time.

In contrast, both the presence and grade of scapular notching has been reported to be directly correlated with the length of follow-up. In a retrospective review of 448 patients who underwent reverse shoulder arthroplasty (RSA), Lévigne et al[13] reported scapular notching in 48% of patients 1 year postoperatively, 60% of patients 2 years postoperatively, and 68% of patients 3 years postoperatively; however, scapular notch evolution varied from patient to patient. The authors described three groups of patients: those in whom scapular notching never developed, those with scapular notching that stabilized within 2 years, and those with scapular notching that continued to progress

Table 1
Rate of Scapular Notching for Reverse Shoulder Prostheses With a Medialized Center of Rotation

Authors (Year)	No. of Shoulders	Mean Patient Follow-up in Months	Rate of Scapular Notching (%)	Rate of Scapular Notching Greater than Grade 2 (%)
Sirveaux et al[7] (2004)	80	45	64	16
Werner et al[5] (2005)	48	38	96	46
Boileau et al[17] (2006)	45	40	68	11
Simovitch et al[12] (2007)	77	44	44	18
Karelse et al[19] (2008)	27	43	59	26
Stechel et al[16] (2010)	59	48	87	5
Kempton et al[18] (2011)	43 (no glenoid tilt)	30	77	23
	28 (inferior glenoid tilt)	24	61	4
Lévigne et al[13] (2011)	461	51	68	23
Weighted mean rate of scapular notching		**46**	**68**	**20**

Adapted with permission from Roche CP, Marczuk Y, Wright TW, et al: Scapular notching and osteophyte formation after reverse shoulder replacement: Radiological analysis of implant position in male and female patients. *Bone Joint J* 2013;95(4):530-535.

after 3 years. The authors reported an increase in grade 3 and grade 4 scapular notching at longer postoperative follow-ups. Similarly, Favard et al[26] reported that the rate of grade 3 and grade 4 scapular notching increased from 35% at 5-year follow-up to 49% at 9-year follow-up.

Scapular notch evolution also may be secondary to polyethylene wear-related osteolysis.[8,27] Scratching and abrasion were the most common damage modes in retrieved RTSA components, and all modes of damage were greatest in the inferior quadrant of the humeral polyethylene component[28] (**Figure 2**). Inferior-quadrant wear is consistent with impingement of the humeral polyethylene component at the lateral edge of the scapula. Nyffeler et al[27] suggested that repetitive contact between the polyethylene component and bone may result in polyethylene wear, chronic inflammation, osteolysis, and loosening of the implant. Boileau et al[17] suggested that grade 3 and grade 4 scapular notching cannot be caused by mechanical impingement

alone and instead is attributable to osteolysis secondary to wear debris. Irlenbusch et al[29] reported the results of 113 patients who had RTSA with the use of a prosthesis that had inverted bearing materials (polyethylene glenoid, metal humeral component). Although limited by short-term follow-up, the authors reported no signs of polyethylene-induced osteolysis after 2 years.

The effect of scapular notching on implant survivorship is unknown. In a small series of only five patients, Delloye et al[30] attributed glenosphere loosening in two patients to the progression of scapular notching. In a retrospective review of 32 RSAs in 30 patients, Vanhove and Beugnies[31] reported one case of glenoid loosening that was related to scapular notching. For this reason, the authors concluded that the long-term outcomes of patients who have grade 3 or grade 4 scapular notching are a matter of concern. Lévigne et al[13] reported that glenoid radiolucent lines were more common if scapular notching was present; however, the authors

did not suggest that failed glenoid fixation was a result of the progression of scapular notching. Nonetheless, the association between scapular notching and radiolucencies adjacent to an implant is a concern, and longer term follow-up is required to better understand the consequences.

The clinical relevance of scapular notching also is unclear. Lévigne et al[13] reported no relationship between scapular notching and pain or Constant-Murley Shoulder Outcome scores at a mean follow-up of 51 months. Similarly, Werner et al,[5] Boileau et al,[3] and other studies[4,32] reported no correlation between scapular notching and clinical outcomes. In a retrospective review of 527 RSAs in 506 patients, Favard et al[26] reported that scapular notching, no matter the grade, did not influence clinical outcomes. More recently, Al-Hadithy et al[14] reported no association between the progression of scapular notching and Constant assessment or Oxford Shoulder Scale scores 24 and 60 months postoperatively.

© 2016 AAOS Instructional Course Lectures, Volume 65

In contrast, several authors have associated scapular notching with poorer functional outcomes, lower patient satisfaction, and more limited shoulder motion. Sirveaux et al[7] reported that patients with more severe notching (grade 3 or grade 4) had lower postoperative Constant assessment scores. Simovitch et al[12] reported that patients with scapular notching had lower Constant assessment scores, a decreased subjective shoulder score, decreased shoulder strength, and decreased postoperative range of motion compared with patients who did not have scapular notching. Lévigne et al[13] reported that scapular notching was accompanied by decreases in strength and forward elevation.

Predictors of Scapular Notching and How to Avoid It

Because of the prevalence of scapular notching and its potential correlation with poorer clinical outcomes, many surgeons have sought to identify predictors associated with its development. Predictors of scapular notching are categorized into several different groups. Lévigne et al[8] reported several patient-specific risk factors for scapular notching, including rotator cuff arthropathy with a decreased acromiohumeral distance, glenoids that have superior erosion, and MRI evidence of Goutallier grade 3 and grade 4 fatty infiltration of the infraspinatus. More active patients also had a slightly higher incidence of scapular notching compared with less active patients (74% and 64%, respectively). In a study of the relationship between scapular pillar anatomy and scapular notching, Berhouet et al[33] were unable to determine a specific scapular shape at high risk for scapular notching. In contrast, Paisley et al[34] reported that patients with a

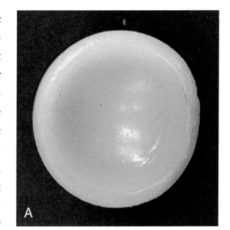
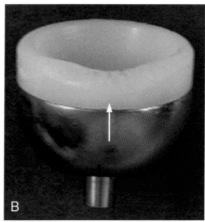
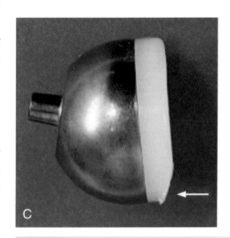
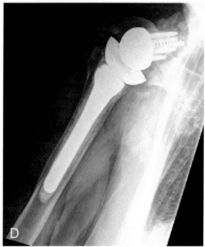

Figure 2   Images show damage modes of polyethylene components. **A,** Photograph shows a retrieved humeral polyethylene component that has abrasions consistent with surface wear. **B** and **C,** Photographs show a retrieved humeral polyethylene component with wear (arrows) in the inferior quadrant that is consistent with an adduction deficit. **D,** AP radiograph of the shoulder that contained the implant shown in panels B and C demonstrates scapular notching. (Reproduced with permission from Nam D, Kepler CK, Nho SJ, Craig EV, Warren RF, Wright TM: Observations on retrieved humeral polyethylene components from reverse total shoulder arthroplasty. *J Shoulder Elbow Surg* 2010;19[7]:1003-1012.)

shorter scapular neck (8.9 mm) had a higher risk of scapular notching compared with patients who had a longer scapular neck (12.1 mm).

Surgical technique also is a risk factor. Lévigne et al[13] reported that the superolateral approach was associated with a higher incidence of scapular notching (86%) compared with the deltopectoral approach (56%). Lévigne et al[8] reported that the superolateral approach tended to place the glenosphere in a superior position with a superior tilt.[13] Irlenbusch et al[29] reported that glenosphere overhang was 2.9 mm in procedures performed with the deltoid-split approach and 4.5 mm in procedures performed with the deltopectoral approach. Similarly, Melis et al[35] reported that scapular notching was more common with the superolateral approach compared with the deltopectoral approach.

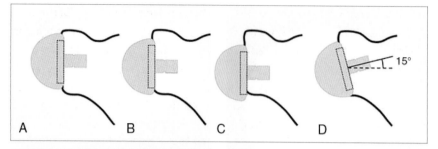

Figure 3 Illustration shows the four positions of a glenoid component. **A,** The inferior glenoid is uncovered. **B,** The glenosphere is flush with the inferior glenoid rim. **C,** The glenosphere has inferior overhang. **D,** The glenosphere has inferior tilt. (Reproduced with permission from Nyffeler RW, Werner CM, Gerber C: Biomechanical relevance of glenoid component positioning in the reverse Delta III total shoulder prosthesis. *J Shoulder Elbow Surg* 2005;14[5]:524-528.)

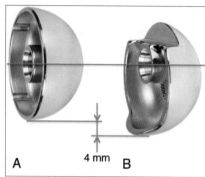

Figure 4 Photograph shows a concentric glenosphere (**A**) and an eccentric glenosphere (**B**). (Reproduced with permission from De Biase CF, Ziveri G, Delcogliano M, et al: The use of an eccentric glenosphere compared with a concentric glenosphere in reverse total shoulder arthroplasty: Two-year minimum follow-up results. *Int Orthop* 2013;37[10]:1949-1955.)

Numerous strategies to reduce impingement and subsequent notching have been proposed. These strategies focus on glenoid height[10] and tilt,[36] increased lateral offset with either glenoid bone grafting[21] or a modified prosthesis,[37] and inclination of the humeral component.[38]

Glenoid Height

Inferior overhang of the glenosphere allows for a space between the glenosphere and the scapular neck, which may decrease scapular notching. Using a computer model that evaluated six different methods to prevent scapular notching, de Wilde et al[39] concluded that inferior glenosphere overhang was the most effective method to prevent scapular notching. Similarly, Gutiérrez et al[38] used a computer model and reported that inferior positioning of the glenosphere was associated with increased range of impingement-free motion.

In a cadaver model study, Nyffeler et al[10] demonstrated that maximum adduction was achieved with inferior overhang of the glenosphere beyond the glenoid rim (**Figure 3**). The authors reported that distalization of the glenoid by 2 mm and 4 mm increased the adduction angle before impingement by 11° and 24°, respectively. Middernacht et al[40] reported that lowering the position of a 36-mm glenosphere by 2 mm increased the adduction angle by 13°. Simovitch et al[12] reported that the craniocaudal position of the glenosphere was the most important predictor of scapular notching. More recently, several authors have demonstrated the importance of inferior overhang. At 2-year follow-up, Bigorre et al[41] reported scapular notching in 65.5% of shoulders that had less than 3 mm of glenosphere overhang and 39.6% of shoulders that had more than 2 mm of glenosphere overhang. In a retrospective review, Li et al[25] reported no scapular notching in 37 patients with inferior offset between 2 and 4 mm. Because inferior glenosphere overhang must be maximized without compromising fixation in the glenoid bone stock, eccentric glenospheres have been developed.

Eccentric Glenosphere

Chou et al[42] biomechanically demonstrated that, compared with a concentric glenosphere, a similarly positioned eccentric glenosphere increased the degree of impingement-free adduction (**Figure 4**). In a biomechanical study that investigated the effect of eccentric glenospheres on micromotion at the glenosphere baseplate-bone interface, Poon et al[43] reported that micromotion was increased in glenospheres that had eccentric designs compared with concentric designs; however, the increase in micromotion was small and well within the accepted limit for osseous ingrowth in uncemented prostheses.

In a retrospective review of 25 patients who had a 4-mm eccentric glenosphere, De Biase et al[22] reported no inferior scapular notching at a mean follow-up of 27.5 months. In a study of 47 patients who underwent RTSA with an eccentric glenosphere component, Mizuno et al[44] reported that the eccentric design of the glenosphere reduced the severity of, but did not prevent, scapular notching. In a randomized controlled trial that compared concentric and eccentric glenospheres, Poon et al[45] reported that eccentric glenospheres trended toward a lower rate of scapular notching compared with concentric glenospheres (4.3% versus 14.8%) but failed to reach statistical significance. The rate of scapular notching observed in both concentric and eccentric glenospheres was markedly lower than the rate of scapular notching reported in many previous clinical series,[3-5-8,12,13,16,19,20,25,36,37] which the authors attributed to improved surgical technique because scapular notching did not develop in patients in either group who had more than 3.5 mm of overhang.

Glenosphere Tilt and Size

Many biomechanical studies have investigated the value of inferior glenosphere tilt. In a study of the effect of glenosphere inclination on component stability, Gutiérrez et al[46] reported that glenospheres that were implanted with 15° of inferior tilt generated the most compression, least tension, and smallest amount of micromotion at the baseplate-bone interface. In a cadaver model study, Nyffeler et al[10] reported that glenospheres that were implanted with 15° of inferior inclination increased both abduction and adduction impingement-free range of motion compared with glenospheres that were implanted in a neutral position. Gutiérrez et al[38] used a computer model to demonstrate that inferior glenoid tilt was associated with increased impingement-free range of motion. Despite these findings, clinical studies have failed to associate inferior glenosphere tilt with a decreased incidence of scapular notching. In a randomized trial of 42 patients who received a glenosphere component that was placed in either a neutral position or 10° of inferior inclination, Edwards et al[36] reported

that scapular notching occurred in 15 of 20 patients (75%) in the inferior tilt group and in 19 of 22 patients (86%) in the neutral group. The authors concluded that inferior tilt does not decrease scapular notching. Kempton et al[18] reported similar results in a retrospective review of 71 shoulders.

Glenosphere size also is believed to influence scapular notching. Using a computer model, Gutiérrez et al[38] reported that an increase in glenosphere diameter resulted in improved impingement-free range of motion. Compared with the humeral neck-shaft angle, the glenosphere position and tilt, and the center of rotation, the glenosphere diameter had the smallest effect on the adduction deficit. Similarly, using a sawbones model, Gutiérrez et al[47] reported that an increased glenosphere diameter decreased inferior impingement; however, the glenosphere diameter was less important than the humeral neck-shaft angle, glenosphere position, and center of rotation.

Lateral Offset

There is a direct correlation between increased lateral offset and increased glenoid baseplate motion.[48-50] Harman et al[50] reported that a lateralized center of rotation substantially increased torque at the glenoid bone-implant surface, which resulted in a failure rate of 12% by 33 months postoperatively. A more medialized center of rotation addresses this problem by converting shear forces into compressive forces at the glenoid bone-implant interface and, thus, decreasing torque and baseplate motion; however, a medialized center of rotation also is associated with an increased rate of scapular notching.[3]

In an attempt to reduce scapular notching, several authors have returned

to a more lateralized center of rotation. Lateralization of the center of rotation may in fact decrease the incidence of scapular notching and may allow for greater impingement-free range of motion. Gutierrez et al[38] reported that lateralization of the center of rotation increased impingement-free adduction (**Figure 5**). Frankle et al[37] reported good clinical outcomes and Cuff et al[23] reported no instances of scapular notching in studies in which a prosthesis with a center of rotation closer to an anatomic location was used. In a study that attempted to lateralize the glenoid component of 42 patients who underwent bony increased-offset RSA by increasing the length of the scapular neck with the use of bony autograft, Boileau et al[21] reported scapular notching in 19% of patients. In a retrospective study that compared patients who underwent a standard Grammont-style RTSA with patients who underwent a bony increased-offset RSA, Athwal et al[51] reported no difference in range of motion, strength, and clinical outcome scores; however, there was a significantly higher rate of scapular notching in the standard RTSA group compared with the offset RSA group (75% versus 40%, respectively). Valenti et al[20] reduced the rate of scapular notching to zero at 2-year follow-up by increasing lateral offset in both the glenosphere and the humeral component. The design of the glenosphere and baseplate allowed for a lateralization of 8.5 mm, and the design of the humeral component added 4 mm of additional lateralization. Kempton et al[18] also reported decreased rates of scapular notching with increased lateral offset; however, de Wilde et al[39] reported that lateralization may be less important if the glenosphere is placed in an inferior

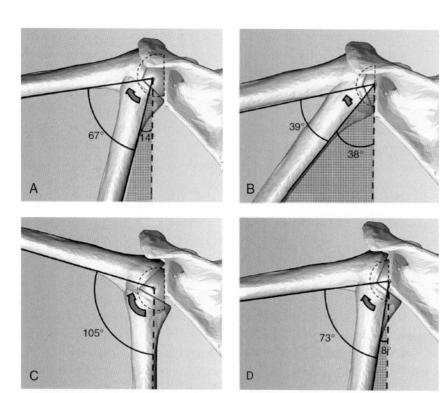

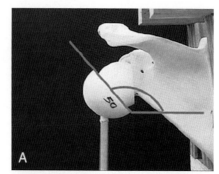

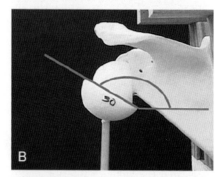

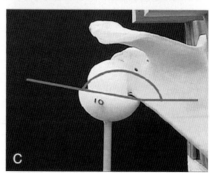

Figure 5 Illustration demonstrates the effects of lateral offset of the center of rotation and the location of the glenosphere on impingement-free range of abduction motion and the adduction deficit associated with a 36-mm glenosphere, a 150° humeral neck-shaft angle, and no glenosphere tilt. **A,** A superiorly positioned glenosphere with 10 mm of lateral offset. **B,** A superiorly positioned glenosphere with no offset. **C,** An inferiorly positioned glenosphere with 10 mm of lateral offset. **D,** An inferiorly positioned glenosphere with no offset. The shaded regions represent the adduction deficit. The range of motion (arrows) is from the point of inferior impingement to the point of superior impingement. (Adapted with permission from Gutiérrez S, Comiskey CA IV, Luo ZP, Pupello DR, Frankle MA: Range of impingement-free abduction and adduction deficit after reverse shoulder arthroplasty: Hierarchy of surgical and implant-design-related factors. *J Bone Joint Surg Am* 2008;90[12]: 2606-2615.)

Figure 6 Photographs of a bone model demonstrate different humeral neck-shaft angles. **A,** 130°. **B,** 150°. **C,** 170°. (Reproduced with permission from Gutiérrez S, Levy JC, Frankle MA, et al: Evaluation of abduction range of motion and avoidance of inferior scapular impingement in a reverse shoulder model. *J Shoulder Elbow Surg* 2008;17[4]:608-615.)

position. The authors reported that 1 mm or more of inferior positioning nullifies the benefit of lateralization on maximum adduction.

Neck-Shaft Angle and Humeral Component Version

The normal mean neck-shaft angle of the humerus is between 135° and 140°. The humeral neck inclination of a Grammont-style humeral component is 155°. As the humeral neck-shaft angle increases, the polyethylene cup assumes a more horizontal position, which potentially increases mechanical contact between the implant and the inferior scapular neck[39] (**Figure 6**). Using a computer model, Gutiérrez et al[38] evaluated the effect of the humeral neck-shaft angle, glenosphere position, glenosphere tilt, the center of rotation, and glenosphere size on impingement-free abduction and adduction. The authors reported that the primary factor that affected the adduction deficit was the humeral neck-shaft angle, and that a decreased humeral neck-shaft angle (ie, a more varus stem) resulted in substantially less inferior scapular impingement. Using a saw-bones model, Gutiérrez et el[47] evaluated the effect of glenosphere diameter, center of rotation offset, glenosphere position, and the humeral neck-shaft angle on range of motion and inferior scapular impingement. The authors reported that the humeral

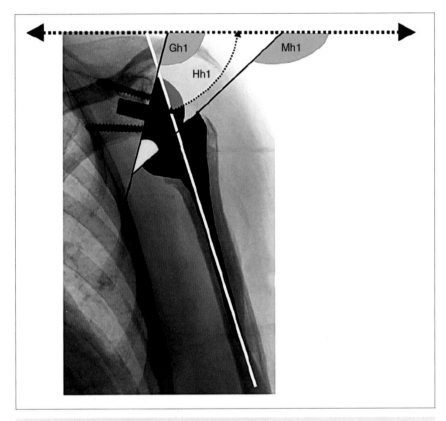

Figure 7   AP radiograph of a shoulder demonstrates the glenometaphyseal angle (yellow shaded region). The glenometaphyseal angle is formed by the glenoid baseplate and the proximal rim of the humeral metaphysis, which represents the relationship between the glenosphere and the humeral component. The dashed line with arrows represents a horizontal line parallel to the floor. Gh1 represents the angle formed by the glenoid baseplate and the dashed line with arrows. Mh1 represents the angle between the proximal humeral metaphysis and the dashed line with arrows. Hh1 represents the angle between the humeral diaphysis (white line) and the dashed line with arrows. (Reproduced with permission from Falaise V, Levigne C, Favard L; SOFEC: Scapular notching in reverse shoulder arthroplasties: The influence of glenometaphyseal angle. *Orthop Traumatol Surg Res* 2011;97[suppl 6]: S131-S137.)

neck-shaft angle had the largest effect on inferior scapular impingement, followed by the glenosphere position. Increased lateral offset had the largest effect on range of motion, followed by the glenosphere position. The authors concluded that a lateralized center of rotation and inferior positioning of the glenosphere provides greater potential range of motion, and a prosthesis that has a decreased neck-shaft angle allows for increased impingement-free adduction. In a retrospective review of 65 shoulders with a minimum follow-up of 1 year, Kempton et al[18] reported that prostheses with a smaller neck-shaft angle (143°) and lateralized center of rotation (2.5 mm) had a significantly reduced incidence of scapular notching (16.2%) compared with prostheses that had a larger neck-shaft angle (155°) and no offset, which had a 60.7% rate of scapular notching.

Falaise et al[52] introduced the concept of the glenometaphyseal angle (**Figure 7**), which corresponds with the relationship between the glenoid component and the humeral component. The authors reported a correlation between a decreased glenometaphyseal angle and a decreased rate of scapular notching. Likewise, in a retrospective review of 133 shoulders in 121 patients, Bigorre et al[41] reported a correlation between the glenometaphyseal angle and scapular notching. The authors reported that a glenometaphyseal angle of more than 28° resulted in a 72.2% rate of scapular notching, and a glenometaphyseal angle of less than or equal to 28° resulted in a 26.5% rate of scapular notching.

Humeral retroversion also can be modified to prevent scapular notching. Stephenson et al[53] reported that humeral components that were placed between 20° and 40° of retroversion most closely restored a functional arc of motion without impingement. In a cadaver model study, Berhouet et al[54] reported that humeral components that were placed between 10° to 20° of retroversion most effectively avoided inferior scapular impingement; however, this finding was not statistically significant and should not be adopted into current practice without further study. Berhouet et al[55] also demonstrated that anterior, posterior, medial, and lateral positioning of the humeral tray had no effect on the incidence of scapular notching.

Summary

Scapular notching is the erosion of the inferior scapular neck as a consequence of mechanical impingement between the humeral component and the lateral scapular pillar. Osteolysis secondary to polyethylene wear debris may contribute to the progression of scapular notching. Scapular notching is categorized according to the Sirveaux classification. Although scapular notching tends to develop early in the postoperative period, the radiographic progression of scapular notching remains controversial. The clinical relevance of scapular notching also is debated; however, with longer follow-up, it is likely that the evolution and clinical effect of scapular notching will be better understood.

Surgeons should be aware of several preoperative predictors for scapular notching. Patient-specific risk factors for scapular notching include a decreased acromiohumeral distance, superior glenoid wear, fatty infiltration of the infraspinatus, and a short scapular neck. Surgical technique also influences the rate of scapular notching, and numerous strategies, including inferior positioning of the glenosphere, inferior tilt of the glenosphere, and increasing the size of the glenosphere, have been proposed to minimize its development. A lateralized center of rotation and decreased humeral neck-shaft angle also decrease the incidence of scapular notching. Rather than embracing a major, singular change, scapular notching is most effectively minimized with the simultaneous adoption of many of the previously discussed strategies.

References

1. Edwards TB, Boulahia A, Kempf JF, Boileau P, Nemoz C, Walch G: The influence of rotator cuff disease on the results of shoulder arthroplasty for primary osteoarthritis: Results of a multicenter study. *J Bone Joint Surg Am* 2002;84(12):2240-2248.

2. Gerber C, Pennington SD, Nyffeler RW: Reverse total shoulder arthroplasty. *J Am Acad Orthop Surg* 2009;17(5):284-295.

3. Boileau P, Watkinson DJ, Hatzidakis AM, Balg F: Grammont reverse prosthesis: Design, rationale, and biomechanics. *J Shoulder Elbow Surg* 2005;14(1, suppl S):147S-161S.

4. Wall B, Nové-Josserand L, O'Connor DP, Edwards TB, Walch G: Reverse total shoulder arthroplasty: A review of results according to etiology. *J Bone Joint Surg Am* 2007;89(7):1476-1485.

5. Werner CM, Steinmann PA, Gilbart M, Gerber C: Treatment of painful pseudoparesis due to irreparable rotator cuff dysfunction with the Delta III reverse-ball-and-socket total shoulder prosthesis. *J Bone Joint Surg Am* 2005;87(7):1476-1486.

6. Cuff D, Pupello D, Virani N, Levy J, Frankle M: Reverse shoulder arthroplasty for the treatment of rotator cuff deficiency. *J Bone Joint Surg Am* 2008;90(6):1244-1251.

7. Sirveaux F, Favard L, Oudet D, Huquet D, Walch G, Molé D: Grammont inverted total shoulder arthroplasty in the treatment of glenohumeral osteoarthritis with massive rupture of the cuff: Results of a multicentre study of 80 shoulders. *J Bone Joint Surg Br* 2004;86(3):388-395.

8. Lévigne C, Boileau P, Favard L, et al: Scapular notching in reverse shoulder arthroplasty. *J Shoulder Elbow Surg* 2008;17(6):925-935.

9. Wierks C, Skolasky RL, Ji JH, McFarland EG: Reverse total shoulder replacement: Intraoperative and early postoperative complications. *Clin Orthop Relat Res* 2009;467(1):225-234.

10. Nyffeler RW, Werner CM, Gerber C: Biomechanical relevance of glenoid component positioning in the reverse Delta III total shoulder prosthesis. *J Shoulder Elbow Surg* 2005;14(5):524-528.

11. Nicholson GP, Strauss EJ, Sherman SL: Scapular notching: Recognition and strategies to minimize clinical impact. *Clin Orthop Relat Res* 2011;469(9):2521-2530.

12. Simovitch RW, Zumstein MA, Lohri E, Helmy N, Gerber C: Predictors of scapular notching in patients managed with the Delta III reverse total shoulder replacement. *J Bone Joint Surg Am* 2007;89(3):588-600.

13. Lévigne C, Garret J, Boileau P, Alami G, Favard L, Walch G: Scapular notching in reverse shoulder arthroplasty: Is it important to avoid it and how? *Clin Orthop Relat Res* 2011;469(9):2512-2520.

14. Al-Hadithy N, Domos P, Sewell MD, Pandit R: Reverse shoulder arthroplasty in 41 patients with cuff tear arthropathy with a mean follow-up period of 5 years. *J Shoulder Elbow Surg* 2014;23(11):1662-1668.

15. Roche CP, Marczuk Y, Wright TW, et al: Scapular notching and osteophyte formation after reverse shoulder replacement: Radiological analysis of implant position in male and female patients. *Bone Joint J* 2013;95(4):530-535.

16. Stechel A, Fuhrmann U, Irlenbusch L, Rott O, Irlenbusch U: Reversed shoulder arthroplasty in cuff tear arthritis, fracture sequelae, and revision arthroplasty. *Acta Orthop* 2010;81(3):367-372.

17. Boileau P, Watkinson D, Hatzidakis AM, Hovorka I: Neer Award 2005: The Grammont reverse shoulder prosthesis: results in cuff tear arthritis, fracture sequelae, and revision arthroplasty. *J Shoulder Elbow Surg* 2006;15(5):527-540.

18. Kempton LB, Balasubramaniam M, Ankerson E, Wiater JM: A radiographic analysis of the effects of glenosphere position on scapular notching following reverse total shoulder arthroplasty. *J Shoulder Elbow Surg* 2011;20(6):968-974.

19. Karelse AT, Bhatia DN, De Wilde LF: Prosthetic component relationship of the reverse Delta III total shoulder prosthesis in the transverse plate of the body. *J Shoulder Elbow Surg* 2008;17(4):602-607.

20. Valenti P, Sauzières P, Katz D, Kalouche I, Kilinc AS: Do less medialized reverse shoulder prostheses increase motion and reduce notching? *Clin Orthop Relat Res* 2011;469(9):2550-2557.

21. Boileau P, Moineau G, Roussanne Y, O'Shea K: Bony increased-offset reversed shoulder arthroplasty: Minimizing scapular impingement while maximizing glenoid fixation. *Clin Orthop Relat Res* 2011;469(9):2558-2567.

22. De Biase CF, Delcogliano M, Borroni M, Castagna A: Reverse total shoulder arthroplasty: Radiological and clinical

result using an eccentric glenosphere. *Musculoskelet Surg* 2012;96(suppl 1): S27-S34.

23. Cuff D, Clark R, Pupello D, Frankle M: Reverse shoulder arthroplasty for the treatment of rotator cuff deficiency: A concise follow-up, at a minimum of five years, of a previous report. *J Bone Joint Surg Am* 2012;94(21):1996-2000.

24. Giuseffi SA, Streubel P, Sperling J, Sanchez-Sotelo J: Short-stem uncemented primary reverse shoulder arthroplasty: Clinical and radiological outcomes. *Bone Joint J* 2014;96(4):526-529.

25. Li X, Dines JS, Warren RF, Craig EV, Dines DM: Inferior glenosphere placement reduces scapular notching in reverse total shoulder arthroplasty. *Orthopedics* 2015;38(2):e88-e93.

26. Favard L, Levigne C, Nerot C, Gerber C, De Wilde L, Mole D: Reverse prostheses in arthropathies with cuff tear: Are survivorship and function maintained over time? *Clin Orthop Relat Res* 2011;469(9):2469-2475.

27. Nyffeler RW, Werner CM, Simmen BR, Gerber C: Analysis of a retrieved delta III total shoulder prosthesis. *J Bone Joint Surg Br* 2004;86(8):1187-1191.

28. Nam D, Kepler CK, Nho SJ, Craig EV, Warren RF, Wright TM: Observations on retrieved humeral polyethylene components from reverse total shoulder arthroplasty. *J Shoulder Elbow Surg* 2010;19(7):1003-1012.

29. Irlenbusch U, Kääb MJ, Kohut G, Proust J, Reuther F, Joudet T: Reversed shoulder arthroplasty with inversed bearing materials: 2-year clinical and radiographic results in 101 patients. *Arch Orthop Trauma Surg* 2015;135(2):161-169.

30. Delloye C, Joris D, Colette A, Eudier A, Dubuc JE: Mechanical complications of total shoulder inverted prosthesis. *Rev Chir Orthop Reparatrice Appar Mot* 2002;88(4):410-414.

31. Vanhove B, Beugnies A: Grammont's reverse shoulder prosthesis for rotator cuff arthropathy: A retrospective study of 32 cases. *Acta Orthop Belg* 2004;70(3):219-225.

32. Walch G, Bacle G, Lädermann A, Nové-Josserand L, Smithers CJ: Do the indications, results, and complications of reverse shoulder arthroplasty change with surgeon's experience? *J Shoulder Elbow Surg* 2012;21(11):1470-1477.

33. Berhouet J, Garaud P, Slimane M, et al: Effect of scapular pillar anatomy on scapular impingement in adduction and rotation after reverse shoulder arthroplasty. *Orthop Traumatol Surg Res* 2014;100(5):495-502.

34. Paisley KC, Kraeutler MJ, Lazarus MD, Ramsey ML, Williams GR, Smith MJ: Relationship of scapular neck length to scapular notching after reverse total shoulder arthroplasty by use of plain radiographs. *J Shoulder Elbow Surg* 2014;23(6):882-887.

35. Melis B, DeFranco M, Lädermann A, et al: An evaluation of the radiological changes around the Grammont reverse geometry shoulder arthroplasty after eight to 12 years. *J Bone Joint Surg Br* 2011;93(9):1240-1246.

36. Edwards TB, Trappey GJ, Riley C, O'Connor DP, Elkousy HA, Gartsman GM: Inferior tilt of the glenoid component does not decrease scapular notching in reverse shoulder arthroplasty: Results of a prospective randomized study. *J Shoulder Elbow Surg* 2012;21(5):641-646.

37. Frankle M, Siegal S, Pupello D, Saleem A, Mighell M, Vasey M: The Reverse Shoulder Prosthesis for glenohumeral arthritis associated with severe rotator cuff deficiency: A minimum two-year follow-up study of sixty patients. *J Bone Joint Surg Am* 2005;87(8):1697-1705.

38. Gutiérrez S, Comiskey CA IV, Luo ZP, Pupello DR, Frankle MA: Range of impingement-free abduction and adduction deficit after reverse shoulder arthroplasty: Hierarchy of surgical and implant-design-related factors. *J Bone Joint Surg Am* 2008;90(12):2606-2615.

39. de Wilde LF, Poncet D, Middernacht B, Ekelund A: Prosthetic overhang is the most effective way to prevent scapular conflict in a reverse total shoulder prosthesis. *Acta Orthop* 2010;81(6):719-726.

40. Middernacht B, De Roo PJ, Van Maele G, De Wilde LF: Consequences of scapular anatomy for reversed total shoulder arthroplasty. *Clin Orthop Relat Res* 2008;466(6):1410-1418.

41. Bigorre N, Lancigu R, Bizot P, Hubert L: Predictive factors of scapular notching in patients with reverse shoulder arthroplasty. *Orthop Traumatol Surg Res* 2014;100(7):711-714.

42. Chou J, Malak SF, Anderson IA, Astley T, Poon PC: Biomechanical evaluation of different designs of glenospheres in the SMR reverse total shoulder prosthesis: Range of motion and risk of scapular notching. *J Shoulder Elbow Surg* 2009;18(3):354-359.

43. Poon PC, Chou J, Young D, Malak SF, Anderson IA: Biomechanical evaluation of different designs of glenospheres in the SMR reverse shoulder prosthesis: Micromotion of the baseplate and risk of loosening. *Shoulder & Elbow* 2010;2(2):94-99.

44. Mizuno N, Denard PJ, Raiss P, Walch G: The clinical and radiographical results of reverse total shoulder arthroplasty with eccentric glenosphere. *Int Orthop* 2012;36(8):1647-1653.

45. Poon PC, Chou J, Young SW, Astley T: A comparison of concentric and eccentric glenospheres in reverse shoulder arthroplasty: A randomized controlled trial. *J Bone Joint Surg Am* 2014;96(16):e138.

46. Gutiérrez S, Greiwe RM, Frankle MA, Siegal S, Lee WE III: Biomechanical comparison of component position and hardware failure in the reverse shoulder prosthesis. *J Shoulder Elbow Surg* 2007;16(3, suppl):S9-S12.

47. Gutiérrez S, Levy JC, Frankle MA, et al: Evaluation of abduction range of motion and avoidance of inferior scapular impingement in a reverse shoulder model. *J Shoulder Elbow Surg* 2008;17(4):608-615.

48. Virani NA, Harman M, Li K, Levy J, Pupello DR, Frankle MA: In vitro and finite element analysis of glenoid bone/baseplate interaction in the reverse shoulder design. *J Shoulder Elbow Surg* 2008;17(3):509-521.

49. Hopkins AR, Hansen UN, Bull AM, Emery R, Amis AA: Fixation of the reversed shoulder prosthesis. *J Shoulder Elbow Surg* 2008;17(6):974-980.

50. Harman M, Frankle M, Vasey M, Banks S: Initial glenoid component fixation in "reverse" total shoulder arthroplasty: A biomechanical evaluation. *J Shoulder Elbow Surg* 2005; 14(1, suppl S):162S-167S.

51. Athwal GS, MacDermid JC, Reddy KM, Marsh JP, Faber KJ, Drosdowech D: Does bony increased-offset reverse shoulder arthroplasty decrease scapular notching? *J Shoulder Elbow Surg* 2015;24(3):468-473.

52. Falaise V, Levigne C, Favard L; SOFEC: Scapular notching in reverse shoulder arthroplasties: The influence of glenometaphyseal angle. *Orthop Traumatol Surg Res* 2011; 97(6, suppl):S131-S137.

53. Stephenson DR, Oh JH, McGarry MH, Rick Hatch GF III, Lee TQ: Effect of humeral component version on impingement in reverse total shoulder arthroplasty. *J Shoulder Elbow Surg* 2011;20(4):652-658.

54. Berhouet J, Garaud P, Favard L: Evaluation of the role of glenosphere design and humeral component retroversion in avoiding scapular notching during reverse shoulder arthroplasty. *J Shoulder Elbow Surg* 2014;23(2):151-158.

55. Berhouet J, Kontaxis A, Gulotta L, et al: Effects of the humeral tray component positioning for onlay reverse shoulder arthroplasty design: A biomechanical analysis. *J Shoulder Elbow Surg* 2015;24(4):569-577.

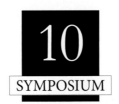

Emerging Indications for Reverse Shoulder Arthroplasty

Ekaterina Urch, MD

Joshua S. Dines, MD

David M. Dines, MD

Abstract

Historically, reverse shoulder arthroplasty was reserved for older, low-demand patients in whom rotator cuff arthropathy was diagnosed. Other common indications included sequelae of previously treated proximal humerus fractures, failed anatomic total shoulder arthroplasty, tumor resection, and rheumatoid arthritis in the elderly population. Unpredictable implant durability and high complication rates have limited the use of reverse shoulder arthroplasty to a narrow group of patients. Over the past decade, however, research has led to an improved understanding of the biomechanics behind reverse shoulder prostheses, which has improved implant design and surgical techniques. Consequently, orthopaedic surgeons have slowly begun to expand the indications for reverse shoulder arthroplasty to include a wider spectrum of shoulder pathologies. Recent studies have shown promising results for patients who undergo reverse shoulder arthroplasty for the treatment of acute proximal humerus fractures, massive rotator cuff tears without arthropathy, primary osteoarthritis, and chronic anterior dislocation, as well as for younger patients who have rheumatoid arthritis. These data suggest that, with judicious patient selection, reverse shoulder arthroplasty can be an excellent treatment option for a growing patient cohort.

Instr Course Lect 2016;65:157–170.

Grammont et al[1] introduced modern reverse shoulder arthroplasty (RSA) in the 1980s as an alternative to anatomic total shoulder arthroplasty (TSA). The procedure was originally designed for older, low-demand patients who had a pseudoparalytic, severely rotator cuff–deficient shoulder. Grammont et al[1] introduced key design elements, including a convex, articular, weight-bearing surface located at the neck of the glenoid and a concave, supported, articulating surface with a medialized and distalized center of rotation. This resulted in an inherently stable, semiconstrained system that both compensates for and bypasses the deficient rotator cuff while taking advantage of the intact deltoid muscle.[2,3]

Historical Indications

Since its introduction, RSA has been advocated for elderly (older than 65 years), low-demand patients who have a functioning deltoid muscle. Based on these basic prerequisites, a core group of well-established indications for RSA have emerged, the most classic of which is rotator cuff tear arthropathy. In patients with rotator cuff tear arthropathy, the disrupted force-couple mechanism leads to superior glenohumeral

Dr. J.S. Dines or an immediate family member has received royalties from Biomet; is a member of a speakers' bureau or has made paid presentations on behalf of Arthrex; serves as a paid consultant to or is an employee of Arthrex, CONMED Linvatec, and Ossur; and serves as a board member, owner, officer, or committee member of the American Shoulder and Elbow Surgeons. Dr. D.M. Dines or an immediate family member has received royalties from Biomet; serves as a paid consultant to or is an employee of Wright Medical Technology; has received nonincome support (such as equipment or services), commercially derived honoraria, or other non-research–related funding (such as paid travel) from Biomet; and serves as a board member, owner, officer, or committee member of the American Shoulder and Elbow Surgeons. Neither Dr. Urch nor any immediate family member has received anything of value from or has stock or stock options held in a commercial company or institution related directly or indirectly to the subject of this chapter.

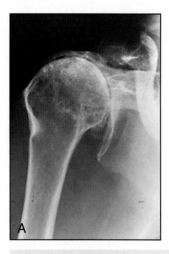
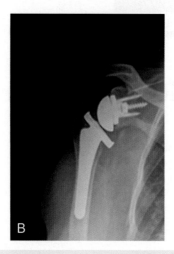
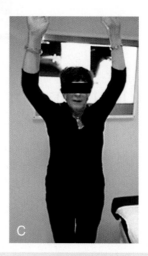
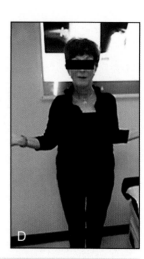

Figure 1 **A,** Preoperative AP radiograph of the shoulder of a patient who had severe rotator cuff tear arthropathy with anterosuperior escape. **B,** Postoperative AP radiograph demonstrates that the patient was treated with a reverse shoulder prosthesis. Postoperative photographs show that forward elevation (**C**) and external rotation (**D**) of the affected shoulder are nearly symmetric to the unaffected side.

instability, which subsequently results in the exertion of abnormal forces on the articular surface, the acromion, and the coracoid. In severe cases, the loss of the subscapularis muscle may lead to anterior and superior escape of the humeral head. Likewise, the loss of the compressive action of the rotator cuff leaves the deltoid unopposed and results in pseudoparalysis, which is defined as the "inability to actively elevate the arm in the presence of free passive range of motion and in the absence of a neurologic lesion."[3] The reverse shoulder prosthesis addresses the inherent instability and muscular deficiencies that accompany rotator cuff tear arthropathy and allows the patient to regain a substantial amount of function[4-11] (**Figure 1**). Similar instability challenges are seen in patients in whom anatomic TSA has failed. In such cases, RSA is a reliable salvage treatment option for both older and younger patients.[12-14]

The management of sequelae of chronic proximal humerus fractures that were treated either conservatively or surgically and the treatment of acute complex fractures in patients who are at risk for tuberosity failure are now both well-established applications of RSA.[15] Common complications after surgical fixation include tuberosity nonunion or malunion, failed hardware, and osteonecrosis of the humeral head. Until recently, tuberosity malunion presented a difficult problem for orthopaedic surgeons. Historically, surgical management of tuberosity malunion required a substantial corrective osteotomy as well as an unconstrained shoulder replacement; however, outcomes after this procedure are fair at best.[16] Recent literature has revealed that, in such cases, RSA effectively addresses problems such as proximal bone loss and rotator cuff deficiency.[17,18] Studies have shown substantial reduction in pain, improvement in function, and a high degree of satisfaction in patients who undergo RSA for the treatment of failed primary fixation.[16,19-21]

RSA also has been successfully applied in the field of orthopaedic oncology. Glenohumeral reconstruction is a dependable option for patients who are left without a rotator cuff or greater tuberosity after tumor resection.[22-24] Similarly, poor tissue quality in patients who have rheumatoid arthritis frequently leads to an incompetent rotator cuff. These patients have been reported to benefit substantially after RSA.[25-27]

A functioning deltoid is essential for the successful implementation of a reverse shoulder prosthesis. Therefore, patients who have axillary nerve dysfunction or an incompetent deltoid are poor candidates for the procedure. Other contraindications include active infection, neuropathic shoulder joints, and large glenoid defects that are not amenable to bone grafting.

Complications

Although the results reported with RSA in both Europe and, more recently, the United States are encouraging, indications for the procedure have largely remained static. This is attributed to the relatively high complication rate associated with RSA, which ranges from 7% to as high as 67%.[2,28,29] Unsurprisingly, complication rates after revision RSA have been reported to be significantly higher than complication rates after primary RSA.[30]

Complications not specific to RSA include superficial and deep infections, hematoma formation, nerve injury, and fracture. Infection rates after RSA range from 1% to 10%.[7,9,10,31-33] Historically, the risk for infection was thought to be higher in patients who have rheumatoid arthritis; however, recent studies suggest that this may not be the case.[26,33] Patients who undergo RSA for the treatment of failed hemiarthroplasty or failed anatomic TSA and patients who are younger than 65 years have the highest risk for infection.[33] Postoperative hematoma occurs in 1% to 20% of patients who undergo RSA and is attributed to the increased potential for dead space in a severely deficient rotator cuff.[4,7,9] Nerve injury after RSA is usually transient but occurs more frequently than after anatomic shoulder arthroplasty.[34] Nerve injury after RSA is attributed to intraoperative traction (especially during glenoid exposure), retractor placement, and relative lengthening of the arm. Intraoperative periprosthetic fractures that involve either the glenoid or humerus are another complication seen in patients who undergo RSA.[2,8,35] Common causes of intraoperative fracture include the failure to start the baseplate reamer before contact is made with the glenoid and reaming of an osteoporotic glenoid face beyond the subchondral bone. Humeral fractures may be caused by excessive torque on the arm during glenoid preparation or aggressive reaming in canal preparation.

Complications unique to RSA include scapular notching, instability, baseplate failure, component dissociation, and acromial and/or deltoid insufficiency. Inferior scapular notching results from impingement of the humeral polyethylene insert against the lateral scapular pillar just inferior to the glenosphere. Historically, scapular notching was nearly ubiquitous, occurring in 51% to 96% of patients after RSA.[2,9,10,36,37] Although the etiology of scapular notching is multifactorial, glenosphere position and the neck-shaft angle of the humeral component are the most important contributing factors.[38] Although conflicting data exist,[39] most evidence suggests that superior placement and tilt of the glenosphere, an acute neck-shaft angle, and medialization of the glenoid vault are independent risk factors for scapular notching.[36,38] Particulate polyethylene debris secondary to mechanical impingement may aggravate scapular notching, which can lead to osteolysis and a potential loss of fixation. Clinically, high-grade scapular notching has been associated with decreased range of motion and lower Constant assessment scores;[9,36] however, recent improvements in implant designs have decreased the incidence of high-grade scapular notching.

The incidence of instability after RSA has been reported as high as 31%.[8,9,25,29] Dislocation is commonly anterior and may be attributed to poor soft-tissue tension, the subscapularis, improper component positioning, inadequate bone stock, poor component design, and axillary nerve or deltoid dysfunction;[40,41] however, the stabilizing effect of the subscapularis remains controversial, with data to both support and refute the importance of subscapularis repair in patients who undergo RTSA.[42] The most substantial risk factor for instability of a reverse shoulder prosthesis is revision surgery, especially for a failed anatomic TSA.[43]

Baseplate failure, which is defined as loosening of the baseplate that detaches it from the glenoid, has been reported in 11.7% to 40% of patients after RSA.[6,44] Improper seating of the baseplate on the glenoid, lack of bony ingrowth, bony fixation (central peg), and glenoid component tilt all are potential causes of baseplate failure.[45,46]

Finally, acromial insufficiency fractures have been reported in approximately 4% of patients after RSA.[47] The underlying etiology of acromial insufficiency fractures is attributed to relative lengthening of the arm and the subsequent increase in deltoid tension, which leads to suboptimal clinical outcomes with low Constant assessment scores and poor overall patient satisfaction.

Modern Implant Design

Over the past decade, there has been a surge in research to improve component designs and surgical techniques, the goal of which is to minimize the incidence of mechanical complications and, thus, enhance the durability of prostheses. An improved understanding of the biomechanics behind reverse shoulder prostheses has led to improvements in technology and implant designs. For example, inferior placement of the glenosphere is important to minimize the risk of scapular notching.[48] In a study of 82 patients who underwent RSA with an eccentric, inferiorly offset glenosphere, Li et al[49] reported that 73 patients (89%) had no evidence of scapular notching at a mean follow-up of 26.3 months. Inferior offset of the glenosphere also improves impingement-free range of motion[37,38,50] (**Figure 2**). Likewise, increased caudal tilt of the glenosphere decreases the incidence of scapular notching and improves range of motion.[6,36,38,51] In a retrospective

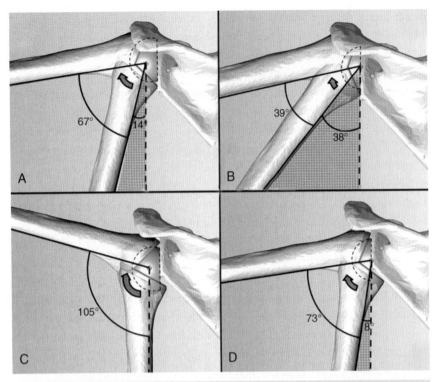

Figure 2 Illustration demonstrates the effects of lateral offset of the center of rotation and of the location of the glenosphere on impingement-free range of abduction motion. **A,** A superiorly positioned glenosphere with 10 mm of lateral offset. **B,** A superiorly positioned glenosphere with no offset. **C,** An inferiorly positioned glenosphere with 10 mm of lateral offset. **D,** An inferiorly positioned glenosphere with no offset. The shaded regions represent the adduction deficit. The range of motion (arrows) is from the point of inferior impingement to the point of superior impingement. (Adapted with permission from Gutiérrez S, Comiskey CA IV, Luo ZP, Pupello DR, Frankle MA: Range of impingement-free abduction and adduction deficit after reverse shoulder arthroplasty: Hierarchy of surgical and implant-design-related factors. *J Bone Joint Surg Am* 2008;90[12]:2606-2615.)

review of 76 patients who were treated with a prosthesis that had a 4-mm offset lateralized glenoid and a more vertical (135° neck) humeral stem, Valenti et al[52] reported no scapular notching at a mean follow-up of 44 months. Implant stability may improve as a result of the increased compressive joint reaction forces created by lateralized offset.[53,54]

Recent attention has focused on the positioning and design of the humeral implant and its effect on impingement. For example, in a study that used a computer model to evaluate the biomechanical effect of humeral tray positioning

after RSA, Berhouet et al[55] reported that the placement of the humeral tray 5 mm posterior to the humeral shaft resulted in reduced superior impingement and increased range of motion. Other studies have reported that a more varus humeral neck-shaft angle (ie, 135° or 145° instead of 155°) resulted in a larger impingement-free arc of motion.[52,56] However, Oh et al[56] reported that an overly aggressive neck-shaft angle (135°) may decrease the stability of the implant in internal rotation, which suggests that a more moderate adjustment (ie, 145°) may be warranted.

Press-fit RSA systems have emerged as a promising design option and have reported results comparable with widely used cemented systems.[57,58] An uncemented system offers the advantages of simplified surgical technique, long-lasting biologic fixation, preserved bone stock, and decreased complexity of revision surgery.

Emerging Indications

Recent advances in implant design and an improved understanding of the biomechanics behind reverse shoulder prostheses have led to a growing list of surgical indications for RSA. In 2011, one-third of an estimated 66,485 TSAs performed in the United States were RSAs.[59] Although epidemiologic data on RSA are limited, it can be logically assumed that the number of RSAs performed over the past decade has increased substantially and continues to grow. A key factor to this growth is, undeniably, the expansion of indications to include a larger cohort of patients.

Complex Proximal Humerus Fractures

Proximal humerus fractures account for roughly 5% of all fractures treated in the United States.[17] Most proximal humerus fractures are fragility fractures that occur in elderly patients.[60] Traditionally, hemiarthroplasty has been the preferred surgical procedure for the treatment of proximal humerus fractures that are not amenable to internal fixation; however, studies have reported inconsistent outcomes after hemiarthroplasty.[61,62] If successful tuberosity healing occurs, patients report excellent pain relief and functional outcomes; however, if tuberosity migration, malunion, nonunion, reabsorption, or humeral stem osteolysis occur, patients are left with weakness,

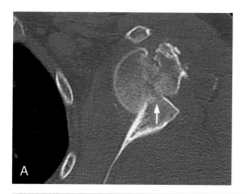
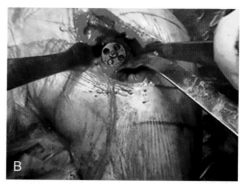
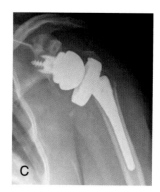

Figure 3   Images demonstrate the use of reverse shoulder arthroplasty for the treatment of a 78-year-old woman who had a four-part anterior proximal humerus fracture-dislocation. **A,** Preoperative axial CT scan demonstrates the four-part anterior proximal humerus fracture-dislocation and an associated fracture of the anterior-inferior glenoid (arrow). **B,** Intraoperative photograph shows the implantation of a 25-mm reverse shoulder mini-baseplate. **C,** Postoperative AP radiograph demonstrates a well-positioned reverse shoulder prosthesis. (Reproduced with permission from Jones KJ, Dines DM, Gulotta L, Dines JS: Management of proximal humerus fractures utilizing reverse total shoulder arthroplasty. *Curr Rev Musculokelet Med* 2013;6[1]:63-70.)

stiffness, and a substantial impediment in function.[16,61,63,64] The likelihood of complications is higher in older patients who have other medical comorbidities, such as diabetes, peripheral vascular disease, osteoporosis, and a history of smoking.

These challenges have led to a rising interest in RSA as the primary treatment option for patients who have acute complex proximal humerus fractures. Although tuberosity healing has been reported to lead to superior clinical results in RSA, it has not been reported to be a prerequisite for a good functional outcome.[60,65,66] In a retrospective study of 30 patients with proximal humerus fractures who underwent RSA, Valenti et al[67] reported no loosening or glenoid notching at a mean follow-up of 22.5 months. The authors reported that patients attained a mean forward elevation of 112°, a mean abduction of 97°, and a mean Constant assessment score of 54.9. The authors concluded that outcomes for patients with proximal humerus fractures who are treated with RSA are more predictable than those

for patients with proximal humerus fractures who are treated with hemiarthroplasty. In a prospective randomized controlled study that compared the outcomes of hemiarthroplasty with those of RSA for the treatment of patients who had proximal humerus fractures, Sebastiá-Forcada et al[68] reported that the 31 patients who were treated with RSA had significantly higher Constant assessment and University of California-Los Angeles shoulder rating scores compared with the 31 patients who were treated with hemiarthroplasty. Likewise, the patients who were treated with RSA had significantly greater forward elevation (120.3° versus 79.8°) and abduction (112.9° versus 78.7°) than their hemiarthroplasty counterparts. Similarly, Ross et al[69] reported good clinical and radiologic outcomes for elderly patients who were treated with RSA for three- and four-part proximal humerus fractures and fracture-dislocations (**Figure 3**).

Although recent data on RSA for the treatment of proximal humerus fractures are compelling, some studies

paint a less optimistic picture. In a systematic review of surgically treated proximal humerus fractures, Gupta et al[70] reported no difference in clinical outcomes between patients who were treated with RSA and patients who were treated with hemiarthroplasty. The similarity in outcomes between RSA and hemiarthroplasty occurred despite a 15.4% tuberosity nonunion rate for patients who were treated with hemiarthroplasty. In a systematic review that compared the outcomes of RSA and hemiarthroplasty for the treatment of proximal humerus fractures, Ferrel et al[71] reported improved forward flexion (118° versus 108°) and a lower revision rate (0.93%) at short-term to midterm follow-up for patients who were treated with RSA; however, the authors found no significant clinical difference in either American Shoulder and Elbow Surgeons Subjective Shoulder Scale or Constant assessment scores between RSA and hemiarthroplasty. These studies emphasize that although compelling evidence exists to support the use of RSA for the treatment of complex proximal humerus fractures, diligent patient selection remains critical to ensure the best possible outcomes.

Massive Rotator Cuff Tear Without Arthropathy

The rotator cuff uses a concavity-compression mechanism to dynamically stabilize the unconstrained glenohumeral joint, which centers the humeral head on the glenoid. In the presence of a massive rotator cuff tear, the concavity-compression mechanism is disrupted. The stable fulcrum around which the deltoid works is compromised, and the muscle is no longer able to effectively rotate the humeral head on the glenoid. Instead, as the deltoid fires, the humeral head is pulled superiorly, and glenohumeral motion is compromised, which results in pseudoparalysis. Pseudoparalysis is defined as active shoulder elevation of less than 90° in the presence of full passive anterior elevation.[9] Substantial rotator cuff tendon retraction, glenohumeral joint instability, and fatty infiltration of muscle are common findings in chronic rotator cuff tears. Patients who have pseudoparalysis experience substantial loss of function and impairment in activities of daily living. Historically, treatment options for massive rotator cuff tears included nonsurgical management, arthroscopic débridement, partial rotator cuff repair, muscle tendon transfers, and hemiarthroplasty.[72,73] Unfortunately, outcomes after these procedures are unpredictable and often leave patients with residual pain and limited function.[72,74-80]

The biomechanics of the reverse shoulder prosthesis makes it an attractive alternative for the treatment of patients who have massive rotator cuff tears. The inherent design of the reverse shoulder prosthesis blocks superior migration of the humeral head, which restores joint stability and places tension on the deltoid. This, in turn, reestablishes the deltoid fulcrum and restores forward elevation. In a study of 58 patients with painful pseudoparesis who were treated with the use of the Delta III reverse shoulder prosthesis (DePuy Synthes), Werner et al[9] reported significant improvements in patient satisfaction, Constant assessment scores, and forward elevation. Although the authors reported a complication rate of 50%, complications did not affect overall patient outcomes. In a study of 40 patients who were treated with RSA after failed rotator cuff surgery, Boileau et al[81] reported improved function for all patients. Forward elevation increased from 56° to 123° in patients who had pseudoparalytic shoulders; however, patients with preserved forward elevation whose main complaint was pain ("copers") had worse outcomes than their pseudoparalytic counterparts. Forward elevation decreased from 146° to 122° in patients who had preserved forward elevation, and 27% of patients who had preserved forward elevation were dissatisfied with their outcome. The authors also noted that the outcomes for patients who were treated with RSA after failed rotator cuff repair were inferior to the outcomes for patients who were treated with primary RSA for massive rotator cuff tears. Mulieri et al[82] evaluated the indications for and outcomes of 60 RSAs in 58 patients who had massive rotator cuff tears without glenohumeral arthritis. The study consisted of three patient groups: patients who had less than 90° of arm elevation without anterosuperior escape, patients who had less than 90° of arm elevation with anterosuperior escape, and patients who had an irreparable rotator cuff tear and pain with retained motion (greater than 90° of arm elevation). All three patient groups had significantly improved postoperative pain and function scores. Despite a 20% complication rate, implant survivorship was 90.7% at a mean follow-up of 52 months.

RSA may also be a practical option for younger patients who have irreparable rotator cuff tears. Ek et al[83] reported significant subjective improvement and a substantial gain in overall function in patients younger than 65 years who were treated with RSA for massive irreparable rotator cuff tears with and without glenohumeral arthritis. At a mean follow-up of 93 months, the authors reported significant improvements in Constant assessment scores, active forward elevation, pain scores, and strength. The authors reported a complication rate of 37.5% and failure rate of 15%; however, overall function scores did not differ between patients who had complications and those who did not ($P > 0.4$). Other studies have reported similar significant improvements in function for patients younger than 60 years who were treated with RSA for rotator cuff tears;[84,85] however, they noted that younger patients were more likely to be dissatisfied with the procedure, which highlights the importance of patient education and selection. Currently, the authors of this chapter believe the best indications for RSA in the setting of a rotator cuff tear without arthropathy are patients with a massive rotator cuff in whom primary repair will likely fail, patients with pseudoparalysis who have rotator cuff weakness on examination ("noncopers"; **Figure 4**), and patients who have potentially repairable rotator cuff tears with concomitant dynamic instability (anterosuperior escape).

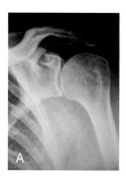
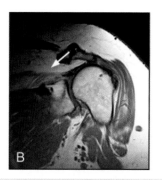
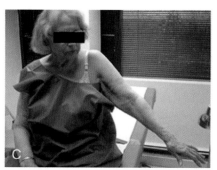
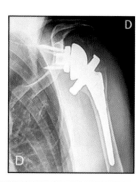

Figure 4   Images demonstrate the use of reverse shoulder arthroplasty for the treatment of a patient who had a massive rotator cuff tear without arthropathy. **A,** Preoperative AP radiograph of the left shoulder demonstrates mild glenohumeral arthritis. **B,** Preoperative axial MRI of the same shoulder reveals a retracted rotator cuff tear with fatty degeneration (arrow). **C,** Photograph shows that, on clinical examination, the patient had limited forward elevation, which is consistent with pseudoparalysis. **D,** Postoperative AP radiograph demonstrates a well-positioned reverse shoulder prosthesis.

Primary Osteoarthritis With Glenoid Bone Loss

TSA has been successful for the treatment of primary glenohumeral arthritis, with 5-, 10-, and 20-year survival rates reported to be 94.2%, 90.2%, and 81.4%, respectively.[86] However, in approximately 15% of patients who have glenohumeral osteoarthritis, substantial posterior glenoid wear leads to a biconcave glenoid and concomitant posterior humeral head subluxation.[87] This glenoid morphology, termed the Walch B2 glenoid, causes a substantial problem for shoulder stability, functional outcomes, and component survivorship after TSA.[88,89] Common techniques to address the glenoid retroversion and bone loss associated with the B2 glenoid include eccentric reaming and bone grafting of the glenoid; however, eccentric reaming presents a technical challenge because it is limited by preoperative glenoid retroversion and may lead to loss of bone stock as a result of the narrowing of the medial glenoid vault.[90] Because of these challenges, TSA outcomes for patients who have a B2 glenoid are dismal. In a review of 92 anatomic TSAs that were performed in patients who had a B2 glenoid, Walch

et al[89,91] reported a revision rate of 16.3% and a glenoid loosening rate of 20.6% at a minimum follow-up of 5 years. The authors reported that preoperative posterior humeral head subluxation greater than 80% and glenoid version of at least 27° were associated with an approximately 50% risk of posterior dislocation or loosening.

The inherent constrained biomechanics of the reverse shoulder prosthesis have allowed orthopaedic surgeons to explore its use in patients who have primary osteoarthritis with substantial glenoid bone loss. Wall et al[10] reviewed the results of 240 RSAs, 33 of which were for the treatment of posterior glenoid bone loss and concomitant humeral head subluxation, based on surgical indication. At a mean follow-up of 38 months, the mean Constant assessment score improved from 24.7 to 65.1, and mean active elevation improved from 77° to 115°. Mizuno et al[92] retrospectively reviewed 27 patients who underwent RSA for the treatment of primary glenohumeral arthritis and a B2 glenoid. Of the 27 patients, 10 underwent glenoid bone grafting to address posterior glenoid erosion. At a mean follow-up of 54 months, the

mean Constant assessment score improved from 31 to 76, and no posterior instability was observed. Complications were reported in four patients (15%), and included three patients with neurologic complications and one patient with early glenoid loosening (**Figure 5**). Although longer follow-up is necessary to determine the ultimate durability of RSA for this patient population, the current literature suggests that RSA may be a suitable treatment for patients who have glenohumeral osteoarthritis with associated posterior instability and glenoid bone loss.

Chronic Anterior Dislocation

Patients who have chronic anterior glenohumeral dislocation present a surgical challenge to orthopaedic surgeons. Substantial soft-tissue contractures and bony deficiencies in the form of a massive rotator cuff tear, an irreparable subscapularis, nonunited greater tuberosity fractures, and humeral and glenoid bone loss are common findings of chronic anterior dislocation.[93] Over the past decade, several studies on the outcomes of anatomic TSA for the treatment of patients with chronic anterior dislocation reported that recurrent

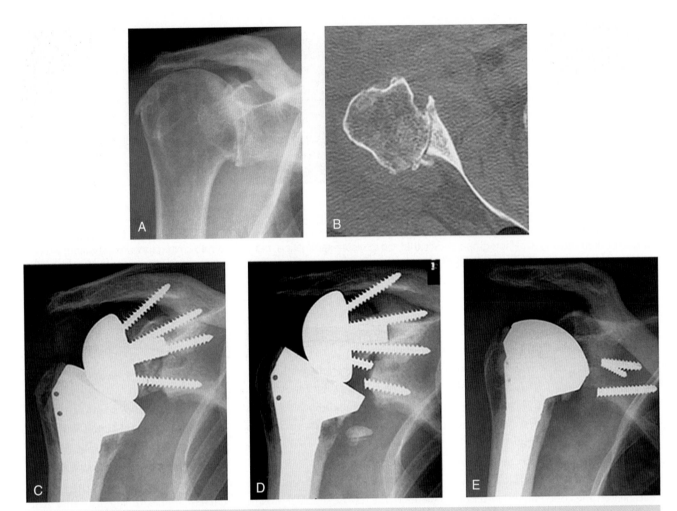

Figure 5   Images demonstrate the use of reverse shoulder arthroplasty for the treatment of a 76-year-old woman who had primary glenohumeral arthritis. **A,** Preoperative AP radiograph demonstrates primary glenohumeral arthritis. **B,** Preoperative axial CT scan demonstrates severe posterior glenoid erosion and posterior humeral head subluxation. **C,** Postoperative AP radiograph taken after the glenoid was reconstructed with the use of structural iliac crest autograft demonstrates that the central peg of the glenoid baseplate was not anchored in the native glenoid. **D,** AP radiograph taken 4 months postoperatively demonstrates superior migration of the humeral component. **E,** Radiograph taken after hemiarthroplasty was performed. (Reproduced with permission from Mizuno N, Denard PJ, Raiss P, Walch G: Reverse total shoulder arthroplasty for primary glenohumeral osteoarthritis in patients with a biconcave glenoid. *J Bone Joint Surg Am* 2013;95[14]:1297-1304.)

instability, glenoid loosening, and graft subsidence all led to a high rate of failure.[94-98] Although research is limited on the outcomes of RSA for the treatment of patients with chronic anterior dislocation, recent reports are favorable. In a review of 21 patients who were treated with single-stage RSA and bone grafting for a long-standing anterior shoulder dislocation, Werner et al[99] reported that Constant assessment scores significantly improved from 5.7 to 57.2 at a mean follow-up of 4.9 years (**Figure 6**). Of the 21 patients, two (9.5%) required revision surgery for baseplate loosening. Because the combination of RSA and bone grafting has been successful for the management of cavitary glenoid defects,[51,100] the technique is quickly emerging as an improved treatment option for shoulders with chronic anterior dislocation.

Rheumatoid Arthritis in Younger Patients

Traditionally, TSA with an unconstrained implant has been the treatment of choice for patients who have rheumatoid arthritis. Although good pain relief has been reported in patients with rheumatoid arthritis who were treated with TSA, improvements in shoulder motion and overall function were found to be less satisfactory,[101-104] which can be

© 2016 AAOS Instructional Course Lectures, Volume 65

explained by the poor quality of tissue intrinsic to patients who have rheumatoid arthritis. As many as 25% to 50% of patients who undergo shoulder arthroplasty for rheumatoid arthritis are found to have concomitant rotator cuff tears at the time of surgery.[101,102,105,106] In addition to poor tissue quality, glenoid bony erosion and poor bone quality predispose patients who have rheumatoid arthritis to component loosening and failure.

RSA has emerged as a promising alternative treatment option to anatomic TSA for the management of patients who have rheumatoid arthritis. In a study of 21 patients with rheumatoid arthritis who underwent RSA, Holcomb et al[27] reported significantly improved shoulder function and pain scores at a minimum follow-up of 2 years. In addition, forward elevation, external rotation, and internal rotation all improved significantly, with 18 of the 21 patients reporting good or excellent outcomes. Similarly, in a study of 18 patients with glenohumeral arthritis (with and without rotator cuff deficiency) who were treated with RSA, Young et al[26] reported that the mean Constant assessment score improved from 22.5 to 64.9 at a mean follow-up of 3.8 years. The authors also reported significant improvement in active forward elevation (77.5° to 138.6°) and in external rotation with the arm in 90° of abduction (16.9° to 46.1°). Iatrogenic fracture that involved the acromion, acromial spine, coracoid, or greater tuberosity was reported in 4 of the 18 patients (22%); however, no cases of infection, component loosening, or dislocation were reported. In a retrospective review of 19 patients with glenohumeral arthritis who were treated with RSA, Hattrup et al[107]

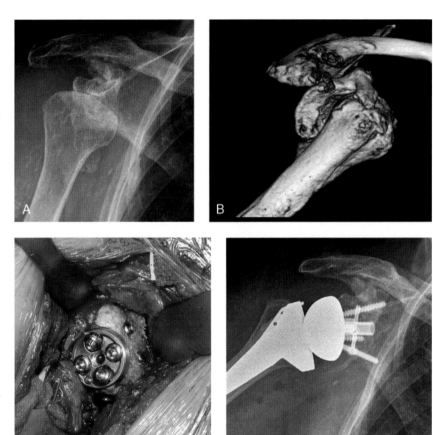

Figure 6   Images demonstrate the use of single-stage reverse shoulder arthroplasty and bone grafting for the treatment of a patient who had a long-standing anterior shoulder dislocation. **A,** Preoperative AP radiograph demonstrates the long-standing anterior shoulder dislocation. **B,** Three-dimensional CT reconstruction was used to evaluate the glenoid bone defect. **C,** Intraoperative photograph taken after the insertion of a glenoid baseplate and grafting of the glenoid bone with resected humeral head, which was secured with two additional 3.5-mm cortical screws. **D,** Postoperative AP radiograph demonstrates a well-positioned reverse shoulder prosthesis. (Reproduced with permission from Werner BS, Böhm D, Abdelkawi A, Gohlke F: Glenoid bone grafting in reverse shoulder arthroplasty for long-standing anterior shoulder dislocation. *J Shoulder Elbow Surg* 2014;23[11]:1655-1661.)

reported significant improvement in pain and function at a mean follow-up of 37 months. Iatrogenic fractures were the most common complication, but no evidence of glenoid loosening was reported. The results of these studies suggest that RSA provides good restoration of function in patients who are debilitated by rheumatoid arthritis. Because of the recent advances in technology and surgical techniques, RSA

may be applicable to younger patients who have rheumatoid arthritis, which can enable them to return to normal activities and remain maximally active.

Summary

Compared with the anatomic total shoulder prosthesis, the reverse shoulder prosthesis offers superior fixation and glenohumeral stability for patients who have soft-tissue or bony deficiencies. An improved understanding of the biomechanics involved in RSA has led to important advances in implant design and surgical techniques, which has resulted in improved implant durability and better reported functional outcomes. Consequently, orthopaedic surgeons have begun to expand their indications for RSA to include the primary treatment of common glenohumeral pathologies. Likewise, RSA is emerging as a dependable treatment option for patients who have atypical, complicated indications. Despite recent data, complication rates associated with RSA remain high, and a reliable salvage procedure for managing failed RSA has yet to be discovered; therefore, it is imperative for surgeons to evaluate each potential RSA patient in an individualized manner and carefully consider each patient's comorbidities, functional demands, and expectations. Patients who emerge as optimal candidates for the procedure can expect substantial, lasting functional improvements.

References

1. Grammont PM, Trouilloud P, Laffay JP, Deries X: Study and development of a new shoulder prosthesis. *Rhumatologie* 1987;39:407-418.

2. Boileau P, Watkinson DJ, Hatzidakis AM, Balg F: Grammont reverse prosthesis: Design, rationale, and biomechanics. *J Shoulder Elbow Surg* 2005;14(1, suppl S):147S-161S.

3. Gerber C, Pennington SD, Nyffeler RW: Reverse total shoulder arthroplasty. *J Am Acad Orthop Surg* 2009;17(5):284-295.

4. Boileau P, Watkinson D, Hatzidakis AM, Hovorka I: Neer Award 2005: The Grammont reverse shoulder prosthesis: results in cuff tear arthritis, fracture sequelae, and revision arthroplasty. *J Shoulder Elbow Surg* 2006;15(5):527-540.

5. Boulahia A, Edwards TB, Walch G, Baratta RV: Early results of a reverse design prosthesis in the treatment of arthritis of the shoulder in elderly patients with a large rotator cuff tear. *Orthopedics* 2002;25(2):129-133.

6. Frankle M, Siegal S, Pupello D, Saleem A, Mighell M, Vasey M: The reverse shoulder prosthesis for glenohumeral arthritis associated with severe rotator cuff deficiency: A minimum two-year follow-up study of sixty patients. *J Bone Joint Surg Am* 2005;87(8):1697-1705.

7. Cuff D, Pupello D, Virani N, Levy J, Frankle M: Reverse shoulder arthroplasty for the treatment of rotator cuff deficiency. *J Bone Joint Surg Am* 2008;90(6):1244-1251.

8. Valenti P, Boutens D, Nerot C, et al: Delta 3 reversed prosthesis for osteoarthritis with massive rotator cuff tear: Long-term results (>5 years), in Walch G, Boileau P, Molé D, eds: *2000 Shoulder Prosthesis: Two to Ten Year Follow-up*. Montpellier, France, Sauramps Medical, 2001, pp 253-259.

9. Werner CM, Steinmann PA, Gilbart M, Gerber C: Treatment of painful pseudoparesis due to irreparable rotator cuff dysfunction with the Delta III reverse-ball-and-socket total shoulder prosthesis. *J Bone Joint Surg Am* 2005;87(7):1476-1486.

10. Wall B, Nové-Josserand L, O'Connor DP, Edwards TB, Walch G: Reverse total shoulder arthroplasty: A review of results according to etiology. *J Bone Joint Surg Am* 2007;89(7):1476-1485.

11. Gerber C, Pennington SD, Lingenfelter EJ, Sukthankar A: Reverse Delta-III total shoulder replacement combined with latissimus dorsi transfer: A preliminary report. *J Bone Joint Surg Am* 2007;89(5):940-947.

12. Patel DN, Young B, Onyekwelu I, Zuckerman JD, Kwon YW: Reverse total shoulder arthroplasty for failed shoulder arthroplasty. *J Shoulder Elbow Surg* 2012;21(11):1478-1483.

13. Walker M, Willis MP, Brooks JP, Pupello D, Mulieri PJ, Frankle MA: The use of the reverse shoulder arthroplasty for treatment of failed total shoulder arthroplasty. *J Shoulder Elbow Surg* 2012;21(4):514-522.

14. Black EM, Roberts SM, Siegel E, Yannopoulos P, Higgins LD, Warner JJ: Reverse shoulder arthroplasty as salvage for failed prior arthroplasty in patients 65 years of age or younger. *J Shoulder Elbow Surg* 2014;23(7):1036-1042.

15. Voos JE, Dines JS, Dines DM: Arthroplasty for fractures of the proximal part of the humerus. *Instr Course Lect* 2011;60:105-112.

16. Boileau P, Trojani C, Walch G, Krishnan SG, Romeo A, Sinnerton R: Shoulder arthroplasty for the treatment of the sequelae of fractures of the proximal humerus. *J Shoulder Elbow Surg* 2001;10(4):299-308.

17. Jobin CM, Galdi B, Anakwenze OA, Ahmad CS, Levine WN: Reverse shoulder arthroplasty for the management of proximal humerus fractures. *J Am Acad Orthop Surg* 2015;23(3):190-201.

18. Mansat P, Bonnevialle N: Treatment of fracture sequelae of the proximal humerus: Anatomical vs reverse shoulder prosthesis. *Int Orthop* 2015;39(2):349-354.

19. Levy J, Frankle M, Mighell M, Pupello D: The use of the reverse shoulder prosthesis for the treatment of failed hemiarthroplasty for proximal humeral fracture. *J Bone Joint Surg Am* 2007;89(2):292-300.

20. Alentorn-Geli E, Guirro P, Santana F, Torrens C: Treatment of fracture sequelae of the proximal humerus: Comparison of hemiarthroplasty and reverse total shoulder arthroplasty. *Arch Orthop Trauma Surg* 2014;134(11):1545-1550.

21. Zafra M, Uceda P, Flores M, Carpintero P: Reverse total shoulder replacement for nonunion of a fracture of the proximal humerus. *Bone Joint J* 2014;96(9):1239-1243.

22. Kapur RA, McCann PA, Sarangi PP: Reverse geometry shoulder replacement for proximal humeral metastases. *Ann R Coll Surg Engl* 2014;96(7):e32-e35.

23. De Wilde L, Sys G, Julien Y, Van Ovost E, Poffyn B, Trouilloud P: The reversed Delta shoulder prosthesis in reconstruction of the proximal

humerus after tumour resection. *Acta Orthop Belg* 2003;69(6):495-500.

24. De Wilde LF, Plasschaert FS, Audenaert EA, Verdonk RC: Functional recovery after a reverse prosthesis for reconstruction of the proximal humerus in tumor surgery. *Clin Orthop Relat Res* 2005;430:156-162.

25. Rittmeister M, Kerschbaumer F: Grammont reverse total shoulder arthroplasty in patients with rheumatoid arthritis and nonreconstructible rotator cuff lesions. *J Shoulder Elbow Surg* 2001;10(1):17-22.

26. Young AA, Smith MM, Bacle G, Moraga C, Walch G: Early results of reverse shoulder arthroplasty in patients with rheumatoid arthritis. *J Bone Joint Surg Am* 2011;93(20):1915-1923.

27. Holcomb JO, Hebert DJ, Mighell MA, et al: Reverse shoulder arthroplasty in patients with rheumatoid arthritis. *J Shoulder Elbow Surg* 2010;19(7):1076-1084.

28. Groh GI, Groh GM: Complications rates, reoperation rates, and the learning curve in reverse shoulder arthroplasty. *J Shoulder Elbow Surg* 2014;23(3):388-394.

29. Sirveaux F, Favard L, Oudet D, Huquet D, Walch G, Molé D: Grammont inverted total shoulder arthroplasty in the treatment of glenohumeral osteoarthritis with massive rupture of the cuff: Results of a multicentre study of 80 shoulders. *J Bone Joint Surg Br* 2004;86(3):388-395.

30. Saltzman BM, Chalmers PN, Gupta AK, Romeo AA, Nicholson GP: Complication rates comparing primary with revision reverse total shoulder arthroplasty. *J Shoulder Elbow Surg* 2014;23(11):1647-1654.

31. Cheung EV, Sperling JW, Cofield RH: Infection associated with hematoma formation after shoulder arthroplasty. *Clin Orthop Relat Res* 2008;466(6):1363-1367.

32. Hattrup SJ: Early complications with the delta reverse shoulder arthroplasty: Influence of the learning curve. *J Shoulder Elbow Surg* 2007;16(2):e55.

33. Morris BJ, O'Connor DP, Torres D, Elkousy HA, Gartsman GM, Edwards TB: Risk factors for periprosthetic infection after reverse shoulder arthroplasty. *J Shoulder Elbow Surg* 2015;24(2):161-166.

34. Lädermann A, Lübbeke A, Mélis B, et al: Prevalence of neurologic lesions after total shoulder arthroplasty. *J Bone Joint Surg Am* 2011;93(14):1288-1293.

35. Wierks C, Skolasky RL, Ji JH, McFarland EG: Reverse total shoulder replacement: Intraoperative and early postoperative complications. *Clin Orthop Relat Res* 2009;467(1):225-234.

36. Simovitch RW, Zumstein MA, Lohri E, Helmy N, Gerber C: Predictors of scapular notching in patients managed with the Delta III reverse total shoulder replacement. *J Bone Joint Surg Am* 2007;89(3):588-600.

37. Lévigne C, Boileau P, Favard L, et al: Scapular notching in reverse shoulder arthroplasty. *J Shoulder Elbow Surg* 2008;17(6):925-935.

38. Gutiérrez S, Levy JC, Frankle MA, et al: Evaluation of abduction range of motion and avoidance of inferior scapular impingement in a reverse shoulder model. *J Shoulder Elbow Surg* 2008;17(4):608-615.

39. Edwards TB, Trappey GJ, Riley C, O'Connor DP, Elkousy HA, Gartsman GM: Inferior tilt of the glenoid component does not decrease scapular notching in reverse shoulder arthroplasty: Results of a prospective randomized study. *J Shoulder Elbow Surg* 2012;21(5):641-646.

40. Gallo RA, Gamradt SC, Mattern CJ, et al: Instability after reverse total shoulder replacement. *J Shoulder Elbow Surg* 2011;20(4):584-590.

41. Cheung E, Willis M, Walker M, Clark R, Frankle MA: Complications in reverse total shoulder arthroplasty. *J Am Acad Orthop Surg* 2011;19(7):439-449.

42. Clark JC, Ritchie J, Song FS, et al: Complication rates, dislocation, pain, and postoperative range of motion after reverse shoulder arthroplasty in patients with and without repair of the subscapularis. *J Shoulder Elbow Surg* 2012;21(1):36-41.

43. Wall B, Walch G, Jouve F, Mottier F: The reverse shoulder prosthesis for revision of failed total shoulder arthroplasty, in Walch G, Boileau P, Molé D, eds: *Reverse Shoulder Arthroplasty: Clinical Results, Complications, Revision*. Montpellier, France, Sauramps Medical, 2006, pp 231-242.

44. Delloye C, Joris D, Colette A, Eudier A, Dubuc JE: Mechanical complications of total shoulder inverted prosthesis. *Rev Chir Orthop Reparatrice Appar Mot* 2002;88(4):410-414.

45. Gutiérrez S, Greiwe RM, Frankle MA, Siegal S, Lee WE III: Biomechanical comparison of component position and hardware failure in the reverse shoulder prosthesis. *J Shoulder Elbow Surg* 2007;16(3, suppl):S9-S12.

46. Holcomb JO, Cuff D, Petersen SA, Pupello DR, Frankle MA: Revision reverse shoulder arthroplasty for glenoid baseplate failure after primary reverse shoulder arthroplasty. *J Shoulder Elbow Surg* 2009;18(5):717-723.

47. Walch G, Wall B, Mottier F: Complications and revision of the reverse prosthesis: A multicenter study of 457 cases, in Walch G, Boileau P, Molé D, eds: *Reverse Shoulder Arthroplasty: Clinical Results, Complications, Revision*. Montpellier, France, Sauramps Medical, 2006, pp 335-352.

48. Nyffeler RW, Werner CM, Gerber C: Biomechanical relevance of glenoid component positioning in the reverse Delta III total shoulder prosthesis. *J Shoulder Elbow Surg* 2005;14(5):524-528.

49. Li X, Dines JS, Warren RF, Craig EV, Dines DM: Inferior glenosphere placement reduces scapular notching in reverse total shoulder arthroplasty. *Orthopedics* 2015;38(2):e88-e93.

50. Gutiérrez S, Comiskey CA IV, Luo ZP, Pupello DR, Frankle MA: Range of impingement-free abduction and adduction deficit after reverse shoulder arthroplasty: Hierarchy of surgical and implant-design-related factors. *J Bone Joint Surg Am* 2008;90(12):2606-2615.

51. Boileau P, Moineau G, Roussanne Y, O'Shea K: Bony increased-offset reversed shoulder arthroplasty: Minimizing scapular impingement while maximizing glenoid fixation. *Clin Orthop Relat Res* 2011;469(9):2558-2567.

52. Valenti P, Sauzières P, Katz D, Kalouche I, Kilinc AS: Do less medialized reverse shoulder prostheses increase motion and reduce notching? *Clin Orthop Relat Res* 2011;469(9):2550-2557.

53. Henninger HB, Barg A, Anderson AE, Bachus KN, Burks RT, Tashjian RZ: Effect of lateral offset center of rotation in reverse total shoulder arthroplasty: A biomechanical study. *J Shoulder Elbow Surg* 2012;21(9):1128-1135.

54. Costantini O, Choi DS, Kontaxis A, Gulotta LV: The effects of progressive lateralization of the joint center of rotation of reverse total shoulder implants. *J Shoulder Elbow Surg* 2015;24(7):1120-1128.

55. Berhouet J, Kontaxis A, Gulotta LV, et al: Effects of the humeral tray component positioning for onlay reverse shoulder arthroplasty design: A biomechanical analysis. *J Shoulder Elbow Surg* 2015;24(4):569-577.

56. Oh JH, Shin SJ, McGarry MH, Scott JH, Heckmann N, Lee TQ: Biomechanical effects of humeral neck-shaft angle and subscapularis integrity in reverse total shoulder arthroplasty. *J Shoulder Elbow Surg* 2014;23(8):1091-1098.

57. Giuseffi SA, Streubel P, Sperling J, Sanchez-Sotelo J: Short-stem uncemented primary reverse shoulder arthroplasty: Clinical and radiological outcomes. *Bone Joint J* 2014;96(4):526-529.

58. Wiater JM, Moravek JE Jr, Budge MD, Koueiter DM, Marcantonio D, Wiater BP: Clinical and radiographic results of cementless reverse total shoulder arthroplasty: A comparative study with 2 to 5 years of follow-up. *J Shoulder Elbow Surg* 2014;23(8):1208-1214.

59. Schairer WW, Nwachukwu BU, Lyman S, Craig EV, Gulotta LV: National utilization of reverse total shoulder arthroplasty in the United States. *J Shoulder Elbow Surg* 2015;24(1):91-97.

60. Jones KJ, Dines DM, Gulotta L, Dines JS: Management of proximal humerus fractures utilizing reverse total shoulder arthroplasty. *Curr Rev Musculoskelet Med* 2013;6(1):63-70.

61. Antuña SA, Sperling JW, Cofield RH: Shoulder hemiarthroplasty for acute fractures of the proximal humerus: A minimum five-year follow-up. *J Shoulder Elbow Surg* 2008;17(2):202-209.

62. Khmelnitskaya E, Lamont LE, Taylor SA, Lorich DG, Dines DM, Dines JS: Evaluation and management of proximal humerus fractures. *Adv Orthop* 2012;2012:861598.

63. Mighell MA, Kolm GP, Collinge CA, Frankle MA: Outcomes of hemiarthroplasty for fractures of the proximal humerus. *J Shoulder Elbow Surg* 2003;12(6):569-577.

64. Noyes MP, Kleinhenz B, Markert RJ, Crosby LA: Functional and radiographic long-term outcomes of hemiarthroplasty for proximal humeral fractures. *J Shoulder Elbow Surg* 2011;20(3):372-377.

65. Bufquin T, Hersan A, Hubert L, Massin P: Reverse shoulder arthroplasty for the treatment of three- and four-part fractures of the proximal humerus in the elderly: A prospective review of 43 cases with a short-term follow-up. *J Bone Joint Surg Br* 2007;89(4):516-520.

66. Klein M, Juschka M, Hinkenjann B, Scherger B, Ostermann PA: Treatment of comminuted fractures of the proximal humerus in elderly patients with the Delta III reverse shoulder prosthesis. *J Orthop Trauma* 2008;22(10):698-704.

67. Valenti P, Katz D, Kilinc A, Elkholti K, Gasiunas V: Mid-term outcome of reverse shoulder prostheses in complex proximal humeral fractures. *Acta Orthop Belg* 2012;78(4):442-449.

68. Sebastiá-Forcada E, Cebrián-Gómez R, Lizaur-Utrilla A, Gil-Guillén V: Reverse shoulder arthroplasty versus hemiarthroplasty for acute proximal humeral fractures: A blinded, randomized, controlled, prospective study. *J Shoulder Elbow Surg* 2014;23(10):1419-1426.

69. Ross M, Hope B, Stokes A, Peters SE, McLeod I, Duke PF: Reverse shoulder arthroplasty for the treatment of three-part and four-part proximal humeral fractures in the elderly. *J Shoulder Elbow Surg* 2015;24(2):215-222.

70. Gupta AK, Harris JD, Erickson BJ, et al: Surgical management of complex proximal humerus fractures—a systematic review of 92 studies including 4500 patients. *J Orthop Trauma* 2015;29(1):54-59.

71. Ferrel JR, Trinh TQ, Fischer RA: Reverse total shoulder arthroplasty versus hemiarthroplasty for proximal humeral fractures: A systematic review. *J Orthop Trauma* 2015;29(1):60-68.

72. Field LD, Dines DM, Zabinski SJ, Warren RF: Hemiarthroplasty of the shoulder for rotator cuff arthropathy. *J Shoulder Elbow Surg* 1997;6(1):18-23.

73. Green A: Chronic massive rotator cuff tears: Evaluation and management. *J Am Acad Orthop Surg* 2003;11(5):321-331.

74. Bokor DJ, Hawkins RJ, Huckell GH, Angelo RL, Schickendantz MS: Results of nonoperative management of full-thickness tears of the rotator cuff. *Clin Orthop Relat Res* 1993;294:103-110.

75. Kempf JF, Gleyze P, Bonnomet F, et al: A multicenter study of 210 rotator cuff tears treated by arthroscopic acromioplasty. *Arthroscopy* 1999;15(1):56-66.

76. Warner JJ, Parsons IM IV: Latissimus dorsi tendon transfer: A comparative analysis of primary and salvage reconstruction of massive, irreparable rotator cuff tears. *J Shoulder Elbow Surg* 2001;10(6):514-521.

77. Gartsman GM: Massive, irreparable tears of the rotator cuff: Results of operative debridement and subacromial decompression. *J Bone Joint Surg Am* 1997;79(5):715-721.

78. Galatz LM, Ball CM, Teefey SA, Middleton WD, Yamaguchi K: The outcome and repair integrity of completely arthroscopically repaired large and massive rotator cuff tears. *J Bone Joint Surg Am* 2004;86(2):219-224.

79. Iannotti JP, Hennigan S, Herzog R, et al: Latissimus dorsi tendon transfer for irreparable posterosuperior rotator cuff tears: Factors affecting outcome. *J Bone Joint Surg Am* 2006;88(2):342-348.

80. Walch G, Edwards TB, Boulahia A, Nové-Josserand L, Neyton L, Szabo

I: Arthroscopic tenotomy of the long head of the biceps in the treatment of rotator cuff tears: Clinical and radiographic results of 307 cases. *J Shoulder Elbow Surg* 2005;14(3):238-246.

81. Boileau P, Gonzalez JF, Chuinard C, Bicknell R, Walch G: Reverse total shoulder arthroplasty after failed rotator cuff surgery. *J Shoulder Elbow Surg* 2009;18(4):600-606.

82. Mulieri P, Dunning P, Klein S, Pupello D, Frankle M: Reverse shoulder arthroplasty for the treatment of irreparable rotator cuff tear without glenohumeral arthritis. *J Bone Joint Surg Am* 2010;92(15):2544-2556.

83. Ek ET, Neukom L, Catanzaro S, Gerber C: Reverse total shoulder arthroplasty for massive irreparable rotator cuff tears in patients younger than 65 years old: Results after five to fifteen years. *J Shoulder Elbow Surg* 2013;22(9):1199-1208.

84. Sershon RA, Van Thiel GS, Lin EC, et al: Clinical outcomes of reverse total shoulder arthroplasty in patients aged younger than 60 years. *J Shoulder Elbow Surg* 2014;23(3):395-400.

85. Muh SJ, Streit JJ, Wanner JP, et al: Early follow-up of reverse total shoulder arthroplasty in patients sixty years of age or younger. *J Bone Joint Surg Am* 2013;95(20):1877-1883.

86. Singh JA, Sperling JW, Cofield RH: Revision surgery following total shoulder arthroplasty: Analysis of 2588 shoulders over three decades (1976 to 2008). *J Bone Joint Surg Br* 2011;93(11):1513-1517.

87. Walch G, Ascani C, Boulahia A, Nové-Josserand L, Edwards TB: Static posterior subluxation of the humeral head: An unrecognized entity responsible for glenohumeral osteoarthritis in the young adult. *J Shoulder Elbow Surg* 2002;11(4):309-314.

88. Iannotti JP, Norris TR: Influence of preoperative factors on outcome of shoulder arthroplasty for glenohumeral osteoarthritis. *J Bone Joint Surg Am* 2003;85(2):251-258.

89. Walch G, Moraga C, Young A, Castellanos-Rosas J: Results of anatomic nonconstrained prosthesis in primary osteoarthritis with biconcave glenoid. *J Shoulder Elbow Surg* 2012;21(11):1526-1533.

90. Denard PJ, Walch G: Current concepts in the surgical management of primary glenohumeral arthritis with a biconcave glenoid. *J Shoulder Elbow Surg* 2013;22(11):1589-1598.

91. Walch G, Young AA, Melis B, Gazielly D, Loew M, Boileau P: Results of a convex-back cemented keeled glenoid component in primary osteoarthritis: Multicenter study with a follow-up greater than 5 years. *J Shoulder Elbow Surg* 2011;20(3):385-394.

92. Mizuno N, Denard PJ, Raiss P, Walch G: Reverse total shoulder arthroplasty for primary glenohumeral osteoarthritis in patients with a biconcave glenoid. *J Bone Joint Surg Am* 2013;95(14):1297-1304.

93. Hyun YS, Huri G, Garbis NG, McFarland EG: Uncommon indications for reverse total shoulder arthroplasty. *Clin Orthop Surg* 2013;5(4):243-255.

94. Cheng SL, Mackay MB, Richards RR: Treatment of locked posterior fracture-dislocations of the shoulder by total shoulder arthroplasty. *J Shoulder Elbow Surg* 1997;6(1):11-17.

95. Sperling JW, Pring M, Antuna SA, Cofield RH: Shoulder arthroplasty for locked posterior dislocation of the shoulder. *J Shoulder Elbow Surg* 2004;13(5):522-527.

96. Hill JM, Norris TR: Long-term results of total shoulder arthroplasty following bone-grafting of the glenoid. *J Bone Joint Surg Am* 2001;83(6):877-883.

97. Matsoukis J, Tabib W, Guiffault P, et al: Primary unconstrained shoulder arthroplasty in patients with a fixed anterior glenohumeral dislocation. *J Bone Joint Surg Am* 2006;88(3):547-552.

98. Scalise JJ, Iannotti JP: Bone grafting severe glenoid defects in revision

shoulder arthroplasty. *Clin Orthop Relat Res* 2008;466(1):139-145.

99. Werner BS, Böhm D, Abdelkawi A, Gohlke F: Glenoid bone grafting in reverse shoulder arthroplasty for long-standing anterior shoulder dislocation. *J Shoulder Elbow Surg* 2014;23(11):1655-1661.

100. Melis B, Bonnevialle N, Neyton L, et al: Glenoid loosening and failure in anatomical total shoulder arthroplasty: Is revision with a reverse shoulder arthroplasty a reliable option? *J Shoulder Elbow Surg* 2012;21(3):342-349.

101. Trail IA, Nuttall D: The results of shoulder arthroplasty in patients with rheumatoid arthritis. *J Bone Joint Surg Br* 2002;84(8):1121-1125.

102. Levy O, Funk L, Sforza G, Copeland SA: Copeland surface replacement arthroplasty of the shoulder in rheumatoid arthritis. *J Bone Joint Surg Am* 2004;86(3):512-518.

103. Fuerst M, Fink B, Rüther W: The DUROM cup humeral surface replacement in patients with rheumatoid arthritis. *J Bone Joint Surg Am* 2007;89(8):1756-1762.

104. Betts HM, Abu-Rajab R, Nunn T, Brooksbank AJ: Total shoulder replacement in rheumatoid disease: A 16- to 23-year follow-up. *J Bone Joint Surg Br* 2009;91(9):1197-1200.

105. Fink B, Singer J, Lamla U, Rüther W: Surface replacement of the humeral head in rheumatoid arthritis. *Arch Orthop Trauma Surg* 2004;124(6):366-373.

106. Rozing PM, Brand R: Rotator cuff repair during shoulder arthroplasty in rheumatoid arthritis. *J Arthroplasty* 1998;13(3):311-319.

107. Hattrup SJ, Sanchez-Sotelo J, Sperling JW, Cofield RH: Reverse shoulder replacement for patients with inflammatory arthritis. *J Hand Surg Am* 2012;37(9):1888-1894.

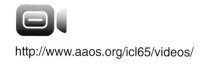

http://www.aaos.org/icl65/videos/

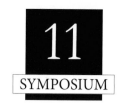

11

Reverse Shoulder Arthroplasty for Trauma: When, Where, and How

Benjamin W. Szerlip, DO
Brent J. Morris, MD
T. Bradley Edwards, MD

Abstract

Reverse shoulder arthroplasty has become increasingly popular for the treatment of complex shoulder injuries, including proximal humerus fractures and fixed glenohumeral dislocation, in the elderly population. The early to midterm results of reverse shoulder arthroplasty for the treatment of proximal humerus fractures are promising compared with the results of unconstrained humeral head replacement, and patients may have more predictable improvement with less dependence on bone healing and rehabilitation. However, long-term follow-up is needed, and surgeons must be familiar with various complications that are specific to reverse shoulder arthroplasty. To achieve optimal patient outcomes for the management of traumatic shoulder injuries, surgeons must have a comprehensive understanding of the current implant options, indications, and surgical techniques for reverse shoulder arthroplasty.

Instr Course Lect 2016;65:171–180.

Reverse shoulder arthroplasty was initially developed for the treatment of arthritis in a rotator cuff-deficient shoulder.[1] The nonanatomic prosthesis used for reverse shoulder arthroplasty improved function and decreased pain.[2]

The indications for reverse shoulder arthroplasty continue to expand as it is used to treat a broad spectrum of shoulder pathologies that may not be adequately addressed by anatomic shoulder arthroplasty. These shoulder pathologies include traumatic injuries, such as fixed glenohumeral dislocations and proximal humerus fractures, which may potentially require prosthetic replacement.

Proximal humerus fractures are the third most common fracture in patients older than 65 years.[3] The incidence of proximal humerus fractures is expected to substantially increase over the next 20 years as the growth rate of this patient population increases.[4] Although many proximal humerus fractures can be treated nonsurgically with satisfactory results, displaced or comminuted proximal humerus fractures are often treated surgically. Definitive management may be challenging because of the lack of consensus on appropriate surgical treatment as well as the technical demands that are required to achieve an optimal functional outcome.[5]

The three primary surgical options for the treatment of proximal humerus fractures are open reduction and internal fixation (ORIF), hemiarthroplasty, and reverse shoulder arthroplasty.

Dr. Morris or an immediate family member serves as a paid consultant to or is an employee of Tornier. Dr. Edwards or an immediate family member has received royalties from Tornier, OrthoHelix, and Shoulder Options; is a member of a speakers' bureau or has made paid presentations on behalf of Tornier; serves as a paid consultant to or is an employee of Kinamed and Tornier; has received research or institutional support from Tornier; has received nonincome support (such as equipment or services), commercially derived honoraria, or other non-research–related funding (such as paid travel) from Tornier; and serves as a board member, owner, officer, or committee member of the American Shoulder and Elbow Surgeons. Neither Dr. Szerlip nor any immediate family member has received anything of value from or has stock or stock options held in a commercial company or institution related directly or indirectly to the subject of this chapter.

Although each procedure may have different indications, tuberosity position and healing are critical for ORIF and hemiarthroplasty. Although results of reverse shoulder arthroplasty for the treatment of proximal humerus fractures are improved if union is achieved, union is not the sole director of outcome. ORIF of complex humerus fractures in the elderly population is challenging and may result in an increased incidence of rotator cuff pathology and osteoporotic bone. Failure rates for patients older than 60 years who are treated with ORIF range from 13% to 20%.[6-10] Even with the use of locking plates to provide a fixed angle construct for ORIF, the rate of secondary screw cutout has been as high as 57%.[11,12]

The use of hemiarthroplasty for the treatment of displaced three- and four-part proximal humerus fractures, as first described by Neer in 1953,[13] may provide some pain relief, but has shown inconsistent results for range of motion, recovery of shoulder function, and tuberosity healing.[14-21] Although Grammont has used reverse shoulder arthroplasty for the treatment of proximal humerus fractures since the late 1980s,[22] the procedure was not introduced in the United States until 2004. The prosthesis for reverse shoulder arthroplasty has an increased deltoid lever arm and places less biomechanical stress on the healing tuberosities, which may deliver more consistent functional results. Several studies have reported the short-term results of reverse shoulder arthroplasty for the treatment proximal humerus fractures.[23-27]

Older patients who have a fixed glenohumeral dislocation present several challenges, including soft-tissue contracture, glenohumeral arthritis, and bone deficiency in both the humeral head and the glenoid. In a study of 11 patients with fixed anterior shoulder dislocations who were treated with anatomic total shoulder arthroplasty, Matsoukis et al[28] reported seven complications in five patients, including four patients (36%) with anterior instability of the shoulder. Older patients who have fixed posterior dislocations are at a decreased risk for recurrent instability. In a study of 32 patients with fixed posterior shoulder dislocations who were treated with anatomic total shoulder arthroplasty, Wooten et al[29] reported three patients with recurrence (9%) in the early postoperative period; however, 13 patients had unsatisfactory outcomes according to a modified Neer rating system, and 9 patients underwent revision surgery for various reasons. The outcomes from these studies suggest that anatomic total shoulder arthroplasty for fixed dislocation is difficult and can lead to complications, and the overall satisfaction rate for patients who undergo anatomic total shoulder arthroplasty for fixed dislocation is inferior compared with that of patients who undergo the same procedure for primary osteoarthritis.

Indications

Traditionally, the indications for hemiarthroplasty in the management of proximal humerus fractures are four-part fractures, three-part fractures in older patients who have osteoporotic bone, fracture-dislocations, head-splitting fractures, and fractures that involve more than 40% of the articular surface.[30-32] These fracture patterns are at an increased risk for complications with traditional ORIF because of the tenuous fixation of fracture fragments in osteoporotic bone and the high rates of osteonecrosis. Hertel et al[33] reported

that the most relevant predictors of humeral head ischemia were the length of dorsomedial metaphyseal extension, the integrity of the medial hinge, and the basic fracture pattern. The authors reported that proximal humerus fractures with metaphyseal head extension less than 8 mm, a medial hinge disruption greater than 2 mm, and an anatomic neck fracture pattern had a positive predictive value of 97% for humeral head ischemia. This may explain why valgus-impacted four-part fractures are relatively unlikely to result in osteonecrosis and may be amenable to nonsurgical treatment.

Reverse shoulder arthroplasty for proximal humerus fractures is typically reserved for older patients with severe osteopenia or comminution who would otherwise be indicated for a hemiarthroplasty (**Figure 1**). Patients with preexisting rotator cuff pathology who sustain proximal humerus fractures that require surgical treatment also are candidates for reverse shoulder arthroplasty rather than hemiarthroplasty. The contraindications for reverse shoulder arthroplasty for proximal humerus fractures are similar to those for conventional shoulder arthroplasty. Active infection is an absolute contraindication, and poor overall health is a relative contraindication. Although there is no absolute minimum age for reverse shoulder arthroplasty, ORIF should be attempted whenever possible for a physiologically young patient, even with a comminuted fracture. Both hemiarthroplasty and reverse shoulder arthroplasty should be approached with caution if the patient is unable to participate in a rehabilitation program to facilitate an optimal outcome. Deltoid insufficiency that results from permanent axillary nerve

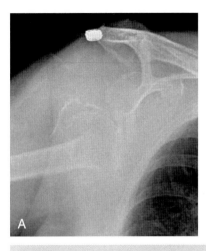
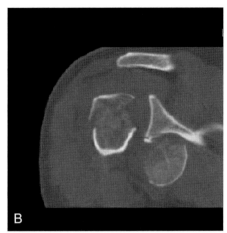

Figure 1   A, AP radiograph demonstrates a four-part proximal humerus fracture-dislocation with osteopenia. **B,** Coronal CT scan demonstrates an anatomic neck fracture-dislocation.

palsy is a contraindication specific to reverse shoulder arthroplasty; however, this contraindication does not apply to transient or subclinical axillary nerve palsy, which can occur in patients who have proximal humerus fractures.

Shoulder arthroplasty may be required for older patients who have chronic (fixed) shoulder dislocations or in the presence of a humeral defect that involves more than 40% of the articular surface.[28,29] For anatomic arthroplasty, if stability in posterior dislocations is not restored with humeral head replacement alone, then posterior capsular plication may be necessary. Augmentation of the glenoid with bone graft may be necessary in anterior dislocations if the humeral head is unstable or if the glenoid deficiency is extensive. The options for glenoid bone graft include an autograft from the native humeral head, iliac crest autograft, coracoid transfer, or a distal tibia allograft. Given the poor outcomes and high rate of complications with anatomic shoulder arthroplasty, the authors of this chapter have found reverse shoulder arthroplasty to be a valuable alternative to anatomic shoulder

arthroplasty for the treatment of fixed dislocation in the older patient. One of the authors of this chapter (T.B.E.) performed reverse shoulder arthroplasty in 21 older patients who had fixed shoulder dislocation (20 anterior and 1 posterior).[34] Only two complications (recurrent dislocation and infection) in one patient were reported at a minimum 2-year follow-up, and active elevation improved from 20° preoperatively to 100° postoperatively.[34]

Influence of Tuberosity Healing on Outcomes for Fracture Patients

Although reverse shoulder arthroplasty for the treatment of proximal humerus fractures is less contingent on a functional rotator cuff or the healing of the tuberosities[24] for active forward elevation than hemiarthroplasty for the treatment of proximal humerus fractures, it is critical that the correct position and stable fixation of the greater tuberosity is achieved during humeral hemiarthroplasty to attain active range of motion and optimal clinical outcome.[15,17,18,20,35] Boileau et al[15] reported that the major

risk factors for poor outcomes after hemiarthroplasty for the treatment of proximal humerus fractures were female sex, age older than 75 years, incorrect prosthetic height or version, and poor initial positioning of the greater tuberosity. The authors reported that the failure to restore the greater tuberosity within 10 mm below or 5 mm above the apex of the humeral head was correlated with superior migration of the humeral prosthesis, shoulder stiffness, and low patient satisfaction.[15] This may explain the bimodal distribution of outcomes reported after hemiarthroplasty and why pain relief is more predictable than mobility.[14] Correct position and healing of the greater tuberosity is crucial to restore external rotation, regardless of whether hemiarthroplasty or reverse shoulder arthroplasty is used. Compared with hemiarthroplasty, reverse shoulder arthroplasty has the theoretical biomechanical advantage of direct compression on the glenosphere during shoulder elevation, which potentially decreases the torque placed on the tuberosities and promotes healing.[36]

Fracture-Specific Implants

Although reverse shoulder arthroplasty has rapidly gained acceptance as a treatment option for complex proximal humerus fractures, tuberosity healing is still an important factor to achieve optimal results; therefore, humeral implants have been specifically designed to address this clinical need. Humeral implant features include a low-profile metaphysis for positioning of the greater tuberosity, a proximal hydroxyapatite coating, and a window into the metaphysis for additional bone graft that may facilitate union between the tuberosity fragments[22] (**Figure 2**). The diaphyseal portion of the humeral implant is

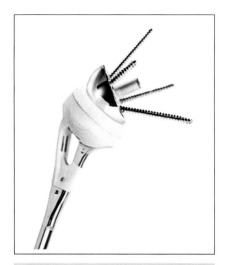

Figure 2 Photograph of a fracture-specific humeral stem for reverse shoulder arthroplasty. (Courtesy of Tornier, Bloomington, MN.)

smooth for cementation, which allows the surgeon to gain the appropriate humeral height and provides rotational stability if there is metaphyseal bone loss.

Reverse Shoulder Arthroplasty Versus Hemiarthroplasty

Several studies have recently compared reverse shoulder arthroplasty for the treatment of proximal humerus fractures with hemiarthroplasty for the treatment of proximal humerus fractures.[23,27,37,38] Namdari et al[39] performed a systematic review that compared the outcomes of reverse shoulder arthroplasty for the treatment of proximal humerus fractures with those of hemiarthroplasty with the use of a fracture-specific stem for the treatment of proximal humerus fractures. Shoulder outcome scores and mobility measurements were similar between the two groups; however, the overall complication rate for the reverse shoulder arthroplasty group was 19.4% compared with

5.6% for the hemiarthroplasty group. The revision surgery rates did not differ between the two groups, which suggest that clinical complications were treated nonsurgically. In a systematic review that compared the outcomes of reverse shoulder arthroplasty for the treatment of older adults who had proximal humerus fractures with those of hemiarthroplasty for the treatment of older adults who had proximal humerus fractures, Mata-Fink et al[40] reported improved forward flexion and functional outcome scores for the reverse shoulder arthroplasty group compared with those for the hemiarthroplasty group; however, the complication rates were not appreciably higher for the reverse shoulder arthroplasty group. Gallinet et al[37] retrospectively compared 40 patients with three- or four-part proximal humerus fractures who were treated with reverse shoulder arthroplasty or hemiarthroplasty. Tuberosity fixation was not routinely performed in the reverse shoulder arthroplasty group. The reverse shoulder arthroplasty group had higher postoperative Constant assessment scores and better forward flexion and abduction than the hemiarthroplasty group; however, both internal and external rotation measurements were decreased in the reverse shoulder arthroplasty group, which emphasizes the importance of tuberosity healing for the restoration of external rotation. Furthermore, it is difficult to accurately compare the overall performance of reverse shoulder arthroplasty with hemiarthroplasty with respect to the treatment of proximal humerus fractures if tuberosity fixation was not attempted for reverse shoulder arthroplasty.[25,37,41,42] Although recent results of reverse shoulder arthroplasty for the treatment proximal humerus fractures are promising,[23,27,37,43] future studies are necessary to determine if reverse shoulder arthroplasty leads to improved functional outcomes and better tuberosity healing compared with hemiarthroplasty. Furthermore, more studies are necessary to determine if the outcomes and tuberosity healing of hemiarthroplasty versus reverse shoulder arthroplasty are influenced by surgeon technique and experience.

Technique
Surgical Approach
Similar to standard shoulder arthroplasty, the patient should be positioned in the modified beach-chair position. Care must be taken to position the patient sufficiently near the edge of the table to allow for full extension of the surgical arm for humeral preparation. The two primary surgical approaches for reverse shoulder arthroplasty are the standard deltopectoral approach and the anterosuperior approach. Each approach has certain benefits and limitations. The anterosuperior approach uses a deltoid split, which improves access to the greater tuberosity; however, the approach requires deltoid detachment and may result in dehiscence. In addition, extensibility is limited during humeral shaft exposure if humeral shaft comminution is present. The authors of this chapter prefer to use the deltopectoral approach because it provides reliable access to the fracture fragments and uncompromised glenoid exposure after tuberosity mobilization.

An incision is begun at the tip of the coracoid process and is extended distally, approximating the deltopectoral interval. The cephalic vein, which is used as a guide to identify the deltopectoral interval, is retracted laterally with the deltoid. The pectoralis major tendon is then identified, and the superior 1 cm may be incised to enhance exposure.

Technique for Fracture Cases

The long head of the biceps tendon is used to identify the greater and lesser tuberosity fragments, which are mobilized with the use of a Cobb elevator. After the lesser tuberosity is identified with its subscapularis attachment, the subscapularis tendon is tagged with two stay sutures to gain control of the fracture fragment. The sutures are placed at the tendon-bone interface and not through the bone. The head fragment is exposed, removed, and preserved for later bone grafting. The greater tuberosity is then gently mobilized with a Lahey clamp, and a double-loaded free needle is used to pass two nonabsorbable sutures through the bone-tendon interface of the greater tuberosity, one superiorly through the infraspinatus tendon and one inferiorly through the teres minor tendon. Any tendon attachment to both the greater and lesser tuberosities, including the supraspinatus, is preserved. After control of the greater and lesser tuberosity fracture fragments is attained, the biceps tendon is tenotomized and, later, tenodesed to the pectoralis major tendon.

Attention is then turned to glenoid exposure and preparation. Anterior and posterior glenoid retractors are placed to retract the lesser and greater tuberosity fragments, respectively. A Hohmann retractor is then placed inferiorly on the glenoid to retract the humeral shaft inferiorly. A capsular release is performed to optimize glenoid exposure, and the long head of the triceps is released from the glenoid to avoid a traction osteophyte that can occur with reverse shoulder arthroplasty. After adequate glenoid exposure has been attained, the

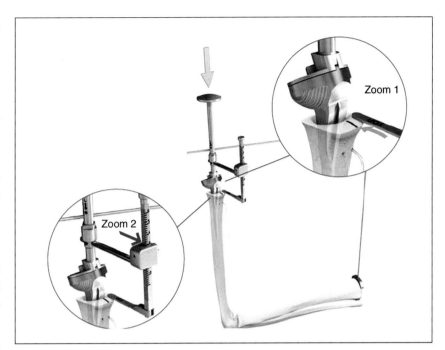

Figure 3   Illustration of a height gauge, which is used to reproduce humeral height. Electrocautery is used to make a mark at the lateral fin of the stem, which will serve as a landmark for retroversion of the final implant. Double-loaded sutures are placed in the diaphysis to serve as a vertical support. (Courtesy of Tornier, Bloomington, MN.)

remaining labrum and the stump of the long head of biceps are removed. The glenoid is then prepared and instrumented in a standard fashion.

With the glenoid retractors removed, the arm is adducted and extended to deliver the diaphysis into the wound. The implant diameter is determined with the use of diaphyseal reamers, and a humeral trial is placed in 20° of retroversion. The ideal humeral height is determined by reducing the implant with the thinnest polyethylene insert available and applying axial traction to the arm. This may cause the humeral diaphysis to move distally on the stem and increase the overall height of the prosthesis that extends from the medial humeral calcar. The ideal amount of traction, or humeral length, is identified if good stability and no gaping between the glenosphere and polyethylene are

noted throughout range of motion. It is important that this part of the procedure be performed under full relaxation by anesthesia. A height gauge is then used to measure the determined humeral height on insertion of the final humeral component. The trial humeral component is removed, and 2-mm drill holes are placed on each side of the bicipital groove distal to the fracture. Two sutures are placed in these holes and used for vertical fixation of the tuberosities to the humeral shaft (**Figure 3**). A cement restrictor is placed, and the final humeral implant is cemented in place at the previously determined height and in 20° of retroversion. The authors of this chapter do not recommend uncemented implants because older patients with proximal humerus fracture may have metaphyseal bone deficiency, which can compromise humeral implant fixation.

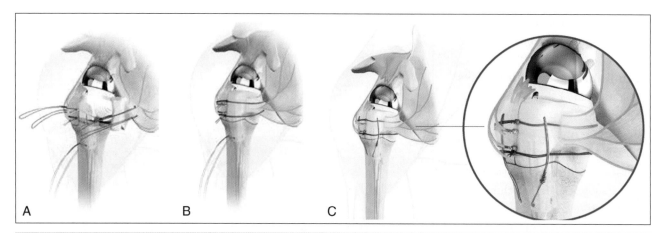

Figure 4 Illustrations demonstrate tuberosity fixation. **A,** The arm is placed in neutral rotation. A clamp is used to gently pull the greater tuberosity anteriorly, which reduces the greater tuberosity to the prosthesis. Two horizontal cerclage sutures (one superior and one inferior) are then tied to secure the greater tuberosity to the prosthesis. **B,** The two remaining horizontal sutures, which had initially been passed through the posterior rotator cuff tendon and around the prosthetic neck, are then passed through the subscapularis tendon. One suture runs through the superior portion of the lesser tuberosity, and the other suture runs through the inferior portion of the lesser tuberosity. Both sutures are passed from inside to outside and are then tied. **C,** Final tightening of the double-loaded sutures that were previously placed through the diaphysis creates a vertical support. The shroud goes behind the infraspinatus tendon, in front of the subscapularis tendon, and is then tied. (Courtesy of Tornier, Bloomington, MN.)

Antibiotic-impregnated bone cement is used because it has been shown to prevent postoperative infection after primary reverse shoulder arthroplasty.[44] After trialing is performed and stability is ensured throughout a full range of motion, the appropriate size polyethylene component is selected. There are two important steps before reduction with final implants. First, one limb of each of the four sutures through the greater tuberosity fragment has to be passed along the medial side of the implant for later tuberosity fixation. Second, if a fracture-specific implant is being used, then the bone graft should be placed in the metaphysis of the component.

After the final implant has been reduced, tuberosity fixation is performed, which is critical for restoration of active external rotation. The ideal construct for tuberosity management uses six sutures (four horizontal cerclage sutures and two vertical tension band sutures) that securely fix the tuberosities to one

another as well as the prosthesis and the diaphysis. This tuberosity management technique provides optimal interfragmentary stability and can be used for both hemiarthroplasty and reverse shoulder arthroplasty.[45,46] One suture from the superior set of greater tuberosity sutures and one suture from the inferior set of greater tuberosity sutures are tied around the medial aspect of the implant to secure the greater tuberosity to the prosthesis (**Figure 4, A**). Next, the final sutures from the superior and inferior sets of greater tuberosity sutures that were previously passed around the medial side of the implant are now passed through the subscapularis tendon at the superior and inferior aspect of the lesser tuberosity. These sutures are tied to secure the lesser tuberosity to the implant and the greater tuberosity (**Figure 4, B**). The authors of this chapter prefer lesser tuberosity repair and healing because it can potentially improve implant stability and ultimate function; however, lesser tuberosity

repair in reverse shoulder arthroplasty for the treatment of proximal humerus fractures is somewhat controversial, and future studies are necessary to clarify this debate. Finally, the sutures that were previously placed through the drill holes in the humeral diaphysis are passed in a vertical cerclage fashion (one anteriorly based and the other posteriorly based) to secure the tuberosities to the diaphysis. The authors of this chapter prefer to use a Nice knot, which is a racking hitch knot, with the cerclage sutures to optimize tuberosity reduction.[47] Additional bone graft may be placed in the area at which the diaphysis and tuberosities meet to promote healing (**Figure 4, C**).

Technical Considerations for Fixed Dislocation

The same deltopectoral approach is used for fixed anterior dislocation; however, the humeral head and shaft may be retracted anteriorly when gaining access to the glenoid. The authors of this chapter prefer to use an osteoto-mized humeral head if deficiency of the anterior glenoid is present (**Figure 5**). A short uncemented stem is implanted in a manner similar to that for reverse shoulder arthroplasty for cuff tear arthropathy. Tuberosity management or a fracture-specific stem are not neces-sary. Soft-tissue contracture may often occur with chronic fixed dislocations. Surgeons must be prepared to address contractures with a larger than normal humeral head cut and soft-tissue releas-es so that appropriate implant tension can be achieved and stable shoulder range of motion can be restored.

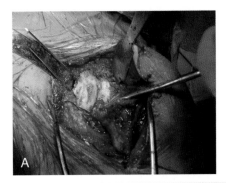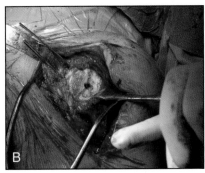

Figure 5   Intraoperative photographs of a patient who has a fixed anterior shoulder dislocation. **A,** Anterior bone deficiency of the glenoid is present. **B,** Glenoid architecture is restored with the use of an osteotomized humeral head.

Summary

Reverse shoulder arthroplasty for the management of complex shoulder pa-thologies, including comminuted prox-imal humerus fractures and chronic dislocations, has rapidly gained pop-ularity. Reverse shoulder arthroplasty has a lower complication rate and better results than unconstrained arthroplasty for the treatment of fixed glenohumeral dislocations. Recent results of reverse shoulder arthroplasty for the treat-ment of fractures are promising and, when compared with results of hemi-arthroplasty for the treatment of frac-tures, have shown improved functional outcomes for older patients who have poor bone quality; however, because long-term follow-up is needed, reverse shoulder arthroplasty for the treatment of proximal humerus fractures should be reserved for older patients with se-vere osteopenia or comminution who are not amenable to another treatment option. Regardless of whether hemi-arthroplasty or reverse shoulder arthro-plasty is used, correct positioning and healing of the tuberosities are crucial to obtain a good outcome. Surgeons

must be familiar with various features that are specific to each implant and in-strumentation system to restore optimal humeral length and version.

References

1. Grammont PM, Baulot E: Delta shoulder prosthesis for rotator cuff rupture. *Orthopedics* 1993;16(1):65-68.

2. Boulahia A, Edwards TB, Walch G, Baratta RV: Early results of a reverse design prosthesis in the treatment of arthritis of the shoulder in elderly patients with a large rotator cuff tear. *Orthopedics* 2002;25(2):129-133.

3. Baron JA, Karagas M, Barrett J, et al: Basic epidemiology of fractures of the upper and lower limb among Ameri-cans over 65 years of age. *Epidemiology* 1996;7(6):612-618.

4. Kannus P, Palvanen M, Niemi S, Parkkari J, Järvinen M, Vuori I: Osteoporotic fractures of the proximal humerus in elderly Finnish persons: Sharp increase in 1970-1998 and alarming projections for the new millennium. *Acta Orthop Scand* 2000;71(5):465-470.

5. Petit CJ, Millett PJ, Endres NK, Dill-er D, Harris MB, Warner JJ: Manage-ment of proximal humeral fractures: Surgeons don't agree. *J Shoulder Elbow Surg* 2010;19(3):446-451.

6. Hawkins RJ, Kiefer GN: Internal fixation techniques for proximal hu-meral fractures. *Clin Orthop Relat Res* 1987;223:77-85.

7. Lee CW, Shin SJ: Prognostic factors for unstable proximal humeral fractures treated with locking-plate fixation. *J Shoulder Elbow Surg* 2009;18(1):83-88.

8. Neer CS II: Displaced proximal humeral fractures: II. Treatment of three-part and four-part dis-placement. *J Bone Joint Surg Am* 1970;52(6):1090-1103.

9. Owsley KC, Gorczyca JT: Fracture displacement and screw cutout after open reduction and locked plate fixation of proximal humeral fractures [corrected]. *J Bone Joint Surg Am* 2008;90(2):233-240.

10. Zyto K, Ahrengart L, Sperber A, Törnkvist H: Treatment of dis-placed proximal humeral fractures in elderly patients. *J Bone Joint Surg Br* 1997;79(3):412-417.

11. Jost B, Spross C, Grehn H, Gerber C: Locking plate fixation of fractures of the proximal humerus: Analysis of complications, revision strategies and outcome. *J Shoulder Elbow Surg* 2013;22(4):542-549.

12. Ricchetti ET, Warrender WJ, Abboud JA: Use of locking plates in the treatment of proximal humerus fractures. *J Shoulder Elbow Surg* 2010; 19(2, suppl):66-75.

13. Neer CS, Brown TH Jr, McLaugh-lin HL: Fracture of the neck of the humerus with dislocation of the head fragment. *Am J Surg* 1953;85(3):252-258.

14. Antuña SA, Sperling JW, Cofield RH: Shoulder hemiarthroplasty for acute fractures of the proximal humerus: A minimum five-year follow-up. *J Shoulder Elbow Surg* 2008;17(2):202-209.

15. Boileau P, Krishnan SG, Tinsi L, Walch G, Coste JS, Molé D: Tuberosity malposition and migration: Reasons for poor outcomes after hemiarthroplasty for displaced fractures of the proximal humerus. *J Shoulder Elbow Surg* 2002;11(5):401-412.

16. Goldman RT, Koval KJ, Cuomo F, Gallagher MA, Zuckerman JD: Functional outcome after humeral head replacement for acute three- and four-part proximal humeral fractures. *J Shoulder Elbow Surg* 1995;4(2):81-86.

17. Kralinger F, Schwaiger R, Wambacher M, et al: Outcome after primary hemiarthroplasty for fracture of the head of the humerus: A retrospective multicentre study of 167 patients. *J Bone Joint Surg Br* 2004;86(2):217-219.

18. Mighell MA, Kolm GP, Collinge CA, Frankle MA: Outcomes of hemiarthroplasty for fractures of the proximal humerus. *J Shoulder Elbow Surg* 2003;12(6):569-577.

19. Prakash U, McGurty DW, Dent JA: Hemiarthroplasty for severe fractures of the proximal humerus. *J Shoulder Elbow Surg* 2002;11(5):428-430.

20. Solberg BD, Moon CN, Franco DP, Paiement GD: Surgical treatment of three and four-part proximal humeral fractures. *J Bone Joint Surg Am* 2009;91(7):1689-1697.

21. Zyto K, Wallace WA, Frostick SP, Preston BJ: Outcome after hemiarthroplasty for three- and four-part fractures of the proximal humerus. *J Shoulder Elbow Surg* 1998;7(2):85-89.

22. Sirveaux F, Roche O, Molé D: Shoulder arthroplasty for acute proximal humerus fracture. *Orthop Traumatol Surg Res* 2010;96(6):683-694.

23. Boyle MJ, Youn SM, Frampton CM, Ball CM: Functional outcomes of reverse shoulder arthroplasty compared with hemiarthroplasty for acute proximal humeral fractures. *J Shoulder Elbow Surg* 2013;22(1):32-37.

24. Bufquin T, Hersan A, Hubert L, Massin P: Reverse shoulder arthroplasty for the treatment of three- and four-part fractures of the proximal humerus in the elderly: A prospective review of 43 cases with a short-term follow-up. *J Bone Joint Surg Br* 2007;89(4):516-520.

25. Cazeneuve JF, Cristofari DJ: Grammont reversed prosthesis for acute complex fracture of the proximal humerus in an elderly population with 5 to 12 years follow-up. *Orthop Traumatol Surg Res* 2014;100(1):93-97.

26. Gallinet D, Adam A, Gasse N, Rochet S, Obert L: Improvement in shoulder rotation in complex shoulder fractures treated by reverse shoulder arthroplasty. *J Shoulder Elbow Surg* 2013;22(1):38-44.

27. Garrigues GE, Johnston PS, Pepe MD, Tucker BS, Ramsey ML, Austin LS: Hemiarthroplasty versus reverse total shoulder arthroplasty for acute proximal humerus fractures in elderly patients. *Orthopedics* 2012;35(5):e703-e708.

28. Matsoukis J, Tabib W, Guiffault P, et al: Primary unconstrained shoulder arthroplasty in patients with a fixed anterior glenohumeral dislocation. *J Bone Joint Surg Am* 2006;88(3):547-552.

29. Wooten C, Klika B, Schleck CD, Harmsen WS, Sperling JW, Cofield RH: Anatomic shoulder arthroplasty as treatment for locked posterior dislocation of the shoulder. *J Bone Joint Surg Am* 2014;96(3):e19.

30. Cadet ER, Ahmad CS: Hemiarthroplasty for three- and four-part proximal humerus fractures. *J Am Acad Orthop Surg* 2012;20(1):17-27.

31. Nho SJ, Brophy RH, Barker JU, Cornell CN, MacGillivray JD: Innovations in the management of displaced proximal humerus fractures. *J Am Acad Orthop Surg* 2007;15(1):12-26.

32. Voos JE, Dines JS, Dines DM: Arthroplasty for fractures of the proximal part of the humerus. *J Bone Joint Surg Am* 2010;92(6):1560-1567.

33. Hertel R, Hempfing A, Stiehler M, Leunig M: Predictors of humeral head ischemia after intracapsular fracture of the proximal humerus. *J Shoulder Elbow Surg* 2004;13(4):427-433.

34. Williams M, Stanley R, Cores Z, Edwards T, Elkousy H, Gartsman G: Reverse total shoulder arthroplasty as treatment for fixed anterior shoulder dislocation. Presented at the 10th International Congress on Surgery of the Shoulder. LaBahia Salvador, Brazil, September 16-20, 2007.

35. Loew M, Heitkemper S, Parsch D, Schneider S, Rickert M: Influence of the design of the prosthesis on the outcome after hemiarthroplasty of the shoulder in displaced fractures of the head of the humerus. *J Bone Joint Surg Br* 2006;88(3):345-350.

36. Aaron D, Parsons BO, Sirveaux F, Flatow EL: Proximal humeral fractures: Prosthetic replacement. *Instr Course Lect* 2013;62:155-162.

37. Gallinet D, Clappaz P, Garbuio P, Tropet Y, Obert L: Three or four parts complex proximal humerus fractures: Hemiarthroplasty versus reverse prosthesis. A comparative study of 40 cases. *Orthop Traumatol Surg Res* 2009;95(1):48-55.

38. Young SW, Segal BS, Turner PC, Poon PC: Comparison of functional outcomes of reverse shoulder arthroplasty versus hemiarthroplasty in the primary treatment of acute proximal humerus fracture. *ANZ J Surg* 2010;80(11):789-793.

39. Namdari S, Horneff JG, Baldwin K: Comparison of hemiarthroplasty and reverse arthroplasty for treatment of proximal humeral fractures: A systematic review. *J Bone Joint Surg Am* 2013;95(18):1701-1708.

40. Mata-Fink A, Meinke M, Jones C, Kim B, Bell JE: Reverse shoulder arthroplasty for treatment of proximal humeral fractures in older adults: A systematic review. *J Shoulder Elbow Surg* 2013;22(12):1737-1748.

41. Cazeneuve JF, Cristofari DJ: Grammont reversed prosthesis for acute complex fracture of the proximal humerus in an elderly population with 5 to 12 years follow-up. *Rev Chir Orthop Reparatrice Appar Mot* 2006;92(6):543-548.

42. Klein M, Juschka M, Hinkenjann B, Scherger B, Ostermann PA: Treatment of comminuted fractures of the proximal humerus in elderly

patients with the Delta III reverse shoulder prosthesis. *J Orthop Trauma* 2008;22(10):698-704.

43. Lenarz C, Shishani Y, McCrum C, Nowinski RJ, Edwards TB, Gobezie R: Is reverse shoulder arthroplasty appropriate for the treatment of fractures in the older patient? Early observations. *Clin Orthop Relat Res* 2011;469(12):3324-3331.

44. Nowinski RJ, Gillespie RJ, Shishani Y, Cohen B, Walch G, Gobezie R: Antibiotic-loaded bone cement reduces deep infection rates for primary reverse total shoulder arthroplasty: A retrospective, cohort study of

501 shoulders. *J Shoulder Elbow Surg* 2012;21(3):324-328.

45. Boileau P, Walch G, Krishnan SG: Tuberosity osteosynthesis and hemiarthroplasty for four-part fractures of the proximal humerus. *Techniques in Shoulder and Elbow Surgery* 2000;1(2):96-109.

46. Sirveaux F, Navez G, Roche O, Mole D, Williams MD: Reverse prosthesis for proximal humerus fracture: Technique and results. *Techniques in Shoulder and Elbow Surgery* 2008;9(1):15-22.

47. Boileau P, Rumian A: The doubled-suture Nice knot: A non-slipping and secure fixation of bone fragments

and soft tissues usable in open and arthroscopic surgery, in Boileau P, ed: *Shoulder Concepts 2010: Arthroscopy and Arthroplasty*. Montpellier, Frances, Sauramps Medical, 2010, pp 245-251.

Video Reference

Szerlip BW, Morris BJ, Edwards TB: Video. *Reverse Shoulder Arthroplasty for Trauma: When, Where, and How*. Houston, TX, 2015.

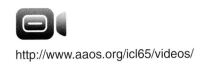

All Things Clavicle: From Acromioclavicular to Sternoclavicular and All Points in Between

Gordon I. Groh, MD
Mark A. Mighell, MD
Carl J. Basamania, MD
W. Ben Kibler, MD

Abstract

The clavicle is the most frequently injured bone in the human body. In most cases, fractures that occur in the midshaft of the clavicle can be managed nonsurgically. An increasing number of studies suggest that displaced midshaft clavicle fractures have improved outcomes after surgical management, and equivalent outcomes can be achieved with both plating and intramedullary techniques. Distal clavicle fractures are managed according to the disruption of the coracoclavicular ligaments. Fractures with disruption of the ligaments usually will require fixation, whereas fractures with intact ligaments may be treated with closed management. Multiple techniques of reconstruction appear to yield similar outcomes; however, hook-plating techniques result in the highest complication rates. The evaluation process for acromioclavicular joint injuries is moving from a static two-dimensional evaluation to a three-dimensional evaluation that involves an assessment for scapular dyskinesis. Surgical reconstruction is indicated for patients who exhibit scapular dyskinesis. Anterior sternoclavicular injuries can typically be managed nonsurgically, whereas posterior sternoclavicular dislocations always require urgent surgical management. Newer techniques of ligament reconstruction for sternoclavicular injuries yield improved biomechanical stability.

Instr Course Lect 2016;65:181–196.

Clavicular fractures and dislocations account for 44% of all shoulder girdle injuries.[1] Although the diagnosis of clavicular fractures and dislocations is rarely problematic, treatment algorithms have evolved in response to a renewed evaluation of clinical outcomes for these injuries. Historically, multiple treatment options have been used to manage clavicular fractures and dislocations, and there is some concern that the increased incidence of higher-energy injuries may skew

previous data. Surgeons should be familiar with the current treatment recommendations for clavicular fractures and dislocations.

Midshaft Clavicle Fractures

Midshaft fractures account for 80% of all clavicular fractures. Until recently, most clavicular fractures were treated conservatively; however, recent studies have reported improved outcomes with the surgical fixation of displaced clavicle fractures.

Nonsurgical Management

Early studies reported high rates of healing with the nonsurgical management of clavicular fractures, despite substantial displacement and subsequent malunion.[1,2] However, the recent literature has refuted these early studies. Hill et al[3] reported a nonunion rate of 15% and unsatisfactory outcomes in 31% of patients with displaced midshaft clavicle fractures who were treated nonsurgically. The authors reported that final shortening of more than 2 cm had a negative effect on patient outcomes. McKee et al[4] reported that previously unrecognized deficits were detected by patient-based outcome measures and objective muscle strength testing after the nonsurgical treatment of displaced midshaft clavicle fractures.

Surgical Versus Nonsurgical Management

The Canadian Orthopaedic Trauma Society[5] compared the surgical and nonsurgical treatment of displaced midshaft clavicle fractures. The society reported that open reduction and internal fixation (ORIF) of displaced midshaft clavicle fractures resulted in earlier healing rates (16.4 weeks versus 28.4 weeks) and lower nonunion rates (2.2% versus 15.1%) compared with nonsurgical management.[5] Although surgical treatment provided better functional outcome scores and fewer symptomatic malunions than nonsurgical management, ORIF had a 12% complication rate; however, most complications were associated with local irritation and prominent hardware. McKee et al[6] evaluated the short-term follow-up of patients who had surgical versus nonsurgical treatment of displaced midshaft clavicle fractures and reported that surgical treatment resulted in a lower nonunion rate (1% versus 14.5%), fewer symptomatic malunions

(zero versus 8.5%), and a quicker return to activity compared with nonsurgical treatment.

Surgical Indications

The primary goal in the treatment of midshaft clavicle fractures is to restore shoulder function. The absolute indications for surgical treatment in healthy patients are open injuries, neurologic or vascular compromise, and posteriorly displaced medial clavicle fractures or dislocations. The relative indications for surgical treatment include widely displaced fractures, shortening of more than 2 cm, substantial comminution, unacceptable cosmesis, multiply injured trauma patients, predicted functional deficits, and painful nonunion or malunion.

Surgical Techniques

During fixation of clavicular fractures, the surgeon should be aware of the adjacent neurovascular structures. Robinson[7] performed an anatomic study and reported that the subclavian vein was consistently within 4.8 mm of the medial one-third of the clavicle. In addition, the authors reported that both the brachial plexus and the subclavian artery were within 2 cm of the medial one-third of the clavicle. These neurovascular structures diverge from the

clavicle in more lateral injuries. The authors stressed the importance of the careful use of clamps, drills, and depth gauges if working around the medial and middle thirds of the clavicle.

Plate Fixation

A curvilinear incision is made over the anterior aspect of the clavicle, and full-thickness skin and subcutaneous flaps are raised. The supraclavicular nerves are exposed with scissor dissection to prevent postoperative hyperesthesia. The platysma is incised longitudinally along the clavicle to allow for a full-thickness fascial layer over the plate at the time of closure. Currently, there is no consensus on plate position for clavicular fracture healing. Early studies reported higher plate bending load to failure with superior plating[8] (**Figure 1**), whereas anteroinferior plating was reported to withstand higher bending loads.[9] Furthermore, biomechanical data reveal no differences in torsional and axial loads between superior and anteroinferior plating.[8] Some authors support superior plating for fractures that have inferior comminution, whereas other authors advocate anteroinferior plating because they believe that such plating allows for reduced plate prominence, longer screw length, and less risk of neurovascular injury during drilling; however, lung structures may be at risk with anterior to posterior drilling.[8-10]

Technique

For transverse and short, oblique midshaft fractures that are not amenable to interfragmentary screw fixation, a 2-mm drill is used to make pilot holes for the placement of pointed reduction forceps. These forceps are used to maintain reduction during plate

Dr. Groh or an immediate family member has received royalties from DJ Orthopaedics; serves as a paid consultant to or is an employee of DePuy, DJ Orthopaedics, and UPex; has stock or stock options held in UPex; has received research or institutional support from DePuy and Integra LifeSciences; and serves as a board member, owner, officer, or committee member of the American Academy of Orthopaedic Surgeons. Dr. Mighell or an immediate family member has received royalties from DJ Orthopaedics and UPex (Newclip Technics); is a member of a speakers' bureau or has made paid presentations on behalf of DJ Orthopaedics, Stryker, and UPex (Newclip Technics); serves as a paid consultant to or is an employee of DJ Orthopaedics and Stryker; has stock or stock options held in UPex (Newclip Technics); has received research or institutional support from Biomet, BioMimetic Therapeutics, and DJ Orthopaedics; and serves as a board member, owner, officer, or committee member of the Foundation for Orthopaedic Research and Education. Dr. Basamania or an immediate family member has received royalties from DePuy; is a member of a speakers' bureau or has made paid presentations on behalf of DePuy and Sonoma Orthopedic Products; serves as a paid consultant to or is an employee of Biomet, BioPoly, DePuy, Invuity, and Sonoma Orthopedic Products; and has stock or stock options held in Invuity. Dr. Kibler or an immediate family member serves as an unpaid consultant to AlignMed; has stock or stock options held in AlignMed; and serves as a board member, owner, officer, or committee member of the Arthroscopy Association of North America.

placement. For comminuted fractures, mini-fragment screws (either 2.0 mm or 2.7 mm) are used to achieve interfragmentary compression before the placement of a precontoured neutralization plate. For true transverse fracture patterns, superior plating allows for better compression across the fracture.

Results

Plate fixation requires a fairly large, noncosmetic incision, considerable soft-tissue stripping, and a risk of damage to the supraclavicular nerves. There also is a risk of damage to the clavicular blood supply, which has been shown to be entirely periosteal without any endosteal contribution. Because of the larger incision, there also is an increased risk of infection, with rates reported as high as 18%.[11] Wijdicks et al[12] reported that nearly 90% of patients who have precontoured plate fixation report local prominence pain and discomfort. The removal of the plate requires an additional large incision and, because of stress shielding of the bone and stress risers that result from multiple screw holes, potentially leaves the bone at risk for refracture (**Figure 2**). A cadaver model study reported substantial weakening of the clavicle after the removal of a plate compared with a normal clavicle; however, there was no substantial weakening after the removal of an intramedullary device.[9]

Overall, most of the complications after plate fixation of clavicular fractures are implant related, with major complications ranging up to 64%.[12] An additional technical problem with plate fixation is whether the plate matches the anatomy of the clavicle or the clavicle is made to match the plate. Huang et al[13] reported a very poor fit of precontoured plates, especially in females. Finally,

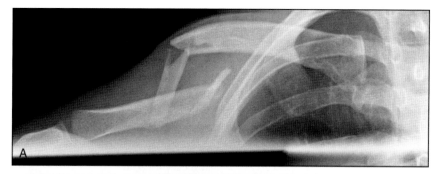

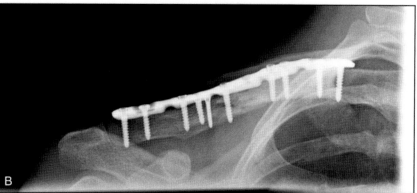

Figure 1   **A,** Preoperative AP radiograph demonstrates a comminuted midshaft clavicle fracture. **B,** Postoperative AP radiograph taken 8 weeks after fixation with a superior plating technique demonstrates fracture union.

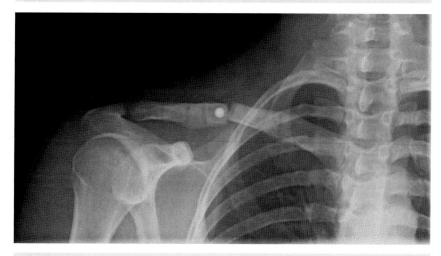

Figure 2   AP radiograph demonstrates a posthardware removal fracture. (Courtesy of Thomas Hackett, MD, Vail, CO.)

there is a risk of major neurovascular injury because of screw penetration in the medial clavicle.[14]

Intramedullary Fixation

The first report in 1930 of intramedullary fixation used beef bone.[15]

Küntscher[16] described the technique for intramedullary fixation in his 1945 textbook. The primary advantage of intramedullary fixation is that it minimizes soft-tissue dissection. It also preserves the periosteal blood supply, has better resistance to repetitive bending,

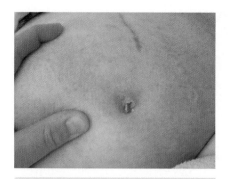

Figure 3 Clinical photograph shows a prominent Hagie pin that caused skin breakdown. (Reproduced with permission from Strauss EJ, Egol KA, France MA, Koval KJ, Zuckerman JD: Complications of intramedullary Hagie pin fixation for acute midshaft clavicle fractures. *J Shoulder Elbow Surg* 2007;16[3]:280-284.)

and promotes callus healing rather than direct osteon healing. There is minimal stress shielding because intramedullary fixation uses a load-sharing device rather than a load-sparing device, such as a plate. The device can be inserted through small cosmetic incisions and can easily be removed without the need for general anesthesia. Theoretically, it is easier to achieve an anatomic reduction with intramedullary fixation because, by definition, its intramedullary position in both major fragments means that the fracture is anatomically aligned.

However, potential complications exist with intramedullary fixation. The most common problem is painful hardware[17,18] (**Figure 3**). Because of the small size of the intramedullary canal of the clavicle, with an average canal diameter in the mid-clavicle of 6 mm, there are limited options in terms of the size of the intramedullary device.[19,20] Smooth fixation devices are prone to migration and loss of fixation.[21,22] The intramedullary technique also requires fluoroscopy, which increases patient exposure to radiation. There also is the

problem of trying to place a straight, rigid intramedullary fixation device into a curved bone[19] in addition to concerns for length and rotation control in comminuted fractures.[22] Another concern with intramedullary fixation is that many of these devices need to be removed, which necessitates a second surgical procedure.

Several devices have been described for intramedullary fixation, including elastic nails,[21,22] screws, Knowles pins,[23] the Rockwood pin,[24-26] and new hybrid devices that allow both rigid and flexible fixation.[27] The primary advantage of the hybrid device is that it allows a greater length of fixation compared with a straight device and has interlocking fixation for use in comminuted fractures, in which length and rotational control may be key issues (**Figure 4**).

Technique
Intramedullary fixation can be achieved by placing the patient in either the supine or beach-chair position. If the patient is placed in a beach-chair position, the torso is aligned approximately 45° relative to the floor. The fluoroscopy unit can then be aligned parallel to the floor, allowing a 40° to 45° cephalic tilt view of the clavicle, which is the best view to assess the contour of the clavicle (**Figure 5**). The surgeon can achieve a "near AP view" of the lateral fragment by extending the patient's arm (**Figure 6**) and a "near axillary view" of the lateral fragment by forward flexing the patient's arm (**Figure 7**).

A small (2.5 to 5 cm) incision is made directly over the fracture site. Care is taken to protect the middle branch of the supraclavicular nerve, which is often close to the fracture (**Figure 8**). The fixation device can be inserted by retrograde pinning into the medial fragment

and out through the anterior cortex of the medial fragment, and then passing the pin antegrade into the lateral fragment. Conversely, the pin can be passed antegrade out though the posterolateral cortex of the lateral fragment and then passed in a retrograde fashion into the medial fragment after the fracture is reduced.

The most important aspect of the lateral fixation intramedullary technique is to ensure that the intramedullary device exits the posterior lateral clavicle in the proper position. To achieve the ideal pin placement within the intramedullary canal, the device should exit the posterior lateral clavicle approximately halfway between the conoid tubercle and the acromioclavicular (AC) joint. The intramedullary device should exit at the "equator" of the clavicle (**Figures 6** and **7**), which allows for the longest possible fixation in the intramedullary canal. Furthermore, this exit point is protected by both the conoid and trapezoid ligaments and minimizes any potential for a stress riser. If the pin exits too superiorly, it may result in apex superior angulation at the fracture site if the device is passed into the medial fragment canal. Conversely, if the pin exits too inferiorly in the posterior lateral cortex, it may cause apex inferior angulation at the fracture site.[19] Comminuted fragments can then be cerclaged into place by leaving the fragments attached to their soft-tissue envelope and passing a large absorbable suture through this soft tissue and around the clavicle. An elevator may be placed beneath the clavicle to protect the underlying neurovascular structures (**Figure 9**).

Postoperatively, patients are allowed to remove the sling as soon as comfort allows. Because of the concern for a lack of rotation control with most

© 2016 AAOS Instructional Course Lectures, Volume 65

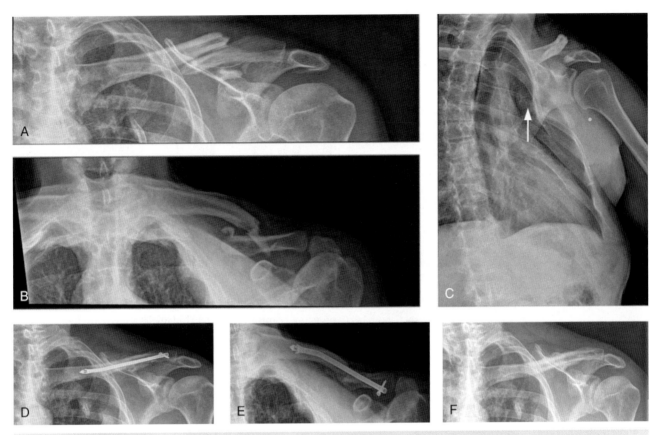

Figure 4 Radiographs demonstrate intramedullary fixation with the use of a hybrid device in a patient who had a midshaft clavicle fracture. AP (**A**) and 45° cephalic tilt (**B**) views demonstrate a substantially shortened and comminuted midshaft fracture of the left clavicle. **C,** Chest view of the same patient demonstrates multiple segmental rib fractures. AP (**D**) and 45° cephalic tilt (**E**) views taken 6 weeks postoperatively demonstrate the hybrid fixation device and bridging callous. **F,** AP view taken 5 months postoperatively demonstrates hardware removal.

intramedullary devices, patients are typically told not to raise their hand higher than shoulder level for at least 4 to 6 weeks postoperatively.

Results

In a study of patients with displaced midshaft clavicle fractures who were treated with intramedullary fixation, major complications, such as bone-healing problems and deep infections, were relatively low at 8.6%. Minor complications, such as delayed union and superficial wound infections, were higher at 17.2%.[18] Few studies directly compare intramedullary fixation with plate and screw fixation.[21,22] In a study of active duty military patients, Wenninger et al[28] reported that although the healing rates for patients who had plate fixation were equal to those for patients who had intramedullary fixation, the overall complication rate for the plate fixation group was 31% compared with 9% for the intramedullary fixation group. In a study that compared plate and screw fixation with elastic intramedullary fixation, Wijdicks et al[21] reported a 14% implant failure rate for the plate fixation group compared with a 2.1% failure rate in the elastic intramedullary fixation group. The authors also reported a refracture rate of 7% in the plate fixation group compared with zero in the elastic intramedullary fixation group and a major revision surgery rate of 11.6% in the plate fixation group compared with 2.1% in the elastic intramedullary fixation group. In a study that compared plate fixation with intramedullary fixation in older patients, Lee et al[23] reported that there were significantly fewer complications, shorter hospital stays, less hardware pain, and less narcotic use for patients who had intramedullary fixation. In a study of patients with displaced and shortened clavicle fractures who were treated with a hybrid intramedullary fixation device, King et al[27] reported that union was achieved in all patients, and there were no noted problems with prominent or painful hardware, which may be found with other intramedullary devices.

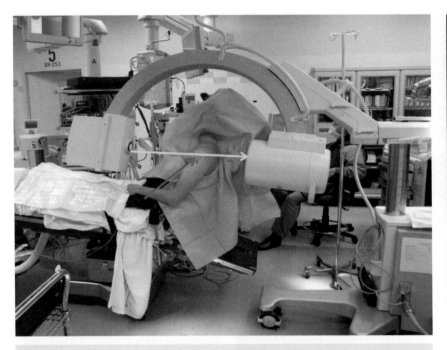

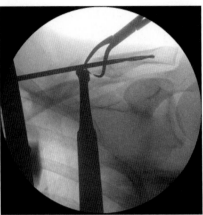

Figure 6 AP equivalent fluoroscopic image taken with the patient's arm in extension demonstrates the ideal exit point of the intramedullary device at the equator of the clavicle.

Figure 5 Clinical photograph shows the positioning of the fluoroscopy unit for intramedullary fixation. The yellow arrow represents the beam of the fluoroscopy unit, which is positioned parallel to the floor. The red arrow represents the torso of the patient, which is positioned at a 45° angle to the floor. This positioning results in an equivalent of a 45° cephalic tilt image, which is helpful for viewing the curvature of the clavicle.

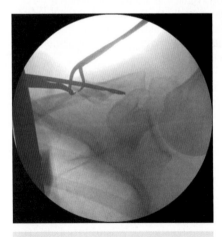

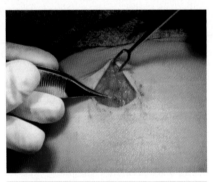

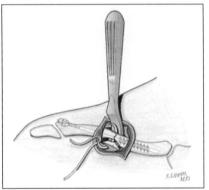

Figure 7 Axillary equivalent fluoroscopic image taken with the patient's arm in forward flexion demonstrates the drill in the lateral fragment. Note the position of the intramedullary device halfway between the conoid tubercle and the acromioclavicular joint.

Figure 8 Intraoperative photograph shows the middle branch of the supraclavicular nerve above the distal end of the medial clavicle fracture fragment.

Figure 9 Illustration shows cerclage of the butterfly fragments using No. 1 absorbable suture. A crego elevator is placed deep to the clavicle to protect the underlying neurovascular structures. (Reproduced with permission from Basamania CJ, Rockwood CA Jr: Fractures of the clavicle, in Rockwood CA Jr, Matsen FA III, Wirth MA, Lippitt SB, eds: *The Shoulder*, ed 4. Philadelphia, PA, Saunders, 2009, pp 381-451.)

Two systematic reviews of studies that compared intramedullary fixation with plate and screw fixation reported that the functional outcomes of the two types of fixation were equivalent; however, most of the studies showed a lower complication rate for patients who were treated with intramedullary fixation.[29,30] In a meta-analysis of randomized controlled studies that compared intramedullary fixation with plate fixation for the management of midshaft clavicle fractures, Duan et al[31] reported no differences in treatment effects between plate fixation and intramedullary fixation; however, plate fixation was associated with more side effects.

Medial Clavicle Fractures

Because of the infrequence of medial clavicle fractures, a paucity of data exist with regard to epidemiology and treatment paradigms. These injuries, as separate entities from sternoclavicular (SC) dislocations or medial physeal fractures of the clavicle, pose a considerable risk to the underlying neurovascular structures. If coupled with high-velocity injuries, fractures of the medial clavicle are associated with high rates of thoracic and cervical injuries.[32] Surgeons should have a keen understanding of the underlying anatomic structures and a high index of suspicion for comorbid conditions.

Epidemiology

Throckmorton and Kuhn[32] reported that many medial clavicle fractures occur in males (80%), are related to vehicular trauma (84%), and are a part of multisystem trauma (90%). The authors reported that medial clavicle fractures occur in patients who are a mean age of 46.3 years, with a wide age range (19 to 88 years). The authors reported a high rate of concomitant thoracic trauma, with 73% of patients having a rib fracture and 42% having either a hemothorax, pneumothorax, or hemopneumothorax. In addition, 36% of patients sustained an intracranial injury (closed head injury or hemorrhage), 26% of patients suffered cervical spine injuries, and 45% of patients had other upper extremity injuries. Importantly, 22% of the medial clavicle fractures were seen on CT scans but not on plain radiographs. Surgical management was reserved for open fractures and fractures with associated neurovascular injury. Postacchini et al[33] reported a 2% incidence of medial clavicle fractures during an 11-year time span. The authors reported that 72.7% of those medial clavicle fractures were displaced in patients who had a bimodal age distribution (18 to 30 years and 50 to 80 years).

Nonsurgical Management

Throckmorton and Kuhn[32] reported high rates of union with the nonsurgical treatment of medial clavicle fractures. Fifty-one of 55 patients who had medial clavicle fractures were treated nonsurgically, and the remaining 4 patients were surgically treated for open fractures. At final follow-up, 47% of patients had no pain, 25% of patients had mild pain, 22% of patients had moderate pain, and 6% of patients had severe pain.

Surgical Management

Low et al[34] reported on a small cohort of five patients who were treated with ORIF for isolated, displaced medial clavicle fractures. These fractures were closed and included shortening and deformity as the result of high-energy trauma. The authors excluded all patients with open physes. Each patient was treated with a medial clavicle plate. At final follow-up, all fractures were united, and each patient had full, active range of shoulder motion. The authors acknowledged that CT scans were helpful for preoperative planning.

Bartoníček et al[35] reported outcomes on a series of five patients who had medial clavicle fractures. Three of the patients (aged 19 to 31 years) were treated with cerclage wire fixation for fracture fragment displacement of more than 2 cm. At final follow-up, each surgically treated patient had full extremity range of motion, visual analog scale scores of zero at rest and with activity, and Disabilities of the Arm, Shoulder and Hand questionnaire scores higher than 24. The two other patients were older, lower-demand individuals who were treated nonsurgically. These patients had decreased shoulder motion, higher visual analog scale scores with activity, and worse Disabilities of the Arm, Shoulder and Hand questionnaire scores than the patients who were treated surgically.

Results

Early surgical fixation of displaced clavicle fractures has been reported to reduce malunion and nonunion. Several studies report that shortening of more than 2 cm is associated with an increased risk of nonunion and poorer functional outcomes.[3,4,36] Other studies report decreased strength about the shoulder after 2 cm of clavicular shortening.[37,38]

The goals in the treatment of clavicular malunions and nonunions are to restore clavicular length, improve shoulder function, and improve cosmesis. Clavicular length can be assessed on high-quality plain radiographs and CT scans. In addition, CT provides accurate digital assessment of fracture length and orientation. Fracture malunions and nonunions with more than 2 cm of shortening may require osteotomy and the placement of cortical graft. For cases of atrophic nonunion, an iliac crest bone graft and an anteroinferior plate construct may be considered. In rare cases, a short superior positioning plate is used to hold the graft in place and establish length before the placement of the anterior plate.

Lateral Clavicle Fractures

Fractures of the lateral third of the clavicle account for approximately 10% to 15% of all clavicular fractures.[39] Nonunion occurs in approximately 40% of

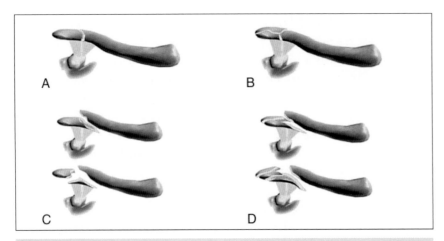

Figure 10 Illustrations show the Robinson classification system of distal clavicle fractures (type 3). **A,** Type 3A1 extra-articular cortical alignment fracture. **B,** Type 3A2 intra-articular cortical alignment fracture. **C,** Type 3B1 extra-articular displaced fractures. **D,** Type 3B2 intra-articular displaced fractures. (Reproduced with permission from Robinson CM: Fractures of the clavicle in the adult: Epidemiology and classification. *J Bone Joint Surg Br* 1998;80[3]:476-484.)

patients who are treated nonsurgically; however, some studies have shown that only one-third of these patients have a symptomatic nonunion that requires surgical intervention. The asymptomatic nonunions seem to occur mostly in elderly patients.[4]

Many different classification systems for lateral clavicle fractures have been suggested; most are based on the integrity of the coracoclavicular (CC) ligaments[7,39,40] (**Figure 10**). If the conoid ligament is damaged, the fracture is considered unstable and at a higher risk for nonunion. Because of this high nonunion rate, Neer[40] recommended surgical treatment for most lateral clavicle fractures. Other authors have recommended nonsurgical treatment for most of fractures in middle-aged and older patients.[41] The most effective treatment for younger patients has yet to be determined.

Nonsurgical Management

Nonsurgical management is indicated for most Neer type I, type III, and nondisplaced type II fractures (Robinson type 3A fractures). Treatment consists of placement of the arm in a sling for 2 to 3 weeks with passive and passive-assisted range of motion. The patient may begin active range of motion after he or she is pain free and signs of healing and consolidation are present on follow-up radiographs.[39,42]

Surgical Management

Some of the surgical treatment considerations for lateral clavicle fractures are the relatively poor bone stock in the metaphyseal bone of the distal fragment and the size of the distal fragment, which can substantially compromise fixation. In addition, the differential motion between the clavicle and the acromion and coracoid limits their use for additional fixation. Furthermore, the bone of the acromion can be quite thin and is easily compromised with screw fixation.

Several different surgical techniques have been described for the management of lateral clavicle fractures, including cerclage suture around the clavicle and the coracoid, suture fixation of the fracture fragments, plate and screw fixation, transacromial fixation with either plates or pins, CC screw fixation or suture anchor fixation, plate fixation, and hybrid fixation with the use of both clavicular plates and CC fixation. A cadaver model study that compared suture fixation with cerclage and CC suture, distal clavicle locking plates, distal clavicle locking plates with suture augmentation, and distal clavicle hook plates showed no significant differences in ultimate load to failure for unstable distal clavicle fractures.[43] Another cadaver model study reported that greater fracture stability was achieved with the combination of coracoid suture fixation and locking clavicle plate constructs than with either method alone.[44]

Results

Specific issues are associated with different types of surgical treatment. Cerclage fixation around the clavicle and the coracoid requires a large exposure, which leads to potential damage of the subcoracoid structures, and can erode through the clavicle and the coracoid (**Figure 11**). Transacromial fixation that violates the AC joint is associated with a high failure rate. Coracoclavicular screw fixation is associated with difficult placement and the need for removal because of differential motion between the clavicle and the scapula. Suture anchor fixation also is associated with potentially difficult placement and the potential for damage to the clavicle and the coracoid with later reinjury.[45-47]

In a meta-analysis of fixation techniques for distal clavicle fractures, Stegeman et al[48] reported that union was achieved in 98% of patients, with similar functional outcomes between the

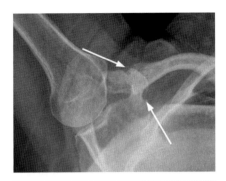

Figure 11 Stryker notch radiograph demonstrates erosion (arrows) of the coracoid and clavicle from permanent sutures.

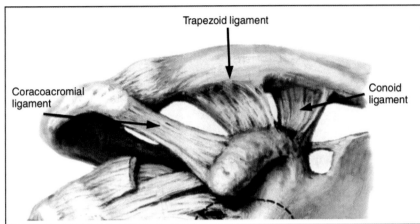

Figure 12 Illustration shows the ligamentous structure of the acromioclavicular joint and coracoid.

techniques previously mentioned; however, complications occurred in 22% of patients who were treated surgically. Compared with suture anchor fixation, hook-plate fixation and intramedullary fixation were associated with an 11-fold and a 24-fold increased risk of major complications, respectively. Complication rates for the other fixation methods were as follows: Kirschner wire plus tension band wiring (20%), CC stabilization (4.8%), intramedullary fixation (2.4%), and interfragmentary fixation (6.3%).[48] Numerous complications have been reported with hook-plate fixation, especially medial peri-implant fractures, acromial erosion, and dislocation of the fixation device.[46,49] Because of these complications, it is typically recommended that the device be removed as soon as healing has been achieved.[49]

AC Joint Injuries
Three-Dimensional Anatomy and Biomechanics

The AC joint is the apex of a triangular support system that maximizes scapulohumeral rhythm and three-dimensional (3D) shoulder girdle functional capability (**Figure 12**). AC joint stability, which is maintained by several aspects of the anatomy, is key to the function of the support system. Clavicular bony length maximizes strut function.[45,50] The CC ligaments control clavicular and scapular motions in an inferior-superior (vertically oriented conoid) and lateral tilt (diagonally oriented trapezoid) direction and, because of their staggered anterior and posterior clavicular attachments, help control clavicular rotation. The posterosuperior AC ligament, which attaches approximately 5 mm from the end of the distal clavicle, controls anterior-posterior motions. This anatomic integrity allows the clavicular-scapular screw axis to guide the relative scapular-clavicular motion running through the AC joint.[45,50,51]

Pathoanatomy and Pathomechanics

AC joint injuries occur from a directed force on the posterior acromion, which drives it downward and anteriorly. The AC ligaments either tear or avulse from the clavicle, but remain attached to the acromion. The CC ligament injury propagates on the inferior clavicle through the trapezoid and then the conoid, usually in the midsubstance. If the screw axis is disrupted, the scapula can translate into a variable amount of inferior, anterior, and medial positions relative to the clavicle. Scapulohumeral rhythm is altered, and the support system is destabilized so that optimal shoulder girdle function can be compromised. Functional consequences include pain, rotator cuff weakness, decreased arm flexion and abduction, muscle spasm, and glenohumeral joint symptoms.

3D Evaluation and Treatment

A literature review of current practices for the assessment and treatment of AC injuries reveals that most surgeons use the Rockwood classification, a two-dimensional method that involves only the static inferior-superior position of two bones. This method has been reported to be unreliable and does not always result in consistent treatment recommendations.[52] Other types of imaging and a dynamic clinical examination can help assess the extent of the 3D injury and suggest treatment options and techniques to restore 3D function. A plain or weighted radiograph often does not estimate the extent of 3D injury and has not been

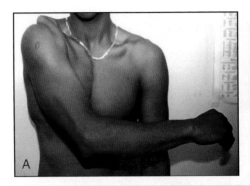 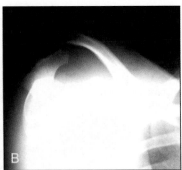

Figure 13   **A,** Clinical photograph shows the cross-body adduction maneuver. **B,** Cross-body adduction radiograph demonstrates an acromioclavicular joint injury.

shown to be reliable for the accurate diagnosis.[52] A cross-body adduction radiograph can better estimate the amount of possible translation and better identify the degree of AC separation (**Figure 13**).

The clinical examination can help assess the dynamics of scapular translation, demonstrate the functional consequences of the AC injury, and help determine the treatment indications, especially for Rockwood type III lesions. The clinical examination can be performed after acute symptoms are minimized, approximately 7 to 10 days after the injury. The clinical examination is based on the assessment of normal or abnormal scapular positioning and motion as an indicator of AC and CC ligament integrity. Abnormal motion, which results from the loss of ligament integrity, can be reliably identified in all 3D directions by observing the medial border of the scapula at rest or with arm elevation. Altered motion is termed dyskinesis.[53,54] The effect of dyskinesis on arm flexion and abduction can be demonstrated, and any improvement with scapular stabilization can further demonstrate the functional consequences. Occasionally, the joint can be manually reduced, and its effect on arm motion can be shown.

If the joint is reducible or there is no observable dyskinesis, rehabilitation that emphasizes scapular retraction can usually produce satisfactory functional results. This "low-grade" scapular position is usually seen in patients who have type I and II lesions and in approximately one-third of patients who have type III lesions.[55] Observable dyskinesis represents more biomechanical disruption and a generally less favorable functional result. This "high-grade" scapular position is seen in two-thirds of patients who have type III lesions and in most patients who have type V lesions. Based on these findings, the International Society of Arthroscopy, Knee Surgery and Orthopaedic Sports Medicine Upper Extremity Committee modified the Rockwood classification of the often controversial type III injuries into types IIIA (no dyskinesis) and IIIB (dyskinesis evident).[56] This "low-grade/high-grade" classification method can help establish more mechanically determined surgical indications, and surgical treatment can then be tailored to restore the demonstrated alterations specific to each individual patient.

Surgical treatment should restore all elements for structural integrity and should be based on adequate clavicle length, high-strength biology that is anatomically positioned on the clavicle, and both CC and AC ligament reconstruction. The preferred technique of the authors of this chapter includes mobilization of the native AC ligaments from their displaced position on the inferior clavicle (**Figure 14, A**); anatomic placement of two 4-mm drill holes in the clavicle, which are centered on the identifiable conoid tubercle and the trapezoid ridge (**Figure 14, B**); and passage of a semitendinosis allograft along with five strands of No. 2 polydioxanone suture, which act as an internal strut, around the coracoid and through the drill holes, and anatomic manual reduction of the joint. Next, the polydioxanone suture is tied, and the graft is sutured over the clavicle; the native AC ligaments are reanchored on the anterior and posterior clavicle; and the graft tails are docked into the dorsal acromion with sutures that are passed through the tails and two 2-mm drill holes to the lateral acromial border. The same technique can be used for both acute and chronic dislocations of the AC joint. The source of the graft (allograft versus autograft) is dependent on the surgeon's preference.

SC Joint Injuries

SC joint injuries are rare. Rowe and Marble[57] reported that SC injuries comprise only 3% of all shoulder girdle injuries. The rarity of SC dislocations should not be confused with these injuries being innocuous. The hilar structures, which are in close proximity to the SC joint, are at risk for possible traumatic injury.[58]

The SC joint is freely mobile. It functions in almost all planes, including rotation.[59] The surrounding ligaments (the intra-articular disk ligament, the costoclavicular ligaments, the capsular ligaments, and the interclavicular ligament) lend integrity to this small incongruous joint (**Figure 15**). Spencer and Kuhn[60] emphasized the importance of the anterior and posterior capsular ligaments, which provide anteroposterior and rotational stability for the SC joint.

Signs and Symptoms

The ligaments of the SC joint are intact in a patient who has a mild sprain. The patient reports pain and tenderness to palpation over the joint. There may be swelling, but no instability is noted. Severe pain and deformity are present in a patient who has a dislocation of the SC joint. Anterior SC injures may manifest as prominence of the medial clavicle. This prominence is more easily appreciated if the patient is supine. Posterior SC dislocations, which are rarer,[61] elicit a higher level of pain complaints from patients. The corner of the sternum may be appreciated if the medial clavicle is displaced posteriorly. Swelling may prevent assessment of the SC joint injury.[62] Patients who have posterior displacement may report shortness of breath, difficulty in swallowing, tingling or numbness, decreased circulation in the ipsilateral extremity, or venous engorgement, all of which may arise from the compression of structures within the mediastinum. Posterior SC dislocations or associated injuries may render patients medically unstable.

Radiographic Evaluation

Routine radiographs of the SC joint are difficult to interpret. CT is a far superior technique compared with conventional radiographs to identify any problems in the SC joint (**Figure 16**). The examination should also include CT of the chest to identify any associated injuries. In children and young adults, MRI is

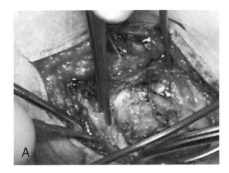
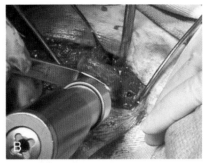

Figure 14   Clinical photographs show the surgical technique for the treatment of an acromioclavicular injury. **A,** The displaced native acromioclavicular ligaments are mobilized. **B,** 4-mm holes are drilled in the clavicle for the placement of a semitendinosis graft.

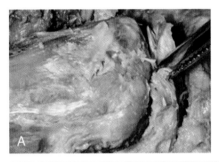
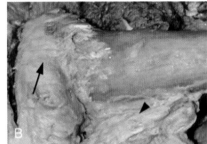

Figure 15   Photographs show the ligamentous structures of the sternoclavicular joint. **A,** The intra-articular disk ligament (held by forceps) that is attached to the right medial clavicle appears normal after removal of the capsular ligaments. **B,** The anterior sternoclavicular capsular ligament (arrow) and the rhomboid appearance of the costoclavicular ligament (arrowhead) shown with the left medial clavicle. (Reproduced from Groh GI, Wirth MA: Management of traumatic sternoclavicular joint injuries. *J Am Acad Orthop Surg* 2011;19[1]:1-7.)

especially helpful to distinguish a dislocation from a physeal injury. Because of its speed, availability, and ability to image bone, CT is the imaging study of choice in acute cases.

Treatment

Anterior Strains/Subluxations

The use of ice and analgesic agents for the initial treatment of SC injuries is advocated. Subluxations may be reduced by directing the shoulder posterior and medial. Support of the injury with a clavicle strap or sling and swathe is typically beneficial. The patient is protected from injury with immobilization for 6 weeks.

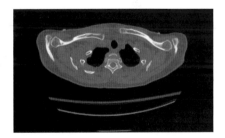

Figure 16   CT scan demonstrates a right posterior sternoclavicular dislocation. The normal position of the left clavicle also is shown.

Anterior Dislocations

Closed reduction of anterior SC dislocations is the current treatment of choice; however, there is still some controversy with regard to management.[63,64]

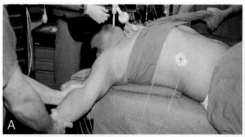
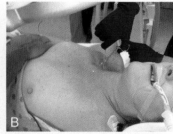

Figure 17 Clinical photographs show techniques for closed reduction of posterior sternoclavicular dislocations. **A,** Traction technique. **B,** Towel-clamp technique.

Closed reduction may be performed with sedation, local anesthesia, or general anesthesia. The patient is placed supine on a table. Pressure is placed posteriorly on the medial clavicle. If the joint remains reduced, the patient is immobilized in either a figure-of-8 or Velpeau-type sling for 6 weeks to allow healing. Unfortunately, most anterior SC dislocations are unstable after closed reduction; however, if the procedure is successful, patients have improved cosmesis. Although numerous methods of open reduction have been described for the treatment of anterior SC dislocations,[65-67] most authors do not recommend open reduction for these unstable injuries and, instead, opt for observation.

Posterior Dislocations

A careful history and physical examination of posterior SC dislocations and a low threshold for the use of CT is recommended. Patients who have mediastinal involvement require prompt consultation with a thoracic or cardiothoracic surgeon.

Closed Reduction

While under sedation or general anesthesia, the patient is placed supine on the surgical table. Initially, gentle traction is applied to the abducted extremity in line with the clavicle as an assistant, who steadies the patient, applies countertraction. The traction on the arm is slowly increased as the arm is brought into extension (**Figure 17, A**). If reduction is achieved via the traction technique, it is typically stable.[68] An immediately available thoracic surgeon is recommended for closed reductions.

If traction techniques are not successful, then the skin is surgically prepped, and a sterile towel clamp is used to grasp the clavicle percutaneously (**Figure 17, B**). The clamp will not penetrate the dense cortical bone of the clavicle; instead, it is used to grasp completely around the clavicle. Traction through the affected limb in combination with lifting of the clavicle anteriorly will usually reduce the dislocation. The reduction should be confirmed with intraoperative radiographs. The authors of this chapter recommend that the patient be immobilized in a figure-of-8 clavicle strap or sling for 4 weeks to allow soft-tissue healing. Groh et al[68] reported high rates of success with closed reduction that was performed as late as 10 days after posterior SC dislocation.

Open Reduction

Open reduction of the SC joint should always be performed with the assistance of a thoracic surgeon or with a thoracic surgeon present. The procedure is performed under general anesthesia, with the patient positioned supine and a bolster placed between the scapulae. A 5- to 7-cm anterior incision that parallels the superior border of the medial clavicle and extends down over the sternum is made. If enough of the anterior capsule has been preserved and is undamaged from the initial injury, the reduction will be stable.

Instability of the medial clavicle can be addressed by various surgical techniques.[65-67] In a biomechanical study, Spencer and Kuhn[60] described a figure-of-8 reconstruction technique that used a semitendinosus graft (**Figure 18**). This reconstruction technique provided an initial stiffness close to that of an intact SC joint. Rockwood et al[69] resected the medial clavicle and secured the residual clavicle anatomically to the periosteum of the first rib with No. 5 nonabsorbable suture to address instability (**Figure 19**). If the repair is tenuous, it may be augmented with the reconstruction technique described by Spencer and Kuhn.[60] A figure-of-8 clavicle splint is used for 4 weeks after all open reductions or resections and is followed by the use of a sling for an additional 6 to 8 weeks. After 12 weeks, patients are allowed to gradually increase the use of the arm for activities of daily living.

Complications of surgical management include postoperative infection, loss of reduction, and posttraumatic arthritis.[70-74] The most serious complications have arisen from the use of pins that cross the SC joint. The tremendous torque that is applied to these pins cause migration and fatigue failure of the hardware. The literature is replete with reports of the migration of intact or broken pins and wires into the heart and the mediastinum.[75-90]

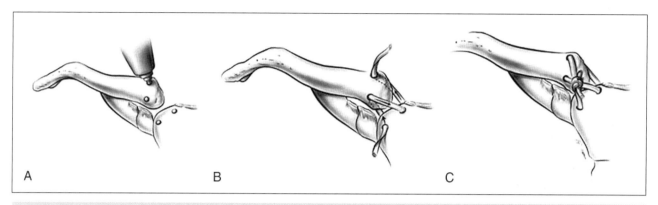

Figure 18   Illustrations show the semitendinosus figure-of-8 reconstruction technique described by Spencer and Kuhn.[60] **A,** Drill holes are placed in the clavicle and manubrium. The semitendinosus graft is woven through the drill holes in a figure-of-8 fashion (**B**) and sutured into position (**C**), which provides stability that is comparable with an intact sternoclavicular joint. (Reproduced from Groh GI, Wirth MA: Management of traumatic sternoclavicular joint injuries. *J Am Acad Orthop Surg* 2011;19[1]:1-7.)

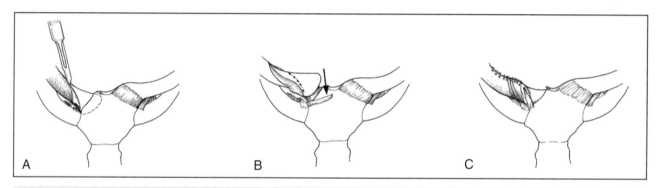

Figure 19   Illustrations show resection of the medial clavicle. **A,** The medial end of the clavicle is exposed subperiosteally. **B,** Drill holes are made at the intended site of the osteotomy to facilitate excision of the medial clavicle. Note the preservation of the capsular ligament (arrow). **C,** The capsular ligament is secured to the medial clavicle with sutures that exit the superior cortex of the clavicle. Closure of the periosteal sleeve and fixation to the costoclavicular ligaments is accomplished with the use of multiple No. 5 nonabsorbable sutures. (Reproduced from Groh GI, Wirth MA: Management of traumatic sternoclavicular joint injuries. *J Am Acad Orthop Surg* 2011;19[1]:1-7.)

Summary

Nonsurgical management remains the mainstay for nondisplaced and minimally displaced clavicle fractures. Recent studies have reported that substantial shoulder dysfunction may result from the nonsurgical management of displaced clavicle fractures. Early treatment with meticulous surgical technique will lead to predictable results and good functional outcomes.

The AC joint functions in three dimensions; therefore, an AC joint injury may alter function in three dimensions. The evaluation of an AC injury from a 3D perspective, often with the use of scapular position and motion as an indication of the altered biomechanics of the joint, can result in a more comprehensive and accurate assessment of the injury and can help guide treatment recommendations, with good treatment outcomes for patients who are treated surgically.

SC joint injuries are rare. Most SC injuries are anterior and typically treated symptomatically. Injuries of the hilar structures, which are in close proximity to the SC joint, may be associated with posterior injuries of the SC joint. The potential for both early and late damage to the hilar structures require that SC joint injures be carefully evaluated and treated.

References

1. Rowe CR: An atlas of anatomy and treatment of midclavicular fractures. *Clin Orthop Relat Res* 1968;58(59):29-42.

2. Neer CS II: Nonunion of the clavicle. *J Am Med Assoc* 1960;172:1006-1011.

3. Hill JM, McGuire MH, Crosby LA: Closed treatment of displaced middle-third fractures of the clavicle gives poor results. *J Bone Joint Surg Br* 1997;79(4):537-539.

4. McKee MD, Pedersen EM, Jones C, et al: Deficits following nonoperative treatment of displaced midshaft clavicular fractures. *J Bone Joint Surg Am* 2006;88(1):35-40.

5. Canadian Orthopaedic Trauma Society: Nonoperative treatment compared with plate fixation of displaced midshaft clavicular fractures: A multicenter, randomized clinical trial. *J Bone Joint Surg Am* 2007;89(1):1-10.

6. McKee RC, Whelan DB, Schemitsch EH, McKee MD: Operative versus nonoperative care of displaced midshaft clavicular fractures: A meta-analysis of randomized clinical trials. *J Bone Joint Surg Am* 2012;94(8):675-684.

7. Robinson CM: Fractures of the clavicle in the adult: Epidemiology and classification. *J Bone Joint Surg Br* 1998;80(3):476-484.

8. Iannotti MR, Crosby LA, Stafford P, Grayson G, Goulet R: Effects of plate location and selection on the stability of midshaft clavicle osteotomies: A biomechanical study. *J Shoulder Elbow Surg* 2002;11(5):457-462.

9. Partal G, Meyers KN, Sama N, et al: Superior versus anteroinferior plating of the clavicle revisited: A mechanical study. *J Orthop Trauma* 2010;24(7):420-425.

10. Collinge C, Devinney S, Herscovici D, DiPasquale T, Sanders R: Anterior-inferior plate fixation of middle-third fractures and non-unions of the clavicle. *J Orthop Trauma* 2006;20(10):680-686.

11. Jeray KJ: Acute midshaft clavicular fracture. *J Am Acad Orthop Surg* 2007;15(4):239-248.

12. Wijdicks FJ, Van der Meijden OA, Millett PJ, Verleisdonk EJ, Houwert RM: Systematic review of the complications of plate fixation of clavicle fractures. *Arch Orthop Trauma Surg* 2012;132(5):617-625.

13. Huang JI, Toogood P, Chen MR, Wilber JH, Cooperman DR: Clavicular anatomy and the applicability of precontoured plates. *J Bone Joint Surg Am* 2007;89(10):2260-2265.

14. Bain GI, Eng K, Zumstein MA: Fatal air embolus during internal fixation of the clavicle: A case report. *JBJS Case Connect* 2013;3(1):e24.

15. Brockway A: Use of the intramedullary beef-bone graft in open reductions of the clavicle. *J Bone Joint Surg Am* 1930;12(3):656-662.

16. Küntscher G: *Technik der Marknagelung.* Leipzig, Germany, Thieme, 1945.

17. Wijdicks FJ, Houwert RM, Millett PJ, Verleisdonk EJ, Van der Meijden OA: Systematic review of complications after intramedullary fixation for displaced midshaft clavicle fractures. *Can J Surg* 2013;56(1):58-64.

18. Millett PJ, Hurst JM, Horan MP, Hawkins RJ: Complications of clavicle fractures treated with intramedullary fixation. *J Shoulder Elbow Surg* 2011;20(1):86-91.

19. Mathieu PA, Marcheix PS, Hummel V, Valleix D, Mabit C: Anatomical study of the clavicle: Endomedullary morphology. *Surg Radiol Anat* 2014;36(1):11-15.

20. Bachoura A, Deane AS, Kamineni S: Clavicle anatomy and the applicability of intramedullary midshaft fracture fixation. *J Shoulder Elbow Surg* 2012;21(10):1384-1390.

21. Wijdicks FJ, Houwert M, Dijkgraaf M, et al: Complications after plate fixation and elastic stable intramedullary nailing of dislocated midshaft clavicle fractures: A retrospective comparison. *Int Orthop* 2012;36(10):2139-2145.

22. Frigg A, Rillmann P, Perren T, Gerber M, Ryf C: Intramedullary nailing of clavicular midshaft fractures with the titanium elastic nail: Problems and complications. *Am J Sports Med* 2009;37(2):352-359.

23. Lee YS, Lin CC, Huang CR, Chen CN, Liao WY: Operative treatment of midclavicular fractures in 62 elderly patients: Knowles pin versus plate. *Orthopedics* 2007;30(11):959-964.

24. Marlow WJ, Ralte P, Morapudi SP, Bassi R, Fischer J, Waseem M: Intramedullary fixation of diaphyseal clavicle fractures using the Rockwood clavicle pin: Review of 86 cases. *Open Orthop J* 2012;6:482-487.

25. Payne DE, Wray WH, Ruch DS, Zura RD, Moorman CT: Outcome of intramedullary fixation of clavicular fractures. *Am J Orthop (Belle Mead NJ)* 2011;40(6):E99-E104.

26. Boehme D, Curtis RJ Jr, DeHaan JT, Kay SP, Young DC, Rockwood CA Jr: Non-union of fractures of the midshaft of the clavicle: Treatment with a modified Hagie intramedullary pin and autogenous bone-grafting. *J Bone Joint Surg Am* 1991;73(8):1219-1226.

27. King PR, Ikram A, Lamberts RP: The treatment of clavicular shaft fractures with an innovative locked intramedullary device. *J Shoulder Elbow Surg* 2015;24(1):e1-e6.

28. Wenninger JJ Jr, Dannenbaum JH, Branstetter JG, Arrington ED: Comparison of complication rates of intramedullary pin fixation versus plating of midshaft clavicle fractures in an active duty military population. *J Surg Orthop Adv* 2013;22(1):77-81.

29. Barlow T, Beazley J, Barlow D: A systematic review of plate versus intramedullary fixation in the treatment of midshaft clavicle fractures. *Scott Med J* 2013;58(3):163-167.

30. Lenza M, Buchbinder R, Johnston RV, Belloti JC, Faloppa F: Surgical versus conservative interventions for treating fractures of the middle third of the clavicle. *Cochrane Database Syst Rev* 2013;6:CD009363.

31. Duan X, Zhong G, Cen S, Huang F, Xiang Z: Plating versus intramedullary pin or conservative treatment for midshaft fracture of clavicle: A meta-analysis of randomized controlled trials. *J Shoulder Elbow Surg* 2011;20(6):1008-1015.

32. Throckmorton T, Kuhn JE: Fractures of the medial end of the clavicle. *J Shoulder Elbow Surg* 2007;16(1):49-54.

33. Postacchini F, Gumina S, De Santis P, Albo F: Epidemiology of clavicle fractures. *J Shoulder Elbow Surg* 2002;11(5):452-456.

34. Low AK, Duckworth DG, Bokor DJ: Operative outcome of displaced medial-end clavicle fractures in adults. *J Shoulder Elbow Surg* 2008;17(5):751-754.

35. Bartoníček J, Fric V, Pacovský V: Displaced fractures of the medial end of the clavicle: Report of five cases. *J Orthop Trauma* 2010;24(4):e31-e35.

36. Eskola A, Vainionpää S, Myllynen P, Pätiälä H, Rokkanen P: Surgery for ununited clavicular fracture. *Acta Orthop Scand* 1986;57(4):366-367.

37. Nowak J, Holgersson M, Larsson S: Sequelae from clavicular fractures are common: A prospective study of 222 patients. *Acta Orthop* 2005;76(4):496-502.

38. Ledger M, Leeks N, Ackland T, Wang A: Short malunions of the clavicle: An anatomic and functional study. *J Shoulder Elbow Surg* 2005;14(4):349-354.

39. Banerjee R, Waterman B, Padalecki J, Robertson W: Management of distal clavicle fractures. *J Am Acad Orthop Surg* 2011;19(7):392-401.

40. Neer CS II: Fracture of the distal clavicle with detachment of the coracoclavicular ligaments in adults. *J Trauma* 1963;3:99-110.

41. Rokito AS, Zuckerman JD, Shaari JM, Eisenberg DP, Cuomo F, Gallagher MA: A comparison of nonoperative and operative treatment of type II distal clavicle fractures. *Bull Hosp Jt Dis* 2002-2003;61(1-2):32-39.

42. Robinson CM, Cairns DA: Primary nonoperative treatment of displaced lateral fractures of the clavicle. *J Bone Joint Surg Am* 2004;86(4):778-782.

43. Bishop JY, Roesch M, Lewis B, Jones GL, Litsky AS: A biomechanical comparison of distal clavicle fracture reconstructive techniques. *Am J Orthop (Belle Mead NJ)* 2013;42(3):114-118.

44. Rieser GR, Edwards K, Gould GC, Markert RJ, Goswami T, Rubino LJ: Distal-third clavicle fracture fixation: A biomechanical evaluation of fixation. *J Shoulder Elbow Surg* 2013;22(6):848-855.

45. Oki S, Matsumura N, Iwamoto W, et al: Acromioclavicular joint ligamentous system contributing to clavicular strut function: A cadaveric study. *J Shoulder Elbow Surg* 2013;22(10):1433-1439.

46. Bisbinas I, Mikalef P, Gigis I, Beslikas T, Panou N, Christoforidis I: Management of distal clavicle fractures. *Acta Orthop Belg* 2010;76(2):145-149.

47. Martetschläger F, Horan MP, Warth RJ, Millett PJ: Complications after anatomic fixation and reconstruction of the coracoclavicular ligaments. *Am J Sports Med* 2013;41(12):2896-2903.

48. Stegeman SA, Nacak H, Huvenaars KH, Stijnen T, Krijnen P, Schipper IB: Surgical treatment of Neer type-II fractures of the distal clavicle: A meta-analysis. *Acta Orthop* 2013;84(2):184-190.

49. Klein SM, Badman BL, Keating CJ, Devinney DS, Frankle MA, Mighell MA: Results of surgical treatment for unstable distal clavicular fractures. *J Shoulder Elbow Surg* 2010;19(7):1049-1055.

50. Debski RE, Parsons IM III, Fenwick J, Vangura A: Ligament mechanics during three degree-of-freedom motion at the acromioclavicular joint. *Ann Biomed Eng* 2000;28(6):612-618.

51. Sahara W, Sugamoto K, Murai M, Yoshikawa H: Three-dimensional clavicular and acromioclavicular rotations during arm abduction using vertically open MRI. *J Orthop Res* 2007;25(9):1243-1249.

52. Ng CY, Smith EK, Funk L: Reliability of the traditional classification systems for acromioclavicular joint injuries by radiography. *Shoulder Elbow* 2012;4(4):266-269.

53. Kibler WB, Sciascia A: Current concepts: Scapular dyskinesis. *Br J Sports Med* 2010;44(5):300-305.

54. Kibler WB, Sciascia A, Wilkes T: Scapular dyskinesis and its relation to shoulder injury. *J Am Acad Orthop Surg* 2012;20(6):364-372.

55. Gumina S, Carbone S, Postacchini F: Scapular dyskinesis and SICK scapula syndrome in patients with chronic type III acromioclavicular dislocation. *Arthroscopy* 2009;25(1):40-45.

56. Bak K, Mazzocca A, Beitzel K, et al: Copenhagen consensus on acromioclavicular disorders, in Arce G, Bak K, Shea KP, et al, eds: *Shoulder Concepts 2013: Consensus and Concerns. Proceedings of the ISAKOS Upper Extremity Committees 2009-2013.* Heidelberg, Germany, Springer, 2013, pp 51-67.

57. Rowe C, Marble H: Fractures and other injuries, in Cave EF, ed: *Shoulder Girdle Injuries.* Chicago, IL, Year Book Medical Publishers, 1958, pp 258-259.

58. Groh GI, Wirth MA: Management of traumatic sternoclavicular joint injuries. *J Am Acad Orthop Surg* 2011;19(1):1-7.

59. Bearn JG: Direct observations on the function of the capsule of the sternoclavicular joint in clavicular support. *J Anat* 1967;101(pt 1):159-170.

60. Spencer EE Jr, Kuhn JE: Biomechanical analysis of reconstructions for sternoclavicular joint instability. *J Bone Joint Surg Am* 2004;86(1):98-105.

61. Nettles JL, Linscheid RL: Sternoclavicular dislocations. *J Trauma* 1968;8(2):158-164.

62. Rockwood CA Jr, Wirth MA: Disorders of the sternoclavicular joint, in Rockwood CA Jr, Matsen FA III, Wirth MA, Lippitt SB, eds: *The Shoulder,* ed 4. Philadelphia, PA, Saunders, 1998, pp 527-560.

63. Féry A, Sommelet J: Sternoclavicular dislocations: Observations on the treatment and result of 49 cases. *Int Orthop* 1988;12(3):187-195.

64. de Jong KP, Sukul DM: Anterior sternoclavicular dislocation: A long-term follow-up study. *J Orthop Trauma* 1990;4(4):420-423.

65. Bankart AS: An operation for recurrent dislocation (subluxation) of the sternoclavicular joint. *Br J Surg* 1938;26(102):320-323.

66. Key JA, Conwell HE: *The Management of Fracture, Dislocations, and Sprains,* ed 5. St. Louis, MO, CV Mosby, 1951, pp 458-461.

67. Burrows HJ: Tenodesis of subclavius in the treatment of recurrent dislocation of the sterno-clavicular joint. *J Bone Joint Surg Br* 1951;33(2):240-243.

68. Groh GI, Wirth MA, Rockwood CA Jr: Treatment of traumatic posterior sternoclavicular dislocations. *J Shoulder Elbow Surg* 2011;20(1):107-113.

69. Rockwood CA Jr, Groh GI, Wirth MA, Grassi FA: Resection arthroplasty of the sternoclavicular joint. *J Bone Joint Surg Am* 1997;79(3):387-393.

70. Wirth MA, Rockwood CA Jr: Complications following repair of the sternoclavicular joint, in Bigliani LU, ed: *Complications of Shoulder Surgery.*

Baltimore, MD, Williams & Wilkins, 1993, pp 139-153.

71. Brown JE: Anterior sternoclavicular dislocation: A method of repair. *Am J Orthop* 1961;31:184-189.

72. Eskola A, Vainionpää S, Vastamäki M, Slätis P, Rokkanen P: Operation for old sternoclavicular dislocation: Results in 12 cases. *J Bone Joint Surg Br* 1989;71(1):63-65.

73. Lunseth PA, Chapman KW, Frankel VH: Surgical treatment of chronic dislocation of the sterno-clavicular joint. *J Bone Joint Surg Br* 1975;57(2):193-196.

74. Omer GE Jr: Osteotomy of the clavicle in surgical reduction of anterior sternoclavicular dislocation. *J Trauma* 1967;7(4):584-590.

75. Buckerfield CT, Castle ME: Acute traumatic retrosternal dislocation of the clavicle. *J Bone Joint Surg Am* 1984;66(3):379-385.

76. Rubinstein ZJ, Morag B, Itzchak Y: Percutaneous removal of intravascular foreign bodies. *Cardiovasc Intervent Radiol* 1982;5(2):64-68.

77. Liu HP, Chang CH, Lin PJ, et al: Migration of Kirschner wire from the right sternoclavicular joint into the main pulmonary artery: A case report. *Changgeng Yi Xue Za Zhi* 1992;15(1):49-53.

78. Salvatore JE: Sternoclavicular joint dislocation. *Clin Orthop Relat Res* 1968;58:51-55.

79. Clark RL, Milgram JW, Yawn DH: Fatal aortic perforation and cardiac tamponade due to a Kirschner wire migrating from the right sternoclavicular joint. *South Med J* 1974;67(3):316-318.

80. Gerlach D, Wemhöner SR, Ogbuihi S: 2 cases of pericardial tamponade caused by migration of fracture wires from the sternoclavicular joint. *Z Rechtsmed* 1984;93(1):53-60.

81. Leonard JW, Gifford RW Jr: Migration of a Kirschner wire from the clavicle into the pulmonary artery. *Am J Cardiol* 1965;16(4):598-600.

82. Richman KM, Boutin RD, Vaughan LM, Haghighi P, Resnick D: Tophaceous pseudogout of the sternoclavicular joint. *AJR Am J Roentgenol* 1999;172(6):1587-1589.

83. Smolle-Juettner FM, Hofer PH, Pinter H, Friehs G, Szyskowitz R: Intracardiac malpositioning of a sternoclavicular fixation wire. *J Orthop Trauma* 1992;6(1):102-105.

84. Worman LW, Leagus C: Intrathoracic injury following retrosternal dislocation of the clavicle. *J Trauma* 1967;7(3):416-423.

85. Jelesijević V, Knoll D, Klinke F, Sine K, Dittrich H: Penetrating injuries of the heart and intrapericardial blood vessels caused by migration of a Kirschner pin after osteosynthesis. *Acta Chir Iugosl* 1982;29(suppl 2):274-277.

86. Pate JW, Wilhite JL: Migration of a foreign body from the sternoclavicular joint to the heart: A case report. *Am Surg* 1969;35(6):448-449.

87. Song HK, Guy TS, Kaiser LR, Shrager JB: Current presentation and optimal surgical management of sternoclavicular joint infections. *Ann Thorac Surg* 2002;73(2):427-431.

88. Nordback I, Markkula H: Migration of Kirschner pin from clavicle into ascending aorta. *Acta Chir Scand* 1985;151(2):177-179.

89. Sethi GK, Scott SM: Subclavian artery laceration due to migration of a Hagie pin. *Surgery* 1976;80(5):644-646.

90. Schechter DC, Gilbert L: Injuries of the heart and great vessels due to pins and needles. *Thorax* 1969;24(2):246-253.

Video Reference

Kibler WB: Video. *AC Joint Reconstruction*. Lexington, KY, 2015.

© 2016 AAOS Instructional Course Lectures, Volume 65

Adult Reconstruction: Hip and Knee

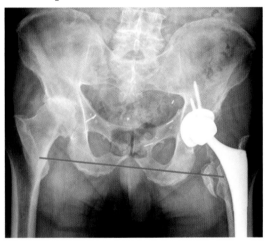

Adult Reconstruction
Hip and Knee

Preventing Hospital Readmissions and Limiting the Complications Associated With Total Joint Arthroplasty

Stephen Yu, MD
Kevin L. Garvin, MD
William L. Healy, MD
Vincent D. Pellegrini Jr, MD
Richard Iorio, MD

Abstract

Total joint arthroplasty is a highly successful surgical procedure for patients who have painful arthritic joints. The increasing prevalence of total joint arthroplasty is generating substantial expenditures in the American healthcare system. Healthcare payers, specifically the Centers for Medicare and Medicaid Services, currently target total joint arthroplasty as an area for healthcare cost-savings initiatives, which has resulted in increased scrutiny surrounding orthopaedic care, health resource utilization, and hospital readmissions. Identifying the complications associated with total hip and total knee arthroplasty that result in readmissions will be critically important for predictive modeling and to decrease the number of readmissions after total joint arthroplasty. In addition, improving perioperative optimization, providing seamless episodic care, and intensifying posthospital coordination of care may decrease the number of unnecessary hospital readmissions. Identified modifiable risk factors that substantially contribute to poor clinical outcomes after total joint arthroplasty include morbid obesity; poorly controlled diabetes and nutritional deficiencies; Staphylococcus aureus *colonization; tobacco use; venous thromboembolic disease; cardiovascular disease; neurocognitive, psychological, and behavioral problems; and physical deconditioning and fall risk. Both clinical practice and research will be enhanced if defined total joint arthroplasty complications are standardized and stratification schemes are used to identify high-risk patients. Subsequently, clinical intervention will be warranted to address modifiable risk factors before proceeding with total joint arthroplasty.*

Instr Course Lect 2016;65:199–210.

Total joint arthroplasty (TJA) is a highly successful surgical procedure that is used to treat patients who have painful, arthritic joints. The prevalence of TJA has increased considerably, and an estimated two million Americans are expected to undergo total hip arthroplasty (THA) or total knee arthroplasty

(TKA) in 2020.[1] The rising number of joint arthroplasty procedures in the United States generates substantial expenditures in the American healthcare system, and healthcare payers are currently targeting TJA for healthcare cost-savings initiatives. The Centers for Medicare and Medicaid Services (CMS)

has targeted orthopaedics, specifically TJA, for evaluation and has begun penalizing hospitals that have high readmission rates.

Jencks et al[2] analyzed Medicare claims data from 2003 and 2004 to determine the frequency and patterns of rehospitalization. Of the 11,855,702

Table 1

Complications and Adverse Events After Total Hip Arthroplasty (THA) as Developed by The Hip Society

Complication	Definition
Bleeding	Postoperative bleeding requiring surgical treatment
Wound complication	Failure of wound healing requiring revision surgery or a change in THA protocol
Thromboembolic disease	Symptomatic thromboembolic event requiring more intensive, nonprophylactic anticoagulant or anti-thrombotic treatment during the first 3 months after index THA
Neural deficit	Postoperative neural deficit (sensory or motor) related to index THA
Vascular injury	Intraoperative vascular injury requiring surgical repair, bypass grafting, or stenting (compartment syndrome or amputation should be recorded)
Dislocation/instability	Dislocation of the femoral head out of the acetabulum or recurrent symptomatic subluxation of the hip joint (direction of instability and type of treatment should be recorded)
Periprosthetic fracture	Periprosthetic fracture of the proximal femur or the acetabulum (intraoperative fracture or postoperative fracture should be recorded; surgical or nonsurgical treatment should be recorded)
Abductor muscle disruption	Symptomatic abductor dysfunction that was not present before the surgery, associated with a positive Trendelenburg sign and use of an ambulatory assist (eg, cane, crutch, walker) for treatment of limp or weakness (nonsurgical management should be recorded)
Deep periprosthetic joint infection	A deep periprosthetic joint infection can be diagnosed if there is a sinus tract communicating with the prosthesis, or a pathogen is isolated by culture from at least two separate tissue or fluid samples obtained from the affected prosthetic joint, or four of the following six criteria exist: elevated ESR and serum CRP level; elevated synovial WBC count; elevated synovial PMN count; presence of purulence in the affected joint; isolation of a microorganism in one culture of periprosthetic tissue or fluid; or >5 neutrophils/high-power field in five high-power fields observed from histologic analysis of periprosthetic tissue at 400× magnification
Heterotopic ossification	Symptomatic heterotopic ossification 1 year after surgery associated with stiffness, reduced range of motion, and Brooker radiographic grade III or IV
Bearing surface wear	Wear of the bearing surface that is symptomatic or requires surgery
Osteolysis	Expansile lytic lesion adjacent to one of the implants that is ≥1 cm in any one dimension or increasing in size on serial radiographs/CT
Implant loosening	Implant loosening confirmed intraoperatively or identified radiographically as a change in implant position or a progressive, radiolucent line at the bone-cement or bone-implant interface
Cup-liner dissociation	Dissociation of the cup liner from the acetabular cup
Implant fracture	Implant fracture (specific implant should be recorded)
Revision surgery	Return to the operating room related to index THA (reasons for revision surgery should be recorded)
Revision	Revision of one or more of the THA implants (acetabular cup, acetabular liner, femoral head, femoral stem)
Readmission	Admission to the hospital for any reason during the first 90 days after THA (reasons for admission and relation to index THA should be recorded)
Death	Death occurring for any reason during the first 90 days after THA (cause of death and relation to index THA should be recorded)

CRP = C-reactive protein, ESR = erythrocyte sedimentation rate, PMN = polymorphonuclear neutrophil, WBC = white blood cell.

Dr. Garvin or an immediate family member serves as an unpaid consultant to TRAK Surgical, and serves as a board member, owner, officer, or committee member of the American Academy of Orthopaedic Surgeons, the American Orthopaedic Association, The Hip Society, and The Knee Society. Dr. Healy or an immediate family member has received royalties from DePuy. Dr. Pellegrini or an immediate family member has received research or institutional support from the Department of Defense, the Agency for Healthcare Research and Quality, and the Patient-Centered Outcomes Research Institute; has received royalties from DePuy; serves as a paid consultant to DePuy; and serves as a board member, owner, officer, or committee member of the American Orthopaedic Association, the Accreditation Council for Graduate Medical Education, the Association of American Medical Colleges, the Council of Faculty and Academic Societies, Health Volunteers Overseas/Orthopaedics Overseas, the Hip Society, and the South Carolina Orthopaedic Association. Dr. Iorio or an immediate family member has received research or institutional support from OrthoSensor and Pacira Pharmaceuticals, and serves as a board member, owner, officer, or committee member of The Hip Society and the American Association of Hip and Knee Surgeons. Neither Dr. Yu nor any immediate family member has received anything of value from or has stock or stock options held in a commercial company or institution related directly or indirectly to the subject of this chapter.

© 2016 AAOS Instructional Course Lectures, Volume 65

Table 2

Complications and Adverse Events After Total Knee Arthroplasty (TKA) as Developed by The Knee Society

Complication	Definition
Bleeding	Postoperative bleeding requiring surgical treatment
Wound complication	Failure of wound healing requiring revision surgery or a change in TKA protocol
Thromboembolic disease	Symptomatic thromboembolic event requiring more intensive, nonprophylactic anticoagulant or antithrombotic treatment during the first 3 months after index TKA
Neural deficit	Postoperative neural deficit (sensory or motor) related to index TKA
Vascular injury	Intraoperative vascular injury requiring surgical repair, bypass grafting, or stenting (compartment syndrome or amputation should be recorded)
Medial collateral ligament injury	Intraoperative or early postoperative medial collateral ligament injury requiring repair, reconstruction, a change in prosthetic constraint, revision surgery, or TKA protocol
Instability	Symptomatic instability reported by the patient and confirmed by laxity on physical examination as defined by The Knee Society Score
Malalignment	Symptomatic malalignment reported by the patient and confirmed radiographically with angular deformity in the coronal plane >10° from the mechanical axis
Stiffness	Limited ROM as reported by the patient and demonstrated in a physical examination with extension limited to 15° short of full extension or flexion <90° (not applicable if preoperative arc of motion <75°)
Deep periprosthetic joint infection	A deep periprosthetic joint infection can be diagnosed if there is a sinus tract communicating with the prosthesis, or a pathogen is isolated by culture from at least two separate tissue or fluid samples obtained from the affected prosthetic joint, or four of the following six criteria exist: elevated ESR and serum CRP level; elevated synovial WBC count; elevated synovial PMN count; presence of purulence in the affected joint; isolation of a microorganism in one culture of periprosthetic tissue or fluid; or >5 neutrophils/high-power field in five high-power fields observed from histologic analysis of periprosthetic tissue at 400× magnification
Periprosthetic fracture	Periprosthetic fracture of the distal femur, proximal tibia, or patella (surgical or nonsurgical treatment should be recorded)
Extensor mechanism disruption	Disruption of the extensor mechanism (surgical repair and/or extensor lag should be recorded)
Patellofemoral dislocation	Dislocation of the patella from the femoral trochlea (direction of instability should be recorded)
Tibiofemoral dislocation	Dislocation of the tibiofemoral joint (direction of instability should be recorded)
Bearing surface wear	Wear of the bearing surface that is symptomatic or requires surgery
Osteolysis	Expansile lytic lesion adjacent to one of the implants that is >1 cm in any one dimension or increasing in size on serial radiographs/CT
Implant loosening	Implant loosening confirmed intraoperatively or identified radiographically as a change in implant position or a progressive, radiolucent line at the bone-cement or bone-implant interface
Implant fracture or tibial insert dissociation	Implant fracture or dissociation of the tibial insert from the tibial implant
Revision surgery	Return to the operating room related to index TKA (reasons for revision surgery should be recorded)
Revision	Revision of one or more of the TKA implants (femur, tibia, tibial insert, patella)
Readmission	Admission to the hospital for any reason during the first 90 days after TKA (reasons for admission and relation to index TKA should be recorded)
Death	Death occurring for any reason during the first 90 days after TKA (cause of death and relation to index TKA should be recorded)

CRP = C-reactive protein, ESR = erythrocyte sedimentation rate, PMN = polymorphonuclear neutrophil, ROM = range of motion, WBC = white blood cell.

Data from Healy WL, Della Valle CJ, Iorio R, et al: Complications of total knee arthroplasty: Standardized list and definitions of the Knee Society. *Clin Orthop Relat Res* 2013;471(1):215-220 and Parvizi J, Zmistowski B, Berbari EF, et al: New definition for periprosthetic joint infection: From the Workgroup of the Musculoskeletal Infection Society. *Clin Orthop Relat Res* 2011;469(11):2992-2994.

Medicare beneficiaries, 19.6% were 30-day readmissions, 70% of whom were readmitted because of a medical condition. The cost of rehospitalization or readmission was $17.4 billion.

Section 3025 of the Affordable Care Act added Section 1886(q) to the Social Security Act, which established the Hospital Readmission Reduction Program that was effective October 1, 2012.[3] The Hospital Readmission Reduction Program expanded and, since 2014, patients admitted for elective TJA have been closely monitored for 30-day readmissions. Hospitals that have unacceptable readmission rates are fined or receive a readmission payment adjustment factor. Similar to payment reductions implemented for readmitted patients who have cardiopulmonary disease, the first-year payment reduction in orthopaedics is anticipated to be 1% in the 2015 fiscal year, 2% in the 2016 fiscal year, and 3% in the 2017 fiscal year for hospitals that have unacceptable readmission rates. The CMS projects that 20% of readmissions are preventable, which represents an estimated annual savings of more than $2 billion.

Identification of the complications associated with TJA that result in hospital readmission is critically important for predictive modeling and to decrease the number of TJA readmissions. In addition, improving perioperative optimization, providing seamless episodic care, and intensifying posthospital coordination of care may result in a decreased number of unnecessary hospital readmissions.

Defining the Complications

Prevention of hospital readmissions requires an understanding of the causes of readmission. Frequently, postoperative complications, both medical and surgical, are associated with readmissions; however, until recently, complications after THA and TKA have not been well defined. In 2011, The Hip Society established a THA complications work group to standardize complications for THA. The goal of the work group was to develop a list of minimum necessary THA complications and adverse events that would result in the accurate reporting of outcomes. A further goal was to develop standardized definitions for TJA complications and adverse events.

The Hip Society defined and endorsed 19 THA complications.[4] The list of THA complications is not comprehensive, and it excludes several conditions that could not be logistically included (**Table 1**). Similarly, The Knee Society published complications associated with TKA[5,6] (**Table 2**). With a standardized, well-defined list of TJA complications, the rates of TJA will likewise approach a value that is more universally accepted. Definitions outlined by both The Hip Society and The Knee Society are used to report the incidences derived from the CMS Limited Dataset[4] (**Table 3**). In addition, the severity of complications may vary. Stratification of complications increases clinical applicability and improves the clarity of research, as evidenced by other surgical specialties, such as general surgery[7] and hip preservation.[8] A modification of the hip preservation stratification system was used to stratify these complications (**Table 4**).

Identifying High-risk Patients

It is logical to assume that identification and correction of modifiable risk factors associated with TJA complications will result in a reduction in hospital readmissions. Kansagara et al[9] reported the risk factors predictive of hospital readmission and grouped them into six categories: medical comorbidities, mental health, illness severity, prior medical use, functional status, and socioeconomic factors. Most studies on readmission risk factors, however, do not use all six of these categories. Mednick et al[10] reported that the risk of revision surgery after THA increased with the number of preoperative comorbidities, morbid obesity, a history of corticosteroid use, and low preoperative serum albumin levels in patients who had postoperative surgical site infection (SSI), thromboembolic events, and sepsis (**Table 5**).

TJA patients commonly have risk factors and comorbidities that increase the risk of complications and adverse outcomes (**Table 6**). A logical step to decrease the risk of readmission includes identifying the factors that are modifiable and determining whether the modifications result in a lower risk of readmission. Risk factors for infection have been well established in TJA patients[11,12] (**Table 7**). Maoz et al[11] identified eight modifiable risk factors that substantially contribute to poor clinical outcomes after TJA: morbid obesity; poorly controlled diabetes and nutritional deficiencies; *Staphylococcus aureus* colonization; tobacco use; venous thromboembolic disease (VTED); cardiovascular disease; neurocognitive, psychological, and behavioral problems; and physical deconditioning and fall risk.

Modifiable Risk Factors
Obesity
The link between obesity, diabetes, metabolic syndrome, and osteoarthritis is well documented.[13,14] As obesity rates rise and patients continue to live longer, the need for TJA will increase.[14] The

Table 3

Incidence of Complications of Total Hip and Knee Arthroplasty Using Definitions Derived by The Hip Society and The Knee Society

Complication	Incidence[a]	
	TKA (%)	THA (%)
Thromboembolic disease	4.54	4.86
Deep periprosthetic joint infection	2.74	3.15
Instability/ dislocation	0.43	3.86
Bleeding	1.02	1.35
Wound complication	0.90	0.52
Periprosthetic fracture	0.14	0.83
Implant loosening	0.23	0.53
Implant fracture/ tibial insert dissociation	0.18	0.44
Neural deficit	0.06	0.10
Bearing surface wear	0.04	0.07
Osteolysis	0.03	0.07
Vascular injury	<0.01	<0.01
Stiffness	15.98	NA
Extensor mechanism disruption	0.10	NA
Medial collateral ligament injury	<0.01	NA
Leg-length discrepancy	NA	1.15
Heterotopic ossification	NA	0.17
Abductor muscle disruption	NA	0.04

NA = not applicable, THA = total hip arthroplasty, TKA = total knee arthroplasty.

[a]Data adapted from Clair AJ, Inneh IA, Iorio R, et al: Can administrative data be used to analyze complications following total joint arthroplasty? *J Arthroplasty* 2015; 30(9 suppl):17-20 and Healy WL, Della Valle CJ, Iorio R, et al: Complications of total knee arthroplasty: Standardized list and definitions of the Knee Society. *Clin Orthop Relat Res* 2013;471(1):215-220.

Table 4

Stratification of Total Hip Arthroplasty Complications

Grade	Description
I	Complication requires no treatment. No change in routine care.
II	Complication requires slight change in care with low-intensity outpatient treatment (nonsurgical management).
III	Complication requires unplanned surgical treatment, prolonged admission, or readmission (surgical treatment).
IV	Complication associated with a life-threatening or limb-threatening event that requires immediate invasive treatment.
V	Death

Adapted from Sink EL, Leunig M, Zaltz I, Gilbert JC, Clohisy J; Academic Network for Conservational Hip Outcomes Research Group: Reliability of a complication classification system for orthopaedic surgery. *Clin Orthop Relat Res* 2012;470(8):2220-2226.

Table 5

Risk Factors Associated With Hospital Readmission

Factors	Description
Demographics	Morbid obesity ($\geq$40 kg/m^2)
Comorbidities	Corticosteroid use preoperatively
Complications	Surgical site infection
	Pulmonary embolism
	Deep vein thrombosis
	Sepsis
Laboratory	Low serum albumin level

Adapted from Mednick RE, Alvi HM, Krishnan V, Lovecchio F, Manning DW: Factors affecting readmission rates following primary total hip arthroplasty. *J Bone Joint Surg Am* 2014;96(14): 1201-1209.

Table 6

Comorbidity Prevalence in Total Hip Arthroplasty Patients

Risk Factors	Prevalence (%)
Musculoskeletal comorbidities	73.8
Hypertension	60.1
Hyperlipidemia	55.3
Tobacco use	22.0
Diabetes	19.2
Depressive disorders	14.5
Morbid obesity	13.8
Ischemic heart disease	13.5
Dysrhythmias	10.8
Valve disease	7.8
Cerebrovascular disease	4.4
Congestive heart failure	2.8

Table 7

Characteristics of Patients Who Have Multiple Risk Factors for Surgical Site Infections That Require Intervention

Total Knee Arthroplasty[a]	Total Hip Arthroplasty[b]
BMI >40 kg/m² and active tobacco use	BMI >40 kg/m² and active tobacco use
BMI >30 kg/m² and active tobacco use	Revision and active tobacco use
Revision and active tobacco use	*S aureus*, revision, and active tobacco use
Staphylococcus aureus, revision, and active tobacco use	*S aureus*, BMI >30 kg/m², and active tobacco use
S aureus, BMI >30 kg/m², and active tobacco use	

BMI = body mass index.
[a]Adapted from Crowe B, Payne A, Evangelista PJ, et al: Risk factors for infection following total knee arthroplasty: A series of 3836 cases from one institution. *J Arthroplasty* 2015 [Epub ahead of print].
[b]Maoz G, Phillips M, Bosco J, et al: The Otto Aufranc Award: Modifiable versus nonmodifiable risk factors for infection after hip arthroplasty. *Clin Orthop Relat Res* 2015;473(2):453-459.

rising incidence of obesity is occurring parallel with the increasing demand for TJA. In the United States, the age-adjusted prevalence of obesity in 2010 was 36% for both men and women, which is a major healthcare concern.[15]

Patients who are obese tend to have higher pain scores, experience slower recovery from pain, and have greater difficulty with functional restoration.[14] Substantial evidence suggests that although patients who are obese often experience improvements after TJA with regard to mobility, pain, and lower limb function, they have an increased risk for immediate and long-term postoperative complications, including infection (both superficial and deep).[13] Contributing factors that lead to increased infection rates include longer surgical time, difficult surgical exposure, decreased vascularization of adipose tissue, and weakened immune response.[13,14] Infection becomes even more difficult if these factors are combined with coexisting immunosuppressive morbidities, such as diabetes.

Obesity has consistently been proven to contribute independently to poorer outcomes, higher costs, and decreased overall patient satisfaction. Gillespie and Porteous[13] reviewed TKA implant survivorship differences between nonobese and obese patients at 7 years (98.7% versus 87.8%, respectively) and at 10 years (98.5% versus 92.7%, respectively) postoperatively. The differences between nonobese and obese patients younger than 60 years were even more impressive (88.6% versus 59.5%, respectively). Bozic et al[16] estimated that the cost of managing these outcomes for the year after the 90-day perioperative period was more than $11,000 per patient.

Preoperative management of obesity is an important component of surgical optimization. Although obesity has been linked to many deleterious effects, the process of preoperative weight-loss management remains controversial. Historically, bariatric surgery has been successful in substantially reducing the body mass index (BMI) of patients who are morbidly obese; however, the clinical effects and timing of bariatric surgery remain unclear in the literature. Severson et al[17] reported that patients who underwent bariatric surgery more

than 2 years before undergoing TKA had shorter anesthesia times, decreased surgical times, and decreased tourniquet times; however, 90-day complication rates and outcomes did not differ substantially. Inacio et al[18] failed to detect any statistical differences in postoperative complications between TJA patients who underwent bariatric surgery and TJA patients who were candidates for but did not undergo bariatric surgery. The authors suggested that bariatric surgery was associated with a higher revision rate and, thus, may not provide the expected dramatic improvements in surgical outcomes.[18]

Obesity is a major risk factor for both intraoperative and postoperative adverse events. Despite these risks, there is no absolute BMI cutoff point that isolates patients at high risk. A cutoff BMI of 40 kg/m² may be reasonable; however, Toman et al[19] identified a BMI of 37.5 kg/m² as a predictor for tibial failure after TKA. Consequently, morbid obesity should be identified as a factor for increased risk and poor outcomes after TJA, and preoperative intervention is warranted. Although there is conflicting literature on the effect and timing of bariatric surgery, it is evident that patients with obesity who participate in nonsurgical weight reduction benefit from both a surgical and functional outcome perspective. Emerging evidence that correlates the severity of obesity with outcomes will result in a more stratified approach for TJA patients who are obese.

Diabetes

Diabetes mellitus (DM) is an important surgical risk factor that may considerably increase the risk of perioperative complications.[20-22] Approximately 8% of all patients who undergo TJA in the

United States have received a diagnosis of DM (type 1 or type 2),[22] which represents a sizable population of at-risk patients.

Patients with uncontrolled DM have a higher risk of complications compared with patients who have controlled DM and patients without DM. Patients with uncontrolled DM who undergo TJA have a substantially increased odds ratios (ORs) of cerebrovascular accident (OR = 4.1), urinary tract infection (OR = 2.5), paralytic ileus (OR = 2.4), infection (OR = 2.3), postoperative hemorrhage (OR = 1.8), transfusion (OR = 1.8), and death (OR = 2.7) compared with patients without DM who undergo TJA.[20] These findings accentuate the importance of controlling a patient's DM prior to TJA to substantially reduce his or her risk of complications.

Perioperative hemoglobin A1c has been used to predict the risk of complications; however, studies have reported an insignificant correlation between perioperative hemoglobin A1c and the risk for infection in patients with DM who underwent TJA.[20,21] Instead, perioperative hyperglycemia was reported to be a more effective measure of risk in TJA patients. Hyperglycemia may result after the administration of dextrose-containing fluids, surgical stress, and underlying, uncontrolled DM.[20] Perioperative hyperglycemia may be a more accurate predictor of complication risk, specifically of postoperative infection. Patients with postoperative infections have been reported to have increased blood glucose levels both preoperatively and postoperatively. Moreover, hyperglycemia levels higher than 200 mg/dL on the first postoperative day result in a twofold increased risk of infection. Even patients without DM have a threefold increased risk of

infection if their blood glucose levels are higher than 140 mg/dL.[23] Thus, increased perioperative blood glucose levels indicate an increased risk of complications after TJA. Specific attention to tighter control of glucose levels during the perioperative period is essential to TJA patient management and may decrease complications and readmissions by improving patient outcomes.

S aureus Colonization

Methicillin-sensitive *S aureus* (MSSA) and methicillin-resistant *S aureus* (MRSA) detection and decolonization are modalities of SSI prevention that have gained momentum. Twenty percent to 30% of the population are persistent nasal carriers of MSSA, and 1% to 5% of the population are carriers of MRSA;[24] correspondingly, *S aureus* is the most common organism responsible for SSIs in patients who undergo TJA.[25] Typically, patients are screened for MSSA/MRSA via a nasal swab up to 3 months before surgery. Patients determined to be carriers are instructed to shower with chlorhexidine and apply 2% intranasal mupirocin ointment twice daily up to 1 week before the day of surgery. For MRSA, both a cephalosporin and a glycopeptide are recommended to cover the normal pathogens associated with a periprosthetic joint infection and the increased risk for an infection by MRSA.

Maoz et al[11] reported the effects of a staphylococcal detection and decolonization protocol to decrease SSIs. For primary THA, factors that substantially increased the risk of SSI included tobacco use, American Society of Anesthesiologists scores higher than 2, BMI greater than or equal to 40, and surgical time longer than 115 minutes. For

primary TKA, substantial predictors of SSI included female sex, tobacco use, concomitant pulmonary disease, and MSSA/MRSA colonization. Patients who had multiple risk factors, including *S aureus* colonization, had a further increased risk for SSIs (**Table 5**).

Specifically targeting MRSA colonization has been an effective prevention scheme.[25] Mehta et al[25] reported that implementation of a preoperative staphylococcal decolonization protocol resulted in a drop in the MRSA prevalence density rate from 1.23 per 1,000 patient days to 0.83 per 1,000 patient days. Decolonization strategies have been successful, and clinical outcomes have positively correlated with a decreased prevalence of colonization. In a study that compared the effect of a MRSA decolonization protocol on the rate of SSIs in patients who underwent primary TJA, Hadley et al[26] reported that staphylococcal decolonization led to a 13% decrease in deep SSIs. The literature supports the implementation of *S aureus* decolonization protocols to reduce the risk of SSIs.

S aureus decolonization protocols also are cost effective. Courville et al[27] analyzed the cost effectiveness of preoperative mupirocin use to prevent *S aureus* colonization. The authors reported that empirical treatment with mupirocin ointment or the use of a screen-and-treat strategy before TJA resulted in substantial cost savings by reducing the number of SSIs. Recent studies report similar results and confirm that these prevention programs lead to decreased rates of infection, complications, and readmission.[25,27]

Tobacco Use

Tobacco dependence, a relevant and leading cause of death in the United

States, results in an estimated cost of $183 billion per year in medical care and lost productivity.[28] Despite efforts to control and raise awareness on the harmful effects of tobacco, 21% to 24% of patients who undergo THA or TKA are active tobacco users.[29]

The harmful effects of tobacco are well documented. Møller et al[30] reported that tobacco use was the single most important risk factor for the development of postoperative complications, including increased wound-related and cardiopulmonary complications, intensive care unit admission, and increased length of hospital stay. In a study that examined the effect of tobacco use and BMI on the length of hospital stay and the risk of short-term postoperative complications, Sadr Azodi et al[31] reported an increased risk of 43% and 56%, respectively. Furthermore, Lavernia et al[32] reported that the cost burden of treating patients who actively use tobacco is substantially higher; tobacco users accrued higher hospital costs compared with nonsmokers ($35,628 versus $30,706, respectively).

With much data illustrating the deleterious effects of tobacco use, it is reasonable to assume that the implementation of a strong preoperative tobacco cessation intervention program may lead to both clinical and economic benefits. Møller et al[33] conducted the first randomized clinical trial on the risk-reducing effects of tobacco cessation intervention programs for patients who underwent THA or TKA. The authors reported that preoperative tobacco cessation programs begun 6 to 8 weeks before surgery substantially reduced postoperative complications, with the risk reduction most evident in wound-related complications. The Gold Standard Program for Tobacco Cessation, which includes education, counseling, and nicotine replacement therapy, resulted in reduced risks for TJA and had continued positive effects on the cessation rate 1 year postoperatively.[33] Thomsen et al[34] reported similar results in a meta-analysis of 11 randomized clinical trials on the effects of tobacco cessation interventions, which included TJA patients. In addition to proven health benefits, tobacco cessation offers a substantial economic incentive for both the patient and the hospital. In a study on the cost effectiveness of an intensive tobacco dependence intervention that was based on self-determination theory, Katz et al[28] reported that the overall incremental cost-effectiveness ratio was a savings of $1,258 per quality-adjusted life-year.

Preoperative tobacco cessation programs in TJA patients have demonstrated that the successful management of a patient's smoking status is beneficial to his or her health and clinical outcomes as well as cost-beneficial for the patient, payer, and hospital as well as for society overall. Surgeons who explain that cessation or decreased tobacco use can help achieve improved TJA results may provide further motivation for patients who have previously failed cessation efforts. The implementation of a strong tobacco cessation initiative, especially for elective TJA patients, can be a worthwhile measure with respect to both outcomes and cost effectiveness.

Venous Thromboembolic Disease

Perioperative cardiac events, stroke, and VTED are the predominant major nonorthopaedic complications after TJA. Contemporary thromboprophylaxis has reduced the overall rate of symptomatic deep vein thrombosis to less than 5% after THA and less than 20% after TKA, whereas symptomatic pulmonary emboli (PE) occur in 1% to 2% of TJA patients, with fatal PE in 0.1% to 0.5% of TJA patients. However, symptomatic in-hospital thromboembolic events (0.53%), namely deep vein thrombosis (0.26%) and PE (0.14%), represent less than 15% of all venous thromboembolisms (VTEs; 2% to 5%) that occur after THA; even with contemporary anticoagulation prophylaxis, 85% of events occur after discharge.[35] Many new anticoagulation agents have been introduced since the last National Institutes of Health conference on VTED more than 25 years ago; however, the evidence for prevention of fatal PE after TJA has changed very little. Randomized clinical trials have reported a dramatic reduction in lower limb clots after the use of potent new anticoagulants, without a similar reduction in fatal PE. Specifically, newer anticoagulants (ie, fractionated heparins, synthetic pentasaccharides, and factor Xa and direct thrombin inhibitors) have all demonstrated substantial efficacy in the reduction of VTED if used for primary chemoprophylaxis after TJA. Despite their efficacy, these newer anticoagulants also have been uniformly associated with a substantial perioperative bleeding risk. Other prophylactic agents, specifically low-intensity warfarin and aspirin, have been associated with a prevalence of residual venographic clot that is up to five times greater than that of newer agents; however, they offer comparable clinical PE rates, with the benefit of a twofold to threefold reduction in major bleeding complications.[36]

The American Academy of Orthopaedic Surgeon clinical practice guidelines suggest that patients who have a high risk for VTE and cardiovascular disease should undergo preoperative screening to determine whether vena cava filter placement or more aggressive or attentive prophylaxis is warranted.[37] However, specific details on the extent and duration of chemoprophylaxis for this high-risk patient population have yet to be determined. The ideal VTE prophylaxis is a balance between the risk of death from PE and major hemorrhage, the morbidity of bleeding associated with anticoagulation, and the preferences and risk tolerances of individual patients. A standardized, risk-stratified approach is necessary to individualize thromboprophylaxis management and, thereby, effectively lower the complication rate in high-risk TJA patients while preventing complications that are associated with overly aggressive anticoagulation measures in lower-risk patients.

Cardiovascular Disease

Careful attention is required for the management of an aging population with increasingly prevalent cardiovascular disease. Perioperative cardiovascular events (eg, myocardial infarction, stroke, VTE) are a major cause of morbidity, mortality, and increased length of hospital stay in patients who undergo orthopaedic procedures.[38] Despite a relatively low incidence in the general joint arthroplasty population, cardiovascular complications are detrimental to outcomes and carry a substantial cost burden to the healthcare system. Consequently, high-risk patients must be carefully managed, and a perioperative strategy should be implemented to optimize these patients before surgery.

The perioperative use of beta blockers has been reported to reduce postoperative myocardial infarction and death after TJA.[39] By combating the catecholamine surge experienced from surgery, beta blockers help blunt increased myocardial oxygen demand. In a high-risk patient cohort with comorbidities such as coronary artery disease, this supply-demand mismatch is further exacerbated. Urban et al[39] reported that the prophylactic use of beta blockers in TKA was associated with a reduced prevalence and duration of postoperative myocardial necrosis. Because most patients who undergo TJA already have a substantial cardiac risk, a more aggressive approach to perioperative medical and cardiac management is likely to be beneficial.[39]

Neurocognitive, Psychological, and Behavioral Problems

Studies have reported strong evidence that modifiable psychological risk factors are associated with low treatment adherence and poor outcomes in patients who have musculoskeletal disorders.[40,41] It is estimated that approximately 30% of TJA patients report high psychological distress before surgery. In addition, adverse surgical outcomes may have a substantial physiologic, functional, and psychological effect, which further complicates a patient's postoperative course.[41]

Psychological factors, such as catastrophizing (ie, imagining the worst), negative mood, perceived disability, negative pain beliefs, and low self-efficacy, have been reported to be predictive of outcomes, such as pain relief, function, and quality of life, in patients who undergo TJA.[42] Poorly compensated individualized pain beliefs and emotional responses are important determinants of patient-centered outcomes and should be included in a preoperative risk modification program. Pain, especially if catastrophically expressed, also has been identified as an important psychological issue with regard to TJA. Witvrouw et al[42] reported that catastrophizing and depression predicted a longer postoperative length of hospital stay. Berge et al[43] reported that patients had a substantially reduced overall pain experience if enrolled in a preoperative pain management program that included arthritis education and cognitive behavioral therapy (CBT).

CBT, which is derived from well-established modes of psychotherapy, may be effectively used to address modifiable psychological risk factors in patients who have musculoskeletal disease. CBT increases patients' sense of self-efficacy and empowers them to take control of their pain and pain-related distress as well as diverts a focus on pain in favor of meaningful activities.[43] Keefe et al[44] reported positive effects, including improved coping skills, reduced intensity of perceived pain, and decreased psychological disability, in patients with osteoarthritis who underwent CBT. It is reasonable to conclude that TJA patients may benefit from some type of psychological intervention if ineffective psychological coping skills put them at risk for poor outcomes. Screening tools, such as the Medical Outcomes Study 12-Item Short Form, the Mental Component Summary, or the Pain Catastrophizing Scale, can identify at-risk patients. Patients may then be offered CBT to better address concerns, positively modify their outlook toward their upcoming surgery, and, perhaps, influence outcomes and satisfaction rates.

Physical Deconditioning and Comorbidities That Affect Ambulation

Preoperative physical conditioning, as measured by ambulatory status, other joint involvement, and general mobility, is an important predictor of outcomes after TJA.[45] Patients who have disabilities and coexisting musculoskeletal, rheumatologic, and neuromuscular diseases that lead to ambulatory mobility problems have an increased risk for extended inpatient hospital and rehabilitation stay.[45] Osteoarthritis can be a debilitating disease; therefore, it is important for orthopaedic surgeons to address any limiting factors that affect a patient's ability to exercise and rehabilitate before and after TJA surgery.

Programs that are designed to increase preoperative physical conditioning, also known as prehabilitation, have been reported to increase postoperative function and independence and hasten return to preoperative levels of function as well as decrease the length of hospital stay and need for inpatient rehabilitation. Snow et al[46] reported that the use of preoperative physical therapy (PT) was associated with a 29% decrease in postacute care services in TJA patients. This resulted in an adjusted cost savings of $1,215 per patient episode, which stemmed from a reduction in the use of skilled nursing facilities, inpatient rehabilitation, and home healthcare services.

Although the concept of prehabilitation may seem beneficial in theory, convincing patients who have arthritis to participate in PT may provoke unnecessary pain and, thus, reduce their compliance and the effectiveness of the program. In addition, the endorsement of preoperative PT sessions limits the amount of possible postoperative PT sessions that are covered by certain payer services, such as Medicare. The greatest clinical and cost benefit is experienced during the preoperative clinical encounter in which the orthopaedic surgeon determines the patients who will substantially benefit from prehabilitation and then prescribes targeted, individualized therapy to address specific areas of deficiency, such as preoperative range of motion or vastus medialis obliquus muscle atrophy. The use of a one-time educational session, instructional videos, or referrals to websites helps increase patient participation and is cost beneficial. Thorstensson et al[47] reported that an individualized home exercise program designed by an orthopaedic surgeon and a physiotherapist in which the patient was strongly encouraged to participate at his or her own self-driven pace resulted in high patient participation and satisfaction rates.

Stratifying Patients Who Have Risk Factors for Hospital Readmission

Because comprehensive studies have reported that it is very difficult to decrease readmissions for high-risk patients, the authors of this chapter recommend stratifying patients based on their readmission risk factors so that their hospital readmission is risk-adjusted and the hospital and surgeon are not penalized for or discouraged from providing care for the high-risk patient population. A recent study detailed the results of Medicare's Quality Improvement Organizations' attempt to reduce readmissions in 14 communities by improving care transition.[48] Despite improvements in care transitions for the patients in these communities, the study failed to demonstrate an improvement or a significant difference in the rate of all-cause readmission (as a proportion of hospital discharges). Brown et al[49] reported that the unexpected result teaches an important lesson: "targeting the performance of one medical care service can change a behavior that can affect the performance of other services."

Summary

Robust evidence shows that a comprehensive program that focuses on the risk factors associated with hospital readmission may result in fewer hospital readmissions. Large multi-institutional studies are encouraged to determine if these programs are successful and that there are not unintended consequences of this program. Difficult medical problems can be managed in the curent healthcare system, and complex surgery can be performed successfully in high-risk patients. It is imperative that the payment system not be incentivized to avoid high-risk patients as the value proposition is encouraged so that all stakeholders are rewarded for optimizing the risk profile.

Although some modifiable risk factors may be long-standing and recalcitrant to change, patients may express a renewed interest in addressing them if any of the risk factors stands in the way of TJA, a procedure patients hope will result in dramatic changes in pain, physical function, and quality of life. The prospect of undergoing TJA may provide surgeons with an opportunity (ie, teachable moment) to identify and manage modifiable risk factors through shared decision making. All primary care and specialty physicians who are involved in the preadmission clearance process can participate in decreasing risk factors preoperatively. The concept of a perioperative orthopaedic surgical home to optimize patients preoperatively is a logical way to address high-risk patients. By implementing risk factor optimization programs, it may be possible to decrease complications after TJA surgery and lower readmission rates.

References

1. Kurtz SM, Ong KL, Lau E, Bozic KJ: Impact of the economic downturn on total joint replacement demand in the United States: Updated projections to 2021. *J Bone Joint Surg Am* 2014;96(8):624-630.

2. Jencks SF, Williams MV, Coleman EA: Rehospitalizations among patients in the Medicare fee-for-service program. *N Engl J Med* 2009;360(14):1418-1428

3. Centers for Medicare and Medicaid Services: Readmission reduction program. 2014. Available at: http://www.cms.gov/Medicare/Medicare-Fee-for-Service-Payment/AcuteInpatientPPS/Readmissions-Reduction-Program.html. Accessed February 14, 2014.

4. Clair AJ, Inneh IA, Iorio R, et al: Can administrative data be used to analyze complications following total joint arthroplasty? *J Arthroplasty* 2015;30(9 suppl):17-20.

5. Healy WL, Della Valle CJ, Iorio R, et al: Complications of total knee arthroplasty: Standardized list and definitions of the Knee Society. *Clin Orthop Relat Res* 2013;471(1):215-220.

6. Parvizi J, Zmistowski B, Berbari EF, et al: New definition for periprosthetic joint infection: From the Workgroup of the Musculoskeletal Infection Society. *Clin Orthop Relat Res* 2011;469(11):2992-2994.

7. Clavien PA, Barkun J, de Oliveira ML, et al: The Clavien-Dindo classification of surgical complications: Five-year experience. *Ann Surg* 2009;250(2):187-196.

8. Sink EL, Leunig M, Zaltz I, Gilbert JC, Clohisy J; Academic Network for Conservational Hip Outcomes Research Group: Reliability of a complication classification system for orthopaedic surgery. *Clin Orthop Relat Res* 2012;470(8):2220-2226.

9. Kansagara D, Englander H, Salanitro A, et al: Risk prediction models for hospital readmission: A systematic review. *JAMA* 2011;306(15):1688-1698.

10. Mednick RE, Alvi HM, Krishnan V, Lovecchio F, Manning DW: Factors affecting readmission rates following primary total hip arthroplasty. *J Bone Joint Surg Am* 2014;96(14):1201-1209.

11. Maoz G, Phillips M, Bosco J, et al: The Otto Aufranc Award: Modifiable versus nonmodifiable risk factors for infection after hip arthroplasty. *Clin Orthop Relat Res* 2015;473(2):453-459.

12. Crowe B, Payne A, Evangelista PJ, et al: Risk factors for infection following total knee arthroplasty: A series of 3836 cases from one institution. *J Arthroplasty* 2015 [Epub ahead of print].

13. Gillespie GN, Porteous AJ: Obesity and knee arthroplasty. *Knee* 2007;14(2):81-86.

14. Kerkhoffs GM, Servien E, Dunn W, Dahm D, Bramer JA, Haverkamp D: The influence of obesity on the complication rate and outcome of total knee arthroplasty: A meta-analysis and systematic literature review. *J Bone Joint Surg Am* 2012;94(20):1839-1844.

15. Flegal KM, Carroll MD, Kit BK, Ogden CL: Prevalence of obesity and trends in the distribution of body mass index among US adults, 1999-2010. *JAMA* 2012;307(5):491-497.

16. Bozic KJ, Stacey B, Berger A, Sadosky A, Oster G: Resource utilization and costs before and after total joint arthroplasty. *BMC Health Serv Res* 2012;12:73.

17. Severson EP, Singh JA, Browne JA, Trousdale RT, Sarr MG, Lewallen DG: Total knee arthroplasty in morbidly obese patients treated with bariatric surgery: A comparative study. *J Arthroplasty* 2012;27(9):1696-1700.

18. Inacio MC, Paxton EW, Fisher D, Li RA, Barber TC, Singh JA: Bariatric surgery prior to total joint arthroplasty may not provide dramatic improvements in post-arthroplasty surgical outcomes. *J Arthroplasty* 2014;29(7):1359-1364.

19. Toman J, Iorio R, Healy WL: All-polyethylene and metal-backed tibial components are equivalent with BMI

of less than 37.5. *Clin Orthop Relat Res* 2012;470(1):108-116.

20. Marchant MH Jr, Viens NA, Cook C, Vail TP, Bolognesi MP: The impact of glycemic control and diabetes mellitus on perioperative outcomes after total joint arthroplasty. *J Bone Joint Surg Am* 2009;91(7):1621-1629.

21. Adams AL, Paxton EW, Wang JQ, et al: Surgical outcomes of total knee replacement according to diabetes status and glycemic control, 2001 to 2009. *J Bone Joint Surg Am* 2013;95(6):481-487.

22. Bolognesi MP, Marchant MH Jr, Viens NA, Cook C, Pietrobon R, Vail TP: The impact of diabetes on perioperative patient outcomes after total hip and total knee arthroplasty in the United States. *J Arthroplasty* 2008;23(6, suppl 1):92-98.

23. Mraovic B, Suh D, Jacovides C, Parvizi J: Perioperative hyperglycemia and postoperative infection after lower limb arthroplasty. *J Diabetes Sci Technol* 2011;5(2):412-418.

24. Wertheim HF, Vos MC, Ott A, et al: Risk and outcome of nosocomial Staphylococcus aureus bacteraemia in nasal carriers versus non-carriers. *Lancet* 2004;364(9435):703-705.

25. Mehta S, Hadley S, Hutzler L, Slover J, Phillips M, Bosco JA III: Impact of preoperative MRSA screening and decolonization on hospital-acquired MRSA burden. *Clin Orthop Relat Res* 2013;471(7):2367-2371.

26. Hadley S, Immerman I, Hutzler L, Slover J, Bosco J: Staphylococcus aureus decolonization protocol decreases surgical site infections for total joint replacement. *Arthritis* 2010;2010:924518.

27. Courville XF, Tomek IM, Kirkland KB, Birhle M, Kantor SR, Finlayson SR: Cost-effectiveness of preoperative nasal mupirocin treatment in preventing surgical site infection in patients undergoing total hip and knee arthroplasty: A cost-effectiveness analysis. *Infect Control Hosp Epidemiol* 2012;33(2):152-159.

28. Katz I, Williams G, Niemiec C, Fiscella K: Cost-effectiveness of intensive tobacco dependence intervention based on self-determination theory. *Am J Manag Care* 2011;17(10):e393-e398.

29. Singh JA, Houston TK, Ponce BA, et al: Smoking as a risk factor for short-term outcomes following primary total hip and total knee replacement in veterans. *Arthritis Care Res (Hoboken)* 2011;63(10):1365-1374.

30. Møller AM, Pedersen T, Villebro N, Munksgaard A: Effect of smoking on early complications after elective orthopaedic surgery. *J Bone Joint Surg Br* 2003;85(2):178-181.

31. Sadr Azodi O, Bellocco R, Eriksson K, Adami J: The impact of tobacco use and body mass index on the length of stay in hospital and the risk of post-operative complications among patients undergoing total hip replacement. *J Bone Joint Surg Br* 2006;88(10):1316-1320.

32. Lavernia CJ, Sierra RJ, Gomez-Marin O: Smoking and joint replacement: Resource consumption and short-term outcome. *Clin Orthop Relat Res* 1999;367:172-180.

33. Møller AM, Villebro N, Pedersen T, Tønnesen H: Effect of preoperative smoking intervention on postoperative complications: A randomised clinical trial. *Lancet* 2002;359(9301):114-117.

34. Thomsen T, Tønnesen H, Møller AM: Effect of preoperative smoking cessation interventions on postoperative complications and smoking cessation. *Br J Surg* 2009;96(5):451-461.

35. Januel JM, Chen G, Ruffieux C, et al: Symptomatic in-hospital deep vein thrombosis and pulmonary embolism following hip and knee arthroplasty among patients receiving recommended prophylaxis: A systematic review. *JAMA* 2012;307(3):294-303.

36. Pellegrini VD Jr: Osgood Lecture: Prevention of pulmonary embolism after total joint arthroplasty. Who knows best? *The Orthopaedic Journal at Harvard Medical School* 2008;10.

37. American Academy of Orthopaedic Surgeons: Clinical Practice Guideline on Preventing Venous Thromboembolic Disease in Patients Undergoing Elective Hip and Knee Arthroplasty. Rosemont, IL, American Academy of Orthopaedic Surgeons, 2011. http://www.aaos.org/research/guidelines/VTE/VTE_full_guideline.pdf.

38. Ackland GL, Harris S, Ziabari Y, Grocott M, Mythen M; SOuRCe Investigators: Revised cardiac risk index and postoperative morbidity after elective orthopaedic surgery: A prospective cohort study. *Br J Anaesth* 2010;105(6):744-752.

39. Urban MK, Markowitz SM, Gordon MA, Urquhart BL, Kligfield P: Postoperative prophylactic administration of beta-adrenergic blockers in patients at risk for myocardial ischemia. *Anesth Analg* 2000;90(6):1257-1261.

40. Jack K, McLean SM, Moffett JK, Gardiner E: Barriers to treatment adherence in physiotherapy outpatient clinics: A systematic review. *Man Ther* 2010;15(3):220-228.

41. Ayers DC, Franklin PD, Trief PM, Ploutz-Snyder R, Freund D: Psychological attributes of preoperative total joint replacement patients: Implications for optimal physical outcome. *J Arthroplasty* 2004;19(7, suppl 2):125-130.

42. Witvrouw E, Pattyn E, Almqvist KF, et al: Catastrophic thinking about pain as a predictor of length of hospital stay after total knee arthroplasty: A prospective study. *Knee Surg Sports Traumatol Arthrosc* 2009;17(10):1189-1194.

43. Berge DJ, Dolin SJ, Williams AC, Harman R: Pre-operative and post-operative effect of a pain management programme prior to total hip replacement: A randomized controlled trial. *Pain* 2004;110(1-2):33-39.

44. Keefe FJ, Caldwell DS, Williams DA, et al: Pain coping skills training in the management of osteoarthritic knee pain: A comprehensive study. *Behav Ther* 1990;21:49-62.

45. Carpenter I, Bobby J, Kulinskaya E, Seymour G: People admitted to hospital with physical disability have increased length of stay: Implications for diagnosis related group reimbursement in England. *Age Ageing* 2007;36(1):73-78.

46. Snow R, Granata J, Ruhil AV, Vogel K, McShane M, Wasielewski R: Associations between preoperative physical therapy and post-acute care utilization patterns and cost in total joint replacement. *J Bone Joint Surg Am* 2014;96(19):e165.

47. Thorstensson CA, Garellick G, Rystedt H, Dahlberg LE: Better management of patients with osteoarthritis: Development and nationwide implementation of an evidence-based supported osteoarthritis self-management programme. *Musculoskeletal Care* 2015;13(2):67-75.

48. Brock J, Mitchell J, Irby K, et al: Association between quality improvement for care transitions in communities and rehospitalizations among Medicare beneficiaries. *JAMA* 2013;309(4):381-391.

49. Brown JR, Sox HC, Goodman DC: Financial incentives to improve quality: Skating to the puck or avoiding the penalty box? *JAMA* 2014;311(10):1009-1010.

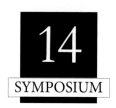

Contemporary Strategies for Rapid Recovery Total Hip Arthroplasty

Jeffrey B. Stambough, MD
Paul E. Beaulé, MD, FRCSC
Ryan M. Nunley, MD
John Clohisy, MD

Abstract

Over the past several years, rapid recovery protocols for total hip arthroplasty have evolved in parallel with advancements in pain management, regional anesthesia, focused rehabilitation, and the patient selection process. As fiscal pressures from payers of health care increase, surgical outcomes and complications are being scrutinized, which evokes a sense of urgency for arthroplasty surgeons as well as hospitals. The implementation of successful accelerated recovery pathways for total hip arthroplasty requires the coordinated efforts of surgeons, practice administrators, anesthesiologists, nurses, physical and occupational therapists, case managers, and postacute care providers. To optimize performance outcomes, it is important for surgeons to select patients who are eligible for rapid recovery. The fundamental tenets of multimodal pain control, regional anesthesia, prudent perioperative blood management, venous thromboembolic prophylaxis, and early ambulation and mobility should be collectively addressed for all patients who undergo primary total hip replacement.

Instr Course Lect 2016;65:211–224.

Dr. Beaulé or an immediate family member has received royalties from Corin USA and MicroPort; is a member of a speakers' bureau or has made paid presentations on behalf of Medacta International and Smith & Nephew; serves as a paid consultant to or is an employee of Corin USA, DePuy, Medacta International, and Smith & Nephew; and has received research or institutional support from Corin USA and DePuy. Dr. Nunley or an immediate family member has received royalties from MicroPort; serves as a paid consultant to or is an employee of Biocomposites, Cardinal Health, DePuy, Smith & Nephew, MicroPort, Medtronic, Polaris Surgical, and Integra LifeSciences; has received research or institutional support from Biomet, Stryker, Smith & Nephew, Medical Compression Systems, DePuy, and Synthes; and serves as a board member, owner, officer, or committee member of the American Association of Hip and Knee Surgeons, the Missouri State Orthopaedic Association, and the Southern Orthopaedic Association. Dr. Clohisy or an immediate family member serves as a paid consultant to or is an employee of MicroPort and Smith & Nephew, and has received research or institutional support from Pivot Medical, Smith & Nephew, and Zimmer. Neither Dr. Stambough nor any immediate family member has received anything of value from or has stock or stock options held in a commercial company or institution related directly or indirectly to the subject of this chapter.

Since its implementation in the United States in the 1960s, total hip arthroplasty (THA) has been considered one of the most successful surgical advances in modern medicine because of its ability to predictably alleviate hip pain, increase ambulatory function, and improve quality of life.[1] As healthcare reform and bundled payment for care structures change the landscape for the practice of medicine and surgery, surgeons must continually strive to achieve value-based care. Fiscal pressures and penalties that incentivize highly efficient surgery with shorter inpatient stays are now in place.[2-4] This paradigm shift places emphasis on patient satisfaction and the quality of care while attempting to minimize costs and complications.[5]

Because of changes in surgical techniques, perioperative pain management, and functional recovery times, surgical teams have markedly reduced the overall hospital length of stay (LOS), with national averages currently between

1 and 3 days.[6,7] Clinical care and rapid recovery teams require the coordinated and concerted efforts of surgeons, anesthesiologists, nurses, physical and occupational therapists, case managers, social workers, and patients' families to work most effectively. As a result, rapid recovery pathways have served as an industrial model to streamline the patient care process.[7,8] Because many institutions have accepted and implemented rapid recovery protocols in either the hospital or short-term surgical care setting, the authors of this chapter found it necessary to update and review various aspects of the rapid recovery process for THA.

Patient Selection and Education

The most important factor for the successful implementation of a rapid recovery program is patient selection. A patient's willingness to fully participate in the rapid recovery process is necessary for its success. A discussion of patient expectations is initiated by the surgeon at the first outpatient clinical visit and is followed by an open dialogue that pertains to the patient's understanding and ability to invest in his or her own recovery.[9] Topics such as discharge criteria and anticipated hospital LOS are discussed with the patient at this time.

The anesthesia team should perform a complete medical workup to stratify surgical risk and answer the patient's questions about anesthesia options. The patient's medical history should be obtained and requisite laboratory testing should be performed to uncover any potential comorbidities. Based on an in-depth preoperative assessment, Meding et al[10] reported that 2.5% of total joint patients (45 of 1,438) were deemed unacceptable surgical candidates, with cardiac problems being the most common new diagnosis made. An in-depth preoperative assessment also provides surgeons with the opportunity to more thoroughly screen for and address nutritional deficiencies, smoking status, and other modifiable risk factors.[11-13] The creation of a center for preoperative assessment and planning where patients have the opportunity to meet with an anesthesiologist and ask questions is one way in-depth preoperative information can be gathered; anesthesiologists can convey the advantages of spinal anesthesia to patients, mitigate patient fears of the unknown, and communicate changes in surgical plans on the day of surgery.

Patient education programs have been shown to reduce hospital LOS and support active participation in early recovery activities.[14,15] Patient education sessions may be performed passively, through pamphlets and handouts, to address the most common patient questions, or actively, through telephone calls or preoperative education classes, to dynamically engage patients and include them in the preoperative discussion. Anxiety before surgery can negatively affect a patient's ability to understand and retain information.[16] The management of patient expectations with preoperative education is associated with less anxiety about surgery and improvements in postoperative patient-reported outcomes.[17-19] Many institutions have endorsed joint arthroplasty preoperative education classes that are led by a designated orthopaedic joint arthroplasty nurse or educator because they clearly delineate patient expectations, reinforce the messages of the surgical team, and review the entire expected hospital course. It may also be valuable for patients to have a designated joint coach who can attend the preoperative education classes with them and provide an additional level of accountability and support throughout the recovery process. Because of preexisting comorbidities or baseline functional limitations, not every patient will achieve a shortened hospital LOS;[20] however, the authors of this chapter believe that the basic tenets of rapid recovery THA, such as early mobility and enhanced pain management protocols, should be used for all patients who undergo THA.

Anesthesia and Perioperative Pain Management

General anesthesia and patient-controlled analgesia were hallmarks of traditional intraoperative and postoperative processes for THA; however, they caused substantial adverse effects, including constipation, dehydration, nausea, vomiting, urinary retention, gastrointestinal ileus, heart attack, delirium, delayed wound healing, and respiratory depression.[21-24] Furthermore, the reliance on narcotic medication has introduced concerns for both short- and long-term tolerance, and narcotic medication has recently been reported to be ineffective for relieving pain that is associated with movement.[25] Because of these concerns, a fundamental shift to spinal anesthesia and multimodal, nonnarcotic pain management strategies as first-line considerations to preemptively prevent pain before the onset of major postoperative discomfort has taken place in THA care pathways.

Compared with general or epidural anesthesia techniques, single-dose spinal anesthesia has been linked to reduced blood loss, decreased rates of thromboembolism, and fewer concerns with respect to airway management.[26] Single-dose spinal anesthesia uses a local anesthetic solution (either lidocaine or bupivacaine) that can be neuraxially administered based on a patient's body mass index and according to the depth and length of the required anesthesia.[27] The authors of this chapter use spinal anesthesia composed of a 10- to 15-mg dose of 0.75% bupivacaine, which if mixed with a small amount of an opioid adjuvant, creates a synergistic effect that allows for a lower overall dose of each individual component.[28] A short-acting sedative (ie, propofol) and intravenous (IV) antiemetics (eg, ondansetron and/or metoclopramide) should be judiciously used intraoperatively in combination with adequate hydration to provide sedation and to limit perioperative nausea and vomiting, which have been shown to be the most common reason for patient dissatisfaction.[21,29,30] The authors of this chapter recommend the infusion of at least 4 L of fluid throughout the perioperative period to expedite the perioperative recovery process.[31,32]

Perioperative multimodal pain management can be conceptualized as a three-pronged approach to address preoperative, intraoperative, and postoperative pain. Various medication combinations should be used at each point along the surgical pathway. The preoperative goals should be to eliminate or wean any narcotic use and to develop a baseline pain receptor familiarity so that an overwhelming nociceptive stimulus is avoided during and after surgery, thereby decreasing postoperative narcotic consumption.[33] Preemptive medications should be initiated days to weeks before surgery to have the greatest effect. A preoperative multimodal regimen that counteracts both inflammatory and neurogenic causes of pain is initiated to diminish central nervous system excitability and to reduce the amount of postoperative medication consumption and the hospital LOS.[30,34,35] Preoperative multimodal pain options include NSAIDs, such as naproxen or celecoxib; a selective cyclooxygenase-2 inhibitor; and gamma-aminobutyric acid analogs, such as gabapentin or pregabalin, all of which act on peripheral and central nonopioid pain pathways. The morning of surgery, the patient should receive a series of medications in the preoperative holding suite as part of the multimodal pain management protocol; these may include both narcotic and nonnarcotic medications as well as IV fluids and antiemetics. Similar to other authors,[36-38] the authors of this chapter use a combination of oral acetaminophen (1000 mg), gabapentin (600 mg), celecoxib (100 mg), and oxycodone (5 mg).

Intraoperative goals for pain control should focus on multiple receptor system modulation to prevent pain and avoid sensitization. The anesthesiologist should administer both IV acetaminophen (1000 mg) and ketorolac (15 mg) during the procedure. At the time of closure, pericapsular injections that include a combination of local anesthetic, NSAIDs, and/or narcotics or steroids should be used.[39] Solovyova et al[40] reported that local capsular infiltration alone, which consists of ketorolac, ropivacaine, and epinephrine, at time of closure is equivalent to local capsular infiltration in combination with continuous infusion at time of closure with respect to medication consumption and pain scores. The authors of this chapter inject both the deep and superficial pericapsular tissues with a 60-mL mixture of 100 mg of 1% bupivacaine, 15 mg of ketorolac, and 100 µg of epinephrine. The injection of ropivacaine solution alone into the pericapsular tissues may provide early functional benefits that allow patients to participate in physical therapy 8 to 10 hours after surgery.[41] Corticosteroids can be included in the pericapsular injection based on the drug's primary mechanisms of action to reduce the local inflammatory response; however, few studies have reported additional benefits of corticosteroids with respect to pain relief and improved outcomes.[42,43] Some surgeons are hesitant to include corticosteroids in pericapsular injections because of the theoretic increased risk of infection if they are applied directly to the surgical area.

Liposomal bupivacaine suspension is an alternative intraoperative pain management solution that has gained traction as a nonnarcotic adjuvant.[44] Liposomal bupivacaine is slowly injected into the intra-articular and surrounding tissue spaces at the time of capsular closure and can provide up to 72 hours of anesthesia if used synergistically with complementary treatment modalities.[45] Because high-level studies with large sample sizes and without industry bias are lacking, the efficacy and cost-effectiveness of liposomal bupivacaine in reducing morphine-equivalent consumption has not yet been proven.[46,47]

Efforts to address postoperative pain begin in the postanesthesia care unit. Current postoperative protocols stress the administration of pain medications on a scheduled rather than an as-needed basis.[39] This ensures that patients do not fall behind in their pain control and prevents a pain crisis that may inhibit physical therapy participation and delay timely discharge. After transfer to the postanesthesia care unit,

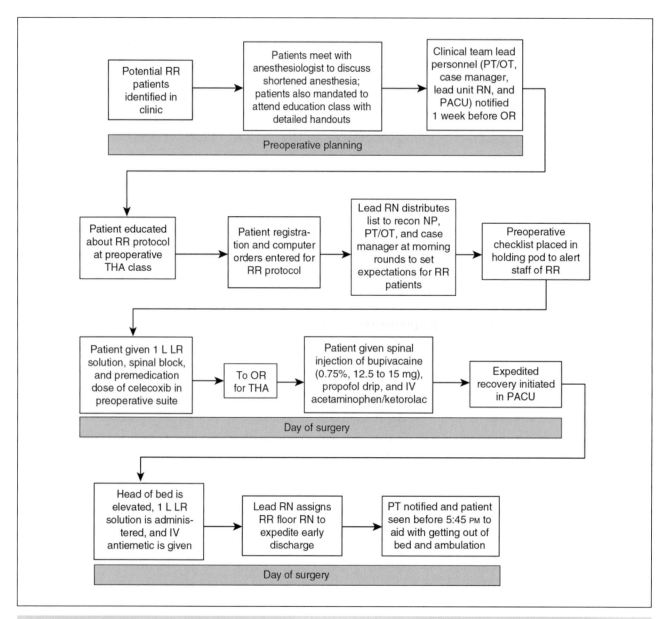

Figure 1 Algorithm demonstrates an overview of a current rapid recovery (RR) protocol for total hip arthroplasty (THA). IV = intravenous, LR = lactated Ringer, OR = operating room, OT = occupational therapist, PACU = postanesthesia care unit, PT = physical therapist, RN = registered nurse, recon NP = adult reconstructive nurse practitioner.

the head of the bed should be elevated to 45°, and the patient should be given a 1-L lactated Ringer solution, 10 mg of IV metoclopramide, and 10 mg of dexamethasone to combat nausea and postoperative inflammation. The first of three postoperative doses of IV ketorolac and celecoxib are administered. The authors of this chapter have implemented a rapid recovery protocol that

highlights the importance of having all members of the rapid recovery team work toward the common goals of improved patient care and early discharge in a clear, delineated fashion (**Figure 1**). After transfer to the inpatient floor, the patient should be given oral acetaminophen (650 mg), oxycodone (5 mg), ketorolac (30 mg for patients ≤65 years; 15 mg for patients

>65 years), celecoxib (200 mg for patients ≤65 years; 100 mg for patients >65 years), and ondansetron (4 to 8 mg) at predetermined intervals for the first 24 hours after surgery. After postoperative day 1, the patient is transitioned to the scheduled administration of hydrocodone (5 mg)/acetaminophen (325 mg) every 4 hours, with hydroxyzine (25 mg) and/or cyclobenzaprine (5 to 10 mg)

available for breakthrough pain, if necessary.

Selective peripheral nerve blockade, with or without indwelling catheters, is an appealing option for postoperative pain management because the motor blockade does not cause muscle weakness. Although peripheral nerve blockade is not as commonly used for THA as it is for total knee arthroplasty, its popularity is rising as the number of dedicated regional anesthesiology block teams increase[48] and as anesthesiologists become more adept with evolving catheter and nerve stimulation technologies.[49] The two most common nerves in the hip that are amenable for peripheral blockade are the sciatic and femoral nerves, which may be targeted together via a lumbar plexus block or independently.[27,50] Currently, there are a paucity of studies that have examined the long-term outcomes of such peripheral nerve blockades. Compared with historical protocols, Pagnano et al[51] reported early improvements in patient satisfaction and the ability to ambulate for patients who had a lumbar plexus blockade in combination with multimodal pain management.

Surgical Approach

Over the past 15 years, the surgical techniques for THA have evolved in parallel with the acceptance and institution of accelerated recovery pathways that stress earlier return of functionality and shorter inpatient hospital stays.[52] Landmark studies, such as Berger et al,[53] have advocated minimally invasive THA techniques as safe and efficacious for patient recovery. Regardless of the approach preferred, surgeons should uphold the principles of musculotendinous unit preservation and conscientious soft-tissue dissection to

afford patients the ability to bear weight without limitations immediately after hip replacement and to reduce blood loss.[54]

The modified minimally invasive anterolateral (Watson-Jones) approach for THA uses the intermuscular interval between the tensor fascia lata and the gluteus medius.[55] Reduced soft-tissue dissection is achieved with this minimally invasive approach via an 8-cm incision that is made from the anterior superior iliac spine and proceeds in an anterolateral fashion toward the trochanteric crest of the anterior tubercle of the greater trochanter. The purported benefits of the modified minimally invasive anterolateral approach are immediate weight bearing without restrictions in the postoperative period as well as a reduced risk of dislocation, which is a result of posterior capsule, abductor, and short external rotator preservation.[56,57] Unfortunately, the modified minimally invasive anterolateral approach has no proven short-term benefits in gait kinematics or hip range of motion compared with conventional transgluteal approaches.[58] In a randomized controlled trial of 90 patients, Repantis et al[59] reported that patients who underwent THA with the modified minimally invasive anterolateral approach had no significant differences in general health outcomes, walking endurance, or reported visual analog pain scores at 4-year follow-up compared with patients who had THA with the conventional modified anterolateral approach.[59] The modified minimally invasive anterolateral approach is not without complications. Unis et al[60] examined the median 9-month postoperative MRIs of patients who underwent THA with the modified minimally invasive anterolateral approach and

reported that 74% of patients exhibited partial superior gluteal nerve denervation, and 42% of patients exhibited fat replacement in the tensor fascia lata.

The minimally invasive posterior approach for THA is similar to the standard posterolateral approach for THA; however, the minimally invasive posterior approach uses an incision that is less than or equal to 10 to 12 cm, which preserves the gluteus maximus and quadratus femoris insertions and pays meticulous attention to the repair of the posterior capsule. This minimally invasive posterior approach has been proven to be powerful and can generate both cosmetic and earlier perceived functional benefits in properly selected patients.[61] The minimally invasive posterior approach also is inherently extensile in nature, so if problems, such as limited hip mobility, heterotopic ossification, or other unexpected difficulties, are encountered, it can be easily converted to a larger approach for improved visualization.[62] Midterm results reported for the minimally invasive posterior approach are promising and, if used as part of a comprehensive THA program, have been associated with reduced hospital LOS, reduced narcotic requirements, and early ambulation.[63]

The direct anterior or Hueter approach for THA is viewed by some surgeons as the ideal approach for a rapid recovery pathway because it uses a true internervous plane, which allows for complete muscle preservation of the hip abductors.[64,65] Drawbacks of the direct anterior approach include an increased learning curve and pressure to use expensive surgical equipment (specialized surgical table, specialized retractors, fluoroscopy, etc.); however, some authors have reported excellent results with the use of a flat-top radiolucent surgical table and a single-shot AP pelvis radiograph.[66,67] The proposed benefits of the direct anterior approach include more precise acetabular cup positioning, reduced blood loss, and less muscle dysfunction in the early recovery period.[68] Because most studies have conflicting or inconsistent postoperative protocols for THA and because postoperative protocols for THA vary based on the surgical technique used, no differences have been found between the anterior and posterior surgical approaches for THA with respect to hospital LOS.[69]

In the experience of the authors of this chapter, either the direct anterior or minimally invasive posterior approaches can be used to deliver a desired, predictable outcome for the rapid recovery patient. Data from a randomized controlled trial by Barrett et al[70] suggested that the direct anterior approach for THA was superior to the posterolateral approach for THA with respect to 3-month pain and functional scores and the ability to ascend stairs; however, the statistical differences between the surgical approaches disappeared after 3 months.[70] In a matched cohort study, Zawadsky et al[71] reported that at 6-week follow-up, patients who underwent THA with the direct anterior approach had better pain scores and were less likely to use an assistive device than patients who underwent THA with the minimally invasive posterior approach. However, Poehling-Monaghan et al[72] reported that there were no appreciable clinical differences between the direct anterior and minimally invasive posterior approaches with respect to gait pattern, pain levels, ability to perform activities of daily living, or muscle strength at 2 days, 2 weeks, and 2 months postoperatively. Similarly, the authors of this chapter have not found

any differences between the direct anterior and posterolateral approaches with respect to acetabular cups positioned outside the traditional Lewinnek safe zone.[73,74]

The current literature supports the use of any of the three previously discussed surgical approaches for rapid recovery protocols because there is no evidence of significant difference in hospital LOS ($P = 0.7$) or physical, mental, and activity outcome scores at 1-year follow-up ($P > 0.55$).[75] The authors of this chapter recommend that surgeons choose the approach that they are most comfortable with because the safe and consistent use of one approach will afford each patient the best possible outcome.

Anticoagulation and Blood Management

To minimize complications and maximize functional return, it is imperative that any modern rapid recovery protocol limit intraoperative autologous blood loss and prevent postoperative thrombotic sequelae. Transfusions are not without complications;[76,77] therefore, the implementation of tactics to limit blood loss are not only beneficial to the patient, but also cost effective. In a study of data from the Nationwide Inpatient Sample, Saleh et al[78] reported that allogeneic transfusion after THA was associated with increased hospital LOS of one-half day, increased cost of $1,730, and 28% increased odds of discharge to an extended care facility.

The authors of this chapter firmly advocate the judicious use of allogeneic blood products in a rapid recovery setting. It is crucial for the surgeon to take into account the patient's symptoms in the decision of whether to transfuse. Preoperatively, a complete blood count

should be performed to screen for anemia; if hemoglobin levels are less than 12 g/dL, the patient should be referred to a primary care physician or hematologist, evaluated, and treated.[79] In an observational cohort of THA patients, Robinson et al[80] reported a 55% reduction in blood transfusion without an increase in postoperative complications if the determination to give a blood transfusion was based on patient symptoms. Overall, the hemoglobin value that triggered blood transfusion was reduced from 7.9 g/dL to 7.3 g/dL over the 6-year study.[80]

In addition to stringent transfusion protocols, other strategies to limit intraoperative blood loss should be used. Antifibrinolytic agents, namely tranexamic acid (TXA), are regularly used in the perioperative setting. Antifibrinolytic agents act along the fibrinolysis pathway to inhibit the breakdown of stable clots, which helps patients achieve relative hemostasis. The application of TXA has been well accepted in the THA literature. Numerous prospective and retrospective studies have reported that IV or topical TXA formulations limit total intraoperative blood loss, reduce the requirement for subsequent allogeneic transfusion, and curtail the postoperative decrease in hemoglobin levels.[81-84] For patients who have contraindications for antithrombotics, such as recent stroke or kidney failure, the authors of this chapter, similar to Chang et al,[85] have found it safe to administer a high dose of topical TXA (3 g in 100 mL saline) at the time of closure, after capsular reattachment. The authors of this chapter have not seen a rise in postoperative complications, such as stroke, deep vein thrombosis, or infection, since they implemented a TXA protocol in 2011. The implementation of TXA protocols in the setting of accelerated care pathways has reduced transfusion rates more than 60%, which has contributed to an estimated cost savings between 53% and 57% of the previous cost for total hip arthroplasty care.[86] Some studies do not support the use of a bipolar sealer for primary THA because there is not sufficient evidence that it reduces blood loss to justify its increased cost per case.[87,88] Furthermore, drains are not regularly placed for primary THA because their use has been linked to increased healthcare costs, increased estimated blood loss, and an increased amount of blood transfused.[89]

How to best prevent venous thromboembolism and its sequelae is another postoperative blood management concern. Historically, chemoprophylactic agents, including warfarin or enoxaparin, were solely used to prevent deep vein thrombosis; however, these pharmaceutical anticoagulants were often associated with increased bleeding and wound complications, which resulted in hospital readmission.[90-93] Mechanical prophylaxis has gained renewed interest as an alternative to chemical prophylactic agents because it has better adverse event profiles.[94] Mobile compression devices prevent clot formation by increasing the pulsatility and velocity of venous blood flow in the lower limbs, which releases a cascade of endothelial-derived relaxing substances.[95] Because imminent changes in reimbursement policies will place greater emphasis on patient-reported outcomes and overall treatment costs, recent research has focused on patient convenience and the ease of use of various prophylactic mechanisms. McAsey et al[96] reported that 94.7% of patients who were treated concurrently with regular-strength aspirin (325 mg) were satisfied with the use of a mobile compression device for 10 days after THA. In a prospective multicenter study of patients who underwent arthroplasty of a lower-extremity joint, Colwell et al,[97] using deep vein thrombosis and/or pulmonary embolism at 3-month follow-up as primary symptomatic end points, proved the noninferiority of mobile compression devices used with or without aspirin compared with standard chemical prophylactic agents. Compared with enoxaparin, mobile compression devices are associated with a substantial projected cost savings component with respect to major bleeding complications.[98] To prevent deep vein thrombosis, the authors of this chapter recommend the use of a mobile compression device for 10 days and 325 mg of aspirin taken twice per day for 6 weeks.[91]

Preparation for Discharge

Rehabilitation and discharge disposition in the immediate postoperative phase are two of the biggest factors that influence THA outcomes.[99,100] Preoperative knowledge of discharge barriers or the likelihood that the patient will require discharge to an extended care facility allows the clinical team to make earlier arrangements and thus, does not negatively affect hospital LOS.

The role of prehabilitation, or preoperative exercise and muscle strengthening programs, as a potential area of intervention to improve postoperative outcomes and reduce postoperative recovery costs has been investigated.[101] Early results reported difficulties as a result of the lack of uniform implementation practices and the additional cost for home therapy providers;[102] however, two retrospective studies reported that preoperative core and leg muscle strengthening programs improved quadriceps muscle strength and the odds of a home discharge by 18% and 25%, respectively,[103] as well as decreased the hospital LOS.[104] Crowe and Henderson[105] reported that patients who participated in prearthroplasty rehabilitation achieved discharge criteria earlier and had a shorter hospital LOS than patients who did not participate in prearthroplasty rehabilitation.[105] In a small prospective randomized series, Wang et al[106] reported substantial functional improvement in stride length, gait cadence, and walking distance at 3 months and 6 months postoperatively for patients who were assigned a standardized 8-week preoperative exercise program.

Patients should begin routine physical therapy on postoperative day 1 or, in increasingly common circumstances, on the day or evening of surgery. To be cleared for discharge, patients must demonstrate safety in navigating stairs, dressing oneself, bed mobility, walking more than 70 m with or without assistive devices, and maintaining hip precautions.[107-109] In a retrospective study of nearly 332 THA patients, Vincent et al[110] reported that women and patients older than 85 years had a longer hospital LOS and were less likely to be discharged home after physical therapy than men and younger patients. In a study that controlled for surgical variables such as nausea and vomiting, Chen et al[111] reported that patients who received immediate rehabilitation on the day of hip replacement surgery (postoperative day zero) had a significantly shorter hospital LOS (2.8 days) compared with patients who did not receive immediate rehabilitation on the day of hip replacement surgery (3.7 days) ($P = 0.02$).

Over the past decade, attempts have been made to create an algorithm that can predict patients' outcomes and, thus, identify patients who are acceptable candidates for rapid recovery based on preoperative factors that influence the likelihood of readmission. Oldmeadow et al[112] generated the Risk Assessment and Prediction Tool (RAPT) for use in Australia to predict whether patients had a low, intermediate, or high risk of discharge to an extended care facility after total joint arthroplasty. The RAPT accurately predicted the risk of discharge to an extended care facility for 89% of patients based on preoperative factors that included sex, age, walking distance, the use of a walking aid, caregiver status, community support, and patient expectations.[112] Subsequently, Oldmeadow et al[113] performed a follow-up study with the use of the RAPT and reported that its use, combined with focused physical therapy, resulted in reduced hospital LOS and more patients discharged home. Barsoum et al[114] devised a Predicting Location after Arthroplasty Nomogram for use in the United States to predict the likelihood that a patient would not be discharged home after THA. The authors used a regression model of 17 surgical and patient variables to allow for a composite determination of discharge destination probability that was based on each variable's weight in the model.[114] Bozic et al[115] reported that 29% of patients across three academic, high-volume joint centers were discharged to extended care facilities after total joint arthroplasty. The authors identified older age (>40 years), higher American Society of Anesthesiologists class, Medicare insurance, and female sex as predictors for discharge to an extended care facility after total

joint arthroplasty.[115] These prognostic models require further investigation in a variety of academic and community settings before they can be universally adopted.

Rapid Recovery Outcomes and Future Directions

The goals of rapid recovery efforts are to reduce hospital LOS; maximize patient satisfaction and outcomes; and minimize healthcare costs, readmissions, and complications.[4,116,117] The most up-to-date literature supports the notion that the successful implementation of both the clinical and logistical aspects of accelerated recovery pathways is associated with a reduced hospital LOS.[7,118-120] In a study of the incremental changes made to rapid recovery protocols for primary THA, Stambough et al[121] reported that modern rapid recovery protocols were associated with a 50% decrease in hospital LOS without an associated rise in readmission rates. The overall 90-day readmission rate of 2.68% reported by Stambough et al[121] was slightly less than the overall 90-day readmission rates reported by other studies (range, 4.4% to 6.5%).[122-124] Two separate studies reported that patients who were discharged home after THA had a significantly lower rate of 90-day readmission compared with patients who were discharged to an extended care facility after THA (1.4% versus 5.1%, respectively, $P = 0.002$ and 2.4% versus 5.2%, respectively, $P < 0.001$).[125,126] Patients who were discharged to an extended care facility after THA had higher odds of hospital readmission within the 90-day postoperative window (odds ratio = 1.9, 95% confidence interval, 1.2 to 3.2; $P = 0.008$) than patients who were discharged home after THA.[126]

Early results suggest that rapid recovery protocols for THA have improved quality of life and patient satisfaction scores. In a large retrospective cohort study of 370 fast-track THA patients from Denmark, Husted et al[127] reported that 85% of patients were satisfied with their outcomes after 1 year, with a mean visual analog scale score of 9.4 out of 10. In a separate study, Husted et al[118] reported that patients' perceptions with respect to the availability of and communication by the surgical team were associated with a shorter hospital LOS and higher reported quality of life ratings. If patients' goals are met via prompt rehabilitation, prospective pain control, and goal setting, then an expectation is established that positively affects the perception of care.

As bundled payment for care initiatives become more common, punitive measures will be implemented to penalize hospital systems that fail to keep hospital readmissions below a set level;[128] therefore, novel tactics are being developed to prevent patient complications and protect against negative outcomes. Edwards et al[129] reported that the implementation of an outpatient support service that maintains frequent communication with patients at set intervals and can escalate communication, depending on individual patient concerns, resulted in a twofold reduction in hospital readmission rates. Gainsharing incentive programs that negotiate implant and device prices also are being explored as a method to control the overall episode of care costs for THA.[130]

Although rapid recovery programs offer enormous potential for both patients and hospital systems, they are not without limitations or shortcomings. Several multicenter studies have reported an association between patient outcomes and surgery volume, both at the hospital and surgeon level.[131-133] Higher surgeon volume was linked to reduced complication rates, reduced hospital readmission rates, reduced hospital LOS, and an increased likelihood of discharge home, and higher hospital volume was linked to reduced hospital readmission rates and improved survivorship.[132,133] The upfront expense to implement and standardize a rapid recovery protocol may not be cost efficient for smaller volume community hospitals.[7] In addition, patients who do not meet initial fast-track recovery requirements in the early postoperative setting because of generalized weakness, dizziness, excessive nausea or vomiting, or symptomatic anemia that requires transfusion will fail the rapid recovery process and likely incur a longer hospital stay.[134]

Sweeping healthcare reforms, including accountable care organizations and bundled payment for care initiatives, are forthcoming; however, present-day incentives are not necessarily in line with the optimization of patient outcomes. In some US states, Medicare and Medicaid payment structures for THA currently discourage early patient discharge (same day of surgery or postoperative day 1). Because Medicare standards still pay based on an optimal 3-day postoperative stay, hospitals that adhere to rapid recovery protocols are not able to fully collect on services rendered.[135] Large scale system inefficiencies such as this are a substantial problem because Medicare is currently the largest payer of all total joint arthroplasty (approximately 65%). Rapid recovery programs will not reach their full potential until all parties unite to contain costs and optimize patient outcomes in an efficient manner. Successful rapid recovery pathways will ensure a seamless transition for THA patients beyond the hospital stay, where there is ample opportunity for better care coordination.[136]

Summary

Rapid recovery efforts use a coordinated team-based approach to improve upon practices that optimize patient outcomes, enhance efficiency, and reduce costs. Open communication between the patient and the surgical team, appropriate preoperative patient education, and close postoperative surveillance will help establish realistic expectations and empower the patient, which will promote greater patient satisfaction and allow for early detection of potential complications. Regardless of eventual discharge disposition, contemporary efforts for rapid recovery THA must include multimodal pain control, regional anesthesia, prudent perioperative blood management, venous thromboembolic prophylaxis, and early ambulation and mobility.

References

1. Harris WH, Sledge CB: Total hip and total knee replacement (2). *N Engl J Med* 1990;323(12):801-807.

2. Hussey PS, Eibner C, Ridgely MS, McGlynn EA: Controlling U.S. health care spending—separating promising from unpromising approaches. *N Engl J Med* 2009;361(22):2109-2111.

3. Berwick DM: Making good on ACOs' promise—the final rule for the Medicare shared savings program. *N Engl J Med* 2011;365(19):1753-1756.

4. Miller DC, Ye Z, Gust C, Birkmeyer JD: Anticipating the effects of accountable care organizations for inpatient surgery. *JAMA Surg* 2013;148(6):549-554.

5. Nwachukwu BU, Hamid KS, Bozic KJ: Measuring value in orthopaedic surgery. *J Bone Joint Surg Rev* 2013;1(1):e2.

6. Berger RA: Total hip arthroplasty using the minimally invasive two-incision approach. *Clin Orthop Relat Res* 2003;417:232-241.

7. Kim S, Losina E, Solomon DH, Wright J, Katz JN: Effectiveness of clinical pathways for total knee and total hip arthroplasty: Literature review. *J Arthroplasty* 2003;18(1):69-74.

8. Gregor C, Pope S, Werry D, Dodek P: Reduced length of stay and improved appropriateness of care with a clinical path for total knee or hip arthroplasty. *Jt Comm J Qual Improv* 1996;22(9):617-628.

9. Pour AE, Parvizi J, Sharkey PF, Hozack WJ, Rothman RH: Minimally invasive hip arthroplasty: What role does patient preconditioning play? *J Bone Joint Surg Am* 2007;89(9):1920-1927.

10. Meding JB, Klay M, Healy A, Ritter MA, Keating EM, Berend ME: The prescreening history and physical in elective total joint arthroplasty. *J Arthroplasty* 2007;22(6, suppl 2):21-23.

11. Cross MB, Yi PH, Thomas CF, Garcia J, Della Valle CJ: Evaluation of malnutrition in orthopaedic surgery. *J Am Acad Orthop Surg* 2014;22(3):193-199.

12. Rai J, Gill SS, Kumar BR: The influence of preoperative nutritional status in wound healing after replacement arthroplasty. *Orthopedics* 2002;25(4):417-421.

13. Møller AM, Pedersen T, Villebro N, Munksgaard A: Effect of smoking on early complications after elective orthopaedic surgery. *J Bone Joint Surg Br* 2003;85(2):178-181.

14. Yoon RS, Nellans KW, Geller JA, Kim AD, Jacobs MR, Macaulay W: Patient education before hip or knee arthroplasty lowers length of stay. *J Arthroplasty* 2010;25(4):547-551.

15. McGregor AH, Rylands H, Owen A, Doré CJ, Hughes SP: Does preoperative hip rehabilitation advice improve recovery and patient satisfaction? *J Arthroplasty* 2004;19(4):464-468.

16. McDonald S, Page MJ, Beringer K, Wasiak J, Sprowson A: Preoperative education for hip or knee replacement. *Cochrane Database Syst Rev* 2014;5:CD003526.

17. Scott CE, Bugler KE, Clement ND, MacDonald D, Howie CR, Biant LC: Patient expectations of arthroplasty of the hip and knee. *J Bone Joint Surg Br* 2012;94(7):974-981.

18. Daltroy LH, Morlino CI, Eaton HM, Poss R, Liang MH: Preoperative education for total hip and knee replacement patients. *Arthritis Care Res* 1998;11(6):469-478.

19. Giraudet-Le Quintrec JS, Coste J, Vastel L, et al: Positive effect of patient education for hip surgery: A randomized trial. *Clin Orthop Relat Res* 2003;414:112-120.

20. Callaghan JJ, Pugely A, Liu S, Noiseux N, Willenborg M, Peck D: Measuring rapid recovery program outcomes: Are all patients candidates for rapid recovery. *J Arthroplasty* 2015;30(4):531-532.

21. Berger RA, Sanders SA, Thill ES, Sporer SM, Della Valle C: Newer anesthesia and rehabilitation protocols enable outpatient hip replacement in selected patients. *Clin Orthop Relat Res* 2009;467(6):1424-1430.

22. Albert TJ, Cohn JC, Rothman JS, Springstead J, Rothman RH, Booth RE Jr: Patient-controlled analgesia in a postoperative total joint arthroplasty population. *J Arthroplasty* 1991;6(suppl):S23-S28.

23. Lamplot JD, Wagner ER, Manning DW: Multimodal pain management in total knee arthroplasty: A prospective randomized controlled trial. *J Arthroplasty* 2014;29(2):329-334.

24. Post ZD, Restrepo C, Kahl LK, van de Leur T, Purtill JJ, Hozack WJ: A prospective evaluation of 2 different pain management protocols for total hip arthroplasty. *J Arthroplasty* 2010;25(3):410-415.

25. Clarke H, Woodhouse LJ, Kennedy D, Stratford P, Katz J: Strategies aimed at preventing chronic post-surgical pain: Comprehensive perioperative pain management after total joint replacement surgery. *Physiother Can* 2011;63(3):289-304.

26. Ritchie PH: Anesthesia and analgesia for total knee replacement and total hip replacement. New York, NY, Hospital for Special Surgery, January 18, 2010. Available at: www.hss.edu/professional-conditions_anesthesia-analgesia-for-total-knee-hip-replacement.asp. Accessed January 19, 2015.

27. Horlocker TT, Kopp SL, Pagnano MW, Hebl JR: Analgesia for total hip and knee arthroplasty: A multi-modal pathway featuring peripheral nerve block. *J Am Acad Orthop Surg* 2006;14(3):126-135.

28. Choi PT, Bhandari M, Scott J, Douketis J: Epidural analgesia for pain relief following hip or knee replacement. *Cochrane Database Syst Rev* 2003;3:CD003071.

29. Singelyn FJ, Ferrant T, Malisse MF, Joris D: Effects of intravenous patient-controlled analgesia with morphine, continuous epidural analgesia, and continuous femoral nerve sheath block on rehabilitation after unilateral total-hip arthroplasty. *Reg Anesth Pain Med* 2005;30(5):452-457.

30. Mallory TH, Lombardi AV Jr, Fada RA, Dodds KL, Adams JB: Pain management for joint arthroplasty: Preemptive analgesia. *J Arthroplasty* 2002;17(4, suppl 1):129-133.

31. Gan TJ, Soppitt A, Maroof M, et al: Goal-directed intraoperative fluid administration reduces length of hospital stay after major surgery. *Anesthesiology* 2002;97(4):820-826.

32. Doherty M, Buggy DJ: Intraoperative fluids: How much is too much? *Br J Anaesth* 2012;109(1):69-79.

33. Al-Mujadi H, A-Refai AR, Katzarov MG, Dehrab NA, Batra YK, Al-Qattan AR: Preemptive gabapentin reduces postoperative pain and opioid demand following thyroid surgery. *Can J Anaesth* 2006;53(3):268-273.

34. Kashefi P, Honarmand A, Safavi M: Effects of preemptive analgesia with celecoxib or acetaminophen on post-operative pain relief following lower extremity orthopedic surgery. *Adv Biomed Res* 2012;1:66.

35. Duellman TJ, Gaffigan C, Milbrandt JC, Allan DG: Multi-modal, pre-emptive analgesia decreases the length of hospital stay following total joint arthroplasty. *Orthopedics* 2009;32(3):167.

36. Ranawat AS, Ranawat CS: Pain management and accelerated rehabilitation for total hip and total knee arthroplasty. *J Arthroplasty* 2007;22(7, suppl 3):12-15.

37. Berger RA: A comprehensive approach to outpatient total hip arthroplasty. *Am J Orthop (Belle Mead NJ)* 2007;36(9, suppl):4-5.

38. Berend KR, Lombardi AV Jr, Mallory TH: Rapid recovery protocol for peri-operative care of total hip and total knee arthroplasty patients. *Surg Technol Int* 2004;13:239-247.

39. Dorr LD, Raya J, Long WT, Boutary M, Sirianni LE: Multimodal analgesia without parenteral narcotics for total knee arthroplasty. *J Arthroplasty* 2008;23(4):502-508.

40. Solovyova O, Lewis CG, Abrams JH, et al: Local infiltration analgesia followed by continuous infusion of local anesthetic solution for total hip arthroplasty: A prospective, randomized, double-blind, placebo-controlled study. *J Bone Joint Surg Am* 2013;95(21):1935-1941.

41. Krenzel BA, Cook C, Martin GN, Vail TP, Attarian DE, Bolognesi MP: Posterior capsular injections of ropivacaine during total knee arthroplasty: A randomized, double-blind, placebo-controlled study. *J Arthroplasty* 2009;24(6, suppl):138-143.

42. Salerno A, Hermann R: Efficacy and safety of steroid use for postoperative pain relief: Update and review of the medical literature. *J Bone Joint Surg Am* 2006;88(6):1361-1372.

43. Liu W, Cong R, Li X, Wu Y, Wu H: Reduced opioid consumption and improved early rehabilitation with local and intraarticular cocktail analgesic injection in total hip arthroplasty: A randomized controlled clinical trial. *Pain Med* 2011;12(3):387-393.

44. Broome CB, Burnikel B: Novel strategies to improve early outcomes following total knee arthroplasty: A case control study of intra articular injection versus femoral nerve block. *Int Orthop* 2014;38(10):2087-2089.

45. Domb BG, Gupta A, Hammarstedt JE, Stake CE, Sharp K, Redmond JM: The effect of liposomal bupivacaine injection during total hip arthroplasty: A controlled cohort study. *BMC Musculoskelet Disord* 2014;15:310.

46. Barrington JW, Halaszynski TM, Sinatra RS, Expert Working Group on Anesthesia and Orthopaedics Critical Issues in Hip and Knee Replacement Arthroplasty FT: Perioperative pain management in hip and knee replacement surgery. *Am J Orthop (Belle Mead NJ)* 2014;43(4, suppl):S1-S16.

47. Andersen LØ, Otte KS, Husted H, Gaarn-Larsen L, Kristensen B, Kehlet H: High-volume infiltration analgesia in bilateral hip arthroplasty: A randomized, double-blind placebo-controlled trial. *Acta Orthop* 2011;82(4):423-426.

48. Schwenk ES, Baratta JL, Gandhi K, Viscusi ER: Setting up an acute pain management service. *Anesthesiol Clin* 2014;32(4):893-910.

49. Enneking FK, Chan V, Greger J, Hadzić A, Lang SA, Horlocker TT: Lower-extremity peripheral nerve blockade: Essentials of our current understanding. *Reg Anesth Pain Med* 2005;30(1):4-35.

50. Hogan MV, Grant RE, Lee L Jr: Analgesia for total hip and knee arthroplasty: A review of lumbar plexus, femoral, and sciatic nerve blocks. *Am J Orthop (Belle Mead NJ)* 2009;38(8):E129-E133.

51. Pagnano MW, Hebl J, Horlocker T: Assuring a painless total hip arthroplasty: A multimodal approach emphasizing peripheral nerve blocks. *J Arthroplasty* 2006; 21(4, suppl 1):80-84.

52. Berry DJ, Berger RA, Callaghan JJ, et al: Minimally invasive total hip arthroplasty: Development, early results, and a critical analysis. Presented at the Annual Meeting of the American Orthopaedic Association, Charleston, South Carolina, USA, June 14, 2003. *J Bone Joint Surg Am* 2003;85(11):2235-2246.

53. Berger RA, Jacobs JJ, Meneghini RM, Della Valle C, Paprosky W, Rosenberg AG: Rapid rehabilitation and recovery with minimally invasive total hip arthroplasty. *Clin Orthop Relat Res* 2004;429:239-247.

54. Goosen JH, Kollen BJ, Castelein RM, Kuipers BM, Verheyen CC: Minimally invasive versus classic procedures in total hip arthroplasty: A double-blind

randomized controlled trial. *Clin Orthop Relat Res* 2011;469(1):200-208.

55. Bertin KC, Röttinger H: Anterolateral mini-incision hip replacement surgery: A modified Watson-Jones approach. *Clin Orthop Relat Res* 2004;429:248-255.

56. Chen D, Berger RA: Outpatient minimally invasive total hip arthroplasty via a modified Watson-Jones approach: Technique and results. *Instr Course Lect* 2013;62:229-236.

57. Pflüger G, Junk-Jantsch S, Schöll V: Minimally invasive total hip replacement via the anterolateral approach in the supine position. *Int Orthop* 2007;31(suppl 1):S7-S11.

58. Pospischill M, Kranzl A, Attwenger B, Knahr K: Minimally invasive compared with traditional transgluteal approach for total hip arthroplasty: A comparative gait analysis. *J Bone Joint Surg Am* 2010;92(2):328-337.

59. Repantis T, Bouras T, Korovessis P: Comparison of minimally invasive approach versus conventional anterolateral approach for total hip arthroplasty: A randomized controlled trial. *Eur J Orthop Surg Traumatol* 2015;25(1):111-116.

60. Unis DB, Hawkins EJ, Alapatt MF, Benitez CL: Postoperative changes in the tensor fascia lata muscle after using the modified anterolateral approach for total hip arthroplasty. *J Arthroplasty* 2013;28(4):663-665.

61. Pagnano MW, Trousdale RT, Meneghini RM, Hanssen AD: Patients preferred a mini-posterior THA to a contralateral two-incision THA. *Clin Orthop Relat Res* 2006;453:156-159.

62. Wenz JF, Gurkan I, Jibodh SR: Mini-incision total hip arthroplasty: A comparative assessment of perioperative outcomes. *Orthopedics* 2002;25(10):1031-1043.

63. Inaba Y, Dorr LD, Wan Z, Sirianni L, Boutary M: Operative and patient care techniques for posterior mini-incision total hip arthroplasty. *Clin Orthop Relat Res* 2005;441:104-114.

64. Siguier T, Siguier M, Brumpt B: Mini-incision anterior approach does not increase dislocation rate: A study

of 1037 total hip replacements. *Clin Orthop Relat Res* 2004;426:164-173.

65. Matta JM, Shahrdar C, Ferguson T: Single-incision anterior approach for total hip arthroplasty on an orthopaedic table. *Clin Orthop Relat Res* 2005;441:115-124.

66. Bender B, Nogler M, Hozack WJ: Direct anterior approach for total hip arthroplasty. *Orthop Clin North Am* 2009;40(3):321-328.

67. Leunig M, Faas M, von Knoch F, Naal FD: Skin crease 'bikini' incision for anterior approach total hip arthroplasty: Surgical technique and preliminary results. *Clin Orthop Relat Res* 2013;471(7):2245-2252.

68. Nakata K, Nishikawa M, Yamamoto K, Hirota S, Yoshikawa H: A clinical comparative study of the direct anterior with mini-posterior approach: Two consecutive series. *J Arthroplasty* 2009;24(5):698-704.

69. Sharma V, Morgan PM, Cheng EY: Factors influencing early rehabilitation after THA: A systematic review. *Clin Orthop Relat Res* 2009;467(6):1400-1411.

70. Barrett WP, Turner SE, Leopold JP: Prospective randomized study of direct anterior vs postero-lateral approach for total hip arthroplasty. *J Arthroplasty* 2013;28(9):1634-1638.

71. Zawadsky MW, Paulus MC, Murray PJ, Johansen MA: Early outcome comparison between the direct anterior approach and the mini-incision posterior approach for primary total hip arthroplasty: 150 consecutive cases. *J Arthroplasty* 2014;29(6):1256-1260.

72. Poehling-Monaghan KL, Kamath AF, Taunton MJ, Pagnano MW: Direct anterior versus miniposterior THA with the same advanced perioperative protocols: Surprising early clinical results. *Clin Orthop Relat Res* 2015;473(2):623-631.

73. Lewinnek GE, Lewis JL, Tarr R, Compere CL, Zimmerman JR: Dislocations after total hip-replacement arthroplasties. *J Bone Joint Surg Am* 1978;60(2):217-220.

74. Nam D, Sculco PK, Su EP, Alexiades MM, Figgie MP, Mayman DJ: Acetabular component positioning in

primary THA via an anterior, posterolateral, or posterolateral-navigated surgical technique. *Orthopedics* 2013;36(12):e1482-e1487.

75. Meneghini RM, Smits SA: Early discharge and recovery with three minimally invasive total hip arthroplasty approaches: A preliminary study. *Clin Orthop Relat Res* 2009;467(6):1431-1437.

76. Stramer SL: Current risks of transfusion-transmitted agents: A review. *Arch Pathol Lab Med* 2007;131(5):702-707.

77. Ponnusamy KE, Kim TJ, Khanuja HS: Perioperative blood transfusions in orthopaedic surgery. *J Bone Joint Surg Am* 2014;96(21):1836-1844.

78. Saleh A, Small T, Chandran Pillai AL, Schiltz NK, Klika AK, Barsoum WK: Allogenic blood transfusion following total hip arthroplasty: Results from the nationwide inpatient sample, 2000 to 2009. *J Bone Joint Surg Am* 2014;96(18):e155.

79. Froimson M: Perioperative management strategies to improve outcomes and reduce cost during an episode of care. *J Arthroplasty* 2015;30(3):346-348.

80. Robinson PM, Obi N, Harrison T, Jeffery J: Changing transfusion practice in total hip arthroplasty: Observational study of the reduction of blood use over 6 years. *Orthopedics* 2012;35(11):e1586-e1591.

81. Wang C, Xu GJ, Han Z, et al: Topical application of tranexamic acid in primary total hip arthroplasty: A systemic review and meta-analysis. *Int J Surg* 2015;15:134-139.

82. Yue C, Kang P, Yang P, Xie J, Pei F: Topical application of tranexamic acid in primary total hip arthroplasty: A randomized double-blind controlled trial. *J Arthroplasty* 2014;29(12):2452-2456.

83. Oremus K, Sostaric S, Trkulja V, Haspl M: Influence of tranexamic acid on postoperative autologous blood retransfusion in primary total hip and knee arthroplasty: A randomized controlled trial. *Transfusion* 2014;54(1):31-41.

84. Konig G, Hamlin BR, Waters JH: Topical tranexamic acid reduces blood loss and transfusion rates in total hip and total knee arthroplasty. *J Arthroplasty* 2013;28(9):1473-1476.

85. Chang CH, Chang Y, Chen DW, Ueng SW, Lee MS: Topical tranexamic acid reduces blood loss and transfusion rates associated with primary total hip arthroplasty. *Clin Orthop Relat Res* 2014;472(5):1552-1557.

86. Harris RN, Moskal JT, Capps SG: Does tranexamic acid reduce blood transfusion cost for primary total hip arthroplasty? A case-control study. *J Arthroplasty* 2015;30(2):192-195.

87. Barsoum WK, Klika AK, Murray TG, Higuera C, Lee HH, Krebs VE: Prospective randomized evaluation of the need for blood transfusion during primary total hip arthroplasty with use of a bipolar sealer. *J Bone Joint Surg Am* 2011;93(6):513-518.

88. Marulanda GA, Ulrich SD, Seyler TM, Delanois RE, Mont MA: Reductions in blood loss with a bipolar sealer in total hip arthroplasty. *Expert Rev Med Devices* 2008;5(2):125-131.

89. Bjerke-Kroll BT, Sculco PK, McLawhorn AS, Christ AB, Gladnick BP, Mayman DJ: The increased total cost associated with post-operative drains in total hip and knee arthroplasty. *J Arthroplasty* 2014;29(5):895-899.

90. Lieberman JR: American College of Chest Physicians evidence-based guidelines for venous thromboembolic prophylaxis: The guideline wars are over. *J Am Acad Orthop Surg* 2012;20(6):333-335.

91. Jacobs JJ, Mont MA, Bozic KJ, et al: American Academy of Orthopaedic Surgeons clinical practice guideline on: Preventing venous thromboembolic disease in patients undergoing elective hip and knee arthroplasty. *J Bone Joint Surg Am* 2012;94(8):746-747.

92. Colwell CW Jr, Froimson MI, Mont MA, et al: Thrombosis prevention after total hip arthroplasty: A prospective, randomized trial comparing a mobile compression device with low-molecular-weight heparin. *J Bone Joint Surg Am* 2010;92(3):527-535.

93. Burnett RS, Clohisy JC, Wright RW, et al: Failure of the American College of Chest Physicians-1A protocol for lovenox in clinical outcomes for thromboembolic prophylaxis. *J Arthroplasty* 2007;22(3):317-324.

94. Colwell CW Jr: Thrombosis prevention in lower extremity arthroplasty: Mobile compression device or pharmacological therapy. *Surg Technol Int* 2014;25:233-238.

95. Vanhoutte PM, Boulanger CM, Mombouli JV: Endothelium-derived relaxing factors and converting enzyme inhibition. *Am J Cardiol* 1995;76(15):3E-12E.

96. McAsey CJ, Gargiulo JM, Parks NL, Hamilton WG: Patient satisfaction with mobile compression devices following total hip arthroplasty. *Orthopedics* 2014;37(8):e673-e677.

97. Colwell CW Jr, Froimson MI, Anseth SD, et al: A mobile compression device for thrombosis prevention in hip and knee arthroplasty. *J Bone Joint Surg Am* 2014;96(3):177-183.

98. Cost-effectiveness Writing Committee: Cost-effectiveness of venous thromboembolism prophylaxis with a new mobile device after total hip arthroplasty. *J Arthroplasty* 2012;27(8):1513-1517.e1.

99. Schweppe ML, Seyler TM, Plate JF, Swenson RD, Lang JE: Does surgical approach in total hip arthroplasty affect rehabilitation, discharge disposition, and readmission rate? *Surg Technol Int* 2013;23:219-227.

100. Barbieri A, Vanhaecht K, Van Herck P, et al: Effects of clinical pathways in the joint replacement: A meta-analysis. *BMC Med* 2009;7:32.

101. Salmon P, Hunt GR, Murthy BV, et al: Patient evaluation of early discharge after hip arthroplasty: Development of a measure and comparison of three centres with differing durations of stay. *Clin Rehabil* 2013;27(9):854-863.

102. Rivard A, Warren S, Voaklander D, Jones A: The efficacy of preoperative home visits for total hip replacement clients. *Can J Occup Ther* 2003;70(4):226-232.

103. Rooks DS, Huang J, Bierbaum BE, et al: Effect of preoperative exercise on measures of functional status in men and women undergoing total hip and knee arthroplasty. *Arthritis Rheum* 2006;55(5):700-708.

© 2016 AAOS Instructional Course Lectures, Volume 65

104. Coudeyre E, Jardin C, Givron P, Ribinik P, Revel M, Rannou F: Could preoperative rehabilitation modify postoperative outcomes after total hip and knee arthroplasty? Elaboration of French clinical practice guidelines. *Ann Readapt Med Phys* 2007;50(3):189-197.

105. Crowe J, Henderson J: Pre-arthroplasty rehabilitation is effective in reducing hospital stay. *Can J Occup Ther* 2003;70(2):88-96.

106. Wang AW, Gilbey HJ, Ackland TR: Perioperative exercise programs improve early return of ambulatory function after total hip arthroplasty: A randomized, controlled trial. *Am J Phys Med Rehabil* 2002;81(11):801-806.

107. Kolk S, Minten MJ, van Bon GE, et al: Gait and gait-related activities of daily living after total hip arthroplasty: A systematic review. *Clin Biomech (Bristol, Avon)* 2014;29(6):705-718.

108. Unver B, Kahraman T, Kalkan S, Yuksel E, Karatosun V, Gunal I: Test-retest reliability of the stair test in patients with total hip arthroplasty. *Hip Int* 2015;25(2):160-163.

109. Tayrose G, Newman D, Slover J, Jaffe F, Hunter T, Bosco J III: Rapid mobilization decreases length-of-stay in joint replacement patients. *Bull Hosp Jt Dis (2013)* 2013;71(3):222-226.

110. Vincent HK, Alfano AP, Lee L, Vincent KR: Sex and age effects on outcomes of total hip arthroplasty after inpatient rehabilitation. *Arch Phys Med Rehabil* 2006;87(4):461-467.

111. Chen AF, Stewart MK, Heyl AE, Klatt BA: Effect of immediate postoperative physical therapy on length of stay for total joint arthroplasty patients. *J Arthroplasty* 2012;27(6):851-856.

112. Oldmeadow LB, McBurney H, Robertson VJ: Predicting risk of extended inpatient rehabilitation after hip or knee arthroplasty. *J Arthroplasty* 2003;18(6):775-779.

113. Oldmeadow LB, McBurney H, Robertson VJ, Kimmel L, Elliott B: Targeted postoperative care improves discharge outcome after hip or knee arthroplasty. *Arch Phys Med Rehabil* 2004;85(9):1424-1427.

114. Barsoum WK, Murray TG, Klika AK, et al: Predicting patient discharge disposition after total joint arthroplasty in the United States. *J Arthroplasty* 2010;25(6):885-892.

115. Bozic KJ, Wagie A, Naessens JM, Berry DJ, Rubash HE: Predictors of discharge to an inpatient extended care facility after total hip or knee arthroplasty. *J Arthroplasty* 2006; 21(6, suppl 2):151-156.

116. Van Citters AD, Fahlman C, Goldmann DA, et al: Developing a pathway for high-value, patient-centered total joint arthroplasty. *Clin Orthop Relat Res* 2014;472(5):1619-1635.

117. Kocher RP, Adashi EY: Hospital readmissions and the Affordable Care Act: Paying for coordinated quality care. *JAMA* 2011;306(16):1794-1795.

118. Husted H, Hansen HC, Holm G, et al: What determines length of stay after total hip and knee arthroplasty? A nationwide study in Denmark. *Arch Orthop Trauma Surg* 2010;130(2):263-268.

119. Walter FL, Bass N, Bock G, Markel DC: Success of clinical pathways for total joint arthroplasty in a community hospital. *Clin Orthop Relat Res* 2007;457:133-137.

120. Vorhies JS, Wang Y, Herndon J, Maloney WJ, Huddleston JI: Readmission and length of stay after total hip arthroplasty in a national Medicare sample. *J Arthroplasty* 2011;26(6, suppl):119-123.

121. Stambough JB, Nunley RM, Curry MC, Steger-May K, Clohisy JC: Rapid recovery protocols for primary total hip arthroplasty can safely reduce length of stay without increasing readmissions. *J Arthroplasty* 2015;30(4):521-526.

122. den Hartog YM, Mathijssen NM, Vehmeijer SB: Reduced length of hospital stay after the introduction of a rapid recovery protocol for primary THA procedures. *Acta Orthop* 2013;84(5):444-447.

123. Lavernia CJ, Villa JM: Readmission rates in total hip arthroplasty: A granular analysis? *J Arthroplasty* 2015;30(7):1127-1131.

124. Zmistowski B, Restrepo C, Hess J, Adibi D, Cangoz S, Parvizi J: Unplanned readmission after total joint arthroplasty: Rates, reasons, and risk factors. *J Bone Joint Surg Am* 2013;95(20):1869-1876.

125. Ramos NL, Karia RJ, Hutzler LH, Brandt AM, Slover JD, Bosco JA: The effect of discharge disposition on 30-day readmission rates after total joint arthroplasty. *J Arthroplasty* 2014;29(4):674-677.

126. Bini SA, Fithian DC, Paxton LW, Khatod MX, Inacio MC, Namba RS: Does discharge disposition after primary total joint arthroplasty affect readmission rates? *J Arthroplasty* 2010;25(1):114-117.

127. Husted H, Holm G, Jacobsen S: Predictors of length of stay and patient satisfaction after hip and knee replacement surgery: Fast-track experience in 712 patients. *Acta Orthop* 2008;79(2):168-173.

128. Froimson MI, Rana A, White RE Jr, et al: Bundled payments for care improvement initiative: The next evolution of payment formulations. AAHKS Bundled Payment Task Force. *J Arthroplasty* 2013; 28(8, suppl):157-165.

129. Edwards PK, Levine M, Cullinan K, Newbern G, Barnes CL: Avoiding readmissions-support systems required after discharge to continue rapid recovery? *J Arthroplasty* 2015;30(4):527-530.

130. Healy WL, Iorio R: Implant selection and cost for total joint arthroplasty: Conflict between surgeons and hospitals. *Clin Orthop Relat Res* 2007;457:57-63.

131. Bozic KJ, Maselli J, Pekow PS, Lindenauer PK, Vail TP, Auerbach AD: The influence of procedure volumes and standardization of care on quality and efficiency in total joint replacement surgery. *J Bone Joint Surg Am* 2010;92(16):2643-2652.

132. Katz JN, Phillips CB, Baron JA, et al: Association of hospital and surgeon volume of total hip replacement with functional status and satisfaction three years following surgery. *Arthritis Rheum* 2003;48(2):560-568.

133. Katz JN, Losina E, Barrett J, et al: Association between hospital and surgeon procedure volume and outcomes of total hip replacement in the United States Medicare population. *J Bone Joint Surg Am* 2001;83(11):1622-1629.

134. Husted H: Fast-track hip and knee arthroplasty: Clinical and organizational aspects. *Acta Orthop Suppl* 2012;83(346):1-39.

135. Lavernia CJ, Villa JM: Rapid recovery programs in arthroplasty: The money side. *J Arthroplasty* 2015;30(4):533-534.

136. Iorio R: Strategies and tactics for successful implementation of bundled payments: Bundled payment for care improvement at a large, urban, academic medical center. *J Arthroplasty* 2015;30(3):349-350.

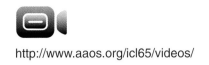

Preventing Leg Length Discrepancy and Instability After Total Hip Arthroplasty

Peter K. Sculco, MD

Matthew S. Austin, MD

Carlos J. Lavernia, MD

Aaron G. Rosenberg, MD

Rafael J. Sierra, MD

Abstract

Restoration of equal leg lengths and dynamic hip stability are essential elements of a successful total hip arthroplasty. A careful clinical examination, a preoperative plan, and appropriate intraoperative techniques are necessary to achieve these goals. Preoperative identification of patients at risk for residual leg length discrepancy allows surgeons to adjust the surgical approach and/or the type of implant and provide better preoperative patient education. The use of larger femoral heads, high-offset stem options, and enhanced soft-tissue repairs have improved impingement-free range of motion as well as dynamic hip stability and have contributed to an overall reduction in dislocation. Methods for accurate leg length restoration and component positioning include anatomic landmarks, intraoperative radiographs, intraoperative calipers, stability testing, and computer-assisted surgery. If recurrent instability occurs after total hip arthroplasty, the underlying cause for dislocation should be identified and treated; this may include the use of semiconstrained dual-mobility or fully constrained liners, depending on abductor function. Surgeons should be aware of the clinical and surgical techniques for achieving leg length equalization and dynamic hip stability in total hip arthroplasty.

Instr Course Lect 2016;65:225–242.

Total hip arthroplasty (THA) is one of the most successful and cost-effective orthopaedic procedures for patients who have end-stage hip arthritis and provides pain relief, restoration of function, and improved quality of life.[1,2] Surgical complications after THA are infrequent and include aseptic loosening, infection, osteolysis, fracture, and substantial leg length discrepancy (LLD) and dislocation; the latter two complications are the most common causes for litigation and revision surgery, respectively.[3] This revision burden is costly for hospitals and causes substantial distress for both patients and surgeons. Historically, the dislocation rate after primary THA was as high as 10%. Modern surgical techniques and implants have reduced the dislocation rate to 3%.[4-7] Variables that affect the risk of dislocation include patient factors, surgical technique, surgeon experience, and implant design; the cause of dislocation is often multifactorial.[8,9]

Leg length equalization after THA optimizes functional results and overall patient satisfaction. The incidence of LLD after THA varies between 1% and 27% and depends on the definition of a substantial LLD.[10-12] Currently, there is no consensus on what constitutes a substantial LLD. Some surgeons believe that anything more than 2 cm constitutes a substantial LLD; others believe that any difference that negatively affects patient function constitutes a substantial LLD. An LLD of more than 1 cm has been reported to negatively affect a patient's walking capacity and increase his or her incidence of limp and low back pain;[13-15] however, other studies have reported that an LLD of more than 1 cm has no effect on patient-reported outcomes.[16,17] Regardless of the effect of LLD on function, patients who are able to detect an increase in leg length may be dissatisfied with or not tolerate a shoe lift. In extreme cases, substantial LLD may require revision surgery and result in potential litigation.[12,18-20]

Leg length restoration and hip stability are interconnected because dynamic hip stability must be achieved via accurate soft-tissue balancing without excessive lengthening. Multiple techniques are available to achieve this goal. It is important for surgeons to identify patient risk factors, create a preoperative surgical plan, and use appropriate surgical techniques to minimize the risk of hip instability and LLD after THA. In addition, surgeons should be aware of the nonsurgical and surgical options for the treatment of postoperative instability.

Preoperative Evaluation

A thorough preoperative history and physical examination will help surgeons identify patients at risk for postoperative LLD and hip instability. A history of trauma, infection, childhood growth plate arrest, congenital dysplasia, and prior surgery may produce extra- or intra-articular leg length differences. In addition, patients who perceive that their surgical leg is longer than their nonsurgical leg when it is, in fact, equal to or shorter than their nonsurgical leg have an increased risk of perceiving a postoperative LLD and should be counselled on this risk preoperatively.

Patient-specific factors that increase the risk for instability after THA include female sex, increasing age, obesity, a diagnosis of osteonecrosis or a femoral neck fracture, neuromuscular and cognitive disorders (ie, cerebral palsy, Parkinson disease, muscular dystrophy, dementia), hyperlaxity (including Marfan syndrome and Ehlers-Danlos syndrome), and alcoholism.[4,13-15,21-24] In addition, patients who have had spinal surgery, particularly spinopelvic fusion with fixed pelvic tilt, may have a higher risk for postoperative instability.[25] Surgeons who recognize the host factors that contribute to an increased risk of

LLD and instability are able to educate patients preoperatively and make adjustments to the surgical approach, implant design, and postoperative plan to minimize this risk.

Physical Examination

The physical examination should begin with an assessment for the presence of a Trendelenburg gait, in which the patient's center of mass translates over the affected hip to reduce joint reactive forces. In addition, any sign of spasticity, rigidity, or imbalance secondary to a neuromuscular condition should be noted. With the patient in the standing position, skeletal abnormalities, such as scoliosis or ankylosing spondylitis, that affect the coronal and sagittal position of the pelvis can be identified and addressed to preoperatively plan for leg length equalization and optimal acetabular component position. A compensatory scoliosis may develop in the presence of a leg length inequality but is often flexible and corrects if the leg lengths are equalized with a calibrated block that is placed under the shorter leg. Pelvic obliquity is considered flexible if the iliac wings are level in cases in which the leg lengths are equalized with a spacer block or in cases in which the patient is placed in a seated position.

Supine examination includes hip range of motion testing and assessment for any hip or knee contractures. A hip abduction contracture abducts the leg, and the pelvis compensates with inferior translation on the ipsilateral side so that the foot can make contact with the ground during the stance phase of gait. In contrast, an adduction contracture, which brings the affected leg toward the midline, causes an elevation of the ipsilateral pelvis. A distal sensory examination should rule out peripheral

Dr. Austin or an immediate family member has received royalties from Zimmer; is a member of a speakers' bureau or has made paid presentations on behalf of DePuy and Zimmer; serves as a paid consultant to Zimmer; and serves as a board member, owner, officer, or committee member of the American Association of Hip and Knee Surgeons and the American Academy of Orthopaedic Surgeons. Dr. Lavernia or an immediate family member has received royalties from MAKO Surgical and Stryker; serves as a paid consultant to or is an employee of MAKO Surgical and Stryker; has stock or stock options held in Johnson & Johnson, Stryker, Symmetry Medical (Telcomet), Wright Medical Technology, and Zimmer; and serves as a board member, owner, officer, or committee member of the American Association of Hip and Knee Surgeons and the Florida Orthopaedic Society. Dr. Rosenberg or an immediate family member has received royalties from Zimmer; is a member of a speakers' bureau or has made paid presentations on behalf of Zimmer; serves as a paid consultant to or is an employee of Zimmer; and has stock or stock options held in Zimmer. Dr. Sierra or an immediate family member has received royalties from Biomet; is a member of a speakers' bureau or has made paid presentations on behalf of Biomet; serves as a paid consultant to or is an employee of Biomet; has received research or institutional support from DePuy, Johnson & Johnson, Zimmer, Stryker, and Biomet; and serves as a board member, owner, officer, or committee member of the Mid-America Orthopaedic Society, the M.E. Müeller Foundation of North America, and the American Association of Hip and Knee Surgeons. Neither Dr. Sculco nor any immediate family member has received anything of value from or has stock or stock options held in a commercial company or institution related directly or indirectly to the subject of this chapter.

neuropathy, which increases the risk of gait imbalance.

Clinical Leg Length Measurements

Leg length can be described as either true leg length or apparent leg length. True leg length is the actual length of the femur and tibia and is measured from the anterior superior iliac spine to the medial malleolus. Apparent leg length is measured from the umbilicus to the medial malleolus, and any factor that affects the functional position of the limb, such as a pelvic obliquity and soft-tissue contracture around the hip, is included in this measurement. Apparent, or functional leg length, reflects a patient's perceived LLD because it represents the position of the limb relative to the contralateral side. Some patients may have a combination of true and apparent LLD that contributes to an overall perception of leg length inequality. Block testing, in which a patient stands on blocks of a known thickness until the two legs feel equal, helps to quantify apparent LLD.[26]

Although leg length restoration is an important component of a successful THA, it is imperative for surgeons to educate patients that a postoperative LLD may be necessary to achieve a dynamically stable hip. Patients also should be informed that they may perceive leg length differences in the early postoperative period despite having equal true leg lengths. Patients who are at risk for the perception of postoperative LLD are those who perceive their preoperative leg lengths to be equal in cases in which their surgical leg is shorter and those who perceive their surgical leg to be longer in cases in which it is equal to the contralateral side. Patients with preoperative flexible

pelvic obliquity also have an increased risk for the perception of postoperative LLD because the surgical leg will feel longer immediately after surgery; however, this will improve over time as residual pelvic tilt resolves and soft-tissue contractures progressively relax. A symptomatic but minor LLD that persists 3 to 6 months after surgery can be treated with a shoe raise.[27] Conversely, a fixed pelvic obliquity secondary to chronic spine pathology will not correct over time and should not be addressed with either excessive shortening or lengthening during THA.[12]

Radiographic Assessment

Standing AP pelvic and femoral radiographs as well as frog-lateral or cross-table lateral radiographs should be obtained for all patients who undergo THA. The leg is internally rotated approximately 15° to remove femoral anteversion and avoid underestimation of femoral offset. A marker of known size placed at the level of the proximal femur allows for magnification correction and accurate preoperative planning. The best way to determine radiographic LLD is to draw a line across two fixed reference points on an AP pelvis radiograph. The three most common radiographic reference points are the inferior aspect of the obturator foramen, the inferior aspect of the ischial tuberosities, and the acetabular teardrop, which is a radiographic sign that represents the floor of the infracondyloid fossa. The distance between this line and a fixed point on the femur, such as the proximal part of the lesser trochanter, can be compared with that of the contralateral hip. The difference between these two distances is the true leg length inequality; however, the measurement is only accurate if the

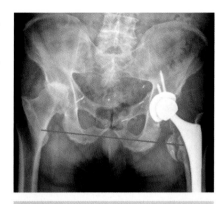

Figure 1   AP pelvic radiograph demonstrates a substantial extra-articular leg-length discrepancy (approximately 12 mm; red line) secondary to lengthening after a previous total hip arthroplasty.

leg lengths are equal below the chosen reference point, there is no substantial hip contracture, and the two limbs are in the same position (not excessively rotated, adducted, or abducted relative to one another). LLD can be either intra-articular or extra-articular. Normally, intra-articular LLD is caused secondary to cartilage wear and loss of joint space. The cause of extra-articular LLD can be multifactorial but is often secondary to leg lengthening after a previous THA (**Figure 1**). Meermans et al[28] reported that, of the three most common radiographic reference points, the acetabular teardrop was the most reproducible and accurate for calculating preoperative LLD. If a patient has distorted pelvic anatomy that makes identification of these landmarks difficult, the incorporation of more than one measurement method may improve measurement accuracy.

Preoperative Templating

The anatomic landmarks on an AP pelvic radiograph that are helpful in templating the placement of the acetabular component include the radiographic acetabular teardrop, the ilioischial line,

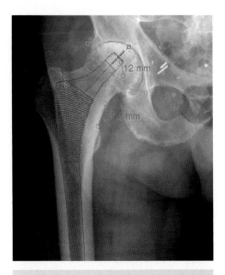

Figure 2 AP radiograph demonstrates planned lengthening to correct a 12-mm extra-articular leg-length discrepancy. The position of the templated femoral stem (red) proximal to the center of rotation of the templated acetabular component (green) represents the amount the limb will be lengthened. The location of the femoral neck osteotomy in relation to the top of the lesser trochanter is measured and reproduced intraoperatively.

and the superolateral ridge of the acetabulum, with the inferomedial aspect of the cup placed slightly inferior but in close approximation to the radiographic acetabular teardrop[29] (**Figure 2**). Using these anatomic landmarks, the cup position and component size are determined. The center of rotation (COR) of the acetabular component as well as the amount, in millimeters, of superolateral component overhang with the cup in 40° to 45° of abduction should be marked and measured on the AP pelvis radiograph. Eggli et al[30] reported that the mean difference between the planned and actual position of the COR of the acetabular component was 2.5 mm ± 1.1 mm vertically and 4.4 mm ± 2.1 mm horizontally. Achieving bleeding bone in most of the acetabulum without proximal reaming

through the subchondral bone will likely allow for COR restoration that most accurately matches the preoperative template.[29]

Femoral templating helps in selection of the implant size and position that will optimally restore hip biomechanics. Templated leg lengthening is easily performed on an AP radiograph. The vertical difference between the COR of the acetabular component and the COR of the femoral component indicates the amount that the leg will need to be lengthened or shortened. Most commonly in THA, the COR of the femoral component will be proximal to the COR of the acetabular component, and the amount of planned lengthening will be equal to the difference between these two points (**Figure 2**). After the position of the stem is determined for the desired leg length, the location of the neck osteotomy is marked on the template and measured, in millimeters, from the top of the lesser trochanter (**Figure 2**). Another preoperative method to assess lengthening includes drawing a line perpendicular to the tip of the greater trochanter and observing at which point the line passes through the femoral head. This can be checked intraoperatively after trial components have been inserted to determine if the center of the head is proximal to, distal to, or in line with the templated line.[29]

Appropriate prosthetic size, which depends on the type of implant and the patient's proximal femoral morphology, also should be estimated. Femoral offset refers to the distance between the COR of the hip and the center of the femoral canal. Component offset, either standard or extended, is selected based on which implant best recreates femoral offset (**Figure 3**). Restoration of femoral offset is essential to a dynamically

stable hip and optimal biomechanics. Failure to re-create appropriate offset increases the risk of postoperative instability.[31] In addition, if appropriate offset is not restored, inadvertent leg lengthening may occur to achieve hip stability. If a patient has a substantial external rotation contracture or femoral head deformity, the contralateral hip can be used for preoperative templating.

Surgical Approaches
Anterior Approach
The direct anterior approach, which has gained increased interest in recent years, exposes the hip via the interval between the sartorius and tensor fascia lata.[32-34] The anterior approach is performed with the patient placed in the supine position, which allows direct leg length measurements to be made. In addition, intraoperative fluoroscopy can assist with component positioning, leg lengthening, and offset. An AP radiograph of the nonsurgical hip can be overlaid on an AP radiograph of the surgical hip with the acetabular component and trial femoral stem in place to assess for accurate restoration of hip biomechanics.[34] The piriformis and conjoined tendon should be preserved; however, a cadaver model study reported that the piriformis and conjoined tendon were partially released at least 50% of the time during femoral mobilization.[35] The reported dislocation rate with the anterior approach is between 0.6% and 1.3%, with a mean LLD of 3.9 mm, which makes the approach reliable for leg length equalization and stability.[20,32,36] A disadvantage of the anterior approach is that it involves a more difficult femoral exposure; this exposure is associated with a learning curve in which an increased risk of complications, including intraoperative femur fracture, may occur.[37,38]

Anterolateral, Direct Lateral, or Hardinge Approach

The direct lateral, or Hardinge, approach displaces the anterior third of the gluteus medius tendon anteriorly with the vastus lateralis, which allows for an anterior hip dislocation that preserves the short external rotators and posterior capsule. The direct lateral approach can be performed with the patient placed in either the supine or lateral decubitus position.[39,40] The anterolateral approach is associated with a low risk of postoperative instability, as shown by Mallory et al,[40] in which a 0.79% dislocation rate was reported in 1,518 THAs. If performed with the patient placed in the supine position, direct leg length measurement is facilitated. The relationship between the tip of the greater trochanter and the center of the femoral head is commonly used as a guide to restore leg length. A disadvantage of the anterolateral approach is that it violates the abductor mechanism, which may be associated with an increased risk of postoperative limp and heterotopic bone formation.[30] Damage to the superior gluteal nerve also may occur if the gluteus medius dissection extends more than 5 cm proximal to the tip of the greater trochanter;[41] however, the gluteal nerve may improve spontaneously without clinically apparent abductor insufficiency.[42]

Posterolateral or Posterior Approach

The posterolateral approach is the most commonly used approach for THA in North America. The posterolateral approach protects the abductor musculature while providing excellent visualization of the acetabulum and femur. Historically, the short external rotators and posterior capsule were not repaired with this approach, and the loss of soft tissue checkrein, in conjunction with the use of small femoral heads (<28 mm), led to unacceptably high dislocation rates.[15] Masonis and Bourne[43] reported a sixfold higher dislocation rate for THAs performed with the posterior approach compared with THAs performed with the direct lateral approach. The introduction of enhanced posterior soft-tissue repair for the posterolateral approach, including a transosseous repair through the greater trochanter or a side-to-side repair of the superior capsule and minimus, restores posterior soft-tissue tension, and several studies have reported a dramatic reduction in the dislocation rate from 4% to less than 1%.[44-47] Currently, with the use of larger femoral head sizes and enhanced repair of the short external rotators and capsule, all three approaches have dislocation rates between 1% and 2%.[7,48-50]

Computer-Assisted Surgery

Computer-assisted surgery (CAS) can be used with all surgical approaches to the hip. Several studies have reported no difference between computer-assisted and conventional THA with respect to leg length equalization.[36,51,52] Lambers et al[51] reported no difference between computer-assisted and conventional THA techniques, with a mean postoperative LLD of 3.9 mm for computer-assisted THA compared with a mean postoperative LLD of 4.2 mm for conventional THA. A study that compared imageless computer-assisted THA with conventional THA with the use of an intraoperative caliper also reported no difference in leg length accuracy, with a mean postoperative LLD of 3.0 mm for computer-assisted THA compared with a mean postoperative LLD of

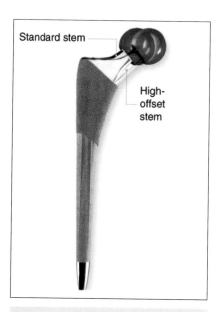

Figure 3 Photograph comparing a standard uncemented femoral stem and a high-offset uncemented femoral stem shows lateralization of the center of rotation of the femoral head without a change in the length of the vertical neck, which allows for an isolated increase in offset without an adjustment in leg length. (Courtesy of Smith & Nephew, Memphis, TN.)

2.9 mm for conventional THA.[52] In a comparison of computer-assisted posterior THA, conventional posterior THA, and direct anterior THA, Nam et al[36] reported no difference in postoperative LLD (3.8 mm, 3.9 mm, and 3.9 mm, respectively). This retrospective study demonstrated that all three surgical techniques, which used three different methods for leg length restoration (navigation, measured femoral neck osteotomy, and intraoperative fluoroscopy), were equally accurate in leg length restoration. In addition, Poehling-Monaghan et al[53] compared a direct anterior approach for THA that used fluoroscopy with a conventional posterior approach for THA and reported no difference in postoperative LLD. The authors concluded that there was no systematic advantage of intraoperative fluoroscopy for improving leg length, offset, or cup positioning compared with a method that relies on careful preoperative templating.

CAS and robotic-assisted surgery have been developed to improve the accuracy of acetabular component placement within what Lewinnek described as the safe zone.[54-56] A recent meta-analysis reported that CAS improved the precision of cup placement by reducing the number of outliers from the desired alignment.[57] Although CAS may increase the probability of cup placement within the safe zone, there is little evidence that this translates into improved long-term clinical outcomes and a reduction in the dislocation rate; therefore, at this time, CAS is not recommended for widespread use.[58-60]

Surgical Technique
Acetabular Component Positioning

Correct positioning of both the acetabular and femoral components will enhance overall hip biomechanics and maximize impingement-free range of motion, which may reduce the risk of postoperative dislocation.[61] Although the optimal target for acetabular inclination and anteversion for each patient is not known, the generally accepted safe zone for acetabular cup positioning is 40° ± 10° of inclination and 20° ± 10° of anteversion.[56] The orientation of the pelvis on the surgical table affects the perceived acetabular component position. If the patient is placed in the lateral decubitus position, his or her pelvis may be substantially adducted, anteverted, or retroverted in relation to the floor.[62] External reference alignment guides that are positioned on the open face of the acetabular component are influenced by changes in pelvic

positioning and must be incorporated into the assessment of component orientation. Anatomic landmarks that assist in accurate cup placement, including the transverse acetabular ligament (TAL), the acetabular sulcus on the ischium, the most lateral prominence of the superior pubic rami (anterior wall), and the superolateral dome of the acetabulum, are independent of patient positioning.[63,64] The TAL has been reported to be a reliable guide for component version.[63] The TAL, which traverses the inferior aspect of the condyloid fossa and reflects the native version of the acetabulum, can be identified in almost all patients. Acetabular component version should be parallel, or more slightly anteverted, to the orientation of the TAL. In a study of 1,000 THAs that were performed with the posterior approach and the use of the TAL as a version guide, Archbold et al[63] reported a dislocation rate of 0.6%, which supported the efficacy of the TAL as a version guide for acetabular component positioning.

In addition to the TAL, the anterior and posterior walls also guide appropriate acetabular component anteversion. A cup without adequate anteversion will be prominent anteriorly and extend beyond the anterior wall. Retroversion with acetabular component prominence has been associated with iliopsoas tendinitis and increased groin pain.[65] Acetabular retroversion, particularly if combined with reduced femoral component anteversion, increases the risk of posterior hip dislocation, particularly after THA is performed with the posterior approach. Superior acetabular component overhang can be estimated based on the preoperative template and provides an intraoperative guide for component inclination. The inclination

of the native acetabulum is approximately 60°; therefore, the acetabular component should usually have a few millimeters of superior uncoverage.[66]

Acetabular osteophytes must be identified preoperatively and intraoperatively because rim osteophytes may be confused with the true acetabular rim, which can lead to inaccurate cup positioning. Superior osteophytes are easily identified on an AP pelvis radiograph, and anterior osteophytes are best identified on a cross-table lateral radiograph. The location of the TAL can be used as an anatomic landmark to identify the true acetabular rim, and excess bone that extends peripherally can be safely removed with an osteotome.

Patel et al[67] used computer models to determine the ideal acetabular and femoral component position that would produce the greatest degree of impingement-free range of motion. The authors recommended that both femoral offset and native femoral anteversion be restored in patients without distorted proximal femoral anatomy to minimize impingement-free range of motion. Optimal acetabular component position was defined as 45° of inclination and 20° of anteversion or matching the natural acetabular anteversion (parallel to the TAL). In addition, the authors concluded that the rim of the cup should not protrude beyond the anterior margin of the acetabulum, and that the posterior protrusion of the cup should be limited to 5 mm to prevent impingement during activities of daily living.

Intraoperative Radiography

Intraoperative radiography is commonly used for THA that is performed with the direct anterior approach, but it has more recently been used for THA approaches that are performed with the patient in the lateral decubitus position. Beamer et al[68] reported that the use of intraoperative radiography in both primary and revision surgery substantially improved placement of the cup in the safe zone for both anteversion and inclination. In a separate study, intraoperative radiographs changed component positioning in 50% of patients and reduced the incidence of component malposition and leg length inequality to 1.5%.[69] Intraoperative radiography also has been reported to help reduce LLDs, as shown by Hofmann et al,[70] in which the use of intraoperative radiographs was associated with a mean postoperative LLD of 0.3 mm and no LLD more than 6 mm. These studies support the use of intraoperative radiographs, which may be helpful if anatomic landmarks are difficult to identify and preoperative templating does not accurately reflect intraoperative findings.

The Effect of Pelvic Tilt on Acetabular Component Position

Pelvic tilt, which reflects the position of the pelvis in relation to the femurs, is classified as either anterior or posterior. The position of the pelvis varies between the sitting and standing positions. The pelvis tilts backward (posterior pelvic tilt) as it progresses to a sitting position. DiGioia et al[71] reported substantial variation in pelvic orientation in the same patient at different time intervals and between different patients as well as a wide range of pelvic mobility. Some patients had a 70° difference in pelvic orientation between the sitting and standing positions, whereas other patients had only a 6° difference in pelvic orientation between the two positions. The effect of THA on pelvic tilt is still unclear. Parratte et al[72] reported

significant variation in pelvic tilt before and after THA, with 31% of patients who had more than a 5° change in pelvic tilt. The authors concluded that because it is difficult to predict postoperative pelvic tilt, preoperative planning based on preoperative pelvic tilt is unreliable. Conversely, Blondel et al[73] reported that 95% of patients had less than a 5° difference between preoperative pelvic tilt and pelvic tilt measured at a 3-year follow-up. Similarly, Murphy et al[74] reported a high correlation between preoperative and postoperative pelvic tilt in both the standing and supine positions. Although the results supported the use of preoperative planning that incorporated preoperative pelvic tilt, the authors could not provide an optimal cup orientation on an individual patient basis that would optimize hip stability and impingement-free range of motion and minimize contact pressures in different functional positions. Unique patients who have extreme degrees of fixed pelvic tilt, such as those with ankylosing spondylitis or spinopelvic fusion, may have a higher risk for dislocation if the component is placed with the use of anatomic landmarks; therefore, component adjustments that are based on pelvic tilt should be considered. Outside of these extreme scenarios, more research is necessary before patient-specific adjustments in acetabular component positioning can be based on pelvic tilt alone.

Femoral Component Positioning

The femoral component size and positioning should accurately restore femoral offset, rotation, and leg length. Both leg length and offset contribute to abductor tension and overall hip stability and function. The proximal-distal

position of the femoral stem in relation to the COR of the acetabular component determines the amount the limb will be lengthened (**Figure 2**). Several methods are available to determine the appropriate femoral stem position and, often, the tip of the greater trochanter or lesser trochanter are used as reference points. The center of the femoral head can be compared with the tip of the greater trochanter preoperatively and then compared again after insertion of the femoral stem. If a larger uncemented femoral stem than that determined preoperatively is required, and this increases the vertical neck distance, the leg will be inadvertently lengthened unless compensatory adjustments are made to the modular femoral head. For all surgical approaches, the preoperative template determines the neck resection level in relation to the lesser trochanter, which can then be reproduced intraoperatively. Woolson et al[75] used the technique of templating the femoral neck resection as a guide for femoral stem positioning and reported accurate leg length restoration in 97% of patients; however, such accuracy also requires accurate recreation of the COR of the acetabular component. **Figure 4** demonstrates the postoperative radiograph of a patient with a 12-mm extra-articular LLD who underwent THA that was performed with the posterior approach. The equalization of leg lengths was achieved with planned leg lengthening and with adjustments in the location of the femoral neck osteotomy.

Femoral offset is defined as the distance from the COR of the femoral head to a line that bisects the long axis of the femur. Femoral offset recreates optimal hip biomechanics, specifically the abductor lever arm, and restores soft-tissue tension and overall hip

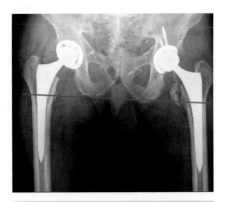

Figure 4 Postoperative AP radiograph demonstrates accurate restoration of leg length (red line), offset, and the acetabular center of rotation.

stability. Appropriate femoral offset has been reported to enhance hip motion and reduce the risk of dislocation.[76] Most modern implant systems offer both standard and high-offset femoral stem options. Femoral component systems either offer direct lateralization, which increases femoral offset without affecting leg length, or change the neck-shaft angle, which increases femoral offset while decreasing vertical neck length. It is important that surgeons understand the specific changes between standard and high-offset stems and the effect on vertical neck length to ensure accurate intraoperative adjustments. The best way to assess whether a patient requires a standard or high-offset stem is during preoperative templating. Femoral templates can help determine whether a standard or high-offset stem best restores femoral offset. After both the femoral and acetabular components have been templated, the overall change in femoral offset can be determined based on the medial-lateral position of the COR of the acetabular and femoral components. If the COR of the femoral component is medial to the COR of the acetabular component, hip offset will be increased.

Rotational alignment of the femoral stem influences the amount of hip motion before impingement. Femoral anteversion contributes to combined anteversion and, if excessive (as seen in some patients who have developmental hip dysplasia), can contribute to hip instability. Native femoral version is the angle formed by a line that is drawn through the midpoint of the medial calcar and a line perpendicular to the center of the distal femur (as estimated by the position of the tibia). Femoral anteversion is usually between 10° and 15° but may vary widely.[77] In patients who have excessive femoral anteversion, a cemented or modular stem may be necessary to reduce native femoral anteversion.

The Role of Combined Anteversion in Hip Stability

Maximizing impingement-free range of motion requires accurate positioning of both the acetabular and femoral components (also known as combined anteversion), with a safe zone between 25° and 50°. Studies that evaluate cup positioning and dislocation risk do not address the importance of femoral version in achieving hip stability. Komeno et al[78] used CT to compare the combined anteversion values of 20 dislocated and 18 nondislocated THAs. The authors reported that dislocation occurred if combined anteversion was outside the safe zone rather than if excessive anteversion was present in either the cup or the stem alone. Dorr et al[79] reported wide variability in native femoral stem version, with values ranging from 17° of retroversion to 28° of anteversion. In a study of native version values in patients who had end-stage osteoarthritis, Merle et al[66] reported that the mean femoral version was

13° ± 10° (range, −7° to 57°). The femur first technique prepares the femur to better appreciate femoral version. The acetabular component is then adjusted based on femoral version to achieve a combined anteversion between 25° and 50°. Adjustments to femoral component anteversion are limited to approximately five degrees of freedom for tapered stems and less for metaphyseal-filling stems.[79] Zhang et al[80] reported on 35 patients (47 hips) with developmental dysplasia who underwent THA with the use of regular uncemented stems. The authors adjusted the cup anteversion to compensate for high femoral anteversion and to maintain a combined anteversion within the safe zone. No dislocations occurred during the 4- to 7-year follow-up period. For most patients, native femoral and acetabular version will produce a combined anteversion value within the desired range.

Soft-Tissue Balancing and Intraoperative Trialing

Accurate soft-tissue balancing reduces the risk of postoperative instability. As previously discussed, inadequate femoral offset reduces soft-tissue tension and increases the risk of dislocation. If stability is achieved via leg lengthening before appropriate offset has been achieved, substantial leg lengthening may occur. Fackler and Poss[81] reported that patients with dislocation had a notable loss of offset (mean, 5.2 mm) compared with patients with stable hips who had a mean difference in offset of only 0.02 mm. Early concerns about the use of lateralized stems for trochanteric pain and loosening have not been validated.[82]

Intraoperative tests to assess hip stability and tension include the shuck test and the drop-kick test. The shuck test involves manual distraction of the prosthesis at the point at which the femoral head will not clear the inferior margin of the acetabular component. The drop-kick test places the patient's hip in extension and flexes the patient's knee to 90° while the surgeon assesses for the amount of recoil. Both tests are highly dependent on surgical approach, type of anesthetic (spinal versus general), and surgeon experience.[31]

An assessment of intraoperative range of motion identifies areas of impingement or positions that may compromise prosthetic stability during activities of daily living. For THA performed with the posterior approach, the most commonly used tests include: (1) extension and external rotation of the femur to assess for posterior prosthetic impingement; (2) observation of the patient's position of sleep (45° of hip flexion and adduction) to assess for posterior subluxation; and (3) hip flexion to 90° and internal rotation until at least 70° before dislocation. For the anterior and anterolateral approaches, both of which dislocate the hip anteriorly, the most common intraoperative tests are leg extension and external rotation testing to assess for posterior impingement as well as the shuck test.

In addition to accurate component positioning, the use of an elevated liner or a larger femoral head size can improve dynamic hip stability. Sultan et al[83] reported an additional 8° of internal rotation stability with the use of a 32-mm femoral head versus a 28-mm femoral head and a 9° improvement in hip stability with the use of a 15° elevated liner, with no evidence of impingement. These intraoperative assessments coupled with proper preoperative templating should help surgeons

restore proper hip offset, leg length, and dynamic hip stability with excellent impingement-free range of motion.

Measuring Leg Length and Offset

An effective method to assess leg length equality intraoperatively involves comparing the surgical leg with the nonsurgical leg both before the procedure and after the trial components are in place.[84] In a series of 410 hips that were treated with primary THA with the use of preoperative templating and the nonsurgical leg as a guide for leg length, the mean postoperative LLD was 4 mm, and only two patients perceived a postoperative LLD.[84] Other intraoperative reference methods for leg length assessment include the femoral neck resection, the distance from the lesser trochanter to the center of the femoral head, and the juxtaposition of the resected femoral head over the femoral trial to confirm that the COR has been restored.[85]

Intraoperative calipers also have been developed to measure changes in leg length and offset but have not been reported to substantially reduce mean postoperative LLD. Steinmann pins, placed in either the ilium or the infracondyloid groove, can serve as pelvic reference points; however, pins may move during surgery or be difficult to place as a result of inferior acetabular osteophytes.[26,86,87] Intraoperative calipers measure from a fixed point on the pelvis to a fixed point on the femur, with measurements obtained before dislocation and after trial reduction.[88,89] Intraoperative calipers are accurate if the limb is in the same position before the hip dislocation and after the trial reduction.[90] The downside of intraoperative calipers is that they are associated

with a learning curve, increased surgical time, and potential expenses, with variable improvements in reducing LLD.[89]

Implant-related Factors
Head Size

Several studies have demonstrated the beneficial effect of a larger head size on hip stability. Larger head sizes have improved head-to-neck ratios, which reduces component impingement and an increased jump-distance. In a randomized controlled trial that examined femoral head size and dislocation, Howie et al[91] reported that 36-mm femoral heads had a significantly lower dislocation rate than 28-mm femoral heads (0.8% versus 4.4%, respectively) at a minimum 1-year follow-up. In addition, several large registry databases have confirmed the clinical benefit of large head sizes on dislocation rates.[92] Several studies have reported decreased dislocation rates for all THA approaches as femoral head size increased from 22 mm to 32 mm.[5,93-95] The disadvantages of a larger femoral head size include the use of thin polyethylene (PE). Fortunately, the increased volumetric wear noted with the use of larger heads and conventional PE has not been reported with the use of highly cross-linked PE.[96]

Liners

Acetabular liners may be lipped, face changing, or lateralizing, each of which has benefits and drawbacks associated with achieving improved hip stability. Lateralized acetabular liners move the acetabular COR away from the midpoint of the pelvis, which slightly increases soft-tissue tension. A lateralized liner may be beneficial to stability if femoral component offset has been maximized and soft-tissue tension is still insufficient.

Compared with neutral liners, elevated liners come in contact with a greater portion of the femoral head during internal rotation of the leg. In a review of more than 5,000 THAs, Cobb et al[97] compared neutral liners with 10° elevated rim liners and reported a significant reduction in the rate of dislocation in the elevated liner group compared with the neutral liner group (2.19% versus 3.85%, respectively) at a 2-year follow-up. A potential drawback of elevated rim liners is an increased risk of femoral neck-liner impingement in the area of elevation, which, theoretically, results in an increase in wear, osteolysis, and possible cup loosening. In a follow-up study on the same patient cohort, Cobb et al[98] did not report an increased rate of loosening or osteolysis associated with the use of elevated rim liners. In addition, a recent analysis from the New Zealand Joint Registry demonstrated that elevated rim liners were associated with a significant decrease in the risk of revision for instability after THA; this was still significant after controlling for femoral head size, surgical approach, age, and sex, which confirms the efficacy of elevated rim liners in reducing dislocation.[99]

Dual-Mobility Devices

The dual-mobility (DM) implant was developed to reduce the incidence of dislocation in patients who are at risk for instability after THA. A DM acetabular component is a tripolar design in which a standard sized femoral head (22 mm or 28 mm) is captured within a larger PE liner, which articulates with a highly polished metal implant that is porous coated and fixed to acetabular bone. In theory, the benefit of the DM design is increased hip range of motion before impingement. The large PE liner

increases the head-neck ratio, acting as a large femoral head, and subsequently increases jump-distance, which reduces the risk of dislocation. Several studies have demonstrated a low dislocation rate for various DM designs that were used in both primary and revision THA.[100-104]

A disadvantage of DM devices is their unique failure mode of intraprosthetic dislocation, which occurs as conventional PE wear at the head-liner interface decreases the ability of the PE liner to contain the inner femoral head. Philippot et al[105] reported a 3.6% incidence (14 of 384 THAs) of inner bearing dislocation at a 15-year follow-up, which is higher than the dislocation rate in conventional contemporary THA; however, the DM designs in this study used conventional rather than highly cross-linked PE liners. Current generation DM devices, which use highly cross-linked PE liners, demonstrate a 97% reduction in wear.[106] Regardless, the long-term survivorship of the newer generation DM bearings is not known; therefore, the use of DM devices should be limited to older, lower demand patients or those who have a high risk for postoperative instability.

Management of Instability

Dislocation after THA is categorized as either early (0 to 6 months), intermediate (6 months to 5 years), or late (after 5 years), with each time point associated with underlying etiologies and risk for recurrence.[107] An early dislocation is usually successfully treated with closed reduction, whereas a late dislocation often requires surgical management. Early and intermediate dislocations may be secondary to patient risk factors, such as female sex or neurologic impairment, or surgeon factors, such as component

malposition. A late dislocation may be the result of loss of abductor function, severe PE wear, osteolysis with trochanteric avulsion, or long-standing component malposition.[108] Surgical treatment is usually recommended after a third dislocation. The surgical treatments for recurrent instability include exchange of the modular components (femoral head and acetabular liner); acetabular revision; the use of a DM device; or the use of a constrained implant. In salvage-type situations, soft-tissue reinforcement, greater trochanteric advancement, and the use of a constrained tripolar device may be necessary.[109-114] Jo et al[115] reported that the long-term outcomes of patients who underwent THA for the treatment of instability included a 34.5% recurrent dislocation rate and a 45.9% reoperation rate, which demonstrates difficulty in the treatment of this challenging patient group. The authors reported that the failure rate increased in patients who had two or more previous surgeries, who had a revised femoral head size less than 36 mm, and who were treated with cup retention.[115]

Clinical Workup for Recurrent Instability

The clinical work-up for recurrent dislocation involves determining the underlying cause for instability. Information on the previous surgical approach and implant details should be obtained. The clinical history should identify patient risk factors for dislocation as well as note the direction of the dislocation (if known), the number of previous dislocations, and the months or years since the index procedure. The physical examination should evaluate leg lengths, abductor function, and peripheral sensation. In addition, if clinically indicated, infection should be ruled out with the use of inflammatory markers and hip aspiration.[116] Metal ion levels should be obtained in any patient who has a modular neck or metal-on-metal articulation because adverse soft-tissue reactions may compromise the abductor musculature and predispose patients to dislocation.

Standard AP pelvic, lateral hip, and cross-table lateral radiographs allow for the evaluation of acetabular retroversion, PE wear, greater trochanteric avulsion, and substantial LLD. CT is usually not required but can provide more information on femoral component version and combined acetabular and femoral version.

Component Revision

Acetabular component malposition with recurrent instability requires acetabular component revision. Component malposition can be diagnosed with plain radiographs, with CT, or during an intraoperative examination. Cementing a constrained implant into a malpositioned cup should be avoided because it has an unacceptably high rate of failure.[117] Indications for the revision of well-fixed femoral components include excessive version contributing to hip instability that cannot be compensated for on the acetabular side as well as soft-tissue tension that cannot be restored with the use of modular femoral head lengths and offset liners.[118,119]

An isolated liner exchange has a high rate of failure (34%) and may result from the failure to recognize and revise a malpositioned acetabular component.[120] Well-positioned implants with inadequate soft-tissue tension may be successfully treated with an increase in femoral head size and modular femoral head length.[5,108] Increasing femoral

head size increases the head-neck ratio, jump-distance, and range of motion before impingement, all of which contribute to improved hip stability.[95] In a level I randomized clinical trial, Garbuz et al[121] evaluated 184 patients who underwent revision THA and received either a 32-mm femoral head (92 patients) or a 36-mm and 40-mm femoral head (92 patients). The dislocation rate was 1.1% (1 of 92 patients) in the 36-mm and 40-mm femoral head group, and the dislocation rate was 8.7% (8 of 92 patients) in the 32-mm femoral head group. The authors concluded that a large femoral head (36 mm or 40 mm) substantially reduces the rate of dislocation in patients who undergo revision THA. In a separate level I randomized study, Howie et al[91] evaluated 644 patients who underwent revision THA with either a 28-mm or 36-mm bearing. The authors reported that the dislocation rate for patients who received a 36-mm bearing was 4.9%, and the dislocation rate for patients who received a 28-mm bearing was 12.2%. Similarly, in a retrospective analysis of 539 hips that were revised for instability, the lowest rate of re-revision and redislocation occurred if a femoral head larger than 36 mm was used in addition to cup revision.[115] These three studies clearly demonstrate the beneficial effect of a large femoral head with respect to dislocation rates after revision THA.

For many years, DM devices have been used for the treatment of recurrent instability after THA. In a series of 180 THAs with recurrent instability that were revised to DM cups, Mertl et al[122] reported that the survival rate, with revision surgery for any cause as the end point, was 92.6% at a minimum 8-year follow-up. In a study of 54 patients who were revised for instability to

a DM implant, Guyen et al[123] reported a 5.5% redislocation rate at a minimum 2-year follow-up. Both of these studies support the use of an unconstrained DM design for the surgical treatment of hip instability.

A constrained tripolar acetabular device is the final salvage option for recurrent instability. A constrained liner provides inherent stability if the soft tissues around the hip are unable to provide adequate tension. A constrained liner is best indicated in low-demand patients who have well-positioned components with neurologic impairment or hip abductor deficiency that contributes to their instability or in patients who have persistent intraoperative instability without a discernable cause.[109,124-130] Reported contraindications of constrained tripolar acetabular devices include high-demand patients, acute dislocation, insufficient acetabular bone structure, acute infection, skeletal immaturity, and neurologic spasticity.[131] Constrained acetabular liners reduce range of motion before impingement, thereby increasing bony stressors, which may accelerate wear, osteolysis, and, possibly, component failure. In a study of 43 failed tripolar constrained devices, Guyen et al[117] reported four types of failure based on location: bone-implant interface, constrained liner pull-out from the metal shell, breakage of the titanium locking ring, and dislocation of the femoral head at the inner bearing.

Callaghan et al[125] reported only two constrained tripolar liner failures (94% success rate) and no recurrent dislocation at a short-term follow-up of 3.9 years. Similarly, in a study of 85 hips that were treated with a constrained tripolar implant, Su and Pellicci[127] reported a 97.6% survival rate at a

4.8-year follow-up. Unfortunately, longer term follow-up has demonstrated that the increased stresses associated with component constraint lead to an increase in late complications and a need for revision surgery. Berend et al[130] reported that the overall failure rate for constrained acetabular components was 42.1% at a follow-up of 10.7 years, with a device failure rate of 29% and a revision surgery rate for aseptic loosening of 8.3%. In a study of 81 patients who underwent THA with the use of a constrained device that allowed for more range of motion and increased lever out strength, Berend et al[129] reported a 98.8% success rate at short-term follow-up; however, long-term data for this device are not currently available. The current evidence supports the use of constrained liners in the treatment of recurrent instability in the setting of abductor dysfunction and a well-fixed, well-positioned acetabular component.[125]

Soft-tissue augmentation is a less commonly used strategy for the treatment of recurrent instability. Reconstruction options include the use of an Achilles tendon allograft, the tensor fascia lata, and a synthetic ligament.[132-134] The indications for soft-tissue augmentation are not well defined but may include deficiency of the hip abductor muscles or hip capsule in the setting of a well-positioned and well-fixed THA.[135] Soft-tissue tensioning also can be achieved with trochanteric osteotomy and advancement. Trochanteric advancement has been advocated for patients who have a well-fixed THA implant. Success rates of 80% have been reported in patients who have recurrent dislocation and well-positioned, well-fixed components.[111,136]

Summary

Accurate restoration of leg length and dynamic hip stability are essential to a successful THA. Risk factors for dislocation should be identified preoperatively, and patients who are at risk for postoperative instability or LLD should be counselled appropriately. The use of larger femoral heads, high-offset stems, and enhanced soft-tissue repairs have contributed to improved soft-tissue tensioning and impingement-free range of motion in THA and has led to decreased dislocation rates with all surgical approaches. Methods for accurate leg length restoration rely on intraoperative radiographs, measured femoral neck osteotomy, intraoperative calipers, and CAS. Accurate stem and cup positioning rely on accurate preoperative templating, anatomic landmarks, intraoperative fluoroscopy, and CAS. Soft-tissue trialing helps identify positions of impingement or laxity, which can be addressed with component reposition, increased offset, or elevated liners. For patients who have recurrent instability, the cause for dislocation should be identified and treated. The use of DM devices is a promising advancement for the treatment of these difficult patients; however, long-term data are still lacking. Because constraint increases the risk of failure at longer term follow-up, constraint should only be considered in well-fixed, well-positioned implants.

References

1. Lavernia CJ, Iacobelli DA, Brooks L, Villa JM: The cost-utility of total hip arthroplasty: Earlier intervention, improved economics. *J Arthroplasty* 2015;30(6):945-949.

2. Chang RW, Pellisier JM, Hazen GB: A cost-effectiveness analysis of total hip arthroplasty for osteoarthritis of the hip. *JAMA* 1996;275(11):858-865.

3. Bozic KJ, Kurtz SM, Lau E, Ong K, Vail TP, Berry DJ: The epidemiology of revision total hip arthroplasty in the United States. *J Bone Joint Surg Am* 2009;91(1):128-133.

4. Woo RY, Morrey BF: Dislocations after total hip arthroplasty. *J Bone Joint Surg Am* 1982;64(9):1295-1306.

5. Berry DJ, von Knoch M, Schleck CD, Harmsen WS: Effect of femoral head diameter and operative approach on risk of dislocation after primary total hip arthroplasty. *J Bone Joint Surg Am* 2005;87(11):2456-2463.

6. Eftekhar NS: Dislocation and instability complicating low friction arthroplasty of the hip joint: 1976. *Clin Orthop Relat Res* 2006;453:1-5.

7. Padgett DE, Warashina H: The unstable total hip replacement. *Clin Orthop Relat Res* 2004;420:72-79.

8. Conroy JL, Whitehouse SL, Graves SE, Pratt NL, Ryan P, Crawford RW: Risk factors for revision for early dislocation in total hip arthroplasty. *J Arthroplasty* 2008;23(6):867-872.

9. Khatod M, Barber T, Paxton E, Namba R, Fithian D: An analysis of the risk of hip dislocation with a contemporary total joint registry. *Clin Orthop Relat Res* 2006;447:19-23.

10. Bhave A, Paley D, Herzenberg JE: Improvement in gait parameters after lengthening for the treatment of limb-length discrepancy. *J Bone Joint Surg Am* 1999;81(4):529-534.

11. Gurney B, Mermier C, Robergs R, Gibson A, Rivero D: Effects of limb-length discrepancy on gait economy and lower-extremity muscle activity in older adults. *J Bone Joint Surg Am* 2001;83(6):907-915.

12. Maloney WJ, Keeney JA: Leg length discrepancy after total hip arthroplasty. *J Arthroplasty* 2004;19(4, suppl 1):108-110.

13. Woolson ST, Rahimtoola ZO: Risk factors for dislocation during the first 3 months after primary total hip replacement. *J Arthroplasty* 1999;14(6):662-668.

14. Lee BP, Berry DJ, Harmsen WS, Sim FH: Total hip arthroplasty for the treatment of an acute fracture of the femoral neck: Long-term results. *J Bone Joint Surg Am* 1998;80(1):70-75.

15. Berry DJ, von Knoch M, Schleck CD, Harmsen WS: The cumulative long-term risk of dislocation after primary Charnley total hip arthroplasty. *J Bone Joint Surg Am* 2004;86(1):9-14.

16. Röder C, Vogel R, Burri L, Dietrich D, Staub LP: Total hip arthroplasty: Leg length inequality impairs functional outcomes and patient satisfaction. *BMC Musculoskelet Disord* 2012;13:95.

17. Whitehouse MR, Stefanovich-Lawbuary NS, Brunton LR, Blom AW: The impact of leg length discrepancy on patient satisfaction and functional outcome following total hip arthroplasty. *J Arthroplasty* 2013;28(8):1408-1414.

18. Parvizi J, Sharkey PF, Bissett GA, Rothman RH, Hozack WJ: Surgical treatment of limb-length discrepancy following total hip arthroplasty. *J Bone Joint Surg Am* 2003;85(12):2310-2317.

19. Austin MS, Hozack WJ, Sharkey PF, Rothman RH: Stability and leg length equality in total hip arthroplasty. *J Arthroplasty* 2003;18(3, suppl 1):88-90.

20. Edeen J, Sharkey PF, Alexander AH: Clinical significance of leg-length inequality after total hip arthroplasty. *Am J Orthop (Belle Mead NJ)* 1995;24(4):347-351.

21. Dudda M, Gueleryuez A, Gautier E, Busato A, Roeder C: Risk factors for early dislocation after total hip arthroplasty: A matched case-control study. *J Orthop Surg (Hong Kong)* 2010;18(2):179-183.

22. Soong M, Rubash HE, Macaulay W: Dislocation after total hip arthroplasty. *J Am Acad Orthop Surg* 2004;12(5):314-321.

23. Sadr Azodi O, Adami J, Lindström D, Eriksson KO, Wladis A, Bellocco R: High body mass index is associated with increased risk of implant dislocation following primary total hip replacement: 2,106 patients followed for up to 8 years. *Acta Orthop* 2008;79(1):141-147.

24. Ekelund A, Rydell N, Nilsson OS: Total hip arthroplasty in patients 80 years of age and older. *Clin Orthop Relat Res* 1992;281:101-106.

25. Seyler TM: Impact of lumbar arthrodesis on outcomes after elective total hip arthroplasty. Presented at the 46th Annual Meeting of the Eastern Orthopaedic Association, Maui, Hawaii, June 17-20, 2015.

26. Ranawat CS, Rodriguez JA: Functional leg-length inequality following total hip arthroplasty. *J Arthroplasty* 1997;12(4):359-364.

27. Clark CR, Huddleston HD, Schoch EP III, Thomas BJ: Leg-length discrepancy after total hip arthroplasty. *J Am Acad Orthop Surg* 2006;14(1):38-45.

28. Meermans G, Malik A, Witt J, Haddad F: Preoperative radiographic assessment of limb-length discrepancy in total hip arthroplasty. *Clin Orthop Relat Res* 2011;469(6):1677-1682.

29. Della Valle AG, Padgett DE, Salvati EA: Preoperative planning for primary total hip arthroplasty. *J Am Acad Orthop Surg* 2005;13(7):455-462.

30. Eggli S, Pisan M, Müller ME: The value of preoperative planning for total hip arthroplasty. *J Bone Joint Surg Br* 1998;80(3):382-390.

31. Charles MN, Bourne RB, Davey JR, Greenwald AS, Morrey BF, Rorabeck CH: Soft-tissue balancing of the hip: The role of femoral offset restoration. *Instr Course Lect* 2005;54:131-141.

32. Berend KR, Lombardi AV Jr, Seng BE, Adams JB: Enhanced early outcomes with the anterior supine intermuscular approach in primary total hip arthroplasty. *J Bone Joint Surg Am* 2009;91(suppl 6):107-120.

33. Kennon RE, Keggi JM, Wetmore RS, Zatorski LE, Huo MH, Keggi KJ: Total hip arthroplasty through a minimally invasive anterior surgical approach. *J Bone Joint Surg Am* 2003;85(suppl 4):39-48.

34. Matta JM, Shahrdar C, Ferguson T: Single-incision anterior approach for total hip arthroplasty on an orthopaedic table. *Clin Orthop Relat Res* 2005;441:115-124.

35. Meneghini RM, Pagnano MW, Trousdale RT, Hozack WJ: Muscle damage during MIS total hip arthroplasty: Smith-Petersen versus posterior approach. *Clin Orthop Relat Res* 2006;453:293-298.

36. Nam D, Sculco PK, Abdel MP, Alexiades MM, Figgie MP, Mayman DJ: Leg-length inequalities following THA based on surgical technique. *Orthopedics* 2013;36(4):e395-e400.

37. Seng BE, Berend KR, Ajluni AF, Lombardi AV Jr: Anterior-supine minimally invasive total hip arthroplasty: Defining the learning curve. *Orthop Clin North Am* 2009;40(3):343-350.

38. Woolson ST, Pouliot MA, Huddleston JI: Primary total hip arthroplasty using an anterior approach and a fracture table: Short-term results from a community hospital. *J Arthroplasty* 2009;24(7):999-1005.

39. Hardinge K: The direct lateral approach to the hip. *J Bone Joint Surg Br* 1982;64(1):17-19.

40. Mallory TH, Lombardi AV Jr, Fada RA, Herrington SM, Eberle RW: Dislocation after total hip arthroplasty using the anterolateral abductor split approach. *Clin Orthop Relat Res* 1999;358:166-172.

41. Abitbol JJ, Gendron D, Laurin CA, Beaulieu MA: Gluteal nerve damage following total hip arthroplasty: A prospective analysis. *J Arthroplasty* 1990;5(4):319-322.

42. Kenny P, O'Brien CP, Synnott K, Walsh MG: Damage to the superior gluteal nerve after two different approaches to the hip. *J Bone Joint Surg Br* 1999;81(6):979-981.

43. Masonis JL, Bourne RB: Surgical approach, abductor function, and total hip arthroplasty dislocation. *Clin Orthop Relat Res* 2002;405:46-53.

44. Pellicci PM, Bostrom M, Poss R: Posterior approach to total hip replacement using enhanced posterior soft tissue repair. *Clin Orthop Relat Res* 1998;355:224-228.

45. Suh KT, Park BG, Choi YJ: A posterior approach to primary total hip arthroplasty with soft tissue repair. *Clin Orthop Relat Res* 2004;418:162-167.

46. Tsai SJ, Wang CT, Jiang CC: The effect of posterior capsule repair upon post-operative hip dislocation following primary total hip arthroplasty. *BMC Musculoskelet Disord* 2008;(9):29.

47. Pagnano MW, Trousdale RT, Meneghini RM, Hanssen AD: Slower recovery after two-incision than mini-posterior-incision total hip arthroplasty: Surgical technique. *J Bone Joint Surg Am* 2009;91(suppl 2 pt 1):50-73.

48. Goldstein WM, Gleason TF, Kopplin M, Branson JJ: Prevalence of dislocation after total hip arthroplasty through a posterolateral approach with partial capsulotomy and capsulorrhaphy. *J Bone Joint Surg Am* 2001;83(pt 1, suppl 2):2-7.

49. White RE Jr, Forness TJ, Allman JK, Junick DW: Effect of posterior capsular repair on early dislocation in primary total hip replacement. *Clin Orthop Relat Res* 2001;393:163-167.

50. Demos HA, Rorabeck CH, Bourne RB, MacDonald SJ, McCalden RW: Instability in primary total hip arthroplasty with the direct lateral approach. *Clin Orthop Relat Res* 2001;393:168-180.

51. Lambers A, Jennings R, Bucknill A: Does computer navigation help the surgeon to achieve pre-operative leg length and offset targets in total hip arthroplasty? *Bone Joint J* 2013; 95(supp 15):110.

52. Ogawa K, Kabata T, Maeda T, Kajino Y, Tsuchiya H: Accurate leg length measurement in total hip arthroplasty: A comparison of computer navigation and a simple manual measurement device. *Clin Orthop Surg* 2014;6(2):153-158.

53. Poehling-Monaghan KL, Kamath AF, Taunton MJ, Pagnano MW: Direct anterior versus miniposterior THA with the same advanced perioperative protocols: Surprising early clinical results. *Clin Orthop Relat Res* 2015;473(2):623-631.

54. Beckmann J, Stengel D, Tingart M, Götz J, Grifka J, Lüring C: Navigated cup implantation in hip arthroplasty. *Acta Orthop* 2009;80(5):538-544.

55. Kalteis T, Beckmann J, Herold T, et al: Accuracy of an image-free cup navigation system—an anatomical study. *Biomed Tech (Berl)* 2004;49(9):257-262.

56. Lewinnek GE, Lewis JL, Tarr R, Compere CL, Zimmerman JR: Dislocations after total hip-replacement arthroplasties. *J Bone Joint Surg Am* 1978;60(2):217-220.

57. Gandhi R, Marchie A, Farrokhyar F, Mahomed N: Computer navigation in total hip replacement: A meta-analysis. *Int Orthop* 2009;33(3):593-597.

58. Spencer JM, Day RE, Sloan KE, Beaver RJ: Computer navigation of the acetabular component: A cadaver reliability study. *J Bone Joint Surg Br* 2006;88(7):972-975.

59. Jaramaz B, DiGioia AM III, Blackwell M, Nikou C: Computer assisted measurement of cup placement in total hip replacement. *Clin Orthop Relat Res* 1998;354:70-81.

60. Moskal JT, Capps SG: Improving the accuracy of acetabular component orientation: Avoiding malposition. *J Am Acad Orthop Surg* 2010;18(5):286-296.

61. Paterno SA, Lachiewicz PF, Kelley SS: The influence of patient-related factors and the position of the acetabular component on the rate of dislocation after total hip replacement. *J Bone Joint Surg Am* 1997;79(8):1202-1210.

62. McCollum DE, Gray WJ: Dislocation after total hip arthroplasty: Causes and prevention. *Clin Orthop Relat Res* 1990;261:159-170.

63. Archbold HA, Mockford B, Molloy D, McConway J, Ogonda L, Beverland D: The transverse acetabular ligament: An aid to orientation of the acetabular component during primary total hip replacement. A preliminary study of 1000 cases investigating postoperative stability. *J Bone Joint Surg Br* 2006;88(7):883-886.

64. Sotereanos NG, Miller MC, Smith B, Hube R, Sewecke JJ, Wohlrab D: Using intraoperative pelvic landmarks for acetabular component placement in total hip arthroplasty. *J Arthroplasty* 2006;21(6):832-840.

65. Dora C, Houweling M, Koch P, Sierra RJ: Iliopsoas impingement after total hip replacement: The results of non-operative management, tenotomy or acetabular revision. *J Bone Joint Surg Br* 2007;89(8):1031-1035.

66. Merle C, Grammatopoulos G, Waldstein W, et al: Comparison of native anatomy with recommended safe component orientation in total hip arthroplasty for primary osteoarthritis. *J Bone Joint Surg Am* 2013;95(22):e172.

67. Patel AB, Wagle RR, Usrey MM, Thompson MT, Incavo SJ, Noble PC: Guidelines for implant placement to minimize impingement during activities of daily living after total hip arthroplasty. *J Arthroplasty* 2010;25(8):1275-1281.e1.

68. Beamer BS, Morgan JH, Barr C, Weaver MJ, Vrahas MS: Does fluoroscopy improve acetabular component placement in total hip arthroplasty? *Clin Orthop Relat Res* 2014;472(12):3953-3962.

69. Ezzet KA, McCauley JC: Use of intraoperative X-rays to optimize component position and leg length during total hip arthroplasty. *J Arthroplasty* 2014;29(3):580-585.

70. Hofmann AA, Bolognesi M, Lahav A, Kurtin S: Minimizing leg-length inequality in total hip arthroplasty: Use of preoperative templating and an intraoperative x-ray. *Am J Orthop (Belle Mead NJ)* 2008;37(1):18-23.

71. DiGioia AM, Hafez MA, Jaramaz B, Levison TJ, Moody JE: Functional pelvic orientation measured from lateral standing and sitting radiographs. *Clin Orthop Relat Res* 2006;453:272-276.

72. Parratte S, Pagnano MW, Coleman-Wood K, Kaufman KR, Berry DJ: The 2008 Frank Stinchfield award: Variation in postoperative pelvic tilt may confound the accuracy of hip navigation systems. *Clin Orthop Relat Res* 2009;467(1):43-49.

73. Blondel B, Parratte S, Tropiano P, Pauly V, Aubaniac JM, Argenson JN: Pelvic tilt measurement before and after total hip arthroplasty. *Orthop Traumatol Surg Res* 2009;95(8):568-572.

74. Murphy WS, Klingenstein G, Murphy SB, Zheng G: Pelvic tilt is minimally changed by total hip arthroplasty. *Clin Orthop Relat Res* 2013;471(2):417-421.

75. Woolson ST, Hartford JM, Sawyer A: Results of a method of leg-length equalization for patients undergoing primary total hip replacement. *J Arthroplasty* 1999;14(2):159-164.

76. McGrory BJ, Morrey BF, Cahalan TD, An KN, Cabanela ME: Effect of femoral offset on range of motion and abductor muscle strength after total hip arthroplasty. *J Bone Joint Surg Br* 1995;77(6):865-869.

77. Amuwa C, Dorr LD: The combined anteversion technique for acetabular component anteversion. *J Arthroplasty* 2008;23(7):1068-1070.

78. Komeno M, Hasegawa M, Sudo A, Uchida A: Computed tomographic evaluation of component position on dislocation after total hip arthroplasty. *Orthopedics* 2006;29(12):1104-1108.

79. Dorr LD, Malik A, Dastane M, Wan Z: Combined anteversion technique for total hip arthroplasty. *Clin Orthop Relat Res* 2009;467(1):119-127.

80. Zhang J, Wang L, Mao Y, Li H, Ding H, Zhu Z: The use of combined anteversion in total hip arthroplasty for patients with developmental dysplasia of the hip. *J Arthroplasty* 2014;29(3):621-625.

81. Fackler CD, Poss R: Dislocation in total hip arthroplasties. *Clin Orthop Relat Res* 1980;151:169-178.

82. Mineo R, Berend KR, Mallory TH, Lombardi AV Jr: A lateralized tapered titanium cementless femoral component does not increase thigh or trochanteric pain. *Surg Technol Int* 2007;16:210-214.

83. Sultan PG, Tan V, Lai M, Garino JP: Independent contribution of elevated-rim acetabular liner and femoral head size to the stability of total hip implants. *J Arthroplasty* 2002;17(3):289-292.

84. Iagulli ND, Mallory TH, Berend KR, et al: A simple and accurate method for determining leg length in primary total hip arthroplasty. *Am J Orthop (Belle Mead NJ)* 2006;35(10):455-457.

85. Alazzawi S, Douglas SL, Haddad FS: A novel intra-operative technique to achieve accurate leg length and femoral offset during total hip replacement. *Ann R Coll Surg Engl* 2012;94(4):281-282.

86. Jasty M, Webster W, Harris W: Management of limb length inequality during total hip replacement. *Clin Orthop Relat Res* 1996;333:165-171.

87. Meftah M, Yadav A, Wong AC, Ranawat AS, Ranawat CS: A novel method for accurate and reproducible functional cup positioning in total hip arthroplasty. *J Arthroplasty* 2013;28(7):1200-1205.

88. Matsuda K, Nakamura S, Matsushita T: A simple method to minimize limb-length discrepancy after hip arthroplasty. *Acta Orthop* 2006;77(3):375-379.

89. Shiramizu K, Naito M, Shitama T, Nakamura Y, Shitama H: L-shaped caliper for limb length measurement during total hip arthroplasty. *J Bone Joint Surg Br* 2004;86(7):966-969.

90. Sarin VK, Pratt WR, Bradley GW: Accurate femur repositioning is critical during intraoperative total hip arthroplasty length and offset assessment. *J Arthroplasty* 2005;20(7):887-891.

91. Howie DW, Holubowycz OT, Middleton R; Large Articulation Study Group: Large femoral heads decrease the incidence of dislocation after total hip arthroplasty: A randomized controlled trial. *J Bone Joint Surg Am* 2012;94(12):1095-1102.

92. Jameson SS, Lees D, James P, et al: Lower rates of dislocation with increased femoral head size after primary total hip replacement: A five-year analysis of NHS patients in England. *J Bone Joint Surg Br* 2011;93(7):876-880.

93. Bartz RL, Nobel PC, Kadakia NR, Tullos HS: The effect of femoral component head size on posterior dislocation of the artificial hip joint. *J Bone Joint Surg Am* 2000;82(9):1300-1307.

94. Kung PL, Ries MD: Effect of femoral head size and abductors on dislocation after revision THA. *Clin Orthop Relat Res* 2007;465:170-174.

95. Sariali E, Lazennec JY, Khiami F, Catonné Y: Mathematical evaluation of jumping distance in total hip arthroplasty: Influence of abduction angle, femoral head offset, and head diameter. *Acta Orthop* 2009;80(3):277-282.

96. Burroughs BR, Rubash HE, Harris WH: Femoral head sizes larger than 32 mm against highly cross-linked polyethylene. *Clin Orthop Relat Res* 2002;405:150-157.

97. Cobb TK, Morrey BF, Ilstrup DM: The elevated-rim acetabular liner in total hip arthroplasty: Relationship to postoperative dislocation. *J Bone Joint Surg Am* 1996;78(1):80-86.

98. Cobb TK, Morrey BF, Ilstrup DM: Effect of the elevated-rim acetabular liner on loosening after total hip arthroplasty. *J Bone Joint Surg Am* 1997;79(9):1361-1364.

99. Insull PJ, Cobbett H, Frampton CM, Munro JT: The use of a lipped acetabular liner decreases the rate of revision for instability after total hip replacement: A study using data from the New Zealand Joint Registry. *Bone Joint J* 2014;96(7):884-888.

100. Vielpeau C, Lebel B, Ardouin L, Burdin G, Lautridou C: The dual mobility socket concept: Experience with 668 cases. *Int Orthop* 2011;35(2):225-230.

101. De Martino I, Triantafyllopoulos GK, Sculco PK, Sculco TP: Dual mobility cups in total hip arthroplasty. *World J Orthop* 2014;5(3):180-187.

102. Vigdorchik JM, D'Apuzzo MR, Markel DC, et al: Lack of early dislocation following total hip arthroplasty with a new dual mobility acetabular design. *Hip Int* 2015;25(1):34-38.

103. Combes A, Migaud H, Girard J, Duhamel A, Fessy MH: Low rate of dislocation of dual-mobility cups in primary total hip arthroplasty. *Clin Orthop Relat Res* 2013;471(12):3891-3900.

104. Boyer B, Philippot R, Geringer J, Farizon F: Primary total hip arthroplasty with dual mobility socket to prevent dislocation: A 22-year follow-up of 240 hips. *Int Orthop* 2012;36(3):511-518.

105. Philippot R, Camilleri JP, Boyer B, Adam P, Farizon F: The use of a dual-articulation acetabular cup system to prevent dislocation after primary total hip arthroplasty: Analysis of 384 cases at a mean follow-up of 15 years. *Int Orthop* 2009;33(4):927-932.

106. Stulberg SD: Dual poly liner mobility optimizes wear and stability in THA: Affirms. *Orthopedics* 2011;34(9):e445-e448.

107. von Knoch M, Berry DJ, Harmsen WS, Morrey BF: Late dislocation after total hip arthroplasty. *J Bone Joint Surg Am* 2002;84(11):1949-1953.

108. Pulido L, Restrepo C, Parvizi J: Late instability following total hip arthroplasty. *Clin Med Res* 2007;5(2):139-142.

109. Cameron HU, Smula V: Review of constrained acetabular component in

total hip replacement. *Acta Chir Orthop Traumatol Cech* 1999;66(5):263-265.

110. Clayton ML, Thirupathi RG: Dislocation following total hip arthroplasty: Management by special brace in selected patients. *Clin Orthop Relat Res* 1983;177:154-159.

111. Ekelund A: Trochanteric osteotomy for recurrent dislocation of total hip arthroplasty. *J Arthroplasty* 1993;8(6):629-632.

112. LaPorte DM, Mont MA, Pierre-Jacques H, Peyton RS, Hungerford DS: Technique for acetabular liner revision in a nonmodular metal-backed component. *J Arthroplasty* 1998;13(3):348-350.

113. Lachiewicz PF, Kelley SS: The use of constrained components in total hip arthroplasty. *J Am Acad Orthop Surg* 2002;10(4):233-238.

114. Sioen W, Simon JP, Labey L, Van Audekercke R: Posterior transosseous capsulotendinous repair in total hip arthroplasty: A cadaver study. *J Bone Joint Surg Am* 2002;84(10):1793-1798.

115. Jo S, Jimenez Almonte JH, Sierra RJ: The cumulative risk of re-dislocation after revision THA performed for instability increases close to 35% at 15 years. *J Arthroplasty* 2015;30(7):1177-1182.

116. Spangehl MJ, Masri BA, O'Connell JX, Duncan CP: Prospective analysis of preoperative and intraoperative investigations for the diagnosis of infection at the sites of two hundred and two revision total hip arthroplasties. *J Bone Joint Surg Am* 1999;81(5):672-683.

117. Guyen O, Lewallen DG, Cabanela ME: Modes of failure of Osteonics constrained tripolar implants: A retrospective analysis of forty-three failed implants. *J Bone Joint Surg Am* 2008;90(7):1553-1560.

118. Pierchon F, Pasquier G, Cotten A, Fontaine C, Clarisse J, Duquennoy A: Causes of dislocation of total hip arthroplasty: CT study of component alignment. *J Bone Joint Surg Br* 1994;76(1):45-48.

119. Mian SW, Truchly G, Pflum FA: Computed tomography measurement of acetabular cup anteversion and retroversion in total hip arthroplasty. *Clin Orthop Relat Res* 1992;276:206-209.

120. Carter AH, Sheehan EC, Mortazavi SM, Purtill JJ, Sharkey PF, Parvizi J: Revision for recurrent instability: What are the predictors of failure? *J Arthroplasty* 2011;26(6, suppl):46-52.

121. Garbuz DS, Masri BA, Duncan CP, et al: The Frank Stinchfield Award: Dislocation in revision THA. Do large heads (36 and 40 mm) result in reduced dislocation rates in a randomized clinical trial? *Clin Orthop Relat Res* 2012;470(2):351-356.

122. Mertl P, Combes A, Leiber-Wackenheim F, Fessy MH, Girard J, Migaud H: Recurrence of dislocation following total hip arthroplasty revision using dual mobility cups was rare in 180 hips followed over 7 years. *HSS J* 2012;8(3):251-256.

123. Guyen O, Pibarot V, Vaz G, Chevillotte C, Béjui-Hugues J: Use of a dual mobility socket to manage total hip arthroplasty instability. *Clin Orthop Relat Res* 2009;467(2):465-472.

124. Callaghan JJ, O'Rourke MR, Goetz DD, Lewallen DG, Johnston RC, Capello WN: Use of a constrained tripolar acetabular liner to treat intraoperative instability and postoperative dislocation after total hip arthroplasty: A review of our experience. *Clin Orthop Relat Res* 2004;429:117-123.

125. Callaghan JJ, Parvizi J, Novak CC, et al: A constrained liner cemented into a secure cementless acetabular shell. *J Bone Joint Surg Am* 2004;86(10):2206-2211.

126. Goetz DD, Bremner BR, Callaghan JJ, Capello WN, Johnston RC: Salvage of a recurrently dislocating total hip prosthesis with use of a constrained acetabular component: A concise follow-up of a previous report. *J Bone Joint Surg Am* 2004;86(11):2419-2423.

127. Su EP, Pellicci PM: The role of constrained liners in total hip arthroplasty. *Clin Orthop Relat Res* 2004;420:122-129.

128. Bremner BR, Goetz DD, Callaghan JJ, Capello WN, Johnston RC: Use of constrained acetabular components for hip instability: An average 10-year follow-up study. *J Arthroplasty* 2003;18(7, suppl 1):131-137.

129. Berend KR, Lombardi AV Jr, Welch M, Adams JB: A constrained device with increased range of motion prevents early dislocation. *Clin Orthop Relat Res* 2006;447:70-75.

130. Berend KR, Lombardi AV Jr, Mallory TH, Adams JB, Russell JH, Groseth KL: The long-term outcome of 755 consecutive constrained acetabular components in total hip arthroplasty examining the successes and failures. *J Arthroplasty* 2005; 20(7, suppl 3):93-102.

131. Sikes CV, Lai LP, Schreiber M, Mont MA, Jinnah RH, Seyler TM: Instability after total hip arthroplasty: Treatment with large femoral heads vs constrained liners. *J Arthroplasty* 2008;23(7, suppl):59-63.

132. Barbosa JK, Khan AM, Andrew JG: Treatment of recurrent dislocation of total hip arthroplasty using a ligament prosthesis. *J Arthroplasty* 2004;19(3):318-321.

133. Lavigne MJ, Sanchez AA, Coutts RD: Recurrent dislocation after total hip arthroplasty: Treatment with an Achilles tendon allograft. *J Arthroplasty* 2001;16(8, suppl 1):13-18.

134. Strømsøe K, Eikvar K: Fascia lata plasty in recurrent posterior dislocation after total hip arthroplasty. *Arch Orthop Trauma Surg* 1995;114(5):292-294.

135. Berend KR, Sporer SM, Sierra RJ, Glassman AH, Morris MJ: Achieving stability and lower limb length in total hip arthroplasty. *Instr Course Lect* 2011;60:229-246.

136. Kaplan SJ, Thomas WH, Poss R: Trochanteric advancement for recurrent dislocation after total hip arthroplasty. *J Arthroplasty* 1987;2(2):119-124.

Video References

Lavernia CJ: Video. *The Importance of the Posterior Superior Iliac Spines When Assessing Leg Length.* Coral Gables, FL, 2015.

Lavernia CJ: Video. *An Inexpensive Method to Assess Length.* Coral Gables, FL, 2015.

© 2016 AAOS Instructional Course Lectures, Volume 65

Lavernia CJ: Video. *Placement of the Tool Beneath the Patient.* Coral Gables, FL, 2015.

Lavernia CJ: Video. *Where is the Problem?* Coral Gables, FL, 2015.

Lavernia CJ: Video. *Preoperative Planning.* Coral Gables, FL, 2015.

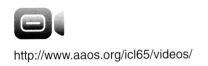

http://www.aaos.org/icl65/videos/

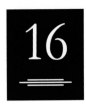

The Difficult Primary Total Knee Arthroplasty

Arthur L. Malkani, MD

Kirby D. Hitt, MD

Sameer Badarudeen, MD, MPH

Courtland Lewis, MD

Jeffrey Cherian, DO

Randa Elmallah, MD

Michael A. Mont, MD

Abstract

Primary total knee arthroplasty (TKA) for the treatment of knee arthritis has substantially increased over the past decade. Because of its success, the indications for primary TKA have expanded to include younger patients who are more active, elderly patients who have multiple comorbidities, and patients who have more complex issues, such as posttraumatic arthritis and severe deformity. TKA also has been used to salvage failed unicondylar arthroplasty and osteotomies about the knee. Exposure may be challenging and outcomes may not be as successful in patients with soft-tissue contractures, such as a stiff knee, who undergo TKA. Bone graft or augments may be required to correct deformity and attain proper knee alignment in patients who have a substantial varus or valgus deformity. TKA is somewhat challenging in patients who have deformity, bone loss, contracture, or multiple comorbidities, or have had prior surgery; therefore, it is necessary for surgeons to be aware of some general principles that may help minimize complications and improve outcomes.

Instr Course Lect 2016;65:243–266.

Severe Varus and Severe Valgus Knee Deformities

Multiple studies have reported that knees aligned in excessive varus or valgus after total knee arthroplasty (TKA) have a greater rate of failure than neutrally aligned knees.[1-6] Ritter et al[6] reported a higher rate of failure in knees with preoperative anatomic alignment greater than 8° of varus or greater than 11° of valgus, even if the knees were corrected to a neutral postoperative alignment. The authors concluded that more advanced preoperative varus and valgus deformities are risk factors for failure independent of postoperative alignment. Inadequate intraoperative balancing of these more severe deformities may account for the higher than expected failure rate. Undercorrection may lead to progressive instability and overload of the polyethylene on the convex side of the deformity. Restoration of neutral limb alignment and the establishment of adequate soft-tissue balance are prerequisites for a successful TKA. During TKA, surgeons not only should restore appropriate alignment but also be familiar with release and balancing techniques, which will help manage severe preoperative varus or valgus deformity, and how each release will affect the flexion-extension balance.

The Severe Varus Knee

Varus is the most commonly seen deformity in patients who undergo primary TKA. Many knees that require replacement have correctable varus deformity, and minimal or no releases are required. Medial releases are often necessary to restore balance and alignment in patients who have rigid, noncorrectable varus deformity. Anatomically, the varus knee is characterized by cartilage

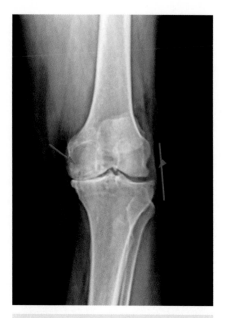

Figure 1   AP radiograph demonstrates a knee that has a type 1 varus deformity with minimal bone loss, minimal or no laxity (arrowhead), no medial contracture (arrow), and no subluxation (line).

and/or tibial bone loss in the medial compartment and associated with proximal tibial varus deformity. Contracture of the medial soft-tissue structures, including the medial collateral ligament (MCL), is frequently present, with flexion contractures and medial subluxation of the femur in patients who have more advanced deformity.

Classification

Varus knee deformities are classified into four separate types.[7] Type 1 deformities have normal convex lateral ligaments, lax concave medial ligaments, and bone loss on the concave side (**Figure 1**). Type 2 deformities have stretched convex lateral ligaments and lax concave medial ligaments, but are correctable. Type 3 deformities have normal convex lateral ligaments, bone loss on the concave side, concave medial ligament contracture, and are noncorrectable. Type 4 deformities have stretched convex lateral ligaments, bone loss on the concave side, and concave medial ligament contracture (**Figure 2**).

Results

Various techniques have been described for management of the varus knee. Verdonk et al[8] used an algorithmic approach to soft-tissue balancing in 359 patients with varus knees who underwent TKA. Of the 359 TKA patients, 255 (71%) were managed with medial capsule and deep MCL release to achieve symmetric gaps. An additional piecrust of the superficial MCL was performed in 87 patients (24%),

with a maximum correction of 6 to 8 mm. A distal release of the superficial MCL was required to achieve balance in 17 patients (5%) who had more severe deformities. There were no significant differences between the groups. Mediolateral stability was assessed at 12-month follow-up, and greater laxity was noted in patients who had superficial MCL release. Meftah et al[9] reported on 34 knees with fixed varus deformity and flexion contracture that underwent TKA with the use of the inside-out technique. This technique involves a posteromedial capsulotomy at the level of the tibial cut and pie-crusting of the superficial MCL. No instability was noted at a mean follow-up of 3.1 years. A mean preoperative coronal alignment of 21.1° of varus was corrected to 4.5° of valgus after surgery, and a semiconstrained TC3 implant, which provided additional varus/valgus constraint via a wider cam post mechanism, was necessary in only two knees.

Dixon et al[10] evaluated a technique of tibial component downsizing and resection of uncapped proximal medial bone in 12 knees with severe varus deformity that underwent TKA. The authors reported that this technique resulted in relative lengthening of the medial ligamentous structures without compromising their integrity, which usually occurs with release techniques. Bellemans et al[11] evaluated a multiple needle puncture technique for balancing the MCL in 35 knees with a mean varus of 12.5° (range, 9° to 23°) that underwent TKA with a posterior-stabilized implant. Successful correction was achieved in 34 knees (97%), with 2- to 4-mm maximal opening in extension and 2- to 6-mm maximal opening in flexion.

Dr. Hitt or an immediate family member has received royalties from Stryker; is a member of a speakers' bureau or has made paid presentations on behalf of Stryker and ConvaTec; has received research or institutional support from Stryker; and has received nonincome support (such as equipment or services), commercially derived honoraria, or other non-research–related funding (such as paid travel) from Stryker. Dr. Malkani or an immediate family member has received royalties from Stryker; is a member of a speakers' bureau or has made paid presentations on behalf of Stryker; serves as a paid consultant to or is an employee of Stryker; has received research or institutional support from Synthes and Stryker; serves as a board member, owner, officer, or committee member of the American Association of Hip and Knee Surgeons. Dr. Lewis or an immediate family member has received research or institutional support from Biomet, and serves as a board member, owner, officer, or committee member of the American Association of Hip and Knee Surgeons, the Connecticut State Medical Society, and the Hartford County Medical Association. Dr. Mont has received royalties from Stryker and Wright Medical Technologies; serves as a paid consultant to or is an employee of DJ Orthopaedics, Janssen Pharmaceutical Companies, Joint Active Systems, Medical Compression Systems, Medtronic, Sage Products, Stryker, TissueGene, and Wright Medical Technologies; has received research or institutional support from DJ Orthopaedics, Joint Active Systems, the National Institutes of Health (NIAMS & NICHD), Sage Products, Stryker, TissueGene, and Wright Medical Technologies; and serves as a board member, owner, officer, or committee member of the American Academy of Orthopaedic Surgeons. None of the following authors nor any immediate family member has received anything of value from or has stock or stock options held in a commercial company or institution related directly or indirectly to the subject of this chapter: Dr. Badarudeen, Dr. Cherian, and Dr. Elmallah.

Surgical Technique

Preoperative Assessment and Approach/Release

A preoperative examination should be performed under anesthesia to determine if the knee is correctable or fixed in flexion and extension. A correctable deformity suggests that minimal or no releases will be required, whereas a fixed deformity will likely require greater focus on soft-tissue balancing and release techniques. The knee should be exposed via the surgeon's preferred approach. The anteromedial capsule and deep MCL should be released back to the semimembranosus bursa. All osteophytes should be removed from the medial femoral condyle. The semimembranosus may have to be released in patients who have associated flexion contracture, but it can be addressed after bony preparation if the deformity persists (**Figure 3**).

Femoral Preparation

Resection of the distal femur is performed in 5° to 7° of valgus. The amount of bone resected off the more normal condyle should be equal to the thickness of the metallic condyle that will be inserted, which is, in most patients, approximately 8 mm. Confirmation with measurement of the resected bone should be performed before further femoral preparation is done. External rotation of the femur can be based off a combination of the anteroposterior axis, the transepicondylar axis, the posterior condylar axis, and mediolateral flexion gap asymmetry. Because primary bone loss in a varus knee is from the tibial plateau, adequate external rotation can be confirmed by verifying that more of the posteromedial condyle than the posterolateral condyle is resected. Rotation also can be confirmed by inspecting the anterior femoral resection footprint before

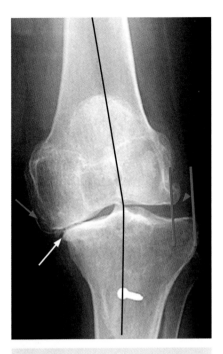

Figure 2   AP radiograph demonstrates a knee that has a type 4 varus deformity with bone loss (white arrow), lateral laxity (arrowhead), medial contracture (red arrow), and subluxation (red lines). The black line represents varus femoral-tibial alignment.

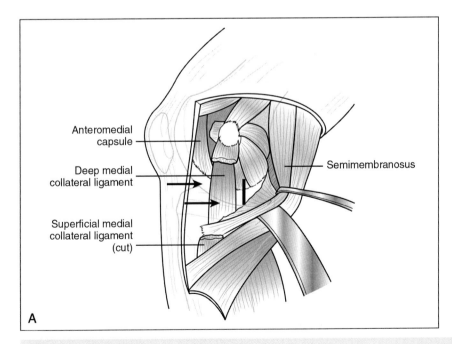

Anteromedial
capsule

Deep medial
collateral ligament

Superficial medial
collateral ligament
(cut)

Semimembranosus

A

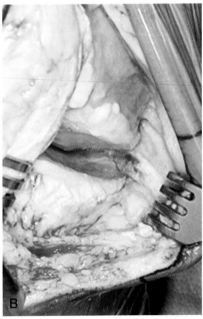

B

Figure 3   Illustration (**A**) and intraoperative photograph (**B**) show medial exposure and release (arrows in panel A) of a passively correctable varus knee deformity. The black line in panel A represents the limits of initial release.

further femoral preparation is done. Excessive external rotation may result in posteromedial laxity in flexion with tightening of the lateral structures, and internal rotation may result in posterolateral laxity in flexion with tightening of the medial structures (**Figure 4**).

Tibial Preparation

Resection of the proximal tibia is performed by referencing approximately two-thirds from anterior to posterior off the more normal lateral tibial plateau, which will ensure that adequate

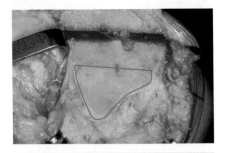

Figure 4 Intraoperative photograph shows assessment of a knee deformity for adequate external rotation. The red outline indicates a "grand piano" anterior femoral resection footprint.

bone is removed (**Figure 5**). If no bone is resected medially, then two options are considered. The resection can be lowered 2 mm to provide a stable medial bone platform for component fixation. If more than 2 mm is required to provide a stable medial platform, then preparation should be made for medial augments by increasing the tibial resection to eliminate the defect and avoid sizing issues between the femur and tibia.

Trialing and Balancing

The trial components are placed and trialing is performed, with assessment of mediolateral stability throughout the range of motion (ROM). If medial tightness is appreciated and a trapezoidal extension space is encountered, the preferred method of medial release of the authors of this chapter includes downsizing the tibial component and resecting the uncapped medial bone, as described by Dixon et al.[10] This technique is limited to implant systems that allow for altered sizing of the femoral and tibial components by at least one

size. A tray that is one size smaller is selected and lateralized to the cortical margin of the lateral tibia. The remaining proximal medial bone that overhangs the medial aspect of the tibial trial is removed flush with the tibial tray (**Figure 6**). The bone to be resected may be outlined with multiple small drill holes to help facilitate removal, which is performed with either osteotomes or a power saw. Release of the semimembranosus that extends posteromedial to include the capsule will provide correction in patients who have an associated flexion contracture. In the rare instance that medial tightness persists, either pie-crusting, a multiple needle puncture technique, or sequential subperiosteal tibial release can be performed. The authors of this chapter prefer the multiple needle puncture technique described by Bellemans et al[11] because minimal release is usually necessary to facilitate balancing and it avoids MCL compromise.

After the trial components are in place, medial-lateral stress testing is performed in flexion and extension to

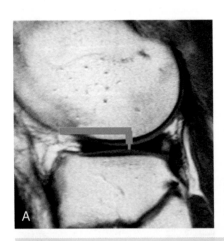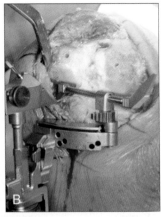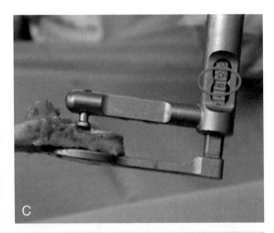

Figure 5 Images demonstrate measurements that should be taken to ensure adequate bone is removed during proximal tibia resection of a varus knee deformity. **A,** Sagittal MRI demonstrates the more normal lateral tibial plateau, which is measured two-thirds posteriorly. The L shape indicates appropriate resection guide placement. **B,** Intraoperative photograph shows measurement of the more normal lateral tibial plateau. **C,** Clinical photograph shows measurement of the tibial resection to ensure enough bone is removed to accommodate the implant. The red circle indicates that tibial resection should be 1 mm less than desired resection because of the thickness of the saw blade.

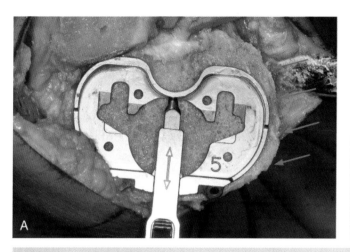
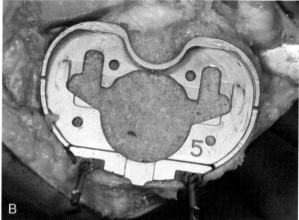

Figure 6 Intraoperative photographs show the medial release technique described by Dixon et al.[10] **A,** Uncapped medial bone (arrows) is present after the tibial baseplate is downsized and lateralized. **B,** The uncapped medial bone is removed flush with the tibial tray.

tension the medial soft-tissue sleeve. Failure of the medial side of the knee to open 1 to 3 mm is an indication that release is necessary and tightness in flexion, extension, or both is present. An 18-gauge needle is used to place multiple punctures in the tightest fibers, which are determined via direct palpation. Serial stress examinations are performed, and the process is repeated until stress examinations reveal a medial opening of approximately 1 to 2 mm in extension and 2 to 3 mm in flexion. If there is medial asymmetric tightness in flexion, then multiple needle punctures of the anterior aspect of the superficial MCL should be performed with the knee in flexion and under tension until correction is achieved. Similarly, if there is medial asymmetric tightness in extension and posteromedial release of the semimembranosus and medial uncapped bone removal have not corrected the deformity, then multiple needle punctures of the posterior aspect of the MCL should be performed with the knee in extension and under tension. Some residual lateral laxity may be present in patients who had attenuated lateral soft tissue preoperatively. Small

amounts of lateral laxity are well tolerated if the overall mechanical alignment has been corrected from the preoperative varus position.

Complications

Asymmetric extension and/or flexion instability may result from improper ligament balancing, which is commonly caused by persistently tight medial structures. The surgeon should critically assess for medial tightness, which presents as lateral opening or inadequate opening (1 mm or less) on the medial side in flexion and extension with stress testing. Internal rotation of the femoral component with the knee in flexion will result in a tight medial gap. For patients who have asymmetric flexion laxity, the surgeon should reevaluate if appropriate femoral rotation was attained. Failure to correct medial tightness may lead to progressive varus deformity from attenuated lateral structures, with an increased load on the implant and polyethylene.

Flexion instability may result from the failure to address differential flexion/extension gaps if the medial structures are released. Release of the

MCL will affect flexion more than extension; therefore, if medial release techniques are being used for balancing, they must be performed sequentially to avoid flexion instability. Overall flexion and extension laxity must be evaluated, and if any instability is present, it needs to be addressed.

Various release techniques may place the MCL in jeopardy of iatrogenic transection or overrelease. With any medial release technique, sequential stepwise releases and frequent checking of soft-tissue balance can help prevent these complications. If the MCL is completely released or too incompetent to affect balancing, then a constrained condylar implant should be used.

The Severe Valgus Knee

A successful TKA requires correction of deformity and restoration of anatomic alignment. Achieving coronal alignment and balance during TKA in patients who have severe valgus deformity is surgically challenging. Although various techniques have been described to treat patients who have severe valgus deformity, there is no consensus among surgeons.[12-22] Valgus deformity is seen

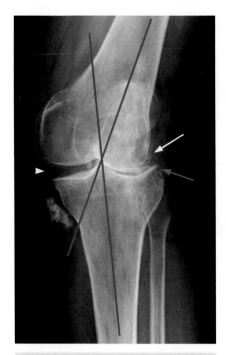

Figure 7 AP radiograph demonstrates a knee that has a type 2 valgus deformity with bone loss (white arrow), medial laxity (arrowhead), and lateral contracture (red arrow). The blue lines represent valgus femoral-tibial alignment.

in approximately 10% of patients who undergo TKA.[23] Severe valgus deformity is characterized by bone loss, primarily of the lateral condyle (both distally and posteriorly) and the central and posterior tibial plateau combined with contracted lateral soft tissues and medial soft-tissue stretching. Lateral knee stabilizers include the lateral collateral ligament (LCL), the iliotibial band (ITB), the posterolateral capsule, and the popliteus tendon. Cadaver model studies have shown that the LCL and popliteus tendon contribute to stability throughout ROM, but that their contributions are more in flexion than extension. The ITB and posterolateral capsule provide stability mainly in flexion.[24] Surgeons should understand the functions of these anatomic structures so that a sequential release

can be performed during balancing of the valgus knee. The release sequence for the valgus knee is more complicated than medial releases for the varus knee, partly because normal exposure is not a part of the necessary releases; attempts at increased exposure may result in overrelease of already attenuated medial structures.

Classification

Valgus knee deformities are classified into three separate types.[7] Type 1 deformities have minimal valgus, minimal lateral soft-tissue contracture, and minimal medial soft-tissue stretching. Type 2 deformities have more substantial deformity (>10°) and medial soft-tissue stretching (**Figure 7**). Type 3 deformities have severe osseous deformity and an incompetent medial soft-tissue sleeve.

Results

Insall et al[25] described their technique of posterolateral release, which included release of the ITB, LCL, popliteus tendon, and posterolateral capsule. The authors reported high rates of instability with this technique and the need for a more constrained prosthesis, and alternative options were developed. In a study of 60 knees with greater than 10° of valgus deformity that were treated with posterolateral release, Miyasaka et al[21] reported excellent correction and survival of the prosthesis at a 14.1-year follow-up; however, a 24% instability rate led the authors to develop alternative lateral release methods.

McAuley et al[26] reported that resection of the LCL and popliteus tendon during valgus deformity correction was associated with higher rates of revision surgery. Meftah et al[9] reported that preservation of the LCL and popliteus

tendon via an inside-out technique with horizontal release of the posterolateral capsule followed by pie-crusting of the ITB had good results. Similar results have been reported for the inside-out technique in combination with additional LCL release.[20] Both Healy et al[27] and Krackow et al[13] have recommended medial soft-tissue advancement in combination with lateral soft-tissue releases for the treatment of severe valgus deformity. Reported drawbacks of this technique include nonunion at the MCL advancement site, increased surgical time, and delayed mobilization.

Surgical Technique
Preoperative Assessment and Approach/Release

A preoperative examination should be performed under anesthesia to determine if the knee is correctable or fixed in flexion and extension. A correctable deformity suggests that minimal or no releases will be required, whereas a fixed deformity will likely require greater focus on soft-tissue balancing and release techniques. Some authors have advocated the lateral approach for the treatment of valgus knees; however, because it is difficult to obtain exposure with this technique, its acceptance has been limited. Care should be taken to avoid overzealous medial release. Medial release should be taken no further than the mid coronal plane (**Figure 3**). Forceful flexion and external rotation of the tibia, which helps provide adequate exposure in a varus knee, should be avoided in a valgus knee to prevent potential stretching of already compromised medial structures. All lateral osteophytes should be removed. Any necessary releases should be performed after bone preparation. Contracture of the posterior cruciate ligament (PCL) is not an infrequent finding in more severe knee deformities that undergo TKA, and balancing or releasing of the PCL is often necessary to complete the balancing efforts. If the surgeon attempts to preserve an intact PCL, critical assessment is mandatory during trialing to identify excessive tightness. A tight PCL may be addressed by either selectively balancing or releasing and converting to a cruciate-sacrificing or cruciate-substituting implant.

Patellar maltracking and the need for lateral retinacular release are common findings seen in TKA for the treatment of severe valgus deformity. Attention to appropriate femoral and tibial rotation should reduce the need for lateral release. Patellofemoral tracking should be assessed with the use of a no-thumbs technique. If lateral maltracking is present, the surgeon should assess if there were patellar tracking problems preoperatively, which would suggest that a lateral release may be indicated. If no tracking problems were noted preoperatively but are seen after trialing, then malalignment of the components should be assessed and, if present, corrected.

Femoral Preparation

The initial femoral intramedullary entry hole should be located medial to the anteroposterior axis and in the notch directly anterior to the PCL attachment to take into account the lateral bow of the distal femur in a valgus knee. For severe valgus deformities, a 3°- to 5°-valgus resection of the distal femur is preferred to prevent undercorrection and reduce stress on the already compromised medial structures. The amount of bone resected off the more normal medial condyle should be equal to the thickness of the metallic

medial condyle. No distal bone will be resected laterally in patients who have more severe lateral condyle deformities. Similar to a cavitary defect, more severe lateral condyle deformities can be managed with cement or bone grafting because anterior and posterior chamfer contact will provide the necessary implant stability. Surgeons should resist the temptation to resect to the level of the deficient lateral side because it can create flexion-extension balancing challenges and can raise the joint line, which will result in midflexion instability. Because of lateral condyle deficiencies, rotational alignment should be based off the anteroposterior and epicondylar axes; this helps avoid internal rotation of the femoral component, which is often associated with posterior condyle referencing. The initial anterior femoral resection footprint should be inspected as a secondary check to confirm appropriate rotation (**Figure 4**).

Tibial Preparation

Tibial resection is performed with extramedullary alignment guides that are placed at a 90° angle to the longitudinal axis of the tibia. Because of the valgus bow of the tibial shaft in a severe valgus knee, intramedullary alignment should be used with caution and checked with extramedullary guides. The degree of posterior slope is based on the particular implant design and whether the PCL is retained or sacrificed. As a general rule, the slope should be approximately 0° in posterior cruciate-substituting and cruciate-sacrificing designs. If the PCL is retained, the slope can vary between 3° and 5°, based on implant manufacturers. Resection of the tibia in a valgus knee is performed by referencing off the medial tibial plateau, with underresection of 2 to 3 mm because

of medial soft-tissue attenuation and to prevent the need for unusually thick tibial inserts.

In severe valgus deformity, the PCL may be contracted and may limit correction. Sequential release of the PCL or substitution may be required. It is the experience of one of the authors of this chapter (K.D.H.) that during proper femoral rotation, a valgus knee is more commonly balanced in flexion and tight laterally in extension. The flexion gap is balanced by adjusting the tibial insert thickness. The knee is then placed in extension, and balance is checked medially and laterally. If the knee is tight laterally in flexion only, which is rare, then the surgeon must evaluate for possible femoral rotational errors. If rotation is satisfactory, then the LCL is released via pie-crusting, a micropuncture technique, or incremental release off the femur. Internal rotation contracture that is associated with lateral tightness in flexion is best managed with release of the popliteus tendon. Likewise, a knee that is tight laterally in flexion and extension is addressed initially with release of the LCL, popliteus tendon, or both via a sequential release technique. Any remaining or isolated extension tightness laterally is addressed with pie-crusting of the ITB or release of the posterolateral capsule (**Figure 8**). More extensive release of the ITB may be required for knees with external tibial rotation contracture, which is more commonly seen in patients who have rheumatoid arthritis (RA). Serial examinations and medial-lateral stress testing should be performed until the knee opens 2 to 3 mm medially and 2 to 4 mm laterally in flexion and 1 to 2 mm medially and 1 to 3 mm laterally in extension. If instability persists after performing

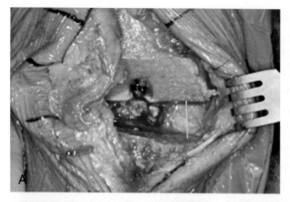
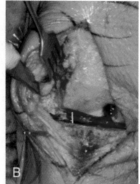
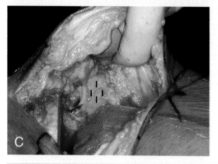
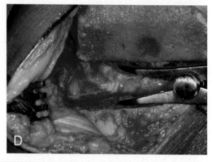

Table 1
Causes of Knee Stiffness

Severe osteoarthritis

Rheumatoid arthritis

Psoriatic arthritis

Complex regional pain syndrome

Severe pain

Posttraumatic arthritis

Neuromuscular disorder

Prior infection

Prior surgery

Figure 8 Intraoperative photographs show evaluation of medial and lateral compartment gaps and releases for lateral extension tightness. **A,** The medial side of the knee opens sufficiently (line) if valgus stress applied. **B,** The lateral side of the knee fails to open sufficiently (line) if varus stress applied. **C,** The iliotibial band is pie-crusted (black lines) if lateral extension tightness is present. **D,** The posterolateral capsule is released if lateral extension tightness persists. The red line represents the area of the posterolateral capsule to be released.

soft-tissue balancing with these release techniques, then a more constrained implant should be used. The level of constraint is based on the availability and function of the collateral ligaments. Higher levels of constraint are necessary as instability increases. A hinged device may be necessary only in patients in whom the collateral ligaments are completely incompetent.

Complications

Correction of valgus deformity and release of the lateral structures may result in stretching of the peroneal nerve. Peroneal palsy has been reported in 0.6% to 4% of patients after TKA for the treatment of valgus deformity.[13,20,21,28] Based on cadaver model studies and MRI, the minimum distance from the posterolateral capsule to the common peroneal nerve is between 6 and 11 mm, with a mean distance of 13 to 15 mm.[29] Guidelines for the prevention and management of neurovascular injuries have been published.[30] As part of informed consent, TKA patients who have a valgus knee deformity should be counseled on the possibility of postoperative peroneal nerve palsy as well as the potential need for bracing and possible permanent neurologic deficit.

Conclusions

Currently, the evidence in the literature is not sufficient to determine the best soft-tissue release technique for the correction of varus or valgus deformity.

However, the literature has reported that minimal, sequential releases provide good, reproducible results as opposed to more extensive release techniques, which result in instability, loosening, and revision surgery. Meticulous surgical technique to restore alignment and balance in TKA can help patients who have varus or valgus deformity achieve the results they deserve.

The Stiff Knee

A stiff knee is a knee that has ROM less than 50°.[31] Because full extension is necessary for normal knee function, a stiff knee may be quite functionally debilitating. In addition, approximately 70° of knee flexion is necessary in the swing phase of the gait cycle, 90° is necessary for stair descending, and approximately 110° is necessary for cycling.[32] The most important predictor of ROM after TKA is preoperative ROM.[33] Preoperative knee stiffness is associated with higher rates of postoperative complications and early TKA failure.

There are several potential causes of knee stiffness (**Table 1**). It is important for surgeons to identify the etiology of a stiff knee because it may have a substantial effect on the management and outcome of a planned TKA. Knee stiffness also may be a sign of an indolent

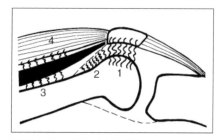

Figure 9 Illustration demonstrates the four components of an extension contracture of the knee. 1 = Fibrosis and shortening of the medial and lateral parapatellar retinacula and obliteration of the gutters. 2 = Adhesions from the deep surface of the patella to the femoral condyles and in the supracondylar gutter, as in intra-articular fibrosis and patellofemoral ankylosis. 3 = Fibrosis of the vastus intermedius with scarring to the rectus femoris muscle and to the front of the femur. 4 = Fibrosis and shortening of the rectus femoris. (Reproduced with permission from Bellemans J, Steenwerckx A, Brabants K, Victor J, Lammens J, Fabry G: The Judet quadricepsplasty: A retrospective analysis of 16 cases. *Acta Orthop Belg* 1996;62[2]:79-82.)

Table 2
Causes of Fixed Flexion Deformity

Inflammatory arthritis

Immobility

Advanced osteoarthritis

Hemophilia

Neuromuscular disorder

Table 3
Potential Pitfalls of Inadequate Total Knee Arthroplasty Exposure in a Stiff Knee

Patellar tendon rupture

Tibial tubercle avulsion

Flexion-extension mismatch

Difficult soft-tissue balancing

Component malposition

Collateral ligament avulsion

infection, underlying reflex sympathetic dystrophy, or a neuromuscular disorder, all of which require additional workup before arthroplasty should be considered.

Pathoanatomy

Knee stiffness may be associated with an extension contracture, a flexion contracture, or a combination of both. The presence of a bony block, heterotopic ossification, and patella baja also may limit knee ROM. The pathology of an extension contracture of the knee consists of four major components[34,35] (**Figure 9**).

Flexion deformities are common in patients who have osteoarthritis. Approximately two-thirds of knees that undergo TKA have some amount of flexion deformity. The common causes of fixed flexion deformity are listed in **Table 2**. The presence of a preoperative flexion deformity increases the risk of a postoperative residual flexion deformity.[33] A fixed flexion deformity of more than 20° is considered a severe deformity. A knee that cannot be fully extended during ambulation requires constant energy expenditure to contract the quadriceps so it can bear weight and keep the knee stable.[36,37] In addition, fixed flexion deformity may result in functional limb-length discrepancy, shortened stride length, altered kinematics of the spine, and a contralateral knee.

Ankylosis can be either bony or fibrous and can occur in either flexion or extension. Although a bony ankylosis may resolve pain, it can cause severe functional disability. The causes of knee ankylosis include healed pyogenic and tuberculous infection, RA, ankylosing spondylitis, and posttraumatic arthritis. The presence of ankylosis increases the risk of inadequate exposure, patellofemoral ankylosis, difficulty in exposure and identification of the joint space, and compromised collateral and cruciate ligaments.

Preoperative Assessment and Approach/Release

The surgical approach for TKA in a stiff knee is challenging because routine patellar eversion and flexion are difficult to achieve, which usually makes exposure inadequate. Preoperative planning should document ROM, the location of prior scars, neurovascular status, and angular deformities as well as plan for the type of prosthesis to be used. **Table 3** lists the potential pitfalls of inadequate TKA exposure in a stiff knee. If infection is a possibility, the preoperative workup should include knee aspiration and the measurement of C-reactive protein levels and erythrocyte sedimentation rate.

For very stiff knees in which exposure is difficult, it may be necessary to enhance exposure with the use of the standard medial parapatellar approach, an additional proximal extension of the quadriceps tendon, and a lateral retinacular release. After a medial arthrotomy is performed, adhesions at the suprapatellar pouch and medial and lateral gutters are released. Careful subperiosteal elevation of the deep MCL along the proximal tibia (usually from the posteromedial corner anterior to the semimembranosus tendon insertion) followed by external rotation of the tibia may facilitate mobilization of the patella. If the knee cannot be flexed to 90° after these steps are performed, then other extensile exposures are warranted (**Table 4**). The quadriceps snip and MCL slide are more utilitarian exposures.

Table 4
Extensile Surgical Exposures for Total Knee Arthroplasty in a Stiff Knee

Extension	Available Approach(es)
Proximal	Quadriceps snip
	V-Y quadriceps turndown
Medial	Medial collateral ligament slide
	Medial femoral peel
	Medial epicondyle oste-otomy
Distal	Tibial tubercle osteotomy

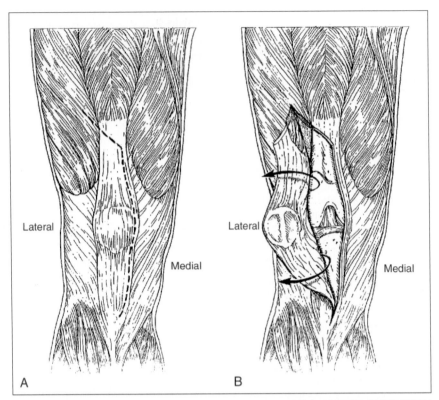

Figure 10 Illustrations demonstrate the quadriceps snip approach. **A,** The standard parapatellar approach with added proximal lateral extension (dashed line). **B,** Eversion (arrows) of the extensor mechanism after the quadriceps snip. (Reproduced from Barrack RL: Specialized surgical exposure for revision total knee: Quadriceps snip and patellar turndown. *Instr Course Lect* 1999;48:149-152.)

Quadriceps Snip

The quadriceps snip, also called a rectus snip, was popularized by Insall.[38,39] The quadriceps snip involves a proximal extension of the arthrotomy along the quadriceps tendon and at its musculotendinous junction. The incision is obliquely directed approximately 30° to 45° (in line with the fibers of vastus lateralis) in the proximal-lateral direction (**Figure 10**). The obliquely directed incision helps preserve lateral superior genicular blood flow to the patella and insertion of the vastus lateralis tendon. Patellar mobilization can be further aided with the addition of a lateral retinacular release, which is placed longitudinally, approximately 1 cm away from the lateral border of the patella to preserve its blood supply. Other advantages of the quadriceps snip include the absence of postoperative rehabilitation restrictions and the avoidance of extensor lag, which is common with other extensile exposures. The quadriceps snip can be converted to a more extensile V-Y quadriceps turndown, if necessary.[40,41]

The outcome of TKAs performed with the quadriceps snip is largely equivalent to those performed with the standard medial parapatellar approach.

Barrack et al[42] reported that the outcomes of 31 patients who underwent a quadriceps snip and 63 patients who underwent a medial parapatellar incision for revision TKA were equivalent. The equivalent outcomes included objective, functional, and total Knee Society scores; ROM; extension lag; patellofemoral pain; and patient satisfaction. In a study that compared Western Ontario and McMaster Universities Osteoarthritis Index function, pain, stiffness, and satisfaction scores between 50 patients who underwent a rectus snip and 57 patients who underwent a standard medial parapatellar approach, Meek et al[43] reported no negative effect from a rectus snip at a mean follow-up of 40.5 months.

V-Y Quadriceps Turndown

Insall modified the Coonse and Adams approach, which involves a standard medial parapatellar arthrotomy, by extending the incision at the apex of the arthrotomy inferolaterally (at a 45° angle over the lateral retinaculum) to the tibia[40,41] (**Figure 11**). The V-Y quadriceps turndown is indicated for knees with severe stiffness; however, there is an increased risk of quadriceps necrosis and an increased incidence of extensor lag postoperatively.

MCL Slide

A subperiosteal MCL slide may be performed to facilitate external rotation of the tibia and help mobilize the patella.[44] Although varus knees require

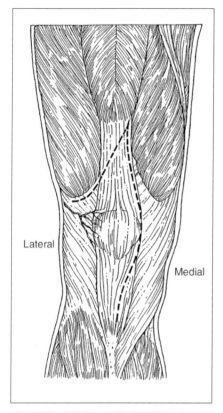

Figure 11   Illustration demonstrates the V-Y quadriceps turndown. The medial dashed line represents the standard parapatellar approach. The lateral dashed line represents the V-Y quadriceps turndown. (Reproduced from Barrack RL: Specialized surgical exposure for revision total knee: Quadriceps snip and patellar turndown. *Instr Course Lect* 1999;48:149-152.)

more distal and posterior elevation of the deep MCL, valgus knees require only minimal a MCL slide.

Medial Femoral Peel

Femoral peel or a more limited medial femoral peel may be used to improve exposure.[44] Subperiosteal elevation of the origin of the MCL and the surrounding soft tissue may be performed to improve visualization of the medial and posterior distal femur. If necessary, subperiosteal elevation of the origin of the LCL may be performed on the lateral side. It is important for the surgeon to maintain the integrity of the soft-tissue sleeve to avoid varus or valgus instability.

Medial Epicondyle Osteotomy

Although it is rarely used, a medial epicondyle osteotomy may be performed in patients who have severe varus and flexion deformities, if necessary. In patients who have cystic lesions or osteolysis, care should be taken to avoid the inadvertent creation of uncontained femoral cavitary defects.[45]

Tibial Tubercle Osteotomy

Tibial tubercle osteotomy was popularized by Whiteside and Ohl and can be used in a stiff knee that has patellar ligament contracture as well as for difficult stem extraction and tubercle malposition.[46,47] The technique involves an osteotomy approximately 8 cm long and 2 cm wide. The osteotomy is developed, and the fragment is booked open, with care taken to keep the lateral soft-tissue sleeve intact. The osteotomy is rigidly repaired with cables or wires, and patients have no postoperative restrictions on rehabilitation.

Results

Barrack[41] described a stepwise approach to gain access to a stiff knee during TKA. This approach involves making a long incision to identify the normal tissue plane. A standard medial parapatellar incision is then made, and the MCL is elevated subperiosteally. The medial and lateral gutters as well as the suprapatellar pouch are then developed. A lateral release can be performed to obtain adequate flexion if minor stiffness is present. A quadriceps snip can be performed if difficulties are encountered. If a quadriceps snip is insufficient, then it can be converted to a V-Y quadriceps turndown.

Bellemans et al[48] obtained excellent results with the use of an algorithm for the treatment of flexion contractures during TKA. Progression from one step in the algorithm to the next was necessary if full extension was not achieved. Step one involved removal of osteophytes, ligament balancing, and overresection of the distal femur by 2 mm. Step two involved posterior capsule release and, if necessary, gastrocnemius release. Step three consisted of additional resection of the distal femur up to 4 mm. Step four, which was performed if the previous three steps failed, involved transection of the hamstring insertion. The authors applied this algorithm to 130 patients who had moderate to severe flexion contractures (ie, more than 15° and more than 30° of contracture, respectively), and reported that 63 patients attained full extension after step one, 37 patients attained full extension after step two, 21 patients attained full extension after step three, and nine patients attained full extension after step four. All patients had full extension at final follow-up except for 13 patients who had a mild flexion contracture of less than 5°, five patients who had a flexion contracture between 5° and 10°, and two patients who had a flexion contracture of more than 10°.

Outcomes

In a study of 84 knees with preoperative stiffness and ROM that ranged from 0° to 20°, 26 of which underwent a modified V-Y quadriceps turndown and 55 of which underwent a quadriceps snip with a lateral release, Rajgopal[31] et al reported a significant improvement in the mean postoperative arc of motion (75°) at a mean follow-up of 9 years.

The authors reported that complications included skin necrosis, superficial wound infection, and peroneal nerve palsy. Bhan et al[49] reported on a series of 90 stiff knees or ankylosed knees that underwent TKA; all of the knees had a preoperative arc of motion less than 50°, and 26 of the knees were ankylosed. The authors reported that ROM improved 1° to 94° in the stiff knees and 3° to 77° in the ankylosed knees. Complications included wound necrosis (7% of the stiff knees, 50% of the ankylosed knees), partial avulsion of the patellar tendon, femoral condyle fracture, hematoma, and peroneal nerve palsy. The ankylosed knees required a V-Y quadriceps turndown and a constrained condylar prosthesis. In a study of 37 knees with a mean preoperative fixed flexion deformity of 78° that underwent TKA, Lu et al[50] reported that, at a mean follow-up of 4.3 years, the mean postoperative fixed flexion deformity was 7° and the postoperative arc of motion was 82°. Seven patients required manipulation under anesthesia, three patients developed transient peroneal nerve palsy, and one patient developed vascular insufficiency. Other complications included delayed wound healing and infection.

In a study of 86 stiff knees that underwent TKA with a constrained condylar or posterior stabilized prosthesis, Kim and Kim[51] reported substantial improvements in Knee Society and Western Ontario and McMaster Universities Osteoarthritis Index scores. A V-Y quadriceps turndown was required in 47% of the knees. ROM improved from 40° preoperatively to 102° postoperatively. Complications included skin necrosis (6%), infection (3%), late quadriceps tendon rupture (2.3%), and aseptic loosening of the

tibial component (1.2%). The same authors[52] reported on a series of 99 ankylosed knees that underwent TKA with a constrained condylar or posterior stabilized prosthesis. The authors reported significant improvements in mean postoperative Western Ontario and McMaster Universities Osteoarthritis Index, Knee Society, and Hospital for Special Surgery scores. Comparing the two studies, the authors reported that the ankylosed knees[52] required a V-Y quadriceps turndown at a higher frequency (73%) compared with the stiff knees[51] (47%). Complications included persistent flexion deformity, skin necrosis (17%), infection (3%), quadriceps tendon rupture (2%), periprosthetic fracture (1%), and aseptic loosening (1%).[52] In all knees that required a V-Y quadriceps turndown, a significant extension lag developed, with a mean extension lag of 15°.[52]

Conclusions

TKA can be challenging in patients who have a stiff knee. It is important for surgeons to preoperatively identify the pathoanatomy or etiology of the stiffness. Careful preoperative planning is paramount to avoid intraoperative problems and postoperative complications. A standard medial parapatellar approach can be used in most patients. A more extensile approach can be used if additional exposure is required. Stiff knees that undergo TKA have a higher risk of complications, especially wound healing complications. The expectations of patients who undergo TKA for the treatment of a stiff knee should be tempered, especially with respect to postoperative ROM and the increased likelihood of postoperative complications.

TKA After Failed Osteotomy or Unicondylar Arthroplasty

Both tibial osteotomy and unicondylar arthroplasty play a role in the surgical treatment of isolated medial compartment osteoarthritis. If either procedure fails, then revision to TKA is more technically challenging and has a higher risk of requiring re-revision surgery than primary tricompartmental arthroplasty. Preoperative planning is essential before conversion of a failed osteotomy to TKA to determine and address the extent of the deformity, the extent of soft-tissue contracture, prior skin incisions, and retained hardware. In certain patients, the surgeon may choose to perform a two-stage conversion with initial hardware removal. The bone loss encountered after removal of a failed implant and loss of the femoral condyle that assists with femoral component rotation are challenges that need to be addressed with regard to failed unicondylar arthroplasty.

Anatomic and Kinematic Considerations

Osteotomy

Conversion to TKA most commonly occurs after a failed proximal tibia closing wedge osteotomy. A tibial osteotomy incision is often lateral, which presents a challenge with regard to the adequacy of the skin bridge, especially if an L-shaped incision was used for the antecedent surgery. A minimum 7-cm skin interval between the prior incision and a medial parapatellar incision should be available. Modern fixation hardware from the index surgery may be challenging to remove. Occasionally, a carbide-tipped high-speed burr may be necessary to remove an osseoingrown device. Lateralization of the tibial tubercle with concomitant patellar

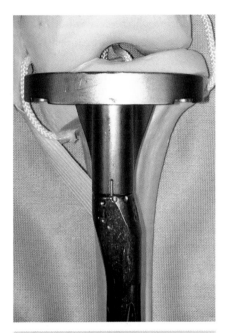

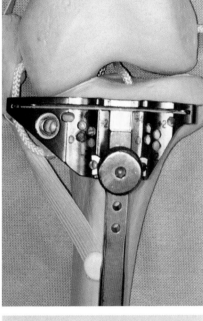

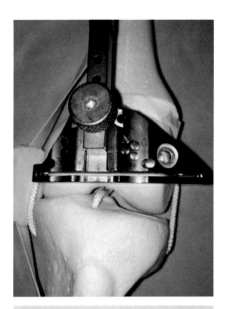

Figure 12   Photograph of a bone model shows relative translation of the tibial diaphysis, which may occur after high tibial osteotomy.

Figure 13   Photograph of a bone model shows increased medial plateau resection, which is used to reestablish the mechanical axis.

Figure 14   Photograph of a bone model shows increased lateral distal condyle resection, which may occur after distal femoral opening wedge osteotomy.

tendon contracture and patella baja will likely result in difficult patellar eversion; therefore, great care is necessary to protect the extensor mechanism. Patients who have tibial shaft offset caused by relative translation of the joint surface compared to the distal tibia may require the use of an offset stem, especially if greater constraint is required (**Figure 12**). To perform a bone cut perpendicular to the mechanical axis, relatively increased medial plateau resection may be necessary (**Figure 13**), which makes restoration of collateral ligament balance and extension/flexion gap balancing difficult.

A proximal tibia opening wedge osteotomy would be expected to decrease patellar-related issues; however, patella baja is common and must be anticipated if conversion to TKA is performed. Alteration in the tibial slope has been reported after proximal tibia opening wedge osteotomy and

should be anticipated and corrected at the time of TKA to avoid sagittal plane instability. Coronal plane stability and extension/flexion gap balancing difficulties after proximal tibia opening wedge osteotomy are similar to those seen after proximal tibia closing wedge osteotomy.

A failed varus-producing distal femoral opening wedge osteotomy for the treatment of a valgus knee can be readily converted to a TKA unless there has been substantial overcorrection. If overcorrection has been performed, increased lateral condyle extension resection may result (**Figure 14**), which makes restoration of collateral ligament balance a challenge that is comparable to valgus osteotomy.

Unicondylar Arthroplasty
Revision of failed unicondylar arthroplasty to TKA is not as predictably simple as some unicondylar arthroplasty

advocates suggest. With any revision arthroplasty, adequate backup with stem extensions, tibial augments, and semiconstrained polyethylene inserts is essential (**Figure 15**). Deficient tibial bone stock is the rule rather than the exception for tibial component loosening with subsidence or even a well-fixed step-cut tibial component that is undergoing revision surgery for opposite compartment wear. With any open arthrotomy knee surgery, concomitant patellar tendon contracture and/or patella baja are common findings. If a posterior referencing total knee system is used, femoral component rotation is a concern (**Figure 16**). If possible, the femoral component should be left in situ to ensure appropriate distal femoral resection, and posterior condyle augmentation may be required to allow for correct component rotation. It is important that joint-line height is restored to ensure optimal kinematics and patellar tracking.

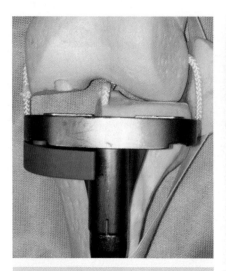

Figure 15 Photograph of a bone model with a stemmed tibial component that has build-up blocks, which can be used if tibial bone loss occurs after unicondylar revision arthroplasty.

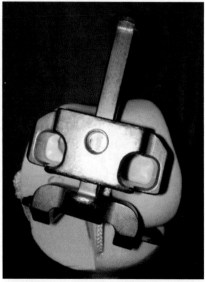

Figure 16 Photograph of a bone model shows potential femoral malrotation, which may occur after unicondylar revision arthroplasty.

Surgical Approach

The surgical approach should be decided, and inventory should be checked to ensure adequate primary and backup instrumentation. The most lateral incision possible should be made, if possible (>7 cm for L-shaped incision or cross at 90°). A lateral retinacular approach to TKA is suboptimal in this instance. The surgeon should protect the patellar tendon. A Kirschner wire may be inserted into the tibial tendon/tibial tubercle, if necessary, to avoid avulsion. The patella should be everted with care. The surgeon should prepare for hardware removal, altered tibial slope (sagittal instability), collateral imbalance (coronal instability), tibial bone deficiency (tibial collapse or step-cut tibial design), offset tibial stem extension, and joint line elevation in the face of patella baja.

Results

Both high tibial osteotomy and unicondylar arthroplasty for the treatment of medial compartment arthrosis have been extensively studied and reported in the literature. Based on meta-analyses of the literature, survivorship for patients who underwent high tibial osteotomy and patients who underwent unicondylar arthroplasty was equivalent (91.0% and 91.5%, respectively, at 5- to 8-year follow-up and 84.4% and 86.9%, respectively, at 9- to 12-year follow-up).[53] Two recent studies found that patient-reported outcomes were better for patients who underwent unicondylar arthroplasty compared with patients who underwent high tibial osteotomy; however, the functional advantage of unicondylar arthroplasty did not remain after 12 years.[53,54] Equivalent return to activity has been reported with both procedures.[55,56] There appears to be an increase in the use of unicondylar arthroplasty compared with high tibial osteotomy, particularly among younger surgeons.[57,58] Recent arthroplasty registry reports, in particular from Finland and New Zealand, demonstrate inferior survivorship at 10- to 15-year follow-up for patients who underwent unicondylar arthroplasty for the treatment of medial compartment arthrosis compared with those who underwent TKA for the treatment of medial compartment arthrosis.[59,60] Although some individuals argue that this may be the result of a lower threshold for revision surgery, the allegations have not been substantiated. There does not appear to be a difference at 5-year follow-up between conversion from failed lateral closing wedge osteotomy to TKA and conversion from failed medial opening wedge osteotomy to TKA with respect to functional outcomes or survivorship.[61,62] Survivorship for TKA after failed high tibial osteotomy was reported to be comparable with survivorship for primary TKA in a retrospective cohort study with a mean follow-up of 14 years[63] and in a meta-analysis with a mean follow-up of 7 years.[64] A recent registry study, however, reported that survivorship for TKA after failed high tibial osteotomy was worse than survivorship for primary TKA (hazard ratio = 1.40; 95% confidence interval, 1.09-1.81).[65]

Surgeons experienced in performing unicompartmental arthroplasty have reported that revision TKA after failed unicondylar arthroplasty is more complex than primary TKA.[66] A study of the United Kingdom National Joint Registry Database demonstrated that revision TKA after failed unicondylar arthroplasty required thicker tibial inserts and more constrained implants than primary TKA, which suggests that revision TKA after failed unicondylar arthroplasty has a higher level of complexity than primary TKA.[67] In addition, recent reports from the New Zealand Joint Registry and the Swedish Knee Arthroplasty Register demonstrate that survivorship for primary

TKA is higher than survivorship for TKA after failed high tibial osteotomy or failed unicondylar arthroplasty.[68,69]

Complications

Skin edge necrosis, patellar tendon avulsion, sagittal and/or coronal plane instability, as well as femoral component malrotation are all well-described complications of conversion/revision TKA after failed high tibial osteotomy or failed unicondylar arthroplasty.

Conclusions

Tibial valgus or femoral varus osteotomies and unicondylar arthroplasty are reasonable surgical procedures for the treatment of medial compartment gonarthrosis. Relative survivorship of high tibial osteotomy versus unicondylar knee arthroplasty cannot be definitively established because of the different patient populations studied but appears to be comparable. Unicompartmental unicondylar arthroplasty appears to offer higher patient-reported outcomes than high tibial osteotomy, but return to activity is equivalent with both procedures. Based on data from multiple arthroplasty registries, survivorship for conversion from both failed high tibial osteotomy and failed unicondylar arthroplasty to TKA appears to be lower than survivorship for primary TKA.

TKA in Patients With Obesity or Other Comorbidities
Obesity

Over the past two decades, the number of individuals with obesity (body mass index [BMI] more than 20% above ideal body weight or $\geq30\,kg/m^2$) has increased worldwide.[70-72] In 2005, the World Health Organization predicted that approximately 10% of the world population (more than 400 million adults) had obesity. Patients with obesity have a higher risk for the development of osteoarthritis at an earlier age than the general nonobese population.[73-76] TKA is increasingly being offered to patients with obesity who were not previously routinely considered candidates for the procedure. With the projected sevenfold increase in the number of TKAs that will be performed by 2030, the dilemma of how best to treat patients with obesity, and what outcomes to expect, will likely become more common,[77,78] and future surgeons will likely see more patients with obesity in their practice.

Commonly reported negative effects of obesity after TKA include prolonged wound drainage, delayed wound healing, high infection rates, more medical complications, poor mobilization, and a lower tolerance for physical therapy.[79-81] Although there is a broad consensus that obesity is directly associated with these complications, it is unclear based on individual studies whether a specific cutoff exists in which patients above the cutoff are placed at a substantially higher risk.[79-81] D'Apuzzo et al[82] reported that patients with morbid obesity (BMI $>40\,kg/m^2$) may have a higher risk of postoperative infection and wound dehiscence. Other studies have reported that a BMI greater than $40\,kg/m^2$ may be used as a cutoff to gauge treatment options as well as guide patient education and outcome expectations.[83] This consideration is particularly important for surgeons during clinical decision making to determine whether to proceed with arthroplasty.

Implant Survivorship

Implant survivorship at longer follow-up has been reported to be higher in patients who had a BMI less than $30\,kg/m^2$ compared with patients with obesity or morbid obesity.[84,85] Amin et al[84] reported that 5-year implant survivorship (mean follow-up, 3 years; range, 6 months to 6 years), using revision as an end point, was substantially lower in patients with morbid obesity (72.3%) compared with patients who had a BMI of less than $30\,kg/m^2$ (97.6%). A study by McElroy et al[83] also reported that patients with morbid obesity (BMI $\geq40\,kg/m^2$) had a lower implant survivorship than patients with obesity (BMI $\geq30\,kg/m^2$ but $<40\,kg/m^2$) and patients without obesity (BMI $<30\,kg/m^2$) at a mean follow-up of 5 years (88% versus 95% versus 97%, respectively; $P < 0.05$). Conversely, Lizaur-Utrilla et al[86] reported no difference in 7-year implant survivorship (mean follow-up, 7 years; range, 5 to 10 years) between obese ($>30\,kg/m^2$) and nonobese groups ($<30\,kg/m^2$; 89% versus 92%, respectively; $P = 0.439$). In addition, Naziri et al[85] reported no significant differences in implant survivorship between patients with super-obesity and patients without obesity (94% versus 98%) at a short-term follow-up of 5 years (range, 3 to 7 years).

Clinical Outcomes

Improvements in clinical outcomes, as measured by objective and functional Knee Society Scores, have been reported in all patients (controls, obese, morbidly obese, super-obese) after TKA.[87-89] However, Winiarsky et al[90] reported significantly higher postoperative Knee Society Scores in patients without obesity (92 points) compared with patients with obesity (84 points; $P < 0.001$) at a mean follow-up of 5 years (range, 2 to 13 years). A study by Dewan et al[91] reported similar changes in objective and functional Knee Society Scores for a control group (89 and 66 points, respectively) compared with a cohort of patients with morbid obesity (85 and 68 points, respectively) at a mean follow-up of 5 years (range, 2 to 15 years). Naziri et al[85] reported comparable objective Knee Society Scores between patients with super-obesity and patients without obesity; however, functional Knee Society Scores were significantly lower in patients with super-obesity compared with patients without obesity (82 versus 90 points) at a mean follow-up of 5 years (range, 3 to 7 years).

Radiographic Outcomes

A paucity of studies have reported an increase in radiolucent lines in patients with obesity or morbid obesity compared with patients without obesity.[84] Amin et al[84] reported that a significant increase in radiolucent lines was found in patients with morbid obesity compared with patients without morbid obesity (29% versus 7%, respectively; $P = 0.02$) at a mean follow up of approximately 3.2 years (range, 0.5 to 5.5 years). Other studies have shown no significant differences. For example, Dewan et al[91] reported that there was a tendency toward an increase in radiolucent lines in patients with morbid obesity (35%) at a mean follow-up of 5 years (range, 2 to 15 years); however, the increase was not significant compared with a control group (28%).

Complications

Patients with morbid obesity and super-obesity may have a higher incidence of overall postoperative complications compared with patients who have lower BMIs.[82,91,92] A study by Dowsey et al[92] reported that, even at 1-year follow-up

(no range given), there was a higher incidence of complications in patients with morbid obesity (35%) compared with a control group (14%). In addition, Dewan et al[91] reported that patients with obesity had higher complication rates than patients without obesity at a mean follow-up of 5 years (range, 2 to 15 years); however, the difference was not significant (16% versus 15%, respectively; $P = 0.301$). D'Apuzzo et al[82] reported that patients with morbid obesity who underwent TKA had a significantly higher risk of postoperative in-hospital infection, wound dehiscence, genitourinary complications, and postoperative mortality, as well as higher total hospital costs than patients without obesity; however, patients with morbid obesity were not at a higher risk for cardiovascular or thromboembolic complications. Conversely, Krushell and Fingeroth[93] reported that there was no significant difference in the incidence of complications (specifically, revision surgery and patellar fractures) at a long-term follow up of 7.5 years (range, 5.2 to 14.1 years) between patients with morbid obesity and patients without obesity.

Other Comorbidities

Various comorbidities, including hypertension, diabetes, coronary artery disease, chronic renal failure, systemic inflammatory diseases, and immuno-compromising diseases, have been reported to affect the clinical outcomes of primary TKA.[94] Parameters that have been evaluated to determine if various comorbidities affect perioperative and postoperative outcomes include hospital length of stay, discharge disposition, healthcare costs, and postoperative complications.[95] With the rise in healthcare costs, there has been growing interest in

identifying measures that may decrease the economic burden of patients who have comorbidities on the healthcare system. It is known that patients who have preoperative medical comorbidities consume more perioperative resources than patients who do not have preoperative medical comorbidities; this results in higher treatment expenditures for patients with comorbidities.[96] Some studies have suggested that the proper identification and characterization of patients who have preoperative medical comorbidities may result in appropriate perioperative interventions to optimize patients and, thus, reduce their burden on the healthcare system.[97,98]

Clinical Outcomes

Patients who have more comorbidities have been reported to have poorer postoperative TKA outcomes compared with patients who do not have preoperative medial comorbidities.[95,98] In a study of the effects of various medical comorbidities on postoperative outcomes for patients who underwent TKA, Wasielewski et al[95] reported that patients who had a greater number of comorbidities had significantly lower preoperative knee scores compared with patients who had fewer comorbidities (46 points versus 29 points; $P = 0.0001$). In addition, patients who had four or more risk factors had significantly lower Medical Outcomes Study 36-Item Short Form physical component scores ($P = 0.044$) at a 3-month follow-up. As the number of medical comorbidities increased, the hospital length of stay also significantly increased ($P = 0.023$). Similarly, SooHoo et al[98] analyzed 222,684 patients who underwent TKA to determine the effect of comorbidities on postoperative outcomes with the use of the Charleston Comorbidity Index.

The authors reported that an increase in the Charleston Comorbidity Index from 0 to 1 resulted in a 161% increase in the probability of mortality, and that an increase in the Charleston Comorbidity Index to more than 2 resulted in a 519% increase. Similarly, there was an increase in the infection rate from 0.59% to 1.18% as the Charleston Comorbidity Index increased.

Although there is a general correlation between a greater number of medical comorbidities and poorer postoperative outcomes, whether any single factor contributes to this correlation is uncertain because of the contrasting evidence, particularly if each comorbidity is specifically evaluated. For example, a study by Meding et al[99] reported that patients with diabetes mellitus had a higher infection rate and a significantly higher revision surgery rate after TKA compared with patients who did not have diabetes mellitus (1.2% versus 0.7%, respectively; $P > 0.05$, and 3.6% versus 0.4%, respectively; $P < 0.05$). However, a recent study of 40,491 TKA patients reported no significant differences in the incidence of deep infection, revision surgery, and deep vein thrombosis between patients who had diabetes mellitus and those who did not have diabetes mellitus.[100] In a study on the effect of demographic and comorbid factors on activity levels after TKA, Issa et al[101] reported that older age, tobacco use, history of malignancy, cardiovascular disease, lymphatic disease, and renal disease had a significant negative effect on postoperative activity levels.

Conclusions

Patients with obesity or other medical comorbidities may have poorer outcomes compared with patients without obesity or other medical comorbidities if they undergo TKA. However, the effects of these conditions may be synergistic with other factors that may contribute to clinical outcomes. More prospective studies are necessary to better evaluate outcomes in patients with obesity and other comorbidities.

TKA in Patients With Cardiovascular Pathology

Cardiovascular, cerebrovascular, and peripheral vascular diseases are highly prevalent in patients who are candidates for TKA. There are concerns for postoperative risks and mortality in patients who have vascular diseases, and it is unclear if they require specialized preoperative assessments. Complications and risks associated with TKA may also be increased in patients who have vascular diseases if they are being treated with anticoagulants, such as clopidogrel. Although prescription guidelines recommend the discontinuation of clopidogrel 5 days before surgery, there is an increased risk of thromboembolic and cardiovascular events, particularly with lower extremity arthroplasty, if it is withheld for an extended period of time.[102] Whether an anticoagulant should be withheld remains controversial. If an anticoagulant is withheld, the optimal amount of time it should be withheld before surgery and the earliest it can be restarted safely also remain controversial.

Postoperative Outcomes

A patient's cardiac history and anticoagulant use are the most prominent factors that affect postoperative recovery and outcomes. Nandi et al[102] reviewed the relationship between preoperative clopidogrel administration and postoperative bleeding events in 114 patients who underwent total hip or total knee arthroplasty. The arthroplasties were divided into three groups based on the length of time clopidogrel was withheld before surgery: 0 days (n=8), 1 to 4 days (n=17), and 5 or more days (n=89). The authors reported that patients who had clopidogrel withheld for 5 or more days before surgery had fewer postoperative bleeding-related events and lower rates of infection that required revision surgery ($P = 0.014$). In addition, patients who did not discontinue clopidogrel at least 5 days before surgery had a higher incidence of postoperative antibiotic use for wound drainage and/or cellulitis ($P = 0.001$). Jacob et al[103] assessed the perioperative use of clopidogrel in 142 patients who underwent primary or revision total hip or total knee arthroplasty, 24 of whom continued and 118 of whom discontinued clopidogrel use perioperatively. The authors reported no significant difference in postoperative hemoglobin levels between patients who continued clopidogrel perioperatively compared with patients who discontinued clopidogrel perioperatively (9.6 g/dL versus 10.6 g/dL, respectively; $P = 0.06$); however, patients who continued clopidogrel perioperatively were more likely to receive a blood transfusion within 24 hours postoperatively than patients who discontinued clopidogrel preoperatively (31.8% versus 7.7%, respectively; $P = 0.004$). In addition, the authors reported no significant difference in acute coronary events between the two groups of patients ($P = 0.28$).

Singh et al[104] evaluated the occurrence and predictors of cardiac events (eg, myocardial infarction, congestive heart failure, or arrhythmia) and thromboembolic events (deep vein thrombosis or pulmonary embolism) in patients who underwent TKA. The authors reported that 16.7% of patients who had a previous cardiac event (n=514) and 2% of patients who had no prior history of a cardiac event (n=1,094) experienced a cardiac event after TKA. Furthermore, 20.7% of patients who had a previous thromboembolic event (n=121) and 3.6% of patients who had no prior history of a thromboembolic event (n=1,487) experienced a thromboembolic event after TKA. Belmont et al[105] reported that patients who had a history of cardiac disease did not have an increased risk of mortality after TKA but did have an increased risk of minor local complications ($P = 0.01$).

Conclusions

A patient's cardiac history plays an important role in TKA outcomes. It is crucial that surgeons identify these high-risk patients to ensure adequate preoperative management and education. In addition, surgeons should consider if these patients require specialized thromboprophylaxis and management of comorbidities. The literature appears to support the discontinuation of anticoagulants, particularly clopidogrel, before surgery to reduce the risk of postoperative bleeding without increasing the risk of an acute coronary event.[103] However, discontinuation of anticoagulants remains controversial, and there are still advocates for the continuation of anticoagulants to prevent the risk of coronary events. If TKA is performed in patients who continue anticoagulant use, then surgeons must recognize the potential increase in transfusion requirements and the necessity for close postoperative monitoring.

TKA in Patients With Immunosuppression

Immunosuppression presents a challenge for patients who undergo all forms of surgery. A substantial proportion of patients with immunosuppression undergo joint arthroplasty, particularly those with a diagnosis of RA. In addition, patients may be being treated with medications that dampen the immune response, such as corticosteroids, anti-tumor necrosis factors (TNFs), and disease-modifying antirheumatic drugs.[106-109] Several studies have reported no increases in infection risk or impaired wound healing if disease-modifying antirheumatic drugs, such as methotrexate, are continued in the perioperative period.[110,111] It is recommended that other therapies, such as biologics, be withheld at least one dosage cycle before surgery (2 to 4 weeks) until staple or suture removal, to allow for progression of wound healing, or up to 4 weeks postoperatively;[110,112,113] however, data specific to elective orthopaedic surgery are limited.

Patients who have inflammatory arthropathies have a higher incidence of cardiac disease, pulmonary disease, and mortality; therefore, they require extensive preoperative planning, especially if general anesthesia will be used.[106] There also is concern that immunosuppression may affect postoperative recovery, particularly with respect to wound healing and the incidence of postoperative infection. Patients with RA have a significantly higher risk of prosthetic joint infection after TKA compared with patients who have OA (4.2% versus 1.4%, respectively; $P = 0.05$). Active diseases that are associated with swollen joints and elevated inflammatory markers are themselves associated with a higher risk of infection after arthroplasty; however,

the use of immunosuppressant medications, such as disease-modifying antirheumatic drugs, may increase the likelihood of delayed wound healing postoperatively.[106]

In a study on the risk of postoperative complications in patients who were treated with and without methotrexate (n=60 and n=61, respectively) and underwent large joint arthroplasty, Perhala et al[108] reported no significant differences in wound healing and infectious complications between the two groups ($P = 0.366$). Visser et al[109] reported that the risk of infection was higher in patients who were treated with corticosteroids compared with patients who were treated with methotrexate, and recommended that patients who are being treated with methotrexate should continue methotrexate use during the perioperative period. Furthermore, corticosteroid use has been consistently associated with a higher risk of perioperative infection. This increased risk of perioperative infection has been reported with corticosteroid doses of less than 5 mg per day, and the risk increased with the duration of therapy.[106] Patients who are being treated with corticosteroids are at risk for adrenal suppression secondary to prolonged steroid use, particularly if subjected to the stress of surgery. It has been recommended that during the perioperative period, patients who are being treated with corticosteroids receive intravenous hydrocortisone, which should be immediately tapered to the usual preoperative dose after hemodynamic stability is acheived.[114,115] Anti-TNF agents also have been associated with higher rates of surgical site infection and prosthetic joint infections, particularly in the first 6 months of therapy.[106] Gilson et al[107] reported that only steroid use was associated with higher infection rates after total joint arthroplasty ($P = 0.03$); however, TNF-blocker use was a predictor of infection after total joint arthroplasty.

Other immunodeficiency diseases, such as HIV, theoretically pose a risk for patients who undergo arthroplasty. Lin et al[116] evaluated the effect of HIV on outcomes after total hip and knee arthroplasty and reported that there was no difference in the complication rates between HIV-positive and HIV-negative patients who underwent TKA; however, HIV-positive patients had a significantly longer hospital length of stay (more than 4 days) compared with HIV-negative patients (36.4% versus 19.6%, respectively; $P < 0.001$). Furthermore, Capogna et al[117] reported no significant difference in deep infection rates, aseptic loosening, and survivorship ($P = 0.11$, 0.06, and 0.09, respectively) between patients with and without HIV after total joint arthroplasty.

Immunosuppression may pose a risk for patients who undergo arthroplasty; however, these risks can be managed with early preoperative assessment and close postoperative monitoring. The evidence in the literature is inconclusive on steroid use; therefore, the treatment for patients who use steroids should be tailored to each patient's length of use, regular dosing, and risk for adrenal insufficiency on discontinuation.[114] Agents such as methotrexate can be continued in the preoperative period; however, biologic agents, such as anti-TNF drugs, should be discontinued 2 to 4 weeks before surgery and resumed after wound healing is demonstrated (approximately 2 weeks after surgery), or surgery should be planned at the end of a dosing cycle.[106]

Summary

Multiple patient-specific and surgical factors may influence recovery and outcomes after TKA. Minimal releases and meticulous surgical technique may restore alignment and balance in patients who have severe varus and valgus deformities; however, the best technique remains undefined. It is important for surgeons to consider the potential etiology of a stiff knee before surgery because it may substantially affect the management and outcome of TKA. Surgeons may have to perform additional steps, such as a quadriceps snip, to obtain adequate exposure in some patients who have a stiff knee. TKA after failed tibial osteotomy or unicondylar arthroplasty may be challenging because of prior skin incisions, retained hardware, and the presence of deformity and bone loss. In addition, patients who have certain comorbidities, such as morbid obesity, rheumatoid arthritis, and cardiovascular pathology, require careful preoperative assessment because they may be immunosuppressed or have an increased risk of postoperative complications.

References

1. Berend ME, Ritter MA, Meding JB, et al: Tibial component failure mechanisms in total knee arthroplasty. *Clin Orthop Relat Res* 2004;428:26-34.

2. Jeffery RS, Morris RW, Denham RA: Coronal alignment after total knee replacement. *J Bone Joint Surg Br* 1991;73(5):709-714.

3. Morgan SS, Bonshahi A, Pradhan N, Gregory A, Gambhir A, Porter ML: The influence of postoperative coronal alignment on revision surgery in total knee arthroplasty. *Int Orthop* 2008;32(5):639-642.

4. Parratte S, Pagnano MW, Trousdale RT, Berry DJ: Effect of postoperative mechanical axis alignment on the fifteen-year survival of modern, cemented total knee replacements. *J Bone Joint Surg Am* 2010;92(12):2143-2149.

5. Ritter MA, Faris PM, Keating EM, Meding JB: Postoperative alignment of total knee replacement: Its effect on survival. *Clin Orthop Relat Res* 1994;299:153-156.

6. Ritter MA, Davis KE, Davis P, et al: Preoperative malalignment increases risk of failure after total knee arthroplasty. *J Bone Joint Surg Am* 2013;95(2):126-131.

7. Krackow KA: Deformity, in *The Technique of Total Knee Arthroplasty*. St. Louis, MO, CV Mosby, 1990, pp 261-280.

8. Verdonk PC, Pernin J, Pinaroli A, Ait Si Selmi T, Neyret P: Soft tissue balancing in varus total knee arthroplasty: An algorithmic approach. *Knee Surg Sports Traumatol Arthrosc* 2009;17(6):660-666.

9. Meftah M, Blum YC, Raja D, Ranawat AS, Ranawat CS: Correcting fixed varus deformity with flexion contracture during total knee arthroplasty: The "inside-out" technique. AAOS exhibit selection. *J Bone Joint Surg Am* 2012;94(10):e66.

10. Dixon MC, Parsch D, Brown RR, Scott RD: The correction of severe varus deformity in total knee arthroplasty by tibial component downsizing and resection of uncapped proximal medial bone. *J Arthroplasty* 2004;19(1):19-22.

11. Bellemans J, Vandenneucker H, Van Lauwe J, Victor J: A new surgical technique for medial collateral ligament balancing: Multiple needle puncturing. *J Arthroplasty* 2010;25(7):1151-1156.

12. Clarke HD, Scuderi GR: Lateral ligament release for valgus deformity in primary total knee arthroplasty. *Techniques in Knee Surgery* 2003;2(2):74-81.

13. Krackow KA, Jones MM, Teeny SM, Hungerford DS: Primary total knee arthroplasty in patients with fixed valgus deformity. *Clin Orthop Relat Res* 1991;273:9-18.

14. Clarke HD, Fuchs R, Scuderi GR, Scott WN, Insall JN: Clinical results in valgus total knee arthroplasty with the "pie crust" technique of lateral

soft tissue releases. *J Arthroplasty* 2005;20(8):1010-1014.

15. Elkus M, Ranawat CS, Rasquinha VJ, Babhulkar S, Rossi R, Ranawat AS: Total knee arthroplasty for severe valgus deformity: Five to fourteen-year follow-up. *J Bone Joint Surg Am* 2004;86(12):2671-2676.

16. Easley ME, Insall JN, Scuderi GR, Bullek DD: Primary constrained condylar knee arthroplasty for the arthritic valgus knee. *Clin Orthop Relat Res* 2000;380:58-64.

17. Engh GA: The difficult knee: Severe varus and valgus. *Clin Orthop Relat Res* 2003;416:58-63.

18. Whiteside LA: Soft tissue balancing: The knee. *J Arthroplasty* 2002; 17(4, suppl 1):23-27.

19. Ritter MA, Faris GW, Faris PM, Davis KE: Total knee arthroplasty in patients with angular varus or valgus deformities of > or = 20 degrees. *J Arthroplasty* 2004;19(7):862-866.

20. Aglietti P, Lup D, Cuomo P, Baldini A, De Luca L: Total knee arthroplasty using a pie-crusting technique for valgus deformity. *Clin Orthop Relat Res* 2007;464:73-77.

21. Miyasaka KC, Ranawat CS, Mullaji A: 10- to 20-year followup of total knee arthroplasty for valgus deformities. *Clin Orthop Relat Res* 1997;345:29-37.

22. Politi J, Scott R: Balancing severe valgus deformity in total knee arthroplasty using a lateral cruciform retinacular release. *J Arthroplasty* 2004;19(5):553-557.

23. Ranawat AS, Ranawat CS, Elkus M, Rasquinha VJ, Rossi R, Babhulkar S: Total knee arthroplasty for severe valgus deformity. *J Bone Joint Surg Am* 2005;87(pt 2, suppl 1):271-284.

24. Krackow KA, Mihalko WM: Flexion-extension joint gap changes after lateral structure release for valgus deformity correction in total knee arthroplasty: A cadaveric study. *J Arthroplasty* 1999;14(8):994-1004.

25. Insall J, Scott WN, Ranawat CS: The total condylar knee prosthesis: A report of two hundred and twenty cases. *J Bone Joint Surg Am* 1979;61(2):173-180.

26. McAuley JP, Collier MB, Hamilton WG, Tabaraee E, Engh GA: Posterior cruciate-retaining total knee arthroplasty for valgus osteoarthritis. *Clin Orthop Relat Res* 2008;466(11):2644-2649.

27. Healy WL, Iorio R, Lemos DW: Medial reconstruction during total knee arthroplasty for severe valgus deformity. *Clin Orthop Relat Res* 1998;356:161-169.

28. Asp JP, Rand JA: Peroneal nerve palsy after total knee arthroplasty. *Clin Orthop Relat Res* 1990;261:233-237.

29. Bruzzone M, Ranawat A, Castoldi F, Dettoni F, Rossi P, Rossi R: The risk of direct peroneal nerve injury using the Ranawat "inside-out" lateral release technique in valgus total knee arthroplasty. *J Arthroplasty* 2010;25(1):161-165.

30. Hitt K: Prevention and management of neurovascular injuries. *Seminars in Arthroplasty* 2003;14(4):194-202.

31. Rajgopal A, Ahuja N, Dolai B: Total knee arthroplasty in stiff and ankylosed knees. *J Arthroplasty* 2005;20(5):585-590.

32. Bae DK, Yoon KH, Kim HS, Song SJ: Total knee arthroplasty in stiff knees after previous infection. *J Bone Joint Surg Br* 2005;87(3):333-336.

33. Ritter MA, Harty LD, Davis KE, Meding JB, Berend ME: Predicting range of motion after total knee arthroplasty: Clustering, log-linear regression, and regression tree analysis. *J Bone Joint Surg Am* 2003;85(7):1278-1285.

34. Bonnin M, Amendola NA, Bellemans J, MacDonald SJ, Ménétrey J, eds: *The Knee Joint: Surgical Techniques and Strategies.* Paris, France, Springer-Verlag, 2013.

35. Bellemans J, Steenwerckx A, Brabants K, Victor J, Lammens J, Fabry G: The Judet quadricepsplasty: A retrospective analysis of 16 cases. *Acta Orthop Belg* 1996;62(2):79-82.

36. Ritter MA, Lutgring JD, Davis KE, Berend ME, Pierson JL, Meneghini RM: The role of flexion contracture on outcomes in primary total knee arthroplasty. *J Arthroplasty* 2007;22(8):1092-1096.

37. Perry J, Antonelli D, Ford W: Analysis of knee-joint forces during flexed-knee stance. *J Bone Joint Surg Am* 1975;57(7):961-967.

38. Garvin KL, Scuderi G, Insall JN: Evolution of the quadriceps snip. *Clin Orthop Relat Res* 1995;321:131-137.

39. Arsht SJ, Scuderi GR: The quadriceps snip for exposing the stiff knee. *J Knee Surg* 2003;16(1):55-57.

40. Barrack RL: Specialized exposure for revision total knee arthroplasty: Quadriceps snip and patellar turndown. *Instr Course Lect* 1999;48:149-152.

41. Barrack R: Surgical exposure of the stiff knee. *Acta Orthop Scand* 2000;71(1):85-89.

42. Barrack RL, Smith P, Munn B, Engh G, Rorabeck C: The Ranawat Award: Comparison of surgical approaches in total knee arthroplasty. *Clin Orthop Relat Res* 1998;356:16-21.

43. Meek RM, Greidanus NV, McGraw RW, Masri BA: The extensile rectus snip exposure in revision of total knee arthroplasty. *J Bone Joint Surg Br* 2003;85(8):1120-1122.

44. Aglietti P, Windsor RE, Buzzi R, Insall JN: Arthroplasty for the stiff or ankylosed knee. *J Arthroplasty* 1989;4(1):1-5.

45. Jacofsky DJ, Della Valle CJ, Meneghini RM, Sporer SM, Cercek RM; American Academy of Orthopaedic Surgeons: Revision total knee arthroplasty: What the practicing orthopaedic surgeon needs to know. *J Bone Joint Surg Am* 2010;92(5):1282-1292.

46. Whiteside LA: Exposure in difficult total knee arthroplasty using tibial tubercle osteotomy. *Clin Orthop Relat Res* 1995;321:32-35.

47. Whiteside LA, Ohl MD: Tibial tubercle osteotomy for exposure of the difficult total knee arthroplasty. *Clin Orthop Relat Res* 1990;260:6-9.

48. Bellemans J, Vandenneucker H, Victor J, Vanlauwe J: Flexion contracture in total knee arthroplasty. *Clin Orthop Relat Res* 2006;452:78-82.

49. Bhan S, Malhotra R, Kiran EK: Comparison of total knee arthroplasty in stiff and ankylosed knees. *Clin Orthop Relat Res* 2006;451:87-95.

© 2016 AAOS Instructional Course Lectures, Volume 65

50. Lu H, Mow CS, Lin J: Total knee arthroplasty in the presence of severe flexion contracture: A report of 37 cases. *J Arthroplasty* 1999;14(7):775-780.

51. Kim YH, Kim JS: Does TKA improve functional outcome and range of motion in patients with stiff knees? *Clin Orthop Relat Res* 2009;467(5):1348-1354.

52. Kim YH, Kim JS: Total knee replacement for patients with ankylosed knees. *J Bone Joint Surg Br* 2008;90(10):1311-1316.

53. Spahn G, Hofmann GO, von Engelhardt LV, Li M, Neubauer H, Klinger HM: The impact of a high tibial valgus osteotomy and unicondylar medial arthroplasty on the treatment for knee osteoarthritis: A meta-analysis. *Knee Surg Sports Traumatol Arthrosc* 2013;21(1):96-112.

54. Fu D, Li G, Chen K, Zhao Y, Hua Y, Cai Z: Comparison of high tibial osteotomy and unicompartmental knee arthroplasty in the treatment of unicompartmental osteoarthritis: A meta-analysis. *J Arthroplasty* 2013;28(5):759-765.

55. Dettoni F, Bonasia DE, Castoldi F, Bruzzone M, Blonna D, Rossi R: High tibial osteotomy versus unicompartmental knee arthroplasty for medial compartment arthrosis of the knee: A review of the literature. *Iowa Orthop J* 2010;30:131-140.

56. Yim JH, Song EK, Seo HY, Kim MS, Seon JK: Comparison of high tibial osteotomy and unicompartmental knee arthroplasty at a minimum follow-up of 3 years. *J Arthroplasty* 2013;28(2):243-247.

57. Nwachukwu BU, McCormick FM, Schairer WW, Frank RM, Provencher MT, Roche MW: Unicompartmental knee arthroplasty versus high tibial osteotomy: United States practice patterns for the surgical treatment of unicompartmental arthritis. *J Arthroplasty* 2014;29(8):1586-1589.

58. Dietz FR, Kelman MG: Surgeon age as the major factor in recommendation of uni-compartmental knee replacement versus high tibial osteotomy: A case study in orthopaedic decision making. *Iowa Orthop J* 2012;32:22-27.

59. Koskinen E, Eskelinen A, Paavolainen P, Pulkkinen P, Remes V: Comparison of survival and cost-effectiveness between unicondylar arthroplasty and total knee arthroplasty in patients with primary osteoarthritis: A follow-up study of 50,493 knee replacements from the Finnish Arthroplasty Register. *Acta Orthop* 2008;79(4):499-507.

60. Pabinger C, Berghold A, Boehler N, Labek G: Revision rates after knee replacement: Cumulative results from worldwide clinical studies versus joint registers. *Osteoarthritis Cartilage* 2013;21(2):263-268.

61. Preston S, Howard J, Naudie D, Somerville L, McAuley J: Total knee arthroplasty after high tibial osteotomy: No differences between medial and lateral osteotomy approaches. *Clin Orthop Relat Res* 2014;472(1):105-110.

62. Bastos Filho R, Magnussen RA, Duthon V, et al: Total knee arthroplasty after high tibial osteotomy: A comparison of opening and closing wedge osteotomy. *Int Orthop* 2013;37(3):427-431.

63. Meding JB, Wing JT, Ritter MA: Does high tibial osteotomy affect the success or survival of a total knee replacement? *Clin Orthop Relat Res* 2011;469(7):1991-1994.

64. Ramappa M, Anand S, Jennings A: Total knee replacement following high tibial osteotomy versus total knee replacement without high tibial osteotomy: A systematic review and meta analysis. *Arch Orthop Trauma Surg* 2013;133(11):1587-1593.

65. Niinimäki T, Eskelinen A, Ohtonen P, Puhto AP, Mann BS, Leppilahti J: Total knee arthroplasty after high tibial osteotomy: A registry-based case-control study of 1,036 knees. *Arch Orthop Trauma Surg* 2014;134(1):73-77.

66. Springer BD, Scott RD, Thornhill TS: Conversion of failed unicompartmental knee arthroplasty to TKA. *Clin Orthop Relat Res* 2006;446:214-220.

67. Sarraf KM, Konan S, Pastides PS, Haddad FS, Oussedik S: Bone loss during revision of unicompartmental to total knee arthroplasty: An analysis of implanted polyethylene thickness from the National Joint Registry data. *J Arthroplasty* 2013;28(9):1571-1574.

68. Pearse AJ, Hooper GJ, Rothwell AG, Frampton C: Osteotomy and unicompartmental knee arthroplasty converted to total knee arthroplasty: Data from the New Zealand Joint Registry. *J Arthroplasty* 2012;27(10):1827-1831.

69. Robertsson O, W-Dahl A: The risk of revision after TKA is affected by previous HTO or UKA. *Clin Orthop Relat Res* 2015;473(1):90-93.

70. Lahti-Koski M, Seppänen-Nuijten E, Männistö S, et al: Twenty-year changes in the prevalence of obesity among Finnish adults. *Obes Rev* 2010;11(3):171-176.

71. Sturm R: Increases in morbid obesity in the USA: 2000-2005. *Public Health* 2007;121(7):492-496.

72. Mokdad AH, Ford ES, Bowman BA, et al: Prevalence of obesity, diabetes, and obesity-related health risk factors, 2001. *JAMA* 2003;289(1):76-79.

73. Coggon D, Reading I, Croft P, McLaren M, Barrett D, Cooper C: Knee osteoarthritis and obesity. *Int J Obes Relat Metab Disord* 2001;25(5):622-627.

74. Manek NJ, Hart D, Spector TD, MacGregor AJ: The association of body mass index and osteoarthritis of the knee joint: An examination of genetic and environmental influences. *Arthritis Rheum* 2003;48(4):1024-1029.

75. Oliveria SA, Felson DT, Cirillo PA, Reed JI, Walker AM: Body weight, body mass index, and incident symptomatic osteoarthritis of the hand, hip, and knee. *Epidemiology* 1999;10(2):161-166.

76. Tukker A, Visscher TL, Picavet HS: Overweight and health problems of the lower extremities: Osteoarthritis, pain and disability. *Public Health Nutr* 2009;12(3):359-368.

77. Kurtz S, Ong K, Lau E, Mowat F, Halpern M: Projections of primary and revision hip and knee arthroplasty in the United States from 2005 to 2030. *J Bone Joint Surg Am* 2007;89(4):780-785.

78. Mokdad AH, Serdula MK, Dietz WH, Bowman BA, Marks JS, Koplan JP: The spread of the obesity epidemic in the United States, 1991-1998. *JAMA* 1999;282(16):1519-1522.

79. Gillespie GN, Porteous AJ: Obesity and knee arthroplasty. *Knee* 2007;14(2):81-86.

80. Dowsey MM, Choong PF: Early outcomes and complications following joint arthroplasty in obese patients: A review of the published reports. *ANZ J Surg* 2008;78(6):439-444.

81. Samson AJ, Mercer GE, Campbell DG: Total knee replacement in the morbidly obese: A literature review. *ANZ J Surg* 2010;80(9):595-599.

82. D'Apuzzo MR, Novicoff WM, Browne JA: The John Insall Award: Morbid obesity independently impacts complications, mortality, and resource use after TKA. *Clin Orthop Relat Res* 2015;473(1):57-63.

83. McElroy MJ, Pivec R, Issa K, Harwin SF, Mont MA: The effects of obesity and morbid obesity on outcomes in TKA. *J Knee Surg* 2013;26(2):83-88.

84. Amin AK, Clayton RA, Patton JT, Gaston M, Cook RE, Brenkel IJ: Total knee replacement in morbidly obese patients: Results of a prospective, matched study. *J Bone Joint Surg Br* 2006;88(10):1321-1326.

85. Naziri Q, Issa K, Malkani AL, Bonutti PM, Harwin SF, Mont MA: Bariatric orthopaedics: Total knee arthroplasty in super-obese patients (BMI > 50 kg/m2). Survivorship and complications. *Clin Orthop Relat Res* 2013;471(11):3523-3530.

86. Lizaur-Utrilla A, Miralles-Muñoz FA, Sanz-Reig J, Collados-Maestre I: Cementless total knee arthroplasty in obese patients: A prospective matched study with follow-up of 5-10 years. *J Arthroplasty* 2014;29(6):1192-1196.

87. Amin AK, Patton JT, Cook RE, Brenkel IJ: Does obesity influence the clinical outcome at five years following total knee replacement for osteoarthritis? *J Bone Joint Surg Br* 2006;88(3):335-340.

88. Hamoui N, Kantor S, Vince K, Crookes PF: Long-term outcome of total knee replacement: Does obesity matter? *Obes Surg* 2006;16(1):35-38.

89. Mont MA, Mathur SK, Krackow KA, Loewy JW, Hungerford DS: Cementless total knee arthroplasty in obese patients: A comparison with a matched control group. *J Arthroplasty* 1996;11(2):153-156.

90. Winiarsky R, Barth P, Lotke P: Total knee arthroplasty in morbidly obese patients. *J Bone Joint Surg Am* 1998;80(12):1770-1774.

91. Dewan A, Bertolusso R, Karastinos A, Conditt M, Noble PC, Parsley BS: Implant durability and knee function after total knee arthroplasty in the morbidly obese patient. *J Arthroplasty* 2009;24(6, suppl):89-94, 94.e1-94.e3.

92. Dowsey MM, Liew D, Stoney JD, Choong PF: The impact of preoperative obesity on weight change and outcome in total knee replacement: A prospective study of 529 consecutive patients. *J Bone Joint Surg Br* 2010;92(4):513-520.

93. Krushell RJ, Fingeroth RJ: Primary total knee arthroplasty in morbidly obese patients: A 5- to 14-year follow-up study. *J Arthroplasty* 2007;22(6, suppl 2):77-80.

94. Adam RF, Noble J: Primary total knee arthroplasty in the elderly. *J Arthroplasty* 1994;9(5):495-497.

95. Wasielewski RC, Weed H, Prezioso C, Nicholson C, Puri RD: Patient comorbidity: Relationship to outcomes of total knee arthroplasty. *Clin Orthop Relat Res* 1998;356:85-92.

96. Ethgen O, Bruyère O, Richy F, Dardennes C, Reginster JY: Health-related quality of life in total hip and total knee arthroplasty: A qualitative and systematic review of the literature. *J Bone Joint Surg Am* 2004;86(5):963-974.

97. Soohoo NF, Zingmond DS, Lieberman JR, Ko CY: Optimal timeframe for reporting short-term complication rates after total knee arthroplasty. *J Arthroplasty* 2006;21(5):705-711.

98. SooHoo NF, Lieberman JR, Ko CY, Zingmond DS: Factors predicting complication rates following total knee replacement. *J Bone Joint Surg Am* 2006;88(3):480-485.

99. Meding JB, Reddleman K, Keating ME, et al: Total knee replacement in patients with diabetes mellitus. *Clin Orthop Relat Res* 2003;416:208-216.

100. Adams AL, Paxton EW, Wang JQ, et al: Surgical outcomes of total knee replacement according to diabetes status and glycemic control, 2001 to 2009. *J Bone Joint Surg Am* 2013;95(6):481-487.

101. Issa K, Jauregui JJ, Given K, Harwin SF, Mont MA: A prospective, longitudinal study of patient activity levels following total knee arthroplasty stratified by demographic and comorbid factors. *J Knee Surg* 2015;28(4):343-348.

102. Nandi S, Aghazadeh M, Talmo C, Robbins C, Bono J: Perioperative clopidogrel and postoperative events after hip and knee arthroplasties. *Clin Orthop Relat Res* 2012;470(5):1436-1441.

103. Jacob AK, Hurley SP, Loughran SM, Wetsch TM, Trousdale RT: Continuing clopidogrel during elective total hip and knee arthroplasty: Assessment of bleeding risk and adverse outcomes. *J Arthroplasty* 2014;29(2):325-328.

104. Singh JA, Jensen MR, Harmsen WS, Gabriel SE, Lewallen DG: Cardiac and thromboembolic complications and mortality in patients undergoing total hip and total knee arthroplasty. *Ann Rheum Dis* 2011;70(12):2082-2088.

105. Belmont PJ Jr, Goodman GP, Waterman BR, Bader JO, Schoenfeld AJ: Thirty-day postoperative complications and mortality following total knee arthroplasty: Incidence and risk factors among a national sample of 15,321 patients. *J Bone Joint Surg Am* 2014;96(1):20-26.

106. Goodman SM, Figgie M: Lower extremity arthroplasty in patients with inflammatory arthritis: Preoperative and perioperative management. *J Am Acad Orthop Surg* 2013;21(6):355-363.

107. Gilson M, Gossec L, Mariette X, et al: Risk factors for total joint arthroplasty infection in patients receiving tumor necrosis factor α-blockers: A case-control study. *Arthritis Res Ther* 2010;12(4):R145.

108. Perhala RS, Wilke WS, Clough JD, Segal AM: Local infectious complications following large joint replacement in rheumatoid arthritis patients treated with methotrexate versus those not treated with methotrexate. *Arthritis Rheum* 1991;34(2):146-152.

109. Visser K, Katchamart W, Loza E, et al: Multinational evidence-based

recommendations for the use of methotrexate in rheumatic disorders with a focus on rheumatoid arthritis: Integrating systematic literature research and expert opinion of a broad international panel of rheumatologists in the 3E Initiative. *Ann Rheum Dis* 2009;68(7):1086-1093.

110. Grennan DM, Gray J, Loudon J, Fear S: Methotrexate and early postoperative complications in patients with rheumatoid arthritis undergoing elective orthopaedic surgery. *Ann Rheum Dis* 2001;60(3):214-217.

111. Scanzello CR, Figgie MP, Nestor BJ, Goodman SM: Perioperative management of medications used in the treatment of rheumatoid arthritis. *HSS J* 2006;2(2):141-147.

112. Ledingham J, Deighton C; British Society for Rheumatology Standards, Guidelines and Audit Working Group: Update on the British Society for Rheumatology guidelines for prescribing TNFalpha blockers in adults with rheumatoid arthritis (update of previous guideline of April 2001. *Rheumatology (Oxford)* 2005;44(2):157-163.

113. Koike R, Takeuchi T, Eguchi K, Miyasaka N, Japan College of Rheumatology: Update on the Japanese guidelines for the use of infliximab and etanercept in rheumatoid arthritis. *Mod Rheumatol* 2007;17(6):451-458.

114. Hoes JN, Jacobs JW, Boers M, et al: EULAR evidence-based recommendations on the management of systemic glucocorticoid therapy in rheumatic diseases. *Ann Rheum Dis* 2007;66(12):1560-1567.

115. Lee JK, Choi CH: Total knee arthroplasty in rheumatoid arthritis. *Knee Surg Relat Res* 2012;24(1):1-6.

116. Lin CA, Kuo AC, Takemoto S: Comorbidities and perioperative complications in HIV-positive patients undergoing primary total hip and knee arthroplasty. *J Bone Joint Surg Am* 2013;95(11):1028-1036.

117. Capogna BM, Lovy A, Blum Y, Kim SJ, Felsen UR, Geller DS: Infection rate following total joint arthroplasty in the HIV population. *J Arthroplasty* 2013;28(8):1254-1258.

Video References

Hitt KD: Video. *Varus Preoperative Examination*. Temple, TX, 2015.

Hitt KD: Video. *Varus Approach and Osteophyte Removal*. Temple, TX, 2015.

Hitt KD: Video. *Varus Balancing*. Temple, TX, 2015.

Hitt KD: Video. *Varus Micropuncture*. Temple, TX, 2015.

Hitt KD: Video. *Valgus Preoperative Examination*. Temple, TX, 2015.

Hitt KD: Video. *Valgus Approach*. Temple, TX, 2015.

Hitt KD: Video. *Valgus Micropuncture*. Temple, TX, 2015.

SECTION

4

Spine

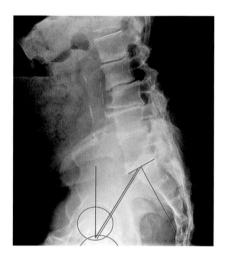

Spine

Treating the Aging Spine

Theodore J. Choma, MD
Glenn Rechtine, MD
Robert A. McGuire, MD
Darrel S. Brodke, MD

Abstract

Demographic trends make it incumbent on orthopaedic spine surgeons to recognize the special challenges involved in caring for older patients with spine pathology. Unique pathologies, such as osteoporosis and degenerative deformities, must be recognized and treated. Recent treatment options and recommendations for the medical optimization of bone health include vitamin D and calcium supplementation, diphosphonates, and teriparatide. Optimizing spinal fixation in elderly patients who have osteoporosis is critical; cement augmentation of pedicle screws is promising. In the management of geriatric odontoid fractures, nonsurgical support with a collar may be considered for low-demand patients, whereas surgical fixation is favored for high-demand patients. Management of degenerative deformity must address sagittal plane balance, which includes consideration of pelvic incidence. Various osteotomies may prove helpful in this setting.

Instr Course Lect 2016;65:269–280.

Between 2012 and 2050, the United States will experience considerable growth in its older population. By 2050, the population older than or equal to 65 years is projected to be 83.7 million, which is nearly double the 43.1 million that was estimated for 2012.[1] In 2012, the total US expenditure for Medicare was $572 billion; growth by 2023 is estimated to be more than $1.1 trillion.[2] As part of the overall surge in cost, orthopaedic surgeons will be faced with unique challenges in caring for an aging patient population; this is particularly true for spine surgeons who are treating a growing number of patients with traumatic or insufficiency spine fractures at the same time that they are treating patients with degenerative deformities and instabilities.

Although many of these challenges currently lack robust evidence to guide optimal treatment, common issues that spine surgeons who care for the aging patient population face, including perioperative bone health, spinal fixation strategies in the osteoporotic spine, odontoid fractures in elderly patients, the role of cement augmentation in elderly patients who have osteoporotic compression fractures, and planning principles in elderly patients who have spine deformity, will need to be addressed.

Medical Management

To a large extent, the perioperative medical treatment of the spine of an

Dr. Choma or an immediate family member serves as a paid consultant to or is an employee of Stryker; has stock or stock options held in Gentis; and serves as a board member, owner, officer, or committee member of AOSpine North America, the Scoliosis Research Society, and the North American Spine Society. Dr. Rechtine or an immediate family member serves as a board member, owner, officer, or committee member of the Cervical Spine Research Society. Dr. McGuire or an immediate family member has received royalties from DePuy; serves as a paid consultant to or is an employee of Synthes; and serves as a board member, owner, officer, or committee member of AOSpine North America. Dr. Brodke or an immediate family member has received royalties from Amedica, DePuy Synthes, and Medtronic; serves as a paid consultant to or is an employee of Amedica; has stock or stock options held in Amedica; and serves as a board member, owner, officer, or committee member of the Cervical Spine Research Society and the Lumbar Spine Research Society.

aging patient includes optimizing medical comorbidities: cardiac, pulmonary, renal, and endocrine. Most of these developments will be managed by a patient's primary team and consultants; however, given the prevalence of bone disease in the aging population, spine surgeons should pay special attention to a patient's bone health.

Evaluation of Bone Health

Women older than 65 years and men older than 70 years benefit from a dual-energy x-ray absorptiometry scan before major surgery such as a spine fusion or joint arthroplasty. The age that triggers the need for a dual-energy x-ray absorptiometry scan is reduced by 5 years for each comorbidity (eg, family history, tobacco use, early hysterectomy, history of fragility fracture). The orthopaedic surgeon who is treating a fragility spine fracture or contemplating spine fusion should order a dual-energy x-ray absorptiometry scan. Studies have reported that, if the orthopaedic surgeon initiates diagnosis and risk stratification, the likelihood that the patient will receive proper treatment increases dramatically.[3]

Routine preoperative evaluation for serum calcium value, 25-hydroxyvitamin D level, intact parathyroid hormone level, and, for males, testosterone level, should be performed. Target serum 25-hydroxyvitamin D levels should be greater than 30 ng/mL.[4] Normal testosterone levels vary for men and decrease with age in adults. It is unlikely that the orthopaedic surgeon is best qualified to make treatment decisions on testosterone supplementation, but based on the results of these evaluations, the patient may be referred for treatment by a metabolic bone expert.

Nutrition

Vitamin D is essential to bone health. Increasingly, vitamin D is being considered a hormone rather than a vitamin because its receptor has been found on the surfaces of many different cell types. For spine patients, the effect of vitamin D on the immune system may be just as important as it is for their bones.[5] Kroner et al[6] reported that "the facts that (i) immune cell functions are critically regulated by bioactive 1,25D; and (ii) immune cells metabolically participate in the generation of 1,25D from serum 25D, clearly document the importance of vitamin D in shaping immune responses."

Routinely recommending vitamin D supplementation for all spine fusion patients (especially those older than 65 years) may be the most efficient way to ensure that a patient will have a sufficient level of vitamin D at the time of surgery.[7] Vitamin D supplementation increases the likelihood of bone healing and may reduce the risk of surgical site infection.[8] A cohort of nursing home residents achieved vitamin D sufficiency with the supplementation of 800 IU/d of cholecalciferol (vitamin D_3).[9] As a fat-soluble vitamin in an increasingly obese elderly population, 1,000 to 2,000 IU/d of vitamin D_3 (available over the counter) is routinely recommended to address deficiency.[10] An alternative treatment algorithm for patients who have severe vitamin D deficiencies (<20 ng/mL) includes the prescription of 50,000 IU/wk of ergocalciferol (vitamin D_2) for 12 weeks followed by a recheck of vitamin D serum levels. Even with moderate sun exposure, 10,000 IU/d of vitamin D_3 can be used without the risk of vitamin D toxicity.[11,12]

Ensuring adequate calcium stores also is important to help prevent orthopaedic surgical complications. The typical choices for oral supplementation are calcium citrate and calcium carbonate. Calcium carbonate typically contains a higher percentage of elemental calcium and tends to be less expensive, but it is associated with more frequent gastrointestinal side effects and is not absorbed without an acidic stomach environment. Patients who take proton pump inhibitors, who require iron or zinc supplementation, who have inflammatory bowel disease, and who cannot take a calcium supplement with meals should be prescribed calcium citrate.[10] Approximately 1,000 mg/d of calcium in divided doses is required for most adults. The US Preventive Services Task Force reviewed the available literature and reported that, although low-dose vitamin D and calcium supplementation has not been reported to reduce the risk of fracture, they have been reported to decrease the risk of falls in those older than or equal to 65 years. The task force also reported insufficient evidence to recommend routine supplementation of more than or equal to 800 IU of vitamin D and more than or equal to 1200 mg of elemental calcium in the elderly population.[13] Clearly this is an area that requires further study. Vitamin D and calcium recommendations from the Institute of Medicine are shown in **Table 1**.[13]

Osteoporosis Medications

Diphosphonates have been reported to have a deleterious effect on fracture healing in some animal models.[14] This same negative effect has not been definitively shown to occur in humans.[15,16] Given these differences, it is difficult to make a strong recommendation on the timing to resume diphosphonate treatment in patients who have osteoporosis and spine fusion or fracture. Denosumab, a receptor activator of nuclear factor-κ B ligand inhibitor, has been reported to have a neutral effect on bone healing; however, it does promote increased bone density and reduction in future fractures.[17]

Teriparatide (ie, recombinant parathyroid hormone) is the only anabolic bone agent currently available; it requires daily subcutaneous injection. Teriparatide can be used for the treatment of patients who have severe osteoporosis or glucocorticoid-induced osteoporosis. It also is the drug of choice for patients with fragility fractures who are already being treated with diphosphonates. In a randomized, blinded trial, Peichl et al[18] reported that teriparatide use was associated with a quicker return of function and fracture healing in patients who had pubic ramus fractures. A pair of prospective studies evaluated teriparatide, diphosphonates, and control groups for pedicle fixation in patients who had degenerative spondylolisthesis; the risk of pedicle screw loosening was dramatically lower and the fusion rate was higher in the parathyroid hormone group.[19,20]

Osteoporosis Treatment After Fragility Fracture

No published data exist on spine surgeon compliance with treatment guidelines; however, a recent study reported that only 19% of patients who had surgically managed hip fractures received treatment within 1 year of fracture.[21] Over the past 15 years, there have been reports on a decline in the rate of osteoporosis treatment after fragility fracture by as much as one-half.[22-24] There may be an opportunity for improvement in this area.

Table 1
Institute of Medicine 2011 Recommended Daily Allowances for Vitamin D and Calcium

Age Group (yr)	Vitamin D	Calcium
Men and women aged 19–70	600 IU	1,000 mg for men 1,200 mg for women
Men and women aged >70	800 IU	1,200 mg

Adapted with permission from U.S. Preventive Services Task Force: Final recommendation statement: Vitamin D and calcium to prevent fractures. Preventive medication. February 2013. Available at: http://www.uspreventiveservicestaskforce.org/Page/Document/UpdateSummaryFinal/vitamin-d-and-calcium-to-prevent-fractures-preventive-medication. Accessed October 16, 2015.

Fixation in the Osteoporotic Spine

The increasing number of aged patients with osteopenia and osteoporosis who generally have a greater demand for an active lifestyle can be vexing for spine surgeons who are contemplating treatment of spinal instability or deformity in this population. Fixation is prone to failure at the bone-implant interface,[25,26] which has led some studies to recommend no surgical options for these older patients. Complications such as proximal junctional failure, pseudarthrosis with rod fracture, screw loosening, and prominent thoracolumbar fixation are well documented in this cohort.[27] To address these challenges, some surgeons have recommended using more points of fixation or protecting the construct with postoperative bracing; however, the evidence for these strategies is weak. There is evidence that larger diameter pedicle screws[28] as well as the addition of laminar hooks[29] improve fixation in osteoporotic vertebrae.

A growing body of literature indicates that pedicle screw augmentation with cement is an effective strategy to improve vertebral fixation in patients who have osteoporosis.[30,31] This effect appears to be maintained whether polymethyl methacrylate or various bioactive cements are used.[32] The augmentation

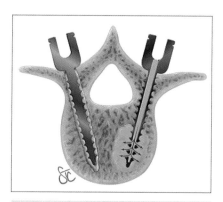

Figure 1   Illustration shows the two options for pedicle screw augmentation with cement: prefilling the pilot hole with cement before screw placement (left) or placing a cannulated screw with fenestrations and injecting cement through the screw (right).

effect also appears to remain substantial whether the cement is placed first and followed by a solid-core screw or the cement is injected through a cannulated pedicle screw[33] (**Figure 1**). It also is probable that pretapping pedicle screw pilot holes further enhances the augmentation effect if cement is used.[34] Although these screw-augmentation techniques are increasing in popularity, particularly in Europe, there is an inherent risk of cement extravasation into the venous system, spinal canal, or disk spaces.[35] Because this risk has been reported only sporadically to date, optimal strategies to mitigate them are not well defined.

Geriatric Odontoid Fractures

Odontoid fractures are the most common cervical spine fracture in adults older than 70 years and are increasing in prevalence.[36,37] At a point of maximal load during falls from a standing height, the presence of weak cortical and scant cancellous bone commonly lead to fractures at the base of the odontoid (ie, type II fractures), which affect treatment decision making. The first treatment decision is the choice between nonsurgical and surgical treatment, followed by the selection of an orthosis or a surgical approach. The fracture morphology, fracture location, angle of the fracture, degree of comminution, and amount of displacement as well as patient factors including the degree of osteoporosis, presence of dysphagia preinjury, and severity of cardiac and pulmonary comorbidities should be taken into account. The patient's social situation and levels of activity and mentation may play a substantial role in decision making. For example, a patient who has dementia and is minimally ambulatory may have such limited rehabilitation potential and/or life expectancy that the risk of surgery is unwarranted.

Nonsurgical Treatment

Nonsurgical treatment of geriatric patients who have odontoid fractures is common but not well studied. The halo vest, a traditional nonsurgical treatment for patients who have odontoid fractures, works relatively well; however, there is a documented nonunion rate in young and older patients who are treated with the vest. A substantially increased rate of morbidity and mortality is a larger problem in elderly patients

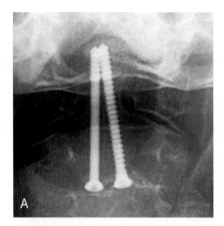 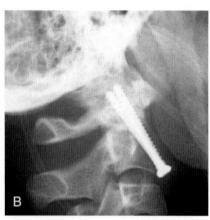

Figure 2 AP (**A**) and lateral (**B**) odontoid radiographs taken after two-screw fixation. Note that the partially threaded screw is placed first to lag the proximal fragment and gain compression at the fracture site. The fully threaded screw is placed second to buttress.

who undergo halo vest treatment.[38,39] Tashjian et al[38] reviewed 78 patients (mean age, 81 years) and reported that the risk of major complications in patients who wore a halo vest was double that of those who did not wear a halo vest (66% versus 36%, respectively) and the risk of mortality in patients who wore a halo vest was double that of those who did not wear a halo vest (42% versus 20%, respectively), both of which were statistically significant. The greatest concern in halo vest treatment is aspiration that may lead to pneumonia. Halo vest treatment should generally be avoided in the elderly population.

A hard cervical collar does not provide as much stability as a halo vest, but it may cause less morbidity.[40] The nonunion rate for hard cervical collars is high; however, if a stable pseudarthrosis is attained, hard cervical collars may be adequate in sedentary elderly patients.[41] Regardless of the treatment, odontoid fractures in elderly patients should be considered a sentinel event that has a fairly high mortality rate. In a review of 322 patients, Chapman et al[42] reported a 30-day mortality rate of 14%, which was markedly higher in the

nonsurgically treated population. In a large prospective study of 159 patients, Fehlings et al[43] reported an 18% mortality rate, which, again, was higher in the nonsurgically treated population. The case series that have reported nonunion rates for halo treatment (range, 10% to 50%) and hard collar (up to 77%) have been too small and heterogeneous from which to draw firm conclusions on comparative effectiveness; however, the use of the halo vest may often lead to union at the cost of a higher risk for morbidity and mortality.[40]

Surgical Treatment

Surgical treatment is divided into two categories: anterior surgery via odontoid screw fixation and posterior surgery via C1-C2 posterior fusion and instrumentation. In the presence of good bone stock and minimal or no comminution at the fracture site, odontoid fixation can be a successful treatment option. Increased failure rates in osteoporotic bone have led some authors to use a two-screw fixation technique[44] (**Figure 2**). Bone or tight fibrous union rates are as high as 90%. Dysphagia is a substantial concern after

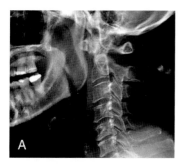
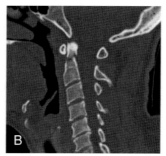
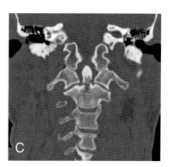
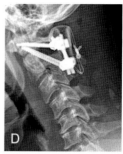

Figure 3 Images demonstrate posterior C1-C2 fusion of a comminuted displaced odontoid fracture. **A,** Lateral radiograph of the cervical spine of a 50-year-old man who had a comminuted displaced odontoid fracture. Note the 6-mm anterior displacement of the proximal fragment at the fracture site. **B,** Sagittal CT scan of the same patient. Note the reverse angle nature of the fracture line with comminution at the fracture site. **C,** Coronal CT scan of the same patient. **D,** Postoperative lateral radiograph of the same patient demonstrates fixation after posterior fusion of C1-C2.

anterior odontoid screw fixation in elderly patients and occurs in as many as 35% of patients postoperatively.[44]

Posterior C1-C2 fusion and instrumentation has become the most common treatment option for geriatric odontoid fractures.[40] In retrospective and prospective cohort studies, the complication and mortality rates associated with surgical treatment are lower than those associated with nonsurgical treatment.[42,43] Fixation can be accomplished with C1-C2 transarticular facet screws if there is adequate space above the vertebral artery notch or with separate C1 lateral mass and C2 pars or pedicle screws (**Figure 3**). Each screw is usually combined with a structural graft between the posterior ring of C1 and the lamina and spinous process of C2. Recent studies suggest improved patient-reported outcomes in active elderly patients who are treated in this fashion.[45]

Nonsurgical Versus Surgical Treatment

Geriatric odontoid fractures are increasingly common and present substantial dilemmas in treatment decision making. Fracture morphology as well as patient factors and comorbidities must be taken into consideration in deciding how to treat patients. Nonsurgical treatment is preferred in sedentary, low-demand elderly patients or if substantial comorbidities preclude surgery. A cervical collar results in less morbidity and mortality than does a halo vest. Surgical stabilization with two odontoid screws may be considered in somewhat younger geriatric patients who have a type II fracture pattern that will be perpendicular to screw trajectory, good bone quality, and minimal comminution; however, these patients are most commonly treated with posterior C1-C2 fusion and instrumentation, which has led to very good functional outcomes in mid- and high-functioning geriatric patients.

Vertebral Compression Fractures

The primary goals for the treatment of vertebral compression fractures are to provide pain relief and improve function by conveying immediate stability to the fracture fragments via cement interdigitation. Early studies were nonrandomized case series, most of which were retrospective, with a few published prospective cohort studies. Diamond et al[46] compared a nonrandomized trial of nonsurgical treatment with vertebroplasty and reported that the patients who were treated with vertebroplasty had more rapid pain relief, more rapid rehabilitation, and a lower complication rate compared with those who underwent nonsurgical treatment; however, the authors reported the benefits of vertebroplasty to be short term only, and that by 6 weeks postoperatively, both groups reported similar pain scores.

Hulme et al[47] performed a systematic review of publications related to vertebroplasty and kyphoplasty. The authors reported that approximately 90% of patients gained some pain relief with either kyphoplasty or vertebroplasty; however, most studies reported very little change in vertebral height restoration. Complications included cement leakage in 9% of patients who were treated with kyphoplasty and 41% of patients who were treated with vertebroplasty, most of whom were asymptomatic. The observation of new fractures at adjacent vertebrae, which was reported in many of the patients in the included studies, was more disconcerting. Similar findings were presented in studies by Taylor et al,[48] Eck et al,[49] and Liu et al,[50] all of which reported no substantial difference between kyphoplasty and vertebroplasty with regard to pain relief, vertebral alignment correction, and functional improvement. Liu et al[50] recommended vertebroplasty based on the higher costs associated with kyphoplasty. Early studies reported that pain relief was similar for both kyphoplasty and vertebroplasty, functional improvement was tied to pain relief, and cement leakage was more frequent with vertebroplasty but might be clinically irrelevant.

In 2011, the American Academy of Orthopaedic Surgeons (AAOS) published its clinical practice guideline on the treatment of insufficiency fractures.[51] The recommendations for cement augmentation were based on two level I prospective randomized studies (concurrently published) that met the inclusion criteria, both of which reported vertebroplasty to be no more effective than sham surgery.[52,53] Kallmes et al[52] reported a trend toward improvement after vertebroplasty; however, no statistical difference was reported during the time the patients were studied. A third study considered by the AAOS guidelines panel correlated kyphoplasty with an early improvement in pain and improved function; however, the authors did not report long-term benefits.[54]

The AAOS clinical practice guideline strongly recommends the use of calcitonin in the first 4 weeks after compression fracture. The AAOS clinical practice guideline recommends against the use of vertebroplasty and weakly recommends the use of kyphoplasty because of its correlation with early pain improvement. At the time the AAOS clinical practice guideline was published, there were no convincing data that the use of cement augmentation for the treatment of insufficiency fractures provided better long-term

benefits compared with nonsurgical treatment.

One of the consistent critiques of the studies by Kallmes et al[52] and Buchbinder et al[53] was that the authors did not adequately assess the acuity of the compression fractures in their study cohorts. It appears that some of the patients in these studies had remote, possibly healed fractures but presented with back pain. Inclusion of such patients may have spuriously indicated no treatment effect for vertebroplasty. Since publication of the AAOS clinical practice guideline, several high-quality studies have reported improved pain relief and quality of life in patients who were treated with vertebroplasty or kyphoplasty.[55-57] Klazen et al[55] prospectively randomized patients who had acute (<6 weeks old) thoracolumbar compression fractures and reported that patients who underwent vertebroplasty had a marked advantage, as measured by the visual analog pain scale, that was maintained 1 year postoperatively compared with those who underwent nonsurgical treatment. There also is evidence of a decreased mortality risk in patients with vertebral body fractures who are treated with cement augmentation. Edidin et al[58] reviewed the US Medicare dataset, which included more than 800,000 patients who had compression fractures, over 4 years. The authors reported a 61% adjusted survival rate for patients who were treated with vertebroplasty or kyphoplasty compared with a 50% survival rate for patients who were treated nonsurgically. Erdem et al[59] reported that patients who have lymphoma and myeloma appear to be particularly good candidates for vertebral augmentation, with improved visual analog pain scale scores, a reduction in narcotic use,

and increased activity levels reported 1 month postoperatively.

Since the AAOS clinical practice guideline was published, there has been compelling evidence that both vertebroplasty and kyphoplasty can improve pain and quality of life; however, additional definitive studies that include a larger number of patients are necessary. Patients who are treated within 3 months of fracture are those who appear to benefit from vertebral augmentation. Most surgical candidates should prove refractory to a trial of nonsurgical treatment.

Management of Thoracolumbar Deformity in the Elderly

There is an increasing number of patients older than 65 years who have spinal stenosis and associated spinal deformity, which has led to a substantial increase in surgical complexity for these patients.[60] Although nonsurgical treatment, including therapeutic exercises, anti-inflammatory medications, and activity modifications, remains the initial and frequently the only treatment required, failure of nonsurgical treatment forces surgeons to make a decision on the next steps. This may necessitate choosing between surgical options, each with its own potential risks and complications.

In general, the outcomes of elderly patients who undergo spinal deformity surgery are equivalent to those of younger patients and closely correlate with preoperative expectations.[61] However, complication rates have ranged from 37% to more than 50% in some studies.[62] Osteoporosis is one of the key comorbidities that affects outcomes, especially if fixation is required. Although bone density changes do not appear to affect fusion rates, they do appear to alter screw fixation and initial spinal stability (the key to deformity correction).

In addition to improving fixation in the osteoporotic spine, less curve correction—while maintaining sagittal and coronal balance—should be the primary goal, and fusion as well as rigid implants should not end at a kyphotic segment. Vertebroplasty placed at the upper instrumented vertebrae (UIV) and the UIV+1 may provide some resistance to proximal junctional failure.[63]

Surgical Options for Spinal Stenosis With Deformity

Initial decision making should seek the minimum level of intervention to accomplish the most functional improvement possible with the least risk of complication. Patients with primary symptoms of spinal stenosis who have a mild deformity (eg, scoliosis <20° without lateral listhesis, minimal stable grade 1 spondylolisthesis) may be treated successfully with decompression alone, with a lower risk of failure and revision than if fusion is added. In a review of Medicare data for patients who had lumbar stenosis, Deyo et al[64] reported that interspinous spacer procedures posed a trade-off: fewer complications at the index procedure but higher rates of revision surgery. The authors also reported that decompression alone was the least costly intervention for patients who had lumbar stenosis compared with interspinous spacers or fusion procedures; however, the addition of fusion should be considered in patients who have loss of lumbar lordosis, higher L3 obliquity, or substantial listhesis, all of which portended a worse prognosis. The extent of fusion and the magnitude of the overall surgery must be weighed against comorbidities

and associated risks. Anterior- and lateral-only surgery are fairly new, and although some authors have reported success in case report series and prospective series, these approaches are somewhat controversial.[65,66] Posterior fusion, or anterior and posterior fusion, remain the most common techniques to manage patients who have severe listhesis as well as sagittal and coronal imbalance. Currently, fusion to the sacrum is often accompanied by fixation to the ilium.[67] Recommendations on how high to go remain elusive.[68] Treatment should be customized to each patient's particular deformity.

A discussion of deformity treatment in adult patients should include an understanding of the elements of sagittal balance as well as how to measure and manage imbalance. Restoration of sagittal balance is critical to good outcomes.[69] The C7 plumb line or sagittal vertical axis (SVA) is the most common way to measure balance; an SVA greater than 4 cm is the definition of imbalance. This does not mean that an SVA greater than 4 cm requires correction; most deformity surgeons aim to bring patients who have substantial imbalance (>10 cm) closer to but not necessarily all the way to an SVA of 5 cm. This effort is made more complex by pelvic tilt and pelvic incidence.[70] Patients with high pelvic incidence have a higher risk of sagittal imbalance, even if the lumbar spine is fixed at normal lordosis. A preoperative understanding of the amount of lordosis required (based on pelvic incidence) is key. Pelvic tilt informs the decision by identifying the extent to which the patient is standing (for the radiograph) in a compensated fashion (ie, pelvic tilt >20° to 25°)[71] (**Figure 4**).

The surgical plan may require the inclusion of an osteotomy for patients

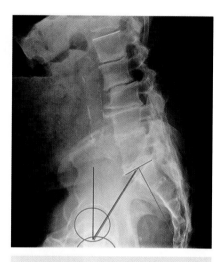

Figure 4   Standing lateral lumbar radiograph demonstrates pelvic incidence of 62° (red lines), lumbar lordosis of 10° (yellow lines), and pelvic tilt of 31° (blue lines).

who have substantial sagittal imbalance, high pelvic tilt, and high pelvic incidence. Smith-Petersen or Ponte osteotomies, with removal of posterior elements and compression of the posterior column (which may lead to distraction of the anterior column), are somewhat easier to accomplish if performed over several levels. These osteotomies can assist in gaining up to 15° or 20° of correction. If a greater change is required, a pedicle subtraction osteotomy, which allows for 25° to 35° of correction, can be performed[70] (**Figure 5**). These procedures can be combined at different levels for additive correction; however, the risk for complications, including high levels of blood loss and neurologic injury, is substantial.

Whether to end an adult deformity construct at L5 or S1 is a topic that is frequently discussed. If the L5-S1 segment appears normal, with no degenerative changes, no listhesis, and no stenosis, and is not involved in the deformity, then it may be reasonable to

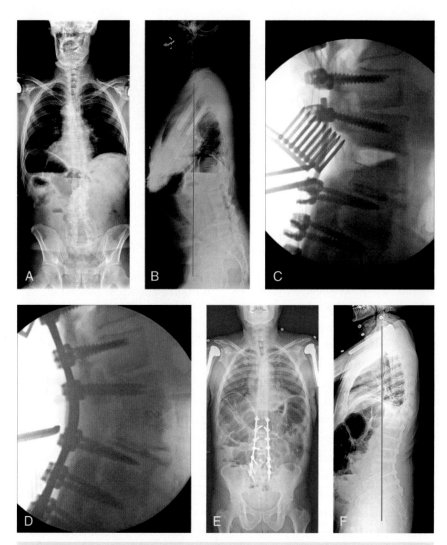

Figure 5 Images demonstrate restoration of sagittal balance. AP (**A**) and lateral (**B**) radiographs of the spine demonstrate scoliosis. Note the sagittal imbalance, with a sagittal vertical axis of 120 mm (red line in panel B). **C** and **D,** Lateral intraoperative fluoroscopic images demonstrate pedicle subtraction osteotomy and reduction. Postoperative AP (**E**) and lateral (**F**) radiographs of the spine demonstrate scoliosis. Note the improved sagittal balance to a sagittal vertical axis of 30 mm (red line in panel F).

the fusion rate by three times, relieves strain on the S1 screws, and protects against screw pullout.[73]

The point at which to stop at the upper end of the construct also is controversial. Although initial studies suggested that crossing the thoracolumbar junction and stopping the construct at T9 or T10 would lead to fewer proximal problems, more recent studies have suggested that this is not the case. Kim et al[74] reported a proximal junctional kyphosis rate of 36% to 55% and a revision surgery rate of 25% whether the construct stopped at L1/L2, T11/T12, or T9/T10. Proximal junctional failure—no matter which specific level is chosen as the UIV—remains a substantial concern. To date, no optimal strategy has emerged to prevent this proximal junctional failure.

Summary

Spinal deformity surgery in elderly patients is increasingly common, with concerns for the management of sagittal and coronal imbalance as well as frequently accompanying spinal stenosis. High complication rates remain a challenge and should be given careful consideration before proceeding with surgery. Nonsurgical treatment is often successful for controlling symptoms. If proceeding with surgery, osteoporosis and the parameters that affect sagittal balance should be identified. Treatment may require an osteotomy, and the levels to include in the fusion should be carefully considered.

References

1. Ortman JM, Hogan H: An aging nation: The older population in the United States, in *Current Population Reports*. Washington, DC, US Census Bureau, 2014, pp 1-28.

exclude the segment from the fusion. The advantages are retained lumbosacral motion, which may allow for more normal gait and less risk of sacroiliac joint degeneration, as well as shorter surgical time and fewer complications, including pseudarthrosis, which is a particularly vexing problem at L5-S1. However, there is a considerable risk of progressive disk degeneration at this level and, in patients who have sagittal imbalance, a risk for recurrence of the imbalance.[72] Therefore, many studies have recommended including the sacrum in a long fusion for the treatment of deformity in adults. Techniques to minimize the rate of pseudarthrosis include the addition of an interbody fusion, the addition of bone morphogenetic protein, and/or fixation to the ilium with iliac bolts or S2 alar-iliac screws. This added fixation increases

© 2016 AAOS Instructional Course Lectures, Volume 65

2. The Daily Briefing: CBO: Medicare spending is slowing faster than expected. February 6, 2013. Available at: https://www.advisory.com/daily-briefing/2013/02/06/cbo-report. Accessed October 16, 2015.

3. Morgan EN, Crawford DA, Scully WF, Noce NJ: Medical management of fragility fractures of the distal radius. *Orthopedics* 2014;37(12):e1068-e1073.

4. Holick MF, Binkley NC, Bischoff-Ferrari HA, et al: Evaluation, treatment, and prevention of vitamin D deficiency: An Endocrine Society clinical practice guideline. *J Clin Endocrinol Metab* 2011;96(7):1911-1930.

5. Carlberg C: The physiology of vitamin D-far more than calcium and bone. *Front Physiol* 2014;5(5):335.

6. Kroner JdeC, Sommer A, Fabri M: Vitamin D every day to keep the infection away? *Nutrients* 2015;7(6):4170-4188.

7. Aspray TJ, Bowring C, Fraser W, et al: National osteoporosis society vitamin D guideline summary. *Age Ageing* 2014;43(5):592-595.

8. Quraishi SA, Bittner EA, Blum L, Hutter MM, Camargo CA Jr: Association between preoperative 25-hydroxyvitamin D level and hospital-acquired infections following Roux-en-Y gastric bypass surgery. *JAMA Surg* 2014;149(2):112-118.

9. Veleva BI, Chel VG, Achterberg WP: Efficacy of daily 800 IU vitamin D supplementation in reaching vitamin D sufficiency in nursing home residents: Cross-sectional patient file study. *BMC Geriatr* 2014;14:103.

10. Ross AC: The 2011 report on dietary reference intakes for calcium and vitamin D. *Public Health Nutr* 2011;14(5):938-939.

11. Vieth R: Vitamin D supplementation, 25-hydroxyvitamin D concentrations, and safety. *Am J Clin Nutr* 1999;69(5):842-856.

12. Vieth R: Vitamin D and cancer mini-symposium: The risk of additional vitamin D. *Ann Epidemiol* 2009;19(7):441-445.

13. U.S. Preventive Services Task Force: Final recommendation statement: Vitamin D and calcium to prevent fractures. Preventive medication. February 2013. Available at: http://www.uspreventiveservicestaskforce.org/Page/Document/UpdateSummaryFinal/vitamin-d-and-calcium-to-prevent-fractures-preventive-medication. Accessed October 16, 2015.

14. Goyal T, Goyal L: Bisphosphonates and direct fracture healing: Area to be explored. *J Pharm Bioallied Sci* 2014;6(4):221.

15. Li YT, Cai HF, Zhang ZL: Timing of the initiation of bisphosphonates after surgery for fracture healing: A systematic review and meta-analysis of randomized controlled trials. *Osteoporos Int* 2015;26(2):431-441.

16. Park YS, Kim HS, Baek SW, Kong DY, Ryu JA: The effect of zoledronic acid on the volume of the fusion-mass in lumbar spinal fusion. *Clin Orthop Surg* 2013;5(4):292-297.

17. Adami S, Libanati C, Boonen S, et al: Denosumab treatment in postmenopausal women with osteoporosis does not interfere with fracture-healing: Results from the FREEDOM trial. *J Bone Joint Surg Am* 2012;94(23):2113-2119.

18. Peichl P, Holzer LA, Maier R, Holzer G: Parathyroid hormone 1-84 accelerates fracture-healing in pubic bones of elderly osteoporotic women. *J Bone Joint Surg Am* 2011;93(17):1583-1587.

19. Ohtori S, Inoue G, Orita S, et al: Teriparatide accelerates lumbar posterolateral fusion in women with postmenopausal osteoporosis: Prospective study. *Spine (Phila Pa 1976)* 2012;37(23):E1464-1468.

20. Ohtori S, Inoue G, Orita S, et al: Comparison of teriparatide and bisphosphonate treatment to reduce pedicle screw loosening after lumbar spinal fusion surgery in postmenopausal women with osteoporosis from a bone quality perspective. *Spine (Phila Pa 1976)* 2013;38(8):E487-E492.

21. Antonelli M, Einstadter D, Magrey M: Screening and treatment of osteoporosis after hip fracture: Comparison of sex and race. *J Clin Densitom* 2014;17(4):479-483.

22. Solomon DH, Johnston SS, Boytsov NN, McMorrow D, Lane JM, Krohn KD: Osteoporosis medication use after hip fracture in U.S. patients between 2002 and 2011. *J Bone Miner Res* 2014;29(9):1929-1937.

23. Wilk A, Sajjan S, Modi A, Fan CP, Mavros P: Post-fracture pharmacotherapy for women with osteoporotic fracture: Analysis of a managed care population in the USA. *Osteoporos Int* 2014;25(12):2777-2786.

24. Balasubramanian A, Tosi LL, Lane JM, Dirschl DR, Ho PR, O'Malley CD: Declining rates of osteoporosis management following fragility fractures in the U.S., 2000 through 2009. *J Bone Joint Surg Am* 2014;96(7):e52.

25. Zhuang XM, Yu BS, Zheng ZM, Zhang JF, Lu WW: Effect of the degree of osteoporosis on the biomechanical anchoring strength of the sacral pedicle screws: An in vitro comparison between unaugmented bicortical screws and polymethylmethacrylate augmented unicortical screws. *Spine (Phila Pa 1976)* 2010;35(19):E925-E931.

26. Yu BS, Zhuang XM, Zheng ZM, Zhang JF, Li ZM, Lu WW: Biomechanical comparison of 4 fixation techniques of sacral pedicle screw in osteoporotic condition. *J Spinal Disord Tech* 2010;23(6):404-409.

27. DeWald CJ, Stanley T: Instrumentation-related complications of multilevel fusions for adult spinal deformity patients over age 65: Surgical considerations and treatment options in patients with poor bone quality. *Spine (Phila Pa 1976)* 2006;31(19, suppl):S144-S151.

28. Kueny RA, Kolb JP, Lehmann W, Püschel K, Morlock MM, Huber G: Influence of the screw augmentation technique and a diameter increase on pedicle screw fixation in the osteoporotic spine: Pullout versus fatigue testing. *Eur Spine J* 2014;23(10):2196-2202.

29. Hasegawa K, Takahashi HE, Uchiyama S, et al: An experimental study of a combination method using a pedicle screw and laminar hook for the osteoporotic spine. *Spine (Phila Pa 1976)* 1997;22(9):958-963.

30. Aydogan M, Ozturk C, Karatoprak O, Tezer M, Aksu N, Hamzaoglu A: The pedicle screw fixation with vertebroplasty augmentation in the surgical treatment of the severe osteoporotic spines. *J Spinal Disord Tech* 2009;22(6):444-447.

31. Sawakami K, Yamazaki A, Ishikawa S, Ito T, Watanabe K, Endo N: Polymethylmethacrylate augmentation of pedicle screws increases the initial fixation in osteoporotic spine patients. *J Spinal Disord Tech* 2012;25(2):E28-E35.

32. Choma TJ, Frevert WF, Carson WL, Waters NP, Pfeiffer FM: Biomechanical analysis of pedicle screws in osteoporotic bone with bioactive cement augmentation using simulated in vivo multicomponent loading. *Spine (Phila Pa 1976)* 2011;36(6):454-462.

33. Choma TJ, Pfeiffer FM, Swope RW, Hirner JP: Pedicle screw design and cement augmentation in osteoporotic vertebrae: Effects of fenestrations and cement viscosity on fixation and extraction. *Spine (Phila Pa 1976)* 2012;37(26):E1628-E1632.

34. Kuhns CA, Reiter M, Pfeiffer F, Choma TJ: Surgical strategies to improve fixation in the osteoporotic spine: The effects of tapping, cement augmentation, and screw trajectory. *Global Spine J* 2014;4(1):47-54.

35. Kerry G, Ruedinger C, Steiner HH: Cement embolism into the venous system after pedicle screw fixation: Case report, literature review, and prevention tips. *Orthop Rev (Pavia)* 2013;5(3):e24.

36. Zusman NL, Ching AC, Hart RA, Yoo JU: Incidence of second cervical vertebral fractures far surpassed the rate predicted by the changing age distribution and growth among elderly persons in the United States (2005-2008). *Spine (Phila Pa 1976)* 2013;38(9):752-756.

37. Smith HE, Kerr SM, Fehlings MG, et al: Trends in epidemiology and management of type II odontoid fractures: 20-year experience at a model system spine injury tertiary referral center. *J Spinal Disord Tech* 2010;23(8):501-505.

38. Tashjian RZ, Majercik S, Biffl WL, Palumbo MA, Cioffi WG: Halo-vest immobilization increases early morbidity and mortality in elderly odontoid fractures. *J Trauma* 2006;60(1):199-203.

39. Majercik S, Tashjian RZ, Biffl WL, Harrington DT, Cioffi WG: Halo vest immobilization in the elderly: A death sentence? *J Trauma* 2005;59(2):350-358.

40. Pal D, Sell P, Grevitt M: Type II odontoid fractures in the elderly: An evidence-based narrative review of management. *Eur Spine J* 2011;20(2):195-204.

41. Chaudhary A, Drew B, Orr RD, Farrokhyar F: Management of type II odontoid fractures in the geriatric population: Outcome of treatment in a rigid cervical orthosis. *J Spinal Disord Tech* 2010;23(5):317-320.

42. Chapman J, Smith JS, Kopjar B, et al: The AOSpine North America Geriatric Odontoid Fracture Mortality Study: A retrospective review of mortality outcomes for operative versus nonoperative treatment of 322 patients with long-term follow-up. *Spine (Phila Pa 1976)* 2013;38(13):1098-1104.

43. Fehlings MG, Arun R, Vaccaro AR, Arnold PM, Chapman JR, Kopjar B: Predictors of treatment outcomes in geriatric patients with odontoid fractures: AOSpine North America multi-centre prospective GOF study. *Spine (Phila Pa 1976)* 2013;38(11):881-886.

44. Dailey AT, Hart D, Finn MA, Schmidt MH, Apfelbaum RI: Anterior fixation of odontoid fractures in an elderly population. *J Neurosurg Spine* 2010;12(1):1-8.

45. Vaccaro AR, Kepler CK, Kopjar B, et al: Functional and quality-of-life outcomes in geriatric patients with type-II dens fracture. *J Bone Joint Surg Am* 2013;95(8):729-735.

46. Diamond TH, Champion B, Clark WA: Management of acute osteoporotic vertebral fractures: A nonrandomized trial comparing percutaneous vertebroplasty with conservative therapy. *Am J Med* 2003;114(4):257-265.

47. Hulme PA, Krebs J, Ferguson SJ, Berlemann U: Vertebroplasty and kyphoplasty: A systematic review of 69 clinical studies. *Spine (Phila Pa 1976)* 2006;31(17):1983-2001.

48. Taylor RS, Taylor RJ, Fritzell P: Balloon kyphoplasty and vertebroplasty for vertebral compression fractures: A comparative systematic review of efficacy and safety. *Spine (Phila Pa 1976)* 2006;31(23):2747-2755.

49. Eck JC, Nachtigall D, Humphreys SC, Hodges SD: Comparison of vertebroplasty and balloon kyphoplasty for treatment of vertebral compression fractures: A meta-analysis of the literature. *Spine J* 2008;8(3):488-497.

50. Liu JT, Liao WJ, Tan WC, et al: Balloon kyphoplasty versus vertebroplasty for treatment of osteoporotic vertebral compression fracture: A prospective, comparative, and randomized clinical study. *Osteoporos Int* 2010;21(2):359-364.

51. Esses SI, McGuire R, Jenkins J, et al: American Academy of Orthopaedic Surgeons clinical practice guideline on: The treatment of osteoporotic spinal compression fractures. *J Bone Joint Surg Am* 2011;93(20):1934-1936.

52. Kallmes DF, Comstock BA, Heagerty PJ, et al: A randomized trial of vertebroplasty for osteoporotic spinal fractures. *N Engl J Med* 2009;361(6):569-579.

53. Buchbinder R, Osborne RH, Ebeling PR, et al: A randomized trial of vertebroplasty for painful osteoporotic vertebral fractures. *N Engl J Med* 2009;361(6):557-568.

54. Wardlaw D, Cummings SR, Van Meirhaeghe J, et al: Efficacy and safety of balloon kyphoplasty compared with non-surgical care for vertebral compression fracture (FREE): A randomised controlled trial. *Lancet* 2009;373(9668):1016-1024.

55. Klazen CA, Lohle PN, de Vries J, et al: Vertebroplasty versus conservative treatment in acute osteoporotic vertebral compression fractures (Vertos II): An open-label randomised trial. *Lancet* 2010;376(9746):1085-1092.

56. Farrokhi MR, Alibai E, Maghami Z: Randomized controlled trial of percutaneous vertebroplasty versus optimal medical management for the relief of pain and disability in acute osteoporotic vertebral compression fractures. *J Neurosurg Spine* 2011;14(5):561-569.

57. Berenson J, Pflugmacher R, Jarzem P, et al: Balloon kyphoplasty versus non-surgical fracture management for treatment of painful vertebral body compression fractures in patients with cancer: A multicentre, randomised controlled trial. *Lancet Oncol* 2011;12(3):225-235.

58. Edidin AA, Ong KL, Lau E, Kurtz SM: Mortality risk for operated and nonoperated vertebral fracture patients in the medicare population. *J Bone Miner Res* 2011;26(7):1617-1626.

59. Erdem E, Samant R, Malak SF, et al: Vertebral augmentation in the treatment of pathologic compression fractures in 792 patients with multiple myeloma. *Leukemia* 2013;27(12):2391-2393.

60. Deyo RA, Mirza SK, Martin BI, Kreuter W, Goodman DC, Jarvik JG: Trends, major medical complications, and charges associated with surgery for lumbar spinal stenosis in older adults. *JAMA* 2010;303(13):1259-1265.

61. Daubs MD, Lenke LG, Cheh G, Stobbs G, Bridwell KH: Adult spinal deformity surgery: Complications and outcomes in patients over age 60. *Spine (Phila Pa 1976)* 2007;32(20):2238-2244.

62. Carreon LY, Puno RM, Dimar JR II, Glassman SD, Johnson JR: Perioperative complications of posterior lumbar decompression and arthrodesis in older adults. *J Bone Joint Surg Am* 2003;85(11):2089-2092.

63. Chiang CK, Wang YH, Yang CY, Yang BD, Wang JL: Prophylactic vertebroplasty may reduce the risk of adjacent intact vertebra from fatigue injury: An ex vivo biomechanical study. *Spine (Phila Pa 1976)* 2009;34(4):356-364.

64. Deyo RA, Martin BI, Ching A, et al: Interspinous spacers compared with decompression or fusion for lumbar stenosis: Complications and repeat operations in the Medicare population. *Spine (Phila Pa 1976)* 2013;38(10):865-872.

65. Dangelmajer S, Zadnik PL, Rodriguez ST, Gokaslan ZL, Sciubba DM: Minimally invasive spine surgery for adult degenerative lumbar scoliosis. *Neurosurg Focus* 2014;36(5):E7.

66. Isaacs RE, Hyde J, Goodrich JA, Rodgers WB, Phillips FM: A prospective, nonrandomized, multicenter evaluation of extreme lateral interbody fusion for the treatment of adult degenerative scoliosis: Perioperative outcomes and complications. *Spine (Phila Pa 1976)* 2010;35(26, suppl):S322-S330.

67. Kim YJ, Bridwell KH, Lenke LG, Rhim S, Cheh G: Pseudarthrosis in long adult spinal deformity instrumentation and fusion to the sacrum: Prevalence and risk factor analysis of 144 cases. *Spine (Phila Pa 1976)* 2006;31(20):2329-2336.

68. Kim HJ, Boachie-Adjei O, Shaffrey CI, et al: Upper thoracic versus lower thoracic upper instrumented vertebrae endpoints have similar outcomes and complications in adult scoliosis. *Spine (Phila Pa 1976)* 2014;39(13):E795-E799.

69. Glassman SD, Bridwell K, Dimar JR, Horton W, Berven S, Schwab F: The impact of positive sagittal balance in adult spinal deformity. *Spine (Phila Pa 1976)* 2005;30(18):2024-2029.

70. Rose PS, Bridwell KH, Lenke LG, et al: Role of pelvic incidence, thoracic kyphosis, and patient factors on sagittal plane correction following pedicle subtraction osteotomy. *Spine (Phila Pa 1976)* 2009;34(8):785-791.

71. Schwab F, Lafage V, Patel A, Farcy JP: Sagittal plane considerations and the pelvis in the adult patient. *Spine (Phila Pa 1976)* 2009;34(17):1828-1833.

72. Edwards CC II, Bridwell KH, Patel A, Rinella AS, Berra A, Lenke LG: Long adult deformity fusions to L5 and the sacrum: A matched cohort analysis. *Spine (Phila Pa 1976)* 2004;29(18):1996-2005.

73. Islam NC, Wood KB, Transfeldt EE, et al: Extension of fusions to the pelvis in idiopathic scoliosis. *Spine (Phila Pa 1976)* 2001;26(2):166-173.

74. Kim YJ, Bridwell KH, Lenke LG, Rhim S, Kim YW: Is the T9, T11, or L1 the more reliable proximal level after adult lumbar or lumbosacral instrumented fusion to L5 or S1? *Spine (Phila Pa 1976)* 2007;32(24):2653-2661.

Avoiding and Managing Intraoperative Complications During Cervical Spine Surgery

Jesse Bible, MD, MHS
Jeffrey A. Rihn, MD
Moe R. Lim, MD
Darrel S. Brodke, MD
Joon Y. Lee, MD

Abstract

The incidence of intraoperative complications during cervical spine surgery is low; however, if they do occur, intraoperative complications have the potential to cause considerable morbidity and mortality. Spine surgeons should be familiar with methods to minimize intraoperative complications. If they do occur, surgeons must be prepared to immediately treat each potential complication to reduce any associated morbidity.

Instr Course Lect 2016;65:281–290.

Complications related to cervical spine surgery can range in incidence as well as associated morbidity and mortality. Complications with a delayed onset, including dysphagia, nonunion, and adjacent-segment disease, are more common than those of immediate onset. Delayed onset complications are associated with reduced relative morbidity and often can be treated nonsurgically. Conversely, intraoperative complications occur much less often but are associated with substantial morbidity and mortality. Given that intraoperative complications are inevitable despite the use of the best surgical techniques, surgeons should be familiar with the risk factors, methods of prevention, and immediate treatment options for such complications, with the goal of mitigating any associated morbidity and mortality. It is important for surgeons to be aware of the potential for intraoperative vertebral artery, neurologic, and esophageal injuries as well as cerebrospinal fluid (CSF) leaks and complications of instrumentation related to cervical spine surgery.

Vertebral Artery Injury
Incidence

Vertebral artery injury is a very rare event but can be associated with considerable morbidity and mortality. In one study, the incidence of injury during anterior cervical spine surgery was 0.3%.[1] In a survey of Cervical Spine Research Society members, the overall incidence of vertebral artery injury in the cervical spine was 0.07% (111 of 163,324 surgeries).[2] Instrumentation of the upper cervical spine (32%), anterior corpectomy (23%), and posterior exposure (12%) were the most common surgical factors associated with vertebral artery injury.

Dr. Rihn or an immediate family member serves as a paid consultant to or is an employee of Pfizer; has received research or institutional support from DePuy; and serves as a board member, owner, officer, or committee member of the North American Spine Society. Dr. Brodke or an immediate family member has received royalties from Amedica, DePuy Synthes, and Medtronic; serves as a paid consultant to or is an employee of Amedica; has stock or stock options held in Amedica; and serves as a board member, owner, officer, or committee member of the Cervical Spine Research Society and the Lumbar Spine Research Society. Dr. Lee or an immediate family member has received research or institutional support from Stryker. Neither of the following authors nor any immediate family member has received anything of value from or has stock or stock options held in a commercial company or institution related directly or indirectly to the subject of this chapter: Dr. Bible and Dr. Lim.

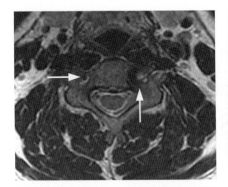

Figure 1 Axial T2-weighted MRI demonstrates a right hypoplastic vertebral artery (horizontal arrow) and medial migration of the left vertebral artery (vertical arrow).

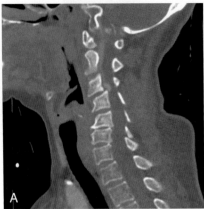

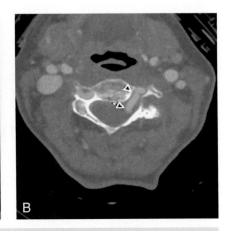

Figure 2 Sagittal (**A**) and axial (**B**) CT scans demonstrate a tortuous vertebral artery (arrowheads) in the spinal canal.

Prevention

Being cognizant of the anatomy of the vertebral artery and being aware of the potential anomalies in the anatomy and course of the vertebral artery is a critical step in preventing vertebral artery injury. The vertebral artery is most susceptible to injury anteriorly at C7, laterally at C3-C6, and posteriorly at C1-C2. After branching from the subclavian artery, the vertebral artery enters through the C6 transverse foramen in 92% to 95% of patients.[3,4] As the vertebral artery ascends from C6 to C3, it moves in a slightly posterior and medial direction and is located approximately 3.3 ± 1.6 mm lateral to the lateral margin of the uncovertebral joints.[3] The vertebral artery deviates 45° laterally through the C2 foramen before traveling posteriorly and medially above the ring of C1. At a distance of 8 to 18 mm from the midline, the vertebral artery abruptly turns superiorly toward the foramen magnum.[5]

Although these numbers may be a helpful reference, they do not replace a careful preoperative examination of the course of the vertebral arteries with the use of all available axial imaging modalities. After noting the level at which the vertebral arteries enter the spine, the medial border of each transverse foramen should be assessed for any medial migration of the arteries (**Figure 1**). A review of 250 consecutive patients' MRI results revealed medial migration of the vertebral artery in 19 patients (7.6%).[4] Other anatomic variations in vertebral arteries include anomalies such as multiluminal or unilaterally hypoplastic arteries and extraforaminal anomalies, which can occur anterior to the transverse processes[6] (**Figures 1** and **2**).

The surgeon must always know the location of the midline throughout any anterior cervical spine surgical procedure. This is reliably done by marking the midline before dissection of the longus colli as well as by identifying the medial portion of the uncovertebral joints and using them as a continuous reference for bone and soft-tissue removal. The monopolar electrocautery device should be set at a low intensity when dissecting laterally under the longus colli to minimize the transduction of heat, which can cause vertebral artery injury, through surrounding structures. Similarly, bipolar electrocautery or transcollation technology can be used for this portion of the surgical

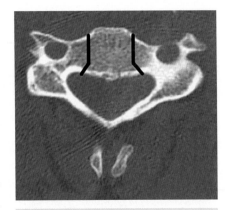

Figure 3 Axial CT scan demonstrates a trumpet-shaped decompression (dark lines) for corpectomy, which allows lateral decompression posterior to the vertebral arteries.

procedure to prevent arterial injuries that are caused by the arcing of energy. Venous bleeding should be controlled with topical hemostatic agents and paddies rather than chased into the lateral vertebral body with the electrocautery device.

Given that the mean interforaminal distance varies from 26 to 29 mm, approximately 15 mm is the recommended width for safe vertebral body removal during corpectomy. An off-center, asymmetric, or oblique corpectomy trough may put the vertebral artery at

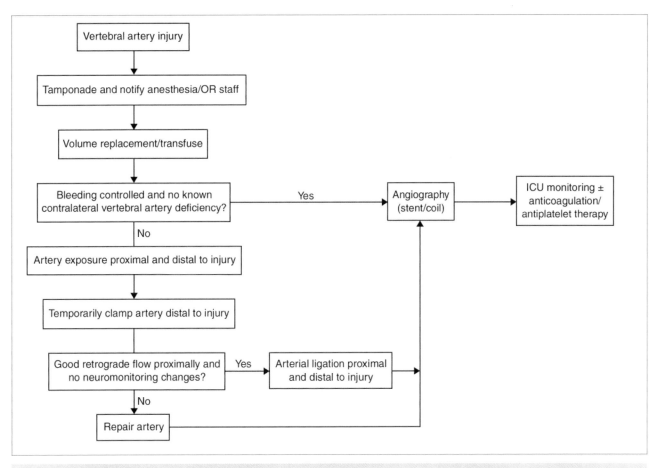

Figure 4   Treatment algorithm for a vertebral artery injury. ICU = intensive care unit, OR = operating room.

risk for injury. In general, the wall of the vertebral body opposite the chief surgeon is more prone to injury secondary to an oblique corpectomy trough. During diskectomies and corpectomies, trumpet laminectomy, which creates a space larger than 15 mm, can be used for optimal lateral decompression of the neural structures (**Figure 3**).

Treatment

The therapeutic goals for the treatment of a vertebral artery injury include control of local hemorrhage, prevention of immediate vertebrobasilar ischemia, and prevention of cerebrovascular complications (**Figure 4**). Efforts should be made immediately after injury to tamponade bleeding with local pressure,

using thromboplastic agents and surgical paddies. Given the theoretical risk of embolization, the use of bone wax or other particulate materials should be avoided if possible. After bleeding is controlled, surgeons should avoid the temptation to definitively treat a vertebral artery injury solely with packing or tamponade because of the risk for delayed hemorrhage or creation of a fistula or pseudoaneurysm.

During the process of tamponade and before any further surgical exploration is attempted, the operating room staff and anesthesiologists should be immediately notified, and the protocol for massive transfusion should be activated because of the potential for 3 to 5 L of rapid blood loss from vertebral

artery injury. Intraoperative consultation with a vascular surgeon also should be considered. In addition, the head of the bed should be immediately returned to the neutral position to ensure that the contralateral vertebral artery will not be mechanically occluded.

At this point, the decision must be made to either have the patient undergo immediate angiography evaluation and possible coil/stent treatment or further surgical exploration with a possible repair or direct ligation. This decision is based on the stability of the patient and area of tamponade; the availability and proximity of angiographic services; the anatomic site and mechanism of injury; and vertebral artery dominance, if it is known. A patient who remains in an

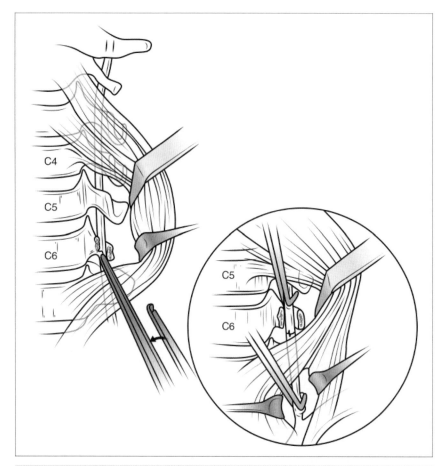

Figure 5 Illustration shows distal control of the left vertebral artery at C7 before it enters the C6 transverse foramen. Inset, the transverse process at the level or levels of injury is then unroofed with a Kerrison rongeur.

be presumed to have a patent circle of Willis or collateral antegrade flow, which allows direct ligation to remain a potentially viable option if the repair is unsuccessful.[7] In addition, any substantial changes in baseline neurologic function should be taken into account when assessing for adequate perfusion.

With clamps in place cephalad and caudal to the injury site, surgical repair is done with 7-0 or 8-0 nonabsorbable polypropylene suture. If repair is unsuccessful or technically impossible, direct ligation with hemoclips should be considered. Blind placement of clamps should be avoided because of the potential for damage to exiting nerve roots. Although most patients who sustain a vertebral artery injury can tolerate unilateral ligation of the injured artery, it poses a grave risk of neurologic compromise in patients who have an absent, hypoplastic, or stenotic contralateral artery. Wallenberg syndrome, cerebellar infarction, cranial nerve palsies, and quadriparesis have been reported in such patients, with death occurring in as many as 12%.[8] The reported incidences of hypoplasia and the absence of the left vertebral artery are 5.7% and 1.3%, respectively, and of the right vertebral artery are 8.8% and 3.1%, respectively.[9]

If arterial injury occurs posteriorly at C1 or C2, direct repair and even ligation may be technically difficult because of poor visualization. If injury occurs during exposure of these cervical vertebrae, an approach similar to that described earlier is taken to expose the artery above and below the site of injury. This may entail removing the lateral masses of C2 and C3 and/or the posterior ring of C1. If injury is noted when drilling or tapping for screw placement, the screw can be placed to plug the drill hole, and bleeding and

unstable state or in whom active bleeding persists despite efforts at hemostasis should not be transported from the operating room to an angiography suite. If the injured vertebral artery is known to be dominant or the contralateral artery is not patent because of prior pathology, repair of the injured artery should be undertaken.

The direct repair or ligation of an injured vertebral artery requires that the ipsilateral artery be clearly exposed above and below the site of injury. For an arterial injury during an anterior procedure, the skin incision can be extended and the sternocleidomastoid muscle partially transected at the level of the arterial injury to create an improved working area. The ipsilateral longus colli is dissected laterally over the transverse processes above and below the site of injury. For distal control of bleeding, the injured vertebral artery is dissected out, and a temporary clamp is applied at the C6-C7 level before the artery enters the C6 transverse foramen (**Figure 5**). For proximal control, the transverse process directly cephalad to the site of injury is unroofed using a 2- or 3-mm Kerrison rongeur, and the intertransversarii muscles are carefully removed. Before a clamp is applied proximally, the presence or absence of retrograde flow from the injury site is determined. If good backfilling of the artery is present, the patient can

© 2016 AAOS Instructional Course Lectures, Volume 65

hemodynamic stability in the surrounding area can be reassessed. After the procedure, the patient should be sent for angiography for potential coiling.

After any vertebral artery injury, the integrity of the repair or ligation is confirmed with angiography. The patient is admitted to the intensive care unit for monitoring for pseudoaneurysm or late hemorrhage. Anticoagulation and/or antiplatelet therapy also should be considered to reduce the risk of vertebrobasilar thromboembolism.

Esophageal Injury
Incidence
The reported incidence of esophageal injury during anterior cervical spine surgery is 0.3% for diskectomy and fusion, 1.6% for corpectomy, and 1.5% for fracture repair.[10] Causes of injury include trauma, erosion by anterior osteophytes, intraoperative injury, and delayed injury from instrument-related erosion (eg, prominent plates or loose screws).

Prevention
The esophagus sits immediately posterior to the longus colli muscle, which requires that retractors be placed around it for visualization of the midline during cervical spine procedures. The use of retractors, as well as the coverage of the posterior esophageal mucosa by only a thin layer of connective tissue, makes injury to the esophagus possible, especially proximally at the Lannier triangle (dorsal midline area just below the cricopharyngeus muscle). The importance of careful manual retraction should be stressed to novice surgical assistants. If self-retaining retractors are placed, special attention should be given to ensure that no esophageal folds protrude into the surgical field, which

make them susceptible to injury from a burr or drill.

Weakened and/or distorted esophageal anatomy can be expected in cases of revision surgery, tumor, or infection. Careful dissection and retraction as well as placement of a nasogastric or orogastric tube to help locate the esophagus during dissection may aid in avoiding esophageal injury.

Evaluation and Treatment
The most important step in the treatment of an esophageal injury is recognizing it initially. Intraoperative injury can sometimes be noted with direct visualization; however, this may be unreliable, especially in patients who have small tears. In a cadaver model study of esophageal perforations, poor sensitivity was reported with reliance only on intraesophageal dye injection (methylene blue/indigo carmine) via a nasogastric tube.[11] Better, although still limited, detection was achieved with the addition of a Foley catheter distal to the suspected area of injury.

In the early postoperative period, a missed intraoperative perforation of the esophagus may present as neck pain, dysphagia, odynophagia, fever, swelling of the neck, wound drainage of food, or subcutaneous emphysema/crepitus. An injury with delayed presentation that was caused by instrument-related erosion presents in a similar manner, with dysphagia or pneumonia of new onset.

The evaluation of an esophageal injury includes radiography with or without CT to assess the position of instrumentation and/or a graft and soft-tissue swelling, pneumomediastinum, or abscess/fluid collection. Contrast esophagoscopy also may be considered but has a false-negative rate of 10%, with barium being slightly more

sensitive than diatrizoate meglumine for the detection of esophageal tears.[12] If, after an initial study that is read as normal, a patient's clinical symptoms raise high suspicion for a tear, direct visualization via surgical exploration may be considered; however, a less invasive method of assessment involves performing serial esophagrams, with surgical exploration performed only after a tear is identified on imaging.

If an esophageal tear is detected during cervical spine surgery, primary repair, which is the standard of care, should be performed, preferably by an otolaryngologist or general surgeon. The patient should refrain from oral foods or liquids (ie, NPO status), with a nasogastric or Dobhoff tube in place, until a swallowing study yields a normal result. In addition, an esophagram is commonly obtained 7 to 10 days after the repair of an esophageal tear. A muscle flap, with a pedicled graft of the sternocleidomastoid muscle most commonly used, may be required to allow for tension-free closure of a delayed or late perforation.

Neurologic Injury
Spinal Cord Injury
Scant literature exists on the incidence of perioperative spinal cord injury in cervical spine surgery; however, a low incidence (<1%) has been reported.[13,14] Spinal cord injury can occur during any phase of the perioperative process and potential causes include hyperextension of the neck during intubation/positioning, hypotension, hematoma, inadequate decompression, interbody graft/cage dislodgement, and surgical trauma. Certain patients, such as those who have severe myelopathy (myelomalacia), spinal instability, and ankylosing spondylitis, and those who undergo

Assessment Checklist	Intervention (If Required)
☐ 1. Electrodes	Reconnect/reposition
☐ 2. MAP >85 mm Hg	Vasopressors/fluid bolus
☐ 3. Body temperature >36.5°C	Raise room temperature, warming blanket/wound irrigation
☐ 4. Different anesthesia agent or bolus	Return to originial agent/reassess after time period
☐ 5. Hemoglobin level >8.0 g/dL (stat ABG): significant EBL	Transfuse
☐ 6. Arm positioning (for upper extremity alerts)	Untape shoulders/check elbows
☐ 7. Explore wound for sites of neural compression, hematoma, bone fragment, hemostatic agent	Remove compressive element
☐ 8. Active distraction or deformity correction	Lessen distraction/correction
☐ 9. Neck position (hyperextension)	Reposition neck
☐10. Instrumentation/cage/graft placement	Radiographically check placement: remove

↓

No improvement

↓

Emergent cervical (± thoracic) MRI to rule out compression (± IV steroids)

Figure 6 Checklist of items for rapid review in the event of a major intraoperative neuromonitoring alert during a cervical spine procedure. ABG = arterial blood gas, EBL = estimated blood loss, IV = intravenous, MAP = mean arterial pressure.

correction of a substantial deformity, may have a particularly high risk for spinal cord injury.

Communication with the operating room staff and anesthesiologists as well as vigilant attention to detail are the keys to avoid a perioperative spinal cord injury. Before intubating the patient, the operating room staff should directly communicate with the anesthesiologists about the severity of any spinal stenosis; this communication should not be restricted to any traumatic instability. A review of the American Society of Anesthesiologists Closed Claims database revealed that 57% of perioperative injuries to the cervical spinal cord occurred in patients who had underlying stenosis and/or herniation, and only 24% of perioperative injuries to the cervical spinal cord occurred in patients who had notable cervical instability.[15] For this reason, fiberoptic intubation, rather than direct laryngoscopy, should be strongly considered in patients who have instability or a tenuous cord

resulting from compressive cord pathology. Furthermore, the mean arterial pressure (MAP) should be kept higher than 85 mm Hg until decompression is performed or the correction of the deformity has been completed.[16] If possible, this pressure also should be maintained during intubation and all subsequent positioning of the patient. Similarly, a cognizant neuromonitoring team can be especially helpful in minimizing neurologic injury. Any signs of lability should be immediately relayed to the operating room staff and anesthesiologists.

The spine surgeon should have a memorized checklist for review in the event of a major neuromonitoring alert to allow for prompt and aggressive management of the source of the alert. When reviewing the list, the surgeon should keep in mind that false-positive neuromonitoring alerts can occur, and that some interventions may cause harm. A typical series of items for swift review include ensuring that the patient

has a MAP higher than 85 mm Hg, a temperature higher than 36.5°C, and a hemoglobin level higher than 8 g/dL as well as determining whether the patient has recently undergone untaping of the shoulders, repositioning of the neck, release of a deformity correction, or removal of an implant (**Figure 6**). Depending on the stage of the cervical spine surgery, aborting the procedure or a wake-up test also may be considered.

Potentially reversible causes for a spinal cord injury that persists postoperatively are investigated with MRI and/or CT. Patients who have a persisting spinal cord injury are admitted to the intensive care unit to maintain a MAP higher than 85 mm Hg as well as a hemoglobin level higher than 10 g/dL for 3 to 5 days and may be treated with intravenous steroids.[17] Peripheral nerve injuries during cervical spine surgery are most often the result of improper positioning, with the most frequent injuries being ulnar neuropathy and brachial plexus injury. Although rare,

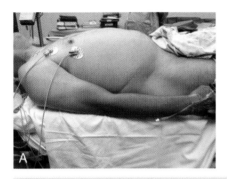 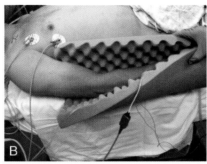 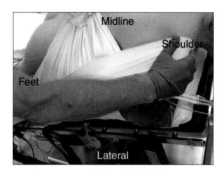

Figure 7   Lateral clinical photographs show an unprotected (**A**) and protected (**B**) ulnar nerve during supine positioning of a patient before the patient's arms are tucked or "papoosed" for anterior cervical procedures. Lines or wires that traverse the medial side of the elbow should be avoided, as seen in panel A.

Figure 8   Clinical photograph demonstrates the use of the surgeon's hand to control desired tension on the shoulder and brachial plexus while securing tape to the surgical table distally for cervical spine procedures.

neuropathy and brachial plexus injury can lead to devastating deficits in upper extremity function.

Ulnar Neuropathy

Ulnar neuropathy, the most common type of perioperative peripheral nerve injury in cervical spine surgery, is responsible for 28% of all claims for anesthesia-related nerve injury.[18] The end result of ulnar neuropathy can include loss of intrinsic hand function and a clawlike deformity of the hand. Preexisting subclinical neuropathy can manifest in the perioperative period if patients who undergo cervical spine surgery are subjected to certain predisposing factors, such as prolonged hypotension. Other patient-related risk factors for perioperative ulnar neuropathy include extreme thinness and obesity, older age, and male sex.[19] Men are more susceptible to direct pressure on the unmyelinated fibers of the ulnar nerve compared with women.[20]

Initial symptoms of ulnar neuropathy in patients who undergo cervical spine surgery are usually noted more than 24 hours postoperatively.[19,21] In a large retrospective study, Warner et al[19] reported a less than 10% instance of ulnar neuropathy in the postoperative

recovery unit. In this study, 47% of ulnar neuropathies presented as sensory deficits, with the remaining 53% presenting as mixed sensory and motor deficits. At 1 year postoperatively, 41% of the patients who had experienced postoperative deficits had persistent deficits. Patients who had mixed deficits were less likely to have a complete recovery (35%) compared with patients who had purely sensory deficits (80%).[19]

Before positioning the arms of the patient in preparation for cervical spine surgery, the elbows of both arms should be wrapped with gel or foam pads, with care taken to ensure that the caudal surfaces of the elbows are adequately protected (**Figure 7**). Similarly, the number of lines and/or wires that traverse the arms should be minimized, especially over the medial side of the elbow.

If no substantial improvements in symptoms of apparent ulnar neuropathy are seen 6 weeks postoperatively, electromyographic testing should be considered and, if necessary, the patient should be referred to a hand specialist.

Brachial Plexus Injury

Brachial plexus injury can result from the stretching or compression of nerves with subsequent ischemia of the vasa

nervorum. During cervical spine procedures, traction injuries are most commonly the result of taping the patient's shoulders to optimally visualize the level of interest on the localizing lateral radiograph. Under general anesthesia, especially with the use of muscle relaxants for intubation, patients have reduced defensive muscle tone, which makes it easy for an inattentive surgeon to apply too much traction. After affixing tape to the shoulder, the surgeon can place one hand over the tape and gently pull the shoulder down until the desired degree of tension is achieved (**Figure 8**). With this hand kept in place over the shoulder, the surgeon can then use the other hand (or ask an assistant) to affix the distal end of the tape to the surgical table. Taping in this manner allows the surgeon to better gauge the tension on the patient's brachial plexus rather than pulling distally using only the affixed tape.

If neuromonitoring is being used and baseline values are recorded before the patient is positioned, they should be recorded before taping to provide the surgical team with a set of baseline values with which to determine whether the tape needs to be relaxed. Likewise, if adequate visualization cannot to obtained without excessive traction, further dissection can be carried cephalad until adequate radiographic localization occurs at a more cephalad level. From this point, the surgeon can manually count down to the cervical level of interest.

In patients in whom a new postoperative deficit is thought to be potentially related to injury of the brachial plexus, an MRI of the cervical spine should be obtained to rule out a compressive disorder masquerading as a plexus injury. Given that most brachial plexus injuries in the setting of cervical spine surgery are traction-related injuries to the upper nerve roots (C5 and C6), patients who manifest signs of such injury may be given a sling for comfort and undergo physical therapy to prevent adhesive capsulitis of the shoulder and/or elbow contractures.

Cerebrospinal Fluid Leaks
Incidence
CSF leaks in the cervical spine are rare. In a retrospective review of 1,994 patients who underwent cervical spine surgery from 1994 through 2005, Hannallah et al[22] reported a 1% (n = 20) incidence of CSF leaks. A 12.5% rate of CSF leakage was reported in patients who underwent ossification of the posterior longitudinal ligament, and a 1.9% rate of CSF leakage was reported in patients who underwent anterior revision procedures. Seventy percent of anterior dural tears were caused by a Kerrison rongeur, and 20% of posterior tears were caused by Bovie electrocautery or from opening of the lamina during laminoplasty. Eleven CSF leaks were treated without repair or lumbar drainage, five CSF leaks were treated with

direct repair, and four CSF leaks were treated without repair but with lumbar drainage. Only one patient (who had no repair or lumbar drainage) required a second operation for persistent CSF leakage.[22]

CSF leaks in cervical trauma also are rare, with higher-energy injuries more likely to cause a dural tear. Common patterns of injury associated with CSF leaks include bilateral facet dislocations and compression-flexion injuries (stages IV and V). Most CSF leaks that are associated with bilateral facet dislocations occur posteriorly and usually do not require repair because of coverage by bone and/or ligamentum flavum of the dural tear through which they occur, which allows the tear to seal itself. In patients who have severe compression-flexion injuries, the retropulsed vertebral body tears into the dura, which causes an anterior CSF leak. These CSF leaks are more likely to be persistent and often require a decompressive corpectomy and direct repair, if possible.

Prevention
Many cervical CSF leaks are unavoidable, particularly in the setting of trauma and ossification of the posterior longitudinal ligament; however, the careful use of Kerrison and pituitary rongeurs is critical to minimize the tears responsible for cervical CSF leaks. During posterior dissection with unipolar electrocautery, special attention should be given to avoid falling into an interlaminar space, especially for patients who have widened interlaminar spaces.

Treatment
Early diagnosis is key, with direct visualization of a CSF leak being

optimal. Occult CSF leaks can be diagnosed based on clear drainage from surgical incision, CT myelography, and/or clinical signs (eg, blurred vision, headaches, light sensitivity, bogginess in the vicinity of the incision).

Treatment strategies for cervical CSF leaks include direct repair, counterpressure, and the placement of diverting drains. Whenever possible, a leak should be directly repaired with a Gore-Tex (Gore Medical) or silk suture. Postoperatively, the head of the patient's bed should be raised to more than or equal to 30° to maintain a low intrathecal pressure. For patients who have posterior cervical CSF leaks, maintaining the head of the bed at 90° may help reduce CSF pressure at the site of the repair. Dural sealants can be used to reinforce leaky repairs; however, the surgeon must be aware of sealant expansion, which can lead to neural compression.

If direct repair of a cervical CSF leak is impossible, autologous fascia, fat, or a collagen matrix can be used as a dural graft. If possible, stay sutures are placed at the corners of the graft, which holds it in place, before a dural sealant further secures the graft. This technique may be valuable for patients who have an anterior cervical CSF leak that cannot be adequately exposed for repair. In such patients, a fascia graft or collagen matrix is laid over the defect and held in place with dural sealant and Gelfoam (Pfizer) before a tricortical bone graft or cage is placed in the usual fashion. More dural sealant can then be added in the lateral gutters.

If a CSF leak cannot be directly repaired, the placement of a lumbar shunt should be considered, with the flow of CSF titrated to 10 mL/h. In addition, a low threshold should be set for lumbar drainage in patients who are ventilator-dependent because positive-pressure ventilation increases intradural pressure, which can potentially cause CSF leaks.

Instrumentation Complications

The increasing use of spinal instrumentation increases the potential for instrumentation complications, especially with a growing osteoporotic patient population. Many surgeons are aware of various spinal instrumentation techniques and the potential for immediate complications associated with the nonanatomic placement of spinal instrumentation; however, it also is important for surgeons to be familiar with salvage or bailout techniques to help mitigate intraoperative spinal instrumentation complications.

Posterior Instrumentation

During posterior subaxial cervical spine procedures, lateral-mass fixation may be tenuous because of poor screw purchase. If the walls of the pilot hole for a screw remain intact, a larger diameter salvage screw can be used with the hope of gaining better purchase; however, this may still provide poor fixation, especially if the superolateral quadrant of a lateral mass sustains a blowout fracture during drilling or screw insertion. For these patients, conversion to a Roy-Camille technique or the use of a transfacet screw can be considered as a salvage procedure. In the Roy-Camille technique for lateral mass fixation with screws, the screw trajectory is more horizontal and perpendicular to the lateral mass, which differs from the parallel articular facet in most other insertion techniques. Transfacet screws provide purchase of the ventral cortex of the

inferior articular process if directed distally across the facet joint. Given the small anteroposterior dimensions and steep surface of this vertebra, failure of a lateral-mass screw inserted at C7 is not an exceedingly rare event; however, pedicle screw placement at this level provides a robust rescue option in this situation. For patients who have poor screw purchase in the atlantoaxial region, supplemental laminar wiring and cortical bone grafting remain viable salvage options. In addition, the use of laminar screws at C2 should be remembered in patients who have a failed pars/pedicle screw or anatomic limitations that are created by the vertebral artery.

Anterior Instrumentation

Anterior osteophytes should be burred down before the placement of an anterior plate in the cervical spine to allow the plate to rest flat against the bone, which provides the best biomechanical environment for screw fixation. If screw purchase is poor, larger diameter and/or longer screws may be placed. Another option to address poor screw purchase in the placement of an anterior plate in the cervical spine is bicortical screw fixation, which can be done via stepwise drilling and the use of a depth gauge under fluoroscopy to avoid catastrophic complications. If anterior fixation remains poor, especially in a patient who has considerable cervical spinal instability, a low threshold should exist for supplemental posterior fixation.

Summary

Intraoperative complications during cervical spine surgery are rare. Surgeons who have a systematic approach for the prevention and immediate management

of intraoperative complications, especially vertebral artery and neurologic injuries, can potentially reduce any associated morbidity.

References

1. Burke JP, Gerszten PC, Welch WC: Iatrogenic vertebral artery injury during anterior cervical spine surgery. *Spine J* 2005;5(5):508-514.

2. Lunardini DJ, Eskander MS, Even JL, et al: Vertebral artery injuries in cervical spine surgery. *Spine J* 2014;14(8):1520-1525.

3. Ebraheim NA, Lu J, Brown JA, Biyani A, Yeasting RA: Vulnerability of vertebral artery in anterolateral decompression for cervical spondylosis. *Clin Orthop Relat Res* 1996;322:146-151.

4. Eskander MS, Drew JM, Aubin ME, et al: Vertebral artery anatomy: A review of two hundred fifty magnetic resonance imaging scans. *Spine (Phila Pa 1976)* 2010;35(23):2035-2040.

5. Ebraheim NA, Xu R, Ahmad M, Heck B: The quantitative anatomy of the vertebral artery groove of the atlas and its relation to the posterior atlantoaxial approach. *Spine (Phila Pa 1976)* 1998;23(3):320-323.

6. Curylo LJ, Mason HC, Bohlman HH, Yoo JU: Tortuous course of the vertebral artery and anterior cervical decompression: A cadaveric and clinical case study. *Spine (Phila Pa 1976)* 2000;25(22):2860-2864.

7. Ye JY, Ayyash OM, Eskander MS, Kang JD: Control of the vertebral artery from a posterior approach: A technical report. *Spine J* 2014;14(6):e37-e41.

8. Shintani A, Zervas NT: Consequence of ligation of the vertebral artery. *J Neurosurg* 1972;36(4):447-450.

9. Bernard, G, Laurian C: *The Vertebral Artery: Pathology and Surgery.* New York, NY, Springer-Verlag GmbH Wien, 1987.

10. Orlando ER, Caroli E, Ferrante L: Management of the cervical esophagus and hypofarinx perforations complicating anterior cervical spine surgery. *Spine (Phila Pa 1976)* 2003;28(15):E290-E295.

11. Taylor B, Patel AA, Okubadejo GO, Albert T, Riew KD: Detection of esophageal perforation using intraesophageal dye injection. *J Spinal Disord Tech* 2006;19(3):191-193.

12. Buecker A, Wein BB, Neuerburg JM, Guenther RW: Esophageal perforation: Comparison of use of aqueous and barium-containing contrast media. *Radiology* 1997;202(3):683-686.

13. Cramer DE, Maher PC, Pettigrew DB, Kuntz C IV: Major neurologic deficit immediately after adult spinal surgery: Incidence and etiology over 10 years at a single training institution. *J Spinal Disord Tech* 2009;22(8):565-570.

14. Graham JJ: Complications of cervical spine surgery: A five-year report on a survey of the membership of the Cervical Spine Research Society by the Morbidity and Mortality Committee. *Spine (Phila Pa 1976)* 1989;14(10):1046-1050.

15. Hindman BJ, Palecek JP, Posner KL, et al: Cervical spinal cord, root, and bony spine injuries: A closed claims analysis. *Anesthesiology* 2011;114(4):782-795.

16. Ryken TC, Hurlbert RJ, Hadley MN, et al: The acute cardiopulmonary management of patients with cervical spinal cord injuries. *Neurosurgery* 2013;72(suppl 2):84-92.

17. Fehlings MG, Tighe A: Spinal cord injury: The promise of translational research. *Neurosurg Focus* 2008;25(5):e1.

18. Cheney FW, Domino KB, Caplan RA, Posner KL: Nerve injury associated with anesthesia: A closed claims analysis. *Anesthesiology* 1999;90(4):1062-1069.

19. Warner MA, Warner ME, Martin JT: Ulnar neuropathy: Incidence, outcome, and risk factors in sedated or anesthetized patients. *Anesthesiology* 1994;81(6):1332-1340.

20. Morell RC, Prielipp RC, Harwood TN, James RL, Butterworth JF: Men are more susceptible than women to direct pressure on unmyelinated ulnar nerve fibers. *Anesth Analg* 2003;97(4):1183-1188.

21. Alvine FG, Schurrer ME: Postoperative ulnar-nerve palsy: Are there predisposing factors? *J Bone Joint Surg Am* 1987;69(2):255-259.

22. Hannallah D, Lee J, Khan M, Donaldson WF, Kang JD: Cerebrospinal fluid leaks following cervical spine surgery. *J Bone Joint Surg Am* 2008;90(5):1101-1105.

Collateral Adverse Outcomes After Lumbar Spine Surgery

Alan H. Daniels, MD

Kenneth Gundle, MD

Robert A. Hart, MD

Abstract

Collateral adverse outcomes are the expected or unavoidable results of a procedure that is performed in a standard manner and typically experienced by the patient. Collateral adverse outcomes do not result from errors, nor are they rare. Collateral adverse outcomes occur as the direct result of a surgical procedure and must be accepted as a trade-off to attain the intended benefits of the surgical procedure. As such, collateral adverse outcomes do not fit into the traditional definition of a complication or adverse event. Examples of collateral adverse outcomes after lumbar spine arthrodesis include lumbar stiffness, postoperative psychological stress, postoperative pain, peri-incisional numbness, paraspinal muscle denervation, and adjacent-level degeneration. Ideally, a comparison of interventions for the treatment of a clinical condition should include information on both the negative consequences (expected and unexpected) and potential benefits of the treatment options. The objective evaluation and reporting of collateral adverse outcomes will provide surgeons with a more complete picture of invasive interventions and, thus, the improved ability to assess alternative treatment options.

Instr Course Lect 2016;65:291–298.

For most surgical interventions, including lumbar spine procedures, the evaluation of adverse events and complications has lagged behind the measurement and reporting of positive outcomes. A complete evaluation of multiple interventions for the treatment of the same clinical condition is fundamental to understand the consequences of each treatment option. Negative outcomes of surgical interventions can be divided into three categories: complications, failure to cure, and collateral adverse outcomes.[1] Complications are defined as a negative deviation from the normal postoperative course. A failure to cure may occur in the absence of complications if an intervention fails to accomplish the desired benefit. Collateral adverse outcomes are negative aftereffects of surgery that are inherent to a procedure.[1]

The authors of this chapter define collateral adverse outcomes as adverse effects that are expected and frequently result from specific procedures but are not equivalent to complications.[1-3] Typically, most patients who experience collateral adverse outcomes do not require further evaluation or treatment, whereas patients who experience

Dr. Daniels or an immediate family member serves as a paid consultant to or is an employee of Osseus and Stryker, and has received nonincome support (such as equipment or services), commercially derived honoraria, or other non-research–related funding (such as paid travel) from DePuy and Stryker. Dr. Hart or an immediate family member has received royalties from DePuy and SeaSpine; is a member of a speakers' bureau or has made paid presentations on behalf of DePuy and Medtronic; serves as a paid consultant to or is an employee of DePuy and Medtronic; has stock or stock options held in Spine Connect; has received research or institutional support from DePuy; and serves as a board member, owner, officer, or committee member of the American Academy of Orthopaedic Surgeons, the American Orthopaedic Association, the Cervical Spine Research Society, the International Spine Study Group, the Lumbar Spine Research Society, the North American Spine Society, the Oregon Association of Orthopaedics, and the Scoliosis Research Society. Neither Dr. Gundle nor any immediate family member has received anything of value from or has stock or stock options held in a commercial company or institution related directly or indirectly to the subject of this chapter.

Table 1
Lumbar Stiffness Disability Index Questionnaire

Choose the statement that best describes the effect of low-back stiffness on your ability to:

1. Bend to your feet to put on your underwear and pants while dressing independently
2. Bend through your waist to put on your socks and shoes
3. Drive a motor vehicle
4. Perform personal hygiene functions after toileting
5. Bend forward to pick up a small object off the floor
6. Get in and out of bed
7. Get in and out of a chair
8. Bathe the lower half of your body
9. Get in and out of an automobile
10. Engage in sexual intercourse

Response options and score for each item

0 = No effect at all
1 = Minor effect
2 = Significant effect
3 = Require assistance
4 = Cannot do at all

Reproduced with permission from Hart RA, Gundle KR, Pro SL, Marshall LM: Lumbar Stiffness Disability Index: Pilot testing of consistency, reliability, and validity. *Spine J* 2013;13(2):157-161.

complications undergo additional monitoring, testing, or treatment because of the effects of the complication. Collateral adverse outcomes should be viewed as inherent to a given treatment and, thus, do not fit the traditional definition of a complication or adverse event. Collateral adverse outcomes also have been termed sequelae.[2] Surgical sequelae of solid-organ transplant procedures have been well described and include the necessity for lifelong immunosuppressant medication after organ transplantation.[2]

Examples of collateral adverse outcomes after lumbar spine surgery include functional limitations, which are caused by lumbar stiffness after fusion procedures;[3-5] postoperative psychological stress;[3,6] postoperative lumbar pain and pain at an autograft bone donor site; muscle denervation; and peri-incisional paresthesia. These collateral adverse outcomes have negative effects on patients, but are, in most cases, expected results of the surgical procedure performed. In general, collateral adverse outcomes are not related to technical errors or medical mismanagement, nor are they rare. Because collateral adverse outcomes are an expected result of some surgical interventions, they must be accepted as a trade-off to attain the intended benefits of the surgical procedure.

Concerns with regard to collateral adverse outcomes are not limited to lumbar spine fusion surgery. Collateral adverse outcomes, including hip abductor weakness after antegrade femoral nailing,[7,8] the necessity of prosthesis wear for ambulation after amputation,[9,10] and body-image and functional changes related to rotationplasty,[11] have been described in patients after orthopaedic trauma and oncology surgery.[7-11] The acceptance of collateral adverse outcomes in patients who undergo surgery for the treatment of trauma or cancer, however, undoubtedly differs from patients who undergo elective interventions to reduce pain and improve function. The collateral adverse outcomes of elective lumbar spine fusion have improved surgeons' understanding of collateral adverse outcomes and have provided surgeons with a more complete picture of the risks and benefits of lumbar spine surgery.

Collateral Adverse Outcomes After Lumbar Spine Surgery
Stiffness After Spinal Fusion

The goal of spinal arthrodesis is to alleviate pain and stabilize the spine affected by various pathologies. The elimination of motion across one or more spinal motion segments is inherent to a successful fusion. It is possible that a clinically successful lumbar spine arthrodesis may result in a decrease in motion that negatively affects a patient's ability to perform activities of daily living (ADLs) that require lumbar mobility. The Lumbar Stiffness Disability Index (LSDI), which is a spine-specific, patient-reported outcome measure, assesses limitations in ADLs that are caused by stiffness after lumbar spine arthrodesis[4,5,12] (**Table 1**). The LSDI consists of 10 questions with regard to the effect of low-back stiffness on a variety of ADLs; the final score ranges from 0 to 100, with higher scores indicating greater disability. The LSDI has excellent internal consistency and retest reliability, and higher LSDI scores correlate with decreased lumbar range of motion as measured on flexion-extension lateral radiographs.[5,12]

An important factor for surgeons to consider in an examination of the aftereffects of spinal fusion is whether patients will detect activity limitations that result from stiffness. In a cross-sectional study of 93 patients who underwent lumbar spine arthrodesis, Hart et al[5] reported that LSDI scores were significantly higher in patients who had five or more spinal level fusions compared with patients who had single-level fusions; however, there was no difference in Oswestry Disability Index (ODI) scores between the two groups. This suggests that patients perceive stiffness as distinct from spine-related pain and disability, with greater effects noted after fusions that include more spinal levels.

An understanding of the effect of changes in stiffness-related activity limitations on patient satisfaction after lumbar fusion is required to address patients' preoperative concerns. Hart et al[4] performed a prospective cohort study of 62 patients who underwent lumbar spine fusion for the treatment of degenerative disk disease, degenerative spondylolisthesis, or spinal deformity. The authors administered the LSDI, ODI, and Medical Outcomes Study 36-Item Short Form (SF-36) as well as a patient-satisfaction survey preoperatively and at a minimum 2-year follow-up. As expected, the ODI scores improved significantly across all arthrodesis levels. Interestingly, patients who underwent a single-level spinal fusion demonstrated a statistically significant decrease in LSDI scores at 2-year follow-up, which indicated fewer functional effects from stiffness after arthrodesis than at baseline. Conversely, there was a consistent trend toward increased LSDI scores as the number of spinal fusion levels increased (**Figure 1**). Patients who underwent five or more spinal level fusions experienced an eight-point increase in their postoperative LSDI scores compared with their preoperative LSDI scores ($P = 0.055$). Most importantly, 91% of patients, including 94% of patients who underwent arthrodesis from the thoracic spine to the pelvis, reported that any increase in stiffness was an acceptable trade-off for their overall pain relief and functional improvement.

Daniels et al[13] compared the LSDI scores of 176 asymptomatic volunteers with the LSDI scores of 693 patients who had an adult spinal deformity

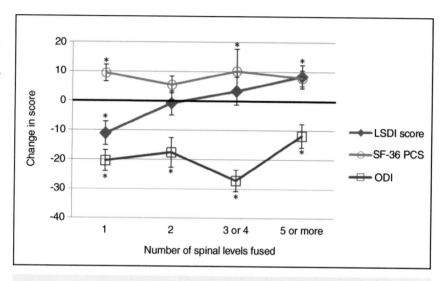

Figure 1   Plot graph shows that the trend toward increased postoperative Lumbar Stiffness Disability Index (LSDI) scores correlate with the number of spinal levels fused. ODI = Oswestry Disability Index, SF-36 PCS = Medical Outcomes Study 36-Item Short Form physical component score. (Reproduced with permission from Hart RA, Marshall LM, Hiratzka SL, Kane MS, Volpi J, Hiratzka JR: Functional limitations due to stiffness as a collateral impact of instrumental arthrodesis of the lumbar spine. *Spine (Phila Pa 1976)* 2014;36[24]:E1468-E1474.)

(ASD). The mean LSDI score for the asymptomatic volunteers was 3.4 ± 6.3 (maximum score = 100), with a significant correlation between increasing age and a higher (worse) LSDI score ($r = 0.30$, $P = 0.0001$), which indicated that stiffness-related disability increases with increasing age, even in patients who do not have symptomatic lumbar spine disease. In the ASD cohort, 301 patients underwent surgery and 392 were treated nonsurgically. The patients with ASD who underwent surgery had significantly higher preoperative LSDI scores than both the patients with ASD who underwent nonsurgical treatment and the asymptomatic volunteers (29.9 versus 17.3 versus 3.4, $P < 0.0001$ for both). Significant correlations were reported between the LSDI and the Scoliosis Research Society-22r Questionnaire pain and function subscales ($r = -0.75$ and -0.76, respectively; $P < 0.0001$ for both) in the patients

who had ASD. The results of this study highlight that patients who have ASD report substantial stiffness-related disability before surgical fusion.

The preoperative stiffness associated with ASD helps explain why some patients who undergo pan-lumbar fusion for the treatment of ASD report 2-year postoperative LSDI scores that are unchanged compared with their preoperative LSDI scores, despite significant improvements in health-related quality-of-life measures (International Spine Study Group, Brighton, CO, unpublished data, 2015). A substantial subset of patients who undergo long-segment spinal fusion, however, report postoperative limitations in dressing and bathing the lower half of their body.[14]

Taken together, these studies demonstrate that stiffness is a specific, patient-reported collateral adverse outcome that may occur after lumbar spine arthrodesis. Beyond radiographic

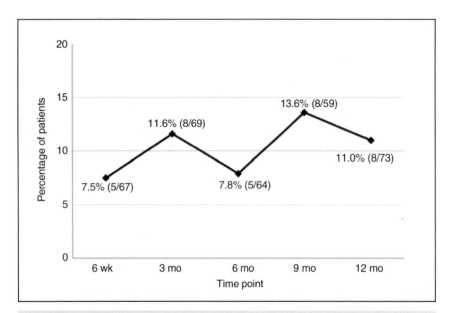

Figure 2 Plot graph shows the incidence of posttraumatic stress in patients in the first year after elective lumbar spine surgery. (Reproduced with permission from Deisseroth K, Hart RA: Symptoms of post-traumatic stress following elective lumbar spinal arthrodesis. *Spine (Phila Pa 1976)* 2012;37[18]: 1628-1633.)

measurements that demonstrate decreased range of motion, some patients perceive increased limitations in ADLs, which are caused by stiffness after lumbar spine fusion, particularly if five or more spinal level fusions are performed. Because fusion is the technical goal of the lumbar spine arthrodesis, stiffness does not represent a complication but, rather, an expected, or collateral, outcome. Surgeons should inform patients of the potential for lumbar stiffness after long-segment arthrodesis; however, it appears that most patients believe that improvements in overall pain and function are more important than the resulting effects of stiffness.

Posttraumatic Stress

Postoperative psychological distress also is an important aftereffect of intensive medical interventions. Symptoms of posttraumatic stress disorder (PTSD) have been reported after elective lumbar fusion[3,6] and musculoskeletal trauma.[3,6,15-17] To assess the incidence and risk factors for the development of PTSD symptoms after elective lumbar arthrodesis, Deisseroth and Hart[6] performed a prospective cohort study at a single tertiary care spine center. A consecutive series of 73 patients who underwent elective lumbar spine arthrodesis were evaluated prospectively with the PTSD Checklist—Civilian Version[18] 6 weeks, 3 months, 6 months, 9 months, and 12 months after surgery. The sex, age, education level, job status, marital status, psychiatric history, surgical approach, estimated blood loss, postoperative intubation, length of intensive care unit and hospital stay, and occurrence of perioperative complications for each patient were analyzed as predictors of PTSD symptoms. The overall incidence of PTSD symptoms that was identified among the elective lumbar fusion patients during at least one time point was 19.2% (14 of 73). The percentage of patients who had

PTSD symptoms at each time point is shown in **Figure 2**. The presence of a prior psychiatric diagnosis was the strongest predictor of postoperative PTSD symptoms (odds ratio = 7.05, $P = 0.002$); however, the occurrence of a complication also was significantly correlated with the development of PTSD symptoms (odds ratio = 4.33, $P = 0.04$).

In a follow-up study of the same patient group, Hart et al[3] performed a prospective assessment to determine the effect of postoperative PTSD symptoms on patient-reported clinical outcomes after lumbar arthrodesis. The authors reported that PTSD symptoms were associated with a statistically significant reduction in surgical benefit as measured by the final and the total change in ODI and SF-36 physical component scores, respectively. The likelihood of reaching minimal clinically important difference for both ODI and SF-36 physical component scores also was reduced in patients who reported PTSD symptoms. Conversely, the presence of a preoperative psychiatric diagnosis was significantly correlated only with the final ODI score. Preoperative SF-36 mental component scores were significantly correlated with the final ODI and SF-36 physical component scores as well as the final change from the preoperative and the likelihood of reaching minimal clinically important difference for SF-36 physical component scores but not for ODI scores.

These studies suggest that postoperative psychological distress is a relatively frequent occurrence after elective lumbar spine fusion and has a clinical effect on patients. Symptoms of PTSD were strongly correlated with reduced clinical benefit among the patients in these studies and appeared to be a stronger predictor of reduced clinical benefit compared with both a major psychiatric diagnosis and preoperative mental component scores. Efforts to reduce the collateral adverse effects of postoperative psychological distress may provide surgeons with an opportunity to enhance patient-reported clinical outcomes after elective spine surgery.

Additional Collateral Adverse Outcomes After Lumbar Spine Surgery

Postoperative pain is almost universal after surgical interventions and is an important collateral adverse outcome after lumbar spinal surgery. Pain at both the lumbar incision site and iliac crest bone graft site may cause substantial physical and psychological stress immediately after surgery and during the prolonged recovery process.[19,20] Buttock paresthesias and peri-incisional numbness are sequelae that also may occur after lumbar spine surgery, especially after long-segment posterior fusion with sacroiliac fixation that results in the disruption of posterior cutaneous innervation.

Although posterior approaches remain an important component of lumbar spine surgical strategy, modern lumbar spine surgery also includes direct anterior, lateral, and oblique approaches. Abdominal wall paralysis, which is caused by division of the abdominal musculature, is a collateral adverse outcome that may occur with the use of an open anterior, oblique, or lateral lumbar approach across multiple spine segments. Abdominal wall paralysis has been reported at the thoracolumbar junction with the use of posterior approaches as well[21] (**Figure 3**) and, presumably, is caused by indirect compression or manipulation of the

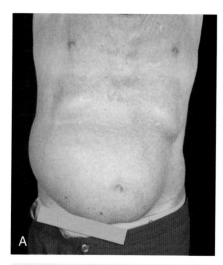 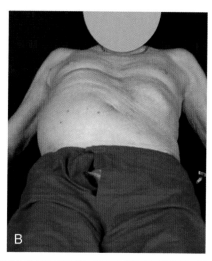

Figure 3   Clinical photographs of the abdomen of a patient in both a standing position (**A**) and lying supine (**B**) show abdominal wall paralysis. (Reproduced with permission from Baker JF, Galbraith JG, Synnott KA: Abdominal wall palsy after spinal surgery. *Spine J* 2014;14[12]:3063-3064.)

segmental roots. Because abdominal wall paralysis is less of an expected result with the use a posterior approach, it would not be considered a collateral adverse outcome.

An additional collateral adverse outcome after lateral lumbar spine surgery is psoas injury. Both open and percutaneous lateral access surgeries include at least some degree of psoas injury,[22] with expected postoperative transient hip flexor weakness that is caused by psoas muscle penetration and/or retraction. Thigh numbness and paresthesias also are common and are believed to be related to femoral cutaneous nerve irritation. Efficient disk space access and preparation are necessary to ensure that hip flexion weakness and thigh paresthesias are temporary collateral adverse outcomes that typically resolve within 3 months after surgery and not permanent adverse events.[23]

Time lost from work and revision surgery are two collateral adverse events that have important psychosocial and economic ramifications. Time loss from work during the recovery process is inherent to most invasive surgical procedures and may be prolonged after lumbar spine fusion, especially in workers compensation patients.[24-26] Revision lumbar spine fusion that results from adjacent-level degeneration also may be considered a collateral adverse outcome because fusion, by intention, increases the mechanical loading and motion of adjacent disks no matter how limited the surgical approach.[27,28] Delineating adjacent-segment degeneration that is caused by natural aging and degenerative processes from adjacent-segment degeneration that is caused by surgical change is virtually impossible; therefore, patients should be counseled that future spinal degeneration may occur with or without the planned surgical intervention.

Discussion

The recent efforts of the authors of this chapter to define and evaluate collateral adverse outcomes after lumbar spine surgery have improved their understanding of the aftereffects of lumbar spine surgery; however, their study and reporting of negative outcomes continues to lag behind the study and reporting of positive outcomes. Clear definitions of collateral outcomes and dedicated attention to their detection are the first steps in clinical research. The authors of this chapter hope that the development and validation of outcome tools, such as the LSDI, may not only answer specific clinical questions but also illustrate the concept of collateral adverse outcomes.

Currently, clinical investigators lack validated, widely accepted tools to record and report collateral outcomes and adverse events after lumbar arthrodesis. Therefore, it is not surprising that clinical researchers who focus on the lumbar spine and other orthopaedic specialties use varied approaches to record and report adverse consequences of treatment.[29-31] Because of this lack of uniform reporting, some studies have used large patient databases as sources for comparative information on the negative effects of spine surgery.[32-35] Patient databases are prone to incomplete and inaccurate data because they are derived from billing and coding information and lack specific information on patient diagnoses, procedures, complications, and ultimate clinical outcomes. Although comparisons of such data may be valid and potentially useful, ultimately, patient databases are not a satisfactory substitute for the direct evaluation and reporting of adverse collateral outcomes.

Efforts to study lumbar stiffness and PTSD symptoms after lumbar spine arthrodesis support the notion that patient-centered tools that are designed to measure collateral adverse outcomes may be helpful to attain a more complete assessment of clinical outcomes after lumbar spine surgery. Future steps should include efforts that weigh the relative effect of further specific collateral outcomes and the development of more general outcome tools that measure the relative perceived negative effects of surgical intervention from the perspective of patients.

Summary

Collateral adverse events are common after lumbar spine surgery and include lumbar stiffness, postoperative psychological stress, postoperative pain, peri-incisional numbness, time loss from work, and adjacent-level degeneration. Future comparisons of interventions for the treatment of specific clinical conditions should include information on both the negative consequences (expected and unexpected) and the potential benefits of treatment options. Additional objective measurement and reporting of collateral and other adverse outcomes of surgery will provide surgeons with a more complete picture of their interventions and, thereby, improve their ability to assess alternative treatments. The potential collateral adverse outcomes of lumbar spine surgery should be clearly presented to any patient who is considering lumbar spine surgery, which may result in more patients who favor nonsurgical management versus surgical intervention.

References

1. Dindo D, Demartines N, Clavien PA: Classification of surgical complications: A new proposal with evaluation in a cohort of 6336 patients and results of a survey. *Ann Surg* 2004;240(2):205-213.

2. Ciesek S, Manns M, Strassburg C: Sequelae of organ transplantation. *Internist (Berl)* 2006;47(3):252, 254-256, 258-260 passim.

3. Hart R, Perry E, Hiratzka S, Kane M, Deisseroth K: Post-traumatic stress symptoms after elective lumbar arthrodesis are associated with reduced clinical benefit. *Spine (Phila Pa 1976)* 2013;38(17):1508-1515.

4. Hart RA, Marshall LM, Hiratzka SL, Kane MS, Volpi J, Hiratzka JR: Functional limitations due to stiffness as a collateral impact of instrumented arthrodesis of the lumbar spine. *Spine (Phila Pa 1976)* 2014;39(24):E1468-E1474.

5. Hart RA, Pro SL, Gundle KR, Marshall LM: Lumbar stiffness as a collateral outcome of spinal arthrodesis: A preliminary clinical study. *Spine J* 2013;13(2):150-156.

6. Deisseroth K, Hart RA: Symptoms of post-traumatic stress following elective lumbar spinal arthrodesis. *Spine (Phila Pa 1976)* 2012;37(18):1628-1633.

7. Archdeacon M, Ford KR, Wyrick J, et al: A prospective functional outcome and motion analysis evaluation of the hip abductors after femur fracture and antegrade nailing. *J Orthop Trauma* 2008;22(1):3-9.

8. Bain GI, Zacest AC, Paterson DC, Middleton J, Pohl AP: Abduction strength following intramedullary nailing of the femur. *J Orthop Trauma* 1997;11(2):93-97.

9. Tsikandylakis G, Berlin Ö, Brånemark R: Implant survival, adverse events, and bone remodeling of osseointegrated percutaneous implants for transhumeral amputees. *Clin Orthop Relat Res* 2014;472(10):2947-2956.

10. Van de Meent H, Hopman MT, Frölke JP: Walking ability and quality of life in subjects with transfemoral amputation: A comparison of osseointegration with socket prostheses. *Arch Phys Med Rehabil* 2013;94(11):2174-2178.

11. Veenstra KM, Sprangers MA, van der Eyken JW, Taminiau AH: Quality of life in survivors with a Van Ness-Borggreve rotationplasty after bone tumour resection. *J Surg Oncol* 2000;73(4):192-197.

12. Hart RA, Gundle KR, Pro SL, Marshall LM: Lumbar Stiffness Disability Index: Pilot testing of consistency, reliability, and validity. *Spine J* 2013;13(2):157-161.

13. Daniels AH, Smith JS, Hiratzka J, et al: Functional limitations due to lumbar stiffness in adults with and without spinal deformity. *Spine (Phila Pa 1976)* 2015. ePub ahead of print.

14. Sciubba DM, Scheer JK, Smith JS, et al: Which daily functions are most affected by stiffness following total lumbar fusion: Comparison of upper thoracic and thoracolumbar proximal endpoints. *Spine (Phila Pa 1976)* 2015;40(17):1338-1344.

15. Helmerhorst GT, Vranceanu AM, Vrahas M, Smith M, Ring D: Risk factors for continued opioid use one to two months after surgery for musculoskeletal trauma. *J Bone Joint Surg Am* 2014;96(6):495-499.

16. Nota SP, Bot AG, Ring D, Kloen P: Disability and depression after orthopaedic trauma. *Injury* 2015;46(2)207-212

17. Vranceanu AM, Hageman M, Strooker J, Ter Meulen D, Vrahas M, Ring D: A preliminary RCT of a mind body skills based intervention addressing mood and coping strategies in patients with acute orthopaedic trauma. *Injury* 2015;46(4):552-557

18. Smith MY, Redd W, DuHamel K, Vickberg SJ, Ricketts P: Validation of the PTSD Checklist-Civilian Version in survivors of bone marrow transplantation. *J Trauma Stress* 1999;12(3):485-499.

19. Heary RF, Schlenk RP, Sacchieri TA, Barone D, Brotea C: Persistent iliac crest donor site pain: Independent outcome assessment. *Neurosurgery* 2002;50(3):510-517.

20. Howard JM, Glassman SD, Carreon LY: Posterior iliac crest pain after posterolateral fusion with or without iliac crest graft harvest. *Spine J* 2011;11(6):534-537.

21. Baker JF, Galbraith JG, Synnott KA: Abdominal wall palsy after spinal surgery. *Spine J* 2014;14(12):3063-3064.

22. Berjano P, Lamartina C: Far lateral approaches (XLIF) in adult scoliosis. *Eur Spine J* 2013;22(suppl 2):242-253.

23. Pumberger M, Hughes AP, Huang RR, Sama AA, Cammisa FP, Girardi FP: Neurologic deficit following lateral lumbar interbody fusion. *Eur Spine J* 2012;21(6):1192-1199.

24. Lavin RA, Tao X, Yuspeh L, Bernacki EJ: Temporal relationship between lumbar spine surgeries, return to work, and workers' compensation costs in a cohort of injured workers. *J Occup Environ Med* 2013;55(5):539-543.

25. Mummaneni PV, Whitmore RG, Curran JN, et al: Cost-effectiveness of lumbar discectomy and single-level fusion for spondylolisthesis: Experience with the NeuroPoint-SD registry. *Neurosurg Focus* 2014;36(6):E3.

26. Oestergaard LG, Christensen FB, Nielsen CV, Bünger CE, Fruensgaard S, Sogaard R: Early versus late initiation of rehabilitation after lumbar spinal fusion: Economic evaluation alongside a randomized controlled trial. *Spine (Phila Pa 1976)* 2013;38(23):1979-1985.

27. Helgeson MD, Bevevino AJ, Hilibrand AS: Update on the evidence for adjacent segment degeneration and disease. *Spine J* 2013;13(3):342-351.

28. Untch C, Liu Q, Hart R: Segmental motion adjacent to an instrumented lumbar fusion: The effect of extension of fusion to the sacrum. *Spine (Phila Pa 1976)* 2004;29(21):2376-2381.

29. Mirza SK, Deyo RA: Systematic review of randomized trials comparing lumbar fusion surgery to nonoperative care for treatment of chronic back pain. *Spine (Phila Pa 1976)* 2007;32(7):816-823.

30. Fenton JJ, Mirza SK, Lahad A, Stern BD, Deyo RA: Variation in reported safety of lumbar interbody fusion: Influence of industrial sponsorship and other study characteristics. *Spine (Phila Pa 1976)* 2007;32(4):471-480.

31. Goldhahn S, Sawaguchi T, Audigé L, et al: Complication reporting in orthopaedic trials: A systematic review of randomized controlled trials. *J Bone Joint Surg Am* 2009;91(8):1847-1853.

32. Irwin ZN, Arthur M, Mullins RJ, Hart RA: Variations in injury patterns, treatment, and outcome for spinal fracture and paralysis in adult versus geriatric patients. *Spine (Phila Pa 1976)* 2004;29(7):796-802.

33. Martin BI, Mirza SK, Comstock BA, Gray DT, Kreuter W, Deyo RA: Are lumbar spine reoperation rates falling with greater use of fusion surgery and new surgical technology? *Spine (Phila Pa 1976)* 2007;32(19):2119-2126.

34. Kalanithi PS, Patil CG, Boakye M: National complication rates and disposition after posterior lumbar fusion for acquired spondylolisthesis. *Spine (Phila Pa 1976)* 2009;34(18):1963-1969.

35. Juratli SM, Mirza SK, Fulton-Kehoe D, Wickizer TM, Franklin GM: Mortality after lumbar fusion surgery. *Spine (Phila Pa 1976)* 2009;34(7):740-747.

SECTION

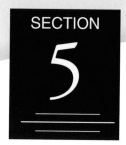

5

Foot and Ankle

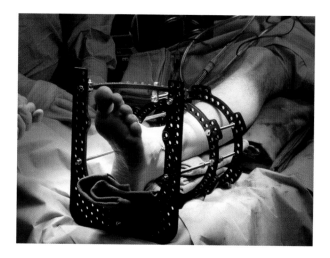

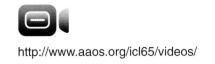

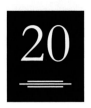

Role of Fresh Osteochondral Allografts for Large Talar Osteochondral Lesions

Christopher E. Gross, MD

Samuel B. Adams Jr, MD

Mark E. Easley, MD

James A. Nunley, MD

Abstract

Osteochondral lesions of the talus, large or small, are challenging for the treating orthopaedic surgeon. These cartilage and bony defects can cause substantial pain and functional disability. Surgical treatment of small osteochondral lesions of the talus has been thoroughly explored and includes retrograde drilling, arthroscopic débridement and marrow stimulation, osteochondral autografting from cartilage/bone unit harvested from the ipsilateral knee (mosaicplasty), and autologous chondrocyte implantation. Although each of these reparative, replacement, or regenerative techniques has varying degrees of success, they may be insufficient for the treatment of large osteochondral lesions of the talus. Large-volume osteochondral lesions of the talus (>1.5 cm in diameter or >150 mm² in area) often involve a sizable portion of the weight-bearing section of the talar dome, medially or laterally. A fresh structural osteochondral allograft is a viable treatment option for large osteochondral lesions of the talus.

Instr Course Lect 2016;65:301–310.

Dr. Adams or an immediate family member is a member of a speakers' bureau or has made paid presentations on behalf of Harvest Technologies; serves as a paid consultant to or is an employee of Biomet, MedShape, Medtronic, Regeneration Technologies, and Stryker; and has stock or stock options held in MedShape. Dr. Easley or an immediate family member is a member of a speakers' bureau or has made paid presentations on behalf of Stryker and Tornier; serves as a paid consultant to or is an employee of DT MedSurg, Exactech, SBI, Tornier, Stryker, and TriMed; serves as an unpaid consultant to Orthofix; has received research or institutional support from Acumed and TriMed; and serves as a board member, owner, officer, or committee member of the American Orthopaedic Foot and Ankle Society. Dr. Nunley or an immediate family member has received royalties from Wright Medical Technology; is a member of a speakers' bureau or has made paid presentations on behalf of Orthofix; serves as a paid consultant to or is an employee of Exactech, DT MedSurg, Stryker, and Tornier; has stock or stock options held in Bristol-Myers Squibb, Merck, and Johnson & Johnson; and has received research or institutional support from the Orthopaedic Research and Education Foundation, Synthes, Integra LifeSciences, Breg, and Tornier. Neither Dr. Gross nor any immediate family member has received anything of value from or has stock or stock options held in a commercial company or institution related directly or indirectly to the subject of this chapter.

Large-volume osteochondral lesions of the talus (OLTs) (>1.5 cm in diameter or >150 mm² in area) often involve a sizable portion of the weight-bearing section of the talar dome, medially or laterally. In addition, they frequently involve the shoulder of the talus. Large OLTs are difficult to treat with standard techniques. OLTs have a poor ability to heal spontaneously, likely because of the relative hypovascularity of the cartilage and a sparse population of chondrocyte progenitor cells. Often, OLTs have a cystic component that is relatively more formidable to treat than a solitary cartilaginous lesion because it requires both cartilage restoration and bony structural support. Fresh structural osteochondral implantation has been used for the treatment of large OLTs.

Clinical Evaluation

Ankle pain carries a broad differential diagnosis (**Table 1**). The surgeon must first obtain a thorough history that

Table 1

Differential Diagnosis of an Osteochondral Lesion of the Talus

Stress fracture of the foot/ankle

Ankle instability

Ankle/subtalar arthritis

Synovitis

Injury to the syndesmosis

Peroneal tendon pathology

Bony or soft-tissue impingement

includes any recent or remote history of trauma or chronic ankle instability and any surgical intervention that has been undertaken about the ankle. Most OLTs can be attributed to a traumatic event; however, atraumatic lesions may occur in up to 24% of cases.[1] OLTs are more commonly seen in the second decade of life and in men (70%).[2] The onset, duration, quality, and severity of the patient's symptoms must be established. The surgeon must document all alleviating or exacerbating factors as well as prior treatment. Frequent symptoms include pain, clicking/catching, stiffness, and pain about the ankle.

Many patients may not be able to tolerate a full examination because of pain or stiffness, but it is imperative to obtain a functional baseline. The entire lower extremity should be examined in both weight-bearing and non–weight-bearing postures because it is critical to assess for mechanical alignment. The physical examination must include range of motion about the ankle and subtalar joints as well as a gait analysis. A gait assessment also is useful to establish a functional baseline. When observing gait, the surgeon should concentrate on the patient's posture, stride length, cadence, and walking speed as well as the duration of the walking cycle.[3] Ankle range of motion should be carefully measured to ensure that compensatory motion from the Chopart joints is not measured and compared with that of the contralateral side. Ankle stability, including the talar tilt and anterior drawer tests in plantar flexion and dorsiflexion, should be measured and compared with that of the opposite ankle.

Imaging

Radiographic imaging should include weight-bearing views (AP, lateral, and mortise/oblique) of the ankle. Hindfoot alignment and foot radiographs also should be considered[4] (**Figure 1**). These views will help the surgeon see early degenerative changes or any malalignment that should be considered during preoperative planning. Often, radiographs may not demonstrate pathology; however, they may detect a cystic component of the lesion if it is sufficiently large.

CT or MRI should be used in a primary role for patients in whom equivocal radiographs are obtained or in a supplemental role during preoperative planning to evaluate the degree of bone loss, osteonecrosis, or subchondral cyst formation (**Figures 2** and **3**). MRI may help identify other bony or soft-tissue lesions; therefore, it should be obtained in patients who have persistent ankle pain without any radiographic abnormality.

No evidence supports the superiority of either CT or MRI in the setting of normal radiographs and a suspicious clinical picture. In a study on the sensitivity and specificity of CT, MRI, and arthroscopy, Verhagen et al[5] reported no significant difference in the diagnosis of OLTs. Conversely, in a study of 14 patients who had OLTs that were not apparent on plain radiographs, Anderson et al[6] reported that CT identified 29% of these lesions, whereas MRI identified all of the lesions.

In characterizing an OLT or in planning surgery, CT is useful in assessing the subchondral bone; however, MRI is better at visualizing the articular surface. In addition, if an OLT is diagnosed on MRI, CT may be useful to determine the appropriate treatment because estimation of the size and stage of the lesion may be obscured on MRI by bone marrow edema.[7] However, MRI is 81% to 92% accurate in staging OLTs.[7-9]

The first widely used radiographic classification of OLTs was developed by Berndt and Harty[10] in 1959 and subsequently modified[10-12] (**Table 2**). OLTs were originally grouped into four stages; however, this classification failed to address any cystic component of the OLT. Stage V was added by Scranton and McDermott[11] in 2001, and Raikin[12] reported treatment of stage VI lesions (ie, >3,000 mm³). The Berndt and Harty[10] classification system may have a poor correlation with what is seen during arthroscopy. In a review of 24 arthroscopically examined OLTs, Pritsch et al[13] reported that 50% of the OLTs classified as Berndt and Harty stage IV had intact cartilage during arthroscopic visualization. The authors described an arthroscopic grading system based on visualization of the cartilage: grade I, intact, firm, shiny cartilage; grade II, intact but soft cartilage; and grade III, frayed cartilage. Ferkel et al[14] expanded this classification system but did not address the subchondral bone. Although several authors have proposed CT or MRI classification

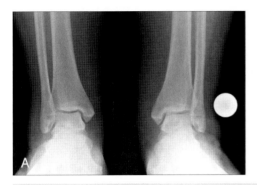
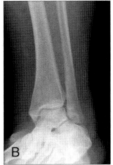
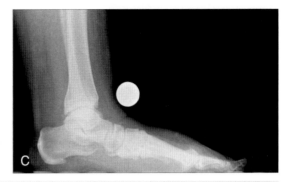

Figure 1   AP (**A**), mortise (**B**), and lateral (**C**) radiographs demonstrate a medial talar dome lesion of a left ankle.

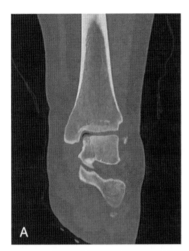
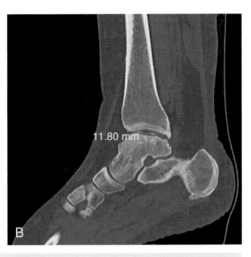

Figure 2   Coronal (**A**) and sagittal (**B**) CT scans demonstrate a medial talar dome osteochondral defect with cystic changes.

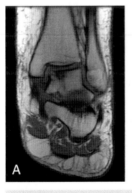
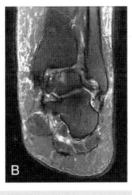
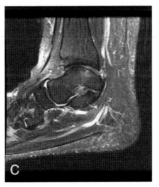

Figure 3   Coronal T1-weighted (**A**), coronal T2-weighted (**B**), and sagittal T2-weighted (**C**) MRIs demonstrate evidence of a medial talar dome osteochondral defect with reactive bone marrow edema and cystic changes.

Table 2
Modified Berndt and Harty[10] Radiographic Classification of Osteochondral Lesions of the Talus

Stage	Radiographic Findings
I	Focal subchondral bone compression
II	Focal subchondral bone compression with partial cartilage detachment
III	Focal subchondral bone compression with complete detachment
IV	Focal subchondral bone compression with complete detachment and displaced
V[11]	Cartilage cap intact, talar dome subchondral cyst
VI[12]	Cystic lesions >3,000 mm³

Nonsurgical Treatment

Some studies recommend a trial of 3 to 6 months of nonsurgical management for all nondisplaced OLTs.[16-18] Nonsurgical therapies include analgesic agents, activity modification, and protected weight bearing (eg, non–weight-bearing cast, controlled ankle movement boot, patellar tendon–bearing brace). However, because quality literature is scarce, no recommendations can be made with regard to the weight-bearing status or appropriate

schemes, their classifications are similar to the original Berndt and Harty[10] classification system.[6,14,15]

Currently, it is unclear whether any classification system helps guide the treating surgeon.

time for and type of immobilization that may be helpful.

Surgical Treatment
Patient Selection

Characteristics of the OLT, including undamaged versus disrupted articular surface, displaced versus nondisplaced, and cystic versus noncystic, must be considered during surgical planning.[19] The patient must understand the inherent risks in receiving an allograft, including disease transmission and allograft rejection, although the actual chances of these complications occurring are minimal. In the practice of the authors of this chapter, the indications for the use of a fresh allograft for the treatment of an OLT include the following: a patient in whom prior arthroscopic techniques or cartilage restoration has failed, a large OLT that involves the shoulder region of the talus, an OLT with a large cystic component, and any lesion larger than 1.5 cm^2 in diameter or larger than 150 mm^2 in area.

To find an appropriate donor talus, the patient's contralateral talus is used as a template and sized on CT. The authors of this chapter attempt to match the size and shape of the allograft as closely as possible to the patient's native anatomy. Specifications are then sent to an agency that obtains allograft tissues. The authors of this chapter use osteochondral allografts obtained from US FDA-approved suppliers who comply with the guidelines of the American Association of Tissue Banks. Both the patient and the surgeon must be prepared to wait an unspecified amount of time and to have a flexible schedule when a graft is available.

The donor talus is sterilely harvested within 24 hours of death. Next, the allograft undergoes disease testing and sterility culturing for approximately 2 weeks. During this time, the donor's medical history is reviewed for factors that may lead to an unacceptable graft, such as high-risk behavior. The graft is maintained at 2°C to 4°C. If the graft is found acceptable, it is then processed and shipped, usually within 3 weeks. The graft typically arrives at the hospital in 1 day. The surgeon must ensure that the graft is from the proper laterality and that the articular cartilage has been left intact on the allograft talus. The authors of this chapter typically obtain a radiograph of the donor talus preoperatively to confirm correct size.

Cartilage Viability

Allograft transplantation prevents long-term joint degeneration by providing viable chondrocytes that have the ability to support themselves. The authors of this chapter prefer to use fresh osteochondral grafts in lieu of fresh-frozen or frozen allografts because of the amount of fresh chondrocytes; however, a recent systematic review[20] of knee osteochondral allografts was unable to report a difference in the failure rate or functional outcomes among the different procurement methods. In the knee literature, fresh osteochondral allografts have been reported to contain viable chondrocytes for up to 17 years after transplantation;[21] however, Enneking and Campanacci[22] and Enneking and Mindell[23] were unable to demonstrate viable chondrocytes 1 year after transplantation. In fact, both studies reported histologic evidence of early cartilage damage.

Chondrocyte viability in fresh allografts decreases with time. At 4 weeks after harvest, osteochondral allografts have a substantial drop in viable chondrocytes, albeit by only 30% from the starting amount.[24] Nonetheless, as soon as the allograft is made available, the transplantation should be scheduled. Williams et al[24] harvested 60 osteochondral plugs from 10 fresh human femoral condyles within 48 hours after the death of the donor. The plugs were stored at 4°C. The specimens were then analyzed at 1 day, 1 week, 2 weeks, and 4 weeks after harvest. Chondrocyte viability and viable cell density remained unchanged up to 2 weeks after harvest. Proteoglycan synthesis remained unchanged until 2 weeks after harvest. No substantial differences were detected in glycosaminoglycan content or compressive or tensile modulus at 4 weeks after harvest.

Surgical Technique
Approaches

Most of the surgical techniques used for smaller OLTs require minimal arthroscopic access. However, if reconstructing larger portions of the talus, the articular surface must be accessed perpendicularly.[12,25-28] Lesions of the anterior or posterior surface of the talus are most easily accessible via a standard anterior or posterior approach for ankle arthrotomy. Depending on the location of the lesion, the talus is either maximally plantarflexed or dorsiflexed to allow for excision of the lesion and allograft transplantation. However, for medial or lateral shoulder lesions, the surgeon needs to perform either a medial malleolar osteotomy or a lateral malleolar osteotomy/anterior talofibular ligament/calcaneofibular ligament release, respectively.

Medial Approach

The preferred approach of the authors of this chapter is the oblique medial malleolar osteotomy. One theoretic concern about this technique is that it breaches the articular surface of the tibial plafond; in practice, however, the authors of this chapter have not experienced any unexpected consequences (eg, accelerated tibial-sided arthritis).

A 5-cm–long incision is made over the medial malleolus longitudinally. Using careful soft-tissue dissection, the superficial neurovascular structures are protected. The posterior tibial tendon is exposed through the flexor retinaculum and protected. Using fluoroscopic guidance, a guide pin or Kirschner wire (K-wire), which is aimed obliquely through the medial malleolar shoulder to the lateral extent of the lesion, is inserted. At this point, the holes for two 4.0-mm partially threaded cancellous screws are drilled. Then, with a saw, the osteotomy is made slightly distal and lateral to the K-wire path. Cold saline is used to mitigate the risk of heat necrosis. Penetration into the articular surface is made with a controlled maneuver using an osteotome. The distal osteotomized medial malleolus is then reflected on a deltoid pedicle.

Anterior Approach

An incision is made 1 cm lateral to the anterior tibial spine, centered over the ankle. The incision should be approximately 6 cm long, two-thirds of which is proximal to the ankle joint and one-third of which is distal to the joint. During the initial incision, care is taken to protect the intermediate cutaneous branch of the superficial peroneal nerve and the anterior neurovascular bundle. The superficial surgical dissection begins by incising the fascia and identifying the plane between the extensor hallucis longus (EHL) and the anterior tibialis tendon (ATT). The EHL is identified distally;

the retinaculum over the sheath is incised to allow for retraction laterally. Alternatively, the ATT sheath can be incised and the tendon moved laterally. The anterior neurovascular bundle is deep to the EHL tendon distally and should be carefully retracted laterally. Typically, the ATT is maintained in its sheath and is retracted medially. The overlying soft tissue is incised to expose the anterior ankle joint capsule. The capsule is reflected medially and laterally. The talus is now fully exposed and visualized. Frequently, a pin distractor is placed (one 2.4-mm pin in the tibia and one 2.4-mm pin in the talus) to enhance visualization.

Lateral Approach

If the talar lesion is lateral, a 6- to 7-cm standard lateral approach is used, centered over the fibula and directed toward the fourth metatarsal. The skin is incised and the subcutaneous tissue is carefully dissected. The inferior extensor retinaculum is identified for later use in the repair. A Freer retractor or hemostat is placed anteriorly between the capsule and the bone, which defines the capsule. The anterior talofibular ligament is then incised, erring on the fibular side so that there is sufficient tissue to pull back up to the fibula for closure. After this step is performed, the talus can be anteriorly translated for the reconstruction. The fibula is rarely osteotomized because so much of the lateral surface of the talus is visible after the lateral ligaments have been released.

Structural Reconstruction

After the lesion is identified, the surgeon should correlate the preoperative imaging with intraoperative visualization of the osteochondral lesion to ensure that the lesion is appreciated.

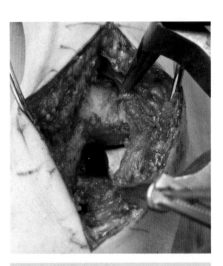

Figure 4   Intraoperative photograph shows that the necrotic section of a talus has been removed using a combination of a microsagittal and a reciprocating saw with cold irrigant.

One or two small K-wires are inserted anterior to posterior into the talus as a guide for removing the OLT. Fluoroscopic imaging should confirm that the guide pin will allow for complete excision of the OLT. Using a combination of a microsagittal and a reciprocating saw (with cold irrigant), the necrotic section of the talus is removed (**Figure 4**). The reciprocating saw is used to create a perfect vertical cut adjacent to the lesion in the talus. A cut is then made perpendicularly approximately 1.5 to 2 cm below the height of the dome of the talus. After the diseased bone and cartilage are removed, the dimensions of the defect are carefully measured with a caliper and ruler.

On a sterile back table, the portion of the allograft talus that corresponds with the defect is carefully measured to match the excised talus. After an outline of the initial cuts is made, both the native talar defects and the allograft talus are again measured (**Figure 5**). The allograft is then cut with a combination of saws. The structural allograft is

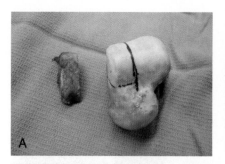
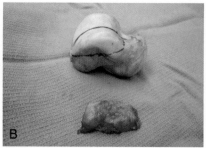
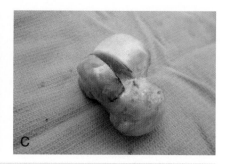

Figure 5 Intraoperative photographs of the talus show that after an outline of the initial cuts is made (**A**), both the native talar defects (**B**) and the allograft talus (**C**) are measured again.

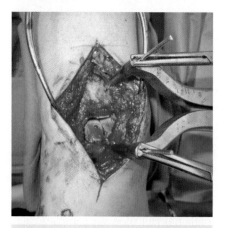

Figure 6 Intraoperative photograph shows the final construct of a talar hemiallograft fixated with one titanium screw.

thoroughly irrigated to reduce potential immunogenicity and is brought to the defect in the talus, where it is trialed. Additional contouring with the use of a small rongeur or power burr is usually necessary. After the allograft has acceptable contours, it can be slightly press-fit into the native talus. Radiographs are checked but may overexaggerate small incongruities; it is best to rely on visual inspection. If imperfections between the inferior surface and the graft-native interface exist, it is best to fill them with crushed cancellous chips. One or two 1.5-mm titanium screws can be used to supplement fixation. It is important that the screw heads be

countersunk (**Figure 6**). The ankle is brought through dorsiflexion and plantar flexion to ensure that the graft fits dynamically and that no impingement exists. The interface between the graft and host is covered with a fibrin sealant. The ankle is then closed in the usual fashion.

If the medial approach is used, the medial malleolus is anatomically reduced, and the reduction is confirmed radiographically. Fixation is performed with two screws and, at times, supplemented with a buttress plate or transverse screw. If the lateral approach is used, the anterior talofibular ligament is anatomically reduced and fixation is accomplished with one 3.5-mm suture anchor while the ankle is held in maximum dorsiflexion and eversion.

Postoperative Protocol

After wound closure, the patient is fitted with a bulky post-mold and sugar tong splint and made non–weight bearing. The patient is usually kept overnight for pain control. Two to 3 weeks postoperatively, the wound is inspected and sutures are removed. Early passive range of motion may be best for the survival of the cartilage;[29] however, this must be balanced with the need for the osteotomy to heal. Therefore, the authors of this chapter fit the patient with

a short leg, non–weight-bearing cast to be worn for an additional 4 weeks. The authors of this chapter split the cast so that the top half may be removed and the patient can perform ankle range-of-motion exercises while lying supine. At 6 weeks postoperatively, the cast is removed, and the patient is fitted with a controlled ankle movement boot. The patient can initiate partial weight bearing and progress to weight bearing as tolerated at 10 to 12 weeks postoperatively. At 3 months postoperatively, the patient is allowed to participate in recumbent cycling and other nonimpact activities. At 6 months postoperatively, the patient may begin more advanced activities.

Outcomes

Few studies exist on osteochondral allografting for OLTs, and there are even fewer studies on osteochondral allografting for larger OLTs. Gross et al[30] studied nine patients who were treated with fresh osteochondral allograft transplantation. Preoperatively, the lesions were at least 1 cm in diameter, with a Berndt and Harty[10] stage IV classification; the authors did not report the mean defect size. Two-thirds of the allografts remained in situ at a mean follow-up of 11 years (range, 4 to 19 years). The grafts in the remaining patients demonstrated radiographic and intraoperative evidence of resorption or fragmentation; all of these patients underwent ankle fusion.

In a study of six patients who had bulk allografting of OLTs (mean defect size, 4.38 cm³; range, 3.54 to 6.70 cm³), Raikin[12] reported satisfactory results in five patients at 23 months postoperatively. Four patients underwent fresh-frozen osteochondral allografting, and the other two patients underwent fresh allograft transplantation. The allografts were fixed with headless dual-pitched screws. The one patient who subsequently underwent ankle fusion had a preoperative CT scan that demonstrated graft incorporation. More recently, Raikin[31] published a study on 15 patients who had large, cystic OLTs (mean defect size, 6.1 cm³; range, 3 to 10 cm³). Surgery was performed via an anterior arthrotomy in 10 patients, a medial malleolar osteotomy in four patients, and a distal fibular osteotomy in one patient. At 54 months postoperatively, 13 allografts remained in situ, with marked improvement in American Orthopaedic Foot and Ankle Society (AOFAS) Ankle-Hindfoot scores and visual analog pain scale scores. Two patients underwent ankle arthrodesis at 32 and 76 months postoperatively.

In a study of 12 ankles that were treated with osteochondral allografting, Görtz et al[32] reported an 83% survival rate at 38 months postoperatively. All patients underwent an anterior arthrotomy with temporary distraction. The mean lesion size was 3.6 cm². Radiographically, all patients demonstrated graft incorporation by 6 months postoperatively. Of the two failures, one patient underwent ankle fusion, and the other patient underwent a revision

allograft, which was functioning well at 7 years postoperatively. Based on the Olerud-Molander Ankle Score, 50% of the surviving grafts had excellent or good outcomes.

In a study of 18 patients who underwent fresh talar allograft implantation, Hahn et al[33] reported that the mean anterior-posterior defect size was 1.9 cm (range, 1.0 to 2.5 cm), and the mean medial-lateral defect size was 1.4 cm (range, 1.0 to 2.0 cm). The fixation methods included bioabsorbable pins, dual-pitched screws, or a combination of the two. A calcium sulfate/demineralized bone matrix, which acted as a grout to fill in incongruences, was used in 85% of the patients. There was a 100% graft incorporation rate seen on plain radiographs and no failures reported in the 13 patients who returned for follow-up (mean, 48 months). There was marked improvement between the patients' preoperative and postoperative pain and activity abilities, as measured by AOFAS Ankle-Hindfoot scores and Foot Function Index scores.

El-Rashidy et al[34] retrospectively reviewed 38 patients who underwent fresh osteochondral allograft transplantation. Each ankle was arthroscopically inspected before the arthrotomy. The mean lesion size was 1.5 cm². An anterior cruciate ligament reamer was used to ream the OLTs to bleeding subchondral bone (10 to 12 mm). At a mean follow-up of 37 months, AOFAS Ankle-Hindfoot scores markedly improved from 52 points to 79 points. Per the authors' protocol, the grafts were harvested from a similar anatomic location in the donor talus to match the anatomy of the recipient talus. Seven patients underwent secondary ankle arthroscopy (four for lateral impingement), which revealed four intact grafts,

three loose grafts, one graft with a 5- to 6-mm area of denuded cartilage, and one graft with diffuse cartilage loss. Of the four patients who had failed grafts, two underwent ankle replacement, one underwent ankle arthrodesis, and one underwent a bipolar total ankle allograft. Postoperative MRI was obtained for 15 of 28 patients at a mean follow-up of 33 months. Using the MRI stability criteria described by De Smet et al,[35] El-Rashidy et al[34] assessed the stability at the allograft-host interface. Ten patients showed no signs of graft instability and had good or fair graft incorporation (defined as ingrowth of bone marrow on T1-weighted MRI). Only three patients had good graft incorporation. Only one patient had evidence of graft collapse/subsidence.

In a study of eight patients who had talar shoulder lesions that were treated with fresh allograft transplantation, Adams et al[36] reported that, at a mean follow-up of 48 months, all grafts were still in place, and patients had improvements in pain and functional outcomes scores (ie, AOFAS Ankle-Hindfoot scores, Lower Extremity Functional Scale scores, visual analog pain scale scores, Short Musculoskeletal Function Assessment scores); however, one-half of the patients required additional surgical procedures, including arthroscopic débridement, removal of medial malleolar hardware, revision medial malleolar osteotomy, and supramalleolar/calcaneal osteotomies for a varus ankle. At final follow-up, radiographs demonstrated no joint-space narrowing or graft subsidence, but 37.5% of the patients had joint degenerative changes. Three patients with medial shoulder grafts had partial radiographic lucency along the lateral interface of the host bone and allograft;

however, these patients were asymptomatic. One patient had superior graft resorption and radiographic lucency along the lateral border of the allograft.

Haene et al[37] used fresh allograft in 17 ankles that had uncontained, large OLTs. The mean volume of the lesions was 3,408 mm^3. Sixteen of the 17 ankles underwent CT at a mean follow-up of 4.1 years. Grafts were not incorporated in two ankles. There was a mean graft subsidence of 0.5 mm. Subchondral cysts and joint-space narrowing were seen in seven ankles. Four ankles were asymptomatic. Two ankles underwent fusion, and one patient had persistent symptoms.

Summary

The use of large osteochondral allografts for the treatment of large symptomatic OLTs can effectively provide pain relief and improve functionality in the midterm. As indications evolve and techniques improve, osteochondral transplantation may stave off ankle fusion or replacement in many patients who have large OLTs. The use and success of osteochondral transplantation hinge on high-quality, thoughtful research in the future.

References

1. Dragoni M, Bonasia DE, Amendola A: Osteochondral talar allograft for large osteochondral defects: Technique tip. *Foot Ankle Int* 2011;32(9):910-916.

2. Chew KT, Tay E, Wong YS: Osteochondral lesions of the talus. *Ann Acad Med Singapore* 2008;37(1):63-68.

3. Chambers HG, Sutherland DH: A practical guide to gait analysis. *J Am Acad Orthop Surg* 2002;10(3):222-231.

4. Reilingh ML, Beimers L, Tuijthof GJ, Stufkens SA, Maas M, van Dijk CN: Measuring hindfoot alignment radiographically: The long axial view is more reliable than the hindfoot alignment view. *Skeletal Radiol* 2010;39(11):1103-1108.

5. Verhagen RA, Maas M, Dijkgraaf MG, Tol JL, Krips R, van Dijk CN: Prospective study on diagnostic strategies in osteochondral lesions of the talus: Is MRI superior to helical CT? *J Bone Joint Surg Br* 2005;87(1):41-46.

6. Anderson IF, Crichton KJ, Grattan-Smith T, Cooper RA, Brazier D: Osteochondral fractures of the dome of the talus. *J Bone Joint Surg Am* 1989;71(8):1143-1152.

7. Lee KB, Bai LB, Park JG, Yoon TR: A comparison of arthroscopic and MRI findings in staging of osteochondral lesions of the talus. *Knee Surg Sports Traumatol Arthrosc* 2008;16(11):1047-1051.

8. Dipaola JD, Nelson DW, Colville MR: Characterizing osteochondral lesions by magnetic resonance imaging. *Arthroscopy* 1991;7(1):101-104.

9. Mintz DN, Tashjian GS, Connell DA, Deland JT, O'Malley M, Potter HG: Osteochondral lesions of the talus: A new magnetic resonance grading system with arthroscopic correlation. *Arthroscopy* 2003;19(4):353-359.

10. Berndt AL, Harty M: Transchondral fractures (osteochondritis dissecans) of the talus. *J Bone Joint Surg Am* 1959;41:988-1020.

11. Scranton PE Jr, McDermott JE: Treatment of type V osteochondral lesions of the talus with ipsilateral knee osteochondral autografts. *Foot Ankle Int* 2001;22(5):380-384.

12. Raikin SM: Stage VI: Massive osteochondral defects of the talus. *Foot Ankle Clin* 2004;9(4):737-744, vi.

13. Pritsch M, Horoshovski H, Farine I: Arthroscopic treatment of osteochondral lesions of the talus. *J Bone Joint Surg Am* 1986;68(6):862-865.

14. Ferkel RD, Zanotti RM, Komenda GA, et al: Arthroscopic treatment of chronic osteochondral lesions of the talus: Long-term results. *Am J Sports Med* 2008;36(9):1750-1762.

15. Hepple S, Winson IG, Glew D: Osteochondral lesions of the talus: A revised classification. *Foot Ankle Int* 1999;20(12):789-793.

16. Bauer M, Jonsson K, Lindén B: Osteochondritis dissecans of the ankle: A 20-year follow-up study. *J Bone Joint Surg Br* 1987;69(1):93-96.

17. McCullough CJ, Venugopal V: Osteochondritis dissecans of the talus: The natural history. *Clin Orthop Relat Res* 1979;144:264-268.

18. Pettine KA, Morrey BF: Osteochondral fractures of the talus: A long-term follow-up. *J Bone Joint Surg Br* 1987;69(1):89-92.

19. McGahan PJ, Pinney SJ: Current concept review: Osteochondral lesions of the talus. *Foot Ankle Int* 2010;31(1):90-101.

20. Chahal J, Gross AE, Gross C, et al: Outcomes of osteochondral allograft transplantation in the knee. *Arthroscopy* 2013;29(3):575-588.

21. Convery FR, Akeson WH, Amiel D, Meyers MH, Monosov A: Long-term survival of chondrocytes in an osteochondral articular cartilage allograft: A case report. *J Bone Joint Surg Am* 1996;78(7):1082-1088.

22. Enneking WF, Campanacci DA: Retrieved human allografts: A clinicopathological study. *J Bone Joint Surg Am* 2001;83(7):971-986.

23. Enneking WF, Mindell ER: Observations on massive retrieved human allografts. *J Bone Joint Surg Am* 1991;73(8):1123-1142.

24. Williams SK, Amiel D, Ball ST, et al: Prolonged storage effects on the articular cartilage of fresh human osteochondral allografts. *J Bone Joint Surg Am* 2003;85(11):2111-2120.

25. Brittberg M, Peterson L, Sjögren-Jansson E, Tallheden T, Lindahl A: Articular cartilage engineering with autologous chondrocyte transplantation: A review of recent developments. *J Bone Joint Surg Am* 2003;85(suppl 3):109-115.

26. Giannini S, Buda R, Grigolo B, Vannini F: Autologous chondrocyte transplantation in osteochondral lesions of the ankle joint. *Foot Ankle Int* 2001;22(6):513-517.

27. Giannini S, Vannini F: Operative treatment of osteochondral lesions of the talar dome: Current concepts review. *Foot Ankle Int* 2004;25(3):168-175.

© 2016 AAOS Instructional Course Lectures, Volume 65

28. Muir D, Saltzman CL, Tochigi Y, Amendola N: Talar dome access for osteochondral lesions. *Am J Sports Med* 2006;34(9):1457-1463.

29. Salter RB, Simmonds DF, Malcolm BW, Rumble EJ, MacMichael D, Clements ND: The biological effect of continuous passive motion on the healing of full-thickness defects in articular cartilage: An experimental investigation in the rabbit. *J Bone Joint Surg Am* 1980;62(8):1232-1251.

30. Gross AE, Agnidis Z, Hutchison CR: Osteochondral defects of the talus treated with fresh osteochondral allograft transplantation. *Foot Ankle Int* 2001;22(5):385-391.

31. Raikin SM: Fresh osteochondral allografts for large-volume cystic osteochondral defects of the talus. *J Bone Joint Surg Am* 2009;91(12):2818-2826.

32. Görtz S, De Young AJ, Bugbee WD: Fresh osteochondral allografting for osteochondral lesions of the talus. *Foot Ankle Int* 2010;31(4):283-290.

33. Hahn DB, Aanstoos ME, Wilkins RM: Osteochondral lesions of the talus treated with fresh talar allografts. *Foot Ankle Int* 2010;31(4):277-282.

34. El-Rashidy H, Villacis D, Omar I, Kelikian AS: Fresh osteochondral allograft for the treatment of cartilage defects of the talus: A retrospective review. *J Bone Joint Surg Am* 2011;93(17):1634-1640.

35. De Smet AA, Ilahi OA, Graf B: Reassessment of the MR criteria for stability of osteochondritis dissecans in the knee and ankle. *Skeletal Radiol* 1996;25(2):159-163.

36. Adams SB Jr, Viens NA, Easley ME, Stinnett SS, Nunley JA II: Midterm results of osteochondral lesions of the talar shoulder treated with fresh osteochondral allograft transplantation. *J Bone Joint Surg Am* 2011;93(7):648-654.

37. Haene R, Qamirani E, Story RA, Pinsker E, Daniels TR: Intermediate outcomes of fresh talar osteochondral allografts for treatment of large osteochondral lesions of the talus. *J Bone Joint Surg Am* 2012;94(12):1105-1110.

Video Reference

Easley ME: Video excerpt: Osteochondral lesions of the talus. *J Am Acad Orthop Surg* 2010;18(10):616-630.

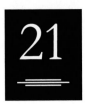

21

Outcomes of Ankle Distraction for the Treatment of Ankle Arthritis

Mai Nguyen, MD
Charles Saltzman, MD
Annunziato Amendola, MD

Abstract

Ankle arthrodesis and total ankle arthroplasty are the most common treatments for end-stage ankle osteoarthritis; however, these surgeries are not ideal for young, active patients because of the nature and long-term consequences of sacrificing the ankle joint. The concept of joint distraction was introduced in the 1970s but has only received clinical support in the past two decades as interest in joint preservation treatments has grown. Ankle distraction preserves the native joint and, thus, does not compromise any future arthroplasty or arthrodesis, if required. The main indication for ankle distraction is severe osteoarthritis, and, with encouraging data, the indications continue to expand. The early results of ankle distraction are promising; however, ankle function after joint distraction declines over time. Careful patient selection is necessary to optimize ankle distraction outcomes and avoid complications.

Instr Course Lect 2016;65:311–320.

End-stage ankle osteoarthritis (OA) is a debilitating condition that causes ankle pain and stiffness.[1] The physical impairment caused by OA of a single lower extremity joint is equivalent to that caused by end-stage kidney disease or heart failure.[2] There are approximately 6 million individuals in the United States who are disabled by posttraumatic OA of the hip, knee, or ankle, with a corresponding estimated annual financial burden of $3.06 billion.[1] Despite the best efforts in fracture management, the most common etiology of ankle OA is previous trauma (70% to 80%).[1] Treatment of posttraumatic ankle OA is complicated because those who are affected by posttraumatic ankle OA tend to be younger, higher demand patients.

Ankle fusion and total ankle replacement have been the mainstays of treatment for end-stage OA of the ankle; however, the long-term complications associated with these joint-sacrificing surgeries, such as the development of adjacent joint arthritis after fusion and implant failure after replacement, have dampened the enthusiasm for their use in younger patients.[3-7] Current options for joint preservation surgeries include realignment osteotomy, allograft replacement, and distraction. Supramalleolar osteotomies are less predictable in patients who have medial malleolar-talar or tibiofibular arthritis that is more than truly isolated, which may cause secondary deformity of the

Dr. Saltzman or an immediate family member has received royalties from Tornier and Zimmer; is a member of a speakers' bureau or has made paid presentations on behalf of Zimmer; serves as a paid consultant to Smith & Nephew, Wright Medical Technology and Zimmer; and serves as a board member, owner, officer, or committee member of the American Board of Orthopaedic Surgery and the Association of Bone and Joint Surgeons. Dr. Amendola or an immediate family member has received royalties from Arthrex, Arthrosurface, and Smith & Nephew; serves as a paid consultant to Arthrex; serves as an unpaid consultant to First Ray; has stock or stock options held in First Ray; and serves as a board member, owner, officer, or committee member of the American Board of Orthopaedic Surgery and the American Orthopaedic Society for Sports Medicine. Neither Dr. Nguyen nor any immediate family member has received anything of value from or has stock or stock options held in a commercial company or institution related directly or indirectly to the subject of this chapter.

hindfoot,[8-10] and bipolar tibiotalar allograft transplantation has been associated with inconsistent outcomes and early failures.[11-13]

In the past two decades, joint distraction with the use of standard external fixator application techniques has emerged as a promising treatment for ankle OA.[14-20] Several biomechanical, animal model, and clinical studies support the use of joint distraction for the diagnosis of cartilage loss and arthrosis.[21-24] Distraction treats patients' symptoms yet keeps arthrodesis and total ankle arthroplasty as viable solutions for patients in whom ankle distraction ultimately fails.

Indications

Ankle distraction is indicated for patients with symptomatic ankle arthritis who are young or have high activity demands that make them less than ideal candidates for total ankle arthroplasty or ankle arthrodesis. There is a disparity in the literature on the ideal age for ankle distraction, with ranges from 55 to 73 years reported. Saltzman et al[23] used 60 years as the upper age limit in a prospective randomized trial.

A thorough history and physical examination should be performed to delineate the underlying disease process. Ankle pain from focal impingement alone does not require ankle distraction. Patients who have ankle pain secondary to inflammatory arthritis, crystal deposition, neuropathic ankle, fibromyalgia, and reflex sympathetic dystrophy should be excluded. Distraction can stretch soft tissue, which leads to exacerbation of neuritis and neurogenic pain; therefore, patients who have scarring in the tarsal tunnel or a history of neuritic issues should be excluded. History of infection around the ankle

demands a thorough work-up, including joint aspiration, to rule out persistent infection. Ankle alignment should be evaluated carefully, both clinically and with radiographs, and substantial malalignment should be addressed separately or simultaneously.

Ideal candidates for ankle distraction are patients with severe diffuse ankle OA who no longer respond to conservative management. Patients should be treated with a course of nonsurgical treatment before surgical intervention is considered. Standard nonsurgical treatment for ankle OA includes the regular use of NSAIDs; unloading methods, such as modified shoe wear, braces, crutches, canes, and walkers; and the judicious use of intra-articular corticosteroid injections. Patients should be counseled on other well-established surgical treatments that are options for severe ankle OA, including total ankle replacement and ankle arthrodesis.

Postoperatively, patients may require upper extremity and contralateral leg strength to help mobility with walking aids. Therefore, ideal patients should have isolated ankle arthritis. Patients should be available for frequent follow-up for close monitoring of the ankle distractor because adjustments may be needed and because pin-site infections as well as irritation are common and must be treated in a timely fashion. Candidates for ankle distraction should be carefully selected to optimize outcomes and minimize complications.

Physical Examination and Radiographic Evaluation

All joints of the lower extremity should be examined. Range of motion, tenderness, swelling, stability, and alignment should be carefully assessed. The physical examination of a potential

candidate for ankle distraction should demonstrate ankle pain, with relatively preserved motion, intact neurovascular status, and only minimal axial or sagittal angular deformity. Plain radiographs should be obtained with standing AP, mortise, and lateral views of the ankle, as well as a standing hindfoot alignment view. The authors of this chapter recommend that the tibial-talar angle be between 84° and 93°, the distal tibial angle be between 78° and 85°, and the calcaneal moment arm be less than 15 mm on hindfoot alignment radiographs.[23]

Surgical Procedure

The procedure is performed with the patient in the supine position. After general anesthesia is administered and prophylactic antibiotics are given, the surgical extremity is prepped and draped in the usual sterile fashion.

Anterior Osteophyte Removal

Osteophyte removal is gaining popularity as an adjunctive procedure that is performed during ankle distraction.[20,23,25] If osteophyte removal is selected, it should be performed before distraction frame application. The authors of this chapter prefer to perform osteophyte removal in all patients because it can effectively eliminate impingement. Osteophyte removal may be performed either arthroscopically or via an open procedure. A tourniquet may be applied over the upper thigh to obtain hemostasis and optimize visibility during arthroscopy. Arthroscopic ankle joint lavage, with removal of any extra-articular anterior osseous osteophytes, is performed with the use of a 4.0-mm arthroscope without joint distraction. Plantar flexion of the ankle should be avoided because it can pull the anterior capsule tightly over the joint and limit accurate and full arthroscopic resection of anterior osteophytes. If the anterior osteophytes are too large to remove arthroscopically, an open incision through an extension of the arthroscopic portals may be made to facilitate removal. The adequacy of the cheilectomy can be determined with resection of the anterior tibial bone spur to the level of the anterior margin of the medial malleolus, visual assessment and removal of any anterior joint impingement, and intraoperative inspection of true lateral fluoroscopic images.

External Fixator Application

The tibial frame is applied with the rings perpendicular to the tibia, and the foot frame is placed in line with the foot. The upper tibial ring is secured with two 5-mm half-pins, and the lower ring is secured with one 5-mm half-pin as well as a crossing thin wire that is tensioned to 110 to 130 lb. The foot frame is then attached with a thin wire that is placed transversely across the talus, two crossing thin wires that are placed across the calcaneus, and two crossing thin wires that are placed across the metatarsals, all of which are tensioned to 70 to 90 lb (**Figure 1**).

Fixed Distraction Versus Motion

Distraction rods with or without hinges may be used, depending on whether a motion or fixed distraction protocol will be used postoperatively. Motion is considered an essential element of cartilage restoration, and several groups of surgeons have added motion to augment distraction.[19,23,25] There is some evidence of better short-term results in patients who are treated with a motion distractor;[23] however, this effect has

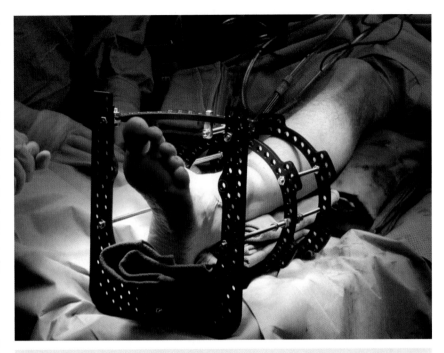

Figure 1   Intraoperative photograph shows an ankle distraction frame.

not been proven in long-term results.[9] If motion distraction is selected, then universal hinges are placed at the level of the tips of the medial and lateral malleoli to approximate the mean location of the ankle joint axis.

Distraction and Postoperative Treatment

Distraction can be performed gradually over the course of 5 days or performed acutely in one sitting.[1,14,25] The authors of this chapter prefer to distract the ankle intraoperatively to 5 mm, which is measured with the use of fluoroscopy, to ensure the adequacy of the frame construct; however, it is safest to then reduce the frame to the nondistracted position and have the patient slowly distract the ankle to the proper length. Distraction distance is measured by using the diameter of the threaded rods as a reference for radiographic magnification. Distraction of the ankle should be assessed with routine radiographic imaging and adjusted

as necessary during close postoperative follow-up (**Figure 2**). The authors of this chapter request that patients return for follow-up at 1, 3, 6, and 9 weeks postoperatively. On the rare occasions that neurapraxia and/or paresthesia occur, the amount of distraction may need to be decreased.[23] Pin care is performed twice a day until the pin sites are dry. If motion is used, patients are instructed to remove the posterior stabilizing bar and use a stockinette that is placed on the foot frame to passively dorsiflex and plantarflex the ankle (20 repetitions, 3 times per day) for weeks 2 through 12. Muscle conditioning is encouraged with the use of a heavy exercise band to attain resisted strengthening of both the dorsiflexor and plantarflexor muscles of the foot (20 repetitions, 3 times per day).

The fixator is removed approximately 3 months after application. The patient is then transitioned to a removable below-the-knee, Velcro-strapped, rocker-bottom boot for 1 month after

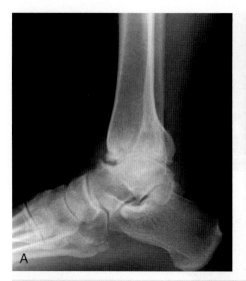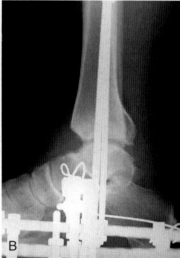

Figure 2 Lateral radiographs of an ankle taken before (**A**) and after (**B**) anterior osteophyte resection and joint distraction.

fixator removal and begins weight bearing in the boot. The patient is gradually allowed to return to full weight bearing without boot immobilization by 6 months after fixator removal.

Results
Short-term Results
van Valburg et al[14] performed ankle distraction in a group of 11 patients to delay ankle fusion. The authors' preliminary results reported improvements in pain (11 of 11 patients), range of motion (6 of 11 patients), and joint-space widening (3 of 6 patients) at a mean follow-up of 20 months. Later, the same group of investigators published comparable results that showed clinical improvement and pain relief in most of the patients 1 to 2 years after ankle distraction[9,14,15,17-20,23,26,27] (**Table 1**). Encouraging results in the Netherlands led to an increased interest in ankle distraction as a treatment for ankle arthritis in the United States. Paley et al,[25] Tellisi et al,[19] and Saltzman et al[23] performed ankle distraction with some variation of

the original surgical techniques used in the Netherlands; similarly, the authors achieved positive results in small cohorts of 23 to 36 patients with a minimum follow-up that ranged from 1 to 2 years.

Randomized Controlled Trials
To rule out the placebo effect, Marijnissen et al[26] performed a randomized trial of 17 patients and a prospective study of 57 patients. The authors randomized eight patients in a control group who underwent arthroscopic débridement alone and randomized nine patients in a treatment group, seven of whom underwent both débridement and distraction and two of whom underwent distraction alone. At a minimum follow-up of 1 year, the authors reported better clinical improvements for the patients in the joint distraction group than for the patients in the débridement-only group. Three patients in whom débridement failed elected to proceed with joint distraction and experienced improvements in pain cessation and function.

Because motion has been accepted as an essential component in cartilage restoration, several investigators believe it provides additional benefits in ankle distraction.[28-30] Saltzman et al[23] performed a randomized controlled trial that compared the outcomes of patients who underwent motion distraction with the outcomes of patients who underwent fixed distraction. Although the results at 2-year follow-up demonstrated that both groups benefited from ankle distraction, patients in the motion group had significantly better Ankle Osteoarthritis Scale (AOS) scores compared with patients in the fixed distraction group.

Intermediate- and Long-term Results
Although the short-term results of ankle distraction are promising, a few intermediate- and long-term follow-up studies have reported less predictable outcomes.[9,17,27] At a follow-up that ranged from 5 to 17 years, Ploegmakers et al[17] reported a 27% failure rate in a cohort of 27 patients who underwent ankle distraction for severe OA. In a cohort of 36 patients who underwent ankle distraction, Nguyen et al[9] reported a 45% conversion rate to total ankle arthroplasty or ankle fusion at a mean follow-up of 8.3 years (SD = 2.2 years). Similarly, in a combined study of patient groups from the Netherlands and Iowa (111 total patients), Marijnissen et al[27] reported a 44% failure rate at a follow-up that ranged from 2 to 17 years.

Predictors of Long-term Results
Using regression analyses, Marijnissen et al[27] determined that sex and preoperative scores were the only factors that

Table 1

Results of Ankle Distraction for the Treatment of Ankle Arthritis

Authors (Year)	Type of Study (No. of Patients)	Mean Patient Age in Years (Range)	Follow-up Range	Results	Outcome Measures	Complications
van Valburg et al[14] (1995)	Retrospective review (11)	35 (20–70)	10–60 months	Pain decreased in all patients; 5 were pain free. Range of movement improved in 55% of patients. Joint space widening was seen in 3 of 6 patients.	Pain Range of motion Radiographs Intra-articular hydrostatic pressure	NR
van Valburg et al[18] (1999)	Prospective study (17)	40 (29–55)	2–8 years	13 patients of 17 (76%) showed improvement on clinical examination, functional questionnaires, and pain scales; effects were progressive in second year of follow-up.	Pain and function based on van Valburg scores Radiographs	Pin-site infection; treated with flucloxacillin Broken wires
Marijnissen et al[26] (2002)	Prospective study (57) Randomized controlled study (17)	44 (18–65)	1–5 years	Significant clinical benefit found in 75% of patients in the prospective study. Joint distraction had significantly better results than débridement. Radiographic evaluation showed increased joint space.	Pain and function based on van Valburg scores Range of motion Radiographs	Pin-site infections in 16 of 57 patients in the prospective study and 3 of 17 patients in the randomized controlled study; effectively treated with antibiotics Broken wires in 8 patients
van Roermund et al[15] (2002)	Case series (50)	NA	1–7 years	75% of patients showed significant clinical improvement. Joint mobility slightly improved.	Pain and function Radiographs	NR
Paley and Lamm[20] (2005)	Case series (20)	NA	2–16 years	18 of 20 patients had good to excellent results. No patients required conversion to ankle fusion or ankle arthroplasty.	Clinical function	NR
Ploegmakers et al[17] (2005)	Retrospective review (27; 22 with follow-up data)	37 (19–55)	7–15 years	16 patients of 22 (73%) showed significant improvement on functional surveys. 6 failures (6 underwent arthrodesis)	Combination of van Valburg and AOS scores	Incomplete Sudeck atrophy

AOFAS = American Orthopaedic Foot and Ankle Society, AOS = Ankle Osteoarthritis Scale, NA = not available, NR = not reported, SF-36 = Medical Outcomes Study 36-Item Short Form.

Table 1 *(continued)*
Results of Ankle Distraction for the Treatment of Ankle Arthritis

Authors (Year)	Type of Study (No. of Patients)	Mean Patient Age in Years (Range)	Follow-up Range	Results	Outcome Measures	Complications
Tellisi et al[19] (2009)	Retrospective case series (25; 23 with follow-up data)	43 (16–73)	12–60 months	Adjuvant procedures, including Achilles tendon lengthening, ankle arthroscopy, arthrotomy, and supramalleolar osteotomy, were performed in some patients. 21 patients of 23 (91%) had improved function. 2 patients underwent ankle fusion.	AOFAS score SF-36 score Range of motion Radiographs	Superficial pin-site infections in 100% of patients; controlled with a single course of oral antibiotics
Saltzman et al[23] (2012)	Prospective randomized controlled trial comparing motion versus fixed distraction (36 total)	42 (18–59)	2 years	Anterior osteophyte was resected. Both groups showed significantly improved AOS scores compared with the scores before treatment. The motion group had significantly better AOS scores than the fixed group.	AOS score SF-36 score Range of motion	43 episodes of pin-tract infection in 19 patients; 4 patients required pin removal, 2 of which had acute osteomyelitis and were treated to resolution with 6 weeks of intravenous antibiotics. 8 patients had numbness and 2 patients had residual numbness 1 patient had symptomatic deep vein thrombosis
Marijnissen et al[27] (2014)	Prospective multicenter study (75) and randomized controlled trial (36)	43 (NR)	2–17 years	44% of patients failed by 12-year follow-up (underwent arthrodesis Sudeck atrophy developed, underwent osteotomy or a second distraction). Female sex and functional disability at baseline predicted worse outcomes.	Failure Pain and functional disability	NR
Nguyen et al[9] (2015)	Prospective study (36; 29 with follow-up data)	42 (18–59)	5–12 years	16 patients of 29 patients (55%) still had native ankle joints whereas 13 patients of 29 (45%) underwent either ankle arthrodesis or total ankle arthroplasty. Radiographs revealed progression of osteoarthritis.	Survival/conversion rate to total ankle or ankle fusion Radiographs	No additional complications from the initial follow-up published by Saltzman et al[23]

AOFAS = American Orthopaedic Foot and Ankle Society, AOS = Ankle Osteoarthritis Scale, NA = not available, NR = not reported, SF-36 = Medical Outcomes Study 36-Item Short Form.

were predictive of outcomes. Tellisi et al[19] reported no significant difference in functional scores among different age groups; however, patients older than 60 years trended toward more improvement than younger patients. Similarly, Nguyen et al[9] reported that older age at the time of surgery was a positive predictor for ankle survival, and that the AOS score at 2-year follow-up was the most predictive factor for intermediate-term survival at a mean follow-up of 8.3 years (SD = 2.2 years). Thus, if AOS scores fail to improve by 2-year follow-up, it is unlikely that patients will eventually benefit from ankle distraction.

Imaging Outcomes

Radiographs obtained at early follow-ups that ranged from 1 to 2 years have shown persistent widening or preservation of the joint space.[14,18,19,26] In a study of three patients who underwent distraction surgery, Lamm and Gourdine-Shaw[31] reported that 13-month follow-up MRIs showed decreased subchondral bone thickness of 0.5 mm and increased cartilage thickness/joint space of 0.5 mm compared with preoperative MRIs. Plain radiographs and CT scans obtained 1 to 2 years after ankle distraction have shown normalization of subchondral bone density, with a decrease in subchondral sclerosis density and an increase in bone density over an area of subchondral cysts.[24,29] In addition, subchondral bone remodeling has been reported to be related to clinical improvement after joint distraction.[32] Radiographs obtained at longer term follow-ups that ranged from 5 to 10 years were consistent with the clinical decline noted at the intermediate-term follow-ups and showed continued progression of ankle OA.[9]

Adjunctive Procedures

Paley et al[20,25] introduced the Baltimore method of ankle distraction, which adds an anatomically located hinge to the ankle distracter that allows the patient to perform range-of-motion exercises. The authors also recommended adjunctive procedures, including osteophyte resection, equinus contracture release, and ankle realignment with supramalleolar osteotomy/tibial lengthening/fibular shortening or lengthening, to increase range of motion, eliminate impingement, and improve stability and alignment. Eleven of 23 patients in their study also received a series of three intra-articular hormone injections.[20] Two patients underwent the distraction procedure twice.[20] At a minimum follow-up of 2 years, 11 patients of 18 (61%) were very satisfied or satisfied with the results. One patient underwent ankle fusion, and one patient underwent total ankle replacement.[25]

Saltzman et al[23] performed ankle arthroscopy with arthroscopic or open débridement of anterior osteophytes in all patients who underwent ankle distraction surgery. The authors reported that patients who underwent motion distraction had better outcomes at 26, 52, and 104 weeks after frame removal compared with patients who underwent fixed distraction; however, a follow-up study of the same group of patients reported that motion distraction did not demonstrate long-term benefits.[9]

Adjuvant procedures, including Achilles tendon lengthening, osteophyte removal, subchondral drilling, and supramalleolar osteotomy, also were advocated by Tellisi et al.[19] At a minimum follow-up of 1 year, 21 patients of the 23 (91%) who underwent ankle distraction reported improved pain, and 17 of 23 patients had

significant improvement in American Orthopaedic Foot and Ankle Society scores. No patients had a loss of motion after distraction. There was no difference in joint space at follow-up compared with preoperative radiographs.

Complications

The most common complication reported after ankle distraction is pin-tract infection, with some studies reporting up to a 100% rate of pin-tract infection.[18,19,23,25,26] Treatments for pin-tract infections vary from oral antibiotics, to intravenous antibiotics, to irrigation and débridement with hardware removal. Nguyen et al[9] reported pin-site infections in 19 of 36 patients who underwent ankle distraction. The authors reported that all of the pin-site infections were treated successfully and that five patients underwent total ankle arthroplasty with no consequences. The detection of pin-site infections requires high vigilance by both patients and physicians so that treatments can be initiated immediately. Other rare complications that may occur after ankle distraction include the need for additional distraction frame adjustments, nerve irritation, reflex sympathetic atrophy, broken wires, and deep vein thrombosis.[17,18,23,25,26]

The Ankle Distraction Effect

The exact mechanism through which ankle distraction alleviates pain is unclear; however, there are several theories that suggest that the potential mechanisms may include mechanical unloading, cartilage repair, and bone cartilage remodeling. Unloading, which is one of the first lines of treatment for ankle OA, helps reduce pain and slow structural damage to the joint. Unloading can be accomplished with modified footwear, bracing, or osteotomy, all of which help correct ankle alignment.[33] Joint distraction, which uses an external frame, allows for a mode of unloading that reduces mechanical stress on the cartilage.[34]

If ankle distraction was achieved with unloading alone, the ankle joints would collapse after removal of the distraction frame. Imaging studies obtained 2 years after distraction frame removal demonstrated persistent joint space widening, which suggests that ankle distraction has a reparative effect on cartilage.[18,32] Ploegmakers et al[17] reported that periarticular osteopenia was induced and subchondral bone sclerosis decreased progressively during 3 months of distraction because load was partially transferred through the fixator frame instead of the bone. Intema et al[32] reported that ankle CT scans obtained 2 years after ankle distractor removal still demonstrated the normalization of subchondral bone, with a decrease in bone density in the sclerotic areas and an increase in bone density in the original cystic areas. The authors reported that the disappearance of subchondral cysts was associated with pain relief, and suggested that the source of pain in OA is cyst generated, perhaps from the increased fluid pressure that the bone senses with cyst development. As the subchondral bone remodels, growth factors are released, which leads to cartilage repair.[34] This bone-cartilage interaction creates an optimal environment for joint remodeling. van Valburg et al[18] reported that persistent joint widening at 2-year follow-up correlated with progressive clinical improvement.

Joint distraction may trigger the cartilage repair process. Mechanical and animal studies have reported that joint distraction is able to alter chondrocyte activity beneficially. Joint distraction results in a temporary relief of mechanical stress on the cartilage and a change in intra-articular fluid pressure, which is important to provide nutrients to the cartilage and promote proteoglycan turnover.[16,22] Studies in animal models, including canine and rabbit models, have shown that joint distraction for OA resulted in a significant change in proteoglycan metabolism toward values similar to those of a normal joint.[24,35] Canine knees that were treated with joint distraction had lower macroscopic and histologic damage scores and less collagen damage compared with a control group, which indicates cartilage repair activity is associated with joint distraction;[24] however, Karadam et al[36] reported no beneficial histologic effects of joint distraction in rabbits that had papain-induced osteoarthrosis.

Summary

The goal of ankle distraction is to relieve pain, improve function, and slow the progression of joint destruction. The outcomes for most patients who undergo joint distraction for the treatment of ankle OA are consistently positive at follow-ups that range from 1 to 2 years; however, a limited number of studies have reported that the long-term outcomes are less predictable. Complications can be minimized with close follow-up, and pin-site infections should be treated in a timely manner. Ankle distraction is a joint-preserving option that does not preclude total ankle arthroplasty or ankle arthrodesis. The authors of this chapter do not know whether ankle distraction alters the outcomes of total ankle replacement or ankle arthrodesis if they are performed after ankle distraction; however, preliminary results suggest that it does not.

Ankle distraction is a versatile surgical technique and may be performed with adjunctive procedures. More research is necessary to understand how the distraction method can be optimized, to determine whether biologic supplemental therapy could be helpful, and to elucidate predictive factors for long-term outcomes so that treatments for ankle OA can be improved.

References

1. Brown TD, Johnston RC, Saltzman CL, Marsh JL, Buckwalter JA: Posttraumatic osteoarthritis: A first estimate of incidence, prevalence, and burden of disease. *J Orthop Trauma* 2006;20(10):739-744.

2. Saltzman CL, Zimmerman MB, O'Rourke M, Brown TD, Buckwalter JA, Johnston R: Impact of comorbidities on the measurement of health in patients with ankle osteoarthritis. *J Bone Joint Surg Am* 2006;88(11):2366-2372.

3. Glazebrook MA, Arsenault K, Dunbar M: Evidence-based classification of complications in total ankle arthroplasty. *Foot Ankle Int* 2009;30(10):945-949.

4. Haddad SL, Coetzee JC, Estok R, Fahrbach K, Banel D, Nalysnyk L: Intermediate and long-term outcomes of total ankle arthroplasty and ankle arthrodesis: A systematic review of the literature. *J Bone Joint Surg Am* 2007;89(9):1899-1905.

5. Saltzman CL, Amendola A, Anderson R, et al: Surgeon training and complications in total ankle arthroplasty. *Foot Ankle Int* 2003;24(6):514-518.

6. Coester LM, Saltzman CL, Leupold J, Pontarelli W: Long-term results following ankle arthrodesis for post-traumatic arthritis. *J Bone Joint Surg Am* 2001;83(2):219-228.

7. Spirt AA, Assal M, Hansen ST Jr: Complications and failure after total ankle arthroplasty. *J Bone Joint Surg Am* 2004;86(6):1172-1178.

8. Pouliquen JC, Beneux J, Judet R, Cogan D: Tibia lengthening in children. Results and complications.

© 2016 AAOS Instructional Course Lectures, Volume 65

Rev Chir Orthop Reparatrice Appar Mot 1978;64(suppl 2):125-128.

9. Nguyen MP, Pedersen DR, Gao Y, Saltzman CL, Amendola A: Intermediate-term follow-up after ankle distraction for treatment of end-stage osteoarthritis. *J Bone Joint Surg Am* 2015;97(7):590-596.

10. Kuhns CA, Emerson ET, Meals RA: Hematoma and distraction arthroplasty for thumb basal joint osteoarthritis: A prospective, single-surgeon study including outcomes measures. *J Hand Surg Am* 2003;28(3):381-389.

11. Bugbee WD, Khanna G, Cavallo M, McCauley JC, Görtz S, Brage ME: Bipolar fresh osteochondral allografting of the tibiotalar joint. *J Bone Joint Surg Am* 2013;95(5):426-432.

12. Meehan R, McFarlin S, Bugbee W, Brage M: Fresh ankle osteochondral allograft transplantation for tibiotalar joint arthritis. *Foot Ankle Int* 2005;26(10):793-802.

13. Kim CW, Jamali A, Tontz W Jr, Convery FR, Brage ME, Bugbee W: Treatment of post-traumatic ankle arthrosis with bipolar tibiotalar osteochondral shell allografts. *Foot Ankle Int* 2002;23(12):1091-1102.

14. van Valburg AA, van Roermund PM, Lammens J, et al: Can Ilizarov joint distraction delay the need for an arthrodesis of the ankle? A preliminary report. *J Bone Joint Surg Br* 1995;77(5):720-725.

15. van Roermund PM, Marijnissen AC, Lafeber FP: Joint distraction as an alternative for the treatment of osteoarthritis. *Foot Ankle Clin* 2002;7(3):515-527.

16. Marijnissen AC, van Roermund PM, van Melkebeek J, Lafeber FP: Clinical benefit of joint distraction in the treatment of ankle osteoarthritis. *Foot Ankle Clin* 2003;8(2):335-346.

17. Ploegmakers JJ, van Roermund PM, van Melkebeek J, et al: Prolonged clinical benefit from joint distraction in the treatment of ankle

osteoarthritis. *Osteoarthritis Cartilage* 2005;13(7):582-588.

18. van Valburg AA, van Roermund PM, Marijnissen AC, et al: Joint distraction in treatment of osteoarthritis: A two-year follow-up of the ankle. *Osteoarthritis Cartilage* 1999;7(5):474-479.

19. Tellisi N, Fragomen AT, Kleinman D, O'Malley MJ, Rozbruch SR: Joint preservation of the osteoarthritic ankle using distraction arthroplasty. *Foot Ankle Int* 2009;30(4):318-325.

20. Paley D, Lamm BM: Ankle joint distraction. *Foot Ankle Clin* 2005;10(4):685-698, ix.

21. Judet R, Judet T: The use of a hinge distraction apparatus after arthrolysis and arthroplasty (author's transl). *Rev Chir Orthop Reparatrice Appar Mot* 1978;64(5):353-365.

22. van Valburg AA, van Roy HL, Lafeber FP, Bijlsma JW: Beneficial effects of intermittent fluid pressure of low physiological magnitude on cartilage and inflammation in osteoarthritis: An in vitro study. *J Rheumatol* 1998;25(3):515-520.

23. Saltzman CL, Hillis SL, Stolley MP, Anderson DD, Amendola A: Motion versus fixed distraction of the joint in the treatment of ankle osteoarthritis: A prospective randomized controlled trial. *J Bone Joint Surg Am* 2012;94(11):961-970.

24. Wiegant K, Intema F, van Roermund PM, et al: Evidence of cartilage repair by joint distraction in a canine model of osteoarthritis. *Arthritis Rheumatol* 2015;67(2):465-474.

25. Paley D, Lamm BM, Purohit RM, Specht SC: Distraction arthroplasty of the ankle—how far can you stretch the indications? *Foot Ankle Clin* 2008;13(3):471-484, ix.

26. Marijnissen AC, Van Roermund PM, Van Melkebeek J, et al: Clinical benefit of joint distraction in the treatment of severe osteoarthritis of the ankle: Proof of concept in an open prospective study and in a randomized

controlled study. *Arthritis Rheum* 2002;46(11):2893-2902.

27. Marijnissen AC, Hoekstra MC, Pré BC, et al: Patient characteristics as predictors of clinical outcome of distraction in treatment of severe ankle osteoarthritis. *J Orthop Res* 2014;32(1):96-101.

28. Buckwalter JA: Effects of early motion on healing of musculoskeletal tissues. *Hand Clin* 1996;12(1):13-24.

29. Buckwalter JA: Activity vs. rest in the treatment of bone, soft tissue and joint injuries. *Iowa Orthop J* 1995;15:29-42.

30. Salter RB: The biologic concept of continuous passive motion of synovial joints: The first 18 years of basic research and its clinical application. *Clin Orthop Relat Res* 1989;242:12-25.

31. Lamm BM, Gourdine-Shaw M: MRI evaluation of ankle distraction: A preliminary report. *Clin Podiatr Med Surg* 2009;26(2):185-191.

32. Intema F, Thomas TP, Anderson DD, et al: Subchondral bone remodeling is related to clinical improvement after joint distraction in the treatment of ankle osteoarthritis. *Osteoarthritis Cartilage* 2011;19(6):668-675.

33. Chiodo CP, McGarvey W: Joint distraction for the treatment of ankle osteoarthritis. *Foot Ankle Clin* 2004;9(3):541-553, ix.

34. Lafeber FP, Intema F, Van Roermund PM, Marijnissen AC: Unloading joints to treat osteoarthritis, including joint distraction. *Curr Opin Rheumatol* 2006;18(5):519-525.

35. van Valburg AA, van Roermund PM, Marijnissen AC, et al: Joint distraction in treatment of osteoarthritis (II): Effects on cartilage in a canine model. *Osteoarthritis Cartilage* 2000;8(1):1-8.

36. Karadam B, Karatosun V, Murat N, Ozkal S, Gunal I: No beneficial effects of joint distraction on early microscopical changes in osteoarthrotic knees: A study in rabbits. *Acta Orthop* 2005;76(1):95-98.

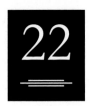

Ankle Arthritis: You Can't Always Replace It

Brandon J. Hayes, MD
Tyler A. Gonzalez, MD, MBA
Jeremy T. Smith, MD
Christopher P. Chiodo, MD
Eric M. Bluman, MD, PhD

Abstract

End-stage arthritis of the tibiotalar joint is disabling and causes substantial functional impairment. End-stage arthritis of the tibiotalar joint is often the residual effect of a previous traumatic injury. Nonsurgical treatment for end-stage arthritis of the ankle includes bracing, shoe wear modifications, and selective joint injections. For patients who fail to respond to nonsurgical modalities, the two primary treatment options are arthroplasty and arthrodesis. Each treatment option has strong proponents who argue the superiority of their treatment algorithm. Although there is no ideal treatment for ankle arthritis, there are high-quality studies that help guide treatment in patients of varying demographics. Many inherent risks are linked with each treatment option; however, the risks of greatest concern are early implant loosening after arthroplasty that requires revision surgery and the acceleration of adjacent joint degeneration associated with arthrodesis.

Instr Course Lect 2016;65:321–330.

Incidence and Etiology

The ankle joint is far less commonly affected by arthritis than other major joints because of differences in articular cartilage, joint motion, and the susceptibility of cartilage to inflammatory mediators.[1] One of the biggest differences between the ankle and the knee is the relatively greater containment and conformity of the ankle joint. The talus is firmly bound on three sides by the fibula, tibial plafond, and medial malleolus as well as their strong ligamentous attachments. This design potentially gives the ankle a better cartilaginous loading profile than the knee, which relies heavily on the menisci for congruent loading. The knee has components of sliding, rolling, and rotation, whereas the ankle is largely a rolling joint that has very little rotation. Interestingly, although the ankle experiences loads similar to the knee or hip and the ankle's contact surface area is less than one-third of that of the knee or hip, the incidence of primary arthritis in the ankle is dramatically less than that in the hip or knee.[2-4]

Trauma is the most common cause of end-stage arthritis of the ankle.[5] Additional causative factors include arthropathies, chronic ankle instability,

Dr. Smith or an immediate family member serves as a board member, owner, officer, or committee member of the American Orthopaedic Foot and Ankle Society. Dr. Chiodo or an immediate family member has received royalties from DJO Global, Arthrex, and Darco; serves as a paid consultant to Zimmer; has stock or stock options held in Johnson & Johnson, Merck, and Zimmer; and serves as a board member, owner, officer, or committee member of the American Academy of Orthopaedic Surgeons, the American Orthopaedic Foot and Ankle Society, and the Massachusetts Orthopaedic Association. Dr. Bluman or an immediate family member serves as a paid consultant to Biomet and Stryker; has stock or stock options held in Extremity Development Corporation and Neutin Orthopedics; has received nonincome support (such as equipment or services), commercially derived honoraria, or other non-research–related funding (such as paid travel) from Rogerson Orthopaedics; and serves as a board member, owner, officer, or committee member of the American Academy of Orthopaedic Surgeons and the American Orthopaedic Foot and Ankle Society. Neither of the following authors nor any immediate family member has received anything of value from or has stock or stock options held in a commercial company or institution related directly or indirectly to the subject of this chapter: Dr. Hayes and Dr. Gonzalez.

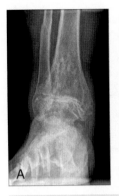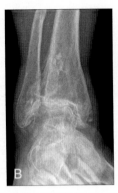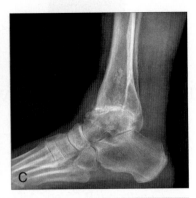

Figure 1 AP (**A**), mortise (**B**), and lateral (**C**) standard weight-bearing radiographs of a patient who has ankle arthritis.

malalignment, and certain medical conditions, such as hemophilia. In a large series from a tertiary referral center, 70% of patients with ankle arthritis had a history of trauma. Inflammatory arthritis was present in approximately 12% of all patients who had ankle arthritis.[5]

The incidence of ankle arthritis is difficult to accurately predict because of its low prevalence and a lack of correlation between radiographic and clinical findings. In a large cadaver model study, the overall incidence of end-stage arthritis was 2%, whereas all cadaver models older than 66 years had at least mild wear patterns.[6] Similarly, in a smaller cadaver model study, Meachim[7] examined 45 randomly selected cadaver models and reported a 5% incidence of full-thickness cartilage loss.

Diagnosis

A patient who has end-stage ankle arthritis often reports considerable limiting pain. It is important to obtain a thorough history to differentiate between the most common causes of ankle arthritis. The examiner should ask about a history of trauma to the extremity, including fracture and recurrent sprains. Other less common

etiologies to inquire about include a history of inflammatory or infectious arthropathies, gout, hemophilia, and neuropathy.

The examiner should clarify the patient's specific discomfort because it often indicates whether the patient has global or focal disease. A history of diffuse ankle pain with activities is more commonly seen with global disease, whereas a more activity-specific complaint suggests focal disease. Pain with activities that require maximal plantar flexion, such as descending stairs or downhill walking, often suggests posterior ankle pathology. If discomfort is anterior and occurs with activities of ankle dorsiflexion, anterior joint disease is a possibility. Subfibular pain may be suggestive of either subtalar or ankle pathology. Posteromedial ankle pain often has a soft-tissue origin.

The examination should begin with simple observations of the patient while he or she is standing. This assessment should include an observation for any residual signs of trauma, such as previous surgical incisions or skin graft sites. The overall alignment of the lower extremity should then be evaluated. It is not uncommon to find deformity through the ankle or subtalar joints. On standing, the heel should fall

into a slight valgus of 5° to 7°. It also is important to evaluate the alignment of the knees. Next, the gait pattern should be assessed, specifically observing for abnormal loading of the foot as it contacts the ground. A neurovascular examination should be performed with the patient seated; neuropathy is not uncommon in this demographic. Motion of the ankle and subtalar joints should be assessed, noting any discomfort and areas of point tenderness. Although it is uncommon for patients to have instability in the setting of arthritis, the ligamentous integrity of all joints should be assessed and documented.

After the physical examination, the patient should undergo a complete weight-bearing radiographic series to further evaluate the extent of his or her arthrosis. Standard three-view, weight-bearing radiographs that include AP, mortise, and lateral ankle views (**Figure 1**) are obtained for all patients at the institution of the authors of this chapter. The authors of this chapter also recommend standard three-view, weight-bearing radiographs of the foot to assess for adjacent joint arthritis. If there is suspicion of hindfoot malalignment, a weight-bearing alignment view, as described by Saltzman and el-Khoury,[8] is obtained. On occasion, CT may be indicated if a deformity is present, talar topography is altered (as in osteonecrosis), or further characterization of the joint is desired.

Treatment
Nonsurgical

The mainstay of initial treatment for ankle arthritis is managing the patient's symptoms nonsurgically. Options for nonsurgical treatment include NSAIDs, bracing, selective joint injection, shoe modifications, and mechanical unloading. NSAIDs can provide sustainable pain relief but may not be tolerated by the patient. Bracing options include the use of a prefabricated carbon-fiber, nonarticulating ankle-foot orthosis or a custom ankle-foot orthosis in an attempt to eliminate motion across the joint. These braces are best suited for a patient who is compliant with regular wear and is not concerned with cosmetic appearances. Selective joint injections, such as NSAIDs, have a widely varied response but can be very helpful for some patients for pain relief. In the experience of the authors of this chapter, some patients experience up to 6 months of pain relief from a single injection. In this subset of patients, long-term satisfactory management can be maintained with serial injections. For patients who receive an injection that provides less than 3 months of pain relief, long-term pain relief is not likely to be attained solely with injections. In these patients, subsequent injections are primarily reserved only for brief reprieves for special upcoming events, such as planned trips or weddings. Shoe modification with the addition of a rocker bottom may help decrease ankle motion. In addition, mechanical unloading of the joint with the use of a cane or other assistive device may be helpful.

Surgical

If nonsurgical measures do not provide adequate symptom relief, two primary treatment options for global end-stage arthritis exist: ankle arthrodesis and total ankle arthroplasty (TAA). Both treatment options have similar good or excellent outcomes (arthroplasty, 69%; arthrodesis, 68%) and similar 1-year postoperative revision surgery rates (arthroplasty, 9%; arthrodesis, 5%).[9,10]

Some clinicians favor arthroplasty because of the risk of nonunion with arthrodesis, which was reported to be 7% in one study.[11] In other studies, the nonunion rate for arthrodesis was reported to be as high as 43% in high-risk subgroups.[12] Furthermore, supporters of arthroplasty note that the risk of adjacent joint disease with arthrodesis, which was reported to be as high as 90%, is increased secondary to the loss of a major motion segment.[13] In the long term, loss of normal ankle motion has been reported to affect a patient's functional status. In a series of 28 patients who considered themselves highly satisfied after ankle arthrodesis, reported functional limitations included difficulty walking on uneven ground (80%), difficulty ascending or descending stairs (75%), and aches after prolonged activity (64%) despite what was considered a successful arthrodesis.[14]

Arthroplasty

Contrary to arguments in favor of TAA, evidence suggests that arthroplasty should be approached with caution. Patient selection for TAA is of utmost importance. Not every patient who has end-stage arthritis is a candidate for TAA. Patients who have acute or chronic joint infections, an insensate foot, severe multiplanar deformity, Charcot arthropathy, osteonecrosis of the talus, and compromised soft tissues are often poor candidates for TAA.[15,16]

Outcomes data for TAA are daunting and somewhat difficult to interpret. Dramatic variations in length of follow-up, patient selection, and definition of failure all make interpretation of these studies a challenge. Reported failure rates range from 2% at short-term follow-up to as high as 55% at long-term

follow-up.[17,18] Haddad et al[10] reported that implant survival rates for patients who underwent ankle arthroplasty were 78% and 77% at 5 years and 10 years postoperatively, respectively, and 1 of every 14 patients required revision surgery. In a study of a mobile-bearing TAA system with longer-term follow-up, Brunner et al[18] reported that the mean implant survival rate was only 45.6% at 14 years postoperatively. The argument often made to counter these high failure rates, most of which occur because of talar component subsidence, is that newer systems preserve more bone, and implants have a more anatomic design. In a study that examined a newer-generation implant system at a mean follow-up of 3.7 years, Adams et al[19] reported that 11% of the ankle implants had been revised or were deemed impending failures. Daniels et al[20] reported that the revision surgery rates of arthrodesis and ankle arthroplasty at a mean follow-up of 5.5 years were 7% and 17%, respectively. In a study on the intermediate- to long-term outcomes of a mobile-bearing TAA system, Daniels et al[21] reported that the revision surgery rate of the metal component was 12% and the failure rate of the polyethylene-bearing component was 18% at a mean follow-up of 4.3 and 5.2 years, respectively.

An advantage of arthrodesis is its ability to avoid the higher risk posed by the anterior incision associated with TAA. Currently, only one total ankle system, the Zimmer Total Ankle System, allows for component implantation via a lateral incision. All other FDA-approved systems require an anterior approach. An anterior approach to the ankle has been associated with wound complications in as many as 7% of patients who undergo TAA.[22-25]

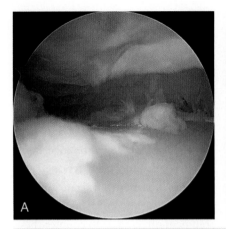
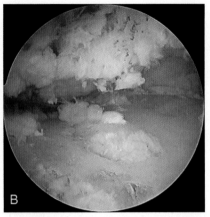
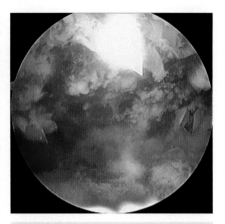

Figure 2 Arthroscopic images demonstrate preparation of an arthritic ankle joint. **A,** On initial arthroscopic evaluation. **B,** After preparation. (Courtesy of Eric Giza, MD, Sacramento, CA.)

Figure 3 Arthroscopic image of an ankle joint after subchondral drilling. Note the vascularity of the tibial and talar surfaces as well as maintenance of articular contours. (Courtesy of Eric Giza, MD, Sacramento, CA.)

Arthrodesis

Numerous techniques for ankle arthrodesis have been described. The authors of this chapter believe that orthopaedic surgeons should be familiar with the advantages and disadvantages of each of the following five techniques.

Arthroscopic-Assisted Technique

Recent advances in arthroscopic equipment and instrumentation have popularized an arthroscopic-assisted fusion technique. Proponents of arthroscopic-assisted fusion report decreased soft-tissue disruption and maintained biology. The main benefit of arthroscopic-assisted fusion is that the rate of union is similar to that of open techniques, with the relative elimination of wound problems that are more commonly seen with open-ankle arthrodesis techniques. The biggest limitations of arthroscopic-assisted fusion are that it is challenging to correct the deformity and it should not be used for patients who have more than 15° of varus or valgus in the coronal plane.[26,27] The authors of this chapter prefer to use arthroscopic-assisted fusion in patients who have nondeformed,

end-stage ankle arthritis and a compromised soft-tissue envelope.

Arthroscopic-assisted arthrodesis has been well described by Ferkel and Hewitt.[26] The patient is positioned supine with the leg held in a padded thigh holder such that the hip is flexed approximately 45°. A noninvasive ankle distractor is applied, and working portals are established in a standard fashion anteromedially, anterolaterally, and posterolaterally. Joint preparation is then begun with the removal of any remaining articular cartilage (**Figure 2**), which can be done with a combination of arthroscopic curettes, periosteal elevators, and shavers. An abrader is then used to resect down to bleeding subchondral bone, taking care not to disrupt the normal contours of the tibia and talus. The final step in joint preparation is to induce channels for vascularized ingrowth with the use of a 2.0-mm burr (**Figure 3**). After joint preparation, guidewires for large cannulated screws are placed.

The authors of this chapter use one of several different fixation constructs, typically with large cannulated screws that are either 6.5 or 7.3 mm in

diameter. In one commonly used construct, a "homerun" screw is placed posterolaterally approximately 2 to 3 cm above the joint line just off the lateral border of the Achilles tendon. The trajectory of this screw is positioned down the long axis of the talar neck. The key consideration in placing this screw is that the talar axis will be slightly medial to the midline. The sural nerve should be protected. A second guidewire is placed in the midaxis of the tibia from the medial side, beginning approximately 2 to 3 cm above the joint line. This guidewire is placed into the talar neck-body junction. The third and final guidewire is directed proximally from the talar neck into the tibia. After all the guidewires are placed, cannulated screws are inserted over the wires in the same sequence as that for the placement of the wires (**Figure 4**). Postoperatively, regardless of technique, the ankle is placed into a well-padded splint, and non–weight-bearing restrictions are implemented. At 2 weeks postoperatively, a wound check is performed, sutures are removed, and the patient is fitted with a

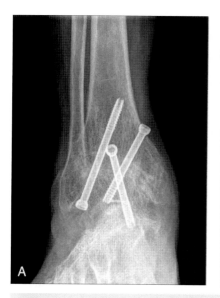

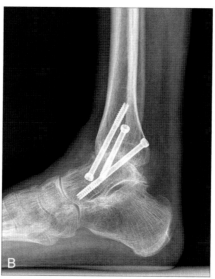

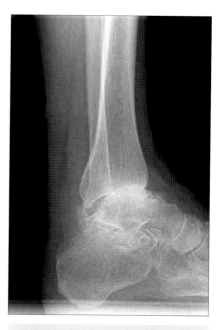

Figure 4 AP (**A**) and lateral (**B**) radiographs of an ankle demonstrate the chapter authors' standard screw configuration for ankle arthrodesis.

Figure 5 Lateral radiograph of an ankle joint demonstrates anterior talar subluxation, which makes less invasive arthrodesis techniques much more difficult.

short leg cast with no weight bearing for a total of 6 to 12 weeks. The duration of restricted weight bearing depends on radiographic signs of union and patient comorbidities. After demonstration of radiographic bony union, the patient is fitted with a walking boot and allowed to progressively begin weight bearing as tolerated. Physical therapy also is begun to assist in strengthening the extremity.

Reported results have been promising for arthroscopic-assisted ankle arthrodesis. In a large multicenter study that compared open ankle arthrodesis with arthroscopic ankle arthrodesis, Townshend et al[28] reported that, compared with the open group, the arthroscopic group had a shorter length of hospital stay (3.7 days versus 2.5 days, respectively) and improved outcomes at 1 year and 2 years postoperatively. In a similar multicenter comparative study, O'Brien et al[29] reported that arthroscopic ankle arthrodesis had shorter surgical and tourniquet times as well as decreased blood loss compared with open ankle arthrodesis. Both studies

reported similar union rates and outcomes 1 year postoperatively.

Miniarthrotomy

Miniarthrotomy, popularized by Paremain et al[30] and Stamatis and Myerson,[31] is a variation on arthroscopic-assisted arthrodesis. Miniarthrotomy is beneficial because it is relatively minimally invasive, which preserves the biology and vascularity of the joint as well as decreases the risk of wound complications. The limitations of miniarthrotomy are similar to those of arthroscopic-assisted arthrodesis and are based on its limited ability to correct larger coronal plane deformities. In addition, it is difficult to adequately reduce an anteriorly subluxated talus with miniarthrotomy (**Figure 5**). The authors of this chapter prefer to use miniarthrotomy in patients who have joints with mild deformity and minimal talar dysplasia.

The surgeon establishes two 1.5-cm working portals, one anteromedial and one anterolateral, in the same

areas where the arthroscopy portals are located. These incisions are made in a longitudinal fashion. The anteromedial incision is placed just medial to the anterior tibial tendon, with care taken to avoid the saphenous nerve and vein. After the anteromedial portal is established, the anterolateral portal is made using spinal needle localization. The anterolateral incision is made, with care taken to protect the superficial peroneal nerve. Visualization is improved by removal of anterior osteophytes and synovial tissue with the use of a rongeur. After clear visualization of the joint is attained, a laminar spreader is introduced through the anterolateral portal (**Figure 6**). Distraction force is applied, and joint preparation is performed in a standard fashion through the anteromedial working portal. The portals then reverse roles, and the anterolateral portal becomes the working portal while the anteromedial portal is used for

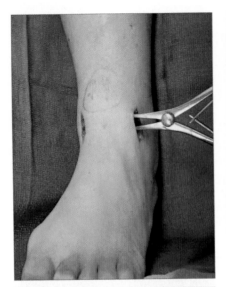

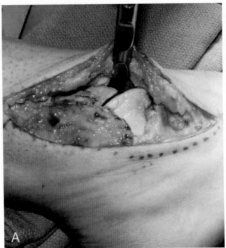

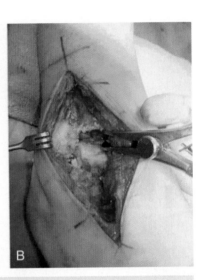

Figure 6 Intraoperative photograph shows a miniarthrotomy performed with the use of working portals and anterolateral placement of the laminar spreader to improve visualization and working room through the anteromedial portal.

Figure 7 Intraoperative photographs show the use of an extensile lateral incision to approach the ankle joint (**A**) and visualization of the ankle joint after resection of the anterior talofibular and calcaneofibular ligaments and joint capsule (**B**).

placement of the laminar spreader and distraction. Some authors report using these portals to perform deformity correction via bone wedge resection; however, in the experience of the authors of this chapter, this is difficult, and an often less-than-ideal correction with marked deformity is reported.[31] The joint is then reduced, and screw fixation is performed as previously discussed in the arthroscopic section. The postoperative protocol also is the same as that described in the arthroscopic section.

The reported results of miniarthrotomy are promising and further supported by the anecdotal clinical experience of the authors of this chapter. Using cadaver models, Miller et al[32] compared the vascular insult after miniarthrotomy with the vascular insult after an open technique. The authors reported that a major contributing blood supply to the fusion site was compromised by

the open technique in 40% of the cadaver models. This was not observed in any of the cadaver models that underwent miniarthrotomy. The authors further evaluated their clinical results in a cohort of 32 patients who underwent fusion with miniarthrotomy. A nonunion occurred in one patient, and two patients had delayed unions. No wound complications occurred, and the only significant postoperative complications were prominent instrumentation and transient ankle inflammation after union, both of which resolved in all patients.[30-32]

Fibular-Sparing Technique
The fibular-sparing technique is a modification of the lateral transfibular approach described by Mann et al.[33] The fibular-sparing technique was designed to maintain an intact fibula. In the classic transfibular approach, the fibula is removed and used as bone graft or as a strut for the fusion. It is the opinion of the senior authors of this chapter (J.T.S., C.P.C., E.M.B.) that removal of the fibula has several disadvantages and

can destabilize the ankle, which may lead to increased rates of nonunion.[10,34] An intact fibula may serve as a guide for proper rotation and positioning of the talus within the mortise, provides additional surface area for fusion, and may block valgus drift in patients who have delayed union. Furthermore, preservation of the fibula enables conversion to TAA, if necessary. The other benefits of the fibular-sparing technique include preparing the joint surfaces in situ as opposed to performing flat cuts and using a single site (ie, fibular window) for autologous bone graft.[11]

In the fibular-sparing approach described by Smith et al,[11] the patient is positioned supine with a stack of towels under the ipsilateral hip. An approximately 12-cm curvilinear incision is made directly over the lateral ankle. The incision is centered at the tip of the fibula and curves distally in line with the base of the fourth metatarsal. Division of the anterior talofibular and calcaneofibular ligaments is performed to allow the talus to rotate out from underneath the mortise (**Figure 7**).

For joint preparation, a sharp curette is used to remove the cartilage. Subchondral tibial and talar bone is then fenestrated with the use of a 4-mm burr that is set at low speed (20,000 rpm) and with continuous saline irrigation. After preparation of the tibia and talus, autogenous bone graft is harvested from the distal fibula through a fibular window. A medium-sized curette is used to harvest cancellous bone. The autograft is then packed onto the prepared tibial and talar surfaces. The ankle is placed in the described optimal position of 0° of dorsiflexion, 5° of hindfoot valgus, and 10° of external rotation.

Fixation is performed with the use of cannulated screws. Two partially threaded screws are passed from lateral to medial as described by Mann et al.[33] One screw with a washer is passed from the base of the talar neck to the tibia. The second screw is inserted from the lateral process of the talus and is directed into the distal tibia posteriorly. Intraoperative fluoroscopy is used to confirm the position of the screws. The postoperative protocol is the same as that described in the arthroscopic section.

Smith et al[11] analyzed 50 consecutive ankle arthrodeses performed with the fibular-sparing technique. At a mean follow-up of 28 months, 38 patients (42 ankles) were reviewed. Ninety-three percent of the patients attained union at a mean follow-up of 12 weeks, and 86% of the patients reported being "completely satisfied" with their outcomes. The mean American Orthopaedic Foot and Ankle Society (AOFAS) ankle-hindfoot score was 84 (out of a possible 86), and the mean Foot Function Index pain score was 1, which indicates no pain. Two ankles (5%) were fused in excessive varus; no patient required

revision surgery for malalignment. All of the patients stated that they would undergo the surgery again.

Anterior Open Plating

Anatomic compression arthrodesis was first described in a study by Holt et al,[35] which reported the benefits of preservation of the bony anatomy, minimal bone resection, and rigid multiplanar screw fixation. Despite these benefits, biomechanical studies have reported that construct stiffness can vary depending on the position of the screws and the quality of the patient's bone.[34] In two cadaver model studies, Thordarson et al[36,37] reported that screw fixation alone was unreliable in cadaver models that had osteoporotic bone. Therefore, to increase construct stiffness, anterior plates may be used to augment multiplanar screw fixation or as an independent fixation method. Mears et al[38] described the use of an anterior tension plate to improve construct stiffness; an anterior tension plate offers improved joint visualization, high fusion rates, and good coverage of instrumentation by soft tissue.[38] In a cadaver model study, Tarkin et al[39] reported that the use of supplemental anterior plating and compression screws increased construct rigidity and limited micromotion at the ankle fusion interface compared with the use of multiplanar lag screws alone. Further studies on fixation with anterior contoured plates alone have reported that rigid construct fixation leads to fusion rates higher than 90%.[40-42] Proponents of the anterior plating technique stress its benefit in patients who have posttraumatic bone loss and/or poor bone quality that requires more rigid fixation than that provided by multiplanar screws alone.[40] An anterior approach to the ankle is

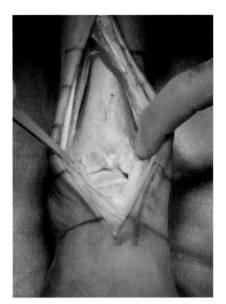

Figure 8   Intraoperative photograph shows a straight anterior approach with visualization of the tibiotalar joint.

used to perform anterior plating. This approach is familiar to most surgeons and allows for enhanced visualization as well as future conversion to TAA, if necessary, because the fibula and medial malleolus are spared in the procedure.

The patient is positioned supine with a stack of towels under the ipsilateral hip. A standard anterior approach to the ankle is performed, and the tibiotalar joint is visualized (**Figure 8**). A laminar spreader can be placed within the ankle joint for distraction and visualization. Meticulous joint preparation is performed with the use of a sharp curette, elevator, chisel, or osteotome. It is important not to disrupt the contour of the tibial plafond and talar dome. After the joint is prepared and the cartilage is removed, a 2.0-mm burr or drill (usually 2.5 mm) may be used to penetrate the subchondral plate and stimulate vascular ingrowth. The ankle is then reduced into the appropriate position and held with the anterior plate. The use of nonlocking or locking plates

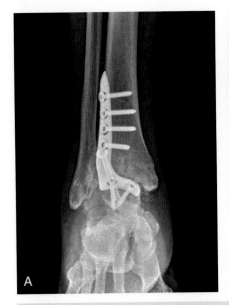 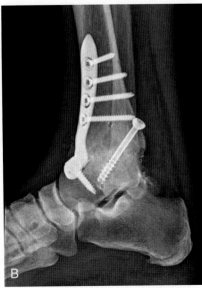

Figure 9 Weight-bearing AP (**A**) and lateral (**B**) radiographs of the ankle demonstrate anterior plating with placement of an additional multiplanar "homerun" screw for additional compression. (Courtesy of James Jastifer, MD, Kalamazoo, MI.)

depends on the quality of the bone and the surgeon's preference for implant design. The senior authors of this chapter (J.T.S., C.P.C., E.M.B.) prefer to use anterior-contoured nonlocking plates for most patients. Many plates are precontoured distally with an anterior bend to fit the anterior talar neck.

Two or three screws are placed first in the talus, followed by similar screws in the tibia using compression techniques specific to each plate design. If additional fixation to increase stability is necessary at this time, multiplanar lag screws may be placed (**Figure 9**). The alignment and position of the instrumentation is checked clinically and fluoroscopically. After acceptable fixation is attained, the wound is copiously irrigated and closed. Closure includes approximation of the extensor retinaculum with No. 1 absorbable suture, followed by subcutaneous closure with No. 3 absorbable suture and skin layer closure with either simple interrupted or horizontal mattress sutures. No

drain is used, and standard postoperative protocol is initiated.

Anterior plating has good outcomes with low complication rates reported in the literature. In a retrospective study of 10 patients who underwent fusion with anterior contoured plates, Guo et al[40] reported that 90% of the patients had fusion at 15 weeks postoperatively, and one patient underwent revision surgery because of screw loosening, which went on to fusion 12 weeks after revision surgery. There were no postoperative wound complications, and all of the patients reported improvements in pain. Rowan and Davey[43] reported a fusion rate of 94% in 33 consecutive patients who underwent fusion with an anterior T-plate. Tibial stress fractures developed and healed without fixation in two patients, and superficial wound infections developed in four patients. Plaass et al[42] used an anterior double-plate system in 29 patients and reported a fusion rate of 100%, an improvement in mean AOFAS scores from 37 to 68, and no

wound complications; 93% of the patients (27 of 29) were satisfied with their outcome and stated that they would undergo the procedure again. The low rates of infection, complication, and nonunion in these studies are similar to those of other reported results for isolated anterior plating as well as combined anterior plating and multiplanar screws.[34,40,41]

External Compression Arthrodesis With the Use of a Circular External Fixator
Ankle arthrodesis with the use of a circular external fixator may be a good option for difficult patients, such as those in whom a previous arthrodesis with or without infection has failed, talar osteonecrosis, soft-tissue compromise, or severe ankle deformity.[44,45]

Various techniques can be used for compression arthrodesis with external fixation rings.[44-47] Joint preparation for arthrodesis depends on the surgeon's preference and patient-specific factors. In patients undergoing revision surgery, prior incisions often must be used. At times, placement of Steinmann pins helps hold the alignment of the ankle while placing the frame. After the joint has been prepared, the frame, which often consists of one or two rings placed orthogonal to the distal tibia and a foot-plate half ring, is applied. Fixation is accomplished with half pins, and tensioned thin wires are placed in a multiplanar fashion. Typically, the tibial ring or rings are applied first, followed by the foot plate. Usually the plantar foot is placed distal to the foot ring. Talar wires can be used to provide increased stability and protect the subtalar joint from compression. The proximal ring or rings are connected to the foot construct by struts, and tibiotalar compression is performed. Wound closure is performed in a standard fashion, and dressings are applied to the pin sites.

The overall results of external compression arthrodesis reported in the literature are good. Hawkins et al[44] used an Ilizarov technique for ankle fusion in 21 patients who had complex distal tibial pathology or failed ankle arthrodesis. Sixty percent of the patients had a good result after solid ankle arthrodesis, with expected functional capacity after fusion and no reports of pain or infection. Twenty percent of the patients had a fair result, which was classified as a solid ankle fusion with marked residual reports of pain or deformity, and 20% of the patients had a poor result, with a residual infection reported in one patient and nonunion reported in three patients. Eylon et al[46] examined 17 patients who underwent either a primary or revision ankle arthrodesis with the use of an Ilizarov frame at a follow-up of 6 years. All of the ankles had a solid fusion, and the mean AOFAS score was 65. In a retrospective review of 91 patients who underwent a complex ankle arthrodesis with the use of the Ilizarov method, Fragomen et al[48] reported a fusion rate of 84% and a mean AOFAS score of 71 at a follow-up of 27 months. In a study of 45 consecutive patients who underwent revision tibiotalar arthrodesis, Easley et al[45] reported that 11 patients underwent repeat internal fixation, 22 patients underwent placement of a ring external fixator, and 12 patients underwent tibiotalocalcaneal arthrodesis. The mean follow-up was 50.3 months, and fusion was attained in 80% of all of the patients and in 87% of the patients (19 of 22) in the ring external fixator group. Current evidence supports the use of ring external fixation in some patients undergoing complex and revision arthrodesis.

Summary

In some patients, global end-stage ankle arthritis can be effectively managed nonsurgically. In patients who have persistent symptoms despite having undergone nonsurgical care, the treating surgeon often faces the difficult decision of whether to fuse or replace the ankle joint. The literature supports both arthrodesis and arthroplasty; however, patient-specific factors, such as medical comorbidities, age, and activity level, influence this decision. The key to a successful outcome is to engage the patient in the decision-making process.

If the surgeon and patient decide that arthrodesis is the preferred treatment, then numerous technical options exist. Questions that aid in determining the most appropriate technique include the following: Is there coronal plane malalignment? Is there sagittal plane translation? Is there talar dysplasia? The more positive responses from these questions, the more the surgeon should consider an extensile approach rather than a less invasive procedure. If the answers are mostly negative, then the surgeon is afforded the option of using a less invasive technique that can potentially preserve the blood supply, decrease the risk of nonunion, and decrease the risk of wound complications. The specific approach must be individualized for each patient. No uniform treatment algorithm exists for this complex pathology.

References

1. Huch K, Kuettner KE, Dieppe P: Osteoarthritis in ankle and knee joints. *Semin Arthritis Rheum* 1997;26(4):667-674.

2. Kimizuka M, Kurosawa H, Fukubayashi T: Load-bearing pattern of the ankle joint: Contact area and pressure distribution. *Arch Orthop Trauma Surg* 1980;96(1):45-49.

3. Ihn JC, Kim SJ, Park IH: In vitro study of contact area and pressure distribution in the human knee after partial and total meniscectomy. *Int Orthop* 1993;17(4):214-218.

4. Brown TD, Shaw DT: In vitro contact stress distributions in the natural human hip. *J Biomech* 1983;16(6):373-384.

5. Saltzman CL, Salamon ML, Blanchard GM, et al: Epidemiology of ankle arthritis: Report of a consecutive series of 639 patients from a tertiary orthopaedic center. *Iowa Orthop J* 2005;25:44-46.

6. Muehleman C, Bareither D, Huch K, Cole AA, Kuettner KE: Prevalence of degenerative morphological changes in the joints of the lower extremity. *Osteoarthritis Cartilage* 1997;5(1):23-37.

7. Meachim G: Cartilage fibrillation at the ankle joint in Liverpool necropsies. *J Anat* 1975;119(pt 3):601-610.

8. Saltzman CL, el-Khoury GY: The hindfoot alignment view. *Foot Ankle Int* 1995;16(9):572-576.

9. SooHoo NF, Zingmond DS, Ko CY: Comparison of reoperation rates following ankle arthrodesis and total ankle arthroplasty. *J Bone Joint Surg Am* 2007;89(10):2143-2149.

10. Haddad SL, Coetzee JC, Estok R, Fahrbach K, Banel D, Nalysnyk L: Intermediate and long-term outcomes of total ankle arthroplasty and ankle arthrodesis: A systematic review of the literature. *J Bone Joint Surg Am* 2007;89(9):1899-1905.

11. Smith JT, Chiodo CP, Singh SK, Wilson MG: Open ankle arthrodesis with a fibular-sparing technique. *Foot Ankle Int* 2013;34(4):557-562.

12. Frey C, Halikus NM, Vu-Rose T, Ebramzadeh E: A review of ankle arthrodesis: Predisposing factors to nonunion. *Foot Ankle Int* 1994;15(11):581-584.

13. Coester LM, Saltzman CL, Leupold J, Pontarelli W: Long-term results following ankle arthrodesis for post-traumatic arthritis. *J Bone Joint Surg Am* 2001;83(2):219-228.

14. Muir DC, Amendola A, Saltzman CL: Long-term outcome of ankle arthrodesis. *Foot Ankle Clin* 2002;7(4):703-708.

15. Gougoulias NE, Khanna A, Maffulli N: History and evolution in total ankle arthroplasty. *Br Med Bull* 2009;89:111-151.

16. Jackson MP, Singh D: Total ankle replacement. *Curr Orthop* 2003;17(4):292-298.

17. Kopp FJ, Patel MM, Deland JT, O'Malley MJ: Total ankle arthroplasty with the Agility prosthesis: Clinical and radiographic evaluation. *Foot Ankle Int* 2006;27(2):97-103.

18. Brunner S, Barg A, Knupp M, et al: The Scandinavian total ankle replacement: Long-term, eleven to fifteen-year, survivorship analysis of the prosthesis in seventy-two consecutive patients. *J Bone Joint Surg Am* 2013;95(8):711-718.

19. Adams SB Jr, Demetracopoulos CA, Queen RM, Easley ME, DeOrio JK, Nunley JA: Early to mid-term results of fixed-bearing total ankle arthroplasty with a modular intramedullary tibial component. *J Bone Joint Surg Am* 2014;96(23):1983-1989.

20. Daniels TR, Younger AS, Penner M, et al: Intermediate-term results of total ankle replacement and ankle arthrodesis: A COFAS multi-center study. *J Bone Joint Surg Am* 2014;96(2):135-142.

21. Daniels TR, Mayich DJ, Penner MJ: Intermediate to long-term outcomes of total ankle replacement with the Scandinavian Total Ankle Replacement (STAR). *J Bone Joint Surg Am* 2015;97(11):895-903.

22. Claridge RJ, Sagherian BH: Intermediate term outcome of the agility total ankle arthroplasty. *Foot Ankle Int* 2009;30(9):824-835.

23. Criswell BJ, Douglas K, Naik R, Thomson AB: High revision and reoperation rates using the Agility™ Total Ankle System. *Clin Orthop Relat Res* 2012;470(7):1980-1986.

24. Hurowitz EJ, Gould JS, Fleisig GS, Fowler R: Outcome analysis of agility total ankle replacement with prior adjunctive procedures: Two to six year followup. *Foot Ankle Int* 2007;28(3):308-312.

25. Saltzman CL, Amendola A, Anderson R, et al: Surgeon training and complications in total

ankle arthroplasty. *Foot Ankle Int* 2003;24(6):514-518.

26. Ferkel RD, Hewitt M: Long-term results of arthroscopic ankle arthrodesis. *Foot Ankle Int* 2005;26(4):275-280.

27. Fitzgibbons TC: Arthroscopic ankle debridement and fusion: Indications, techniques, and results. *Instr Course Lect* 1999;48:243-248.

28. Townshend D, Di Silvestro M, Krause F, et al: Arthroscopic versus open ankle arthrodesis: A multicenter comparative case series. *J Bone Joint Surg Am* 2013;95(2):98-102.

29. O'Brien TS, Hart TS, Shereff MJ, Stone J, Johnson J: Open versus arthroscopic ankle arthrodesis: A comparative study. *Foot Ankle Int* 1999;20(6):368-374.

30. Paremain GD, Miller SD, Myerson MS: Ankle arthrodesis: Results after the miniarthrotomy technique. *Foot Ankle Int* 1996;17(5):247-252.

31. Stamatis E, Myerson MS: The miniarthrotomy technique for ankle arthrodesis. *Tech Foot Ankle Surg* 2002;1(1):8-16.

32. Miller SD, Paremain GP, Myerson MS: The miniarthrotomy technique of ankle arthrodesis: A cadaver study of operative vascular compromise and early clinical results. *Orthopedics* 1996;19(5):425-430.

33. Mann RA, Van Manen JW, Wapner K, Martin J: Ankle fusion. *Clin Orthop Relat Res* 1991;268:49-55.

34. Clare MP, Sanders RW: The anatomic compression arthrodesis technique with anterior plate augmentation for ankle arthrodesis. *Foot Ankle Clin* 2011;16(1):91-101.

35. Holt ES, Hansen ST, Mayo KA, Sangeorzan BJ: Ankle arthrodesis using internal screw fixation. *Clin Orthop Relat Res* 1991;268:21-28.

36. Thordarson DB, Markolf KL, Cracchiolo A III: Arthrodesis of the ankle with cancellous-bone screws and fibular strut graft: Biomechanical analysis. *J Bone Joint Surg Am* 1990;72(9):1359-1363.

37. Thordarson DB, Markolf K, Cracchiolo A III: Stability of an ankle arthrodesis fixed by cancellous-bone

screws compared with that fixed by an external fixator: A biomechanical study. *J Bone Joint Surg Am* 1992;74(7):1050-1055.

38. Mears DC, Gordon RG, Kann SE, Kann JN: Ankle arthrodesis with an anterior tension plate. *Clin Orthop Relat Res* 1991;268:70-77.

39. Tarkin IS, Mormino MA, Clare MP, Haider H, Walling AK, Sanders RW: Anterior plate supplementation increases ankle arthrodesis construct rigidity. *Foot Ankle Int* 2007;28(2):219-223.

40. Guo C, Yan Z, Barfield WR, Hartsock LA: Ankle arthrodesis using anatomically contoured anterior plate. *Foot Ankle Int* 2010;31(6):492-498.

41. Kakarala G, Rajan DT: Comparative study of ankle arthrodesis using cross screw fixation versus anterior contoured plate plus cross screw fixation. *Acta Orthop Belg* 2006;72(6):716-721.

42. Plaass C, Knupp M, Barg A, Hintermann B: Anterior double plating for rigid fixation of isolated tibiotalar arthrodesis. *Foot Ankle Int* 2009;30(7):631-639.

43. Rowan R, Davey KJ: Ankle arthrodesis using an anterior AO T plate. *J Bone Joint Surg Br* 1999;81(1):113-116.

44. Hawkins BJ, Langerman RJ, Anger DM, Calhoun JH: The Ilizarov technique in ankle fusion. *Clin Orthop Relat Res* 1994;303:217-225.

45. Easley ME, Montijo HE, Wilson JB, Fitch RD, Nunley JA II: Revision tibiotalar arthrodesis. *J Bone Joint Surg Am* 2008;90(6):1212-1223.

46. Eylon S, Porat S, Bor N, Leibner ED: Outcome of Ilizarov ankle arthrodesis. *Foot Ankle Int* 2007;28(8):873-879.

47. Salem KH, Kinzl L, Schmelz A: Ankle arthrodesis using Ilizarov ring fixators: A review of 22 cases. *Foot Ankle Int* 2006;27(10):764-770.

48. Fragomen AT, Borst E, Schachter L, Lyman S, Rozbruch SR: Complex ankle arthrodesis using the Ilizarov method yields high rate of fusion. *Clin Orthop Relat Res* 2012;470(10):2864-2873.

The Failed Cavovarus Foot: What Went Wrong and Why?

Jonathan R.M. Kaplan, MD
Mark S. Myerson, MD

The adult cavovarus foot exists on a spectrum and, therefore, requires a thorough evaluation to determine the extent of the deformity and then choose from a multitude of surgical procedures to achieve correction. Regardless of the severity of the deformity, treatment should include an algorithmic approach to adequately achieve a stable, balanced, and plantigrade foot. To prevent failure, the surgeon should evaluate whether the deformity is flexible or rigid, determine the location of the apex or apices of the deformity, evaluate any muscle imbalances occurring about the foot and ankle, and determine the need for additional procedures. A failure to consider these principles and, subsequently, the extent of the deformity often results in recurrence and progression of the deformity.

Instr Course Lect 2016;65:331–342.

Management of the adult cavovarus foot is complex and requires an understanding of not only the etiology of the deformity but also any muscle imbalances occurring about the foot and ankle. The goal of surgical intervention is to attain a plantigrade and balanced foot, which requires a systematic and stepwise treatment algorithm. To accomplish this, it is important for the surgeon to evaluate if the deformity is flexible or rigid, determine the apex (or, in some feet, apices) of the deformity, evaluate any muscle imbalances occurring about the foot and ankle, and determine if ancillary procedures are necessary. A failure to consider these principles and apply appropriate treatment may result in inadequate treatment and recurrence and progression of the deformity.

Treatment of the cavovarus foot begins with a thorough evaluation that includes a clinical examination and appropriate radiographic studies. To determine the true extent of the deformity, it is important for the surgeon to evaluate patients in both the standing and seated positions. There is often variation in the extent of the deformity; therefore, it is important for the surgeon to have a good understanding of its complex three-dimensional nature, including the supinated and varus alignment of the hindfoot, the plantarflexed medial column, and associated forefoot pronation. A patient's gait should be observed to evaluate for associated muscle weakness, particularly a slight footdrop, and any attempted compensation for this weakness with the toe extensors.

Flexibility of the Deformity

Whenever possible, the surgeon should perform osteotomies rather than arthrodesis. After an osteotomy, the foot will be more flexible, and recuperation will generally be easier and quicker compared with more complex hindfoot arthrodesis procedures. The most common error that surgeons have made over the past decades was pushing the envelope with respect to flexibility and performing an osteotomy in cases in which arthrodesis would have been more appropriate. Unfortunately, because of its historically poor outcomes, arthrodesis has been considered a

Dr. Myerson or an immediate family member has received royalties from Biomet, DePuy, and Tornier; serves as a paid consultant to or is an employee of Biomet, BioMedical Enterprises, and Tornier; and serves as an unpaid consultant to Tornier. Neither Dr. Kaplan nor any immediate family member has received anything of value from or has stock or stock options held in a commercial company or institution related directly or indirectly to the subject of this chapter.

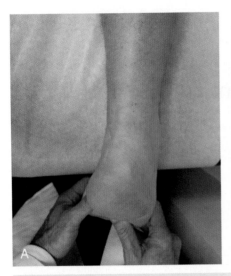
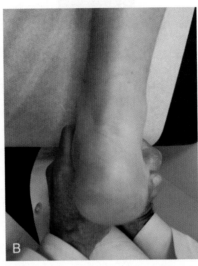

Figure 1   Clinical photographs of the hindfoot of a patient in the prone position. **A,** The hindfoot is in varus alignment without manipulation or correction of the deformity. **B,** Manipulation of the hindfoot into valgus alignment demonstrates a flexible deformity.

salvage procedure; however, the poor outcomes may be related to a failure to consider some of the principles of deformity correction, including muscle balance and a plantigrade foot.[1-4]

Various examination techniques have been used to evaluate the flexibility of the cavovarus foot, including the Coleman block test, a prone examination, and a supine or seated examination.[5-7] Coleman and Chestnut[5] were the first to describe the Coleman block test, in which a block is placed under the lateral column to accommodate the plantarflexed first ray. In forefoot-driven cavus, the initial deformity occurs as the peroneus longus overpowers the tibialis anterior, resulting in a plantarflexed first ray with subsequent cavovarus of the hindfoot. If the varus alignment of the hindfoot corrects with the Coleman block test, then it is considered passively correctable and, in theory, can be treated with an elevation osteotomy of the first metatarsal only. The authors of this chapter, however, have found that this is rarely the case

because the cavovarus foot exists on a spectrum of deformity. Furthermore, the Coleman block test does not reveal the full extent of deformity correction. The authors of this chapter recommend supplementing the Coleman block test with an examination in which the surgeon manually manipulates the hindfoot of a patient in a seated or prone position. If the varus alignment of the hindfoot is correctable, the heel will easily move into valgus alignment with the foot in equinus[7] (**Figure 1**). The extent of deformity correction can be determined with this examination technique and typically consists of osteotomies involving both the hindfoot and the forefoot rather than an isolated first metatarsal osteotomy, which may be mistakenly recommended with the use of only the Coleman block test.

Radiographic studies should include AP, oblique, and lateral views of the foot and an AP view of the ankle. Radiographic abnormalities include an increased calcaneal pitch, an increased Meary angle, and a decreased Hibbs

angle.[8] A hindfoot alignment radiograph also is beneficial for evaluating the extent of malalignment in the coronal plane.[9] In addition to these standard radiographic views, weight-bearing radiographs with the Coleman block may be beneficial for radiographically determining the flexibility of the deformity (**Figure 2**).

The flexible cavovarus foot is amenable to motion-sparing surgical corrections that consist of a combination of hindfoot, midfoot, and forefoot osteotomies in addition to the required tendon transfers. The truly flexible cavovarus foot may not require tendon transfers, but this is not typically the case. In general, the authors of this chapter use a combination of a first metatarsal osteotomy, a calcaneal osteotomy, and a peroneus longus to brevis transfer for milder deformities. With respect to the hindfoot, the calcaneal osteotomy has traditionally been described as either a lateral slide osteotomy or a lateral closing wedge osteotomy.[10] Instead, it should be thought of as a three-dimensional osteotomy that consists of a lateral closing wedge osteotomy combined with a shift both proximally and superiorly (**Figure 3**).[11] The closing wedge osteotomy with lateral shift improves the weight-bearing axis of the hindfoot, and the superior shift accommodates the increased calcaneal pitch. The principle of correction is to start proximally and progress distally, beginning with the calcaneal osteotomy and followed by the midfoot and forefoot osteotomies.

It is essential for the surgeon to recognize the many subtleties of a calcaneal osteotomy, both preoperatively and intraoperatively. As the incision is being made, the surgeon must consider the need for additional procedures, such as peroneal tendon repair or transfer and the possibility of lateral ligament reconstruction. As dissection is carried down to bone, the surgeon must take special care to prevent injury to the adjacent peroneal tendons and the sural nerve. After dissection down to bone, the surgeon must elevate an adequate amount of periosteum to allow for a wedge of bone to be removed. The authors of this chapter prefer to use a saw to perform the wedge resection, with the first cut made perpendicular to the axis of the calcaneus and at a 45° angle to the tuberosity. In general, the second cut is made at a 20° angle to the first cut; however, the angle can be increased or decreased, depending on the amount of correction required. The varus alignment of the hindfoot should be evaluated intraoperatively, with both direct visualization and fluoroscopy, to ensure that no overcorrection (with subsequent valgus alignment of the hindfoot) or undercorrection (with persistent varus alignment) occurs. Bruce et al[12] reported that tarsal tunnel volume is reduced after a lateral calcaneal osteotomy; therefore, prophylactic tarsal tunnel release should be considered for patients who require an extensive lateral shift. Finally, it is important for the surgeon to tamp down any laterally overhanging bone that may cause irritation to the peroneal tendons and persistent postoperative symptomatology.

As the calcaneus is moved into valgus alignment, the eversion produces further plantar flexion of the first metatarsal; therefore, a first metatarsal dorsiflexion osteotomy should be performed to correct the plantarflexed first ray. While the medial column is plantarflexed, the lateral column is both rotated and adducted, and rotational

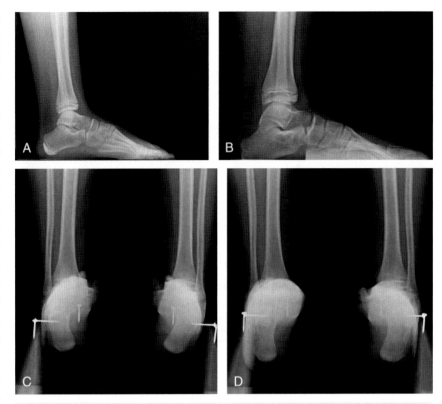

Figure 2   **A,** Lateral weight-bearing radiograph of the foot taken without the Coleman block demonstrates an increased calcaneal pitch, a decreased Meary angle, and a decreased talar declination angle. There also is a rotational deformity about the midfoot and forefoot, with an elevated medial column and metatarsal stacking. **B,** Lateral weight-bearing radiograph of the foot taken with the Coleman block placed under the lateral column demonstrates correction of the plantarflexed first ray and some improvement in the calcaneal pitch, the talar declination angle, and rotational deformity. **C,** Hindfoot alignment weight-bearing radiograph taken without the Coleman block demonstrates bilateral varus alignment of the hindfoot. **D,** Hindfoot alignment weight-bearing radiograph taken with the Coleman block placed under the left lateral column demonstrates improvement in hindfoot alignment compared with the contralateral side.

malalignment must be addressed to prevent persistent lateral column overload. It is important for the surgeon to evaluate the forefoot and determine if the deformity is isolated to the first ray or if it affects the entire forefoot. Cavovarus isolated to the first ray is amenable to correction with a dorsiflexion osteotomy of the first metatarsal; global cavovarus may require a tarsometatarsal truncated-wedge arthrodesis[13] or osteotomies at the bases of all the metatarsals.

Apex of the Deformity

Although motion preservation is desirable, an arthrodesis that produces a stable, plantigrade foot is better than a joint-sparing surgery that fails to completely correct the deformity. Therefore, it is necessary for the surgeon to determine the apex of the deformity in both the sagittal and coronal planes. In addition to arthrodesis, it is important that tendon transfers and ancillary procedures are performed, otherwise the procedure is likely to fail.

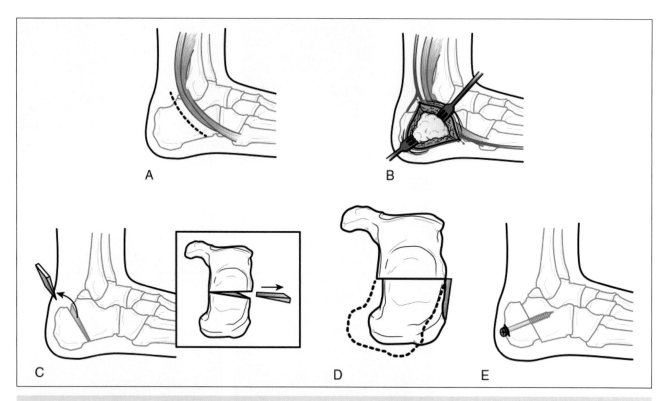

Figure 3   Illustrations demonstrate the steps of a calcaneal osteotomy for surgical correction of a flexible cavovarus foot. **A,** The incision (dashed line) is typically made at a level beneath the peroneal tendons and the sural nerve; however, it should be adjusted based on additional necessary procedures. **B,** The periosteum is elevated, and retractors are used to protect the adjacent soft tissue. **C,** A wedge of bone is removed (arrow) from the lateral calcaneus. Inset shows an axial view of the wedge of bone being removed (arrow) from the lateral calcaneus. **D,** The calcaneal osteotomy is closed, and the tuberosity is simultaneously shifted laterally, proximally, and superiorly (shaded area). The dashed line represents the positioning of the tuberosity before the osteotomy is closed. **E,** After the osteotomy is secured with an appropriately sized screw, the final position of the tuberosity should be more posterior with an improvement in calcaneal pitch.

Because it is difficult to appreciate the apex of the deformity with only a clinical examination, radiographs should be taken in both the coronal and sagittal planes. In the sagittal plane, the apex is classified as anterior if it is located in the midfoot at the intertarsal or tarsometatarsal joints or posterior if it is located in the hindfoot.[14] In the coronal plane, the apex can occur anywhere along the lateral column.

A midfoot arthrodesis is the best technique to correct an anterior-apex deformity because the deformity is located distal to the transverse tarsal joint and because a triple arthrodesis would fail to address the deformity in the sagittal plane. Although a midfoot arthrodesis may be more technically challenging, correction is more accurate if it is performed at the apex of the deformity. Although multiple techniques have been described to correct an anterior-apex deformity, the specific location of the deformity should determine which technique is selected.[13,15-17]

The Cole midtarsal osteotomy and the Japas osteotomy are options to correct a deformity in which the apex occurs at the midtarsal joint. The Cole midtarsal osteotomy is a dorsal closing wedge osteotomy, in which a wedge of bone is removed from one cut through the cuboid joints and navicular and a second cut through the cuboid joints and cuneiforms.[16] Because the Cole midtarsal osteotomy may result in shortening of the foot,[16] the authors of this chapter prefer to use the Japas osteotomy, which is a dorsal wedge osteotomy performed at the naviculocuneiform and cuboid joints. This technique maintains length, allows for multiplanar correction, and, most importantly, is performed at the apex of the deformity.[17] It is important for surgeons who are performing a Japas osteotomy to resect more bone dorsally and medially; this creates a tapered wedge with minimal to no bone removed from the cuboid and allows for dorsiflexion medially, dorsal translation, and lateral rotation.[14] Although less common, if the apex of the deformity in the sagittal plane occurs more distally at the tarsometatarsal joint, it may be more amenable to a Jahss dorsal wedge osteotomy at the tarsometatarsal joints. The Jahss dorsal wedge osteotomy is similar to a midfoot osteotomy, in that more bone is resected dorsally and medially, which allows for correction of both the cavus and the rotational deformity.[13]

Triple arthrodesis supplemented by appropriate soft-tissue balancing with tendon transfers is the best technique to correct a deformity in the hindfoot because the deforming forces typically occur distal to the site of the triple arthrodesis. In addition to the standard triple arthrodesis technique that Ryerson described in 1923, other techniques, including beak triple arthrodesis, have been used specifically to correct posterior-apex cavovarus deformities.[18-20] To perform a beak triple arthrodesis, the surgeon makes an osteotomy through the anterior calcaneus and the talar head-neck region to create a talar beak, which is then used to lock the forefoot under the talus at the level of the navicular. This technique not only improves the cavovarus foot with its apex at the talonavicular joint but also provides additional length to the foot.

Understanding the three-dimensional nature of the cavovarus foot is key because the varus alignment of the hindfoot is corrected with a truncated-wedge resection at the level of the subtalar joint, whereas midfoot rotation is corrected through the transverse tarsal joint. A truncated-wedge resection provides better decompression compared with a triangular-wedge resection because it allows for easier correction of the

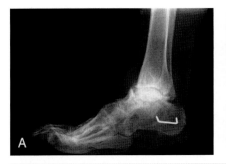
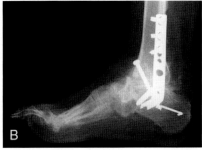

Figure 4　　**A,** Preoperative lateral weight-bearing radiograph of the foot demonstrates cavovarus alignment and increased lateral column overload with hypertrophy and a stress fracture involving the fifth metatarsal base. **B,** Postoperative lateral weight-bearing radiograph of the foot demonstrates correction of the cavovarus alignment and resection of the fifth metatarsal. (Reproduced with permission from Shariff R, Myerson MS, Palmanovich E: Resection of the fifth metatarsal base in the severe rigid cavovarus foot. *Foot Ankle Int* 2014;35[6]:558-565.)

deformity, albeit with slight shortening of the foot.

The authors of this chapter prefer to use two incisions to allow for joint preparation and deformity correction as well as for exposure for associated tendon transfers. The authors first perform a posterior tibial tendon release, which is tagged for later transfer, followed by a plantar fascia release. For a typical cavovarus deformity, the authors first correct the subtalar joint into 5° of valgus alignment; provisionally fix it with a guide pin; and then correct the transverse tarsal joint with rotation, abduction, and dorsiflexion. To correct a more severe deformity in which the apex of the deformity is located directly at the talonavicular joint, the authors use the beak triple arthrodesis technique, in which the navicular is recessed under the head of the talus. The articular surface and the dorsal cortex of the navicular are débrided; a notch is cut in the plantar half of the talar head, and the dorsal half of the talar head is kept intact; and the navicular is slid under the head of the talus. This technique corrects the deformity and preserves the length of the foot without resection of a

large wedge of bone through the transverse tarsal joint. The talonavicular joint is fixed with one medial screw and supplemented by a dorsal, two-hole locking compression plate. It is important for the surgeon to recognize that the cuboid tends to subluxate plantarward, and that a failure to elevate the lateral column may result in persistent lateral column overload. Persistent rotation about the forefoot may exist even after the calcaneocuboid joint is corrected, resulting in an excessively plantar fifth metatarsal base that requires resection.[21] After the beak triple arthrodesis is completed, the surgeon should evaluate the foot to determine if a double-apex deformity—a second deformity in the midfoot or forefoot that also may require arthrodesis—is present. Finally, the authors of this chapter complete the tendon transfers and any necessary ancillary procedures, such as ankle stabilization for lateral instability or fifth metatarsal base resection (**Figure 4**).

Tendon Transfers for Soft-Tissue Balancing

Regardless whether a cavovarus foot is flexible or rigid, adequate soft-tissue

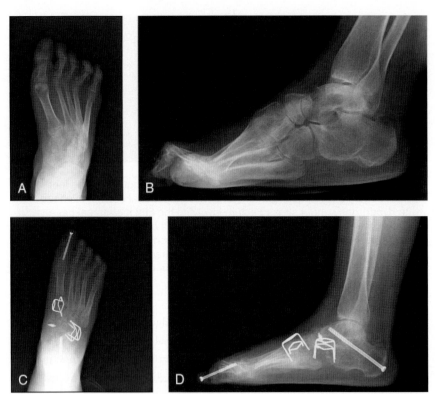

Figure 5 Preoperative AP (**A**) and lateral (**B**) radiographs of the foot demonstrate a double-apex deformity. The posterior apex occurs at the transverse tarsal joint, with an increased calcaneal pitch and a decreased talar declination angle. The second apex occurs distally in the midfoot, with increased medial column height compared with lateral column height and an elevated navicular and medial cuneiform, which suggest over-pull of the tibialis anterior. Postoperative AP (**C**) and lateral (**D**) radiographs of the foot demonstrate improved alignment. The foot is plantigrade with improved correction of both apex deformities. Note the improved talar declination angle, calcaneal pitch, and plantigrade measurement ratio, with an increase in height from the medial cuneiform to the floor and a decrease in height from the fourth metatarsal base to the floor.

balancing with tendon transfers must be performed to achieve a stable, plantigrade foot. As previously discussed, osseous correction alone does not rectify the underlying cause of the deformity, which is a dynamic muscle imbalance that occurs across the hindfoot, midfoot, and forefoot.[22,23] Traditionally, in Charcot-Marie-Tooth disease, the peroneus longus overpowers the weak tibialis anterior, resulting in a plantar-flexed first ray, and the posterior tibial tendon overpowers the weak peroneus brevis, accentuating the elevated arch

and contributing to the varus alignment of the hindfoot.[24,25]

To be adequate for transfer, a tendon should usually have at least grade 4 strength; transfer of a tendon that is not phasic will result in a slight loss of power.[26] Tendon transfer not only augments lost function but also removes the force that contributes to the deformity. This is best illustrated in a transfer of the posterior tibial tendon, which is frequently the major deforming force in the cavovarus foot. Because the posterior tibial tendon has a broad insertion,

inserting on not only the navicular but also more distal secondary attachments, it is important that the tendon is transferred regardless of its exact strength; failure to do so will lead to a recurrence and progression of the deformity because of its insertion distal to the site of arthrodesis. Recurrence and progression of the deformity is common in the treatment of the cavovarus foot because surgeons often mistakenly perceive that a weak posterior tibial tendon will not function as an effective transfer. Although the weak tendon may have only minimal strength, it will still cause recurrent deformity and gradually result in adductovarus of the midfoot.

Transfer of the posterior tibial tendon not only removes the deforming force but also strengthens the already weak eversion. The exact location of the site for insertion of the posterior tibial tendon depends on the extent of the deformity and the strength of the remaining muscles. For example, in a foot with weak dorsiflexion strength, the posterior tibial tendon can be transferred to the lateral cuneiform to maximize dorsiflexion and to minimize inversion or eversion deformity.[27] The cavovarus foot, however, commonly has weak eversion strength as a result of the weak peroneus brevis; therefore, the authors of this chapter recommend a more lateral transfer of the posterior tibial tendon to the cuboid to improve not only dorsiflexion strength but also eversion strength.

The technique used to transfer the posterior tibial tendon is equally important as the location of the insertion site. Transfer of the posterior tibial tendon through the interosseous membrane is more phasic and may maintain a greater amount of strength than a nonphasic transfer. First described by Watkins

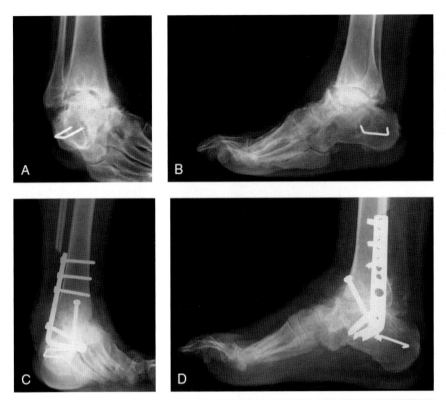

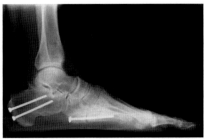

Figure 7   Lateral weight-bearing radiograph of the foot taken after intramedullary screw fixation of a fifth metatarsal base fracture and calcaneal osteotomy to correct varus alignment of the hindfoot. Although screw fixation may be somewhat inadequate, failure likely occurred as a result of persistent lateral column overload, which is evident in the increased plantigrade measurement ratio between the medial cuneiform to floor length and the fourth metatarsal base to floor length.

Figure 6   Preoperative AP (**A**) and lateral (**B**) radiographs of the foot demonstrate varus alignment of the ankle, a recurrent cavovarus foot after triple arthrodesis without transfer of the posterior tibial tendon, and the development of ankle arthritis as well as a hypertrophic reaction at the fifth metatarsal base as a result of persistent lateral column overload. Postoperative AP (**C**) and lateral (**D**) radiographs of the foot demonstrate improvement in the varus alignment of the ankle, the cavovarus foot, and the plantigrade measurement ratio.

et al,[28] this technique was modified by Hsu and Hoffer[29] to a four-incision technique that allows for effective transfer through less invasive incisions. Biomechanically, the interosseous transfer has been shown to provide a greater degree of dorsiflexion compared with subcutaneous transfer; however, this has not been substantiated clinically.[27] The Bridle procedure modifies the transfer of the posterior tibial tendon through the interosseous membrane to the dorsum of the foot by adding a dual anastomosis of the tibialis anterior muscle and the peroneus longus muscle.[30,31] The authors of this chapter often find that an anastomosis is not necessary to achieve muscle balance and, therefore, prefer interosseous transfer without anastomosis.

The peroneus longus should be transferred to the peroneus brevis via a direct tenodesis between the peroneus longus and brevis. This not only decreases the plantar flexion on the first ray but also further augments the weak eversion. The peroneus longus typically is sutured to the peroneus brevis in a side-to-side manner; however, if the peroneus brevis is torn substantially, the peroneus longus can be transferred directly to the fifth metatarsal base. If both the peroneus brevis and longus are torn and the surgeon is not able to transfer the posterior tibial tendon into the cuboid to compensate for lateral weakness, then either a transfer of the flexor digitorum longus or a transfer of the flexor hallucis longus to the fifth metatarsal base should be performed.

A failure to recognize subtle changes in the forefoot is another reason that treatment of the cavovarus foot may not succeed. These subtle changes of the forefoot typically consist of clawing of the hallux as well as the lesser toes and occur if the intrinsic muscles are weak and overpowered by the extrinsic muscles.[32] To correct clawing of the hallux, a modified Jones procedure, in which the extensor hallucis brevis is transferred to the neck of the first metatarsal and the hallux interphalangeal joint is fused, is recommended.[33-36] Although less commonly performed, transfer of the flexor hallucis longus to the dorsal aspect of the base of the proximal phalanx is an effective technique to correct clawing of the hallux.[37,38] Similar

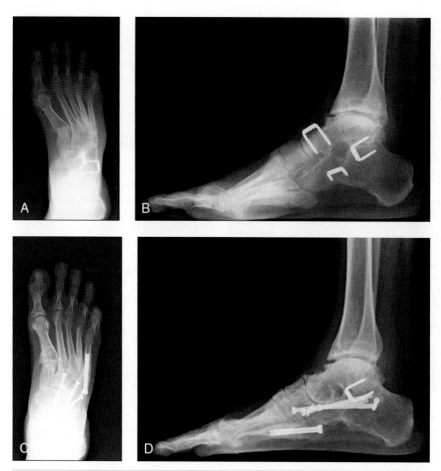

Figure 8 Preoperative AP (**A**) and lateral (**B**) weight-bearing radiographs taken after a failed triple arthrodesis demonstrate a persistent cavovarus foot. Undercorrection is evident with an increase in the calcaneal pitch, a decrease in the Meary angle as well as the talar declination angle, and metatarsal stacking with a fifth metatarsal base fracture as a result of persistent lateral column overload. Postoperative AP (**C**) and lateral (**D**) weight-bearing radiographs of the foot taken after revised triple arthrodesis demonstrate correction of the deformity with improvement in the calcaneal pitch, the talar declination angle, the Meary angle, forefoot rotation, and the plantigrade measurement ratio.

to the modified Jones procedure, the Hibbs procedure involves transferring the overpowering extensor digitorum longus more proximally to the dorsal aspect of the associated metatarsals.[39] For both the modified Jones procedure and the Hibbs procedure, the tendons can be transferred more proximally into the midfoot to the level of the cuneiforms if additional dorsiflexion strength is desired. Similar to hindfoot tendon transfers, the modified Jones procedure

and the Hibbs procedure not only remove the deforming force but also improve dorsiflexion strength.

Ancillary Procedures

The final step in the algorithmic approach for the treatment of the cavovarus foot involves recognizing the need for ancillary procedures. In most cavovarus feet, the plantar fascia is contracted and requires release; however, in some cavovarus feet, the plantar fascial

contracture may also require release of the abductor hallucis tendon and abductor fascia. The cavovarus foot is commonly associated with contracture of the gastrocnemius-soleus complex, which causes an equinus deformity. To completely appreciate the extent of an equinus contracture deformity, it is important for the surgeon to examine the patient in both the seated and standing positions as well as examine the patient's gait. The surgeon should also perform the Silfverskiöld test because it can differentiate between an isolated gastrocnemius contracture that requires gastrocnemius recession and a more global contracture of the gastrocnemius-soleus complex that requires Achilles tendon lengthening.

Regardless whether a cavovarus foot is flexible or rigid, it is important for the surgeon to evaluate the stability of the lateral ligamentous complex; a failure to address instability may compromise correction of the deformity. Generally, correction of the deformity as previously discussed will alleviate stress on the ankle; however, if the instability of the lateral ligamentous complex is substantial, the authors of this chapter perform ligament reconstruction using a modified Chrisman-Snook procedure.[40]

A cavovarus foot always has an increased load along the lateral column. It is important for the surgeon to evaluate the extent of loading because additional procedures may be required to resolve excessive loading, particularly to the fifth metatarsal base. Because the fifth metatarsal rotates under the cuboid in severe deformities, the prominence of the base of the fifth metatarsal will remain despite good correction of the cavovarus foot through the transverse tarsal joint. To avoid excessive pressure and pain, the authors of this chapter recommend resection of the fifth metatarsal base.[21] Because the peroneus brevis does not function in severe deformities, removal of the base of the fifth metatarsal will not compromise the outcome of the procedure. If necessary and as previously discussed, it is still possible to transfer the peroneus longus to the remaining fascia around the base of the fifth metatarsal.

Case Studies

Case 1: Double-Apex Deformity

An example of a double-apex deformity in the sagittal plane is shown in **Figure 5, A** and **B**. The patient had both a posterior and an anterior apex, both of which needed to be addressed to achieve a plantigrade foot. Reconstruction involved a triple arthrodesis to address the posterior apex and a first tarsometatarsal arthrodesis to address the anterior apex (**Figure 5, C** and **D**). Additional procedures included a tibialis anterior tendon transfer to correct the elevated medial column at the midfoot, Achilles tendon lengthening, and a modified Jones procedure.

Case 2: Failure of Triple Arthrodesis Performed Without Tendon Transfer

The patient had progression of a cavovarus foot after undergoing a triple arthrodesis performed by an outside physician. Because the original procedure was performed without appropriate tendon transfers, recurrence of the cavovarus foot and varus alignment of the ankle developed in the patient because of the persistent deforming force from the posterior tibial tendon (**Figure 6, A** and **B**). Treatment for this recurrent, progressive deformity required tibiotalocalcaneal arthrodesis

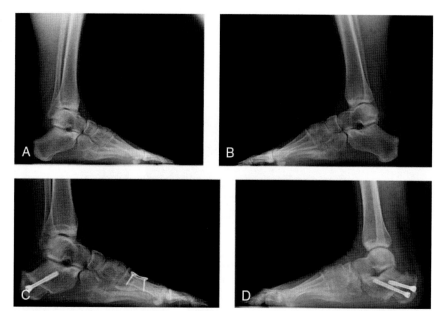

Figure 9 Preoperative lateral weight-bearing radiographs of the left (**A**) and right (**B**) feet demonstrate cavovarus deformities with increased calcaneal pitch, decreased talar declination angles, decreased Meary angles, and varus alignment of the hindfeet, which is evident in the increased visualization of the sinus tarsi and poor visualization of the tibiotalar joint. Postoperative lateral weight-bearing radiographs of the left (**C**) and right (**D**) feet demonstrate improvement in the cavovarus deformities; however, there is a slight undercorrection in the left foot compared with the right foot plus a slight residual increase in the calcaneal pitch and visualization of the sinus tarsi, which suggest varus alignment. There also is an increased plantigrade measurement ratio in the left foot compared with the right foot.

with a concomitant posterior tibial tendon transfer and a fifth metatarsal base resection (**Figure 6, C** and **D**).

Case 3: Persistent Lateral Column Overload

An outside physician treated a patient with intramedullary screw fixation for a fifth metatarsal base fracture and with a lateral calcaneal sliding osteotomy for varus alignment of the hindfoot. Although the patient initially came to the senior author (M.S.M) of this chapter for evaluation of a persistent fifth metatarsal base fracture, she was noted to have hardware failure and persistent lateral column overload as a result of undercorrection of the varus alignment (**Figure 7**).

Case 4: Failed Triple Arthrodesis as a Result of Undercorrection

The patient whose radiographs are shown in **Figure 8, A** and **B** had a persistent cavovarus foot after undergoing a triple arthrodesis performed by an outside physician. In this patient, the cavovarus foot persisted because of undercorrection of the deformity, causing persistent lateral column overload and a subsequent fifth metatarsal base fracture. The treatment required a revised triple arthrodesis with derotation to correct the malalignment, appropriate tendon transfers, and intramedullary screw fixation of the fifth metatarsal base fracture (**Figure 8, C** and **D**).

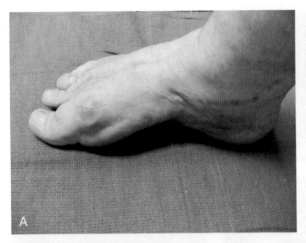

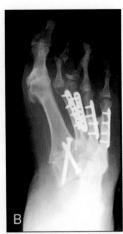

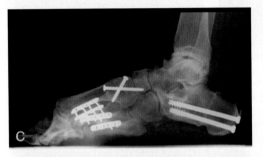

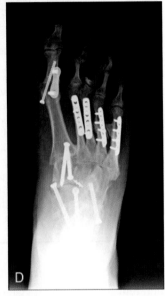

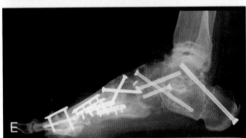

Figure 10   **A,** Clinical photograph shows a cavovarus foot with plantar flexion of the first ray and subsequent elevation of the medial column at the midfoot. Preoperative AP (**B**) and lateral (**C**) radiographs of the foot demonstrate an anterior-apex deformity with flexion at the hallux metatarsophalangeal joint and subsequent elevation of the medial column at the midfoot. Postoperative AP weight-bearing (**D**) and lateral (**E**) radiographs demonstrate a plantigrade foot. There is improvement in the midfoot deformity as well as the flexion deformity of the hallux metatarsophalangeal joint. (Panels B through E reproduced with permission from Zide JR, Myerson MS: Arthrodesis for the cavus foot: When, where, and how? *Foot Ankle Clin* 2013;18[4]:755-767.)

Case 5: Derotational Midfoot Osteotomy After Correction of Varus Alignment of the Hindfoot

The patient underwent a left cavovarus foot reconstruction that consisted of a calcaneal osteotomy, a first metatarsal osteotomy, plantar fascia release, and a peroneus longus to brevis transfer. At a later date, the patient underwent a right cavovarus foot reconstruction that consisted of a calcaneal osteotomy, a midfoot derotational osteotomy, and plantar fascia release. Although the preoperative radiographs (**Figure 9, A** and **B**) demonstrated a similar severity of varus alignment in both feet, the postoperative radiographs (**Figure 9, C** and **D**) demonstrate better correction in the right foot, which is likely a result of the midfoot derotational osteotomy.

Case 6: Inadequate Reconstruction Requiring Triple Arthrodesis

The senior author (M.S.M) of this chapter examined a patient who had undergone a calcaneal osteotomy, a first tarsometatarsal arthrodesis, and osteotomies of the second through fifth metatarsal shafts to correct a cavovarus foot. It was unclear if there was malreduction or malunion of the first tarsometatarsal arthrodesis; however, the procedure resulted in flexion of the hallux and subsequent elevation of the medial column in the midfoot and contracture of the tibialis anterior tendon (**Figure 10, A** through **C**). The treatment required a triple arthrodesis, a lateral transfer of the tibialis anterior, revision of the first tarsometatarsal malunion, and a hallux metatarsophalangeal joint arthrodesis (**Figure 10, D** and **E**).

Case 7: Single-Apex Deformity Requiring Calcaneal and Midfoot Osteotomies

The patient had a flexible, single-apex deformity at the transverse tarsal joint. The treatment required appropriate tendon transfers, plantar fascia release, and both a calcaneal osteotomy and a midfoot osteotomy to achieve a plantigrade foot (**Figure 11**).

Summary

It is important for surgeons to recognize that the cavovarus foot is a complex deformity that exists on a broad

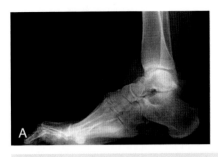
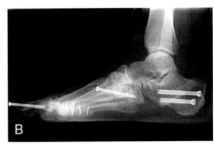

Figure 11 **A,** Preoperative lateral weight-bearing radiograph of the foot demonstrates a posterior-apex deformity at the transverse tarsal joint with an increased calcaneal pitch and decreased talar declination and Meary angles. **B,** Postoperative lateral weight-bearing radiograph of the foot demonstrates improvement in the deformity. The calcaneal pitch is decreased, and the talar declination angle is increased.

spectrum, may present in several ways, and results from a dynamic imbalance across the foot and ankle. Therefore, surgeons should have a stepwise treatment algorithm that allows for extensive and appropriate evaluation of the deformity to ensure adequate treatment and achievement of a stable, plantigrade foot. It is important for surgeons to determine if the deformity is flexible or rigid, the location of the apex (or apices) of the deformity in both the sagittal and coronal planes, the dynamic imbalances that require tendon transfers and soft-tissue balancing, and the presence of associated abnormalities that require ancillary procedures at the time of deformity correction. A failure to consider these principles of the treatment algorithm may result in a failure of deformity correction, recurrence and worsening of the cavovarus foot, and persistent symptomatology.

References

1. Raikin SM: Failure of triple arthrodesis. *Foot Ankle Clin* 2002;7(1):121-133.

2. Wetmore RS, Drennan JC: Long-term results of triple arthrodesis in Charcot-Marie-Tooth disease. *J Bone Joint Surg Am* 1989;71(3):417-422.

3. Wukich DK, Bowen JR: A long-term study of triple arthrodesis for correction of pes cavovarus in Charcot-Marie-Tooth disease. *J Pediatr Orthop* 1989;9(4):433-437.

4. Santavirta S, Turunen V, Ylinen P, Konttinen YT, Tallroth K: Foot and ankle fusions in Charcot-Marie-Tooth disease. *Arch Orthop Trauma Surg* 1993;112(4):175-179.

5. Coleman SS, Chesnut WJ: A simple test for hindfoot flexibility in the cavovarus foot. *Clin Orthop Relat Res* 1977;123:60-62.

6. Price BD, Price CT: A simple demonstration of hindfoot flexibility in the cavovarus foot. *J Pediatr Orthop* 1997;17(1):18-19.

7. Myerson MS: Cavus foot correction, in Myerson MS, ed: *Reconstructive Foot and Ankle Surgery: Management of Complications*, ed 2. Philadelphia, PA, Elsevier, 2010, pp 155-173.

8. Weseley MS, Barenfeld PA, Shea JM, Eisenstein AL: The congenital cavus foot: A follow-up report. *Bull Hosp Jt Dis Orthop Inst* 1982;42(2):217-229.

9. Saltzman CL, el-Khoury GY: The hindfoot alignment view. *Foot Ankle Int* 1995;16(9):572-576.

10. Dwyer FC: Osteotomy of the calcaneum for pes cavus. *J Bone Joint Surg Br* 1959;41(1):80-86.

11. Saxby T, Myerson MS: Calcaneus osteotomy, in Myerson MS, ed: *Current Therapy in Foot and Ankle Surgery*. St. Louis, MO, Mosby Year Book, 1993, pp 159-162.

12. Bruce BG, Bariteau JT, Evangelista PE, Arcuri D, Sandusky M, DiGiovanni CW: The effect of medial and lateral calcaneal osteotomies on the tarsal tunnel. *Foot Ankle Int* 2014;35(4):383-388.

13. Jahss MH: Tarsometatarsal truncated-wedge arthrodesis for pes cavus and equinovarus deformity of the fore part of the foot. *J Bone Joint Surg Am* 1980;62(5):713-722.

14. Zide JR, Myerson MS: Arthrodesis for the cavus foot: When, where, and how? *Foot Ankle Clin* 2013;18(4):755-767.

15. Wilcox PG, Weiner DS: The Akron midtarsal dome osteotomy in the treatment of rigid pes cavus: A preliminary review. *J Pediatr Orthop* 1985;5(3):333-338.

16. Cole WH: The treatment of claw-foot. *J Bone Joint Surg Am* 1940;22(4):895-908.

17. Japas LM: Surgical treatment of pes cavus by tarsal V-osteotomy: Preliminary report. *J Bone Joint Surg Am* 1968;50(5):927-944.

18. Hoke M: An operation for stabilizing paralytic feet. *Am J Orthop Surg* 1921;3:494-507.

19. Ryerson EW: Arthrodesing operations on the feet. *J Bone Joint Surg Am* 1923;5(3):453-471.

20. Siffert RS, Forster RI, Nachamie B: "Beak" triple arthrodesis for correction of severe cavus deformity. *Clin Orthop Relat Res* 1966;45:101-106.

21. Shariff R, Myerson MS, Palmanovich E: Resection of the fifth metatarsal base in the severe rigid cavovarus foot. *Foot Ankle Int* 2014;35(6):558-565.

22. Ward CM, Dolan LA, Bennett DL, Morcuende JA, Cooper RR: Long-term results of reconstruction for treatment of a flexible cavovarus foot in Charcot-Marie-Tooth disease. *J Bone Joint Surg Am* 2008;90(12):2631-2642.

23. Ryssman DB, Myerson MS: Tendon transfers for the adult flexible cavovarus foot. *Foot Ankle Clin* 2011;16(3):435-450.

24. Mann RA, Missirian J: Pathophysiology of Charcot-Marie-Tooth disease. *Clin Orthop Relat Res* 1988;234:221-228.

25. Alexander IJ, Johnson KA: Assessment and management of pes cavus in Charcot-Marie-tooth disease. *Clin Orthop Relat Res* 1989;246:273-281.

26. Jeng C, Myerson M: The uses of tendon transfers to correct paralytic deformity of the foot and ankle. *Foot Ankle Clin* 2004;9(2):319-337.

27. Goh JC, Lee PY, Lee EH, Bose K: Biomechanical study on tibialis posterior tendon transfers. *Clin Orthop Relat Res* 1995;319:297-302.

28. Watkins MB, Jones JB, Ryder CT Jr, Brown TH Jr: Transplantation of the posterior tibial tendon. *J Bone Joint Surg Am* 1954;36(6):1181-1189.

29. Hsu JD, Hoffer MM: Posterior tibial tendon transfer anteriorly through the interosseous membrane: A modification of the technique. *Clin Orthop Relat Res* 1978;131:202-204.

30. Rodriguez RP: The Bridle procedure in the treatment of paralysis of the foot. *Foot Ankle* 1992;13(2):63-69.

31. Richardson DR, Gause LN: The bridle procedure. *Foot Ankle Clin* 2011;16(3):419-433.

32. Olson SL, Ledoux WR, Ching RP, Sangeorzan BJ: Muscular imbalances resulting in a clawed hallux. *Foot Ankle Int* 2003;24(6):477-485.

33. Giannini S, Girolami M, Ceccarelli F, Maffei G: Modified Jones operation in the treatment of pes cavovarus. *Ital J Orthop Traumatol* 1985;11(2):165-170.

34. de Palma L, Colonna E, Travasi M: The modified Jones procedure for pes cavovarus with claw hallux. *J Foot Ankle Surg* 1997;36(4):279-283.

35. Jones R III: The Soldier's foot and the treatment of common deformities of the foot. *Br Med J* 1916;1(2891):749-753.

36. Breusch SJ, Wenz W, Döderlein L: Function after correction of a clawed great toe by a modified Robert Jones transfer. *J Bone Joint Surg Br* 2000;82(2):250-254.

37. Kadel NJ, Donaldson-Fletcher EA, Hansen ST, Sangeorzan BJ: Alternative to the modified jones procedure: Outcomes of the flexor hallucis longus (FHL) tendon transfer procedure for correction of clawed hallux. *Foot Ankle Int* 2005;26(12):1021-1026.

38. Steensma MR, Jabara M, Anderson JG, Bohay DR: Flexor hallucis longus tendon transfer for hallux claw toe deformity and vertical instability of the metatarsophalangeal joint. *Foot Ankle Int* 2006;27(9):689-692.

39. Hibbs RA: An operation for "claw foot." *JAMA* 1919;73(21):1583-1585.

40. Acevedo JI, Myerson MS: Modification of the Chrisman-Snook technique. *Foot Ankle Int* 2000;21(2):154-155.

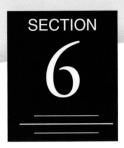

Pediatrics

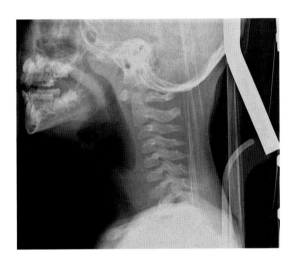

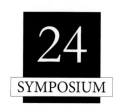

Avoiding Errors in the Management of Pediatric Polytrauma Patients

Kenneth Chin, MD

Joshua Abzug, MD

Donald S. Bae, MD

Bernard D. Horn, MD

Martin Herman, MD

Craig P. Eberson, MD

Abstract

Management of pediatric polytrauma patients is one of the most difficult challenges for orthopaedic surgeons. Multisystem injuries frequently include complex orthopaedic surgical problems that require intervention. The physiology and anatomy of children and adolescent trauma patients differ from the physiology and anatomy of an adult trauma patient, which alters the types of injuries sustained and the ideal methods for management. Errors of pediatric polytrauma care are included in two broad categories: missed injuries and inadequate fracture treatment. Diagnoses may be missed most frequently because of a surgeon's inability to reliably assess patients who have traumatic brain injuries and painful distracting injuries. Cervical spine injuries are particularly difficult to identify in a child with polytrauma and may have devastating consequences. In children who have multiple injuries, the stabilization of long bone fractures with pediatric fixation techniques, such as elastic nails and other implants, allows for easier care and more rapid mobilization compared with cast treatments. Adolescent polytrauma patients who are approaching skeletal maturity, however, are ideally treated as adults to avoid complications, such as loss of fixation, and to speed rehabilitation.

Instr Course Lect 2016;65:345–352.

An estimated 11 million emergency department visits each year are related to pediatric trauma. Most of these visits result from falls, motor vehicle collisions, bicycle accidents, pedestrian-related accidents, sports injuries, or violence. Many of these injuries are orthopaedic in nature: fractures, dislocations, and sprains. Ten percent of all pediatric trauma patients are considered polytrauma patients. Polytrauma patients are those who sustain a life- or limb-threatening injury, injury to more than one organ system, or multiple long bone fractures. The treatment of children with polytrauma may be complex and requires a multidisciplinary team that involves pediatric general surgery, pediatrics, and surgical subspecialty services. Orthopaedic injuries are the second leading cause of long-term morbidity in pediatric polytrauma patients (head trauma is the first).[1] It is imperative that orthopaedic surgeons who care for pediatric polytrauma patients are familiar with the care of orthopaedic injuries in the setting of multiorgan system involvement. In addition, because pediatric polytrauma patients often straddle the line between adolescence and adulthood, pediatric orthopaedic surgeons also should be familiar with some adult surgical techniques.

Effect of Injury on Growth in Children

Differences in the musculoskeletal anatomy between children and adults alter the assessment and treatment of pediatric polytrauma patients. A child's immature skeleton is distinct from an adult's mature skeleton and reacts differently to traumatic forces. Pediatric bone is less dense and more porous compared with adult bone, which means that plastic deformation may occur before complete fracture and that less energy is required to create a fracture. Compared with adult periosteum, pediatric periosteum is thicker, stronger, and more vascular, which limits the degree of fracture displacement and, secondarily, restricts the scope of soft-tissue injury. The increased vascularity also leads to more abundant callus formation and more rapid healing; however, the thick periosteum also may become interposed between fracture fragments, which sometimes makes reduction maneuvers more difficult.

Open physes also differentiate the pediatric skeleton from the adult skeleton. The physis is weaker than the surrounding epiphysis, metaphysis, and supporting ligaments at the distal and proximal ends of the long bones. This leads to fractures that involve the physis, which are eponymously known as Salter-Harris fractures.[2] Fractures that involve the physes have the potential to cause limb-length discrepancy and angular deformity secondary to growth disturbances.

Body proportions and size also differ in a comparison of adults and children. The size and weight of the head is proportionally larger in children than adults. Because a heavier head will hit the ground first, a pediatric cranium is more susceptible to injury.[3] The proportionally increased pediatric head size, in addition to weaker neck muscles, results in more frequent upper cervical fractures and ligamentous injuries. Young children are shorter in height and weigh less than adults, which affects injury patterns. This can be illustrated with an example of the injury pattern in pedestrians who are struck by a car. In adults, the bumper will typically strike the lower leg, which leads to a tibial fracture. The Waddell triad describes the injury pattern in young pedestrians.[4] The bumper will typically strike at the level of the pelvis or thigh, which leads to pelvic or femoral fractures. Next, the torso will strike the leading edge of the hood, which causes thoracoabdominal trauma. Last, the relatively light weight of the child may propel him or her into the air, which creates an opportunity for a third injury, usually if the head strikes the ground.

Pediatric physiology differs from adult physiology. Children have a lower circulating blood volume, so they cannot tolerate as much blood loss with an injury as can adults; however, compared with adults, children have more efficient sympathetic compensatory mechanisms, which can maintain blood pressure even in times of hypovolemia.[4] This means that children may decompensate rapidly, and signs of shock may appear quickly despite normal vital signs. Pediatric patients also have a higher body surface to weight ratio than adults, which makes them more vulnerable to hypothermia.

Primary Orthopaedic Assessment

Initial assessment and resuscitation efforts begin at the scene with first responders. Polytrauma patients are usually transported on a backboard to protect the spine and its neural elements. If pediatric polytrauma patients require immobilization, they should be placed on a pediatric backboard or a modified adult backboard. Because children have a proportionally larger head than adults, they need more space behind the head to achieve a neutral cervical spine position. This can be accomplished with the use of a pediatric backboard that has a recess for the head or an adult backboard that has a lifted pad for the torso. The placement of a child on a regular adult backboard may create a flexed posture of the cervical spine, which may worsen a potential cervical spine injury and possibly lead to neurologic damage (**Figure 1**). After appropriate stabilization, patients are taken to the closest pediatric trauma center. A thorough primary assessment is performed with a brief neurologic examination that prioritizes the airway, breathing, and circulation. After the initial trauma assessment is complete,

Dr. Abzug is a member of a speakers' bureau or has made paid presentations on behalf of Checkpoint Surgical, and serves as a paid consultant to AxoGen. Dr. Bae or an immediate family member has stock or stock options held in Cempra, Johnson & Johnson, Kythera Biopharmaceuticals, and Vivus; and serves as a board member, owner, officer, or committee member of the American Academy of Orthopaedic Surgeons, the American Society for Surgery of the Hand and the Pediatric Orthopaedic Society of North America. Dr. Horn or an immediate family member has stock or stock options held in Johnson & Johnson, and serves as a board member, owner, officer, or committee member of the American Academy of Orthopaedic Surgeons. Dr. Herman or an immediate family member serves as a board member, owner, officer, or committee member of the Pediatric Orthopaedic Society of North America. Dr. Eberson or an immediate family member has received royalties from Globus Medical; is a member of a speakers' bureau or has made paid presentations on behalf of Stryker Spine and Orthofix Spine; serves as a paid consultant to Orthofix; and serves as a board member, owner, officer, or committee member of the Scoliosis Research Society and the Pediatric Orthopaedic Society of North America. Neither Dr. Chin nor any immediate family member has received anything of value from or has stock or stock options held in a commercial company or institution related directly or indirectly to the subject of this chapter.

© 2016 AAOS Instructional Course Lectures, Volume 65

the orthopaedic surgeon may begin the orthopaedic portion of the secondary assessment. It is imperative that the orthopaedic assessment be performed in conjunction with the trauma team because vigilance for life-threatening injuries must be maintained.

Secondary Assessment and Imaging

A thorough secondary assessment should be performed after the primary assessment. The secondary assessment involves a complete history and physical examination and should include a careful orthopaedic and neurologic examination, which is critical if there is a suspected traumatic brain injury or spinal cord injury. The orthopaedic examination should be performed in a systematic stepwise fashion. The axial skeleton is examined first with the spine and pelvis. The cervical spine is manually stabilized, and the cervical collar is removed. The posterior elements of the spine are palpated for tenderness, step-offs, and deformity. After the cervical collar is carefully reapplied, the patient is logrolled laterally to allow access to the spine. The entire thoracic, lumbar, and sacral spine is inspected and palpated. At this time, the skin integrity is examined for abrasions, lacerations, contusions, and penetrating trauma. It is important for the orthopaedic surgeon to understand the difference between hypovolemic shock from blood loss and neurogenic shock from a spinal cord injury, the latter of which presents with bradycardia as opposed to tachycardia. Pediatric polytrauma patients may sustain a spinal cord injury without obvious bony injury (spinal cord injury without radiographic abnormality); it is important for orthopaedic surgeons to be cognizant of the possibility of an

unstable spine with an associated spinal cord injury in the examination of an obtunded patient who has hypotension. Failure to do so may result in further damage to the spinal cord.

The patient is again placed in the supine position, and attention is turned to the pelvis. An external rotation force is applied with posterior compression over the anterior superior iliac spine bilaterally to evaluate for anteroposterior compression injuries, after which an internal rotation force with medial compression of the iliac wings is applied to evaluate for a lateral compression type pelvic injury. If instability is noted on external rotation stress, or if there is unexplained hemodynamic instability, a pelvic binder or circumferential sheet should be applied at the level of the greater trochanters. An unstable pelvis may result in substantial continued blood loss and should be considered in any patient who has unexplained hypovolemic shock after major trauma.

A meticulous examination that includes inspection, palpation, and range of motion of the extremities is performed next. The upper extremities should be examined from the clavicles to the fingertips, and the lower extremities should be examined from the hips to the toes. Careful attention should be given to the soft tissues; abrasions, lacerations, crush injuries, degloving injuries, and compartment tightness are all potential injuries that must be identified. Gross deformities must be gently reduced and splinted before imaging studies are undertaken. Large wounds and open fractures are cleansed and covered with dressings. Any open fracture should be promptly treated with the administration of appropriate intravenous antibiotics and a tetanus booster. Early antibiotic administration

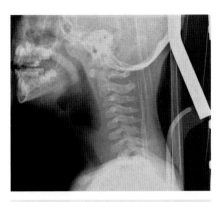

Figure 1 Lateral radiograph of the cervical spine of a 6-year-old child being transported on a standard backboard with the neck positioned in hyperflexion because of a large head-to-body ratio. Note the slight increase in the atlantodens interval with flexion of the cervical spine. A proper pediatric backboard allows the occiput to sit posterior to the shoulders by providing a cutout for the skull or by elevating the torso on pads.

may be the best defense against infection, particularly if formal débridement is not possible because of the patient's condition.[5] High-quality orthogonal radiographs are necessary to evaluate any area with soft-tissue injury, crepitus, deformity, or tenderness and to avoid a missed fracture.

Fracture Management
Damage Control

Damage-control orthopaedics was initially developed in adult orthopaedic trauma protocols. Damage-control concepts promote provisional stabilization of fractures and delayed definitive fixation until a patient's overall condition improves,[6] which allows pulmonary, neurologic, cardiac, and abdominal injuries to be treated first. It is believed that the early definitive fixation of fractures may be a major physiologic stress to patients and can cause a "second hit" that may be harmful to a critically ill patient. Delayed definitive treatment

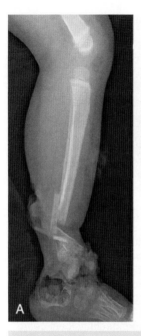
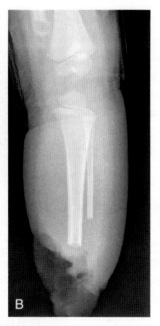
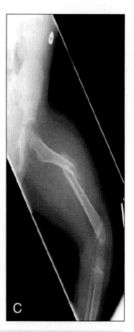

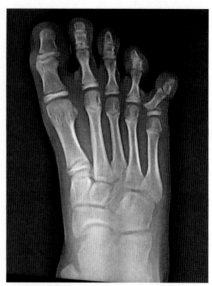

Figure 2 **A,** Lateral radiograph of the tibia of a 2-year-old girl whose leg was run over by a riding lawnmower demonstrates severe soft-tissue and neurovascular injury. **B,** AP radiograph demonstrates that a primary amputation was performed. The girl remained hospitalized for serial débridements before definitive wound closure. On postinjury day 20, her father noted a lump in her thigh. **C,** Lateral radiograph demonstrates a missed femur fracture, which explained the child's extreme need for pain medication.

Figure 3 AP radiograph of the foot of a 12-year-old boy who was a backseat passenger in a motor vehicle accident. He initially sustained a closed head injury and was unresponsive. The foot injury was noticed when he stood up for physical therapy and was unable to put his shoe on because of the deformed toe, which required open reduction to achieve realignment.

allows time for the recovery of visceral injuries, which potentially lowers the risk of acute respiratory distress syndrome and multiorgan failure. Although damage-control protocols have not been studied specifically in pediatric trauma patients, the principles are practiced in most trauma centers. Orthopaedic emergencies, such as compartment syndrome, vascular injuries, or open fractures, must be addressed as soon as possible. Common guidelines for the application of damage-control orthopaedics in the pediatric trauma patient include the triad of death (hypothermia, coagulopathy, acidosis), persistent hemodynamic instability, or a traumatic brain injury with intracranial pressures greater than 30 mm Hg. Orthopaedic surgeons must be comfortable with a variety of rapid

stabilization techniques, such as splinting;[7] emergency department-/intensive care unit-applied external fixators;[8] and various pelvic stabilization techniques, such as rapidly applied external fixators, pelvic C-clamps, and pelvic binders, that are more common in the adult population. There are two main categories of avoidable errors for pediatric polytrauma patients: missed injuries and the undertreatment of fractures.

Avoiding Missed Injury

The primary method to avoid a missed injury is a high degree of suspicion. Distracting injuries are common and may delay detection of otherwise obvious injuries (**Figure 2**). It is equally important to maintain vigilance during hospitalization. The tertiary or even secondary assessment may be sometimes applied

in a cursory manner because of more life-threatening injuries, which may lead to a substantial problem or complication from a missed injury after the primary and more serious issue stabilizes (**Figure 3**).

An additional method to avoid errors is to recognize the fracture patterns that are often seen in children. The previously mentioned Waddell triad alerts the orthopaedic surgeon to look for signs of abdominal injury in patients who have pelvic/upper femur fractures and head injuries. Likewise, patients who have lap belt injuries to the abdomen (pancreatic or small bowel injury) are at a high risk for flexion-distraction (Chance) injuries of the spine and should be examined carefully for this injury (**Figure 4**). In addition, an association exists between closed head injuries and cervical spine fractures. Holly et al[9] reported that approximately 5% of patients who had a moderate or severe head injury also had an associated cervical spine fracture. Of those patients, approximately 58% also sustained a spinal cord injury. The authors reported that a Glasgow Coma Scale score of 8 or less was a significant risk factor for spine injury. Because most children who have head injuries will undergo CT of the head, a CT scan of the cervical spine should be obtained at the same time to avoid missing a subtle bony injury that is not visible on plain radiographs. At some trauma centers, MRI is used to detect occult bone injury and soft-tissue disruption, which may not be visible on CT scans. MRI is particularly helpful in very young patients who have a minimally ossified cervical spine and in obtunded patients who cannot be assessed for painful cervical spine motion or palpation. Compared with CT, MRI requires a longer scan time. Trauma patients often undergo CT of the abdomen and pelvis; therefore, it is easy to add an MRI of the cervical spine. Both CT and MRI play a role in the detection of occult cervical spine injuries.

Definitive Fracture Stabilization

The optimal timing of definitive fracture stabilization has not been completely established. In a retrospective review of 78 pediatric polytrauma patients, Loder et al[10] compared patients who underwent definitive fixation within 3 days of injury with patients who had fixation delayed more than 3 days. The authors reported that patients who had definitive fixation within the first 3 days of injury spent decreased time on mechanical ventilation, had shorter

stays in the intensive care unit, and had shorter overall hospital stays compared with patients who had delayed fixation. Similarly, Letts et al[11] reported fewer complications in patients who underwent earlier treatment compared with patients who had delayed treatment. The path to the operating room is a multidisciplinary decision that is made among the trauma team, anesthesiologist, and orthopaedic surgeon. The surgeon needs to clearly communicate the length of the surgery, estimated blood loss, and patient positioning with the rest of the team because these factors can affect the patient's status and recovery. It is important for orthopaedic surgeons to understand that many children who have a severe head injury will achieve complete or near-complete recovery; it is critical to treat bone injuries in this light to avoid long-term sequelae from fracture healing complications.

Undertreatment of Fractures

Many victims of high-energy injuries are adolescents. Although the age cutoff for care in adult versus pediatric trauma centers is institution dependent, many older adolescents will be treated in a children's hospital setting. It is imperative for the treating orthopaedic surgeon, if he or she is a pediatric orthopaedic surgeon, to view these adolescent patients through the lens of an adult traumatologist. Older adolescents require rigid fixation in the trauma setting to allow for early mobilization (**Figure 5**).

Elastic nail fixation, also known as elastic intramedullary nailing, is a popular and successful method for the management of pediatric long bone fractures; however, the technique may be fraught with complications in older adolescents. Elastic intramedullary

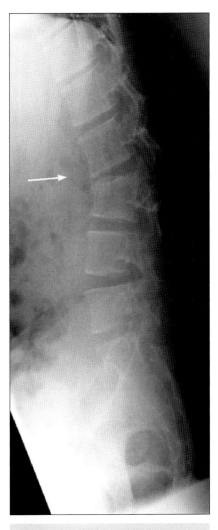

Figure 4 Lateral radiograph of the lumbar spine of a 17-year-old boy who was admitted for a small bowel injury, which required resection, and an open thumb fracture, which was treated with irrigation and débridement. Persistent back pain and foot drop that were noted 2 weeks after injury prompted radiographic assessment and subsequent transfer to a pediatric trauma center, where the patient underwent an uneventful posterior fusion from L2 to L3. He subsequently recovered full neurologic function. The arrow is pointing to focal kyphosis secondary to ligamentous disruption.

nailing is contraindicated for patients who weigh more than 100 lb and may not be appropriate for patients who

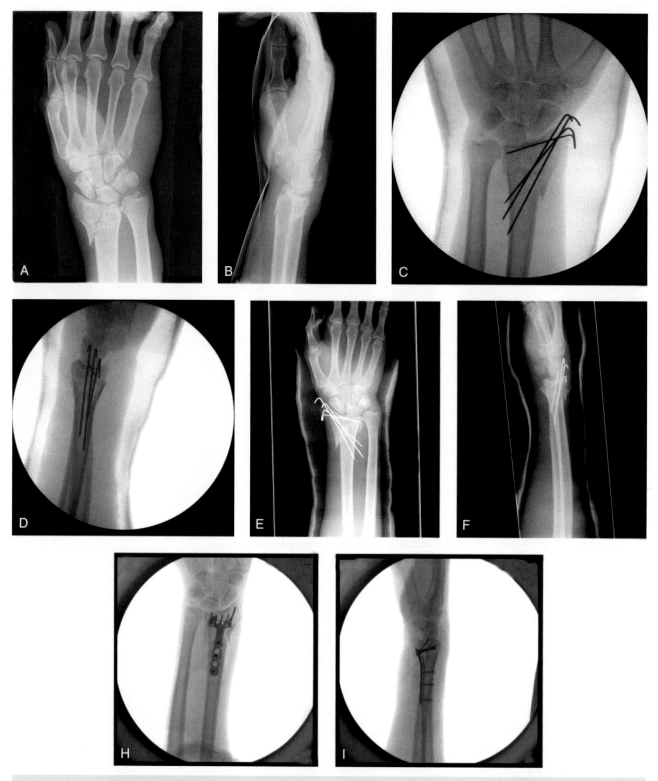

Figure 5 Images of the hand and wrist of a 16-year-old boy who was an unrestrained passenger in a high-speed motor vehicle accident. In addition to pulmonary contusions, the patient sustained bilateral upper extremity injuries. The left wrist sustained a nondisplaced scaphoid fracture. AP (**A**) and lateral (**B**) radiographs demonstrate that the right wrist sustained a comminuted injury. AP (**C**) and lateral (**D**) fluoroscopic images show that the initial treating physician performed closed reduction and percutaneous Kirschner wire fixation. AP (**E**) and lateral (**F**) radiographs obtained at the 7-day follow-up visit demonstrate loss of reduction. AP (**G**) and lateral (**H**) fluoroscopic images show subsequent definitive fixation with standard volar plate fixation.

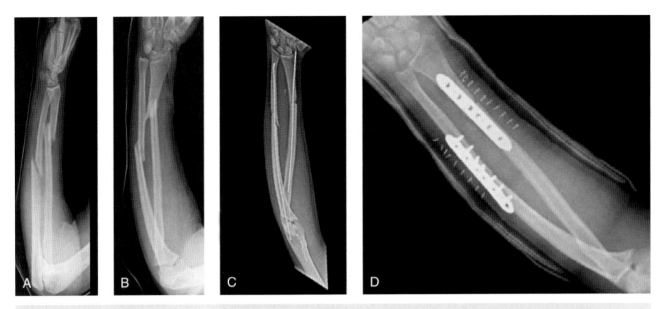

Figure 6   Lateral (**A**) and AP (**B**) radiographs of the arm of a 16-year-old boy who fell from a platform demonstrate a high-energy open forearm fracture of both bones. **C,** AP radiograph taken 2 months after injury demonstrates minimal healing, and it was noted that the patient was beginning to suffer the effects of prolonged immobilization. **D,** AP radiograph demonstrates that compression plating (after intraoperative cultures were negative for infection) yielded rapid healing.

have comminuted fractures; however, recent literature appears to refute this.[12] Based on fracture patterns and patient size, trochanteric entry nails and submuscular plating may be better options for these patients.[13] The authors of this chapter prefer to use trochanteric entry nailing in patients who are nearing skeletal maturity and have an intramedullary canal large enough to accept available trochanteric entry nails (approximately 8 mm or larger). Submuscular plating is a reasonable option for fractures in the proximal subtrochanteric region, fractures within 5 cm of the distal femoral physis, or smaller patients in whom nailing would be difficult; submuscular plating can be used for any patients, regardless of skeletal maturity. Elastic intramedullary nailing also is a successful method for the management of forearm fractures; however, plating may permit earlier mobilization and more reliable healing in older patients

who have additional injuries (**Figure 6**). The authors of this chapter prefer to perform elastic nailing in patients who are more than 2 years from skeletal maturity. The relative indications for plating include comminuted fractures, adolescent patients who are large in size, and patients in whom nails do not permit restoration of a radial bow that is sufficient for normal forearm rotation. Although the choice is clear for very young and very old patients, there is a large middle ground of patients who may be treated in either manner. The final decision should be made by the treating surgeon based on his or her experience and expertise.

Summary

Despite improved injury prevention efforts and an increased focus on child safety, pediatric polytrauma patients continue to present to trauma centers around the world. Specialized pediatric

trauma centers have multidisciplinary teams that are optimized to treat pediatric polytrauma patients who require thorough evaluation and treatment. Several studies have reported that pediatric trauma centers have better outcomes compared with trauma centers that do not have a dedicated team of pediatric specialists.[14-16] By following protocols in the primary and secondary assessment of pediatric polytrauma patients, surgeons can optimize survival rates. Orthopaedic surgeons play a major role on the trauma team. By maintaining attention to detail and recognizing common injury patterns and associations, missed injuries can largely be avoided. The selection of appropriate fixation may help ensure a rapid functional recovery and avoid prolonged disability.

References

1. Marcus RE, Mills MF, Thompson GH: Multiple injury in children. *J Bone Joint Surg Am* 1983;65(9):1290-1294.

2. Salter RB, Harris WR: Injuries involving the epiphyseal plate. *J Bone Joint Surg Am* 1963;45(3):587-622.

3. Wilber JH, Thompson GH, Son-Hing J: The multiply injured child, in Green NE, Swiontowski MF, eds: *Skeletal Trauma in Children,* ed 4. Philadelphia, PA, Saunders Elsevier, 2009, pp 57-83.

4. Waddell JP, Drucker WR: Occult injuries in pedestrian accidents. *J Trauma* 1971;11(10):844-852.

5. Lack WD, Karunakar MA, Angerame MR, et al: Type III open tibia fractures: Immediate antibiotic prophylaxis minimizes infection. *J Orthop Trauma* 2015;29(1):1-6.

6. Pape HC, Giannoudis P, Krettek C: The timing of fracture treatment in polytrauma patients: Relevance of damage control orthopedic surgery. *Am J Surg* 2002;183(6):622-629.

7. Ritterman SA, Daniels AH, Kane PM, Eberson CP, Born CT: J-splint use for temporizing management of pediatric femur fractures: A review of 18 cases. *Pediatr Emerg Care* 2014;30(8):516-520.

8. Lareau CR, Daniels AH, Vopat BG, Kane PM: Emergency department external fixation for provisional treatment of pilon and unstable ankle fractures. *J Emerg Trauma Shock* 2015;8(1):61-64.

9. Holly LT, Kelly DF, Counelis GJ, Blinman T, McArthur DL, Cryer HG: Cervical spine trauma associated with moderate and severe head injury: Incidence, risk factors, and injury characteristics. *J Neurosurg* 2002; 96(3, suppl):285-291.

10. Loder RT: Pediatric polytrauma: Orthopaedic care and hospital course. *J Orthop Trauma* 1987;1(1):48-54.

11. Letts M, Davidson D, Lapner P: Multiple trauma in children: Predicting outcome and long-term results. *Can J Surg* 2002;45(2):126-131.

12. Goodbody CM, Lee RJ, Flynn JM, Sankar WN: Titanium elastic nailing for pediatric tibia fractures: Do older, heavier kids do worse? *J Pediatr Orthop* 2015. ePub ahead of print.

13. Ramseier LE, Janicki JA, Weir S, Narayanan UG: Femoral fractures in adolescents: A comparison of four methods of fixation. *J Bone Joint Surg Am* 2010;92(5):1122-1129.

14. Hall JR, Reyes HM, Meller JL, Loeff DS, Dembek R: The outcome for children with blunt trauma is best at a pediatric trauma center. *J Pediatr Surg* 1996;31(1):72-77.

15. Nakayama DK, Copes WS, Sacco W: Differences in trauma care among pediatric and nonpediatric trauma centers. *J Pediatr Surg* 1992;27(4):427-431.

16. Potoka DA, Schall LC, Gardner MJ, Stafford PW, Peitzman AB, Ford HR: Impact of pediatric trauma centers on mortality in a statewide system. *J Trauma* 2000;49(2):237-245.

Current Strategies for the Management of Pediatric Supracondylar Humerus Fractures: Tips and Techniques for Successful Closed Treatment

Brian Brighton, MD, MPH
Joshua Abzug, MD
Christine Ann Ho, MD
Todd F. Ritzman, MD

Abstract

Pediatric supracondylar humerus fractures are the most commonly encountered type of elbow fractures in children that require surgical fixation. Many pediatric supracondylar humerus fractures can be treated with closed reduction and percutaneous skeletal fixation. In difficult fractures, adjunct pin techniques, such as joystick wires and leverage pins, can be used to help attain a satisfactory and stable reduction before an open approach is used. After the fracture is reduced, optimal pinning, with the use of either crossed or lateral-entry techniques, and fixation that achieves maximal spread at the fracture site as well as bicortical engagement in both fragments are essential to maintain reduction and avoid complications that are associated with malunion. A practical approach as well as several tips and techniques may help surgeons attain and maintain stable closed reduction of pediatric supracondylar humerus fractures.

Instr Course Lect 2016;65:353–360.

Most displaced supracondylar humerus fractures in children can be managed with closed reduction and percutaneous pinning. Clinical practice guidelines for the management of pediatric supracondylar humerus fractures exist, but they do not provide insight into the subtleties of achieving and maintaining successful closed treatment.[1,2] Closed treatment, which uses skin or skeletal traction followed by casting, remains largely historical. Open treatment is indicated for patients who have open fractures, irreducible fractures, or fractures that require exploration or repair of compromised neurovascular structures. Most displaced extension-type and flexion-type supracondylar humerus fractures can be managed with closed reduction and percutaneous pinning; however, there are numerous clinical and biomechanical studies that debate the optimal pinning technique and pin construct. Fracture characteristics, associated injuries, and patient factors are unique to each patient and affect the decisions the treating surgeon makes. The surgical fixation plan to attain

Dr. Brighton or an immediate family member serves as a paid consultant to DePuy, and serves as a board member, owner, officer, or committee member of the Pediatric Orthopaedic Society of North America and the American College of Surgeons. Dr. Abzug or an immediate family member is a member of a speakers' bureau or has made paid presentations on behalf of Checkpoint Surgical, and serves as a paid consultant to AxoGen. Dr. Ho or an immediate family member serves as a board member, owner, officer, or committee member of the Pediatric Orthopaedic Society of North America. Dr. Ritzman or an immediate family member serves as an unpaid consultant to Apto Orthopaedics and the Austin BioInnovation Institute of Akron, and has stock or stock options held in Apto Orthopaedics.

anatomic reduction and stable fixation is equally important as the execution of that plan.

Fracture Reduction

The first step in the management of pediatric supracondylar humerus fractures is attaining an anatomic or near-anatomic reduction with minimal to no rotation. Traditionally, reduction of extension-type fractures begins with the application of initial longitudinal traction through the arm with correction of medial or lateral translation and any varus or valgus coronal malalignment. In patients who have severely displaced fractures with associated ecchymosis in the cubital fossa and skin tenting or puckering, a milking maneuver that was described by Archibeck et al[3] can be performed to reduce the proximal fracture through the interposed brachialis and soft tissue. Next, the surgeon should flex the patient's elbow while applying direct pressure with his or her thumb over the tip of the olecranon process using an anteriorly directed force. Care must be taken to avoid overzealous reduction and conversion to an unstable fracture, which will disrupt the intact posterior hinge. The amount of elbow flexion attained in this step of the reduction may provide the surgeon with a sense of the adequacy of the reduction or the amount of anterior soft-tissue swelling; inadequate anterior translation of the fragment or severe swelling may prevent elbow flexion. Depending on the initial displacement of the fracture, the fracture pattern, and the integrity of the periosteal hinge in the zone of injury, pronation or supination of the forearm after the elbow is flexed may provide additional stability to the reduction.

After a satisfactory reduction is attained, an image intensifier is used to confirm adequate reduction. The reduction is assessed on a Jones radiograph, which is an AP radiograph of the elbow taken through the overlying flexed forearm. A lateral radiograph is obtained by externally rotating the patient's entire arm through the glenohumeral joint while the forearm and elbow are held stationary. Medial and lateral oblique radiographs may help the surgeon judge the adequacy of the reduction of the medial and lateral columns.[4] For flexion-type fractures or rotationally unstable type IV fractures that were described by Leitch et al,[5] reduction of the elbow may be best attained in approximately 90° of flexion and assessed by viewing the fracture on a lateral elbow radiograph taken with an image intensifier.

Generally accepted parameters for adequate closed reduction include no varus or valgus angulation, minimal to no rotation, restoration of the anterior humeral line as viewed on a lateral radiograph, and a few millimeters of mediolateral or anteroposterior translation. In addition, there should be no gap at the fracture site because it may represent an entrapped neurovascular structure or soft-tissue tethering of the adjacent neurovascular structures. Radiographic parameters, such as the Baumann angle, the anterior humeral line, and the lateral shaft-condylar angle, can be used intraoperatively to determine the quality of the initial reduction.[6]

Closed Reduction With Pin-Assisted Techniques

If acceptable closed reduction cannot be attained with the method previously discussed, there are several other techniques that can be performed before

proceeding to open reduction. Several authors have described a joystick technique to gain control of the distal and/or proximal fragments and obtain an acceptable reduction. Novais et al[7] used a laterally placed 2.0-mm pin as a joystick to manipulate the distal fragment and attain successful closed reduction of multidirectionally unstable supracondylar humerus fractures. Basaran et al[8] reported successful outcomes and shorter surgical durations for supracondylar humerus fractures that were managed with a similar joystick technique that involved the lateral placement of a pin in the distal fragment. Parmaksizoglu et al[9] placed a temporary 2.0- to 3.0-mm Kirschner wire (K-wire) lateral to medial below the deltoid in the proximal humerus to obtain control of the proximal fragment, which allowed for easier fracture alignment and lateral pin fixation of supracondylar humerus fractures. Herzog et al[10] used a 2.5-mm Schanz pin that was placed posteriorly in the distal humeral metaphysis to aid in reduction of supracondylar humerus fractures before they were stabilized with K-wires (**Figure 1**).

Pin leverage techniques also have been described to gain control of the distal and/or proximal fragments and obtain an acceptable reduction. Similar to the Kapandji technique of intrafocal pinning for distal radius fractures, pin leverage techniques have been reported to help obtain closed reduction and stabilize pediatric supracondylar humerus fractures.[11-15] A pin is inserted at a posterior starting point cephalad to the distal fracture fragment, advanced into the fracture, and used as a lever to aid in reduction (**Figure 2**). After the fracture is stabilized with lateral-entry pins, the leverage pin may be removed

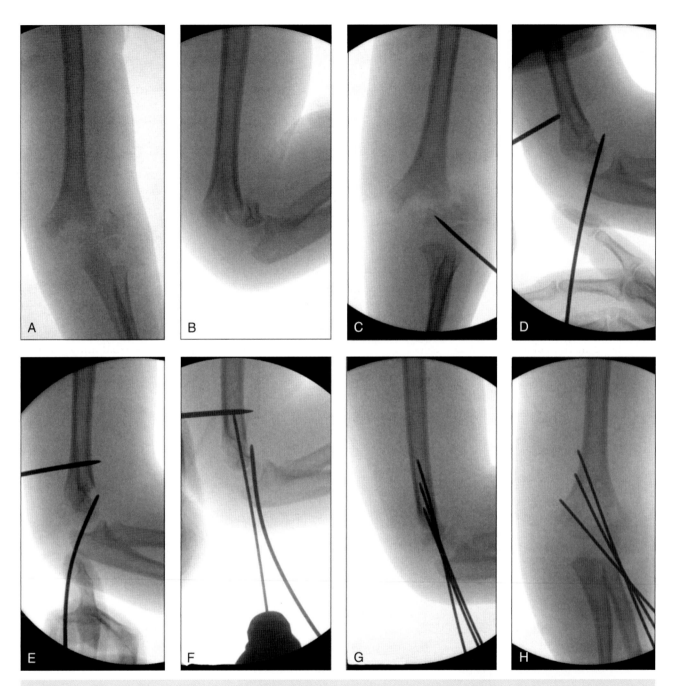

Figure 1   Fluoroscopic images of the left humerus of a 4-year-old girl who had an unstable type IV supracondylar fracture. Treatment consisted of closed reduction and pinning with the use of joystick wires. **A,** AP view demonstrates lateral displacement of the distal fragment. **B,** Lateral view demonstrates a flexion deformity despite an initial reduction attempt. **C,** A 2.0-mm Kirschner wire (K-wire) is placed laterally in the capitellum to control the distal fragment. **D** and **E,** A 2.4-mm K-wire is placed posteriorly in the proximal fragment to help control anterior translation, posterior translation, and rotation of the humeral shaft as well as to correct varus and valgus coronal malalignment. **F,** With the C-arm in a swing through the lateral position, the 2.0-mm K-wire in the distal fragment can be used to correct the extension deformity of the fracture, and an initial fixation K-wire is placed. With the C-arm in the lateral (**G**) and AP (**H**) positions, lateral-entry fixation with three 0.062-inch K-wires is performed after reduction and removal of the joystick wires. (Courtesy of Brian Brighton, MD, MPH, Charlotte, NC.)

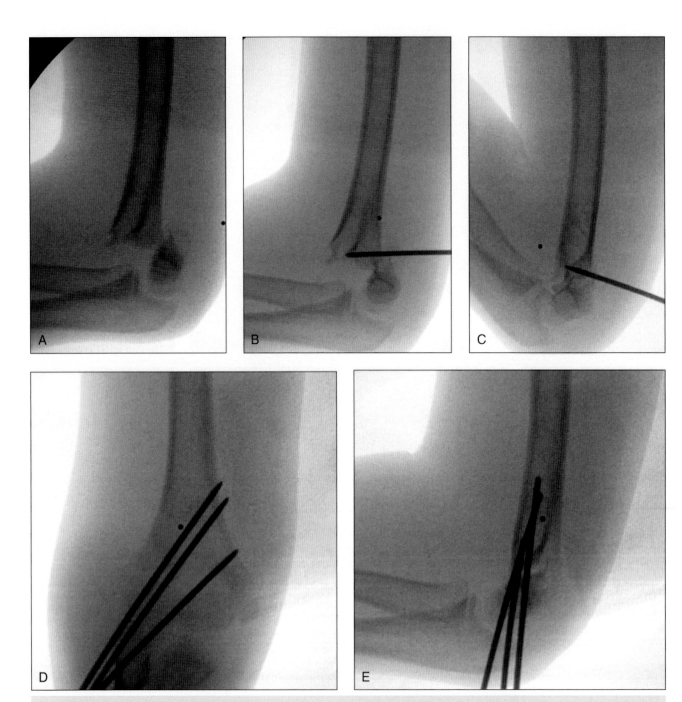

Figure 2   Fluoroscopic images of the right humerus of an 8-year-old girl who had a type III supracondylar fracture. Treatment was with a leverage pin. **A,** Lateral view demonstrates a displaced extension-type supracondylar humerus fracture. **B,** A 2.0-mm pin is placed within the fracture site. **C,** The pin is used as a lever to aid in reduction of the fracture. With the C-arm in the AP (**D**) and lateral (**E**) positions, lateral-entry fixation with three Kirschner wires is performed after reduction and removal of the leverage pin. (Courtesy of Brian Brighton, MD, MPH, Charlotte, NC.)

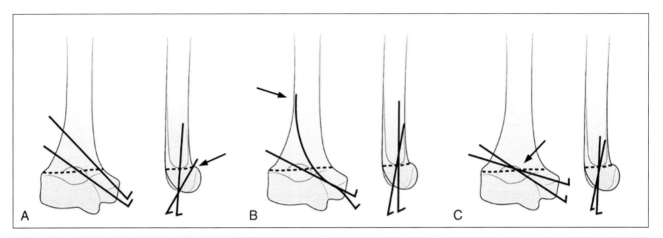

Figure 3   Illustrations demonstrate potential technical errors in closed reduction and percutaneous pinning of supracondylar humerus fractures in children. In each panel, the left image is an AP view and the right image is a lateral view. **A,** Failure to obtain bicortical fixation across the fracture secondary to the pin exiting anteriorly through the fracture site (arrow). **B,** Failure to obtain bicortical fixation across the fracture site secondary to intramedullary pin placement (arrow). **C,** The pins cross the fracture site with a spread of less than 2 mm (arrow). (Reproduced from Abzug JM, Herman MJ: Management of supracondylar humerus fractures in children: Current concepts. *J Am Acad Orthop Surg* 2012;20[2]: 69-77.)

or advanced across the fracture for additional fixation.

Pin Configuration and Placement

There is some controversy on whether crossed pinning or lateral-entry pinning is the ideal pin configuration for the fixation of supracondylar humerus fractures. Several randomized studies and systematic reviews of the literature reported no significant difference in maintenance of reduction or in malunion between the two pinning configurations.[16-19] Early biomechanical studies reported increased torsional strength with crossed-pinning constructs compared with lateral-entry pinning constructs. Divergent lateral pinning constructs had stability to resist extension, varus, and valgus forces that was similar to crossed-pinning constructs but avoided injury to the ulnar nerve.[20,21]

Regardless of the preferred pinning technique, surgeons who treat pediatric supracondylar humerus fractures must

be familiar with the principles for proper placement of both medial and lateral pins. Lateral-entry pins must be placed with the following technical points kept in mind: (1) maximize separation of the pins at the fracture site, (2) engage both the medial and lateral columns proximal to the fracture site, (3) engage adequate fixation in both the proximal and distal fragments, and (4) use a third pin from a lateral-entry starting point if adequate fracture stability is not achieved with two pins.[22] Fracture stability can be assessed intraoperatively by taking the elbow through an arc of motion and rotation under live fluoroscopy. Sankar et al[23] reported that failure to achieve more than 2 mm of pin separation at the fracture site, failure to engage both the proximal and distal fragments, and failure to achieve bicortical fixation were associated with postoperative loss of reduction in patients who were treated with lateral-entry pinning constructs (**Figures 3** and **4**). In a study of 192 patients who had supracondylar humerus fractures, Pennock et al[24] reported that

decreased pin separation at the fracture site was associated with loss of reduction. The authors recommended pin separation of at least 13 mm or one-third of the width of the humerus at the level of the fracture site to prevent loss of reduction.

To achieve adequate pin separation at the fracture site and engage as much bone as possible in the distal fragment with lateral-entry pinning, the surgeon must consider the starting point. In a biomechanical analysis of starting points for supracondylar humerus fractures, Gottschalk et al[25] reported that a capitellar starting point that was paraolecranon or in the capitellum anlage provided increased construct stiffness compared with a direct lateral starting point. Because this starting point may allow the pin to communicate with the joint, the pins should only remain in place for 3 to 4 weeks to lessen the chance of septic arthritis in the event of a pin-tract infection.

Additional construct stability can be attained with the use of larger pin

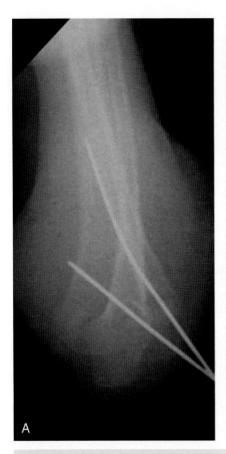

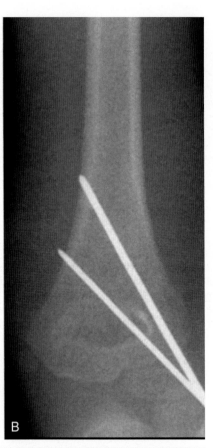

Figure 4 Fluoroscopic images demonstrate a solution for a technical error in the closed reduction and percutaneous pinning of a supracondylar humerus fracture in a child. **A,** Bicortical fixation was not initially achieved with lateral-entry pinning secondary to intramedullary pin placement. **B,** Bicortical fixation was achieved by upsizing the pin to avoid deflection off the medial cortex but maintaining the original lateral-entry starting point. (Courtesy of Brian Brighton, MD, MPH, Charlotte, NC.)

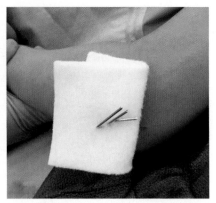

Figure 5 Intraoperative photograph shows postoperative management of lateral-entry Kirschner wires, which are cut and bent over sterile felt before cast application. (Courtesy of Brian Brighton, MD, MPH, Charlotte, NC.)

fixation. In a randomized controlled trial of patients who underwent either medial- and lateral-entry pinning or lateral-entry pinning for the treatment of supracondylar humerus fractures, Kocher et al[19] selected pin size based on patient weight. Patients who weighed 20 kg or less were treated with 1.6-mm pins, and patients who weighed more than 20 kg were treated with 2.0-mm pins. Srikumaran et al[26] reported that patients who had a pin size ratio (defined as the ratio of a pin's diameter to the humeral midshaft cortical thickness) of 1 or higher demonstrated improved maintenance of sagittal alignment on postoperative radiographs. In a stable fracture model, the use of two 2.0-mm pins provided better construct stiffness in internal and external rotation than three 1.6-mm pins.[25] In clinical practice, larger lateral-entry pins, if used in an older or larger child, tend to follow a truer path that resists deflection off the anterior or medial cortex during placement.

If medial pin placement is required, either for medial and lateral-crossed pinning or to add additional fixation in an unstable fracture after two or more lateral-entry pins have been placed, the surgeon must be familiar with the medial pinning technique. Some surgeons recommend that a small incision be made over the medial epicondyle with blunt dissection via the spread of a hemostat to find the medial starting point.[4] Other surgeons suggest that the elbow be extended approximately 60° after two lateral pins have been placed and that the ulnar nerve be palpated and displaced posteriorly before percutaneous pin placement.[27]

The Dorgan technique is a method of crossed pinning in which a high lateral pin is placed in an inferior and medial direction across the fracture site to avoid risk of injury to the ulnar nerve. A risk of injury to the radial nerve at the location at which the pin enters the lateral cortex proximal to the fracture site has been reported as a potential complication with this technique.[28-30]

Postoperative Management

Percutaneous pins are typically bent, cut, and left outside the skin (**Figure 5**). The arm is placed in a splint or a univalved or bivalved cast for immediate postoperative immobilization.

Care should be taken to avoid excessive dressings or cast padding on the antecubital fossa, which may compromise skin or perfusion to the forearm. With stable percutaneous pinning techniques, the elbow can be placed in less than 90° of flexion (range, 45° to 80°), depending on the amount of expected or immediate postoperative swelling. Sterile foam or felt may be placed around the pins to prevent motion at the pin site and skin interface under the postoperative cast or splint, thus, lessening the chance of pin-site irritation or pin loosening.[31] Pins are typically removed in the office 3 to 4 weeks after surgery.

Summary

Most pediatric supracondylar humerus fractures can be managed with closed reduction and percutaneous pinning. Unsatisfactory reduction, unnecessary open reduction, and loss of reduction as a result of inadequate fracture fixation may lead to potential loss of elbow range of motion or cubitus varus. Surgeons who follow the principles of ideal pin constructs and placement for the surgical treatment of pediatric supracondylar humerus fractures will be able to obtain a closed reduction, maintain alignment until healing, and achieve successful postoperative functional outcomes.

References

1. Howard A, Mulpuri K, Abel MF, et al: The treatment of pediatric supracondylar humerus fractures. *J Am Acad Orthop Surg* 2012;20(5):320-327.

2. Mulpuri K, Wilkins K: The treatment of displaced supracondylar humerus fractures: Evidence-based guideline. *J Pediatr Orthop* 2012;32(suppl 2): S143-S152.

3. Archibeck MJ, Scott SM, Peters CL: Brachialis muscle entrapment in displaced supracondylar humerus fractures: A technique of closed reduction and report of initial results. *J Pediatr Orthop* 1997;17(3):298-302.

4. Yen YM, Kocher MS: Lateral entry compared with medial and lateral entry pin fixation for completely displaced supracondylar humeral fractures in children: Surgical technique. *J Bone Joint Surg Am* 2008;90(suppl 2 pt 1):20-30.

5. Leitch KK, Kay RM, Femino JD, Tolo VT, Storer SK, Skaggs DL: Treatment of multidirectionally unstable supracondylar humeral fractures in children: A modified Gartland type-IV fracture. *J Bone Joint Surg Am* 2006;88(5):980-985.

6. Flynn JM, Skaggs DL, Waters PM, eds: *Rockwood and Wilkins' Fractures in Children*, ed 8. Philadelphia, PA, Wolters Kluwer Health, 2014.

7. Novais EN, Andrade MA, Gomes DC: The use of a joystick technique facilitates closed reduction and percutaneous fixation of multidirectionally unstable supracondylar humeral fractures in children. *J Pediatr Orthop* 2013;33(1):14-19.

8. Basaran SH, Ercin E, Bilgili MG, Bayrak A, Cumen H, Avkan MC: A new joystick technique for unsuccessful closed reduction of supracondylar humeral fractures: Minimum trauma. *Eur J Orthop Surg Traumatol* 2015;25(2):297-303.

9. Parmaksizoglu AS, Ozkaya U, Bilgili F, Sayin E, Kabukcuoglu Y: Closed reduction of the pediatric supracondylar humerus fractures: The "joystick" method. *Arch Orthop Trauma Surg* 2009;129(9):1225-1231.

10. Herzog MA, Oliver SM, Ringler JR, Jones CB, Sietsema DL: Mid-America Orthopaedic Association Physician in Training Award: Surgical technique. Pediatric supracondylar humerus fractures: A technique to aid closed reduction. *Clin Orthop Relat Res* 2013;471(5):1419-1426.

11. Sawaizumi T, Takayama A, Ito H: Surgical technique for supracondylar fracture of the humerus with percutaneous leverage pinning. *J Shoulder Elbow Surg* 2003;12(6):603-606.

12. Lee HY, Kim SJ: Treatment of displaced supracondylar fractures of the humerus in children by a pin leverage technique. *J Bone Joint Surg Br* 2007;89(5):646-650.

13. Fahmy MA, Hatata MZ, Al-Seesi H: Posterior intrafocal pinning for extension-type supracondylar fractures of the humerus in children. *J Bone Joint Surg Br* 2009;91(9):1232-1236.

14. Kao HK, Yang WE, Li WC, Chang CH: Treatment of Gartland type III pediatric supracondylar humerus fractures with the Kapandji technique in the prone position. *J Orthop Trauma* 2014;28(6):354-359.

15. Yu SW, Su JY, Kao FC, Ma CH, Yen CY, Tu YK: The use of the 3-mm K-Wire to supplement reduction of humeral supracondylar fractures in children. *J Trauma* 2004;57(5):1038-1042.

16. Tripuraneni KR, Bosch PP, Schwend RM, Yaste JJ: Prospective, surgeon-randomized evaluation of crossed pins versus lateral pins for unstable supracondylar humerus fractures in children. *J Pediatr Orthop B* 2009;18(2):93-98.

17. Gaston RG, Cates TB, Devito D, et al: Medial and lateral pin versus lateral-entry pin fixation for Type 3 supracondylar fractures in children: A prospective, surgeon-randomized study. *J Pediatr Orthop* 2010;30(8):799-806.

18. Brauer CA, Lee BM, Bae DS, Waters PM, Kocher MS: A systematic review of medial and lateral entry pinning versus lateral entry pinning for supracondylar fractures of the humerus. *J Pediatr Orthop* 2007;27(2):181-186.

19. Kocher MS, Kasser JR, Waters PM, et al: Lateral entry compared with medial and lateral entry pin fixation for completely displaced supracondylar humeral fractures in children: A randomized clinical trial. *J Bone Joint Surg Am* 2007;89(4):706-712.

20. Lee SS, Mahar AT, Miesen D, Newton PO: Displaced pediatric supracondylar humerus fractures: Biomechanical analysis of percutaneous pinning techniques. *J Pediatr Orthop* 2002;22(4):440-443.

21. Zionts LE, McKellop HA, Hathaway R: Torsional strength of pin

configurations used to fix supracondylar fractures of the humerus in children. *J Bone Joint Surg Am* 1994;76(2):253-256.

22. Skaggs DL, Cluck MW, Mostofi A, Flynn JM, Kay RM: Lateral-entry pin fixation in the management of supracondylar fractures in children. *J Bone Joint Surg Am* 2004;86(4):702-707.

23. Sankar WN, Hebela NM, Skaggs DL, Flynn JM: Loss of pin fixation in displaced supracondylar humeral fractures in children: Causes and prevention. *J Bone Joint Surg Am* 2007;89(4):713-717.

24. Pennock AT, Charles M, Moor M, Bastrom TP, Newton PO: Potential causes of loss of reduction in supracondylar humerus fractures. *J Pediatr Orthop* 2014;34(7):691-697.

25. Gottschalk HP, Sagoo D, Glaser D, Doan J, Edmonds EW, Schlechter

J: Biomechanical analysis of pin placement for pediatric supracondylar humerus fractures: Does starting point, pin size, and number matter? *J Pediatr Orthop* 2012;32(5):445-451.

26. Srikumaran U, Tan EW, Erkula G, Leet AI, Ain MC, Sponseller PD: Pin size influences sagittal alignment in percutaneously pinned pediatric supracondylar humerus fractures. *J Pediatr Orthop* 2010;30(8):792-798.

27. Edmonds EW, Roocroft JH, Mubarak SJ: Treatment of displaced pediatric supracondylar humerus fracture patterns requiring medial fixation: A reliable and safer cross-pinning technique. *J Pediatr Orthop* 2012;32(4):346-351.

28. Queally JM, Paramanathan N, Walsh JC, Moran CJ, Shannon FJ, D'Souza LG: Dorgan's lateral cross-wiring of supracondylar fractures of the

humerus in children: A retrospective review. *Injury* 2010;41(6):568-571.

29. Gangadharan S, Rathinam B, Madhuri V: Radial nerve safety in Dorgan's lateral cross-pinning of the supracondylar humeral fracture in children: A case report and cadaveric study. *J Pediatr Orthop B* 2014;23(6):579-583.

30. Shannon FJ, Mohan P, Chacko J, D'Souza LG: "Dorgan's" percutaneous lateral cross-wiring of supracondylar fractures of the humerus in children. *J Pediatr Orthop* 2004;24(4):376-379.

31. Seehausen DA, Kay RM, Ryan DD, Skaggs DL: Foam padding in casts accommodates soft tissue swelling and provides circumferential strength after fixation of supracondylar humerus fractures. *J Pediatr Orthop* 2015;35(1):24-27.

Open Reduction Techniques for Supracondylar Humerus Fractures in Children

Jessica Jane Wingfield, MD
Christine Ann Ho, MD
Joshua Abzug, MD
Todd F. Ritzman, MD
Brian Brighton, MD, MPH

Abstract

Supracondylar humerus fractures are the most common elbow fractures in children. Displaced supracondylar humerus fractures that are associated with neurologic and/or vascular injuries should be treated with timely reduction via closed techniques. If closed reduction fails, reduction via open techniques is indicated. There is controversy about which surgical approach yields the best cosmetic and functional outcomes while minimizing postoperative complications. Open reduction, if indicated, has been reported to yield good outcomes in patients in whom closed reduction fails.

Instr Course Lect 2016;65:361–370.

Supracondylar humerus fractures are the most common elbow fractures in children.[1,2] Approximately 95% of supracondylar humerus fractures are classified as extension-type injury patterns that result from forced hyperextension of the elbow after a fall onto an outstretched arm.[3] Supracondylar humerus fractures can be classified based on their direction of displacement in both the sagittal and the coronal planes, which has implications for involvement of the neural or vascular structures. The literature suggests that surgical management with closed reduction techniques and percutaneous pin fixation is the standard of care for Gartland type III fractures.[4-6] Open reduction and percutaneous pin fixation is an acceptable method of treatment for supracondylar humerus fractures that are not amenable to closed reduction;[2,5] however, there is no clear consensus on the preferred surgical approach if open reduction of a displaced supracondylar humerus fracture is indicated.

Indications for Open Reduction

The most commonly reported indication for open reduction is failed treatment via closed reduction.[5] Additional indications for open reduction of supracondylar humerus fractures include débridement of open fractures, compartment syndrome, and neurologic and/or vascular injury that requires open exploration and potential repair.[2,5,7]

Dr. Ho or an immediate family member serves as a board member, owner, officer, or committee member of the Pediatric Orthopaedic Society of North America. Dr. Abzug or an immediate family member is a member of a speakers' bureau or has made paid presentations on behalf of Checkpoint Surgical, and serves as a paid consultant to AxoGen. Dr. Ritzman or an immediate family member serves as an unpaid consultant to Apto Orthopaedics/Austen BioInnovation Institute in Akron, and has stock or stock options held in Apto Orthopaedics. Dr. Brighton serves as a paid consultant to DePuy, and serves as a board member, owner, officer, or committee member of the Pediatric Orthopaedic Society of North American and the American College of Surgeons. Neither Dr. Wingfield nor any immediate family member has received anything of value from or has stock or stock options held in a commercial company or institution related directly or indirectly to the subject of this chapter.

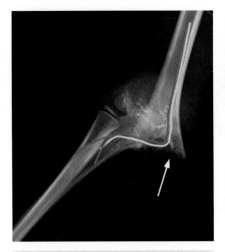

Figure 1 Radiograph demonstrates displacement of the median nerve (yellow line) and brachial artery (red line) in a posterolateral displacement injury pattern. The neurovascular bundle is tented over the metaphyseal spike (arrow).

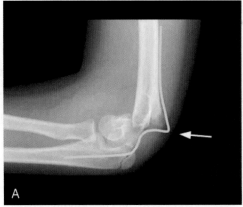
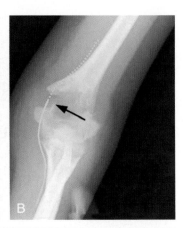

Figure 2 Lateral (**A**) and AP (**B**) radiographs demonstrate displacement of the ulnar nerve (yellow line) in a flexion-type injury pattern. The ulnar nerve is tented around the metaphyseal spike (white arrow). A segment of the ulnar nerve is trapped within the fracture site (black arrow).

The most commonly reported cause of inability to achieve a satisfactory closed reduction is interposition of the brachialis muscle, with buttonholing of the metaphyseal spike through the muscle.[1,7] Entrapment of the brachial artery and neurologic structures, such as the median nerve, has been reported.[1,2] Interposition of the periosteum or joint capsule within the fracture site also has been reported as a common cause of failed closed reduction. Ay et al[7] reported an occurrence rate of 45.8% for proximal fragment metaphyseal spikes that buttonholed through the brachialis muscle and an occurrence rate of 32.7% for capsular interposition in patients who required open reduction after failure of initial closed reduction.

Neurovascular Injury Patterns Based on the Direction of Displacement

Specific implications for neurologic or vascular injury exist based on the displacement direction of the distal fragment and the proximal metaphyseal spike. Some studies advocate selection of a surgical approach based on the direction of displacement.[5] In a series of 65 patients who required open reduction, Reitman et al[5] used a medial approach for posterolaterally displaced fractures as well as flexion-type injuries. A lateral approach was used for posteromedially displaced fractures. Direct posterior displacement was addressed via an anterior cubital fossa approach. The authors reported that the direction of exposure was selected to avoid disruption of the intact periosteum because disruption could further destabilize the fracture or interrupt the blood supply.[5] Furthermore, the direction of displacement has been reported to be a predictor of the nerve injury pattern. Posterolateral displacement is associated with median nerve and anterior interosseous nerve injuries (**Figure 1**). Ulnar nerve injuries most commonly occur in flexion-type deformities (**Figure 2**). Posteromedial displacement is associated with radial nerve injuries[5,7-9] (**Figure 3**). Although posteromedial displacement is the most common injury pattern in patients who have displaced type III injuries, posterolateral displacement appears to be more prevalent in patients who have irreducible fractures.[5,7]

Approaches for Open Reduction

Because of instability and the difficulty in maintaining reduction in supracondylar humerus fractures that require open reduction, it is highly recommended that surgery be performed on a radiolucent arm board or hand table; the use of the image intensifier portion of a C-arm fluoroscopy machine is not recommended. Because the fracture may be too unstable to rotate the arm to obtain a lateral view, it may be necessary to obtain a lateral fluoroscopic view of the fracture by rotating the arc of the fluoroscopy beam to 90°. The surgical table should be rotated to 90° to align the fluoroscopic arm parallel with the bed. The authors of this chapter prefer to position the fluoroscopy machine at the head of the bed so that the C-arm is easily rotated for a lateral fluoroscopic view without the image intensifier hitting the bed (**Figure 4**). A radiolucent arm table or Plexiglass is used for the patient's surgical arm. Especially in

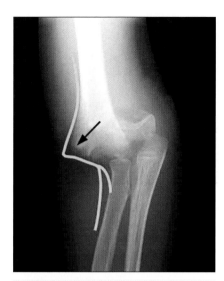

Figure 3   Radiograph demonstrates displacement of the radial nerve (yellow line) in a posteromedial displacement injury pattern. The radial nerve is displaced by the metaphyseal spike (arrow).

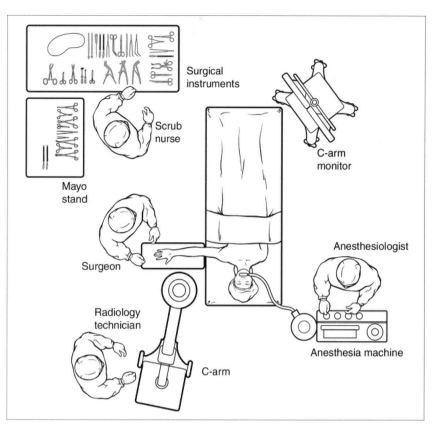

Figure 4   Illustration shows the operating room setup for reduction of supracondylar humerus fractures.

toddlers and small children, the surgical arm must be brought distal enough on the radiolucent table to facilitate complete fluoroscopic visualization. The fluoroscopy arm can then be easily rotated to a lateral view if necessary. Folded towels may be placed under the elbow to elevate the arm from the table, which aids in obtaining a lateral view.

Regardless of the surgical approach used, after the fracture has been opened, reduction and fixation of the fracture is often difficult and problematic because of the complete lack of stability as a result of extensive periosteal stripping. The reduction is often most stable at 90° of flexion, with a small folded towel under the distal fragment and the surgeon's fingers manually holding the reduction of the metaphyseal spike to the distal piece. An assistant must then drive Kirschner wires (K-wires) blind across the fracture site. If provisional fixation can be obtained with this method, the fracture is often stable enough for the surgeon to remove his

or her fingers, hyperflex the elbow, and pin the fracture using traditional closed methods. The provisional K-wires may then be removed. If no assistant is available, two retrograde K-wires can be placed percutaneously into the distal fragment up to the level of the fracture site. The fracture is then reduced and held by the surgeon's fingers while the K-wires are driven across the proximal cortex. Because these fractures tend to be very unstable, the surgeon may prefer to use a cross-pinned configuration rather than an all-lateral pin construct, especially because the ulnar nerve can be visualized and protected in an open approach; however, preference for the use of a cross-pinned configuration versus an all-lateral pin construct is controversial and highly surgeon-dependent.

The literature suggests multiple options for the surgical approach, including anterior, posterior, medial, and lateral approaches as well as variations of these approaches, if open reduction is indicated. The selected approach should allow for reduction that results in anatomic alignment, access to the involved neural and/or vascular structures, and satisfactory cosmetic and functional outcomes while minimizing postoperative complications.[1]

The Chapter Authors' Preference

Similar to Reitman et al,[5] the authors of this chapter prefer to use a surgical approach that is based on the location of the metaphyseal spike and the displacement of the distal fragment. Often, the

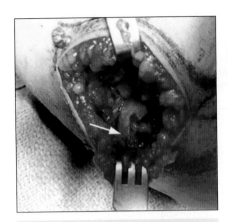

Figure 5 Intraoperative photograph shows the metaphyseal spike (arrow), which is visible immediately after skin incision via a lateral approach. The metaphyseal spike has already performed the dissection.

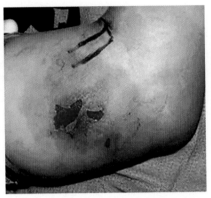

Figure 6 Clinical photograph shows tenuous skin, which should be avoided to minimize wound healing complications.

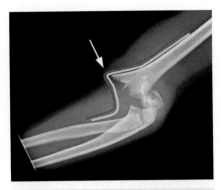

Figure 7 Lateral radiograph demonstrates displacement of the brachial artery (yellow line) and median nerve (red line) in an extension-type injury pattern. The neurovascular bundle is tented over the metaphyseal spike (arrow).

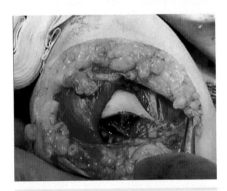

Figure 8 Intraoperative photograph shows the anteromedial approach with median nerve and brachial artery injury from the metaphyseal spike. The biceps muscle belly is visualized lateral to the metaphyseal fragment, which has displaced the neurovascular bundle medially.

dissection has been performed by the metaphyseal spike, and the periosteum has already been disrupted (**Figure 5**). This approach allows for direct visualization of anatomic structures that are trapped or displaced by the metaphyseal spike. Care must be taken in planning the incision to avoid areas of compromised skin. Dissection through already traumatized skin may lead to skin necrosis and complications in wound healing (**Figure 6**).

Anterior Approach

Because most supracondylar humerus fractures are extension-type injuries and because indications for open reduction of these injuries include exploration of the potentially injured neurovascular bundle, the anterior approach has the most utility (**Figure 7**). The incision for the anterior approach is made in a transverse or "lazy S" fashion and centered over the flexion crease of the antecubital fossa. Although the authors of this chapter typically prefer to start with the transverse limb of the incision, the planned "lazy S" skin incision may be extended laterally, medially, proximally,

and distally to gain exposure to structures if necessary. Blunt dissection is used to complete the traumatic exposure down to the level of the proximal metaphyseal fragment. If the soft tissues have been disrupted by the sharp anterior metaphyseal spike of bone, then the dissection has already been performed (**Figure 8**). If this approach is used to extract interposed periosteum or muscle bellies from the fracture site, care should be taken to stay lateral to the biceps tendon to avoid potential iatrogenic neurologic or vascular injury.

The neurovascular bundle, which can be identified proximal to the fracture site and medial to the biceps tendon and muscle belly, should be carefully protected during any deeper dissection to the fracture site (**Figure 9**). Blunt dissection should be performed carefully because the neurovascular bundle can be displaced into a nonanatomic position secondary to the injury. Interposed structures are then freed from the fracture site and reduction is obtained under direct visualization and by palpation.

Reduction may be obtained by applying direct posterior pressure on the proximal fragment while the assistant

pulls traction and flexes the elbow with direct pressure on the olecranon.[7] If there is a substantial amount of proximal displacement and shortening of the distal fragment, traction and length can be obtained by levering a baby Hohmann retractor or Freer elevator on the distal fragment with the tip of the instrument while balancing the shaft of the tool on the proximal metaphysis as a fulcrum. Careful, gentle pressure is required because rough force from

© 2016 AAOS Instructional Course Lectures, Volume 65

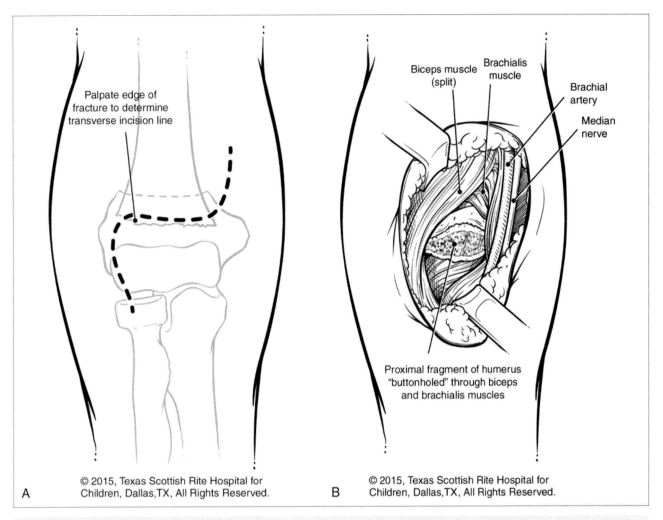

© 2015, Texas Scottish Rite Hospital for Children, Dallas,TX, All Rights Reserved.

© 2015, Texas Scottish Rite Hospital for Children, Dallas,TX, All Rights Reserved.

Figure 9   Illustrations show the anterior approach. **A,** Extension of the transverse skin incision can be attained via a "lazy S" incision (dashed line) if more proximal or distal exposure is required. **B,** Typical appearance after the superficial layer of skin and fat is incised. The metaphyseal spike has already performed the dissection by lacerating the brachialis and biceps brachii muscle bellies. (Copyright Texas Scottish Rite Hospital for Children, Dallas, TX.)

the instrument may lead to iatrogenic fracture of the metaphyseal cortex. In addition, baby Hohmann or other retractors should be used to carefully protect the neurovascular structures during reduction, which will prevent iatrogenic injury.

One advantage of the anterior approach is the ability to extend the incision to expose neurologic and/or vascular structures if they require exploration and/or repair.[7,10,11] The neurovascular bundle can be safely identified proximal to the zone of injury and then carefully dissected to the fracture site. Often, the nerve and artery are intact but are trapped in fascial bands at the fracture site, or the adventitial tissue is kinked in the fracture site; these structures can be simply and gently released from the offending structures.

Some surgeons advocate the use of the anterior approach in patients in whom vascular exploration of the brachial artery is anticipated;[7,10] however, vascular surgery expertise may be required in these patients, and the availability of a surgeon who has experience in end-to-end microanastomosis, vein grafts, and patch grafts should be considered before exploring the avascular hand (**Figure 10**). Although the anterior approach has the most utility for the treatment of supracondylar humerus fractures, great care is required to avoid iatrogenic injury to the anterior neurovascular structures.

Posterior Approach

Posterior triceps-sparing approaches, as well as those that require division of the tricipital aponeurosis, have been

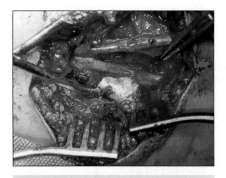

Figure 10 Intraoperative photograph shows the anterior approach via a transverse incision. Proximal is to the left, distal is to the right. The median nerve is trapped within the fracture site. The brachial artery required repair with a patch graft.

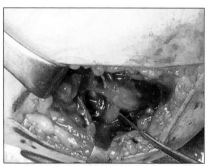

Figure 11 Intraoperative photograph shows the medial approach for a flexion-type supracondylar humerus fracture that was irreducible via closed means. Proximal is to the left, distal is to the right. A Freer elevator is on the ulnar nerve, which is trapped between the metaphysis and the anteriorly displaced distal humerus fragment.

described for the treatment of supracondylar humerus fractures.[12,13] An incision made over the posterior distal humerus favors the medial side of midline. The ulnar nerve should be carefully identified and protected from the dissection. The distal tendinous portion of the triceps is incised and reflected laterally and medially to gain exposure to the distal humerus. The dissection is then carried down to expose the proximal metaphyseal spike. The interposed muscle or structures are removed, and reduction is achieved. The triceps is then reapproximated and repaired.[13] Concerns regarding potential disruption to the blood supply, which may result in osteonecrosis, have been raised with this approach.[13-15] Additional uncertainties include increased rates of postoperative stiffness from adding a posterior dissection to an existing traumatic anterior soft-tissue injury.[13,14,16] Because of these risks and the fact that typical soft-tissue interposition precluding reduction is anterior and remote from this approach, the posterior approach is rarely, if ever, used in the practice of the authors of this chapter.

Lateral Approach

The lateral approach may be used for posteromedially displaced fractures in which the metaphyseal spike is buttonholed in the brachioradialis or lateral fascia. An incision is made over the lateral supracondylar ridge, the fascia is divided, and the plane between the brachioradialis and triceps is identified. The dissection is carried directly down to bone. The triceps can be reflected posteriorly, and the brachioradialis can be carried anteriorly. If an extensile approach is required, the distal intermuscular plane is developed in the Kocher interval between the anconeus and the extensor carpi ulnaris. In adults, dissection of more than 6 cm proximal to the lateral epicondyle is contraindicated to avoid injury to the radial nerve. Because there are no published studies on radial nerve anatomy in children, the authors of this chapter advise surgeons to proceed with caution if the lateral approach is extended proximal to the metaphysis. Hematoma is removed from the fracture site and trapped structures are freed. Reduction is obtained under

direct visualization and confirmed by fluoroscopy.

Medial Approach

The medial approach is useful for posterolaterally displaced fractures and flexion-type fractures that cannot be reduced via closed techniques, typically because of entrapment of the ulnar nerve; the medial approach allows for direct access and visualization of the interposed nerve. The medial epicondyle is palpated as an anatomic landmark, and an incision is made over the medial aspect of the elbow. Dissection is carried down to the level of the ulnar nerve, which is carefully mobilized and protected from the surgical field. The exposure is carried down using blunt dissection until the distal aspect of the proximal fragment is identified by reflecting the brachialis muscle.[16]

Hematoma is removed and any trapped structures are freed (**Figure 11**). Reduction is obtained via traction and manual pressure or via leverage with an elevator if necessary. For flexion-type injuries, folded sterile towels are placed under the olecranon, and the elbow is positioned in extension to assist in reduction of the distal fragment. Reduction is confirmed by direct visualization and palpation and/or fluoroscopy before definitive K-wire fixation is obtained.

Results of Open Reduction

Many studies have reported the functional, cosmetic, and radiographic outcomes of the various surgical approaches for the treatment of supracondylar humerus fractures if open reduction is indicated.[1,4,5,7,10,12,17]

Functional Outcomes

The primary predictor of functional outcome is postoperative range of

© 2016 AAOS Instructional Course Lectures, Volume 65

motion. Flynn et al[18] reported that 0° to 5° of motion loss in the sagittal plane was an excellent outcome, 6° to 10° was a good outcome, 11° to 15° was a fair outcome, and more than 15° was a poor outcome (**Table 1**). Pretell Mazzini et al[1] reported that patients who underwent fixation via the posterior approach had a high frequency of poor outcomes based on the criteria described by Flynn et al.[18] In a study that compared patients who underwent the open posterior triceps-sparing approach with a closed reduction cohort, 48% of patients who underwent open reduction had fair to poor functional outcomes based on the criteria described by Flynn et al[18] and their Baumann angle.[12] Ay et al[7] reported on a series of 61 patients with displaced supracondylar humerus fractures who underwent open reduction via the anterior approach. Using the criteria described by Flynn et al,[18] Ay et al[7] reported that 72.8% of patients had excellent outcomes, 27.2% of patients had good outcomes, and no patients had fair or poor outcomes. In a study of patients who underwent open reduction via the lateral approach, Ersan et al[10] reported that 50% of patients had excellent outcomes and 47.4% of patients had good outcomes based on the criteria described by Flynn et al.[18] In a study of 25 patients who underwent open reduction via the medial approach, Yaokreh et al[4] reported that 76% of patients had excellent or good outcomes. Supracondylar humerus fractures that are treated via open techniques, excluding the posterior approach, demonstrate favorable functional results similar to closed techniques. The original study by Flynn et al[18] of patients with supracondylar humerus fractures who were treated with closed reduction and percutaneous fixation reported that 98%

Table 1
Functional Outcome Criteria

Result	Rating	Cosmetic Factor: Carrying Angle Loss (Degrees)	Functional Factor: Motion Loss (Degrees)
Satisfactory	Excellent	0–5	0–5
	Good	6–10	6–10
	Fair	11–15	11–15
Unsatisfactory	Poor	>15	>15

Adapted with permission from Flynn JC, Matthews JG, Benoit RL: Blind pinning of displaced supracondylar fractures of the humerus in children: Sixteen years' experience with long-term follow-up. *J Bone Joint Surg Am* 1974;56(2):263-272.

of the 52 patients available at long-term follow-up had satisfactory outcomes.[18]

Cosmetic Outcomes

Changes in the carrying angle as well as scar formation are cited as reasons for poor outcomes. The criteria described Flynn et al[18] are the most widely accepted measures of postoperative cosmetic outcomes (**Table 1**). Higher rates of unsatisfactory cosmetic outcomes have been reported in patients who undergo treatment via the posterior and lateral approaches.[1,7,10,12] Aktekin et al[12] reported that 26% of patients who underwent a triceps-sparing technique via the posterior approach had fair or poor cosmetic outcomes based on the criteria described by Flynn et al.[18] Some studies have suggested that the posterior and lateral approaches do not allow surgeons to adequately address medial comminution, which results in coronal plane abnormalities and alterations to the carrying angle.[1] In a study of 32 patients who underwent open reduction via the anterior approach, Ay et al[7] reported excellent cosmetic outcomes, with a low percentage of patients who had postoperative coronal plane deformities. Other studies have reported that 99% of patients had excellent or good

outcomes via the anterior approach.[10] Open reduction via the medial approach has been associated with a lower rate of changes in the carrying angle, with reported rates ranging from 4% to 6%.[4,19]

Scar formation based on the anatomic location of an incision also has been described as a cosmetic outcome. In a study of 84 patients who underwent open reduction and K-wire fixation, Ersan et al[10] reported that hypertrophic scar formation developed in two of the 38 patients who had a lateral incision; no hypertrophic scar formation was reported in the 46 patients who had an anterior cubital fossa incision. Hypertrophic scar formation has been reported in up to 17% of patients who have posteriorly based incisions.[12]

Radiographic Outcomes

Radiographic outcomes assessed in the literature primarily measure radiographic time to union. In a systematic review of seven studies, Pretell Mazzini et al,[1] reported no significant difference between anatomic approaches with regard to radiographic time to union. The authors reported a mean union time of 4.5 weeks for the lateral approach, 4.7 weeks for the medial approach,

4 weeks for the posterior approach, and 4 weeks for the anterior cubital fossa approach. In a study that was not included in the systematic review by Pretell Mazzini et al,[1] 23 patients who underwent open reduction via a posterior triceps-sparing approach had a mean time to union of 7 weeks.[12]

Complications
Infection

In a study of 23 patients who were treated with open reduction via a posterior incision, Aktekin et al[12] reported that a superficial infection that required treatment with oral antibiotics developed in two patients, and wound dehiscence that resolved with local wound care and did not require further surgical treatment developed in two patients. None of these complications occurred in patients who had open fractures. In a systematic review of 226 patients who underwent various surgical techniques, no significant difference in the rate of postoperative infection was reported; however, there was a trend toward a higher rate of postoperative infection in patients who underwent surgery via the medial approach, but it did not reach statistical significance.[1] All reported infections resolved with oral antibiotics alone and did not require surgical treatment.

Iatrogenic Nerve Injury

In a series of 25 patients who underwent open reduction via the medial approach, Yaokreh et al[4] reported no patients with iatrogenic nerve injury. Similarly, in a study of 84 patients, 46 of whom underwent open reduction via an anterior incision, Ersan et al[10] reported no patients with iatrogenic nerve injury. In that same series, 38 patients underwent open reduction via a lateral incision. Postoperative ulnar nerve symptoms developed in one patient; the authors did not use an additional medial incision to facilitate the placement of a medially based pin. The patient's symptoms resolved after pin removal. In a review of 226 patients who underwent open reduction, Pretell Mazzini et al[1] reported a 2.21% rate of iatrogenic nerve injury, with the ulnar nerve most commonly involved. There was no statistically significant difference in the rate of nerve injury among the various approaches; however, there was a trend toward a higher rate of nerve injury for both lateral and posterior incisions in which medially and laterally based pins were commonly used.[1]

Vascular Injury

No iatrogenic vascular injuries have been reported during open reduction procedures for the treatment of supracondylar humerus fractures.

Compartment Syndrome

Compartment syndrome is a very rare complication of supracondylar humerus fractures. In a review of the literature, the authors of this chapter found no reported cases of compartment syndrome in patients who underwent open reduction and percutaneous pin fixation.[2,4,5,7,10,12,17]

Trochlear Osteonecrosis

The authors of this chapter are unaware of any reported cases of trochlear osteonecrosis in patients who underwent open reduction of a supracondylar humerus fracture via an anterior, lateral, or medial approach;[4,7,10] however, there were two reported cases of trochlear osteonecrosis in a study of 23 patients who underwent open reduction via a posterior approach.[12] These two cases of trochlear osteonecrosis support studies that report that a posterior dissection in a pediatric patient places the trochlear blood supply at risk.[3,13,14] Trochlear osteonecrosis results in limited elbow extension after trochlear resorption, which leads to instability, proximal migration of the ulna, and subsequent posterior impingement of the olecranon onto the distal humerus.[12]

Nonunion

The authors of this chapter were unable to find any reported cases of nonunion in pediatric patients with displaced supracondylar humerus fractures who underwent open reduction and percutaneous pin fixation[1,4,5,7,10,12,17]

Summary

Displaced supracondylar humerus fractures are common injuries in the pediatric population. Closed reduction and fixation with percutaneous pins is the first line of treatment for displaced supracondylar humerus fractures. If closed reduction fails, open reduction is indicated and demonstrates favorable outcomes. Multiple surgical approaches, including anterior, posterior, lateral, and medial approaches, as well as variations of these approaches, exist. Many studies advocate the use of the anterior cubital fossa incision because it allows access to potentially injured neural and/or vascular structures and yields consistently good cosmetic and functional outcomes with low complication rates. The posterior approach is associated with the least satisfactory outcomes, with notable limitations in sagittal plane motion as well as reported concerns for trochlear osteonecrosis and cosmetic outcomes. However, no significant differences have been reported among the various open reduction approaches with regard to infection rates, compartment syndrome, time to union, and iatrogenic nerve injury. Some studies advocate for medial or laterally centered incisions based on the displacement direction of the distal fragment to address potential nerve injuries around the displaced metaphyseal spike. Open reduction, if indicated, has been reported to yield good outcomes in patients in whom closed reduction fails.

References

1. Pretell Mazzini J, Rodriguez Martin J, Andres Esteban EM: Surgical approaches for open reduction and pinning in severely displaced supracondylar humerus fractures in children: A systematic review. *J Child Orthop* 2010;4(2):143-152.

2. Koudstaal MJ, De Ridder VA, De Lange S, Ulrich C: Pediatric supracondylar humerus fractures: The anterior approach. *J Orthop Trauma* 2002;16(6):409-412.

3. Tachdjian MO: *Pediatric Orthopedics.* Philadelphia, PA, WB Saunders, 2014, vol 5, pp 1265-1293.

4. Yaokreh JB, Gicquel P, Schneider L, et al: Compared outcomes after percutaneous pinning versus open reduction in paediatric supracondylar elbow fractures. *Orthop Traumatol Surg Res* 2012;98(6):645-651.

5. Reitman RD, Waters P, Millis M: Open reduction and internal fixation for supracondylar humerus fractures in children. *J Pediatr Orthop* 2001;21(2):157-161.

6. Kasser JR: Percutaneous pinning of supracondylar fractures of the humerus. *Instr Course Lect* 1992;41:385-390.

7. Ay S, Akinci M, Kamiloglu S, Ercetin O: Open reduction of displaced pediatric supracondylar humeral fractures through the anterior cubital approach. *J Pediatr Orthop* 2005;25(2):149-153.

8. Brown IC, Zinar DM: Traumatic and iatrogenic neurological complications after supracondylar humerus fractures in children. *J Pediatr Orthop* 1995;15(4):440-443.

9. Campbell CC, Waters PM, Emans JB, Kasser JR, Millis MB: Neurovascular injury and displacement in type III supracondylar humerus fractures. *J Pediatr Orthop* 1995;15(1):47-52.

10. Ersan O, Gonen E, İlhan RD, Boysan E, Ates Y: Comparison of anterior and lateral approaches in the treatment of extension-type supracondylar humerus fractures in children. *J Pediatr Orthop B* 2012;21(2):121-126.

11. Weisel SW: *Operative Techniques in Pediatric Orthopaedics.* Philadelphia, PA, Lippincott Williams & Wilkins, 2010, pp 21-24.

12. Aktekin CN, Toprak A, Ozturk AM, Altay M, Ozkurt B, Tabak AY: Open reduction via posterior triceps sparing approach in comparison with closed treatment of posteromedial displaced Gartland type III supracondylar humerus fractures. *J Pediatr Orthop B* 2008;17(4):171-178.

13. Gruber MA, Healy WA III: The posterior approach to the elbow revisited. *J Pediatr Orthop* 1996;16(2):215-219.

14. Kasser JR, Beaty JH: Supracondylar fractures of the distal humerus, in Beaty JH, Kasser JR, eds: *Rockwood and Wilkins' Fractures in Children,* ed 6. Philadelphia, PA, Lippincott Williams & Wilkins, 2006, pp 543-589.

15. Naji UK, Zahid A, Faheem U: Type III supracondylar fracture humerus: Results of open reduction and internal fixation after failed closed reduction. *Rawal Med J* 2010;35:156-159.

16. Kumar R, Kiran EK, Malhotra R, Bhan S: Surgical management of the severely displaced supracondylar fracture of the humerus in children. *Injury* 2002;33(6):517-522.

17. Kaewpornsawan K: Comparison between closed reduction with percutaneous pinning and open reduction with pinning in children with closed totally displaced supracondylar humeral fractures: A randomized controlled trial. *J Pediatr Orthop B* 2001;10(2):131-137.

18. Flynn JC, Matthews JG, Benoit RL: Blind pinning of displaced supracondylar fractures of the humerus in children: Sixteen years' experience with long-term follow-up. *J Bone Joint Surg Am* 1974;56(2):263-272.

19. Shakir H, Malik FA, Khalid W: Displaced supracondylar fractures of humerus in children treated with open reduction and cross K-wire fixation. *JPMI* 2010;24(4):301-306.

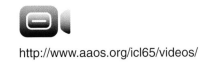

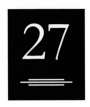

http://www.aaos.org/icl65/videos/

The Difficult Supracondylar Humerus Fracture: Flexion-Type Injuries

Daniel Bouton, MD
Christine Ann Ho, MD
Joshua Abzug, MD
Brian Brighton, MD, MPH
Todd F. Ritzman, MD

Abstract

Although flexion-type supracondylar humerus fractures account for a minority of all supracondylar humerus fractures, they warrant special attention because of their relatively high rate of requirement for open reduction and their potential for ulnar nerve injury or entrapment. The severity of flexion-type supracondylar humerus fractures may be difficult to appreciate on initial radiographs; therefore, surgeons must have a high index of suspicion in the evaluation of a patient who has a suspected flexion-type supracondylar humerus fracture. Nondisplaced or minimally displaced flexion-type supracondylar humerus fractures can be treated with long arm casting. Displaced flexion-type supracondylar humerus fractures require surgical reduction and stabilization. The unique instability of and reduction position for flexion-type supracondylar humerus fractures make reduction and pinning more of a challenge compared with the more common extension-type supracondylar humerus fractures; therefore, special considerations are required in the surgical setup and planning for flexion-type supracondylar humerus fractures.

Instr Course Lect 2016;65:371–378.

The injury pattern of flexion-type supracondylar fractures certainly validates Mercer Rang's statement to "pity the young surgeon whose first case is a fracture around the elbow."[1] The rare injury pattern of flexion-type supracondylar fractures accounts for a minority of pediatric elbow fractures, yet it has a high rate of neurologic injury and a disproportionate requirement for open reduction compared with its more common extension-type counterpart.

Incidence

Although most supracondylar humerus fractures in children are extension-type injuries, flexion-type injuries, which comprise only 2% to 3% of all supracondylar humerus fractures, also exist.[2-4] Compared with extension-type injuries, which tend to occur in younger children, flexion-type injuries tend to occur in older children (mean, 5.8 years

Dr. Ritzman or an immediate family member serves as an unpaid consultant to Apto Orthopaedics and the Austin BioInnovation Institute of Akron, and has stock or stock options held in Apto Orthopaedics. Dr. Ho or an immediate family member serves as a board member, owner, officer, or committee member of the Pediatric Orthopaedic Society of North America. Dr. Abzug or an immediate family member is a member of a speakers' bureau or has made paid presentations on behalf of Checkpoint Surgical, and serves as a paid consultant to AxoGen. Dr. Brighton or an immediate family member serves as a paid consultant to DePuy, and serves as a board member, owner, officer, or committee member of the Pediatric Orthopaedic Society of North America and the American College of Surgeons. Neither Dr. Bouton nor any immediate family member has received anything of value from or has stock or stock options held in a commercial company or institution related directly or indirectly to the subject of this chapter.

versus 7.5 years, respectively); however, there is no consistent sex predisposition to either flexion- or extension-type injuries.[2-11]

Mechanism of Injury

Unlike extension-type injuries, which usually result after a fall onto an outstretched hand, flexion-type injuries most often occur after a fall directly onto the posterior aspect of an elbow. In this type of fall, an anteriorly directed force is generated on the distal fragment, which results in the flexion deformity seen in flexion-type injuries. The distal fragment may be displaced anteriorly and proximally because of the pull of the anterior musculature. Because the ulnar nerve is acutely stretched over the posterior spike of the proximal fragment in flexion-type injuries, it may be at risk for injury.[2,5-7] The ulnar nerve also may become acutely entrapped in the fracture site at the time of closed reduction or in a delayed fashion within the healing callus.[8] Ulnar nerve injury occurs in up to 19% of patients who sustain a flexion-type supracondylar fracture.[2]

Evaluation

The evaluation of a patient who has a flexion-type supracondylar fracture is similar to that of a patient who has any type of injury about the elbow. A detailed history that focuses on the mechanism of injury, location of pain, and presence or absence of any numbness or tingling in the extremity should be obtained. In addition, the surgeon should rule out other possible concomitant injuries. If a splint is already in place, it should be removed to allow for a thorough examination of the entire extremity and to avoid a delayed diagnosis of open fracture patterns. The skin should be inspected for any ecchymosis, lacerations, abrasions, puckering, or open injuries. Adequate perfusion should be confirmed with an examination of warmth, color, radial pulse, and capillary refill. The arm and forearm compartments must be evaluated for supple compressibility to identify signs of compartment syndrome. The examination should evaluate the remainder of the ipsilateral extremity for floating elbow injury patterns or other trauma. A standard neurologic examination, including an assessment of motor, sensory, and sympathetic function, is requisite. Particular care should be taken to assess the function of the ulnar nerve, which is more frequently injured in flexion-type injuries, with a confirmation of sensation in the ulnar one and one-half digits of the hand as well as interossei motor function.

Imaging

AP and lateral elbow radiographs should be obtained if elbow trauma is suspected. If the injury cannot be localized to the elbow, a radiologic examination of the entire extremity may be required. True AP and lateral radiographs of the elbow may be difficult to obtain in patients who have displaced supracondylar fractures, and oblique radiographs can assist with diagnosis and management. In older children, radiographs should be used to rule out intercondylar or intra-articular splits, and CT may aid in preoperative planning if a more complex T-condylar injury pattern is suspected. On the lateral radiograph, flexion-type injuries may vary from a mild angular deformity to complete anterior and proximal displacement of the distal fragment. As with all supracondylar humerus fractures, the Baumann angle and the anterior humeral line should be assessed on the AP and lateral radiographs, respectively. Comparison images of the contralateral elbow can help determine norms if uncertainty about the presence of a mild fracture exists. Because comminution may dictate the optimal pin pattern for surgical fixation, the integrity of the medial and lateral columns also should be scrutinized. Flexion-type supracondylar fractures typically have an obliquity on lateral radiographs that is the opposite of an extension-type injury, with a characteristic fracture line that traverses from anterosuperior to posteroinferior. Because radiographs represent only one point in time, the amount of displacement or instability in a universally unstable injury may be underestimated; anecdotally, often the most unstable fractures that present challenging reductions are not appreciated until an examination is performed under fluoroscopic examination in the operating room secondary to this phenomenon.

Classification

Flexion-type supracondylar humerus fractures are classified similar to extension-type supracondylar humerus fractures. Wilkins modified the Gartland classification for flexion-type injury patterns: flexion-type I supracondylar humerus fractures are nondisplaced; flexion-type II supracondylar humerus fractures have anterior angulation of the distal fragment, with the anterior cortex remaining in continuity but hinged; and flexion-type III supracondylar humerus fractures have a loss in continuity of both the anterior and posterior cortices, with anterior displacement of the distal fragment (**Figure 1**).[2,9] Leitch et al[3] added a type IV injury to the classic Gartland

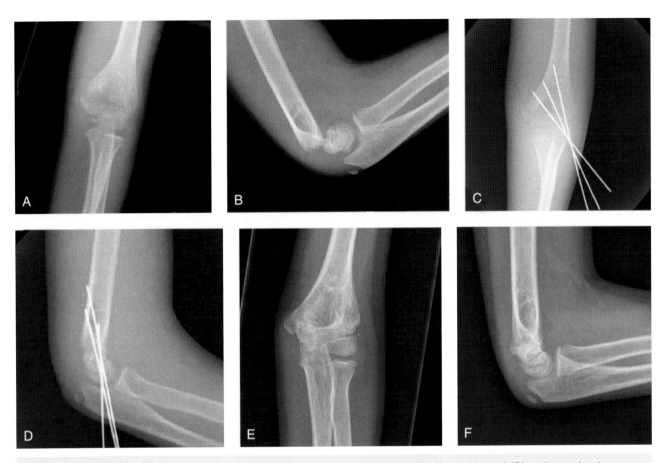

Figure 1   Images show a flexion-type III supracondylar humerus fracture. AP (**A**) and lateral (**B**) radiographs demonstrate the injury. AP (**C**) and lateral (**D**) intraoperative fluoroscopic images show fixation after closed reduction and percutaneous pinning. AP (**E**) and lateral (**F**) radiographs taken at final follow-up demonstrate fracture union.

classification to account for universally unstable flexion-type supracondylar humerus fractures. Flexion-type IV supracondylar humerus fractures notably lack a competent periosteal hinge, which may be attributed to either the injury mechanism itself or iatrogenic over-manipulation of an unstable extension-type fracture, and often are not radiographically confirmed until a fluoroscopic examination is performed under anesthesia.

Management

A treatment algorithm similar to that used for the management of extension-type supracondylar fractures can be applied to the management of flexion-type supracondylar fractures. Nondisplaced

flexion-type I supracondylar fractures can be treated in a long arm cast, with the arm comfortably positioned in approximately 70° to 80° of elbow flexion.[1,10,12] Rarely, minimally displaced, flexion-type II supracondylar fractures can be casted in an extended position if radiographs obtained in the cast confirm that the anterior humeral line intersects the capitellum within acceptable limits. The cast should remain in place for 3 weeks, with repeat radiographs taken 1 and 3 weeks after casting.[4]

Surgical fixation is preferred for most flexion-type II as well as all flexion-type III and flexion-type IV supracondylar fractures. Closed reduction and percutaneous pinning is the surgical treatment of choice for

most patients (**Figure 1**). Flexion-type fractures tend to be more difficult to treat with closed reduction and percutaneous pinning compared with their extension-type counterparts, which is primarily because flexion-type fractures are unstable in the fully flexed position and it is difficult to maintain reduction during the insertion of Kirschner wires.

If closed reduction and percutaneous pinning is unsuccessful, an open reduction may be required. Open reduction is more likely necessary for flexion-type injuries compared with extension-type injuries (31% versus 10%, respectively).[2] An anteromedial approach is preferred over a direct anterior approach because the brachialis is usually intact in flexion-type injuries and needs to be retracted to expose the fracture site, which is more easily achieved with a medial extension to an anterior approach. In addition, the medial extension of the anteromedial approach allows for exploration and mobilization of the ulnar nerve out of the fracture site during open reduction.

Outcomes

Because of the low incidence of flexion-type supracondylar fractures, there is a paucity of literature on the treatment outcomes for flexion-type supracondylar fractures.[2,3,5-12] In a review of the literature, the authors of this chapter found that all of these studies were retrospective reviews that included a limited number of patients (range, 1 to 58) who had flexion-type injury patterns. Furthermore, only four of the studies reported on the use of percutaneous pin fixation, with the rest of the studies reporting on the retrospective results of splint, cast, and skin/skeletal traction treatment.[2,3,5,11] Accordingly, evidence-based treatment recommendations on the timing of surgery, indications for closed versus open reduction, and percutaneous pin construct patterns that are specific to flexion-type supracondylar fractures cannot be derived from a review of the literature.

In a review of 58 patients who had flexion-type supracondylar fractures, Mahan et al[2] reported that 19% of patients with flexion-type supracondylar fractures had a preoperative ulnar nerve injury compared with only 3% of patients in a comparison cohort who had extension-type supracondylar fractures. The authors reported that all of the patients who had flexion-type supracondylar fractures required open reduction with ulnar nerve exploration compared with only 0.3% of the patients who had

extension-type injuries. Furthermore, 31% of patients who had flexion-type fractures required an open approach to facilitate reduction compared with 10% of the patients in the comparison cohort who had extension-type injuries. Both lateral entry and crossed-pin constructs were used. Approximately two-thirds of the flexion-type fractures were fixed with two-pin constructs, and the remaining one-third were fixed with three or more pin constructs. The authors did not report range of motion, radiographic, or patient-reported outcome data at follow-up. In a study of 175 patients who had supracondylar fractures, Fowles and Kassab[5] reported 17 patients who had flexion-type injuries. Nine of the 17 patients who had flexion-type injuries were treated with closed reduction and percutaneous pinning, and three of the patients required open reduction. Good or excellent outcomes were reported in 13 of these 17 patients, with "some limitation of movement" that was attributed to the less optimal results. In a study of 22 patients with displaced flexion-type fractures who were treated with closed reduction and percutaneous pinning, De Boeck[11] reported good or excellent radiographic results in 86.2% of patients at a mean follow-up of 6.3 years. All of these authors report near-ubiquitous spontaneous recovery of ulnar nerve neurapraxia in their studies; however, a report on the timing of neurologic function recovery or recommendations on indications for ulnar nerve exploration cannot be derived from this body of literature.

Preferred Treatment Method of the Authors of this Chapter

Standard AP and lateral elbow radiographs are obtained in patients who

have suspected elbow trauma. Special attention is directed toward evaluation of the distal fragment to rule out T-condylar or intra-articular split fracture patterns in older children or peri-adolescent patients because these fracture patterns may dictate a planned open surgical approach with internal fixation rather than closed reduction and percutaneous pinning. CT is invaluable in diagnosis and surgical planning if intra-articular split fracture patterns are suspected. No advanced imaging is required if a true flexion-type supracondylar fracture is diagnosed.

The experience of the authors of this chapter has verified the unique challenge in the treatment of flexion-type supracondylar fractures. Anticipation of the potential for difficulty in attaining reduction, the probable instability of the fracture reduction, the potential for ulnar nerve entrapment, and the potential need for open reduction dictates a unique preoperative discussion and surgical planning (**Figure 2**). Rather than a sterile-towel and sterile-glove approach, which may be acceptable for extension-type supracondylar fracture pinning, the entire surgical team prepares with full gown and glove as well as full sterile prep and drape for patients who have displaced flexion-type fractures in anticipation of the potential need for conversion to an open reduction (**Figure 3, A**). Even the most severely displaced extension-type III supracondylar fractures will typically have an intact posterior humeral periosteum that contributes to stable reduction in maximal elbow flexion and a subsequent stable platform in the reduced position in which to perform divergent lateral pinning. This is not the case for flexion-type fractures. Reduction of flexion-type fractures typically requires the elbow to be held in mid-flexion or relative extension, which renders percutaneous pinning difficult because landmarks for the percutaneous lateral entry site are obscured with the elbow in extension and there is no stable/locked position of reduction to enable a stable platform for pinning. Accordingly, the authors of this chapter initially place one or two divergent lateral pins in the center of the distal fragment with the elbow in mid-flexion before reduction is performed as described by Leitch et al[3] (**Figure 4**).

The instability of most flexion-type supracondylar fractures precludes lateral imaging with simple external rotation of the reduced humerus; therefore, swing-though lateral images with the C-arm are often required. The patient is positioned supine on the surgical table; the C-arm is positioned parallel with the surgical table to allow for AP and swing-through lateral imaging of the elbow (**Figure 3, B**). Initial correction of length and coronal alignment is attained with traction and direct manipulation of the fragment. Any inability to close the medial column reduction gap warrants consideration of open reduction

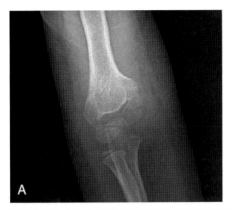
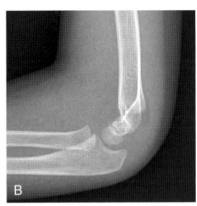

Figure 2   AP (**A**) and lateral (**B**) radiographs demonstrate a flexion-type III supracondylar humerus fracture. Note the medial column gap and associated risk for ulnar nerve entrapment at reduction. Although these static radiographs suggest minimal displacement, extreme instability was noted during reduction.

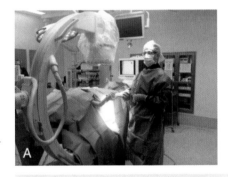
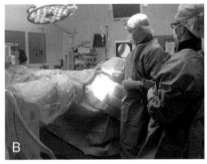

Figure 3   Photographs show the surgical suite setup for pinning of a flexion-type supracondylar fracture. Note the full prep and drape in anticipation of the potential need for open reduction (**A**) and the positioning of the fluoroscopy unit to allow for swing-through lateral imaging at time of pinning (**B**).

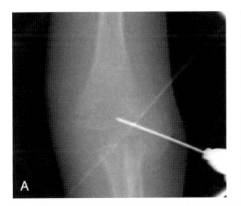
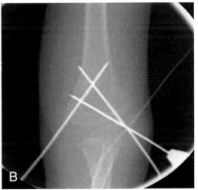
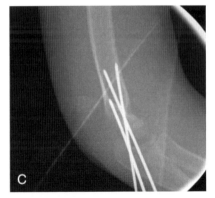

Figure 4   Intraoperative fluoroscopic images show the technique used for percutaneous pinning of a flexion-type supracondylar fracture. **A**, AP view shows the initial lateral pin placement in the distal fragment. Reduction in the coronal plane is followed by swing-through lateral imaging to enable reduction in the sagittal plane, with temporary fixation attained using an initial Kirschner wire that is driven across the fracture site. AP (**B**) and lateral (**C**) views show the final pin construct. Note the closure of the medial fracture gap.

via an anteromedial approach to enable exploration and delivery of the ulnar nerve from fracture site entrapment. The fluoroscopy unit is rotated through to obtain a lateral image, and the fracture is reduced in the sagittal plane with the use of relative elbow extension and direct manipulation of the distal fragment. After satisfactory alignment is attained in both planes, Kirschner wire(s) are driven across the fracture site and through the medial cortex of the proximal fragment. The authors of this chapter prefer to use three divergent lateral Kirschner wires for flexion-type III fractures (**Figure 1**); however, a percutaneous medial pin is routinely added if rotational instability, medial column comminution, or instability are present on live lateral fluoroscopic imaging after lateral pin placement (**Figure 4**). A long arm posterior splint or bivalve long arm cast is applied with the elbow in approximately 70° of flexion.

Follow-up radiographs are obtained 1 week postoperatively to confirm stable alignment; in addition, cast spacers are removed and the cast is overwrapped at this time. Cast and Kirschner wires are removed in the office 3 weeks postoperatively, and radiographs are obtained to confirm early fracture union, after which activities of daily living may be resumed. Routine physical therapy is not prescribed or required. Return to activities is permitted after confirmation of return of range of motion and mature radiographic fracture union, 10 to 12 weeks postoperatively.

Summary

Although flexion-type supracondylar humerus fractures account for a minority of all supracondylar humerus fractures, they warrant special attention because of their unique treatment challenges.

The literature reports a relatively high rate of requirement for open reduction and the potential for ulnar nerve injury or entrapment. Nondisplaced or minimally displaced flexion-type supracondylar humerus fractures can be treated with long arm casting for 3 weeks postoperatively. Displaced flexion-type supracondylar humerus fractures require surgical reduction and stabilization. The unique instability of and reduction position in relative extension for flexion-type supracondylar humerus fractures make reduction and pinning more challenging than the more common extension-type fracture; therefore, special considerations are required for the surgical setup and planning. The authors of this chapter caution against the use of a mini-fluoroscopy unit because frequent swing-through lateral imaging is required for flexion-type fractures. The authors of this chapter also caution against the use of the glove-only pinning technique for the treatment of flexion-type fractures because of the potential need for open reduction to resolve fracture instability or ulnar nerve entrapment. An inability to close the medial fracture gap warrants open reduction of the elbow via an anteromedial approach, with exploration and delivery of the ulnar nerve from fracture site entrapment. Although the treatment of flexion-type supracondylar fractures presents unique challenges for orthopaedic surgeons, reliably good outcomes can be expected with the prompt recognition of flexion-type injury patterns, conscientious preoperative planning, and the use of open reduction via an anteromedial approach in patients who have ulnar nerve entrapment or if reduction cannot be achieved via closed reduction.

References

1. Wenger DR, Pring ME, Rang M: Elbow—distal humerus, in *Rang's Children's Fractures*. Philadelphia, PA, Lippincott Williams & Wilkins, 2005, pp 95-118.

2. Mahan ST, May CD, Kocher MS: Operative management of displaced flexion supracondylar humerus fractures in children. *J Pediatr Orthop* 2007;27(5):551-556.

3. Leitch KK, Kay RM, Femino JD, Tolo VT, Storer SK, Skaggs DL: Treatment of multidirectionally unstable supracondylar humeral fractures in children: A modified Gartland type-IV fracture. *J Bone Joint Surg Am* 2006;88(5):980-985.

4. Kasser JR, Beaty JH: Supracondylar fractures of the distal humerus, in Beaty JH, Kasser JR, eds: *Rockwood and Wilkins' Fractures in Children*, ed 6. Philadelphia, PA, Lippincott Williams & Wilkins, 2006, pp 582-586.

5. Fowles JV, Kassab MT: Displaced supracondylar fractures of the elbow in children: A report on the fixation of extension and flexion fractures by two lateral percutaneous pins. *J Bone Joint Surg Br* 1974;56(3):490-500.

6. Hagen R: Skin-traction-treatment of supracondylar fractures of the humerus in children: A ten-year review. *Acta Orthop Scand* 1964;35:138-148.

7. Royle SG, Burke D: Ulna neuropathy after elbow injury in children. *J Pediatr Orthop* 1990;10(4):495-496.

8. Lalanandham T, Laurence WN: Entrapment of the ulnar nerve in the callus of a supracondylar fracture of the humerus. *Injury* 1984;16(2):129-130.

9. Gartland JJ: Management of supracondylar fractures of the humerus in children. *Surg Gynecol Obstet* 1959;109(2):145-154.

10. el-Ahwany MD: Supracondylar fractures of the humerus in children with a note on the surgical correction of late cubitus varus. *Injury* 1974;6(1):45-56.

11. De Boeck H: Flexion-type supracondylar elbow fractures in children. *J Pediatr Orthop* 2001;21(4):460-463.

12. Nand S: Management of supracondylar fracture of the humerus in children. *Int Surg* 1972;57(11):893-898.

Video Reference

Koerner J, Sabharnal S: Video. Percutaneous Pinning of Supracondylar Humerus Fractures. Philadelphia, PA, 2013.

28

Transphyseal Distal Humerus Fracture

Joshua Abzug, MD
Christine Ann Ho, MD
Todd F. Ritzman, MD
Brian Brighton, MD, MPH

Abstract

Transphyseal distal humerus fractures typically occur in children younger than 3 years secondary to birth trauma, nonaccidental trauma, or a fall from a small height. Prompt and accurate diagnosis of a transphyseal distal humerus fracture is crucial for a successful outcome. Recognizing that the forearm is not aligned with the humerus on plain radiographs may aid in the diagnosis of a transphyseal distal humerus fracture. Surgical management is most commonly performed with the aid of an arthrogram. Closed reduction and percutaneous pinning techniques similar to those used for supracondylar humerus fractures are employed. Cubitus varus caused by a malunion, osteonecrosis of the medial condyle, or growth arrest is the most common complication encountered in the treatment of transphyseal distal humerus fractures. A corrective lateral closing wedge osteotomy can be performed to restore a nearly normal carrying angle.

Instr Course Lect 2016;65:379–384.

Transphyseal distal humerus fractures, which are commonly referred to as transphyseal separations, are uncommon injuries. Transphyseal distal humerus fractures typically occur in children younger than 3 years. Visualization of transphyseal distal humerus fractures on plain radiographs is difficult because most of the distal humerus is composed of cartilage. As a result, these injuries are often mistaken for elbow dislocations; however, elbow dislocations almost never occur in children younger than 3 years because their cartilaginous physis is weaker than their bone-ligament interface, which predisposes them to physeal fractures rather than ligament disruptions and dislocations.

Transphyseal distal humerus fractures can occur during the birthing process (**Figure 1**). Typically, transphyseal distal humerus fractures can result from the forces of labor during a vaginal delivery or from the obstetric maneuvers used to deliver a baby, especially if a shoulder dystocia is present and/or the delivery is traumatic.[1,2] Transphyseal distal humerus fractures also can occur during a cesarean section and may be related to excessive traction.[2,3] Nonaccidental trauma also has been reported as a cause of transphyseal separation.[4-8] In these patients, a rotational force and twisting mechanism are the suspected mechanisms of injury because the physis is biomechanically the weakest location about the distal humerus.[5] In addition, a fall onto an outstretched hand with the elbow extended can result in a transphyseal distal humerus fracture.

Dr. Abzug or an immediate family member is a member of a speakers' bureau or has made paid presentations on behalf of Checkpoint Surgical, and serves as a paid consultant to AxoGen. Dr. Ho or an immediate family member serves as a board member, owner, officer, or committee member of the Pediatric Orthopaedic Society of North America. Dr. Ritzman or an immediate family member is a member of a speakers' bureau or has made paid presentations on behalf of OrthoPediatrics; serves as an unpaid consultant to Apto Orthopaedics/Austen BioInnovation Institute in Akron; and has stock or stock options held in Apto Orthopaedics. Dr. Brighton or an immediate family member serves as a paid consultant to DePuy, and serves as a board member, owner, officer, or committee member of the Pediatric Orthopaedic Society of North America and the American College of Surgeons.

© 2016 AAOS Instructional Course Lectures, Volume 65

379

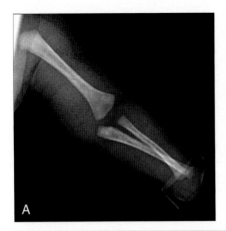 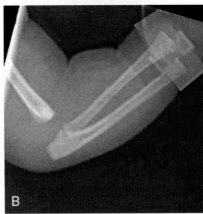

Figure 1 AP (**A**) and lateral (**B**) radiographs of the elbow of a 5-day-old boy who sustained a transphyseal separation during the birthing process. Note that the forearm is not aligned with the humeral shaft. (Courtesy of Joshua Abzug, MD, Baltimore, MD.)

Diagnosis

The presentation of a transphyseal distal humerus fracture varies somewhat based on the age of the child and the index of suspicion for the injury. Misdiagnosis or a delayed diagnosis (even up to 1 week) is quite common.[4,9] Both radiologists and emergency department physicians commonly misdiagnose transphyseal separations as supracondylar humerus fractures, condylar and epicondylar fractures, and suspected infections.[2,4]

In newborns, the index of suspicion for a transphyseal distal humerus fracture must be high. Newborns will initially be irritable and inconsolable. Swelling and/or ecchymosis may be present about the elbow region, and the infant will likely have pseudoparalysis or diminished spontaneous movement of the extremity.[2-4] Neurovascular compromise is rare.

In toddlers, transphyseal distal humerus fractures commonly occur secondary to a fall from a small height, such as from a bed or chair or down the stairs.[2,4] A transphyseal distal humerus fracture also may occur if a child jumps or falls on a younger child's elbow.[2] The child will have pain in the elbow region and limited use of the extremity. Typically, the child will be neurovascularly intact.

Because of the potential association of transphyseal distal humerus fractures with nonaccidental trauma, a detailed discussion on the mechanism of injury and a careful review of the child's medical and fracture history are imperative. Unwitnessed injuries, inconsistent explanations for the mechanism of injury, and a history of multiple injuries should raise concern for nonaccidental trauma. In addition, a complete physical examination to identify other potential injuries, such as bruising, healing burns, bite marks, or any other areas of bony tenderness, is mandatory. If concern for nonaccidental trauma exists, a skeletal survey should be performed and the child-abuse team and social services department should be consulted.

Imaging

Plain radiography is the first-line imaging modality for a patient who has a suspected transphyseal distal humerus fracture. In the case of an infant or toddler who has a suspected injury about the elbow, plain radiographs of the elbow, forearm, and arm should be obtained. It is important to obtain true AP and lateral images of each area, especially the elbow, to appropriately diagnose the injury. "Baby grams," or radiographs of the entire extremity, often lead to missed diagnoses or the inability to completely assess the injury pattern. Radiographs of the elbow should be centered on the elbow; the same is true for centering the forearm and humerus on their respective radiographs.

Because ossification of the distal humerus is not typically present in young children who sustain physeal injuries of the distal humerus, the key to diagnosis of transphyseal distal humerus fractures on plain radiographs is recognizing that the forearm is not aligned with the humeral shaft (**Figures 1** and **2**). The forearm is most commonly displaced posteromedially, unlike most elbow dislocations, which are displaced posterolaterally. If the capitellum ossification center is present, it will be aligned with the shaft of the radius, which makes the diagnosis of a transphyseal distal humerus injury definitive; this is best visualized on AP radiographs. Other potential findings on plain radiographs include soft-tissue swelling and/or signs of joint effusion, such as a posterior fat pad sign. In a study of children with a displaced fracture in whom plain radiographs were obtained within 2 days of injury, Gilbert and Conklin[4] reported a posterior fat pad sign in all of the children; however, none had an anterior fat pad sign.

It is important for orthopaedic surgeons to recognize that transphyseal distal humerus injuries are often missed on

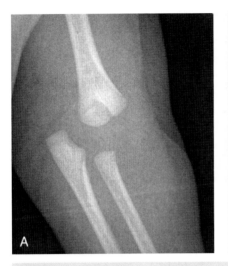

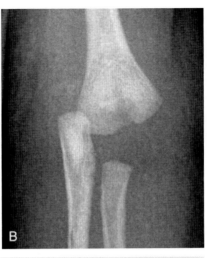

Figure 2   Oblique (**A**) and AP (**B**) plain radiographs of the elbow demonstrate that the forearm is not aligned with the humerus, which is characteristic of a transphyseal distal humerus fracture. (Courtesy of Joshua Abzug, MD, Baltimore, MD.)

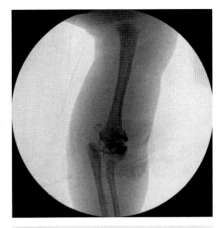

Figure 3   Elbow arthrogram obtained in the operating room demonstrates the full extent of a transphyseal distal humerus fracture. (Courtesy of Joshua Abzug, MD, Baltimore, MD.)

plain radiography, even by radiologists; therefore, orthopaedic surgeons must carefully assess a patient's radiographs rather than relying on the radiology report alone. In a study of 16 children who had distal humeral epiphyseal separation, Supakul et al[2] reported that more than 50% of the fractures (9 of 16) were missed by the initial radiologist. Elbow dislocation was diagnosed in four patients, a supracondylar fracture was diagnosed in three patients, and the radiographs of two patients were interpreted as normal. In addition, the authors noted that true lateral radiographs of the elbow were not obtained in 10 of 16 patients; therefore, the posterior displacement of the radius and ulna could not be recognized. Furthermore, two oblique radiographs of the elbow were obtained in one child; however, the medial and posterior displacement was unapparent on both views.[2] The frequency of misdiagnosed transphyseal distal humerus fractures secondary to inadequate radiographs underscores the importance of obtaining true orthogonal radiographs of the elbow.

Alternative modalities for the assessment of a transphyseal distal humerus fracture include ultrasonography and MRI. Ultrasonography is ideal for diagnosing transphyseal distal humerus injuries because no radiation is used, no sedation is required, and it is relatively quick and inexpensive. Separation of the distal humeral epiphysis from the metaphysis can be identified by noting a lack of cartilage at the distal extent of the humeral metaphysis.[2] Furthermore, the surgeon can perform a dynamic examination to assess the instability of the epiphysis relative to the metaphysis; however, ultrasonography is dependent on the experience and availability of the ultrasonographer and radiologist. MRI requires sedation and is not always readily available; therefore, the authors of this chapter do not routinely use this imaging modality.

Elbow arthrography is another modality that can be used to diagnose a transphyseal distal humerus fracture. Elbow arthrography allows for visualization of the distal articular surface and the proximal radius (**Figure 3**). If

elbow arthrography is performed under anesthesia in the operating room, reduction and stabilization of the fracture can be performed at the same time, if necessary. Elbow arthrography is performed via either a posterolateral or direct posterior approach. In very young children (younger than 3 years), the authors of this chapter have found that it is easier to use a direct posterior approach into the olecranon fossa because it limits any potential scuffing of the articular cartilage if a posterolateral portal is used. Lateral fluoroscopic images can be obtained to ensure appropriate placement of the needle before puncturing the skin. A solution of equal parts saline and contrast is injected into the joint, and the joint is brought through a range of motion. Fluoroscopic images can then be obtained to identify the articular surfaces of the distal humerus and the proximal radius and ulna (**Figure 4**). If closed reduction and pinning are being performed, the arthrogram will aid in visualization of the pin starting points on the capitellum as well as in assessment of the quality

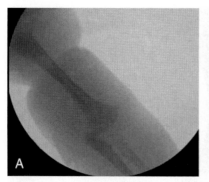
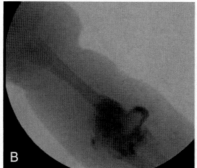
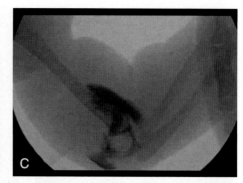

Figure 4 **A,** Intraoperative true AP fluoroscopic image of the elbow of the patient shown in Figure 1 demonstrates lack of alignment of the forearm and humeral shaft. **B** and **C,** Intraoperative arthrograms allow for clear visualization of the articular surface of the distal humerus and aid in the pinning process. (Courtesy of Joshua Abzug, MD, Baltimore, MD.)

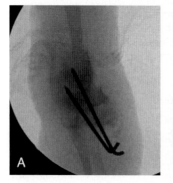
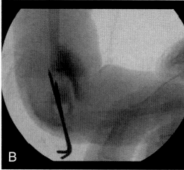
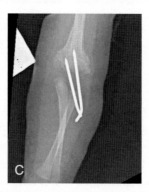
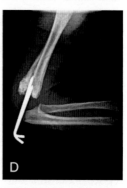

Figure 5 Intraoperative AP (**A**) and lateral (**B**) fluoroscopic images of the elbow of the patient shown in Figures 1 and 4 demonstrate near anatomic alignment after reduction and pinning. Postoperative AP (**C**) and lateral (**D**) radiographs of the elbow obtained 3 weeks postoperatively demonstrate abundant callus formation. (Courtesy of Joshua Abzug, MD, Baltimore, MD.)

of the reduction by allowing for visualization of the anterior humeral line that intersects the capitellum on lateral fluoroscopic images. The condyles can be assessed for anatomic reduction on AP fluoroscopic images (**Figure 5**).

Classification

Transphyseal distal humerus fractures are classified based on the displacement direction of the distal fragment. Posteromedial displacement is the most common injury pattern; however, there have been reports of anterior displacement as well.[9,10] The Salter-Harris classification is used to classify transphyseal distal humerus injuries. Older children (older than 3 years) typically have a metaphyseal piece attached to the distal fragment (Salter-Harris type II injuries), and younger children have pure physeal fractures (Salter-Harris type I injuries).[9] Rarely, intra-articular extension may be present (Salter-Harris type III or type IV injuries); if this occurs, differentiating between a transphyseal distal humerus fracture and a lateral condyle fracture may be difficult, and the addition of arthrography may aid in diagnosis.

Nonsurgical Management

The role of nonsurgical management is limited because transphyseal distal humerus fractures are typically displaced. Gilbert and Conklin[4] treated four patients with immobilization alone, three of whom had residual deformity and one of whom had limited motion and was then lost to follow-up. It is reasonable to treat nondisplaced or minimally displaced injuries in a splint or cast for 2 to 3 weeks. In addition, fractures that have a late presentation are best treated nonsurgically initially, with the understanding that if deformity persists or develops, an osteotomy may be required. Fractures that require reduction are best treated with stabilization after reduction to ensure adequate reduction. Furthermore, maintenance of reduction may prove difficult, especially if swelling is present and then decreases.

© 2016 AAOS Instructional Course Lectures, Volume 65

Surgical Management

Most transphyseal distal humerus fractures are best managed via closed reduction and percutaneous pinning, with the aid of an elbow arthrogram. Reduction parameters for transphyseal distal humerus fractures are similar to those for supracondylar fractures—no cubitus varus is acceptable, the anterior humeral line should bisect the capitellum (visualized on the arthrogram), and no malrotation should be present. The procedure is performed with the patient under general anesthesia. Because of the small size of these children, the procedure is best performed on a radiolucent table or a surgical table with a radiolucent extension to allow for easy fluoroscopic access.

The entire upper extremity is prepped and draped, and an elbow arthrogram is performed (**Figure 4**). After the arthrogram, the direction of displacement is noted, and a closed reduction is performed. The reduction maneuvers for transphyseal distal humerus fractures are similar to those for supracondylar fractures (ie, gentle traction, correction of translation/malrotation, then elbow flexion); however, very little force is typically required. In many patients, the distal fragment can be grasped between the index finger and thumb and then reduced to the remainder of the humeral shaft. Flexion of the elbow aids in maintenance of reduction and allows access to the capitellum for fracture stabilization with pins.

Stabilization of a transphyseal distal humerus fracture can be achieved with smooth pins. Two or three 0.062-inch Kirschner wires are inserted from the lateral side of the elbow in a retrograde fashion. The authors of this chapter prefer to use these large pins in small patients, even neonates, to limit loss of

reduction. The pins should be placed in a divergent manner, ensuring that they penetrate both cortices and have good spread at the fracture site. The arthrogram aids in visualization during the pinning process.

After pin placement, the elbow is extended, and fluoroscopic images are obtained to confirm adequate reduction and pin placement. Additional arthrogram solution may be necessary to aid in visualization of the articular surfaces. Live fluoroscopy is then performed as the elbow is brought through a range of motion, including flexion/extension, and varus/valgus stress is applied to the elbow to ensure its stability. The pins are then bent and cut, the arm is placed in a splint, and the child is awakened from anesthesia (**Figure 5**).

Postoperative Care

The authors of this chapter prefer to admit patients to the hospital overnight to administer 24 hours of intravenous antibiotics and monitor for compartment syndrome. Typically, pain is adequately controlled without the use of narcotics.

Patients are seen 1 week postoperatively, and radiographs are obtained to ensure maintenance of the alignment. At 3 weeks postoperatively, repeat radiographs are obtained to ensure that healing has occurred, and the pins are removed in the office. The child is allowed to perform active range of motion at this time. The authors of this chapter advise parents not to submerge the elbow in water for approximately 5 days after pin removal to limit the risk of infection at the pin tracts.

Patients are observed for at least 2 to 4 years after nonsurgical and surgical management of transphyseal distal humerus fractures because growth disturbance and/or osteonecrosis can

result in progressive deformity. True AP and lateral radiographs of the elbow must be obtained to assess for growth disturbance or osteonecrosis of the trochlea.

Outcomes

With prompt recognition and management, transphyseal distal humerus fracture outcomes are generally excellent, with ultimate return of near-full range of motion if normal growth resumes.[2-4] However, if growth disturbance, osteonecrosis, or malunion occurs as a result of the misdiagnosis of a transphyseal distal humerus fracture, cubitus varus can occur. Loss of motion, if it occurs, does not typically result in functional limitations.[4,9]

Complications

Complications associated with transphyseal distal humerus fractures are similar to those associated with supracondylar fractures of the distal humerus and include cubitus varus, growth disturbance, osteonecrosis, compartment syndrome, decreased range of motion, and neurovascular injuries. Cubitus varus, which is the most common complication, is more commonly associated with transphyseal distal humerus fractures than supracondylar fractures, with reported rates as high as 71% in a series of 21 patients.[11]

Cubitus varus deformity can result from malunion, osteonecrosis of the medial condyle, or growth arrest.[10] Because of the high risk of misdiagnosis as well as the difficulty associated with the assessment and maintenance of reduction of transphyseal distal humerus fractures, malunion is not uncommon. This is especially true for patients who undergo nonsurgical treatment and those who are treated with closed reduction alone. Correction of cubitus varus can be done with the use of a closing wedge osteotomy, which will result in a nearly normal carrying angle.[11] The authors of this chapter prefer to perform a lateral closing wedge osteotomy because the technique is straightforward, union is reliable, the lateral prominence is asymptomatic and often unrecognized, and the complication rate is lower compared with other more complex osteotomies (eg, step-cut or dome osteotomy).[12]

Growth disturbance is a complication somewhat unique to transphyseal distal humerus separations. The forces that cause transphyseal distal humerus fracture can damage the cartilaginous precursor of the distal humerus and its vascular supply, which may lead to abnormal development and growth of the elbow. Typically, growth disturbance manifests as progressive cubitus varus (similar to growth disturbance associated with osteonecrosis of the medial condyle);[10] however, other abnormalities, such as joint irregularities, other angular deformities, and limb-length discrepancy, may occur. Corrective osteotomies and lengthening procedures can be used to address these complications. The practice of the authors of this chapter is to observe these children for several years, even after identification of a growth disturbance, to identify any progressive changes that occur,

with the hope of being able to address all the issues during a single surgical procedure. Furthermore, surgery and postoperative care are more easily undertaken if the extremity is larger and the child is more cooperative, typically after age 5 years.

Summary

Transphyseal distal humerus fractures are rare injuries. Prompt recognition and appropriate treatment, typically via closed reduction and percutaneous pinning with the aid of an arthrogram, usually result in excellent outcomes; however, disruption of the blood supply or growth arrest can result in complications, most commonly cubitus varus. A lateral closing wedge osteotomy can be performed to treat cubitus varus and restore a nearly normal carrying angle.

References

1. Barrett WP, Almquist EA, Staheli LT: Fracture separation of the distal humeral physis in the newborn. *J Pediatr Orthop* 1984;4(5):617-619.

2. Supakul N, Hicks RA, Caltoum CB, Karmazyn B: Distal humeral epiphyseal separation in young children: An often-missed fracture-radiographic signs and ultrasound confirmatory diagnosis. *AJR Am J Roentgenol* 2015;204(2):W192-W198.

3. Kamaci S, Danisman M, Marangoz S: Neonatal physeal separation of distal humerus during cesarean section. *Am J Orthop (Belle Mead NJ)* 2014;43(11):E279-E281.

4. Gilbert SR, Conklin MJ: Presentation of distal humerus physeal separation. *Pediatr Emerg Care* 2007;23(11):816-819.

5. Shrader MW: Pediatric supracondylar fractures and pediatric physeal elbow fractures. *Orthop Clin North Am* 2008;39(2):163-171, v.

6. Nimkin K, Kleinman PK, Teeger S, Spevak MR: Distal humeral physeal injuries in child abuse: MR imaging and ultrasonography findings. *Pediatr Radiol* 1995;25(7):562-565.

7. Hansen M, Weltzien A, Blum J, Botterill NJ, Rommens PM: Complete distal humeral epiphyseal separation indicating a battered child syndrome: A case report. *Arch Orthop Trauma Surg* 2008;128(9):967-972.

8. Merten DF, Kirks DR, Ruderman RJ: Occult humeral epiphyseal fracture in battered infants. *Pediatr Radiol* 1981;10(3):151-154.

9. de Jager LT, Hoffman EB: Fracture-separation of the distal humeral epiphysis. *J Bone Joint Surg Br* 1991;73(1):143-146.

10. Oh CW, Park BC, Ihn JC, Kyung HS: Fracture separation of the distal humeral epiphysis in children younger than three years old. *J Pediatr Orthop* 2000;20(2):173-176.

11. Abe M, Ishizu T, Nagaoka T, Onomura T: Epiphyseal separation of the distal end of the humeral epiphysis: A follow-up note. *J Pediatr Orthop* 1995;15(4):426-434.

12. Kumar K, Sharma VK, Sharma R, Maffulli N: Correction of cubitus varus by French or dome osteotomy: A comparative study. *J Trauma* 2000;49(4):717-721.

© 2016 AAOS Instructional Course Lectures, Volume 65

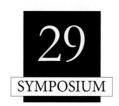

Common Errors in the Management of Pediatric Supracondylar Humerus Fractures and Lateral Condyle Fractures

Gurpal S. Pannu, MD

Craig P. Eberson, MD

Joshua Abzug, MD

Bernard D. Horn, MD

Donald S. Bae, MD

Martin Herman, MD

Abstract

Supracondylar humerus fractures and lateral condyle fractures are the two most common pediatric elbow fractures that require surgical intervention. Although most surgeons are familiar with supracondylar humerus fractures and lateral condyle fractures, these injuries present challenges that may lead to common errors in evaluation and management and, thus, compromise outcomes. It is well agreed upon that nondisplaced supracondylar fractures (Gartland type I) are best managed nonsurgically with cast immobilization. Errors may be made, however, in the treatment of type II fractures because the extent of displacement and instability are difficult to assess. Although some type II fractures are stable after closed reduction, many are not and benefit from closed reduction and percutaneous pinning to prevent late displacement and cubitus varus deformity. Stable fixation must be achieved and errors related to pin placement must be avoided to prevent the failure of type III fractures after closed reduction and percutaneous pinning. Many potential errors and pitfalls also are seen in the management of lateral condyle fractures. Radiographic assessment of displacement can be improved by obtaining an internal oblique view of the elbow. Surgical treatment with closed reduction and percutaneous pinning may be indicated for minimally displaced fractures (2 to 4 mm) that show evidence of increasing displacement over time or demonstrate intra-articular extension on an arthrogram. Displaced fractures are best treated with open reduction and internal fixation. Errors in surgical dissection, fracture reduction, and fixation are common and may result in osteonecrosis, malunion, and nonunion.

Instr Course Lect 2016;65:385–398.

Pediatric Supracondylar Humerus Fractures

Supracondylar humerus fractures represent 85% of all pediatric elbow fractures.[1] The annual incidence of pediatric supracondylar humerus fractures has been reported to be as high as 177 per 100,000, and these injuries are most commonly sustained in children aged 4 to 9 years.[2] In 98% of patients, supracondylar humerus injuries are the result of a fall onto an outstretched hand. Some studies have hypothesized that the increasing incidence of supracondylar humerus fractures may be attributed to recent trends in sports and leisure activities.[3,4] Most of these fractures demonstrate little to no long-term deformity or functional disability; however, loss of motion, deformity of the distal humerus, neurovascular injury,

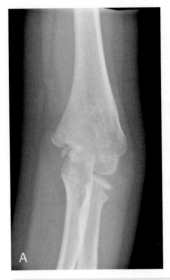
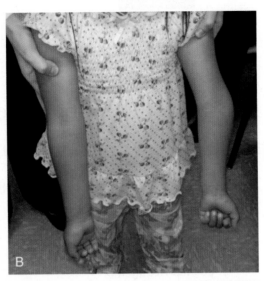

Figure 1 AP radiograph (**A**) and clinical photograph (**B**) of a 6-year-old girl who sustained a type III supracondylar humerus fracture 2 years ago demonstrate posttraumatic cubitus varus with a classic gunstock deformity noted on physical examination.

and Volkmann contracture all are potential complications that may result from supracondylar humerus fractures. It is important that surgeons understand the principles and techniques for the fixation of supracondylar humerus fractures to avoid errors specifically related to the misidentification of unstable fracture patterns and inadequate fixation. Both of these errors may result in malunion, which most commonly results in a cubitus varus deformity (**Figure 1**).

Background

Most supracondylar humerus fractures result after a fall from a height. A hyperextension force after a fall onto an outstretched hand causes the olecranon to act as a fulcrum. The distal humeral attachment of the anterior capsule applies a further anterior tension force. The distal humerus ultimately fails anteriorly, in the relatively thin supracondylar region. This results in the more common extension-type fracture. The less frequently encountered flexion-type

injury occurs after a fall directly onto a flexed elbow.[5,6] The age of the patient tends to correlate with the exact mechanism of injury. In a review of 391 supracondylar humerus fractures, Farnsworth et al[3] reported that children younger than 2 years were most likely to sustain a fracture after falling off a piece of furniture. Older children were much more likely to sustain an injury on playground equipment. Of all supracondylar humerus fractures in children between age 4 and 5 years, 44% occurred in the playground setting. The monkey bars were by far the most dangerous playground equipment, accounting for 25% of fractures in this age group. Less common mechanisms of injury included ground-level falls and bicycle-, skateboard-, and roller-skate–related injuries.

Classification

Gartland[7] initially described extension-type supracondylar humerus fractures based on the degree of displacement. The Gartland classification system is widely used for extension-type fractures, which represent 98% to 99% of all supracondylar humerus fractures.[1,8] Type I fractures typically have a visible fracture line but no displacement. In addition, a radiograph that demonstrates a positive posterior fat pad sign with no identifiable fracture line is often classified as a type I fracture. Type II fractures have an extension deformity of the distal fragment with an intact or hinged posterior cortex, and, essentially, are a greenstick fracture of the distal humerus. Type III fractures are extension-type injuries that result in complete displacement and demonstrate no intact posterior cortex. In addition to classifying the fracture types, the Gartland classification also

Dr. Eberson or an immediate family member has received royalties from Globus Medical; is a member of a speakers' bureau or has made paid presentations on behalf of Stryker Spine and Orthofix Spine; serves as a paid consultant to Orthofix; and serves as a board member, owner, officer, or committee member of the Scoliosis Research Society and the Pediatric Orthopaedic Society of North America. Dr. Abzug is a member of a speakers' bureau or has made paid presentations on behalf of Checkpoint Surgical, and serves as a paid consultant to AxoGen. Dr. Horn or an immediate family member has stock or stock options held in Johnson & Johnson, and serves as a board member, owner, officer, or committee member of the American Academy of Orthopaedic Surgeons. Dr. Bae or an immediate family member has stock or stock options held in Cempra, Johnson & Johnson, Kythera Biopharmaceuticals, and Vivus, and serves as a board member, owner, officer, or committee member of the American Academy of Orthopaedic Surgeons, the American Society for Surgery of the Hand, and the Pediatric Orthopaedic Society of North America. Dr. Herman or an immediate family member serves as a board member, owner, officer, or committee member of the Pediatric Orthopaedic Society of North America. Neither Dr. Pannu nor any immediate family member has received anything of value from or has stock or stock options held in a commercial company or institution related directly or indirectly to the subject of this chapter.

guides treatment. Traditional teaching is that type I fractures are treated in a cast, type II fractures are treated with closed reduction and cast immobilization of the elbow, and type III fractures are best treated with closed reduction and percutaneous pinning (CRPP).

Two proposed modifications of the Gartland classification are worth noting. Wilkins[9] introduced a subset of type II fractures that demonstrate rotational and translational displacement and labeled these as type IIB fractures. Type IIA fractures are generally amenable to reduction and cast immobilization; however, type IIB fractures are best treated with CRPP. Leitch et al[10] added a type IV supracondylar fracture that appears similar to an extension type III fracture on injury radiographs, but exhibits instability in both flexion and extension during reduction. Type IV fractures represent a complete disruption of the posterior periosteal hinge, which normally is intact in type III injuries. A type IV fracture insinuates a high-energy mechanism of injury and requires a modification of the standard CRPP technique that is employed for type III fractures.

Diagnosis

Patients will typically have a swollen, tender elbow after a fall onto an outstretched hand. Point tenderness over the medial and lateral columns suggests a supracondylar humerus fracture. Puckering of the anterior skin often occurs if the proximal fracture fragment pierces the brachialis muscle and engages the deep dermis. The presence of puckering suggests substantial underlying soft-tissue damage. Any bleeding or a punctate wound should be regarded as a sign of an open fracture.[5]

A detailed neurologic and vascular examination is absolutely critical if the patient is examined in the emergency department. The distal pulse, capillary refill, warmth, and color of the injured extremity should be assessed. Neurologic examination includes sensory testing in the radial, ulnar, and median nerve distributions. Sensory examination is best assessed in the first dorsal web space, palmar little finger, and palmar index finger, respectively. Motor examination of the radial/posterior interosseous nerve can be assessed by active wrist, finger, and thumb extension. Active thumb interphalangeal flexion and distal interphalangeal flexion of the index finger test the anterior interosseous nerve. Finally, interossei function assesses the ulnar nerve, and thenar strength tests the recurrent median motor nerve.

The clinician should be suspicious of a developing compartment syndrome if a tense volar forearm compartment, skin puckering, absent pulse, and substantial discomfort with passive flexion and extension of the digits are present. The risk of compartment syndrome is higher with concomitant fracture of the same extremity.

Initial radiographic evaluation consists of AP and lateral elbow radiographs. Because supracondylar humerus injuries most often occur after a fall onto an outstretched hand, the surgeon should obtain radiographs of the entire humerus and forearm to identify any coexisting injury. Although plain radiographs are adequate for the diagnosis and management of most supracondylar humerus fractures, CT may aid in the preoperative planning for a comminuted or intra-articular fracture. MRI does not have a role in the acute management of supracondylar humerus injuries.

Management

Type I Fractures

Nonsurgical management of type I supracondylar humerus fractures is well agreed upon. Cast immobilization with the elbow held in 90° of flexion for 3 to 4 weeks reliably yields excellent outcomes without complications.

Type II Fractures

The management of type II supracondylar fractures is more controversial than the management of type I supracondylar fractures. The Wilkins modification emphasizes the importance of rotation and translation on postreduction instability. An extension-type II fracture pattern without any evidence of rotation or translation may be appropriately treated with closed reduction. It is important that the elbow be immobilized in flexion greater than 90° to decrease the risk of fracture redisplacement. Follow-up radiographs should be obtained 5 to 7 days postoperatively to identify a loss of reduction. A type II fracture with evidence of rotation or translation (Wilkins type IIB) may be similarly treated; however, the risk of displacement in a cast is greater for Wilkins type IIB fractures compared with that for classic Gartland type II and Wilkins type IIA fractures.

Errors for Type II Fractures

Because it may be extremely difficult to confidently exclude a rotational or translational deformity in some type II supracondylar humerus fractures on standard injury radiographs, surgeons commonly underestimate the degree of instability (**Figure 2**). In one study, as many as 25% of type II fractures that were treated with closed reduction and casting lost reduction in the cast after an acceptable closed reduction.[11] If the

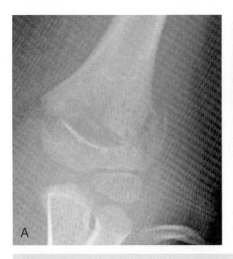
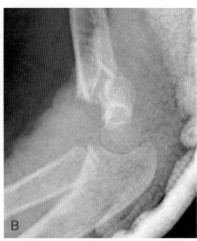

Figure 2   Radiographs of the elbow of a 5-year-old boy who fell from the monkey bars and sustained a type IIB supracondylar humerus fracture. **A,** AP view demonstrates translational and rotational displacement of the distal fragment. **B,** Lateral view demonstrates cortical contact at the fracture site.

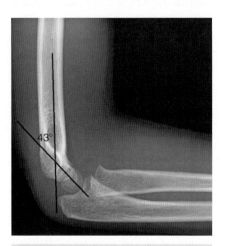

Figure 3   Lateral radiograph of an elbow demonstrates measurement of the shaft-condylar angle that is formed by the intersection of the humeral shaft and condylar axis.

authors of this chapter cannot readily identify a stable fracture pattern (type IIA) on radiographs, then the fracture is examined under fluoroscopy in the operating room. Injuries that are confirmed as type IIA and are stable after closed reduction are casted. Type IIA fractures that have instability and all type IIB fractures are treated with CRPP. CRPP also is indicated for all

type IIA fractures that have medial column comminution, which will result in cubitus varus deformity without reduction and fixation. Published results confirm the safety and efficacy of this approach.[12]

Type III Fractures

CRPP is universally accepted for all type III supracondylar humerus fractures. Surgical fixation of most type III injuries may be delayed for up to 8 to 12 hours, with the most common scenario being overnight admission, careful neurovascular monitoring, and surgery early the next morning. Some type III injuries, including open fractures, fractures associated with an abnormal vascular examination or a complete median nerve palsy, fractures with puckering in the antecubital fossa or severe swelling of the elbow and forearm, and supracondylar fractures that occur concomitantly with an ipsilateral forearm or wrist fracture (floating elbow), require emergency surgical treatment. The fracture is carefully reduced under general anesthesia and with the aid of

fluoroscopic imaging. In practice, acceptable reduction in the coronal plane consists of no varus malalignment and valgus deformity within 5° to 10° of the unaffected elbow's carrying angle. Sagittal alignment is acceptable if the anterior humeral line intersects the capitellum.[13] For children younger than 4 years, the anterior humeral line generally intersects the anterior third of the capitellum. For older children, the anterior humeral line intersects the middle third of the capitellum.[14] Another method to confirm sagittal reduction involves measuring the shaft-condylar angle, which is formed by the intersection of the humeral shaft and condylar axis, on a lateral radiograph (**Figure 3**). This angle should be approximately 40°. Residual translation of the distal fragment, less than 25% in either plane, is acceptable as long as the previously mentioned reduction criteria are met.[5]

After reduction is complete, CRPP is performed. The authors of this chapter generally fix type II supracondylar fractures with two pins and type III fractures with three pins. In general, the authors of this chapter use 5/64-in pins in children older than 8 to 10 years and 0.062-mm pins in children younger than 10 years. All pins are placed laterally, unless severe lateral skin abrasions are present, in which case a medial/lateral cross-pin configuration is used.[12,15] The wires must achieve bicortical fixation and, ideally, span both the medial and lateral columns of the distal humerus. This is best achieved by placing divergent pins that are maximally spread at the fracture site in both the AP and lateral planes (**Figure 4**). Because of the risk of ulnar nerve injury, medial pins are almost never used; however, an exception exists if lateral pins alone do not achieve stability of

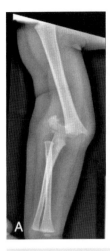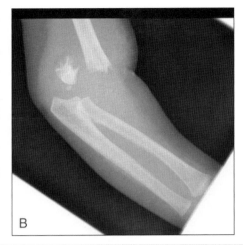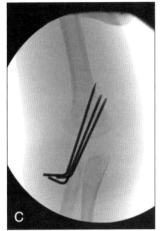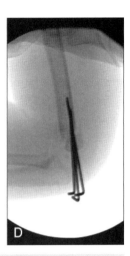

Figure 4   AP (**A**) and lateral (**B**) radiographs of the elbow of a 16-month-old girl who sustained a type III supracondylar humerus fracture after falling off a couch. AP (**C**) and lateral (**D**) fluoroscopic images demonstrate that adequate reduction and ideal pin configuration was achieved with closed reduction and percutaneous pinning.

the fracture, if substantial medial column comminution is present, or in the presence of lateral skin abrasions. Medial pin placement is performed with the elbow held in extension. It is the practice of the authors of this chapter to perform medial pin placement via a small incision that allows for identification of the ulnar nerve so that it may be avoided when driving the pin. After placement, the pins are bent and left outside the skin. After fixation is achieved, the stability of the construct is assessed by flexing and extending the elbow under fluoroscopy.

Errors for Type III Fractures

Two substantial errors must be avoided in the treatment of type III supracondylar humerus fractures: inappropriate delay of care and failure to achieve adequate stability of the fracture. Although there are benefits in delaying surgery until the pediatric orthopaedic team is well rested and assembled in the morning, the surgeon's decision to delay treatment to the next day must be made only after weighing the patient's risks for serious complications, such

as compartment syndrome and neurovascular injury. The decision to delay treatment can only be made after the patient is evaluated by a reliable orthopaedic resident or an attending physician, with care taken to document the patient's skin status, swelling about the elbow and forearm, and the neurovascular examination in detail. The injury types that are best treated emergently were discussed previously. Erring on the side of caution and treating the most severe injuries emergently will help to reduce disastrous complications, such as compartment syndrome, vascular compromise, and limb loss.

The most common error made in the management of type III supracondylar humerus fractures is failing to achieve adequate stability with CRPP (**Figure 5**). The reported loss of reduction after surgical fixation of supracondylar humerus fractures varies in the literature, but has most recently been reported to be 4.2%.[16] In a large series of unstable supracondylar fractures that were treated with CRPP, Sankar et al[17] identified three important technical errors of pin placement seen in

patients in whom reduction was lost. These errors included failure to engage the proximal fragment (eg, if the pin exits the fracture site), lack of bicortical fixation (eg, if the pin fails to engage the medial proximal humerus because of comminution or intramedullary position), and inadequate pin spread across the fracture (eg, if two pins crossing at the fracture site effectively act as one point of fixation, or failure of the pins to engage both the medial and lateral columns) (**Figure 6**). Pennock et al[16] recently published a retrospective review to identify if both patient- and surgeon-related risk factors lead to loss of postoperative fracture reduction. The authors concluded that patient sex, age, fracture severity, medial comminution, the number of pins inserted, and the use of cross-pin versus lateral-only configurations did not substantially affect the rate of reduction loss. The authors reported that the only surgeon-related variable that substantially affected the risk of reduction loss was pin spread at the fracture site. The authors reported that constructs that had only 9.7 mm of pin spread demonstrated a greater rate of displacement compared with those that had 13.7 mm of pin spread. A pin spread that is greater than one-third of the width of the humerus was reported to have a lower risk of reduction loss (**Figure 7**).

In the experience of the authors of this chapter, the rate of reduction loss after CRPP may be decreased if several important factors are carefully assessed. The surgeon should reduce the fracture as anatomically as possible to improve the stability of the pinning construct and facilitate adequate pin placement. For almost all fractures, lateral pin fixation with three pins is adequate to maintain reduction. If stability cannot be achieved after inserting three lateral pins, it is the practice of the authors of this chapter to add a fourth lateral pin or a medial pin, which is placed through the medial epicondyle with the elbow extended. Finally, after pinning, it is important that the surgeon assess all pins individually to rule out the errors described by Sankar et al[17] and then stress the construct under fluoroscopy. In the opinion of the authors of this chapter, this last step is the most important.

Care after CRPP

After CRPP, the arm is placed in a splint or bivalved cast to allow for postsurgical swelling. Patients are instructed to follow up 5 to 7 days postoperatively for a clinical examination and repeat radiographs to assess for a loss of reduction or hardware failure. Pins are removed in the office at 3 or 4 weeks postoperatively after repeat radiographs show healing. After pin removal, patients are encouraged to begin active range of motion of the elbow as tolerated. At 6 to 8 weeks after injury, most patients have regained nearly full range

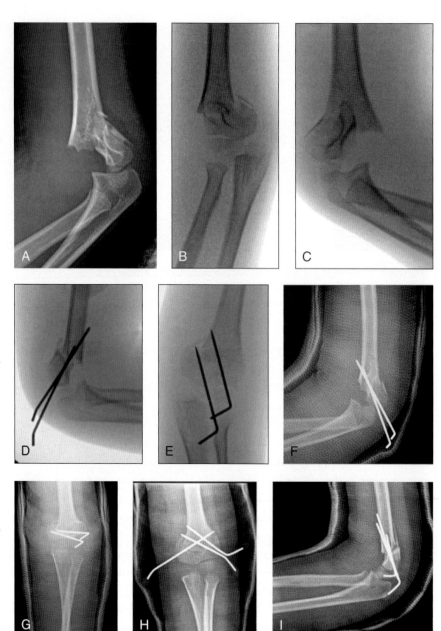

Figure 5   Lateral (**A**), AP (**B**), and oblique (**C**) radiographs of the elbow of a 6-year-old boy who fell off a bunk bed and sustained a displaced supracondylar humerus fracture. Lateral (**D**) and AP (**E**) fluoroscopic images demonstrate inadequate fixation after closed reduction and pinning. Lateral (**F**) and AP (**G**) radiographs taken at 1-week follow-up demonstrate further loss of reduction. AP (**H**) and lateral (**I**) radiographs taken after the patient underwent revised closed reduction and pinning.

of motion; for patients who have not, physical therapy may be ordered, but it generally is not needed. In general, outcomes after successful CRPP of displaced supracondylar fractures are outstanding, with most patients regaining normal function and returning to all activities 3 months after injury.

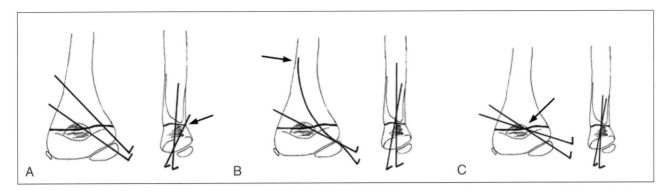

Figure 6   Illustrations show errors in pin configuration. **A,** Failure to engage the proximal fragment, which is evidenced by the pin exiting at the fracture site (arrow). **B,** Failure to achieve bicortical fixation (arrow). **C,** Failure to achieve adequate pin spread at the fracture site (arrow). (Reproduced with permission from Sankar WN, Hebela NM, Skaggs DL, Flynn JM: Loss of pin fixation in displaced supracondylar humeral fractures in children: Causes and prevention. *J Bone Joint Surg Am* 2007;89[4]:713-717.)

Pediatric Lateral Condyle Fractures

After supracondylar humerus fractures, lateral condyle fractures are the most common fracture about the pediatric elbow,[18-22] representing 10% to 20% of all pediatric elbow fractures. Pediatric lateral condyle injuries most commonly occur as a result of varus stress on a hyperextended elbow.[21] Despite the relatively high incidence of lateral condyle fractures, substantial controversy exists regarding optimal treatment. Although it is agreed that substantially displaced fractures are best treated surgically, minimally displaced and nondisplaced lateral condyle fractures present a management challenge. Some studies have reported substantial rates of displacement in attempts to treat seemingly stable lateral condyle fractures with cast immobilization alone.[23-25] The extent and stability of lateral condyle fractures may be difficult to interpret on radiographs, especially in young children who have a largely cartilaginous capitellum. The potential complications of fractures that are inadequately treated or, in some cases, even those treated with appropriate surgical intervention

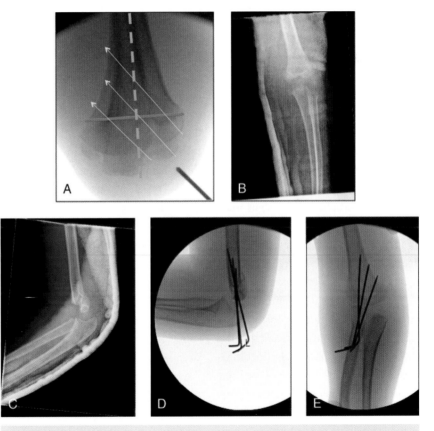

Figure 7   **A,** AP fluoroscopic image demonstrates ideal pin configuration, which consists of engagement of the proximal fragment (solid line), bicortical fixation (dashed line), and adequate pin spread at the fracture site (arrows). AP (**B**) and lateral (**C**) radiographs of the elbow of a 5-year-old boy who sustained a type IIB supracondylar humerus fracture after falling from monkey bars. Postoperative lateral (**D**) and AP (**E**) fluoroscopic images taken after the patient underwent closed reduction and percutaneous pinning demonstrate ideal construct configuration.

include malunion, nonunion, osteonecrosis, premature epiphyseal fusion, and the development of a progressive valgus deformity that results in tardy ulnar nerve palsy.[21] It is important for surgeons to understand the common errors associated with the management of pediatric lateral condyle fractures.

Background

Lateral humeral condyle fractures in children are defined as injuries in which the fracture line travels from the lateral humeral metaphysis distally and medially. The fracture line may exit into the joint either through the capitellar ossification center or medial to it, extending through the trochlear groove or through the cartilaginous trochlea.[21] Lateral humeral condyle injuries may occur after an avulsion injury from a sudden pull of the common extensor muscular attachment, which creates a varus force across the elbow. Alternatively, lateral humeral condyle injuries may result after a violent impaction of the radial head into the lateral humeral condyle and a subsequent valgus force across the elbow.

The most critical errors made in the treatment of lateral humeral condyle injuries are related to the anatomy of the osteocartilaginous distal humerus in a growing child. First, the fracture line often extends into the articular surface after traversing the often-difficult-to-visualize ossification center of the lateral condyle. Jakob et al[26] described a cartilaginous bridge at the joint level that, if intact, anchors the fracture fragment to the distal humeral epiphysis. Using MRI, Horn et al[27] demonstrated that the presence of an intact cartilaginous bridge correlated with fracture stability and subsequent healing; however, the integrity of this cartilage bridge is

impossible to determine on standard radiographs. Second, the common extensor musculature attachment on the lateral humeral metaphysis may act as a deforming force on the fracture fragment, which is likely responsible for the late displacement seen in some fractures that are initially nondisplaced.[20,24,26,28-30] Finally, complete fractures that extend through the articular surface, even if initially nondisplaced, are bathed in synovial fluid that impairs healing. Errors made related to the assessment of fracture displacement, stability, and healing potential are responsible for the most serious lateral condyle fracture complications, including nonunion and malunion.

Classification

Numerous classification systems have attempted to characterize lateral condyle fractures. The Jakob classification[26] defines type I fractures as those that are displaced less than 2 mm and have an intact articular surface. Type II fractures have displacement, but no rotation. Importantly, the cartilage hinge is disrupted. Type III fractures have a displaced and rotated fragment. The Milch[31] classification describes type I lateral condyle fractures as those that exit lateral to the trochlear groove, representing the equivalent of a type IV supracondylar humerus injury. Type II lateral condyle fractures exit medial to the trochlear groove, representing the equivalent of a type II supracondylar humerus injury and, potentially, an unstable elbow joint. Recently, Weiss et al[32] proposed a novel classification system that may be used to guide the treatment of lateral condyle fractures. Type I lateral condyle fractures are described as those that have less than 2 mm of displacement on internal

oblique radiographs. Type II fractures are those that have more than or equal to 2 to 4 mm of displacement on internal oblique radiographs. Type III fractures are those that have more than 4 mm of displacement on internal oblique radiographs (**Figure 8**). The authors recommended surgical treatment for type II and type III lateral condyle fractures; however, treatment recommendations substantially extended beyond the simple classification of the fracture types. Although almost all type III fractures were treated with open reduction and fixation because of articular surface disruption, the authors were able to demonstrate that many type II fractures had an intact articular surface with the use of intraoperative arthrography. For this subgroup of type II fractures, CRPP was an effective treatment.

Diagnosis

Patients will typically have a swollen, tender elbow and a history of a fall onto an outstretched hand. If clinical suspicion for a lateral condyle fracture exists, radiographs of the elbow should be obtained. In addition to standard AP and lateral radiographs, an internal oblique radiograph should be obtained. Song et al[22] reported that an internal oblique radiograph allows for the most accurate assessment of displacement and the fracture pattern. In a comparison of the same fracture on AP and internal oblique radiographs, the authors reported different degrees of displacement in 70% of patients (**Figure 9**). Notably, greater displacement was consistently identified on the oblique radiograph compared with the standard view. An intraoperative arthrogram may help assess articular congruity. Further imaging modalities are generally unnecessary in the initial management of lateral condyle fractures. CT and MRI may be used for treating complications of healing, such as nonunion or growth disturbance.

Management

Type I Fractures

Weiss type I fractures (<2 mm of displacement) are treated with a well-molded long arm cast. The forearm should be supinated and the wrist should be slightly dorsiflexed to minimize the pull of the common extensor musculature on the fracture fragment. It is absolutely imperative that the patient and family be educated on the importance of radiographic follow-up. Pirker et al[23] reported an 11.7% rate of displacement in minimally displaced lateral condyle fractures that were treated with immobilization (**Figure 10**). All but one fracture showed displacement within the first week. Most authors recommend elbow immobilization for a minimum of 6 weeks,[30] with discontinuation of the cast only if an examination and radiographs are consistent with a healed fracture.

Errors for Type I Fractures

Several errors are commonly made in the management of type I fractures. First, the failure to accurately identify the degree of initial displacement on AP and lateral radiographs can be avoided by obtaining an internal oblique radiograph before casting and at all subsequent visits. Second, because casts may obscure the fracture detail and make measurement or identification of change less accurate, follow-up radiographs should be ideally taken without a cast. Finally, although displacement typically occurs within the first week after injury, displacement may occur as long as

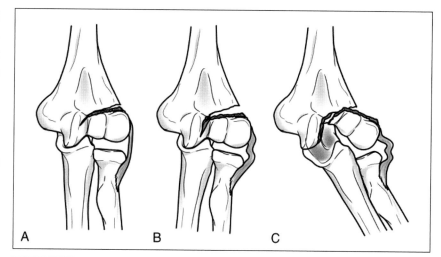

Figure 8   Three-dimensional illustrations show the Weiss classification system of lateral condyle humerus fractures. **A,** Type I fractures have less than 2 mm of displacement. **B,** Type II fractures have more than or equal to 2 to 4 mm of displacement and have a congruent articular surface. **C,** Type III fractures have more than 4 mm of displacement and loss of articular congruency.

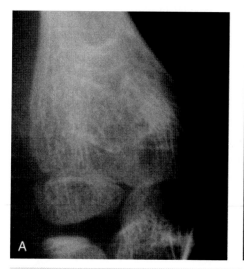
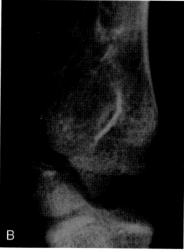

Figure 9   **A,** AP radiograph of the elbow of a 10-year-old boy demonstrates a minimally displaced fracture. **B,** Internal oblique radiograph of the elbow of the same patient demonstrates a substantially displaced fracture through the capitellum. Failure to obtain internal oblique radiographs may result in a gross underestimate of the degree of fracture displacement. (Reproduced with permission from Song KS, Kang CH, Min BW, Bae KC, Cho CH: Internal oblique radiographs for diagnosis of nondisplaced or minimally displaced lateral condyle fractures of the humerus in children. *J Bone Joint Surg Am* 2007;89[1]:58-63.)

2 weeks after injury. For this reason, the authors of this chapter obtain new radiographs weekly for the first 2 or 3 weeks after injury. Any measurable change beyond 2 mm of displacement is suspicious for an unstable fracture, and the authors of this chapter typically treat it surgically.

Type II Fractures

The authors of this chapter generally manage Weiss type II fractures surgically, in a systematic method similar to that described by Weiss et al.[32] Fractures that have more than or equal to 2 to 4 mm of displacement are best managed surgically. The true degree of displacement and joint congruity can be assessed after an intraoperative elbow arthrogram is obtained. If the fracture is hinged laterally but has an intact cartilage bridge, the surgeon may attempt closed reduction with the use of a Kirschner wire as a joystick to facilitate reduction. The wire is then advanced across the fracture site, after which additional wires are placed. Open reduction is used if closed reduction and pinning cannot restore anatomic joint congruity.[33]

Errors for Type II Fractures

Closed reduction and casting cannot be reliably used to manage fractures with more than 2 mm of displacement, which makes inappropriate nonsurgical treatment the first error to avoid in the management of type II fractures. The most substantial surgical error to avoid in the treatment of type II fractures is the acceptance of a suboptimal reduction. As stated previously, many type II fractures can be treated with arthrography-assisted closed reduction and pinning. Although closed reduction may seem to be a better option than open reduction because it is less invasive, joint incongruity and failure to achieve adequate reduction may result in malunion, which represents a much worse outcome for patients. The authors of this chapter err on the side of open reduction if they cannot achieve an anatomic closed reduction or are having difficulty assessing the reduction. The technique used

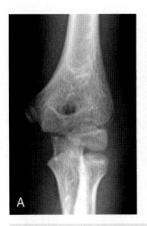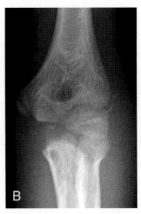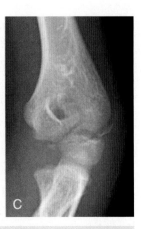

Figure 10   **A,** AP radiograph of the elbow of an 8-year-old boy who fell from monkey bars demonstrates a minimally displaced lateral condyle fracture. Follow-up AP (**B**) and internal oblique (**C**) radiographs taken 1 week after the injury demonstrate characteristic late displacement of the fracture.

for open reduction of type II fractures is identical to that for type III fractures.

Type III Fractures

Fractures that have more than 4 mm of displacement as well as those that have obvious malrotation or substantial anterior or lateral displacement are best treated with open reduction and fixation. The fragment is exposed with a lateral Kocher-type elbow incision, taking care to avoid stripping the posterior soft-tissue attachments. After the anterior joint surface is visualized, anatomic reduction of the joint surface is performed and held in place as wires are introduced, either through the wound or, ideally, percutaneously, to achieve stable fixation. Typically, three wires are necessary to achieve stable fixation. Stability is confirmed before wound closure by visualizing the reduction during elbow flexion and extension. Pins may be bent and cut outside the skin or buried, based on surgeon preference.

Errors for Type III Fractures

Three important errors of open treatment are crucial to avoid. First, excessive posterior stripping of the soft tissue

from the lateral condyle fragment or posterior distal metaphysis may disrupt the blood supply to the fragment, which may lead to osteonecrosis and joint deformity. Posterior dissection should be avoided to minimize this risk. Second, exposure must be extensile enough to allow for visualization of the joint line (**Figure 11**). Confirmation of an anatomic reduction by looking only at the metaphyseal displacement may not always be accurate because comminution or plastic deformation may be present at the fracture site. Third, the pins should be removed no sooner than 4 weeks postoperatively, and the elbow should be immobilized in a long arm cast for 6 to 8 weeks postoperatively. After open reduction, it is critical that radiographic confirmation of healing is obtained before immobilization is discontinued. Although elbow stiffness is a concern, fracture healing is more important than early range of motion.

Complications
Nonunion, Malunion, and Osteonecrosis

Nonunion of a lateral humeral condyle fracture is a serious complication and

                                          © 2016 AAOS Instructional Course Lectures, Volume 65

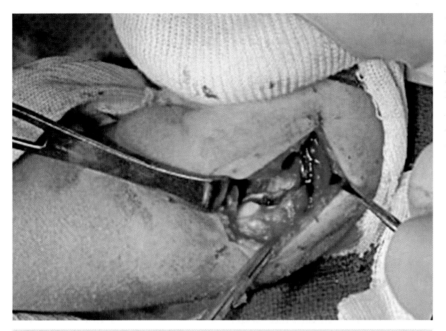

Figure 11   Intraoperative photograph shows open reduction of a displaced lateral condyle fracture. Adequate exposure allows for visualization of joint line congruity, and the avoidance of extensive posterior dissection preserves blood flow to the fracture fragment.

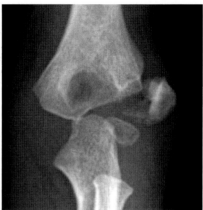

Figure 12   AP radiograph of the elbow of an 8-year-old boy taken 8 months after he sustained a lateral condyle humerus fracture after falling off a bicycle demonstrates a nonunion of the fracture.

may result in a progressive cubitus valgus deformity and subsequent tardy ulnar nerve palsy.[21,34] Patients may have pain and instability up to 15 to 20 years after the initial injury.[21] The relatively high rate of nonunion is likely related to the pull of the extensor musculature on the fracture fragment,[20,24,26,28-30] the intra-articular nature of the fracture with subsequent exposure to synovial fluid, and the relatively tenuous metaphyseal bloody supply[35] (**Figure 12**). Malunion[36] is very uncommon but may manifest as cubitus varus from the healing of a hinged fragment with residual displacement or from joint incongruity that is caused by poor reduction during the surgical fixation of a displaced fracture. Premature cartilage wear can result from osteonecrosis and/or growth disturbance of the distal humerus, which may lead to cartilage insufficiency and joint deformities, most commonly the so-called fishtail deformity.

Lateral Spur Formation

The most common complication in the management of lateral humeral condyle fractures is the formation of a lateral metaphyseal bump, which may be a concern for the patient and family. Pribaz et al[37] reported that a lateral spur developed in 73% of lateral humeral condyle fractures (**Figure 13**). The authors reported that the size of the metaphyseal overgrowth was proportional to the degree of initial displacement. No functional disability or range of motion deficit was reported in patients in whom a lateral spur developed. The patient and family should be counseled on the possible formation of a functionally benign lateral bump.

Managing Complications

The most challenging complications are related to nonunion and malunion of unstable lateral condyle fractures. The best way to avoid nonunion and

malunion is to consider anatomic reduction and stable fixation for fractures with more than 2 mm of displacement.[28,32] Although this may seem to be an aggressive approach, it is the opinion of the authors of this chapter that nonsurgical management is an error to be avoided for lateral condyle fractures with more than 2 mm of displacement. Another critical error to avoid is the failure to confirm radiographic healing at follow-up for all lateral condyle fractures, regardless of initial displacement and the method of treatment. Range of motion returns to normal for most patients, even for those who have incomplete healing or nonunion. The burial of pins for later removal and prolonged cast immobilization, sometimes for as long as 3 to 4 months, are other strategies that have been used to achieve union. If identified early, delayed union is easier to manage than a nonunion associated with progressive valgus deformity and tardy ulnar nerve palsy. Delayed union and nonunions that occur within several months of

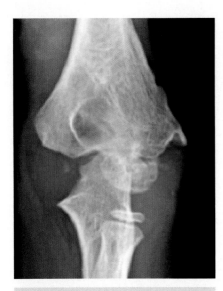

Figure 13 AP radiograph of the elbow of a 9-year-old boy demonstrates a healed lateral condyle fracture. The lateral metaphyseal overgrowth was asymptomatic.

injury may be treated with curettage, bone grafting, and pin or screw fixation, and nonunions diagnosed later also may require osteotomy and ulnar nerve transposition. Some patients who have osteonecrosis and growth disturbances with deformity may be amenable to salvage procedures, such as elbow arthroscopy with chondral procedures or osteotomies.[38] The concerns of families may be allayed more easily if the possibility of lateral spurring and its benign nature are explained before the onset of treatment. Radiographic follow-up is warranted for nearly all patients, regardless of clinical signs and symptoms, at yearly intervals for a minimum of 2 years after surgery to ensure that complications are identified and managed in an appropriate and timely fashion.

Summary

Supracondylar humerus fractures are the elbow fractures that most frequently occur in children. If treated appropriately, most supracondylar humerus fractures confer no long-term functional or cosmetic deformity to the patient. The most common long-term complication of supracondylar humerus fractures, a cubitus varus deformity, frequently results from errors that may be avoided. Closed reduction and cast immobilization of type II fractures that are unstable is a common error that leads to deformity. A type II fracture with any evidence of translation or malrotation is best treated with CRPP. All type III fractures are best treated with CRPP using bicortical pins that are spread widely at the fracture site and should demonstrate stability under fluoroscopic examination. Adherence to these basic surgical principles will, in most patients, allow the surgeon to achieve a stable construct and minimize the risk of postoperative reduction loss.

Pediatric lateral humeral condyle fractures present a challenge for orthopaedic surgeons and are associated with many common management errors. The accurate measurement of displacement and careful surveillance for even subtle changes in fracture reduction are critical steps to prevent malunion and nonunion. Although controversial, it is the opinion of the authors of this chapter that the most crucial mistake made in the management of displaced or unstable lateral humeral condyle fractures with more than or equal to 2 to 4 mm of displacement is failure to achieve anatomic reduction. Errors of technique that should be avoided include excessive posterior stripping of the lateral condyle fragment, inadequate exposure that leads to poor reduction, and inadequate duration of wire fixation and immobilization after surgery. Careful surveillance after injury is imperative and may improve the outcomes of complication management and allow for counseling of families regarding potential problems that may occur.

References

1. Shrader MW: Pediatric supracondylar fractures and pediatric physeal elbow fractures. *Orthop Clin North Am* 2008;39(2):163-171, v.

2. Houshian S, Mehdi B, Larsen MS: The epidemiology of elbow fracture in children: Analysis of 355 fractures, with special reference to supracondylar humerus fractures. *J Orthop Sci* 2001;6(4):312-315.

3. Farnsworth CL, Silva PD, Mubarak SJ: Etiology of supracondylar humerus fractures. *J Pediatr Orthop* 1998;18(1):38-42.

4. Brauer CA, Lee BM, Bae DS, Waters PM, Kocher MS: A systematic review of medial and lateral entry pinning versus lateral entry pinning for supracondylar fractures of the humerus. *J Pediatr Orthop* 2007;27(2):181-186.

5. Beaty JH, Kasser JR, eds: *Rockwood and Wilkins' Fractures in Children,* ed 7. Philadelphia, PA, Lippincott, Williams & Wilkins, 2010.

6. Brubacher JW, Dodds SD: Pediatric supracondylar fractures of the distal humerus. *Curr Rev Musculoskelet Med* 2008;1(3-4):190-196.

7. Gartland JJ: Management of supracondylar fractures of the humerus in children. *Surg Gynecol Obstet* 1959;109(2):145-154.

8. Cheng JC, Lam TP, Maffulli N: Epidemiological features of supracondylar fractures of the humerus in Chinese children. *J Pediatr Orthop B* 2001;10(1):63-67.

9. Wilkins KE: Fractures and dislocations of the elbow region, in Rockwood CA, Wilkins KE, King RE, eds: *Fractures in Children.* Philadelphia, PA, JB Lippincott, 1984, vol 3, pp 363-575.

10. Leitch KK, Kay RM, Femino JD, Tolo VT, Storer SK, Skaggs DL: Treatment of multidirectionally unstable supracondylar humeral fractures in children: A modified Gartland

© 2016 AAOS Instructional Course Lectures, Volume 65

type-IV fracture. *J Bone Joint Surg Am* 2006;88(5):980-985.

11. Parikh SN, Wall EJ, Foad S, Wiersema B, Nolte B: Displaced type II extension supracondylar humerus fractures: Do they all need pinning? *J Pediatr Orthop* 2004;24(4):380-384.

12. Skaggs DL, Hale JM, Bassett J, Kaminsky C, Kay RM, Tolo VT: Operative treatment of supracondylar fractures of the humerus in children: The consequences of pin placement. *J Bone Joint Surg Am* 2001;83(5):735-740.

13. Omid R, Choi PD, Skaggs DL: Supracondylar humeral fractures in children. *J Bone Joint Surg Am* 2008;90(5):1121-1132.

14. Herman MJ, Boardman MJ, Hoover JR, Chafetz RS: Relationship of the anterior humeral line to the capitellar ossific nucleus: Variability with age. *J Bone Joint Surg Am* 2009;91(9):2188-2193.

15. Kocher MS, Kasser JR, Waters PM, et al: Lateral entry compared with medial and lateral entry pin fixation for completely displaced supracondylar humeral fractures in children: A randomized clinical trial. *J Bone Joint Surg Am* 2007;89(4):706-712.

16. Pennock AT, Charles M, Moor M, Bastrom TP, Newton PO: Potential causes of loss of reduction in supracondylar humerus fractures. *J Pediatr Orthop* 2014;34(7):691-697.

17. Sankar WN, Hebela NM, Skaggs DL, Flynn JM: Loss of pin fixation in displaced supracondylar humeral fractures in children: Causes and prevention. *J Bone Joint Surg Am* 2007;89(4):713-717.

18. Bast SC, Hoffer MM, Aval S: Nonoperative treatment for minimally and nondisplaced lateral humeral condyle fractures in children. *J Pediatr Orthop* 1998;18(4):448-450.

19. Beaty JH, Kasser JR: The elbow: Physeal fractures, apophyseal injuries of the distal humerus, osteonecrosis of the trochlea, and t-condylar fractures, in Beaty JH, Kasser JR, eds: *Rockwood*

and Wilkins' Fractures in Children, ed 6. Philadelphia, Lippincott Williams & Wilkins, 2006, pp 591-660.

20. Foster DE, Sullivan JA, Gross RH: Lateral humeral condylar fractures in children. *J Pediatr Orthop* 1985;5(1):16-22.

21. Fontanetta P, Mackenzie DA, Rosman M: Missed, maluniting, and malunited fractures of the lateral humeral condyle in children. *J Trauma* 1978;18(5):329-335.

22. Song KS, Kang CH, Min BW, Bae KC, Cho CH: Internal oblique radiographs for diagnosis of nondisplaced or minimally displaced lateral condylar fractures of the humerus in children. *J Bone Joint Surg Am* 2007;89(1):58-63.

23. Pirker ME, Weinberg AM, Höllwarth ME, Haberlik A: Subsequent displacement of initially nondisplaced and minimally displaced fractures of the lateral humeral condyle in children. *J Trauma* 2005;58(6):1202-1207.

24. Finnbogason T, Karlsson G, Lindberg L, Mortensson W: Nondisplaced and minimally displaced fractures of the lateral humeral condyle in children: A prospective radiographic investigation of fracture stability. *J Pediatr Orthop* 1995;15(4):422-425.

25. Hasler CC, von Laer L: Prevention of growth disturbances after fractures of the lateral humeral condyle in children. *J Pediatr Orthop B* 2001;10(2):123-130.

26. Jakob R, Fowles JV, Rang M, Kassab MT: Observations concerning fractures of the lateral humeral condyle in children. *J Bone Joint Surg Br* 1975;57(4):430-436.

27. Horn BD, Herman MJ, Crisci K, Pizzutillo PD, MacEwen GD: Fractures of the lateral humeral condyle: Role of the cartilage hinge in fracture stability. *J Pediatr Orthop* 2002;22(1):8-11.

28. Badelon O, Bensahel H, Mazda K, Vie P: Lateral humeral condylar fractures in children: A report of 47 cases. *J Pediatr Orthop* 1988;8(1):31-34.

29. Thönell S, Mortensson W, Thomasson B: Prediction of the stability of minimally displaced fractures of the lateral humeral condyle. *Acta Radiol* 1988;29(3):367-370.

30. Launay F, Leet AI, Jacopin S, Jouve JL, Bollini G, Sponseller PD: Lateral humeral condyle fractures in children: A comparison of two approaches to treatment. *J Pediatr Orthop* 2004;24(4):385-391.

31. Milch H: Fractures and fracture dislocations of the humeral condyles. *J Trauma* 1964;4:592-607.

32. Weiss JM, Graves S, Yang S, Mendelsohn E, Kay RM, Skaggs DL: A new classification system predictive of complications in surgically treated pediatric humeral lateral condyle fractures. *J Pediatr Orthop* 2009;29(6):602-605.

33. Song KS, Waters PM: Lateral condylar humerus fractures: Which ones should we fix? *J Pediatr Orthop* 2012;32(suppl 1):S5-S9.

34. Toh S, Tsubo K, Nishikawa S, Inoue S, Nakamura R, Harata S: Long-standing nonunion of fractures of the lateral humeral condyle. *J Bone Joint Surg Am* 2002;84(4):593-598.

35. Tejwani N, Phillips D, Goldstein RY: Management of lateral humeral condylar fracture in children. *J Am Acad Orthop Surg* 2011;19(6):350-358.

36. Skak SV, Olsen SD, Smaabrekke A: Deformity after fracture of the lateral humeral condyle in children. *J Pediatr Orthop B* 2001;10(2):142-152.

37. Pribaz JR, Bernthal NM, Wong TC, Silva M: Lateral spurring (overgrowth) after pediatric lateral condyle fractures. *J Pediatr Orthop* 2012;32(5):456-460.

38. Bauer AS, Bae DS, Brustowicz KA, Waters PM: Intra-articular corrective osteotomy of humeral lateral condyle malunions in children: Early clinical and radiographic results. *J Pediatr Orthop* 2013;33(1):20-25.

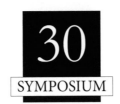

30

SYMPOSIUM

Pediatric Monteggia Fracture-Dislocations: Avoiding Problems and Managing Complications

Kenneth Chin, MD
Scott H. Kozin, MD
Martin Herman, MD
Bernard D. Horn, MD
Craig P. Eberson, MD
Donald S. Bae, MD
Joshua Abzug, MD

Abstract

Monteggia fracture-dislocations typically involve a dislocation of the radial head with an associated fracture of the ulnar shaft. The prompt diagnosis and treatment of these acute injuries result in excellent outcomes. Unfortunately, a Monteggia fracture-dislocation is often missed during diagnostic testing and results in a chronic Monteggia fracture-dislocation. The subsequent timing and treatment of chronic Monteggia fracture-dislocations are debatable because outcomes are suboptimal. Therefore, it is critical that the initial injury be correctly diagnosed and treated as close to the time of injury as possible to ensure excellent outcomes.

Instr Course Lect 2016;65:399–408.

In 1814, Giovanni Monteggia described an injury pattern of the upper extremity that involved a fracture of the proximal one-third of the ulna with an anterior dislocation of the radial head.[1] Since then, the definition of a Monteggia injury has broadened to include any fracture along the ulna that is associated with a radiocapitellar subluxation or dislocation. This injury pattern is seen in both the adult and pediatric populations and is usually sustained after a fall onto an outstretched hand. The mechanism of injury involves an axial load with hyperpronation of the forearm and a

hyperextension moment about the elbow.[2,3] Monteggia fracture-dislocations comprise approximately 1% of all pediatric forearm fractures. Compared with adults, the presentation and treatment options are different in the pediatric population because of the presence of the physis and plastic deformation that may occur about the ulna.[4]

In 1967, Bado[5] classified Monteggia injuries into four types based on the direction of radial head subluxation or dislocation (**Table 1**). In pediatric patients, type I injuries are the most common, followed by type III injuries.

In 1985, Letts et al[6] modified the Bado classification for use in the pediatric population (**Table 2**). Other fracture variants are now considered Monteggia fractures as well, including any ulnar fracture that has a concomitant radial neck fracture, because of the similarity of the injury patterns and the mechanisms of injury.

Acute Monteggia fracture-dislocations should be treated with prompt reduction after the injury is identified. In general, anatomic reduction of the ulna will restore length to the ring of the forearm and will permit

Table 1
Bado Classification of Monteggia Fractures

Type	Injury Pattern
I	Fracture of the proximal or middle third of the ulna with anterior dislocation of the radial head
II	Fracture of the proximal or middle third of the ulna with posterior dislocation of the radial head
II	Fracture of the ulnar metaphysis with lateral dislocation of the radial head
IV	Fracture of the proximal or middle third of the ulna and radius with anterior dislocation of the radial head

Table 2
Letts Classification of Pediatric Monteggia Fractures

Type	Injury Pattern
A	Anterior radial head dislocation and plastic deformation of the ulna with anterior apex deformity
B	Anterior radial head dislocation with greenstick-type fracture of the ulna
C	Anterior radial head dislocation with complete fracture of the ulna
D	Posterior dislocation of the radial head with any fracture of the ulna
E	Lateral dislocation of the radial head with any fracture of the ulna

reduction of the radial head.[7] Occasionally, the annular ligament will slip off the proximal radius like a necktie being pulled over the head, which creates a block to radiocapitellar joint reduction. Awareness of the direction of the radial head dislocation also may help with reduction. Early detection and treatment of a Monteggia injury generally leads to excellent outcomes (**Figure 1**); however, these injuries are not recognized often. A delayed diagnosis that leads to a chronic injury may be very challenging to treat, even for the most experienced surgeons.

Pathoanatomy
The forearm can be described as an elongated ring structure that is composed of the ulna and radius; the two bones are joined distally by the distal radioulnar joint, centrally by the interosseous membrane, and proximally by the proximal radioulnar joint. The proximal radioulnar joint is a complex joint that is stabilized by the elbow capsule, annular ligament, radial collateral ligament, and quadrate ligament. The annular ligament maintains the radial head in congruent alignment within the lesser sigmoid notch of the proximal ulna, with both the distal radioulnar joint and proximal radioulnar joint permitting rotational motion of the forearm. Chronic injury and subsequent instability of these joints may limit pronation and supination and may ultimately lead to long-term arthrosis of the elbow and wrist.

A Monteggia injury is both a bony and ligamentous failure in the forearm, with a fracture or plastic deformation of the ulna combined with a radiocapitellar ligamentous injury that most commonly results in the subluxation or dislocation of the radial head. The radial head subluxation or dislocation involves failure of the annular and quadrate ligaments. The displacement of the radial head may lead to impingement of the surrounding neurovascular structures, specifically the posterior interosseous nerve that lies on the anterior radial neck. Radial nerve palsy is seen in up to 10% of patients who have Monteggia fracture-dislocations.[8]

Acute Injuries
Evaluation
Because many Monteggia injuries are initially misdiagnosed, it is critical for surgeons to understand key points in the evaluation of acute injuries. The correct initial diagnosis of Monteggia fracture patterns is crucial to prevent missed injuries and the development of

Dr. Kozin or an immediate family member serves as a paid consultant to Checkpoint Surgical, and serves as a board member, owner, officer, or committee member of the American Society for Surgery of the Hand. Dr. Herman or an immediate family member serves as a board member, owner, officer, or committee member of the Pediatric Orthopaedic Society of North America. Dr. Horn or an immediate family member has stock or stock options held in Johnson & Johnson, and serves as a board member, owner, officer, or committee member of the American Academy of Orthopaedic Surgeons. Dr. Eberson or an immediate family member has received royalties from Globus Medical; is a member of a speakers' bureau or has made paid presentations on behalf of Stryker Spine and Orthofix Spine; serves as a paid consultant to Orthofix; and serves as a board member, owner, officer, or committee member of the Scoliosis Research Society and the Pediatric Orthopaedic Society of North America. Dr. Bae or an immediate family member has stock or stock options held in Cempra, Johnson & Johnson, Kythera Biopharmaceuticals, and Vivus, and serves as a board member, owner, officer, or committee member of the American Academy of Orthopaedic Surgeons, the American Society for Surgery of the Hand, and the Pediatric Orthopaedic Society of North America. Dr. Abzug is a member of a speakers' bureau or has made paid presentations on behalf of Checkpoint Surgical, and serves as a paid consultant to Axogen. Neither Dr. Chin nor any immediate family member has received anything of value from or has stock or stock options held in a commercial company or institution related directly or indirectly to the subject of this chapter.

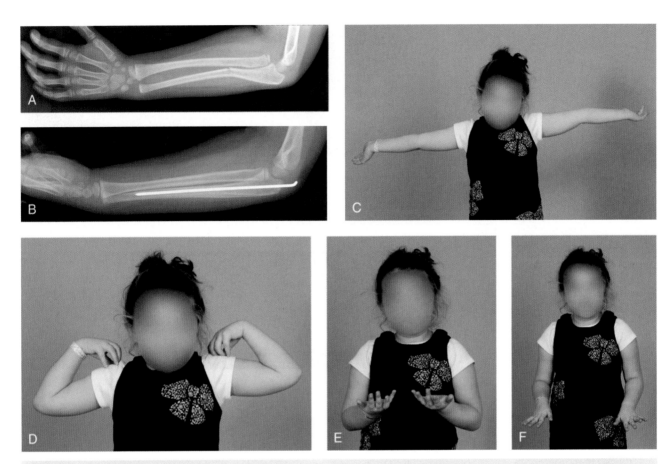

Figure 1   Images of a 5-year-old girl who fell 5 days ago. **A,** Lateral arm radiograph demonstrates plastic deformation and incomplete fracture of the ulna. The radial head is dislocated in an anterior direction. **B,** Lateral arm radiograph taken after closed reduction and intramedullary rodding of the ulna demonstrates reduction of the radial head dislocation. Clinical photographs taken after rod removal show full symmetric elbow extension (**C**), full elbow flexion (**D**), full supination (**E**), and full pronation (**F**). (Courtesy of Shriners Hospitals for Children, Philadelphia, PA.)

chronic Monteggia injuries, which are notoriously challenging to treat.

The clinical suspicion for a Monteggia fracture must be high for any child who has elbow and/or forearm pain and limitations in range of motion, particularly forearm rotation. Most often children have pain, swelling, and, occasionally, deformity about the forearm and/or elbow after a fall onto an outstretched hand. During the physical examination, pain and limited range of motion with elbow flexion and extension as well as forearm supination and pronation are typically present. Palpation along the ulnar shaft may reveal a step-off deformity; however, the only

indication of an injury in patients who have plastic deformation may be tenderness. Careful palpation of the radial head may reveal an obvious dislocation; however, a subtle subluxation may be difficult to identify. A thorough neurovascular examination also must be performed, with special attention paid to the function of the radial and posterior interosseous nerves. The function of these nerves can be assessed by ensuring that the patient is able to extend his or her digits at the metacarpophalangeal joints. In addition to the more common radial and posterior interosseous nerve palsies, median and ulnar nerve deficits have been described.[9-11]

High-quality radiographs of the forearm and elbow are important to correctly diagnose a Monteggia injury. The radiographs should be centered on the appropriate part of the limb (ie, on the midforearm for forearm radiographs and about the elbow for elbow radiographs). A true lateral radiograph of the elbow is often difficult to obtain, especially in an uncooperative child who is in pain (**Figure 2**); however, it is imperative to do so because it has been reported that a Monteggia fracture-dislocation is most commonly missed as a result of inadequate radiographs or the improper interpretation of radiographs.[12] Therefore, repeat radiographs,

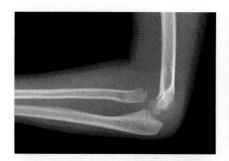

Figure 2 True lateral radiograph demonstrates obvious anterior radial head dislocation. (Courtesy of Shriners Hospitals for Children, Philadelphia, PA.)

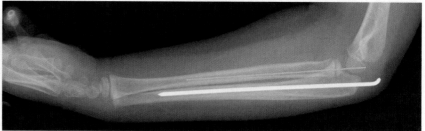

Figure 3 Lateral radiograph demonstrates the radiocapitellar line, which, if drawn down the shaft of the radius, should intersect the center of the capitellum of the distal humerus dislocation. (Courtesy of Shriners Hospitals for Children, Philadelphia, PA.)

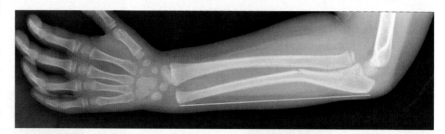

Figure 4 Lateral radiograph demonstrates the ulnar bow sign, which suggests plastic deformation of the ulna. This can be seen by the line drawn from the distal metaphysis of the ulna to the olecranon, which should be straight compared with the ulna. (Courtesy of Shriners Hospitals for Children, Philadelphia, PA.)

sometimes taken with a technologist or parent holding the child's limb, may be necessary to obtain adequate radiographs that allow for a full assessment of the injury.

In addition to a careful analysis of the cortical borders of the ulna and radius, surgeons who suspect a Monteggia injury must systematically review several other radiographic landmarks to identify a fracture. The radiocapitellar line, a straight line drawn down the shaft of the radius, should intersect the center of the capitellum of the distal humerus on all radiographic views of the elbow (**Figure 3**). If the radiocapitellar line does not intersect the center of the capitellum, then a Monteggia fracture-dislocation is present. Although Monteggia fracture-dislocations are classically associated with an ulnar shaft fracture in adults, pediatric patients may not have a complete fracture of the ulna. Instead, children and adolescents may have ulnar plastic deformation or bowing that is unable to be appreciated on radiographs, which is an important reason for a missed diagnosis. The ulnar bow sign can be used to help diagnose plastic deformation of the ulna, which most frequently occurs at the midshaft. A line drawn along the dorsal ulnar shaft from the distal metaphysis of the ulna to the olecranon should appear straight on a true lateral radiograph of the forearm. An uninjured ulna should maintain a straight dorsal border; deviation of the ulna from this line is indicative of plastic deformation[13,14] (**Figure 4**).

Treatment

Closed Reduction

Prompt reduction that results in stability of the fracture fragments and the radiocapitellar joint is the goal of treatment for acute Monteggia fracture-dislocations. In the emergency department, closed reduction may be attempted under conscious sedation. The aid of a minifluoroscopy unit may help confirm radial head reduction and permit assessment of stability after the reduction. To obtain reduction, longitudinal traction is first applied to the forearm, and reduction of the ulnar fracture is performed. Anatomic reduction of the ulnar fracture restores length to the forearm and may result in incidental reduction of the radial head.[15] To achieve reduction of the radiocapitellar joint in Monteggia-type fractures that have an anterior radial head dislocation, the most common type of Monteggia fracture, hyperflexion of the elbow is typically necessary while applying direct pressure on the radial head. Elbow extension may be necessary to reduce rare types of Monteggia fractures that have posterior radial head dislocation. After reduction of the radial head is confirmed via fluoroscopy and the radial head in Monteggia fracture types that have anterior radial head dislocation is stable, a long arm cast or splint is applied with the elbow in 90° to 100°

of flexion and the forearm in maximal supination. Postreduction radiographs are necessary to ensure that reduction was maintained during cast application.

Cast immobilization may be successful as the definitive method of treatment for many acute fractures with an ulnar fracture pattern that is length-stable after reduction. Careful follow-up after reduction is necessary to ensure maintenance of reduction. Injuries that are older than 1 week usually cannot be reduced in a closed fashion and often require surgery.[16] Additional indications for surgery include open Monteggia fractures, Monteggia fractures in which the ulnar fracture is irreducible or unstable after reduction, Monteggia fractures in which the radial head is irreducible or unstable after reduction, and Monteggia fractures that have displaced after cast treatment has been attempted.

Surgical Considerations

Repeat closed reduction may be attempted in the operating room under general anesthesia with the aid of fluoroscopy and adequate relaxation. With the ulna out to length, the radial head is assessed for the position of greatest stability in pronation and supination. An elbow arthrogram may be extremely useful in young children to permit visualization of the entire radial head (**Figure 5**). The arthrogram is performed by mixing equal parts of saline and contrast dye. This mixture is injected into the elbow joint via a posterior injection site located on the olecranon fossa. The elbow is then brought through a range of motion to disperse the dye. Excellent visualization of the entire radial head should be present after injection.

If anatomic reduction of the ulna or radial head fails, it is the practice of the authors of this chapter to approach

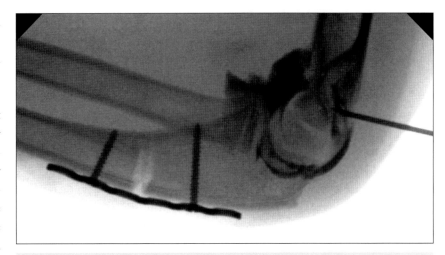

Figure 5   Elbow arthrogram performed via a posterior injection demonstrates enhanced visualization of the entire radial head in a young child. (Courtesy of Shriners Hospitals for Children, Philadelphia, PA.)

the ulna first because reduction of the radial head will often follow suit. Transverse or short oblique fractures of the ulna (length-stable fracture patterns) are treated with anterograde fixation using intramedullary nails that are placed in the ulna via an olecranon starting point (**Figure 1**). Long oblique and comminuted fractures are usually length-unstable fracture patterns, and, therefore, require open reduction and plating. Open reduction and plating is performed via a direct approach to the ulna that exploits the interval between the extensor carpi ulnaris and flexor carpi ulnaris. Plastic deformation of the ulna may be corrected with the application of manual pressure over a bump or with percutaneous osteoclasis. Intramedullary nail fixation may then be performed; however, often no fixation is necessary for this type of ulnar injury.

After stable fixation of the ulna is achieved, it is of paramount importance for the surgeon to assess the integrity of the radiocapitellar joint. If the radial head remains irreducible or subluxated, a lateral Kocher approach is undertaken to examine the joint directly. An

incarcerated annular ligament is often the reason radial head reduction is prevented. The annular ligament may actually be intact and be able to be slipped back over the proximal radius. Alternatively, the ligament may be torn, and a repair may be necessary. Annular ligament reconstruction is almost never necessary in acute Monteggia fractures. Rarely, an osteochondral fragment or the posterior interosseous nerve may impede reduction of the radial head.

Postoperative Care

Radiographs are obtained 1 week after reduction to ensure the maintenance of radial head reduction. The patient's arm is placed in a long arm cast for 4 to 6 weeks or until there is radiographic evidence of ulnar healing. Active range of motion is begun after fracture union, with a gradual return to activities.

Chronic Injuries
Evaluation

A careful history must be obtained from the patient and caregiver to determine the timing of the injury and to rule out the possibility of a congenital radial head dislocation. Distinguishing a chronic Monteggia fracture-dislocation from a congenital radial head dislocation is difficult because both diagnoses may present with similar clinical photographs and radiographic findings: a radial head dislocation with a convex radial head and a hypoplastic capitellum. Patients who have chronic injuries report no symptoms before an injury, and patients who have congenital radial head dislocations often report long-standing deformity and limitation of motion without pain. An arthrogram may help distinguish the two diagnoses if necessary; a congenitally dislocated radial head will be intracapsular, whereas a chronic Monteggia injury will usually be extracapsular.[17] The authors of this chapter find it extremely helpful to retrieve and evaluate the original injury radiographs to identify the ulnar fracture and radial head subluxation/dislocation, which may have been missed at the time of injury.

Monteggia fracture-dislocations are missed 16% to 33% of the time, most frequently if the ulna is plastically deformed as opposed to if a complete fracture is present.[18] Patients with chronic radial head dislocations have symptoms that typically worsen with time. Substantial pain will develop in 60% of patients who have chronic Monteggia fracture-dislocations, and 50% of patients who have chronic Monteggia fracture-dislocations will present with limited range of motion about the elbow.[19] Neglected chronic Monteggia fracture-dislocations that have a radial head dislocation may lead to morphologic and functional changes in the upper extremity. A dislocated radial head undergoes hypertrophic changes to its shape, including a loss of concavity at the articular surface. On the other side of the joint, the capitellum undergoes flattening. Normally, the radial head acts as a static stabilizer to valgus stress at the elbow; however, the morphologic changes caused by chronic Monteggia injuries drive the elbow into cubitus valgus deformity. Subsequently, progressive valgus deformity may place the ulnar nerve on stretch; therefore, a thorough neurovascular examination is essential for patients who have chronic Monteggia fracture-dislocations.

Treatment

The treatment of chronic Monteggia injuries is challenging for the patient, his or her family, and the surgeon. Long-term outcomes of nonsurgical treatment for chronic Monteggia injuries are poor; therefore, the current trend is toward surgical intervention.[20] However, controversy exists with regard to the indications and contraindications for surgical management. Children who experience a longer interval between the initial Monteggia injury and surgical management as well as older children have been reported to have worse outcomes. The best outcomes may be expected in children who have surgery less than 3 years after the original injury or who are younger than 12 years.[19,21] This is likely because the longer the chronicity of the injury, the more dysplastic the radiocapitellar joint becomes, with increasing convexity of the radial head and worsening hypoplastic changes at the capitellum. Treatment of missed Monteggia fracture-dislocations that are older than 3 years can yield acceptable outcomes; however, the surgeon must carefully assess the amount of osseous deformity that is present. Maintenance of radial head concavity and evidence of a congruent capitellum may be indications for reduction of the dislocation, regardless of the time interval after injury or the age of the patient.

Reconstruction

With the exception of advanced deformity and degenerative changes of the radiocapitellar joint, most patients who have chronic Monteggia fractures are treated surgically (**Figure 6**). The primary goal in the surgical treatment of chronic Monteggia injuries is to obtain stable radial head reduction. Reconstruction usually begins with open reduction of the radial head. A temporary Kirschner wire may be driven across the joint to maintain reduction. Next, an ulnar osteotomy is performed at the level of the original fracture, if it is known. If the original fracture location is unknown, then a more proximal ulnar osteotomy is performed, which helps maintain the integrity of the interosseous membrane.[22] The ulna is permitted to sit where it lies and is fixed in situ with the use of a plate-and-screw construct. Maintaining the integrity of the interosseous membrane may help keep the radial head reduced because the interosseous membrane is a secondary stabilizer for the proximal radioulnar joint. After fixation of the ulna is achieved, the radiocapitellar pin is removed, and the stability of the radial head reduction is assessed.

If the radiocapitellar joint remains unstable, then the annular ligament is repaired if there is adequate tissue present, or a ligament reconstruction is performed. The authors of this chapter prefer to reconstruct the annular ligament with a technique described by Seel and Peterson,[23] which uses the flexor carpi radialis because the palmaris longus tendon tends be an inadequate size to perform the procedure as a result of

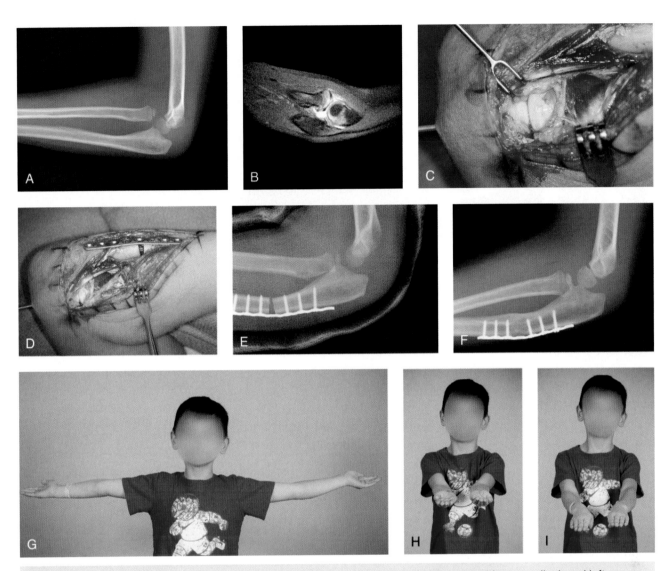

Figure 6   Images of a 6-year-old boy who fell off his bike 3 months ago and was treated for a nondisplaced left supra-condylar fracture. **A,** Lateral elbow radiograph demonstrates frank radial head subluxation. **B,** Sagittal MRI of the elbow demonstrates further delineation of the radial head position, with cartilage compression along the inferior radial head. **C,** Intraoperative photograph of the elbow shows ulnar osteotomy, open reduction of the radiocapitellar joint, and temporary radiocapitellar pinning. **D,** Intraoperative photograph of the elbow shows the ulnar plate in situ. **E,** Postoperative lateral elbow radiograph demonstrates maintenance of radiocapitellar alignment. **F,** Postoperative lateral elbow radiograph demonstrates ultimate healing of the ulnar osteotomy and an aligned radial head. Clinical photographs show full elbow extension (**G**), full supination (**H**), and full pronation (**I**). (Courtesy of Shriners Hospitals for Children, Philadelphia, PA)

its small girth. It is important to avoid overtightening the reconstruction because it may lead to substantial stiffness and a loss of forearm rotation. The authors of this chapter prefer to perform radial head resection and interpositional arthroplasty in patients who have severe dysplasia of the radial head that is not able to be reconstructed. The details of

this salvage procedure are beyond the scope of this chapter.

Postoperative Care

The patient is seen 1 week postoperatively to ensure maintenance of reduction. At this time, the splint that was applied in the operating room is converted to a long arm cast, with the

elbow in 90° of flexion and the forearm in maximal supination. The cast is removed 6 weeks postoperatively, and radiographs are obtained to ensure that union is present at the osteotomy site and that the radial head has maintained its alignment, after which active range of motion is begun. The patient is allowed to return to activities

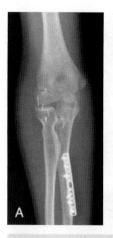
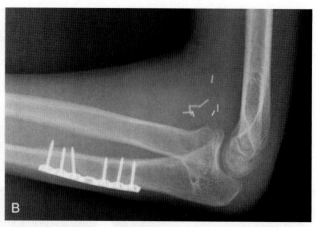

Figure 7 Radiographs of the arm of a 5-year-old boy with a chronic Monteggia fracture-dislocation who underwent open reduction, annular ligament reconstruction, and an ulnar osteotomy. He had persistent pronation and supination limitations after the procedure. **A,** AP view demonstrates a reduced radial head with notching about the radial neck secondary to an overly taut ligament reconstruction. **B,** Lateral view demonstrates similar findings with possible radioulnar synostosis. (Courtesy of Shriners Hospitals for Children, Philadelphia, PA.)

approximately 3 months postoperatively after range of motion and strength have been restored.

Complications

The most important complications for the surgeon to be aware of in the postoperative period include compartment syndrome of the forearm; nerve palsies, especially posterior interosseous palsy; and loss of radiocapitellar joint reduction. To minimize the potential for recurrent subluxation or dislocation, the surgeon should ensure that the radiocapitellar joint is aligned and stable before leaving the operating room. Stiffness that results in a loss of full forearm rotation most commonly is caused by prolonged immobilization. The initiation of range of motion as soon as good radiographic healing is confirmed at the osteotomy site may diminish this risk. An annular ligament reconstruction that is too tight, which will result in notching of the proximal radius, must be considered if a child

is having difficulty regaining motion (**Figure 7**). Uncommon complications, such as heterotopic ossification or myositis ossificans, may develop and lead to stiffness; however, because they are relatively rare complications, the authors of this chapter do not routinely administer prophylaxis.

Summary

Monteggia fracture-dislocations can have excellent outcomes if they are recognized and treated appropriately in the acute setting. Unfortunately, Monteggia fracture-dislocations are frequently missed in the acute setting, which leads to suboptimal outcomes in many children. Surgeons need to have a high index of suspicion for a Monteggia injury in any child who has elbow or forearm pain, and must ensure that adequate radiographs of the forearm and elbow are obtained. The prompt reduction of an acute Monteggia fracture-dislocation is critical to ensure a successful outcome and to prevent chronic Monteggia

injuries, which are more challenging to treat.

References

1. Monteggia GB: *Istituzioni Chirurgiche.* Milano, Italy, Pirotta & Maspero, 1814, vol 5.

2. Kay RM, Skaggs DL: The pediatric Monteggia fracture. *Am J Orthop (Belle Mead NJ)* 1998;27(9):606-609.

3. Speed J, Boyd HB: Treatment of fractures of ulna with dislocation of head of radius. *J Am Med Assoc* 1940;115(20):1699-1705.

4. Boyd HB, Boals JC: The Monteggia lesion: A review of 159 cases. *Clin Orthop Relat Res* 1969;66:94-100.

5. Bado JL: The Monteggia lesion. *Clin Orthop Relat Res* 1967;50:71-86.

6. Letts M, Locht R, Wiens J: Monteggia fracture-dislocations in children. *J Bone Joint Surg Br* 1985;67(5):724-727.

7. Ring D, Jupiter JB, Waters PM: Monteggia fractures in children and adults. *J Am Acad Orthop Surg* 1998;6(4):215-224.

8. Chen WS: Late neuropathy in chronic dislocation of the radial head: Report of two cases. *Acta Orthop Scand* 1992;63(3):343-344.

9. Li H, Cai QX, Shen PQ, Chen T, Zhang ZM, Zhao L: Posterior interosseous nerve entrapment after Monteggia fracture-dislocation in children. *Chin J Traumatol* 2013;16(3):131-135.

10. Engber WD, Keene JS: Anterior interosseous nerve palsy associated with a Monteggia fracture: A case report. *Clin Orthop Relat Res* 1983;174:133-137.

11. Stein F, Grabias SL, Deffer PA: Nerve injuries complicating Monteggia lesions. *J Bone Joint Surg Am* 1971;53(7):1432-1436.

12. Gleeson AP, Beattie TF: Monteggia fracture-dislocation in children. *J Accid Emerg Med* 1994;11(3):192-194.

13. Lincoln TL, Mubarak SJ: "Isolated" traumatic radial-head dislocation. *J Pediatr Orthop* 1994;14(4):454-457.

14. Degreef I, De Smet L: Missed radial head dislocations in children associated with ulnar deformation:

© 2016 AAOS Instructional Course Lectures, Volume 65

Treatment by open reduction and ulnar osteotomy. *J Orthop Trauma* 2004;18(6):375-378.

15. Olney BW, Menelaus MB: Monteggia and equivalent lesions in childhood. *J Pediatr Orthop* 1989;9(2):219-223.

16. Ring D, Waters PM: Operative fixation of Monteggia fractures in children. *J Bone Joint Surg Br* 1996;78(5):734-739.

17. Kosay C, Akcali O, Manisali M, Ozaksoy D, Ozcan C: Congenital anterior dislocation of the radial head: A case with radiographic findings identical to traumatic dislocation. *Eur J Radiol* 2002;43(1):57-60.

18. Dormans JP, Rang M: The problem of Monteggia fracture-dislocations in children. *Orthop Clin North Am* 1990;21(2):251-256.

19. Nakamura K, Hirachi K, Uchiyama S, et al: Long-term clinical and radiographic outcomes after open reduction for missed Monteggia fracture-dislocations in children. *J Bone Joint Surg Am* 2009;91(6):1394-1404.

20. Stoll TM, Willis RB, Paterson DC: Treatment of the missed Monteggia fracture in the child. *J Bone Joint Surg Br* 1992;74(3):436-440.

21. Wang MN, Chang WN: Chronic posttraumatic anterior dislocation of the radial head in children: Thirteen cases treated by open reduction, ulnar osteotomy, and annular ligament reconstruction through a Boyd incision. *J Orthop Trauma* 2006;20(1):1-5.

22. Rahbek O, Deutch SR, Kold S, Søjbjerg JO, Møller-Madsen B: Long-term outcome after ulnar osteotomy for missed Monteggia fracture dislocation in children. *J Child Orthop* 2011;5(6):449-457.

23. Seel MJ, Peterson HA: Management of chronic posttraumatic radial head dislocation in children. *J Pediatr Orthop* 1999;19(3):306-312.

Sports Medicine

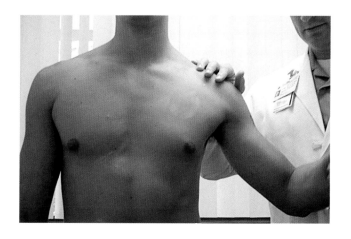

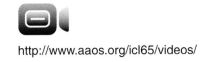

http://www.aaos.org/icl65/videos/

Arthroscopic Management of Anterior, Posterior, and Multidirectional Shoulder Instabilities

Larry D. Field, MD
Richard K.N. Ryu, MD
Jeffrey S. Abrams, MD
Matthew Provencher, MD

Abstract

Arthroscopic shoulder stabilization offers several potential advantages compared with open surgery, including the opportunity to more accurately evaluate the glenohumeral joint at the time of diagnostic assessment; comprehensively address multiple pathologic lesions that may be identified; and avoid potential complications unique to open stabilization, such as postoperative subscapularis failure. A thorough understanding of normal shoulder anatomy and biomechanics, along with the pathoanatomy responsible for anterior, posterior, and multidirectional shoulder instability patterns, is very important in the management of patients who have shoulder instability. The treating physician also must be familiar with diagnostic imaging and physical examination maneuvers that are required to accurately diagnose shoulder instability.

Instr Course Lect 2016;65:411–436.

Arthroscopic shoulder stabilization is a commonly performed and well-accepted orthopaedic procedure for the treatment of patients who have shoulder instability and. Arthroscopic techniques specifically designed to address anterior, posterior, and multidirectional instability (MDI) patterns have been developed and provide reliably successful outcomes for most patients who require surgical intervention.

Arthroscopic Bankart repair has evolved into the procedure of choice for the treatment of symptomatic anterior instability. Numerous risk factors for failure—including sex, age, contact sports participation, and bone loss—have been identified and must be factored into any decision-making process. Often, the loss of static restraint that is normally provided by the anteroinferior labrum is compounded by associated anteroinferior glenoid bone loss (GBL). Acute glenoid rim fracture and attritional GBL largely contribute to recurrent instability by decreasing the contact area between the humeral head and the glenoid and reducing the function of static glenohumeral restraints. In the past decade, the importance of GBL to recurrent glenohumeral instability has been increasingly recognized, and treatment strategies for patients with recurrent instability have focused on addressing the bone in addition to the soft tissues to truly reestablish static restraint to the glenohumeral joint. Patients who have substantial GBL may be best treated with a procedure that allows for grafting of the deficiency. The Latarjet procedure is perhaps the best technique and is widely used to treat medium to large glenoid bone defects. Most often, this procedure is performed via an open approach to the shoulder.

Posterior glenohumeral instability is less common than anterior instability. The diagnosis of posterior glenohumeral instability may be challenging because the symptoms may be vague and often are not localized posteriorly. Recurrent subluxation is more common than frank dislocation, and most patients do not recall a specific traumatic event. Posterior instability pathoanatomy is varied and may include injury to the posterior labrum, capsuloligamentous structures, and the bony glenoid. For patients in whom posterior stabilization is required, arthroscopic techniques designed to address labral and capsular lesions are very effective. The advantages of an arthroscopic approach include its minimally invasive nature as well as its ability to address the variety of pathologic lesions commonly encountered in posterior instability.

A structured trial of nonsurgical management is important for shoulders that are disabled by MDI. The length of nonsurgical management has been debated, and a minimum of 3 to 6 months should be considered before proceeding with surgical intervention. Treatment should include scapular stabilization, rotator cuff strengthening in nonpainful positions, and closed-chain–linked functional exercises to increase functional gains. Surgical options can be considered for patients who do not experience adequate improvement with nonsurgical management. Arthroscopic

stabilization can provide a balanced repair with multiquadrant correction and is widely accepted as a reliable and successful technique for most patients who have MDI.

It is important for surgeons to have a thorough understanding of the history and physical examination findings, pathoanatomy, pertinent diagnostic imaging, surgical indications, and state-of-the-art arthroscopic techniques for the treatment of patients who have anterior instability (with and without substantial associated glenoid and humeral head bone loss), posterior instability, and MDI. In addition, surgeons should be aware of the limitations of and controversies related to arthroscopic shoulder stabilization for each instability pattern.

Anterior Instability

Because of its unparalleled, multiplanar range of motion, the shoulder is uniquely susceptible to traumatic anterior instability. Anterior dislocation represents more than 95% of all shoulder instability episodes.[1] Substantial controversy exists regarding the optimal treatment for patients who have anterior instability. Numerous factors must be considered

to determine the appropriate treatment for patients who have anterior instability, including risk factors such as age, sex, contact sports participation, bone loss, and associated ligamentous laxity.[2-8] If surgery is undertaken, the arthroscopic approach is now widely accepted as the primary intervention of choice.[9] Several studies in the literature have addressed the technical aspects of an arthroscopic Bankart repair, including anchor placement, suture passage and configuration, the number of anchors, adjunctive remplissage, the incorporation of any bony Bankart component, and the essential task of retensioning the glenohumeral ligaments, and the likelihood of success.[10-21]

Pathoanatomy

The stability of the shoulder relies on a complex balance of static and dynamic stabilizers. The role of core and scapular strength on glenohumeral stability has been historically underappreciated but currently occupies a prominent position in the successful treatment of patients who have anterior shoulder instability.[22,23] Much is known about the static stabilizers of the glenohumeral joint, and although the Bankart lesion has been described as the essential lesion, capsular deformation is critical to symptomatic instability, which reinforces the critical task of retensioning the glenohumeral ligaments.[24-26]

Clinical Evaluation

Anterior shoulder instability is usually the direct result of a traumatic event, and the history should provide the diagnosis in most patients; however, distinguishing a posterior event from an anterior event may be challenging. The position of the shoulder in a posterior instability event, namely forward

Dr. Field or an immediate family member is a member of a speakers' bureau or has made paid presentations on behalf of Smith & Nephew; serves as a paid consultant to or is an employee of Mitek and Smith & Nephew; has received research or institutional support from Arthrex, Mitek, and Smith & Nephew; and serves as a board member, owner, officer, or committee member of the American Academy of Orthopaedic Surgeons, the American Orthopaedic Society for Sports Medicine, the American Shoulder and Elbow Surgeons, and the Arthroscopy Association of North America. Dr. Ryu or an immediate family member is a member of a speakers' bureau or has made paid presentations on behalf of Mitek; serves as a paid consultant to or is an employee of MedBridge and Rotation Medical; has stock or stock options held in Rotation Medical; and serves as a board member, owner, officer, or committee member of the American Orthopaedic Society for Sports Medicine and the Arthroscopy Association of North America. Dr. Abrams or an immediate family member has received royalties from ArthroCare; serves as a paid consultant to or is an employee of ArthroCare, ConMed Linvatec, Mitek, and Rotation Medical; serves as an unpaid consultant to Ingen Technologies and KFx Medical; has stock or stock options held in ArthroCare, Cayenne Medical, Ingen Technologies, KFx Medical, and Rotation Medical; and serves as a board member, owner, officer, or committee member of the American Shoulder and Elbow Surgeons and the Arthroscopy Association of North America. Dr. Provencher or an immediate family member has received royalties from Arthrex; serves as a paid consultant to or is an employee of Arthrex and the Joint Restoration Foundation; and serves as a board member, owner, officer, or committee member of the American Academy of Orthopaedic Surgeons, the American Society for Sports Medicine, the American Shoulder and Elbow Surgeons, the Arthroscopy Association of North America, the International Society of Arthroscopy, Knee Surgery, and Orthopaedic Sports Medicine, the San Diego Shoulder Institute, and the Society for Military Orthopaedic Surgeons.

flexion, adduction, and internal rotation, is substantially different from the abducted, externally rotated posture most often encountered in an anterior instability event.

On physical examination, the apprehension test, in which instability, not pain, is the response, should be performed in the abducted, externally rotated stress position, preferably with the patient positioned supine. Typically, the apprehensive response is relieved with the use of a relocation maneuver, in which a posteriorly directed force is applied to the humeral head while the patient's shoulder is maintained in an abducted, externally rotated position. The failure to relieve apprehension and/or an increase in symptoms of pain make anteroinferior instability less likely. Similar apprehensive reactions with the shoulder in lesser degrees of abduction may indicate substantial bone loss because capsular integrity provides the bulk of stability in the maximally abducted and externally rotated position, whereas in lesser degrees of abduction, the integrity of the glenoid rim becomes more salient. The presence of an engaging Hill-Sachs lesion is difficult to determine during physical examination, and substantial crepitus may indicate humeral head bone loss. An evaluation for signs of ligamentous laxity,[27] including the Wynne-Davies signs,[28] is an important element of the physical examination because surgical implications, including additional capsular retensioning, exist if a surgical solution is mandated in patients who have a traumatic dislocation superimposed on generalized ligamentous laxity.[29] Finally, it is very important that the contralateral shoulder be examined for comparison.

Imaging

Standard radiographs, including AP views in internal and external rotation as well as an axillary view are recommended initially; however, an axillary view may be challenging in the acute setting. A loss of the bony contour of the anterior glenoid on the AP view is associated with a loss of bony integrity on the glenoid rim.[2] A posterolateral humeral head defect is best seen on the internal rotation AP view and is consistent with a Hill-Sachs lesion. Additional views, including the Stryker notch view, can be obtained to better assess a Hill-Sachs lesion. The West Point and Bernageau views[30] offer profiles of the anterior glenoid rim to help quantify bone loss.

MRI with contrast is the imaging modality of choice because both the degree of labral pathology and the presence of associated pathology, including rotator cuff and superior labral injuries, can be established. Although bone loss can be appreciated on plain radiographs and MRI, the use of three-dimensional CT, with coronal and sagittal reconstructions and humeral head subtraction views, remains the most reliable imaging modality to accurately assess the degree of glenoid and humeral head bone loss.[31-33]

Treatment Options

Surgical treatment of the unstable shoulder often is considered the definitive intervention; however, nonsurgical management may be appropriate in certain circumstances. Numerous studies from various military academies emphasize the recurrence rates with nonsurgical management of high-risk athletes.[34,35] However, for individuals who do not pursue vigorous recreational activities or have high-risk occupations,

the risk of recurrence may be lower.[36,37] For individuals who have a low risk of recurrence, a program of immobilization to control discomfort, followed by rehabilitation to control strength and range of motion and then a gradual return to activities, is a reasonable alternative to surgery. Furthermore, an early course of immobilization in external rotation may offer a lower risk of recurrence. Proper tensioning of the inferior glenohumeral ligament (IGHL) in external rotation as it attempts to heal forms the rationale behind this conservative immobilization philosophy. To date, this course of treatment remains controversial because mixed results have been reported.[38-41] This treatment regimen may be combined with follow-up evaluations in which a persistent positive apprehension test after nonsurgical management may predict a higher risk of recurrent instability.[42]

Surgical stabilization is the recommended course of treatment for individuals who have a high risk for recurrence. The arthroscopic approach is now the procedure of choice for surgical stabilization; however, long-term studies have reported a substantial failure rate after primary stabilization.[5,14,18,43-45] Alternative surgical approaches have been espoused for primary stabilization, including open Bankart repair and either open or arthroscopic bone block procedures. The Latarjet procedure, although considered an option for failed arthroscopic procedures or for patients who have substantial bone loss, is a viable option for a primary intervention because long-term studies confirm a very low recurrence rate.[46-49] Although the Latarjet procedure is effective, it is technically demanding and associated with high complication rates; if undertaken, appropriate planning and practice must

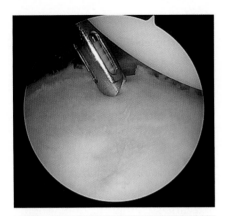

Figure 1 Arthroscopic image of a left shoulder as viewed from the anterosuperior portal. The drill sleeve is placed at the 6-o'clock position from a posterolateral accessory portal.

precede the intervention to minimize the risk of complications.[50]

To avoid failure after an arthroscopic Bankart repair, the mitigation of risk factors is the most coherent strategy in decision making. Intrinsic risk-factor mitigation includes a careful analysis of the bone loss, the age and the sex of the patient, the expectation of a return to contact sports participation, and ligamentous laxity and compliance. If a confluence of risk factors cannot be mitigated, then soft-tissue stabilization may not be an appropriate initial intervention. If addressing technical risk factors, mitigation implies the ability to address not only the primary pathology but also adjunctive measures, such as remplissage, the incorporation of bony Bankart lesions, novel anchor placement, and a robust suturing pattern.

First-Time Dislocations

Many studies have been published on the optimal treatment for a first-time dislocation, and each patient must be individualized to the given circumstances that affect the decision for treatment. Abundant clinical and economic

evidence supports early intervention in patients deemed to have a high risk for recurrent instability.[50-54] Several level I studies have clearly elucidated the benefit of early intervention in not only preventing recurrent instability episodes but also improving quality-of-life parameters.[55-58]

Surgical Technique: Arthroscopic Bankart Repair With Enhanced Techniques

If an arthroscopic soft-tissue Bankart procedure is selected, then the patient is placed in the lateral decubitus position.[59] The surgical table is rotated 90° such that the orthopaedic surgeon can move from back to front around the patient's upper torso without impediment. The table is tilted 10° to 15° to orient the glenoid parallel with the floor.

Dual anterior portals are established, with the anteroinferior portal directly superior to the intra-articular slip of the subscapularis, occupying the lowest portion of the rotator interval, and the anterosuperior portal at the superior border of the interval, directly behind the biceps tendon. A posterior portal is created slightly lateral to and above the equator of the glenoid, thus making the posterior portal the working portal without interference from the glenoid rim. The anterosuperior portal provides a direct view of the anterior glenoid and the IGHLs while allowing for identification of the Bankart lesion and a survey of the shoulder for additional pathology. Concomitant superior labrum anterior to posterior rotator cuff or chondral injuries are not uncommonly discovered in the instability setting. Humeral avulsion of the glenohumeral ligament (HAGL) lesions must be identified because a failure to do so is associated with a higher failure

rate.[60] Although considered the essential lesion, a Bankart lesion alone is not sufficient to cause recurrent instability. Some element of capsular deformation accompanies the primary pathology and must be addressed in addition to the repair of the Bankart defect. To accomplish this, the Bankart lesion must be thoroughly elevated off the glenoid neck, and the subscapularis muscle belly should be clearly visible through the Bankart defect. The IGHL can then easily be shifted in an inferior-to-superior direction, which is a critical step in capsular retensioning. Occasionally, anterior labroligamentous periosteal sleeve avulsion (ALPSA) lesions are encountered, and mobilization of these scarred lesions requires more time and effort. If mobilization is done properly, then the ALPSA lesion floats up to the glenoid rim before repair. Despite good technique, lower success rates have been reported if ALPSA lesions are repaired.[61]

In chronic cases with associated capsular deformation, special consideration must be directed to the inferior capsule. By using an accessory inferolateral portal (1 cm lateral and 2 to 3 cm inferior to the standard posterior portal), an anchor at the 6-o'clock position can be placed at the most inferior aspect of the glenoid (**Figure 1**). A suture hook is used through the standard posterior portal to pass sutures, and the inferior capsule can be directly retensioned. This should be accomplished before repairing the anterior Bankart lesion.

After the inferior capsule has been assessed and treated, instrumentation for anchor placement is positioned through the anteroinferior portal at the lowest anchor site (eg, the 7-o'clock position in a left shoulder). The authors of this chapter recommend that the drill hole for the anchor be placed on the glenoid rim by securing the drill guide immediately adjacent to the articular surface. If difficulty is encountered in securing the drill guide in this position, it is acceptable to advance the guide 2 to 3 mm onto the articular surface to ensure good anchor purchase in the glenoid. The authors of this chapter think this is essential to re-create labral height and reestablish the concavity-compression phenomenon. Care must be taken not to drill out the anchor and suture that were previously placed at the 6-o'clock position. After the double-loaded suture anchor is inserted, a suture hook loaded with No. 1 polydioxanone suture (PDS) is used to penetrate the IGHL 1 to 2 cm inferior and lateral to the anchor. This permits adequate tissue shifting as well as a lateral-to-medial closure. Alternating horizontal mattress and simple sutures with a double-loaded anchor facilitates this configuration and lessens the risk of abutting the articular surface with suture material as range of motion is introduced. Data also indicate that the use of mattress sutures in this setting is associated with a greater return to sporting activities in younger patients.[12] This process is repeated until the anterior labrum is completely repaired and retensioned.

The authors of this chapter use a minimum of three double-loaded anchors with six high-strength sutures. The humeral head should be centered in the glenoid when viewing from the anterosuperior portal. The ability to subluxate or dislocate the shoulder should be corrected. If the capsule is not properly tensioned, then additional capsular tucks can be placed at this time.

If a bony Bankart lesion is present, even chronically, then an attempt should

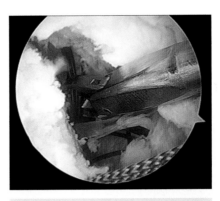

Figure 2   Arthroscopic image of a left shoulder as viewed from the anterosuperior portal. The grasper is passed through the Bankart interval to grasp the polydioxanone suture shuttle that is being passed under the bony Bankart lesion and resting on the subscapularis muscle belly.

be made to incorporate bone into the repair.[15] Passing suture through bone is particularly challenging and is usually successful only in thinner or attenuated bony Bankart lesions. The use of a suture bridge technique[62] to span the bone fragment is warranted if a larger fragment is present. Attempts to simply encircle the fragment with suture from a single anchor are more likely to lead to a nonanatomic position with poor bone contact. After the bony Bankart lesion is sufficiently mobilized, blind passage of the suture hook and wheeling of the PDS shuttle underneath the bony Bankart lesion followed by retrieval of the suture, which rests on the subscapularis muscle belly, from the interval between the glenoid and the labrum can be easily accomplished (**Figure 2**). This suture can then be used to pass the sutures from the medial anchor of the bone bridge construct around the bone fragment with a knotless anchor technique on the glenoid face, which completes the repair. Stabilization of the inferior aspect of the bony Bankart lesion is helpful, but the remaining sutures must

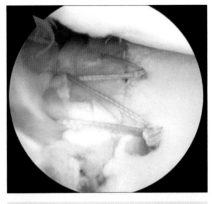

Figure 3   Arthroscopic image shows a large bony Bankart fracture fragment that was secured using a double row anchor technique with the lateral row of knotless anchors placed at the articular margin.

all be passed before the bone fragment is secured (**Figure 3**).

If a substantial Hill-Sachs lesion is present and engages with a deficient glenoid track,[63] then an adjunctive remplissage procedure (tenodesis of the infraspinatus into the Hill-Sachs defect) should be implemented.[10,13] Technically, it is easier to place the anchor into the center of the Hill-Sachs defect and pass sutures through the lateral extent of the infraspinatus tendon before completing the Bankart repair rather than after the Bankart lesion has been repaired and the posterior exposure has been reduced.

Associated ligamentous laxity may need to be addressed. Although arthroscopic rotator interval closure is still controversial in its efficacy for posterior instability and MDI,[64,65] closure of the interval in patients who have anterior instability may act as an internal splint while the lesion is healing. A simple and safe technique for interval closure consists of placing two No. 1 PDSs through the superior rotator interval using the anteroinferior portal cannula, which has

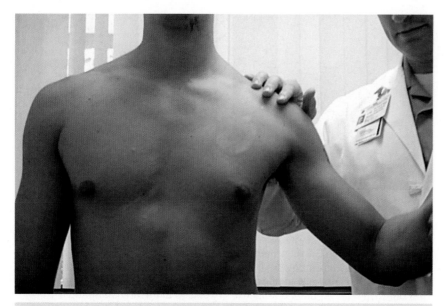

Figure 4 Clinical photograph shows the physical examination for anterior instability.

been withdrawn to the outer capsular margin. An angled retrieval instrument can be passed through the same cannula, piercing the middle glenohumeral ligament to capture the PDSs, which are then tied blindly through the anteroinferior portal cannula to close the interval.

Reconstruction Failures

Recent literature has exposed the worrisome, long-term failure rate associated with arthroscopic Bankart repair.[5,14,18,44,45] The risk factors for failed arthroscopic Bankart repair are male sex, younger age, glenoid bone loss of 25% or more, associated ligamentous laxity, multiple dislocations, contact sports participation, and the length of time between injury and surgery. The Instability Severity Index Score described by Balg and Boileau[2] has been popularized conceptually as a profiling tool; however; its validity is still debated.[66] Furthermore, revision arthroscopic Bankart repair has resulted in inferior results compared with primary

surgery.[16,43,67-69] These data underscore the need for careful patient selection and surgical technique if contemplating and performing an arthroscopic Bankart repair.

Anterior Instability in the Presence of GBL

The most common soft-tissue pathology encountered in the setting of anterior instability is an avulsion of anteroinferior capsular-labral tissue (ie, a Bankart lesion) from the glenoid rim,[69] which is often associated with anteroinferior capsular attenuation.[70] Often, a loss of static restraint that is normally provided by the anteroinferior labrum is compounded by associated anteroinferior GBL. Acute glenoid rim fracture and attritional GBL largely contribute to recurrent instability by decreasing the contact area between the humeral head and the glenoid and by reducing the function of static glenohumeral restraints.[71,72] In the past decade, the importance of GBL to recurrent glenohumeral instability has been

increasingly recognized, and treatment strategies for patients with recurrent instability have focused on addressing the bone in addition to soft tissues to truly reestablish static restraint to the glenohumeral joint.

Physical Examination

During the physical examination, the surgeon should try to differentiate patients who have bony injuries from those who have only soft-tissue lesions. In comparing the affected shoulder with the contralateral side, the surgeon should pay close attention to the degree of instability and expect higher degrees of instability in patients who have GBL compared with patients who have an isolated soft-tissue lesion.[73] Typically, patients with GBL have a greater extent of apprehension and instability in both early and mid-ranges of motion[65,66] (**Figure 4**). Specifically, GBL or bony injuries may be detected with the arm in lesser abduction and external rotation.

Imaging

All patients who have suspected GBL in the setting of anterior shoulder instability should undergo a complete radiographic assessment of the involved shoulder. A displaced bony Bankart fragment or shadow may be seen on projections parallel to the glenoid face, on an axillary or glenoid view, and on a standard AP view.[74] A more accurate diagnosis may be obtained with an apical oblique view,[75] a Didiée view,[76] or a West Point view.[77] To visualize potential associated Hill-Sachs lesions, an AP or Stryker notch view should be obtained with the humeral head internally rotated.[76,78] MRI or magnetic resonance arthrography also is useful to diagnose GBL and is perhaps most revealing if viewing the most lateral aspect of the glenoid on a sagittal view.[78] Currently, CT is the preferred method for quantifying GBL. With recent technology improvements, three-dimensional CT scans may be acquired with the humeral head digitally subtracted. GBL can be quantified in a variety of ways using an en face view; the best-fit circle method is the classic method.[72,79] On the en face view, the inferior two-thirds of the glenoid are outlined with a perfect fit circle that matches the anatomic configuration of the glenoid. The amount of missing bone is calculated as a percentage by dividing the area of the circle that is missing the bone (the bony fragment) by the area of the whole circle (the theoretical glenoid surface)[78] (**Figure 5**). Given the precision of this method, CT with three-dimensional reconstructions is highly recommended if GBL is predicted with plain radiographs, the patient's history, and the physical examination. It is important for surgeons to consider the degree of bone loss on the humeral head (ie, the Hill-Sachs lesion) in analyzing the imaging studies of patients who have GBL, especially in the setting of recurrent instability.[80] Depending on the location and the volume of humeral head bone loss,[81] the humeral head may engage the glenoid during range of motion. GBL treatment may be enough to prevent further engagement of the humeral head, even if the humeral head defect is left untreated.[82]

Anterior Arthroscopic Stabilization

Most patients who have anterior instability with associated GBL are managed surgically. Although nonsurgical treatment modalities are available, surgical intervention is usually warranted given the age, activity level, and demands of the typical patient who has recurrent

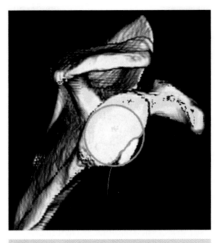

Figure 5   En face three-dimensional CT scan of a left glenoid demonstrates approximately 15% anterior glenoid bone loss (circle and line).

anterior instability with associated GBL.[4] For all patients, an arthroscopic determination of bone loss should be performed to confirm the anticipated degree of GBL as determined by the preoperative imaging analysis. Although the importance of the glenoid articular surface bare spot as a landmark is under debate,[83] arthroscopic measurement of GBL has been well documented and is recommended before any intervention[78] (**Figure 6**). This information is important because the degree of GBL may ultimately be more than anticipated, and, in some patients, it may be necessary to convert from a soft-tissue-only surgical procedure to a reconstruction with bony glenoid augmentation (by means of a Latarjet coracoid transfer, iliac crest bone graft, or structural reconstruction with allograft).

Piasecki et al[78] described treatment options for various degrees of GBL in patients who had anterior shoulder instability after failed nonsurgical management. The authors recommended the following treatment algorithm, depending on the degree of anterior GBL;

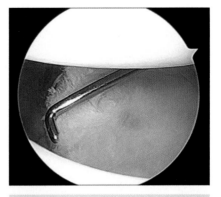

Figure 6   Arthroscopic image of the glenoid taken with the patient in the lateral decubitus position. The arthroscopic probe shows anterior glenoid bone loss of approximately 15%.

however, treatment also depends on if there is a large Hill-Sachs lesion, the type of patient sports participation (if any), and other demographic concerns.

1. If the amount of GBL is less than 15%, then it can typically be incorporated into the repair, and isolated arthroscopic soft-tissue stabilization is generally performed. The surgeon should be aware of an ALPSA lesion. Bernhardson et al[84] reported that patients who have an ALPSA lesion have nearly twice the amount of GBL and substantially more instability events (**Figure 7**). Direct arthroscopic incorporation of the bony fragment should be attempted in all patients.

2. If the amount of GBL is 15% to 25% (**Figure 8**), then there are two options: (a) For low-demand patients, arthroscopic soft-tissue stabilization with fixation of the bone fragment is performed. (b) For higher demand patients, arthroscopic stabilization with bone fragment incorporation is performed. If no bone fragment is available, arthroscopic soft-tissue stabilization plus glenoid reconstruction with either autograft (coracoid

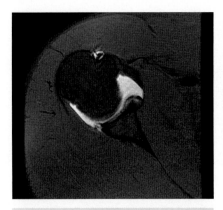

Figure 7 Axial MRI of a right shoulder demonstrates an anterior labral periosteal sleeve avulsion lesion.

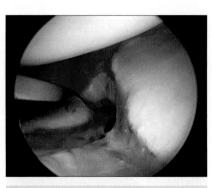

Figure 8 Arthroscopic image of the glenoid taken with the patient in the lateral decubitus position. The arthroscopic elevator shows anterior glenoid bone loss of approximately 20%.

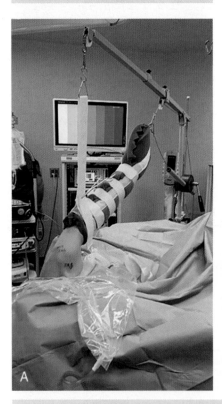

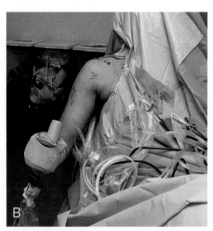

Figure 9 Intraoperative photographs show a left shoulder in the lateral decubitus position (**A**) and the beach-chair position (**B**).

positioning in either the beach-chair or lateral decubitus position is arranged per surgeon preference. A recent systematic review of more than 60 studies reported that the lateral decubitus position provides a slightly lower recurrence rate than the beach-chair position in patients who undergo arthroscopic anterior stabilization (8.5% versus 14.7%, respectively); however, it should be noted that the beach-chair position allows for easier conversion to open procedures if the degree of GBL requires open osseous augmentation[59] (**Figure 9**). The authors of this chapter prefer the lateral decubitus position so that all pathology of the anterior, inferior, and, occasionally, posteroinferior glenoid labrum complex can be more easily accessed and addressed. Regardless of the chosen position, after the patient is positioned appropriately, an examination under anesthesia should be performed; typically, instability in the mid-ranges of motion will be encountered, which supports the anticipated diagnosis of GBL.

Proper portal placement is of utmost importance in the arthroscopic treatment of anterior instability with GBL. The surgeon should pay strict attention to portal location to ensure that the surgical procedure is efficient, which allows for better visualization and adequate spacing for instrumentation during the procedure. The following portals are typically used during arthroscopic instability repair in patients who have GBL.

- The anterosuperior portal is established through the superior portion of the rotator interval. This portal allows for excellent visualization of the anterior aspect of the glenoid.
- The posterior portal is established 1 cm inferior from the posterior

transfer, iliac crest) or allograft (fresh distal tibia allograft [DTA], fresh glenoid allograft) is performed. The surgeon must counsel patients on the possible increased failure rate among contact athletes and the loss of external rotation in throwers if soft-tissue

stabilization alone is performed to treat GBL greater than 20%.[20]

3. If the amount of GBL is greater than 25%, then bone loss must be restored.

For the arthroscopic management of patients who have GBL, patient acromion tip in line with the lateral edge. This portal provides a slight downward trajectory on the glenoid surface to simplify instrumentation usage during the procedure.

- The anterior mid-glenoid portal is established in the rotator interval just superior to the subscapularis tendon. To avoid intra-articular crowding during the procedure, the mid-glenoid portal should have enough skin bridge separation (2 to 3 cm) from the anterosuperior portal.

- The posterolateral portal is established at the 7-o'clock position (in a right shoulder) or the 5-o'clock position (in a left shoulder) and is used for percutaneous anchor placement. Alternatively, a small cannula may be inserted to facilitate glenoid anchor placement and repair along the inferior and posteroinferior aspect of the glenoid. During the creation of this portal, the surgeon must be aware of the axillary nerve, which typically lies 12.5 to 15 mm away from the inferior glenoid rim (ie, the 6-o'clock position)[21] (**Figure 10**).

After all the necessary portals have been established and diagnostic arthroscopy is complete, attention is turned to the repair. In all arthroscopic procedures, every attempt should be made to repair the capsulolabral tissue back to the glenoid with a minimum of three to four anchors below the 3-o'clock position (in a right shoulder) or the 9-o'clock position (in a left shoulder), incorporating the bony fragment whenever possible. Adequate preparation of the glenoid rim and mobilization of the labral tissue are of utmost importance. All soft tissue should be removed from the glenoid rim without injuring the articular cartilage. The rim must be débrided up to

1 to 2 cm medially to initiate bleeding. Débridement of the glenoid rim with a small bone-cutting-type shaver (3.0 to 3.5 mm, using the high-speed reverse setting) may ultimately enhance bone-to-soft-tissue healing. An arthroscopic elevator and an arthroscopic rasp can be used to peel the labrum from the glenoid. If an osseous fragment is present, care should be taken to not destroy the bony fragment during débridement of the labrum. The rasp should be used gently, and, ideally, bone-to-bone healing will be possible in these scenarios. Proper preparation of the labrum and the capsular attachments to the glenoid is indicated by visualization of posterior subscapularis muscle fibers, which confirm sufficient mobilization for the repair.

After the labrum and the glenoid surfaces are prepared, serial suture anchors are placed (45° relative to the glenoid surface, 2 to 3 mm inside the glenoid rim) at the articular cartilage margin to avoid nonanatomic medial scapular neck placement. In most procedures, at least three to four anchors are placed below the equator (the 3-o'clock position in a right shoulder or the 9-o'clock position in a left shoulder). Anchors are placed sequentially from inferior to superior, and the bony fragment is incorporated whenever feasible. Often, 1 to 1.5 cm of capsular tissue is imbricated up to the glenoid rim during passage of the suture material (or suture-tape material if performing a knotless repair construct), which effectively produces a capsular plication to reduce any glenohumeral ligament redundancy. If a standard suture-anchor repair construct is being used, then it is imperative to pull on the sutures before knot tying and after the capsulolabral repair stitch has been placed to

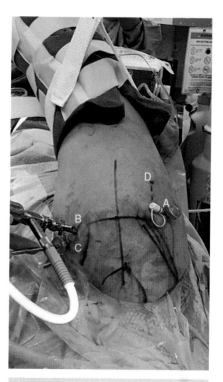

Figure 10   Intraoperative photograph of a right shoulder in the lateral decubitus position shows portal placement. A = standard posterior portal, B = anterosuperior portal, C = midglenoid portal (just above the subscapularis), D = posterolateral portal.

visualize capsular plication and confirm that adequate capsular tissue has been incorporated (**Figure 11**). If there is substantial concomitant posterior laxity, then a posteroinferior anchor can be placed (in the 7-o'clock position in a right shoulder or the 5-o'clock position in a left shoulder) with an associated capsular plication.[85]

Open Bone Augmentation

Options for bony reconstruction include iliac crest bone graft, coracoid transfer (Latarjet procedure), and fresh allograft (DTA or fresh glenoid allograft). The Latarjet procedure is perhaps the best-described technique and is widely used to treat medium to large glenoid bone defects. Most often,

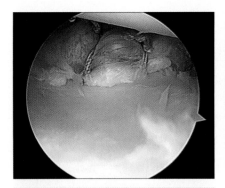

Figure 11 Arthroscopic image of the glenoid taken with the patient in the lateral decubitus position demonstrates the final soft-tissue repair construct with anterior glenoid bone loss of approximately 15%.

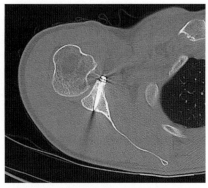

Figure 12 Axial MRI demonstrates a coracoid transfer (Latarjet procedure).

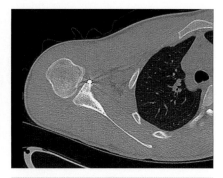

Figure 13 Axial MRI demonstrates anterior glenoid reconstruction with the use of a distal tibia allograft. The glenoid angle is close to anatomic, with no graft lysis and complete incorporation.

this procedure is performed via an open approach to the shoulder.[49,86] More recently, arthroscopic techniques for the Latarjet procedure have been described, particularly in France, and show encouraging outcomes.[87] The Latarjet procedure is an effective technique that provides stability to the glenohumeral joint by reconstructing the natural osseous arc of the glenoid with the patient's own bone (**Figure 12**). In a study that analyzed the long-term outcomes of patients who had a Latarjet procedure for the treatment of anterior glenohumeral instability, Allain et al[88] reported low recurrence rates but the development of early osteoarthritis at a mean follow-up of 14.3 years (range, 10 to 23 years). Although this procedure provides excellent stability, as reported in a variety of short-, medium-, and long-term outcomes studies,[49,88] there are concerns about the possibility of long-term coracoid osteolysis and the risk of developing early glenohumeral arthritis because of the extra-articular, nonanatomic nature of the reconstruction. An alternative to the Latarjet procedure, or for salvage of a failed

Latarjet procedure, is anterior glenoid reconstruction with fresh DTA. Biomechanically, fresh DTA has been reported to provide better joint congruity and lower peak forces within the glenohumeral joint at 60° of abduction and in the abducted externally rotated position compared with Latarjet reconstruction[89] (**Figure 13**). Although the literature is limited to biomechanical data and case reports, the available clinical studies are encouraging, with excellent short-term clinical outcomes reported in three patients.[31] More recently, Provencher et al reported excellent clinical outcomes without recurrent instability in a series of 27 patients at a mean follow-up of 45 months (Matthew Provencher, MD, Boston, MA, unpublished data, 2014). Certainly, further studies with longer follow-up are needed to gain a better understanding of the long-term clinical outcomes of DTA reconstruction, especially with regard to the longevity of the allograft and the ability of the procedure to maintain glenohumeral stability without causing glenohumeral arthritis.[90]

Rehabilitation

Outcomes after surgical management of anterior instability with GBL

depend on thorough planning and coordination among the patient, the physical therapist, and the orthopaedic surgeon. The type of rehabilitation program depends on the degree of instability, the specific procedure performed, the integrity of soft tissue at the time of the repair, the surgeon's comfort level with the quality of the repair, and any associated findings and treatments (eg, biceps tendon tear, rotator cuff tear).[80] Immediately postoperatively, an abduction sling is recommended for most patients who have undergone anterior stabilization to allow the shoulder to remain in a neutral position as the soft tissues heal.[80] Typically, the patient is allowed to begin physical therapy 7 to 10 days after surgery to work on soft-tissue modalities. Passive and active-assisted range-of-motion exercises are usually initiated 4 weeks postoperatively. Full active and passive range of motion should be achieved by 8 weeks postoperatively. Strengthening is allowed at 8 weeks postoperatively, with full return to activities expected by 4 to 6 months postoperatively.

Posterior Instability

Posterior glenohumeral instability is less common than anterior instability and occurs in only 2% to 10% of patients who have shoulder instability.[91-93] The diagnosis may be challenging because the symptoms may be vague and often are not localized posteriorly.[94,95] Frequently, patients report pain rather than instability episodes. Recurrent subluxation is more common than frank dislocation, and most patients do not recall a specific traumatic event.[96,97] Etiologies include acute trauma, chronic repetitive microtrauma, and atraumatic instability.[98] Posterior instability is more common in athletes who repetitively load their shoulders in a flexed and adducted position (eg, weightlifters, football lineman, and rowers). Pathoanatomy is varied and may include injury to the posterior capsuloligamentous structures, the bony glenoid or humerus, the rotator interval, and the rotator cuff.[99-103]

Surgical intervention is indicated for patients with recurrent posterior instability in whom nonsurgical management has failed. Although posterior instability was historically treated with open surgery, this required large surgical dissections, and the reported failure rates ranged from 30% to 70%.[104] These failure rates, along with the technological and technique advances made in arthroscopic surgery, have led to increased use of arthroscopy for the treatment of posterior glenohumeral instability in patients without substantial osseous deficiency. The advantages of an arthroscopic approach include its minimally invasive nature and its ability to address the variety of pathoanatomy seen in patients who have posterior instability.[91,105,106] Various studies have reported that the arthroscopic management of posterior glenohumeral instability can successfully restore shoulder stability.[99,103-112]

Pathoanatomy

The shoulder joint is stabilized by an intricate and sophisticated combination of static and dynamic constraints. The geometric conformity of the articular surfaces, the glenoid labrum, and the capsular ligaments all function as static stabilizers. In addition, bony morphology, including glenoid and humeral version, glenoid inclination, and joint congruency, contribute to static stability and must be considered in the evaluation of patients who have glenohumeral instability. The disruption of these static stabilizers may result from posterior glenoid erosion, excessive glenoid retroversion, glenoid hypoplasia, and excessive humeral retroversion and may predispose patients to posterior instability. The depth and surface area of the glenoid is further increased by the glenoid labrum because it attaches along the margin on the glenoid fossa. The labrum also serves as a stable fibrocartilaginous anchor for the posterior ligaments, including the important posterior band of the IGHL that traverses the posterior shoulder capsule. This posterior capsule has been identified as the thinnest portion of the shoulder capsule and is recognized as an area of relative capsular weakness.[113]

Posterior instability develops secondary to traumatic causes, atraumatic causes, or repetitive microtraumatic insults to the posterior stabilizing structures. The most common cause of posterior instability is a repetitive microtraumatic injury mechanism. Recurrent posterior subluxation is a much more common entity[104] and is seen in patients who have a repetitive microtraumatic injury mechanism. Frank posterior dislocations are more commonly seen in patients who sustain high-energy trauma, seizures, or electrocutions. Athletes are particularly susceptible to repetitive microtraumatic injury, with resultant pathologic changes caused by the demands placed on their posterior stabilizing structures. In addition, these athletes' shoulders tend to become unstable during competition as their dynamic stabilizers fatigue. Thus, athletes with posterior instability have a greater risk for subluxation or even dislocation the longer they participate in an athletic contest.

Athletes who have sustained a traumatic posterior subluxation are at risk for the development of a posterior labral detachment (ie, a reverse Bankart lesion). These labral tears, which can develop after a traumatic injury or as the result of repetitive insult, are important to recognize (**Figure 14**). Posterior labral tears, however, are often much less impressive and may be difficult to identify on diagnostic imaging or at the time of surgical intervention. Specifically, cumulative glenoid rim loading secondary to recurrent shoulder subluxation can lead to the development of a posterior labral crack at the posterior labrum attachment site on the posteroinferior glenoid rim, which has been termed a Kim lesion.[114] In addition, posterior capsular stretching and tearing, including detachment of the lateral capsule from the posterior humeral head (ie, a reverse HAGL), can occur.[101,102]

Clinical Evaluation

Patients with posterior instability often have nonspecific complaints, such as pain and weakness, and more subtle physical findings on examination than those typically exhibited in patients

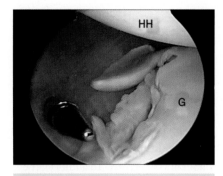

Figure 14 Arthroscopic image shows a posterior labral detachment as viewed from the anterosuperior portal. Assessment of the posterior labral and capsular structures via the anterosuperior portal helps to identify and accurately assess pathology in the posteroinferior aspect of the glenohumeral joint. G = glenoid, HH = humeral head.

who have anterior instability. Examiners should understand the mechanism for posterior instability and be familiar with the sports that commonly place athletes at a higher risk for the development of posterior instability, such as weightlifting, football (especially offensive linemen), hockey, rugby, and wrestling. If patients are asked to detail the arm position that most reproduces or exacerbates their symptoms, they will often position the arm in forward flexion, adduction, and internal rotation.[115] Although patients may report an inciting event that initiated the onset of their symptoms, a specific history of traumatic subluxation or dislocation is usually absent. In addition, reports of pain are common but often difficult to localize; however, patients most commonly report pain along the posterior joint line or the superior aspect of the shoulder. In addition to pain, athletes less often report apprehension during participation in at-risk activities. Some patients also report crepitus or clicking.

The physical examination should always incorporate a bilateral assessment and include visual inspection, palpation, active and passive range of motion, and motor and sensory testing. Patients who have posterior instability generally maintain normal range of motion and strength but will occasionally have tenderness to palpation over the posterior joint line. In addition to a thorough standard shoulder examination, multiple specific provocative tests to assess for posterior instability, including the posterior load and shift test, the jerk test, and the Kim test, can be performed. The Kim test was reported to be 97% sensitive for the detection of posteroinferior labral lesions if combined with the jerk test.[116] To perform the posterior load and shift test, the patient is placed supine on the examination table to stabilize the scapula. The arm is positioned in approximately 20° of abduction and forward flexion. A slight axial load is applied to center the humeral head in the glenoid, and then the examiner attempts to translate the humeral head posteriorly. The examiner notes whether the humeral head can be translated beyond the glenoid rim and if this reproduces the patient's posterior shoulder discomfort. For the jerk test, the patient is placed supine on the examination table to stabilize the scapula. The patient's arm is positioned in 90° of forward flexion with the elbow bent, and the arm is internally rotated across the patient's body. The arm is then slightly adducted, and a posterior axial load is applied along the axis of the humerus. A sudden clunk or jerk is indicative of posterior humeral head subluxation. For the Kim test, the patient is placed in a sitting position with the arm in 90° of abduction. With the examiner holding the patient's elbow

and the lateral aspect of the proximal arm, a simultaneous axial loading force and 45° of upward diagonal elevation is applied to the distal arm, and an inferior and posterior force is applied to the proximal arm. The sudden onset of posterior shoulder pain is considered a positive test. Having the patient sit against the back of a chair to help facilitate the application of a firm axial compression force provides good countersupport for the axial loading of the Kim test.

Imaging

If patients complain of pain and instability, the surgeon should obtain standard AP, axillary, and supraspinatus outlet radiographs. Although these radiographs are often normal in patients who have posterior instability, the combination of these three views allows the surgeon to assess a patient's shoulder for static anterior or posterior humeral head translation, a reverse Hill-Sachs lesion, excessive glenoid retroversion, a reverse bony Bankart lesion, fracture or erosion of the posterior glenoid, and glenoid dysplasia. In addition to radiographs, MRI can be used to achieve a detailed assessment of the soft-tissue or cartilaginous damage that potentially contributes to instability, such as posterior labral tears or lateral capsular detachments. CT also can be used if substantial bony abnormalities are identified on plain radiographs or if such bony lesions are suspected based on the patient's history and physical examination. CT is the best imaging modality available to evaluate the size of reverse Hill-Sachs lesions because it allows the surgeon to determine the percentage of humeral articular cartilage included in the impression fracture.

Treatment Options

An initial nonsurgical course that incorporates several months of activity modification and organized physical therapy to strengthen the dynamic shoulder stabilizers is generally recommended and has had substantial clinical success in certain patients.[104,115,117-119] If conservative management fails to adequately improve a patient's symptoms, then surgery should be considered.

Surgical Technique

Posterior Arthroscopic Stabilization

A complete examination of both shoulders is performed under anesthesia to evaluate for glenohumeral instability. The patient is then placed in the lateral decubitus position. The authors of this chapter prefer the lateral decubitus position because it provides improved access to the posteroinferior quadrant of the shoulder compared with the beach-chair position. The patient's torso is rotated approximately 30° posteriorly, which brings the glenoid parallel to the operating room floor. An axillary roll is placed, and all bony prominences are well padded. An inflatable bean bag is used to stabilize the patient in this position, and the nonsurgical arm is placed on an arm board. The patient's surgical arm is then prepped and draped, placed in approximately 45° of abduction and 10° of flexion, and attached to the traction apparatus. Ten pounds of balanced suspension traction are most often used, with 15 lb reserved for larger patients if 10 lb is insufficient.

The arthroscope is inserted into the posterior viewing portal, and standard glenohumeral diagnostic arthroscopy is performed. An anterior portal is created in an outside-in fashion in the center of the rotator interval. A medium-sized (7.0 mm) plastic cannula is placed in the anterior portal. The arthroscope is then switched to the anterior portal, and a switching stick is placed in the posterior portal. While viewing from the anterior portal, the anterior humeral head is thoroughly evaluated for a reverse Hill-Sachs lesion. Attention is then turned to the posterior capsulolabral structures. Under direct arthroscopic visualization, a cannula is placed over the posterior switching stick. A probe is then inserted through the posterior cannula, and the posterior labrum and capsule are thoroughly evaluated. It is important to note that posterior labral injury may be less dramatic than that commonly seen with anterior Bankart lesions; however, there is often associated posterior capsular injury or redundancy.

After posterior capsuloligamentous pathology is confirmed, the arthroscope is placed back in the posterior portal. An anterosuperior accessory portal is then created in the rotator interval just anterior to the leading edge of the supraspinatus. A 5.5-mm cannula is placed in the anterosuperior accessory portal, and the arthroscope is moved to this cannula. Viewing from the anterosuperior portal allows for complete visualization of the glenoid and associated capsuloligamentous structures. A probe is inserted into the posterior portal cannula and is used to again evaluate the posterior labrum and the posterior capsule. Not infrequently, the orthopaedic surgeon will note injury to both the labrum and the capsule. The labrum may be detached from the posterior glenoid rim, which can occur with or without an associated bony lesion. In addition, the posterior capsule can be torn in its midsubstance or be avulsed from its humeral insertion site (ie, a reverse HAGL).

Access to the posteroinferior glenoid is crucial for success during arthroscopic posterior labral repair. The standard posterior viewing portal is typically too medial for posterior labral elevation, glenoid preparation, and suture anchor insertion. Furthermore, the inferior capsule may be difficult to reach via the standard posterior portal; therefore, an inferior posterolateral accessory working portal (a posterior instability portal) is created. This portal is typically 1 to 2 cm lateral and distal to the standard posterior portal. Because accurate positioning of this portal is critical, it is best localized with a spinal needle while viewing with the arthroscope from the anterosuperior portal (**Figure 15**). The spinal needle position and trajectory should be critically evaluated before the creation of the posterolateral accessory portal. The portal location should allow the surgeon to easily reach the posteroinferior capsule and glenoid as well as provide optimal trajectory for posterior glenoid anchor placement. After localization of the inferior posterolateral accessory portal, a large plastic cannula (7.0 or 8.5 mm) is inserted over a switching stick into this portal.

In patients who have posterior shoulder instability without labral injury, the surgeon may choose to plicate the posterior capsule to the intact labrum; however, in the experience of the authors of this chapter, posterior labral injury is commonly seen, and suture anchor fixation is preferred. To prepare for anchor placement, an elevator is inserted in one of the posterior portals to mobilize the posterior labrum from the glenoid. Alternatively, the elevator can be placed in the mid-glenoid anterior portal if it provides a better trajectory for labral mobilization. The

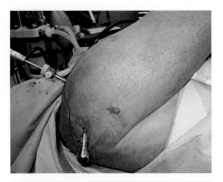

Figure 15 Intraoperative photograph shows the arthroscopic portals typically used for posterior labral repair, as viewed posteriorly with the patient's head to the left. A plastic cannula anterosuperiorly is used primarily to view with an arthroscope but also can be used for labral preparation and suture management as necessary. A metal cannula is in the standard posterior portal. The posterolateral accessory portal, shown here by the spinal needle with the green cap, is distal and lateral to standard posterior portal. This portal is created under direct arthroscopic visualization and is essential for effective posterior labral repair. The posterolateral accessory portal provides the proper trajectory for posterior anchor placement and also allows the orthopaedic surgeon to more easily access the posteroinferior capsule for capsular shift and plication.

surgeon should avoid capsular plication to a frayed and attenuated labrum, even if a complete posterior Bankart lesion is not identified. The labrum should be freed, and a suture anchor technique should be implemented. After the posterior labrum and capsule have been sufficiently mobilized, a rasp is used to gently abrade the labrum and capsule to encourage healing. An arthroscopic shaver or burr is then used to débride the glenoid rim to create a bleeding surface but with every attempt made to preserve bone.

Anchors are then placed via the inferior posterolateral accessory portal while the arthroscope remains in the anterosuperior portal. The inferiormost anchor is placed first, typically in the 7-o'clock position for a right shoulder or the 5-o'clock position for a left shoulder. Anchors are placed at the articular margin of the glenoid and spaced approximately 5 mm apart. Typically, two to four anchors are used, depending on the extent of labral injury. Double-loaded anchors are preferred because of their increased load to failure. After an anchor has been placed, the surgeon prepares for suture passage. Determining the appropriate amount of capsular shift and plication is a challenge and must be assessed on a case-by-case basis. To estimate the necessary amount of capsular shift and plication, the surgeon can use an arthroscopic grasper that provisionally reduces the labrum to the glenoid. The surgeon can then further tension the posterior capsule by pulling it farther superiorly or anteriorly until sufficient capsular tension is attained. The surgeon then attempts to replicate this capsular tension during suture passage and tying. If there is any evidence of inferior capsular laxity in addition to labral pathology, the inferior capsule must be directly addressed with an inferiorly placed anchor.

Sutures are passed through the capsule and the labrum in an inferior-to-superior progression. In this manner, the more difficult inferior suture is passed first, which allows the surgeon to more easily assess the posterior capsular plication achieved with each successive suture. A suture retriever (or suture shuttle) is placed into the joint via the inferior posterolateral accessory portal. The suture retriever is then used to penetrate the posteroinferior

capsule inferior and lateral to the respective glenoid anchor position, thus affecting capsular plication and superior capsular shift. If the inferior capsule is difficult to reach with the suture passer, an arthroscopic grasper or a traction stitch can be used to pull the capsule superiorly. This facilitates suture shuttling as well as tensions the inferior capsule and provides superior capsular shift (**Figure 16**). Care is taken when penetrating the posteroinferior capsule by maintaining direct visualization and limiting the depth of capsular penetration to avoid iatrogenic axillary nerve injury. Passing a suture hook through the capsular tissue and then immediately and carefully supinating allows for penetration of the capsule without plunging, which avoids iatrogenic injury to the surrounding neurovascular structures. After the suture passer penetrates the lateral aspect of the posteroinferior capsule, it is delivered under the torn labrum at the glenoid margin near the respective suture anchor. The suture retriever is deployed to shuttle one inferior anchor suture through the posterior capsule. The suture shuttling steps can be repeated to create a horizontal mattress suture if desired. If a simple suture configuration is used, then the limb passing through the capsule is designated as the tying post. In this manner, the arthroscopic knot rests away from the glenoid, and the redundant capsule is pushed up against the glenoid to act as a bumper to limit posterior humeral head translation. These steps are repeated as necessary for the more superior anchors. Capsular tension is evaluated after each successive knot is tied. The posteroinferior capsule is the location at which most capsular shift and plication should be performed.

Management of Posterior (Reverse) HAGLs

Posterior shoulder instability may be caused by a posterior Bankart lesion, capsular redundancy, and/or a posterior reverse HAGL.[101,102] Reverse HAGL lesions may occur in isolation or in combination with a posterior Bankart lesion.[100]

Several additional surgical steps are needed to repair a reverse HAGL lesion. First, an arthroscopic shaver is used to débride the bone along the posterior humeral neck in the area of the posterior capsular insertion. One or two suture anchors are then placed into the humeral neck at the anatomic insertion of the posterior IGHL and the posterior capsule. Next, the posterior cannula is slightly withdrawn from the shoulder joint so that it is superficial to the joint capsule but deep to the deltoid. A suture retriever is then used through the cannula to penetrate the posterior capsule and retrieve one of the suture limbs from a respective anchor. The penetrator is used to pierce the capsule again and retrieve the other suture, taking care to retrieve this suture from a separate capsular window so that a mattress suture construct is created. The shoulder is then placed in external rotation. The sutures are tensioned while viewing from the glenohumeral joint so the surgeon can confirm that the ligament and the capsule anatomically reduce to the humeral neck. The sutures are then tied extracapsularly in a blind fashion. Standard repair of a posterior Bankart lesion is completed if such a labral lesion also is present. Note that a reverse HAGL is repaired before a posterior Bankart lesion. If posterior Bankart repair was undertaken first, the surgeon could inadvertently plicate the posterior capsule excessively,

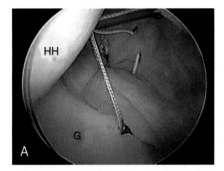
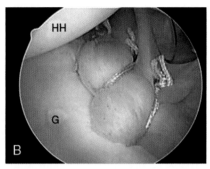

Figure 16   Arthroscopic images show posterior labral repair and capsular plication as viewed from an anterosuperior portal. **A,** The capsular limb of the anchor suture is passed inferior and lateral to its respective anchor. **B,** The sutures are subsequently tied, the capsule is shifted superiorly, and the redundant capsule is plicated to form a labral bumper. Note that anchor placement as well as suture passage and tying proceed in an inferior-to-superior fashion. G = glenoid, HH = humeral head.

which would unintentionally prevent subsequent reduction of the posterior IGHL to its humeral neck insertion site.

Rotator interval closure for patients who have posterior shoulder instability is controversial. Some surgeons use rotator interval plication routinely for patients who have posterior shoulder instability, whereas others use it rarely, stating that excellent results have been reported without rotator interval closure.[105,107,108,120] Selective rotator interval closure is reserved predominantly for patients who have very high or even extreme degrees of posterior instability. These patients often have hyperlaxity and a prominent sulcus sign on physical examination. Thin or poor capsular tissue and/or revision surgery are other potential indications for rotator interval plication.

Rehabilitation

After surgical intervention, the patient's surgical arm is kept in a shoulder immobilizer in approximately 15° of external rotation for 4 weeks postoperatively. The arm is maintained posterior to the patient's trunk to minimize stress on the repair. The patient participates in gentle elbow, wrist, and hand range-of-motion exercises. After 4 weeks, the patient begins active-assisted range-of-motion exercises, including forward elevation in the scapular plane and external rotation with the arm at the side. Internal rotation behind the patient's back also is initiated; however, internal rotation with the arm elevated is prohibited at this time. Limited strengthening exercises also are initiated. At 8 weeks postoperatively, patients progress to more advanced rehabilitation with unrestricted range of motion and comprehensive shoulder and periscapular strengthening. Sport-specific training typically begins 3 to 4 months postoperatively, and a return to collision sports and unrestricted weightlifting is usually allowed after 6 months.

Multidirectional Instability

Patients who have MDI require an accurate diagnosis and selective treatment to avoid continued problems. A review of the literature has identified several areas of concern, including making the correct diagnosis, the duration of nonsurgical treatment methods, and selecting the best surgical procedure to manage patients in whom nonsurgical treatment has failed.[121] Shoulders that have MDI are different from the unidirectionally unstable shoulders described thus far and require additional measures to reduce the risk of failure.[122,123] Physicians often confuse excessive laxity with MDI and, as a result, have determined variable reports of success, both surgically and with nonsurgical techniques.

First defined by Neer and Foster,[124] MDI is uncontrollable and involuntary symptomatic inferior subluxation or dislocation associated with anterior, posterior, or both directions of subluxation. Matsen et al[125] introduced the AMBRI classification, which described shoulders with MDI as having an atraumatic onset; having MDI; commonly being bilateral; being initially managed with rehabilitation; and if failure occurred, then requiring an inferior capsular shift to reduce the size of the inferior capsular pouch. Bidirectional instability was used to describe shoulders that had symptomatic unidirectional instability and laxity in the opposite direction.[126] Patients with bidirectional instability had success with routine unidirectional surgical correction and should not be considered as a subset of patients who have MDI. Additional experience since the original description of MDI has identified subsets of patients with MDI that is caused by repetitive movement patterns or collagen disorders (ie, Ehlers-Danlos and Marfan syndromes, with inadequate ligamentous intrinsic strength). These definitions are very important in reviewing the literature and considering the success or failure of the management of patients who have MDI. Surgeons should be aware that the successful resolution of instability symptoms may be challenging in patients who have pain and are unaware

of subluxation. Identification of the key factors that cause the symptoms is critical to a successful intervention. Inferior symptomatic luxation is an important clinical characteristic of MDI, and the sulcus sign is an important feature of this inferior symptomatic luxation.[114] The reproduction of symptoms with provocative testing should raise suspicion and may help identify symptomatic directions of instability.

History

Patients who have suspected MDI usually report instability. The inferior direction from the original description may be discovered if objects are lifted from the ground. A loss of arm control, a painful click, and potentially a deadarm syndrome are reported in select patients. Additional positions and postures are important to identify associated directions that are symptomatic. Some patients describe pain as disabling, which can originate from compensatory movements, either structural or neurologic, but not necessarily the shoulder instability pattern. Patients who have disabling MDI often develop compensatory mechanisms, such as scapular dyskinesis, in an attempt to minimize their shoulder dysfunction. In fact, compensatory postural changes may lead to additional symptoms of pain, fatigue, and glenohumeral instability.

It is important for the physician to differentiate symptomatic instability from volitional subluxation. Some patients may voluntarily sublux their shoulders for secondary gain, such as attention. Symptomatic instability patterns can develop in these patients, but they are not surgical candidates. A common and substantial distinguishing feature of volitional subluxation

patients is that they often will volunteer to demonstrate their ability to actively sublux their shoulder joints, which often is not associated with noticeable discomfort.

Painful clicking with movements, the identification of positions that reproduce symptoms, and the identification of factors that cause fatigue help identify shoulders that have lost dynamic stability. Proprioception also may be altered in shoulders with MDI.[127] A traumatic event can tip the scale from a minimally symptomatic loose shoulder to a symptomatic shoulder that has MDI. Inferior symptomatic luxation is a distinguishing feature of shoulders that have MDI. Although structural changes can develop in patients who have MDI, the dynamic stabilizers can define success and failure with early management. A review of prior physical therapy is an important part of designing a treatment plan. Failed surgical stabilization is not uncommon in patients who have MDI because of symptomatic recurrence.

Physical Examination

The hallmark of shoulders that have MDI is the sulcus sign. To test for the sulcus sign, the patient is placed in a seated position with the affected forearm resting on his or her lap. The test is positive for the sulcus sign if an inferior directed force creates excessive inferior translation that results in increased acromial-humeral distance (**Figure 17**). Additional features of this test are a click associated with subluxation, with the patient identifying reproduction of his or her symptoms. Although apprehension is uncommon, some highly symptomatic patients may attempt to protect their shoulders from this painful occurrence.

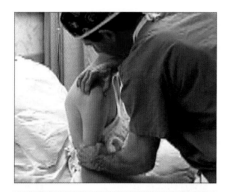

Figure 17   Clinical photograph shows an examiner testing for the sulcus sign with the patient in a seated position. The patient in this photograph shows inferior symptomatic subluxation.

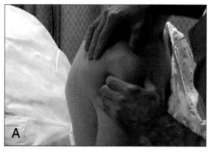
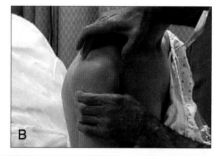

Figure 18   Clinical photographs show an examiner performing the load-and-shift maneuver with the patient in a seated position to test for anterior (**A**) and posterior (**B**) translation.

The sulcus sign has recently been examined with the shoulder in external rotation and has been associated with an enlarged rotator interval, which is commonly found in shoulders with MDI.[128] The additional rotation attempts to pre-tension capsular ligaments to reduce the translation. Persistent sulcus suggests that the capsular ligaments cannot limit the humeral translation. A Gagey sign, or hyperabduction sign, has been used to identify an enlarged inferior capsular pouch.[129] Passive abduction greater than 105° with a stabilized scapula is a positive finding for inferior capsular laxity.[129]

Anterior and posterior translation can be evaluated with the patient placed in the seated or supine position (**Figure 18**). A load-and-shift examination allows for measurement of the translation: grade I to the edge, grade II over the edge with spontaneous reduction, and grade III with dislocation that does not spontaneously reduce.[11] Increased translation should be compared with the opposite shoulder to identify subtle differences. The classic apprehension sign and reduction maneuver are uncommon in patients who have MDI. Shoulders that have MDI

often exhibit increased external and internal rotation with the arm in neutral and with 90° of abduction.

A telling feature of the disabled shoulder can be identified by standing behind the patient and asking him or her to demonstrate the most disabling posture for the shoulder. Winging of the scapula and avoidance of posture because of painful subluxation may help identify the most symptomatic directions (**Figure 19**). Areas of tenderness may include anterior and posterior joint lines. Selective muscle testing includes the cuff, the scapular stabilizers, and the biceps and helps direct physical therapy modalities.

Imaging and Testing

Radiographs can help identify glenoid dysplasia, which may predispose a shoulder to painful subluxation. A true AP radiograph and an axillary radiograph provide the best views. Stress testing films can illustrate increased translation and are helpful if the symptoms are reproduced.[130] An MRI, with or without articular contrast, will often demonstrate an enlarged inferior pouch. Structural damage, including superior labral tears, minimally displaced inferior labral tears, and enlarged intervals, may be found in some shoulders. Electromyography and nerve

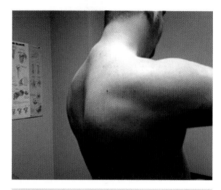

Figure 19   Clinical photograph shows a patient who has scapular winging, which is an abnormal muscle firing pattern that occurs with forward flexing.

conduction velocity are usually normal despite scapular winging, which suggests a dynamic pathologic response, not a neurologic injury. The serratus and long thoracic nerves are not injured or paralyzed, and other muscles may be overactive, which creates scapular rotation that exposes the static ligaments to additional vulnerability.

Treatment

A structured trial of nonsurgical treatment is important for shoulders that are disabled by MDI. The length of nonsurgical treatment has been debated, and a minimum of 3 months should be considered before symptomatic improvement and return to activities are measured.[131] Treatment should include

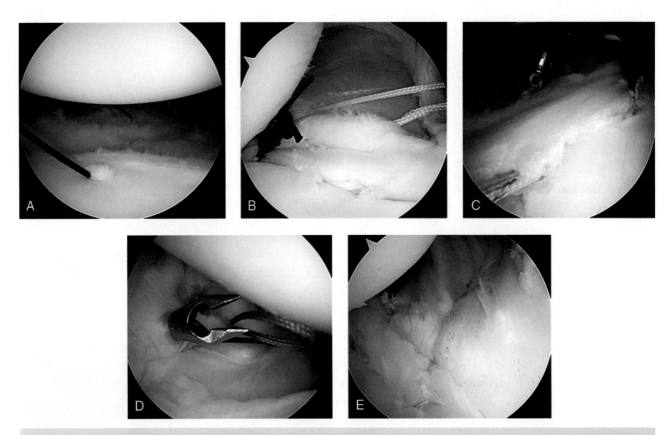

Figure 20 Arthroscopic images show arthroscopic stabilization of a shoulder that has multidirectional instability. **A,** A monofilament suture is placed at the 6-o'clock position after capsular preparation. **B,** A posteroinferior mattress suture is placed between the capsule and labrum. **C,** An anteroinferior suture anchor is placed, and a suture hook is used directly to reduce the inferior pouch. **D,** Rotator interval closure is selectively performed to incorporate the deep and superficial layers of the midcapsular structures and the superior glenohumeral ligament. **E,** The completed inferior capsular shift is demonstrated by wide reinforced tissue adjacent to the glenoid.

scapular stabilization, cuff strengthening in nonpainful positions, and functional closed chain-linked exercises to increase functional gains. Surgical treatment options may be considered for patients who do not improve.

Arthroscopic stabilization can provide a balanced repair with multiquadrant correction. Diagnostic arthroscopy should evaluate the superior labrum, the anterior and posterior capsular labral structures, and the humeral capsular attachments. The rotator interval can be qualified, and the capsular ligaments can be assessed. In chronic cases, the surgeon should evaluate the articular surface of the humerus and the glenoid.

Inferior capsular tensioning begins with the arthroscope in the anterior viewing portal midway between the acromion and the coracoid. After rasping the capsular tissues, a suture hook is introduced through the posterior portal, and a monofilament suture is passed through the capsule and the labrum at the 6-o'clock position (**Figure 20, A**). To minimize the risk of injury to the axillary nerve, the capsule is punctured 1 to 1.5 cm from the labrum, and the suture device is rotated toward the glenoid, which reduces the depth of penetration. The tip of the suture device can grasp the labrum for initial fixation. This suture is tied to begin the plication. A posteroinferior suture anchor is placed

through an accessory portal lateral to the posterior working portal. The suture hook is passed to create a mattress suture through the capsule and under the labrum (**Figure 20, B**). This suture may be tied or left untied until after the anteroinferior anchor is placed to avoid crowding. The anteroinferior portal is developed lateral to the coracoid and allows for proper placement of an anchor 1 cm anterior to the monofilament suture. A suture hook is passed through the same anteroinferior or posterior cannula, and a capsular shift is created by penetrating the pouch inferior and medial to the anchor. A simple or mattress suture may be completed depending on the quality of the tissue (**Figure 20, C**).

The surgeon should select the most symptomatic direction, either anterior or posterior. The capsular plication is continued on the selected side, substituting for soft-braided sutures. Mattress sutures will maximize the width of the paraglenoid fixation and the distance of the knots from the humeral surface. Patients who have insufficient labral tissue or an injury to the labral glenoid interface should undergo suture anchor fixation to maximize the strength of the repair. The opposite capsule is plicated with monofilament sutures to add symmetric tension to the glenohumeral articulation. Using a suture hook, these sutures can be passed and tied in an inferior-to-superior progression. Permanent suture can be used in select shoulders.

The rotator interval is often stretched and may contribute to inferior subluxation. The multiple layers of the rotator interval can be incorporated in the plication. The arthroscope is placed in the posterior portal, and a single large cannula is located in the middle of the interval space. The cannula is partially withdrawn to allow a suture hook to penetrate the deep bursal interval tissue, the upper border of the subscapularis fibers, and the middle glenohumeral ligament. The cannula is withdrawn to allow the superior capsule to cover the cannula. A piercing grasping instrument is passed through the superior ligament parallel to the glenoid, and the suture is retrieved (**Figure 20, D**). This suture may be exchanged for a soft No. 2 braided suture in nonthrowing athletes. A second parallel suture may be placed laterally to further reinforce this region. These stitches can incorporate the coracohumeral ligament to provide additional support to the adducted shoulder. Because overhead throwing

athletes may lose terminal rotation, this step should be avoided; alternatively, absorbable suture material can be used.

Articular portal closure can be performed with the piercing instrument. Withdrawal of the posterior cannula allows the capsule and the infraspinatus to close in front of the opening, which facilitates side-to-side suture being placed in the middle capsular region and tied external to the joint. This will create thickening of the midcapsular tissue and close portals that are potential stress risers for continued stretching deformity forces. A well-centered humeral head resting in the center of the glenoid is the goal of a balanced repair (**Figure 20, E**).

Select patients who have a superior labral tear should undergo suture anchor repair. If a true superior labrum anterior to posterior tear is diagnosed in the initial part of the procedure, the capsular plication bites can be adjusted to avoid overconstraining the joint. Mattress suture repair of the superior labrum will minimize the risk of head abrasion. Anchor placement is posterior to the biceps insertion through an accessory portal at the abraded glenoid neck, not on top of the articular cartilage. The suture hook enters through the anterior portal and pierces the labrum without the capsule (**Figure 21**). Each limb is passed separately in this manner, which allows for a mattress knot fixation.

Patients who have collagen disorders, such as Ehlers-Danlos and Marfan syndromes, may have an increased risk for failure with a purely medially based arthroscopic procedure. An open capsular shift has been presented as an alternative because greater restraints can be created with a laterally based correction. In these patients, success

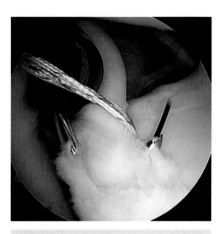

Figure 21 Arthroscopic image shows the repair of a superior labral tear in a patient who had inferior instability.

is problematic with either arthroscopic or open repairs because of collagen changes. Grafting of the capsule can be accomplished with the use of allograft as well as autograft and can be performed arthroscopically as a Gallie procedure, which augments the inferior capsular repair.[132] Suture hooks are used to reinforce the inferior capsule, and suture anchor fixation is recommended to secure the superior ends of the grafted capsule. Delayed rehabilitation is recommended for patients who have collagen disorders.

Postoperative Management

A supportive sling brace is applied with the shoulder placed in reduced internal rotation. The sling is worn for 6 weeks postoperatively, and scapular shrugs are started during this phase. After 6 weeks postoperatively, the patient begins passive forward flexion in the supine position using the opposite extremity to assist. A gradual approach to range of motion should be monitored closely. External rotation to 30° can be assisted in the next 4 weeks, and external rotation to 45° can be assisted in the subsequent 4 weeks. Cross-chest stretching and internal rotation can begin at 8 weeks postoperatively. Placing the hand behind the back and reaching above the waist is delayed to avoid stretching the critical areas of repair. Cuff strengthening begins at 10 weeks postoperatively, and scapular strength continues with resistance. The surgeon should monitor scapular control and coordination and adjust exercises based on the patient's ability to actively flex without winging. Return to sport and work is often delayed 6 to 7 months postoperatively depending on symptomatic improvement, acceptable range of motion, protective strength to the rotator cuff, and scapular core strength.

Results

The success of nonsurgical treatment has been reported in several studies, with emphasis on activity, restrictions, rotator cuff stabilization exercises, and open and closed-chain scapular stability strengthening programs.[117] Misamore et al[131] suggested that many patients will remain symptomatic or have symptomatic relapses and should choose stabilization surgery despite an organized physical therapy approach; however, the patients in this study who had a higher rate of failure for nonsurgical treatment were those who did not maintain a regimen of home exercises. The authors suggested improvement within 3 months as a prognostic finding. Early surgical studies included open surgery with laterally based, overlapping capsule flaps after tenotomy of the rotator cuff and indirect shifting of the inferior capsular pouch. The arthroscopic approach is a medially based correction and can create a balanced direct approach in all four compartments. Successful resolution of symptoms has been reported in 65% to 88% of

patients.[114,132-135] Static stabilizers may improve the proprioception component of instability symptoms, with dynamic stabilization of the scapula and glenohumeral positioning essential for mid- and long-term success.

Very little literature exists on patients who have either Ehlers-Danlos or Marfan syndrome and MDI. The current anecdotal reports suggest early return of laxity with soft-tissue procedures. Capsular grafting may increase the duration of capsular restraint, but laxity is a common outcome. There is a window of opportunity for return to prior functional levels with a dynamic stabilization program that includes core strengthening. Recovery is often prolonged, and return to offending activities is difficult and has had mixed results.[133]

Summary

Anterior instability, posterior instability, and MDI can be successfully and reliably treated arthroscopically. Arthroscopic stabilization has evolved into the procedure of choice for most patients who require surgical intervention for shoulder instability. Patients who have substantial GBL may be best treated with a procedure that incorporates grafting of the bony defect. If arthroscopic surgery is selected, meticulous surgical technique that focuses on the mitigation of risk factors is essential. The integration of newer arthroscopic surgical methods—such as the use of an anchor in the 6-o'clock position, the use of adjunctive Hill-Sachs remplissage if indicated, the inclusion of any bony Bankart or reverse Bankart lesions, the use of an adequate number of suture anchors, the use of supplemental capsular plication, and the use of a robust suturing pattern—may improve surgical outcomes and reduce recurrence rates.

References

1. Simonet WT, Melton LJ III, Cofield RH, Ilstrup DM: Incidence of anterior shoulder dislocation in Olmsted County, Minnesota. *Clin Orthop Relat Res* 1984;186:186-191.

2. Balg F, Boileau P: The instability severity index score: A simple pre-operative score to select patients for arthroscopic or open shoulder stabilisation. *J Bone Joint Surg Br* 2007;89(11):1470-1477.

3. Porcellini G, Campi F, Pegreffi F, Castagna A, Paladini P: Predisposing factors for recurrent shoulder dislocation after arthroscopic treatment. *J Bone Joint Surg Am* 2009;91(11):2537-2542.

4. Burkhart SS, DeBeer JF: Traumatic glenohumeral bone defects and their relationship to failure of arthroscopic Bankart repairs: Significance of the inverted-pear glenoid and the humeral engaging Hill-Sachs Lesion. *Arthroscopy* 2000;16(7):677-694.

5. Voos JE, Livermore RW, Feeley BT, et al: Prospective evaluation of arthroscopic Bankart repairs for anterior instability. *Am J Sports Med* 2010;38(2):302-307.

6. Wasserstein D, Dwyer T, Veillette C, et al: Predictors of dislocation and revision after shoulder stabilization in Ontario, Canada, from 2003 to 2008. *Am J Sports Med* 2013;41(9):2034-2040.

7. Boileau P, Villalba M, Héry JY, Balg F, Ahrens P, Neyton L: Risk factors for recurrence of shoulder instability after arthroscopic Bankart repair. *J Bone Joint Surg Am* 2006;88(8):1755-1763.

8. Mazzocca AD, Brown FM Jr, Carreira DS, Hayden J, Romeo AA: Arthroscopic anterior shoulder stabilization of collision and contact athletes. *Am J Sports Med* 2005;33(1):52-60.

9. Owens BD, Harrast JJ, Hurwitz SR, Thompson TL, Wolf JM: Surgical trends in Bankart repair: An analysis of data from the American Board of Orthopaedic Surgery certification examination. *Am J Sports Med* 2011;39(9):1865-1869.

10. Franceschi F, Papalia R, Rizzello G, et al: Remplissage repair—new frontiers

© 2016 AAOS Instructional Course Lectures, Volume 65

in the prevention of recurrent shoulder instability: A 2-year follow-up comparative study. *Am J Sports Med* 2012;40(11):2462-2469.

11. Bedi A, Ryu RK: Revision arthroscopic Bankart repair. *Sports Med Arthrosc* 2010;18(3):130-139.

12. Ozturk BY, Maak TG, Fabricant P, et al: Return to sports after arthroscopic anterior stabilization in patients aged younger than 25 years. *Arthroscopy* 2013;29(12):1922-1931.

13. Boileau P, O'Shea K, Vargas P, Pinedo M, Old J, Zumstein M: Anatomical and functional results after arthroscopic Hill-Sachs remplissage. *J Bone Joint Surg Am* 2012;94(7):618-626.

14. Castagna A, Markopoulos N, Conti M, Delle Rose G, Papadakou E, Garofalo R: Arthroscopic bankart suture-anchor repair: Radiological and clinical outcome at minimum 10 years of follow-up. *Am J Sports Med* 2010;38(10):2012-2016.

15. Sugaya H, Moriishi J, Kanisawa I, Tsuchiya A: Arthroscopic osseous Bankart repair for chronic recurrent traumatic anterior glenohumeral instability. *J Bone Joint Surg Am* 2005;87(8):1752-1760.

16. McCabe MP, Weinberg D, Field LD, O'Brien MJ, Hobgood ER, Savoie FH III: Primary versus revision arthroscopic reconstruction with remplissage for shoulder instability with moderate bone loss. *Arthroscopy* 2014;30(4):444-450.

17. Ryu RKN, Bedi A: Arthroscopic treatment of traumatic shoulder instability, in Angelo RL, Esch JC, Ryu RKN, eds: *AANA Advanced Arthroscopy: The Shoulder*. Philadelphia, PA, Saunders Elsevier, 2010, pp 106-114.

18. van der Linde JA, van Kampen DA, Terwee CB, Dijksman LM, Kleinjan G, Willems WJ: Long-term results after arthroscopic shoulder stabilization using suture anchors: An 8- to 10-year follow-up. *Am J Sports Med* 2011;39(11):2396-2403.

19. Zhu YM, Lu Y, Zhang J, Shen JW, Jiang CY: Arthroscopic Bankart repair combined with remplissage technique for the treatment of anterior shoulder instability with engaging Hill-Sachs lesion: A report of 49 cases with a minimum 2-year follow-up. *Am J Sports Med* 2011;39(8):1640-1647.

20. Mologne TS, McBride MT, Lapoint JM: Assessment of failed arthroscopic anterior labral repairs: Findings at open surgery. *Am J Sports Med* 1997;25(6):813-817.

21. Brophy RH, Marx RG: The treatment of traumatic anterior instability of the shoulder: Nonoperative and surgical treatment. *Arthroscopy* 2009;25(3):298-304.

22. Provencher CM, Makani A, McNeil JW, Pomerantz ML, Golijanin P, Gross D: The role of the scapula in throwing disorders. *Sports Med Arthrosc* 2014;22(2):80-87.

23. Braun S, Kokmeyer D, Millett PJ: Shoulder injuries in the throwing athlete. *J Bone Joint Surg Am* 2009;91(4):966-978.

24. Turkel SJ, Panio MW, Marshall JL, Girgis FG: Stabilizing mechanisms preventing anterior dislocation of the glenohumeral joint. *J Bone Joint Surg Am* 1981;63(8):1208-1217.

25. Lippitt SB, Vanderhooft JE, Harris SL, Sidles JA, Harryman DT II, Matsen FA III: Glenohumeral stability from concavity-compression: A quantitative analysis. *J Shoulder Elbow Surg* 1993;2(1):27-35.

26. Speer KP, Deng X, Borrero S, Torzilli PA, Altchek DA, Warren RF: Biomechanical evaluation of a simulated Bankart lesion. *J Bone Joint Surg Am* 1994;76(12):1819-1826.

27. Quatman CE, Ford KR, Myer GD, Paterno MV, Hewett TE: The effects of gender and pubertal status on generalized joint laxity in young athletes. *J Sci Med Sport* 2008;11(3):257-263.

28. Wynne-Davies R: Familial joint laxity. *Proc R Soc Med* 1971;64(6):689-690.

29. Castagna A, Borroni M, Delle Rose G, et al: Effects of posterior-inferior capsular plications in range of motion in arthroscopic anterior Bankart repair: A prospective randomized clinical study. *Knee Surg Sports Traumatol Arthrosc* 2009;17(2):188-194.

30. Murachovsky J, Bueno RS, Nascimento LG, et al: Calculating anterior glenoid bone loss using the Bernageau profile view. *Skeletal Radiol* 2012;41(10):1231-1237.

31. Provencher MT, Bhatia S, Ghodadra NS, et al: Recurrent shoulder instability: Current concepts for evaluation and management of glenoid bone loss. *J Bone Joint Surg Am* 2010;92(suppl 2):133-151.

32. Warner JJ, Gill TJ, O'Hollerhan JD, Pathare N, Millett PJ: Anatomical glenoid reconstruction for recurrent anterior glenohumeral instability with glenoid deficiency using an autogenous tricortical iliac crest bone graft. *Am J Sports Med* 2006;34(2):205-212.

33. Provencher MT, Frank RM, LeClere LE, et al: The Hill-Sachs lesion: Diagnosis, classification, and management. *J Am Acad Orthop Surg* 2012;20(4):242-252.

34. Owens BD, Duffey ML, Nelson BJ, DeBerardino TM, Taylor CD, Mountcastle SB: The incidence and characteristics of shoulder instability at the United States Military Academy. *Am J Sports Med* 2007;35(7):1168-1173.

35. Owens BD, Dawson L, Burks R, Cameron KL: Incidence of shoulder dislocation in the United States military: Demographic considerations from a high-risk population. *J Bone Joint Surg Am* 2009;91(4):791-796.

36. Sachs RA, Lin D, Stone ML, Paxton E, Kuney M: Can the need for future surgery for acute traumatic anterior shoulder dislocation be predicted? *J Bone Joint Surg Am* 2007;89(8):1665-1674.

37. Hovelius L, Olofsson A, Sandström B, et al: Nonoperative treatment of primary anterior shoulder dislocation in patients forty years of age and younger: A prospective twenty-five-year follow-up. *J Bone Joint Surg Am* 2008;90(5):945-952.

38. Liavaag S, Brox JI, Pripp AH, Enger M, Soldal LA, Svenningsen S: Immobilization in external rotation after primary shoulder dislocation did not reduce the risk of recurrence: A randomized controlled trial. *J Bone Joint Surg Am* 2011;93(10):897-904.

39. Limpisvasti O, Yang BY, Hosseinzadeh P, Leba TB, Tibone JE, Lee TQ: The effect of glenohumeral position on the shoulder after traumatic

anterior dislocation. *Am J Sports Med* 2008;36(4):775-780.

40. Itoi E, Hatakeyama Y, Kido T, et al: A new method of immobilization after traumatic anterior dislocation of the shoulder: A preliminary study. *J Shoulder Elbow Surg* 2003;12(5):413-415.

41. Whelan DB, Litchfield R, Wambolt E, Dainty KN; Joint Orthopaedic Initiative for National Trials of the Shoulder (JOINTS): External rotation immobilization for primary shoulder dislocation: A randomized controlled trial. *Clin Orthop Relat Res* 2014;472(8):2380-2386.

42. Milgrom C, Milgrom Y, Radeva-Petrova D, Jaber S, Beyth S, Finestone AS: The supine apprehension test helps predict the risk of recurrent instability after a first-time anterior shoulder dislocation. *J Shoulder Elbow Surg* 2014;23(12):1838-1842.

43. Ryu RK, Ryu JH: Arthroscopic revision Bankart repair: A preliminary evaluation. *Orthopedics* 2011;34(1):17.

44. Mohtadi NG, Chan DS, Hollinshead RM, et al: A randomized clinical trial comparing open and arthroscopic stabilization for recurrent traumatic anterior shoulder instability: Two-year follow-up with disease-specific quality-of-life outcomes. *J Bone Joint Surg Am* 2014;96(5):353-360.

45. Weber SC: Arthroscopic Bankart repair: Minimum 10 year follow-up with emphasis on survivorship. Presented at the 33rd Annual Meeting of the Arthroscopy Association of North America, Hollywood, FL, May 1-3, 2014.

46. Dumont GD, Fogerty S, Rosso C, Lafosse L: The arthroscopic Latarjet procedure for anterior shoulder instability: 5-year minimum follow-up. *Am J Sports Med* 2014;42(11):2560-2566.

47. Mizuno N, Denard PJ, Raiss P, Melis B, Walch G: Long-term results of the Latarjet procedure for anterior instability of the shoulder. *J Shoulder Elbow Surg* 2014;23(11):1691-1699.

48. Hovelius L, Sandström B, Sundgren K, Saebö M: One hundred eighteen Bristow-Latarjet repairs for recurrent anterior dislocation of the shoulder prospectively followed for fifteen years: Study

I—clinical results. *J Shoulder Elbow Surg* 2004;13(5):509-516.

49. Bhatia S, Frank RM, Ghodadra NS, et al: The outcomes and surgical techniques of the Latarjet procedure. *Arthroscopy* 2014;30(2):227-235.

50. Bishop JA, Crall TS, Kocher MS: Operative versus nonoperative treatment after primary traumatic anterior glenohumeral dislocation: Expected-value decision analysis. *J Shoulder Elbow Surg* 2011;20(7):1087-1094.

51. Arciero RA, Wheeler JH, Ryan JB, McBride JT: Arthroscopic Bankart repair versus nonoperative treatment for acute, initial anterior shoulder dislocations. *Am J Sports Med* 1994;22(5):589-594.

52. Crall TS, Bishop JA, Guttman D, Kocher M, Bozic K, Lubowitz JH: Cost-effectiveness analysis of primary arthroscopic stabilization versus nonoperative treatment for first-time anterior glenohumeral dislocations. *Arthroscopy* 2012;28(12):1755-1765.

53. Dickens JF, Owens BD, Cameron KL, et al: Return to play following in-season anterior shoulder instability: A prospective multicenter study. Presented at the 2014 Annual Meeting of the American Orthopedic Society for Sports Medicine, Seattle, WA, July 10-13, 2014.

54. Bottoni CR, Wilckens JH, DeBernardino TM, et al: A prospective, randomized evaluation of arthroscopic stabilization versus nonoperative treatment in patients with acute, traumatic, first-time shoulder dislocations. *Am J Sports Med* 2002;30(4):576-580.

55. Jakobsen BW, Johannsen HV, Suder P, Søjbjerg JO: Primary repair versus conservative treatment of first-time traumatic anterior dislocation of the shoulder: A randomized study with 10-year follow-up. *Arthroscopy* 2007;23(2):118-123.

56. Robinson CM, Jenkins PJ, White TO, Ker A, Will E: Primary arthroscopic stabilization for a first-time anterior dislocation of the shoulder: A randomized, double-blind trial. *J Bone Joint Surg Am* 2008;90(4):708-721.

57. Kirkley A, Griffin S, Richards C, Miniaci A, Mohtadi N: Prospective randomized clinical trial comparing

the effectiveness of immediate arthroscopic stabilization versus immobilization and rehabilitation in first traumatic anterior dislocations of the shoulder. *Arthroscopy* 1999;15(5):507-514.

58. Longo UG, Loppini M, Rizzello G, Ciuffreda M, Maffulli N, Denaro V: Management of primary acute anterior shoulder dislocation: Systematic review and quantitative synthesis of the literature. *Arthroscopy* 2014;30(4):506-522.

59. Frank RM, Saccomanno MF, McDonald LS, Moric M, Romeo AA, Provencher MT: Outcomes of arthroscopic anterior shoulder instability in the beach chair versus lateral decubitus position: A systematic review and meta-regression analysis. *Arthroscopy* 2014;30(10):1349-1365.

60. Bokor DJ, Conboy VB, Olson C: Anterior instability of the glenohumeral joint with humeral avulsion of the glenohumeral ligament: A review of 41 cases. *J Bone Joint Surg Br* 1999;81(1):93-96.

61. Ozbaydar M, Elhassan B, Diller D, Massimini D, Higgins LD, Warner JJ: Results of arthroscopic capsulolabral repair: Bankart lesion versus anterior labroligamentous periosteal sleeve avulsion lesion. *Arthroscopy* 2008;24(11):1277-1283.

62. Millett PJ, Braun S: The "bony Bankart bridge" procedure: A new arthroscopic technique for reduction and internal fixation of a bony Bankart lesion. *Arthroscopy* 2009;25(1):102-105.

63. Di Giacomo G, Itoi E, Burkhart SS: Evolving concept of bipolar bone loss and the Hill-Sachs lesion: From "engaging/non-engaging" lesion to "on-track/off-track" lesion. *Arthroscopy* 2014;30(1):90-98.

64. Harryman DT II, Sidles JA, Harris SL, Matsen FA III: The role of the rotator interval capsule in passive motion and stability of the shoulder. *J Bone Joint Surg Am* 1992;74(1):53-66.

65. Rouleau DM, Hébert-Davies J, Djahangiri A, Godbout V, Pelet S, Balg F: Validation of the instability shoulder index score in a multicenter reliability study in 114 consecutive cases. *Am J Sports Med* 2013;41(2):278-282.

66. Franceschi F, Longo UG, Ruzzini L, Rizzello G, Maffulli N, Denaro V: Arthroscopic salvage of failed arthroscopic Bankart repair: A prospective study with a minimum follow-up of 4 years. *Am J Sports Med* 2008;36(7):1330-1336.

67. Abouali JA, Hatzantoni K, Holtby R, Veillette C, Theodoropoulos J: Revision arthroscopic Bankart repair. *Arthroscopy* 2013;29(9):1572-1578.

68. Bartl C, Schumann K, Paul J, Vogt S, Imhoff AB: Arthroscopic capsulolabral revision repair for recurrent anterior shoulder instability. *Am J Sports Med* 2011;39(3):511-518.

69. Hintermann B, Gächter A: Arthroscopic findings after shoulder dislocation. *Am J Sports Med* 1995;23(5):545-551.

70. Urayama M, Itoi E, Sashi R, Minagawa H, Sato K: Capsular elongation in shoulders with recurrent anterior dislocation: Quantitative assessment with magnetic resonance arthrography. *Am J Sports Med* 2003;31(1):64-67.

71. Itoi E, Lee SB, Berglund LJ, Berge LL, An KN: The effect of a glenoid defect on anteroinferior stability of the shoulder after Bankart repair: A cadaveric study. *J Bone Joint Surg Am* 2000;82(1):35-46.

72. Sugaya H, Moriishi J, Dohi M, Kon Y, Tsuchiya A: Glenoid rim morphology in recurrent anterior glenohumeral instability. *J Bone Joint Surg Am* 2003;85(5):878-884.

73. Mologne TS, Provencher MT, Menzel KA, Vachon TA, Dewing CB: Arthroscopic stabilization in patients with an inverted pear glenoid: Results in patients with bone loss of the anterior glenoid. *Am J Sports Med* 2007;35(8):1276-1283.

74. Edwards TB, Boulahia A, Walch G: Radiographic analysis of bone defects in chronic anterior shoulder instability. *Arthroscopy* 2003;19(7):732-739.

75. Garth WP Jr, Slappey CE, Ochs CW: Roentgenographic demonstration of instability of the shoulder: The apical oblique projection. A technical note. *J Bone Joint Surg Am* 1984;66(9):1450-1453.

76. Pavlov H, Warren RF, Weiss CB Jr, Dines DM: The roentgenographic evaluation of anterior shoulder instability. *Clin Orthop Relat Res* 1985;194:153-158.

77. Rokous JR, Feagin JA, Abbott HG: Modified axillary roentgenogram: A useful adjunct in the diagnosis of recurrent instability of the shoulder. *Clin Orthop Relat Res* 1972;82:84-86.

78. Piasecki DP, Verma NN, Romeo AA, Levine WN, Bach BR Jr, Provencher MT: Glenoid bone deficiency in recurrent anterior shoulder instability: Diagnosis and management. *J Am Acad Orthop Surg* 2009;17(8):482-493.

79. Huysmans PE, Haen PS, Kidd M, Dhert WJ, Willems JW: The shape of the inferior part of the glenoid: A cadaveric study. *J Shoulder Elbow Surg* 2006;15(6):759-763.

80. Provencher MT, Ghodadra N, Romeo AA: Arthroscopic management of anterior instability: Pearls, pitfalls, and lessons learned. *Orthop Clin North Am* 2010;41(3):325-337.

81. Yamamoto N, Itoi E, Abe H, et al: Contact between the glenoid and the humeral head in abduction, external rotation, and horizontal extension: A new concept of glenoid track. *J Shoulder Elbow Surg* 2007;16(5):649-656.

82. Metzger PD, Barlow B, Leonardelli D, Peace W, Solomon DJ, Provencher MT: Clinical application of the "glenoid track" concept for defining humeral head engagement in anterior shoulder instability: A preliminary report. *Orthop J Sports Med* 2013;1(2).

83. Kralinger F, Aigner F, Longato S, Rieger M, Wambacher M: Is the bare spot a consistent landmark for shoulder arthroscopy? A study of 20 embalmed glenoids with 3-dimensional computed tomographic reconstruction. *Arthroscopy* 2006;22(4):428-432.

84. Bernhardson AS, Bailey JR, Solomon DJ, Stanley M, Provencher MT: Glenoid bone loss in the setting of an anterior labroligamentous periosteal sleeve avulsion tear. *Am J Sports Med* 2014;42(9):2136-2140.

85. Snyder SJ, Strafford BB: Arthroscopic management of instability of the shoulder. *Orthopedics* 1993;16(9):993-1002.

86. Latarjet M: Treatment of recurrent dislocation of the shoulder. *Lyon Chir* 1954;49(8):994-997.

87. Lafosse L, Lejeune E, Bouchard A, Kakuda C, Gobezie R, Kochhar T: The arthroscopic Latarjet procedure for the treatment of anterior shoulder instability. *Arthroscopy* 2007;23(11):1242.e1-1242.e5.

88. Allain J, Goutallier D, Glorion C: Long-term results of the Latarjet procedure for the treatment of anterior instability of the shoulder. *J Bone Joint Surg Am* 1998;80(6):841-852.

89. Bhatia S, Van Thiel GS, Gupta D, et al: Comparison of glenohumeral contact pressures and contact areas after glenoid reconstruction with Latarjet or distal tibial osteochondral allografts. *Am J Sports Med* 2013;41(8):1900-1908.

90. Provencher MT, Ghodadra N, LeClere L, Solomon DJ, Romeo AA: Anatomic osteochondral glenoid reconstruction for recurrent glenohumeral instability with glenoid deficiency using a distal tibia allograft. *Arthroscopy* 2009;25(4):446-452.

91. Provencher MT, LeClere LE, King S, et al: Posterior instability of the shoulder: Diagnosis and management. *Am J Sports Med* 2011;39(4):874-886.

92. Owens BD, Campbell SE, Cameron KL: Risk factors for posterior shoulder instability in young athletes. *Am J Sports Med* 2013;41(11):2645-2649.

93. Robinson CM, Seah M, Akhtar MA: The epidemiology, risk of recurrence, and functional outcome after an acute traumatic posterior dislocation of the shoulder. *J Bone Joint Surg Am* 2011;93(17):1605-1613.

94. Van Tongel A, Karelse A, Berghs B, Verdonk R, De Wilde L: Posterior shoulder instability: Current concepts review. *Knee Surg Sports Traumatol Arthrosc* 2011;19(9):1547-1553.

95. Lenart BA, Sherman SL, Mall NA, Gochanour E, Twigg SL, Nicholson GP: Arthroscopic repair for posterior shoulder instability. *Arthroscopy* 2012;28(10):1337-1343.

96. Millett PJ, Clavert P, Hatch GF III, Warner JJ: Recurrent posterior shoulder instability. *J Am Acad Orthop Surg* 2006;14(8):464-476.

97. Bradley JP, Tejwani SG: Arthroscopic management of posterior instability. *Orthop Clin North Am* 2010;41(3):339-356.

98. Tannenbaum EP, Sekiya JK: Posterior shoulder instability in the contact athlete. *Clin Sports Med* 2013;32(4):781-796.

99. Savoie FH III, Holt MS, Field LD, Ramsey JR: Arthroscopic management of posterior instability: Evolution of technique and results. *Arthroscopy* 2008;24(4):389-396.

100. Pokabla C, Hobgood ER, Field LD: Identification and management of "floating" posterior inferior glenohumeral ligament lesions. *J Shoulder Elbow Surg* 2010;19(2):314-317.

101. Shah AA, Butler RB, Fowler R, Higgins LD: Posterior capsular rupture causing posterior shoulder instability: A case report. *Arthroscopy* 2011;27(9):1304-1307.

102. Hill JD, Lovejoy JF Jr, Kelly RA: Combined posterior Bankart lesion and posterior humeral avulsion of the glenohumeral ligaments associated with recurrent posterior shoulder instability. *Arthroscopy* 2007;23(3): 327.e1-327.e3.

103. Kim SH, Kim HK, Sun JI, Park JS, Oh I: Arthroscopic capsulolabroplasty for posteroinferior multidirectional instability of the shoulder. *Am J Sports Med* 2004;32(3):594-607.

104. Hawkins RJ, Koppert G, Johnston G: Recurrent posterior instability (subluxation) of the shoulder. *J Bone Joint Surg Am* 1984;66(2):169-174.

105. Wolf EM, Eakin CL: Arthroscopic capsular plication for posterior shoulder instability. *Arthroscopy* 1998;14(2):153-163.

106. Bottoni CR, Franks BR, Moore JH, DeBerardino TM, Taylor DC, Arciero RA: Operative stabilization of posterior shoulder instability. *Am J Sports Med* 2005;33(7):996-1002.

107. Kim SH, Ha KI, Park JH, et al: Arthroscopic posterior labral repair and capsular shift for traumatic unidirectional recurrent posterior subluxation of the shoulder. *J Bone Joint Surg Am* 2003;85(8):1479-1487.

108. Bradley JP, McClincy MP, Arner JW, Tejwani SG: Arthroscopic capsulolabral reconstruction for posterior instability of the shoulder: A prospective study of 200 shoulders. *Am J Sports Med* 2013;41(9):2005-2014.

109. Bahk MS, Karzel RP, Snyder SJ: Arthroscopic posterior stabilization and anterior capsular plication for recurrent posterior glenohumeral instability. *Arthroscopy* 2010;26(9):1172-1180.

110. Williams RJ III, Strickland S, Cohen M, Altchek DW, Warren RF: Arthroscopic repair for traumatic posterior shoulder instability. *Am J Sports Med* 2003;31(2):203-209.

111. Wanich T, Dines J, Dines D, Gambardella RA, Yocum LA: 'Batter's shoulder': Can athletes return to play at the same level after operative treatment? *Clin Orthop Relat Res* 2012;470(6):1565-1570.

112. Abrams JS, Bradley JP, Angelo RL, Burks R: Arthroscopic management of shoulder instabilities: Anterior, posterior, and multidirectional. *Instr Course Lect* 2010;59:141-155.

113. Pagnani MJ, Warren RF: Stabilizers of the glenohumeral joint. *J Shoulder Elbow Surg* 1994;3(3):173-190.

114. Kim SH, Ha KI, Yoo JC, Noh KC: Kim's lesion: An incomplete and concealed avulsion of the posteroinferior labrum in posterior or multidirectional posteroinferior instability of the shoulder. *Arthroscopy* 2004;20(7):712-720.

115. Tibone JE, Bradley JP: The treatment of posterior subluxation in athletes. *Clin Orthop Relat Res* 1993;291:124-137.

116. Kim SH, Park JS, Jeong WK, Shin SK: The Kim test: A novel test for posteroinferior labral lesion of the shoulder—a comparison to the jerk test. *Am J Sports Med* 2005;33(8):1188-1192.

117. Burkhead WZ Jr, Rockwood CA Jr: Treatment of instability of the shoulder with an exercise program. *J Bone Joint Surg Am* 1992;74(6):890-896.

118. Fronek J, Warren RF, Bowen M: Posterior subluxation of the glenohumeral joint. *J Bone Joint Surg Am* 1989;71(2):205-216.

119. Wilk KE, Macrina LC, Reinold MM: Non-operative rehabilitation for traumatic and atraumatic glenohumeral instability. *N Am J Sports Phys Ther* 2006;1(1):16-31.

120. Provencher MT, Bell SJ, Menzel KA, Mologne TS: Arthroscopic treatment of posterior shoulder instability: Results in 33 patients. *Am J Sports Med* 2005;33(10):1463-1471.

121. Schenk TJ, Brems JJ: Multidirectional instability of the shoulder: Pathophysiology, diagnosis, and management. *J Am Acad Orthop Surg* 1998;6(1):65-72.

122. Hawkins RH, Hawkins RJ: Failed anterior reconstruction for shoulder instability. *J Bone Joint Surg Br* 1985;67(5):709-714.

123. Gaskill TR, Taylor DC, Millett PJ: Management of multidirectional instability of the shoulder. *J Am Acad Orthop Surg* 2011;19(12):758-767.

124. Neer CS II, Foster CR: Inferior capsular shift for involuntary inferior and multidirectional instability of the shoulder: A preliminary report. *J Bone Joint Surg Am* 1980;62(6):897-908.

125. Matsen FA III, Thomas SC, Rockwood CA, Wirth MA: Glenohumeral instability, in Rockwood CA, Matsen FA III, eds: *The Shoulder*, ed 2. Philadelphia, PA, WB Saunders, 1998, pp 611-689.

126. Gartsman GM, Roddey TS, Hammerman SM: Arthroscopic treatment of bidirectional glenohumeral instability: Two- to five-year follow-up. *J Shoulder Elbow Surg* 2001;10(1):28-36.

127. Barden JM, Balyk R, Raso VJ, Moreau M, Bagnall K: Dynamic upper limb proprioception in multidirectional shoulder instability. *Clin Orthop Relat Res* 2004;420:181-189.

128. Provencher MT, Dewing CB, Bell SJ, et al: An analysis of the rotator interval in patients with anterior, posterior, and multidirectional shoulder instability. *Arthroscopy* 2008;24(8):921-929.

129. Gagey OJ, Gagey N: The hyperabduction test. *J Bone Joint Surg Br* 2001;83(1):69-74.

130. Hawkins RJ, Abrams JS, Schutte JP: Multidirectional instability of the shoulder: An approach to diagnosis. *Orthop Trans* 1987;11:246.

131. Misamore GW, Sallay PI, Didelot W: A longitudinal study of patients with multidirectional instability of the shoulder with seven- to ten-year follow-up. *J Shoulder Elbow Surg* 2005;14(5):466-470.

132. McIntyre LF, Caspari RB, Savoie FH III: The arthroscopic treatment of multidirectional shoulder instability: Two-year results of a multiple suture technique. *Arthroscopy* 1997;13(4):418-425.

133. Baker CL III, Mascarenhas R, Kline AJ, Chhabra A, Pombo MW, Bradley JP: Arthroscopic treatment of multidirectional shoulder instability in athletes: A retrospective analysis of 2- to 5-year clinical outcomes. *Am J Sports Med* 2009;37(9):1712-1720.

134. Hewitt M, Getelman MH, Snyder SJ: Arthroscopic management of multidirectional instability: Pancapsular plication. *Orthop Clin North Am* 2003;34(4):549-557.

135. Treacy SH, Savoie FH III, Field LD: Arthroscopic treatment of multidirectional instability. *J Shoulder Elbow Surg* 1999;8(4):345-350.

Video Reference

Field LD: Video. *Arthroscopic Management of Shoulder Instabilities: Anterior, Posterior, and Multidirectional*. Jackson, MS, 2015.

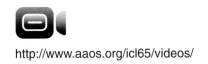

http://www.aaos.org/icl65/videos/

Hip Arthroscopy: Tales From the Crypt

Dean K. Matsuda, MD
Marc J. Philippon, MD
Marc R. Safran, MD
Thomas G. Sampson, MD

Abstract

Complications after hip arthroscopy vary in frequency and severity, even for experienced surgeons. It is important for surgeons to be aware of some of the more dramatic, often unusual, and always memorable (nightmarish) complications of hip arthroscopy and understand how they are caused, how they can be treated, and how they can be prevented.

Instr Course Lect 2016;65:437–446.

Although hip arthroscopy has experienced rapid growth in utilization and indications,[1] it remains a technically challenging procedure. The complication rate after arthroscopy for the treatment of femoroacetabular impingement (FAI), the most common indication, ranges from 1% to 6%, with most complications being of minor severity.[1-4] It is important for surgeons to be aware of interesting, important, and unusual complications that may occur after hip arthroscopy, some of which have not yet been introduced into the orthopaedic literature, and understand how they are caused, how they can be treated, and the lessons that can be learned from them.

Dysplasia Aphasia (Pitfalls in Dysplasia)
Complication and Causation

Anterior hip dislocation is a complication that may occur immediately after hip arthroscopy for the treatment of FAI (**Figure 1**). Matsuda[5] reported an occurrence of anterior hip dislocation in a case study of a woman who underwent hip arthroscopy for the treatment of FAI. This dramatic and rare complication that compromised hip stability was caused by a combination of bone and soft-tissue disruptions. The author performed excessive rim trimming, which removed a radiographic crossover sign but caused iatrogenic dysplasia. Suture cut-through of a severely damaged labrum occurred in attempted labral refixation. Subsequent débridement rather than labral reconstruction was performed, which compromised soft-tissue stability. Capsular stability was adversely affected because supranormal traction was applied to remove a foreign body (detached metallic tip of a radiofrequency wand) from the inferomedial joint, which caused capsular

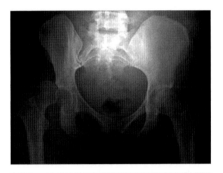

Figure 1 Portable AP radiograph of a pelvis demonstrates a dislocation of a right anterior hip that occurred in the recovery room after hip arthroscopy for the treatment of femoroacetabular impingement. (Reproduced with permission from Matsuda DK: Acute iatrogenic dislocation following hip impingement arthroscopic surgery. *Arthroscopy* 2009;25[4]:400-404.)

attenuation, and the capsulotomy was not repaired.

Treatment

After failed closed reduction attempts in which concentric reduction was achieved but with ongoing instability, an open capsular repair was performed (**Figure 2**). The patient's hip was placed in a brace after surgery; a cam walker prevented hip extension

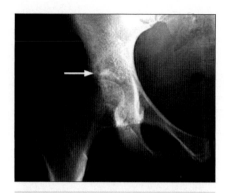

Figure 2 Detail AP radiograph of a pelvis taken after closed reduction and mini-open capsulorrhaphy. The arrow is pointing to the trimmed lateral acetabular rim. (Reproduced with permission from Matsuda DK: Acute iatrogenic dislocation following hip impingement arthroscopic surgery. *Arthroscopy* 2009;25[4]:400-404.)

during ambulation. The patient was given the option of a periacetabular osteotomy; however, rehabilitation was preferred, and the patient anticipated a future total hip arthroplasty. Despite osteoarthrosis, the patient's hip has not redislocated.

Lessons Learned

Surgeons should be wary of patients (particularly female) who have

borderline dysplasia (lateral center-edge angle of 25° and/or acetabular index >10°). Although the patient in the case study had a normal center-edge angle, she had an upsloping sourcil, which suggests borderline dysplasia. Not all radiographic crossover signs should be removed. A crossover sign, although often indicative of focal acetabular overcoverage, may be physiologic in dysplasia, providing needed bony stability. Rim trimming should be carefully monitored to prevent iatrogenic dysplasia. This case led to the development of a fluoroscopic templating technique,[6] which provides more precise arthroscopic rim trimming, and improvements in radiofrequency wand design. Surgeons should avoid excessive distraction (no more than 10 mm), which may cause capsular attenuation. A medial portal, curved devices, and/or suction devices may facilitate foreign or loose body extraction without requiring excessive distraction.[7,8] Arthroscopic capsular repair or plication should be performed in patients who have borderline dysplasia, increased femoral or acetabular anteversion, and/or generalized or focal hyperlaxity.[9]

Likewise, iliopsoas release should not be performed in patients who have a predisposition toward anterior instability.[10] If labral preservation via repair, refixation, or selective débridement is not possible, then labral reconstruction should be considered.[11-14] A large graft (eg, semitendinosus or tubularized iliotibial band) may be appropriate in the replacement of a hypertrophic labrum, which is often seen in dysplasia.[15]

Twist and Shout (Extreme Femoral Version)
Complication and Causation

Persistent bilateral cam FAI is a complication that may occur after hip arthroscopy, even if the hip arthroscopy was performed with well-done femoroplasties. Severe femoral retroversion may cause persistent cam FAI, even if normally sufficient femoroplasties are performed. Although Matsuda et al[16] reported bilateral cam FAI in a case study of a man who had abnormal femoral head-neck morphology, conceptually, femoral retroversion can cause cam FAI in the setting of otherwise normal morphology (eg, normal α angle and normal anterior offset). In this patient, cam FAI persisted even though surgically well-contoured normal head-neck morphology (**Figure 3**) was present in both hips.

Treatment

Bilateral closed derotational osteotomies were performed with the use of an intramedullary saw (**Figure 4**) and stabilized via interlocked rodding.[16] Initial hip arthroscopy confirmed ongoing cam FAI with restricted flexed-hip internal rotation on dynamic testing despite robust femoroplasties. Postosteotomy eradication of ongoing cam impingement was confirmed on static

Dr. Matsuda or an immediate family member has received royalties from ArthroCare and Smith & Nephew; serves as a paid consultant to Biomet; and serves as a board member, owner, officer, or committee member of the American Academy of Orthopaedic Surgeons and Orthopaedics Overseas. Dr. Philippon or an immediate family member has received royalties from Arthrosurface, Bledsoe Brace Systems, CONMED Linvatec, DonJoy, and Smith & Nephew; serves as a paid consultant to MIS and Smith & Nephew; has stock or stock options held in Arthrosurface, Hipco, and MIS; has received research or institutional support from Össur, Siemens, Smith & Nephew, and Vail Valley Medical Center; has received nonincome support (such as equipment or services), commercially derived honoraria, or other or non–research-related funding (such as paid travel) from Smith & Nephew; and serves as a board member, owner, officer, or committee member of the American Orthopaedic Society for Sports Medicine, the International Society for Hip Arthroscopy, and the Steadman Philippon Research Institute. Dr. Safran or an immediate family member has received royalties from ArthroCare, DJ Orthopaedics, and Stryker; is a member of a speakers' bureau or has made paid presentations on behalf of Smith & Nephew; serves as a paid consultant to CONMED Linvatec and Cool Systems; serves as an unpaid consultant to Cool Systems, Cradle Medical, Biomimedica, and Eleven Blade Solutions; has stock or stock options held in Cool Systems, Cradle Medical, Ferring Pharmaceuticals, Biomimedica, and Eleven Blade Solutions; has received research or institutional support from Ferring Pharmaceuticals and Smith & Nephew; and serves as a board member, owner, officer, or committee member of the American Orthopaedic Society for Sports Medicine, the International Society of Arthroscopy, Knee Surgery and Orthopaedic Sports Medicine, and the International Society for Hip Arthroscopy. Dr. Sampson or an immediate family member is a member of a speakers' bureau or has made paid presentations on behalf of Arthrex and Smith & Nephew; serves as a paid consultant to CONMED Linvatec; and serves as a board member, owner, officer, or committee member of the International Society for Hip Arthroscopy.

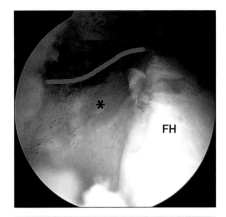

Figure 3 Arthroscopic image of the left hip of a patient who had ongoing cam femoroacetabular impingement as a result of severe femoral retroversion taken immediately before derotational osteotomy demonstrates sufficient previous femoroplasty (asterisk). The line represents sufficient anterior offset. FH = femoral head. (Reproduced with permission from Matsuda DK, Gupta N, Martin HD: Closed intramedullary derotational osteotomy and hip arthroscopy for cam femoroacetabular impingement from femoral retroversion. *Arthrosc Tech* 2014;3[1]:e83-e88.)

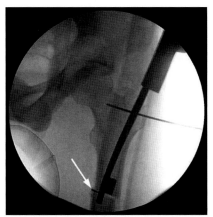

Figure 4 Intraoperative fluoroscopic image of a left proximal femur demonstrates completion of a transverse osteotomy with the use of an intramedullary saw (arrow). (Reproduced with permission from Matsuda DK, Gupta N, Martin HD: Closed intramedullary derotational osteotomy and hip arthroscopy for cam femoroacetabular impingement from femoral retroversion. *Arthrosc Tech* 2014;3[1]:e83-e88.)

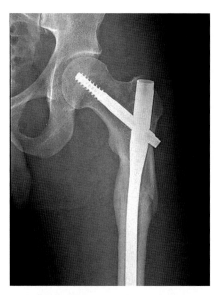

Figure 5 AP radiograph of a left hip demonstrates union after closed derotational osteotomy. (Reproduced with permission from Matsuda DK, Gupta N, Martin HD: Closed intramedullary derotational osteotomy and hip arthroscopy for cam femoroacetabular impingement from femoral retroversion. *Arthrosc Tech* 2014;3[1]:e83-e88.)

and dynamic arthroscopic examinations. The patient was discharged to home the morning after each procedure. Weight-bearing ambulation as tolerated with the use of two crutches was permitted because load-sharing stabilization was provided. Radiographic union of each osteotomy was demonstrated at 3 months postoperatively (**Figure 5**). The patient had improved pain in both hips, and his gait improved from severe outtoeing to a normal foot progression angle.

Lessons Learned

Cam FAI that is caused by extreme retroversion may not be able to be fully corrected with femoroplasty alone, and compensatory excessive femoroplasty may result in iatrogenic fracture. A

consideration of femoral retroversion as well as extreme anteversion, which may cause anterior instability, and their relation to acetabular version (McKibben index normal = 40°) based on a hip examination (relative external to internal rotation in hip extension [eg, prone]) and, possibly, CT or MRI assessment may become a part of routine hip evaluations. Arthroscopic-guided derotational osteotomy is a less invasive approach to reduce cam FAI in patients who have extreme retroversion and to improve anterior stability in patients who have extreme anteversion.[16]

Off With His Head (Excessive Cam Decompression)
Complication and Causation

Iatrogenic overresection of a femoral cam lesion is a complication that may occur in a patient who undergoes

hip arthroscopy for the treatment of FAI. Overaggressive femoroplasty (**Figure 6**) may result in a loss of the labral suction seal, which can be observed during arthroscopic dynamic examination. Excessive cam decompression may increase a patient's susceptibility for femoral neck fracture.

Treatment

An initial surgical assessment revealed extensive bone loss, which resulted from proximal anterior femoral head-neck resection, and subsequent loss of the labral seal at approximately 35° of hip flexion. A 1-cm gap was observed between the labrum and articular surface. A residual cam lesion was noted in the superolateral aspect of the femoral head-neck junction. Revision femoroplasty was performed from the 12 o'clock position to the 9 o'clock

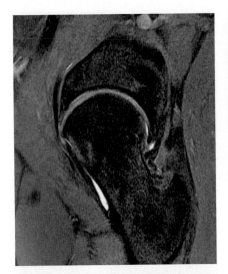

Figure 6 Sagittal MRI of a left hip demonstrates an over-resected femoroplasty.

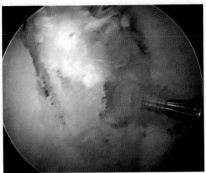

Figure 7 Arthroscopic image demonstrates bone allograft screw fixation.

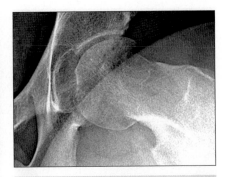

Figure 8 Dunn lateral radiograph taken after arthroscopic bone grafting of a previously overresected anterior femoral head-neck junction.

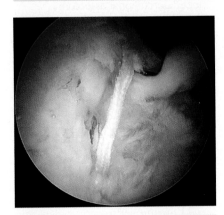

Figure 9 Arthroscopic image of a right anterosuperior acetabulum demonstrates exposed suture from errant suture anchor and chondral damage.

position to reestablish the femoral head-neck offset. The pincer lesion was corrected with acetabuloplasty and subspinal decompression. Labral refixation was performed. Proximal femoral bone loss was reconstructed with a fresh-frozen femoral head allograft (**Figure 7**). Three bone fragments were fixated with four screws and contoured with the use of an arthroscopic burr to cover a surface area of approximately 3 cm × 2 cm. Fluid-seal restoration was

confirmed during dynamic examination. At 7 weeks postoperatively, the patient had minimal pain, and radiographs showed a well-preserved joint space without reabsorption and displacement of the bone graft (Marc J. Philippon, MD, Vail CO, unpublished data, 2015) (**Figure 8**).

Lessons Learned

Precise depth and location are critical to the success of cam decompression. Although underresection is a leading cause of revision hip arthroscopy,[17,18] surgeons should also be vigilant of iatrogenic cortical notching and/or over-resection, which leaves the hip joint devoid of the labral suction seal and increases vulnerability for a femoral neck fracture. Wijdicks et al[19] reported that cam resection with associated cortical notching depths of 4 mm and 6 mm resulted in a significantly lower ultimate load and energy to failure compared with nonresected femurs. In addition, cam resection with an associated cortical notching depth of 6 mm resulted in a significantly lower ultimate load and energy to failure compared with cam resection only. A dynamic intraoperative hip examination that assesses the interaction of the proximal femur with the

acetabular rim can be used to diagnose bony impingement. Periodic dynamic arthroscopic examinations provide crucial feedback on the progression of the osteoplasty and help ensure proper femoral head-neck offset correction and labral fluid-seal retention. Bone grafting with fixation has resulted in successful clinical outcomes after overzealous cam decompression.

Errant Anchors (Intra-articular Anchors)
Complication and Causation

An intra-articularly placed labral repair anchor (**Figure 9**) that causes worsening pain and osteoarthrosis is a complication that may occur after arthroscopy for the treatment of FAI. Recently, Matsuda et al[20] reported a case series on anchor-induced chondral damage of the hip. Although it is desirable for suture anchor placement to be close to the articular cartilage, errant trajectory during acetabular rim drilling and/or anchor placement may cause damage to the acetabular cartilage, which, in this case, occurred with full-thickness chondral violation. The errant trajectory likely resulted from not using a distal-based portal for drilling and/or anchor insertion. Encroachment,

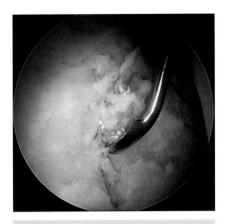

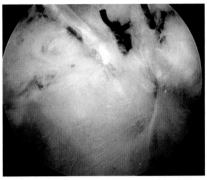

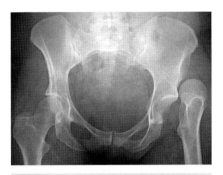

Figure 12   AP radiograph of a pelvis demonstrates a dislocation of a left anterior hip.

Figure 11   Arthroscopic image demonstrates a completed left hip capsular repair.

Figure 10   Arthroscopic image demonstrates anchor removal with the use of an angled curet.

elevation, or frank penetration of the acetabular chondral surface was most likely not visualized during anchor placement (viewing from above the labrum and not checking from within the central compartment). Chondral damage to the acetabular and femoral heads and subsequent osteoarthrosis resulted from iatrogenic wear against the protruding hard anchor.

Treatment

Revision arthroscopy with removal of suture and anchor (**Figure 10**) as well as chondral débridement were performed. The amount of arthritis was too advanced to justify microfracture chondroplasty. Although the patient was doing well 6 months after revision arthroscopy (feels 90% of normal), radiographs showed some progression of joint space narrowing.

Lessons Learned

The surgeon should ensure that the angle of approach is started distally when drilling. The authors of this chapter prefer the midanterior portal[21] or the modified midanterior portal[22] for anchor placement; however, the distal anterolateral accessory portal[21] or the

percutaneous distal portal also may be used. The drill should be intentionally aimed away from the acetabular articular surface. The joint should be visualized when drilling and during placement of anchors. The surgeon should look from the posterolateral compartment when drilling because he or she will be able to see acetabular chondral elevation or movement (**Figure 3**) if unwanted anchor violation is occurring. Tactile and/or auditory changes during drilling also may indicate inadvertent encroachment or violation of the acetabular subchondral bone.[20] The use of curved drill guides and soft suture-based anchors may lessen the occurrence or consequences of intra-articular anchors.

Capsular Massacre (Iatrogenic Instability)
Complication and Causation

Anterior hip instability is a complication that may occur after hip arthroscopy. Despite capsular repair with absorbable suture (**Figure 11**), anterior hip instability may have been caused by preexisting ligamentous laxity, borderline dysplasia, and a sudden jerking motion, which may have compromised the capsular repair suture.

Treatment

The patient's hip dislocated 1 week postoperatively (**Figure 12**) and was treated with closed reduction. No further treatment was required, and the patient was doing well without limitations at 1-year follow-up (Thomas G. Sampson, MD, San Francisco, CA, unpublished data, 2014).

Lessons Learned

Surgeons should be wary of borderline dysplasia (lateral center-edge angle of 25° and/or acetabular index >10°) in female patients. The surgeon should check for both hip and generalized ligamentous laxity. The surgeon should close the capsule and consider using a primary hip stabilizer to help protect against excessive hyperextension and external rotation, both of which may prevent sufficient healing of the anterior capsule and the iliofemoral ligament. Capsular plication may be the key to produce more successful arthroscopic outcomes in patients who have borderline dysplasia.[23] Capsular defects are common after hip arthroscopy[24] and may result in instability or cyst formation (**Figure 13**).

The Rack (Traction Complications)

Complication and Causation

Chondral scuffing, labral damage, neurapraxia, injury to the perineal soft tissues, and compressive neuropathy of the foot are complications that may occur during hip arthroscopy. Insufficient or excessive distraction forces contribute to traction-related complications

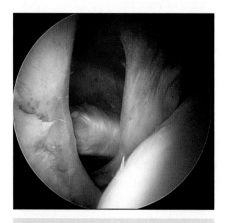

Figure 13 Arthroscopic image demonstrates an anterior capsular defect after arthroscopy for the treatment of femoroacetabular impingement.

during hip arthroscopy. Insufficient distraction, which often occurs during attempted access into a tight joint, may predispose a patient to chondral scuffing and/or labral damage. Conversely, lengthy distraction times with too much force may cause compressive or distractive neurapraxia (**Figure 14**) or perineal injuries (eg, scrotal or labial tears). Applied traction after improper patient positioning also may contribute to these complications. Loss of foot fixation may result from excessive padding and/or insecure strapping.

Treatment

Surgeons should become familiar with the type of distracter being used and optimize its function with proper placement. Surgeons should educate the surgical staff on the proper distraction technique. The patient is placed either in the supine or lateral decubitus position, and the downside bony structures are padded. A perineal post larger than 9 cm is chosen, and the perineal structures are cleared from the post. Padding

to the foot should be just enough to allow for semirigid fixation to the footplate. The amount of heel liftoff in distraction should be tested. The surgeon should understand the patient's laxity index to anticipate the forces necessary for distraction. Preoperative fluoroscopy is performed to map out bony conflicts. The surgeon should anticipate that a difficult hip with global acetabular overcoverage[25] and soft-tissue stiffness will require greater distraction forces. A capsulotomy reduces the necessary distraction forces and provides access for pre-distraction rim trimming. The surgeon should adhere to a predetermined surgical plan to optimize surgical efficiency while minimizing traction time and traction force.

Lessons Learned

Inadequate or excessive traction causes complications in hip arthroscopy. Data on evoked potentials from Telleria et al[26] demonstrated that increased forces were more likely to cause sciatic nerve neurapraxia (**Figure 14**) than the

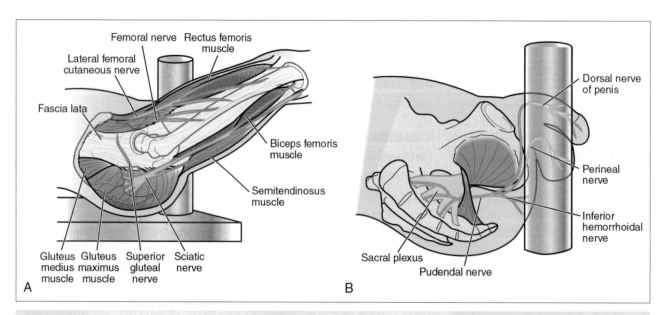

Figure 14 Traction-induced nerve injuries may be caused by distraction mechanisms (**A**) or compressive mechanisms (**B**).

length of time in distraction. Distraction for potential foot pullout problems should be pretested. Structures that are at risk, such as the vulva, scrotum, and penis, should be cleared and protected. If the patient is in the lateral decubitus position, then compressive forces to the downside leg should be minimized with proper padding. Typically, distraction is used for central compartment access and procedures and is released for peripheral compartment procedures, such as femoroplasty; however, the judicious application of partial or full distraction may be indicated during rim trimming (to protect the femoral head from burr-induced damage), lateral femoroplasty (to achieve proximal cam decompression), and suture anchor placement in labral repairs or reconstructions (to avoid inadvertent intra-articular violation). The anticipation of difficult cases and the education of the surgical staff on the proper use of a hip distracter may reduce complications.

The Alien Within (Intra-abdominal Fluid Extravasation)
Complication and Causation

Fluid extravasation into the retroperitoneal space during hip arthroscopy is a complication that can cause severe abdominal pain and abdominal compartment syndrome. Hip arthroscopy is commonly performed with the use of a mechanical pump that has inflow and/or outflow sensors. Extravasation may occur from fluid pressure elevation, imbalance between the inflow and outflow sensors, a lack of outflow sensors, or poor pump calibration. Entering the iliopsoas bursa during tendon release may create a direct conduit to the retroperitoneal space (retroperitoneum).

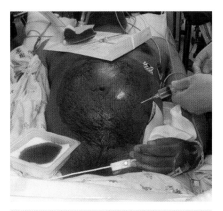

Figure 15 Intraoperative photograph shows the distended abdomen of a patient who had intra-abdominal fluid extravasation after hip arthroscopy. Note the attempted percutaneous paracentesis. The patient was successfully treated with CT-guided paracentesis.

Treatment

It is necessary for surgeons to understand the anatomy of the iliopsoas and its relationship to the hip and the retroperitoneal space. In addition, it is mandatory for surgeons to have a thorough understanding of an arthroscopic pump. The surgical staff and the surgeon must be vigilant of pump operation. If the pump is working unusually hard, immediate attention is necessary to determine if the fluid dynamics are appropriate. If abdominal distention occurs, then the patient's vital signs should be monitored, and the patient's degree of distention should be determined. Surgery should be aborted as soon as possible if the patient has moderate to severe abdominal distention (**Figure 15**). Abdominal compartment syndrome may cause respiratory depression and end-organ failure, which is a potential life-threatening complication.[27,28] It is often necessary to transfer the patient from an outpatient facility to the emergency department and obtain a surgical consult. A radiograph of the

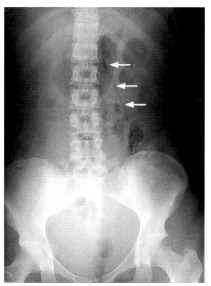

Figure 16 AP radiograph demonstrates a fluid track (arrows) in a patient who had intra-abdominal extravasation immediately after right hip arthroscopy.

kidney, ureter, or bladder (**Figure 16**) and/or CT may detect abnormal retroperitoneal fluid collection. Although clinical observation and analgesic agents are typically sufficient, paracentesis is occasionally indicated. Laparotomy is rarely required.[29]

Lessons Learned

The most common cause of intra-abdominal fluid extravasation and abdominal compartment syndrome is an iliopsoas release that is performed early in the procedure.[29] Therefore, release of the iliopsoas should be performed toward the end of hip arthroscopy. Mechanical pump malfunction, with errant pressure readings below the actual elevated fluid pressure, has been implicated as a cause of intra-abdominal fluid extravasation in at least one patient. Prevention begins with training the surgeon and the entire surgical staff to be keenly aware of pump fluid dynamics (pressures, performance, altered sounds that suggest pump strain or malfunction) and empowering any member of the surgical staff to shut down the pump. The anesthesiologist should alert the surgical team if the patient has any substantial decrease in core body temperature or resistance to respiratory ventilation. In addition, the draped abdomen should be palpated every 15 to 30 minutes, which allows for comparison with the preoperative baseline. This very rare but serious complication merits urgent evaluation and treatment.

The Tell-Tale Heart (Cardiac Arrhythmia From Hip Arthroscopy)
Complication and Causation
Tachycardia, acute pulmonary edema, hypertension, and decreased core temperature are complications that may occur after the administration of room-temperature irrigation fluid during hip arthroscopy. Several factors can contribute to these complications. Potential phrenic nerve irritation and core body temperature drop from possible intra-abdominal extravasation of room temperature fluid may result in cardiac and pulmonary concerns.[30-32]

Treatment
Cardiology was immediately consulted. A transthoracic echocardiogram and a contrast-enhanced echocardiogram were performed, neither of which showed gross abnormalities. An electrocardiogram demonstrated sinus rhythm with nonspecific inferior and lateral ST changes. A chest radiograph indicated diffuse alveolar infiltrates. The patient was taken from the operating room to an imaging suite, and a pulmonary embolism was ruled out via a chest CT pulmonary angiogram. The

patient's lung fields were mostly clear by this time, which suggested resolution of the pulmonary edema. The electrocardiogram normalized after resolution of the pulmonary edema. Laboratory tests, including a hemoglobin and hematocrit blood test, a B-type natriuretic peptide blood test, a troponin test, and a basic metabolic panel blood test, revealed normal results. The patient was transferred to the intensive care unit and remained intubated overnight. The patient was extubated the next morning without incident. The patient had no further complications and was released from the hospital 2 days after arthroscopy (Marc J. Philippon, MD, Vail CO, unpublished data, 2015).

Lessons Learned
Irrigation fluids should be warmed to close to body temperature before they are infused into the hip during arthroscopy.

Summary
Although the title of this chapter suggests levity, surgical complications should not be taken lightly. The hip arthroscopy complications that were previously discussed have varying degrees of occurrence, chronicity, and consequences. Traction-induced complications may be the most common; fortunately, they are typically of limited duration and severity. Although rare, fluid management-related complications may have severe consequences. Potentially lethal complications from abdominal compartment syndrome or cardiopulmonary aberrations may arise from the amount or temperature of arthroscopic hip fluid. Technical errors may cause subtle anchor-induced chondral damage or dramatic hip dislocation, both of which may result in

irreversible joint injury. Sometimes, a near-perfect surgical execution may yield complicated outcomes, as exemplified by a sufficient arthroscopic femoroplasty with ongoing cam FAI from untreated femoral retroversion. Too much of a good thing may be as bad (or worse) than too little, which is seen in cases of overzealous cam resection that then requires bone grafting. The authors of this chapter hope that by sharing these nightmarish experiences, individual and collective learning may help improve patient safety and outcomes for hip arthroscopy.

References
1. Bozic KJ, Chan V, Valone FH III, Feeley BT, Vail TP: Trends in hip arthroscopy utilization in the United States. *J Arthroplasty* 2013; 28(8, suppl):140-143.

2. Park MS, Yoon SJ, Kim YJ, Chung WC: Hip arthroscopy for femoroacetabular impingement: The changing nature and severity of associated complications over time. *Arthroscopy* 2014;30(8):957-963.

3. Oak N, Mendez-Zfass M, Lesniak BP, Larson CM, Kelly BT, Bedi A: Complications in hip arthroscopy. *Sports Med Arthrosc* 2013;21(2):97-105.

4. Matsuda DK, Carlisle JC, Arthurs SC, Wierks CH, Philippon MJ: Comparative systematic review of the open dislocation, mini-open, and arthroscopic surgeries for femoroacetabular impingement. *Arthroscopy* 2011;27(2):252-269.

5. Matsuda DK: Acute iatrogenic dislocation following hip impingement arthroscopic surgery. *Arthroscopy* 2009;25(4):400-404.

6. Matsuda DK: Fluoroscopic templating technique for precision arthroscopic rim trimming. *Arthroscopy* 2009;25(10):1175-1182.

7. Polesello GC, Omine Fernandes AE, de Oliveira LP, Tavares Linhares JP, Queiroz MC: Medial hip arthroscopy portals: An anatomic study. *Arthroscopy* 2014;30(1):55-59.

8. Nho SJ, Freedman RL, Federer AE, et al: Computed tomographic analysis of curved and straight guides for placement of suture anchors for acetabular labral refixation. *Arthroscopy* 2013;29(10):1623-1627.

9. Domb BG, Philippon MJ, Giordano BD: Arthroscopic capsulotomy, capsular repair, and capsular plication of the hip: Relation to atraumatic instability. *Arthroscopy* 2013;29(1):162-173.

10. Sansone M, Ahldén M, Jónasson P, Swärd L, Eriksson T, Karlsson J: Total dislocation of the hip joint after arthroscopy and ileopsoas tenotomy. *Knee Surg Sports Traumatol Arthrosc* 2013;21(2):420-423.

11. Geyer MR, Philippon MJ, Fagrelius TS, Briggs KK: Acetabular labral reconstruction with an iliotibial band autograft: Outcome and survivorship analysis at minimum 3-year follow-up. *Am J Sports Med* 2013;41(8):1750-1756.

12. Matsuda DK, Burchette RJ: Arthroscopic hip labral reconstruction with a gracilis autograft versus labral refixation: 2-year minimum outcomes. *Am J Sports Med* 2013;41(5):980-987.

13. Philippon MJ, Nepple JJ, Campbell KJ, et al: The hip fluid seal—Part I: The effect of an acetabular labral tear, repair, resection, and reconstruction on hip fluid pressurization. *Knee Surg Sports Traumatol Arthrosc* 2014;22(4):722-729.

14. Nepple JJ, Philippon MJ, Campbell KJ, et al: The hip fluid seal—Part II: The effect of an acetabular labral tear, repair, resection, and reconstruction on hip stability to distraction. *Knee Surg Sports Traumatol Arthrosc* 2014;22(4):730-736.

15. Matsuda DK: Arthroscopic labral reconstruction with gracilis autograft. *Arthrosc Tech* 2012;1(1):e15-e21.

16. Matsuda DK, Gupta N, Martin HD: Closed intramedullary derotational osteotomy and hip arthroscopy for cam femoroacetabular impingement

from femoral retroversion. *Arthrosc Tech* 2014;3(1):e83-e88.

17. Ross JR, Larson CM, Adeoye O, Kelly BT, Bedi A: Residual deformity is the most common reason for revision hip arthroscopy: A three-dimensional CT study. *Clin Orthop Relat Res* 2015;473(4):1388-1395.

18. Domb BG, Stake CE, Lindner D, El-Bitar Y, Jackson TJ: Revision hip preservation surgery with hip arthroscopy: Clinical outcomes. *Arthroscopy* 2014;30(5):581-587.

19. Wijdicks CA, Balldin BC, Jansson KS, Stull JD, LaPrade RF, Philippon MJ: Cam lesion femoral osteoplasty: In vitro biomechanical evaluation of iatrogenic femoral cortical notching and risk of neck fracture. *Arthroscopy* 2013;29(10):1608-1614.

20. Matsuda DK, Bharam S, White B, Safran MR, Matsuda NA: Anchor-induced chondral damage of the hip. *J Hip Preserv Surg* 2015;2(1):56-64.

21. Robertson WJ, Kelly BT: The safe zone for hip arthroscopy: A cadaveric assessment of central, peripheral, and lateral compartment portal placement. *Arthroscopy* 2008;24(9):1019-1026.

22. Matsuda DK, Villamor A: The modified mid-anterior portal for hip arthroscopy. *Arthrosc Tech* 2014;3(4):e469-e474.

23. Domb BG, Stake CE, Lindner D, El-Bitar Y, Jackson TJ: Arthroscopic capsular plication and labral preservation in borderline hip dysplasia: Two-year clinical outcomes of a surgical approach to a challenging problem. *Am J Sports Med* 2013;41(11):2591-2598.

24. McCormick F, Slikker W III, Harris JD, et al: Evidence of capsular defect following hip arthroscopy. *Knee Surg Sports Traumatol Arthrosc* 2014;22(4):902-905.

25. Matsuda DK, Gupta N, Hanami D: Hip arthroscopy for challenging deformities: Global pincer

femoroacetabular impingement. *Arthrosc Tech* 2014;3(2):e197-e204.

26. Telleria JJ, Safran MR, Harris AH, Gardi JN, Glick JM: Risk of sciatic nerve traction injury during hip arthroscopy—is it the amount or duration? An intraoperative nerve monitoring study. *J Bone Joint Surg Am* 2012;94(22):2025-2032.

27. Fowler J, Owens BD: Abdominal compartment syndrome after hip arthroscopy. *Arthroscopy* 2010;26(1):128-130.

28. Bartlett CS, DiFelice GS, Buly RL, Quinn TJ, Green DS, Helfet DL: Cardiac arrest as a result of intraabdominal extravasation of fluid during arthroscopic removal of a loose body from the hip joint of a patient with an acetabular fracture. *J Orthop Trauma* 1998;12(4):294-299.

29. Kocher MS, Frank JS, Nasreddine AY, et al: Intra-abdominal fluid extravasation during hip arthroscopy: A survey of the MAHORN group. *Arthroscopy* 2012;28(11):1654-1660.e2.

30. Cho SH, Yi JW, Kwack YH, Park SW, Kim MK, Rhee YG: Ventricular tachycardia during arthroscopic shoulder surgery: A report of two cases. *Arch Orthop Trauma Surg* 2010;130(3):353-356.

31. Board TN, Srinivasan MS: The effect of irrigation fluid temperature on core body temperature in arthroscopic shoulder surgery. *Arch Orthop Trauma Surg* 2008;128(5):531-533.

32. Parodi D, Valderrama J, Tobar C, et al: Effect of warmed irrigation solution on core body temperature during hip arthroscopy for femoroacetabular impingement. *Arthroscopy* 2014;30(1):36-41.

Video Reference

Philippon MJ: Video. *Hip Arthroscopy With Bone Augmentation*. Vail, CO, 2015.

Orthopaedic Medicine

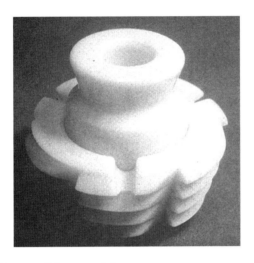

Update on Biomaterials

Paul A. Anderson, MD

Nicholas J. Giori, MD, PhD

Carlos J. Lavernia, MD

Jesus M. Villa, MD

A. Seth Greenwald, DPhil (Oxon)

Abstract

Biomaterials are essential to the use and development of successful treatments for orthopaedic patients. Orthopaedic surgeons need to understand the expected clinical performance and the effects of implants in patients. Recent attempts to improve implant durability have resulted in adverse effects related to biomaterials and their relationship to patients. Examples of these adverse effects in hip arthroplasty include wear and corrosion of metal-on-metal bearings, trunnions, and tapered modular neck junctions. Conversely, polymers and ceramics have shown substantial improvements in durability. Improved implant compositions and manufacturing processes have resulted in ceramic head and acetabular liners with improved material properties and the avoidance of voids, which have, in the past, caused catastrophic fractures. Cross-linking of polyethylene with radiation and doping with antioxidants has substantially increased implant durability and is increasingly being used in joint prostheses other than the hip. Additive manufacturing is potentially a transformative process; it can lead to custom and patient-specific implants and to improvements in material properties, which can be optimized to achieve desired bone responses. Orthopaedic surgeons must understand the material properties and the biologic effects of new or altered biomaterials and manufacturing processes before use. In addition, a clear benefit to the patient must be proven based on superior preclinical results and high-quality clinical investigations before orthopaedic surgeons use new or altered biomaterials.

Instr Course Lect 2016;65:449–466.

Biomaterials are essential for surgical success in orthopaedic surgery. New biomaterials, as well as refinements of current materials, are available. Furthermore, new manufacturing processes are being developed to allow more biomaterial customization at lower costs. Orthopaedic surgeons must stay up to date with these technologies so that proper choices can be made to maximize patient outcomes and reduce potential harm. Orthopaedic surgeons should be knowledgeable about advances in the most important biomaterials, including metals, polymers, and ceramics, as well as new methods of additive manufacturing. It is important that orthopaedic surgeons have a basic understanding of the biomaterials they use and to be up to date with their current applications, advantages, and disadvantages.

Update on Metals
Metal-on-Metal Hip Arthroplasty

Hard-on-hard bearings were popularized in the United States approximately 10 years ago. Polyethylene wear and osteolysis in patients younger than 65 years were the driving forces behind hard-on-hard bearings. Hard-on-hard bearings allowed for the use of larger head sizes and reduced postoperative restrictions. New metallurgical methods, precision machining, and improved design were features that theoretically solved the poor outcomes associated with the prior use of similar bearing couples, such as the McKee-Farrar. Modern metal-on-metal (MOM) bearings exhibit low wear in in vitro testing. In the past 7 years, there has been a sharp decline in the use of MOM bearings for total hip arthroplasty (THA), from 31% in 2007, to 11% in 2010, and to 1% in 2012.[1] The Australian Orthopaedic Association National Joint Arthroplasty Registry provided the first indications that there was a higher rate of failure with MOM bearings.[2] Early failures with the DePuy Articular Surface Replacement MOM hip arthroplasty system triggered one of the largest hip implant recalls in the history of orthopaedics.[3] The exact etiology for these failures is still the subject of much debate. New data are available on wear and subsequent ion release from MOM bearing surfaces, a new disease related to wear of the taper trunnion of the neck, and early failures caused by wear of modular neck implants.

High blood ion levels have been reported to reliably predict accelerated wear of bearing surfaces, and the use of blood ion levels as a monitoring tool has been advocated. Based on the current data available, a chromium (Cr) or cobalt (Co) ion level higher than 4.5 ppb may serve as a threshold to indicate abnormal wear and as a trigger for further investigation, such as a metal artifact reduction sequence MRI.[4] Blood ion levels represent a balance between ion production (from the device) and renal excretion; consequently, they can be affected by renal function. Furthermore, the use of various chromium supplementation products could be an external cause of high serum metal concentration levels.[5]

Thermal treatments of alloys were introduced in postcasting processes to reduce porosity. The high-carbon alloy owes its wear resistance to the presence of a higher fraction (approximately 5% by volume) of carbides (metal-carbon precipitates) in the microstructure; however, postcasting thermal treatments, such as solution heat treatment or hot isostatic pressing, may deplete the alloy of its higher carbide fraction. Carbide depletion is detrimental to the hardness of the material and, consequently, its wear resistance. Double-heat treatment of cast CoCr MOM bearings also has been attempted, and the results indicated that double-heat treatments of MOM bearings may lead to an increased incidence of wear-induced osteolysis.[6]

In a multivariate analysis to determine the mechanisms of failure of 138 femoral head and acetabular cup couples removed from large-head MOM hip replacements, Hart et al[7] reported that 88 acetabular cups (64%) had edge-loading; however, only 43 (31%) of the 138 hips had a cup inclination angle greater than 55°. The data showed that the most important factor responsible for wear rate variation was the presence or absence of edge-loading, even after adjustments for the cup inclination angle. There was a strong positive correlation between acetabular cup alignment and femoral head wear rates and between wear rates and blood CoCr ion levels. Jacobs and Wimmer[8] highlighted the importance of the Hart et al[7] study by concluding that "edge-loading is the most important factor responsible for the variation of wear rate," and that "there was a strong positive correlation between blood metal levels and wear rate." These conclusions are essential to understand the performance of the current generation of MOM hip arthroplasty implants. One of the most important findings mentioned by Jacobs and Wimmer[8] was that 69% of the failures had an acetabular cup inclination angle less than 55°, which indicated that factors other than cup orientation were responsible for the failure. The authors suggested that the contact areas of MOM trunnion modular junctions experienced tribocorrosive processes that could have generated debris

Dr. Anderson or an immediate family member has received royalties from Pioneer Surgical Technology and Stryker; serves as a paid consultant to or is an employee of Aesculap/B. Braun and Stryker; serves as an unpaid consultant to Expanding Orthopedics, SI-BONE, Spartek, and Titan Surgical; has stock or stock options held in Expanding Orthopedics, Pioneer Surgical Technology, SI-BONE, Spartek, and Titan Surgical; and serves as a board member, owner, officer, or committee member of the American Academy of Orthopaedic Surgeons, the American Society for Testing and Materials, the Lumbar Spine Research Society, the North American Spine Society, the International Society for the Advancement of Spine Surgery, and the spine section of the American Association of Neurological Surgeons/Congress of Neurological Surgeons Joint Section on Disorders of the Spine and Peripheral Nerves. Dr. Lavernia or an immediate family member has received royalties from MAKO Surgical and Stryker; has stock or stock options held in Johnson & Johnson, Stryker, Symmetry Medical (Tecomet), Wright Medical Technology, and Zimmer; and serves as a board member, owner, officer, or committee member of the American Association of Hip and Knee Surgeons and the Florida Orthopaedic Society. Dr. Greenwald or an immediate family member has received research or institutional support from Aesculap/B. Braun, Biomedical Development Corporation, Biomet, DePuy, ICONACY Orthopedic Implants, implantcast, Intellirod Spine, LimaCorporate, MatOrtho, Maxx Orthopedics, Medacta, OMNILife Science, Ranier Technology, Smith & Nephew, Total Joint Orthopedics, and Zimmer; and serves as a board member, owner, officer, or committee member of the American Academy of Orthopaedic Surgeons and the Orthopaedic Research and Education Foundation. Neither of the following authors nor any immediate family member has received anything of value from or has stock or stock options held in a commercial company or institution related directly or indirectly to the subject of this chapter: Dr. Giori and Dr. Villa.

© 2016 AAOS Instructional Course Lectures, Volume 65

and contributed to failure (**Figure 1, A** and **B**).

Trunnion Corrosion

To determine if wear and increased corrosion of the MOM bearing articulation and the taper interface could occur simultaneously, Witt et al[5] performed explant analysis of 43 large-diameter CoCr bearings of the same design that were implanted with a titanium stem with the use of a titanium adaptor. The authors investigated the relationship between titanium taper corrosion and CoCr bearing wear by categorizing retrievals into slight or severe corrosion groups via visual inspection of the female taper surface of the adaptor. The authors reported that severe taper corrosion, which was defined as either material deposition or wear, was present in 30% of the retrievals. The global bearing wear rate was significantly higher in the group with severe taper corrosion than in the group with slight corrosion (7.2 mm^3/y versus 3.1 mm^3/y, respectively; $P = 0.023$), as were the serum cobalt levels (40.5 µg/L verus 15.2 µg/L, respectively; $P = 0.024$) and the serum chromium ion concentrations (32.7 µg/L and 12.0 µg/L, respectively; $P = 0.019$). These findings supported the hypothesis that increased friction in the joint articulation is one of the factors responsible for simultaneous articulation and taper damage; however, independent taper or bearing damage also was observed, which suggests that other factors are involved. The most substantial contribution of this study is that titanium taper corrosion and wear, at least in large-head MOM hip arthroplasties, cannot be dissociated. As Hart et al[7] clearly illustrated, the failure mechanisms of MOM implants are extremely complex and involve many factors.

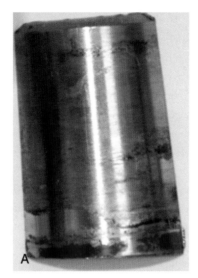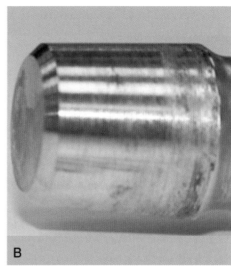

Figure 1 Clinical photographs show examples of trunnions that have corrosion. **A,** A retrieval sample has corrosion (red color) on the distal part of the trunnion. **B,** A retrieval sample has corrosion most noticeably on the distal part of the trunnion. The corrosion on both trunnions is so severe that it is clearly visible without magnification.

Recently, numerous studies on mechanically assisted crevice corrosion at the taper junction have been published. Esposito et al[9] recently conducted a systematic review of the literature (MEDLINE and EMBASE) to summarize failure modes that are associated with modular stems. Of 1,043 articles reviewed, the authors found that 68 articles reported failures that were attributed to modular femoral stems for various modalities, including tribocorrosion-associated adverse local tissue reactions (ALTRs). As suspected, the authors found that in the past 3 years, there was an increase in publications that described ALTRs around modular hip prostheses; some studies attributed the increase in ALTRs to implant design changes, such as larger femoral heads and smaller trunnion. In an analysis of a revision retrieval database that consisted of 85 modular femoral stems that were implanted between 1991 and 2012 and retrieved at revision surgery between 2004 and 2012, Porter et al[10] reported that there was variability in the flexural rigidity of various taper designs, with a long-term tendency toward the modification of trunnions to become shorter, thinner, and more flexible. The authors speculated that this temporal trend may explain, at least in part, why taper corrosion is seen with increasing frequency in modern THAs.

Nassif et al[11] also investigated whether trunnion taper design affects the failure of large-head MOM THAs. Taper damage in 40 retrieved heads was subjectively graded for fretting and corrosion, and wear was determined. The authors compared various taper types (11/13, 12/14, and type 1), and reported that the fretting scores were higher in 11/13 tapers than in type 1 tapers. In general, thicker tapers with longer contact lengths were associated with higher fretting scores, whereas no relationship was found among the three designs with respect to volumetric wear or corrosion scores.

The use of a larger head size is likely to have a substantial effect on taper wear. In a finite element analysis, Elkins et al[12] reported that contact stress and computed wear at the trunnion interface increased with increasing head size. Heads with diameters greater than 40 mm had a substantial increase in wear potential at the trunnion. Cook et al[13] analyzed two cases of uncemented, large-diameter metal-on-polymer modular THAs that required retrieval because of pseudotumor formation as a result of tribocorrosion at the taper interface. The failure analysis revealed a distinct pattern of material loss from the distal end of the head taper and stem trunnion interface. The authors reported that the use of a proximal contacting taper design provided insufficient mechanical locking between the head and the stem, which allowed the head to toggle on the trunnion. The authors also reported that the difference in the taper and the trunnion angles created a crevice between the two components, and that through a combination of various factors (crevice environment, mechanically assisted corrosion, mechanical wear, and erosion), debris and metal ions were released, which resulted in ALTRs. As early as 1987, Cook et al[14] identified manufacturing tolerances of the trunnion-head couple as a major factor in the development of crevice corrosion.

Modular Neck Corrosion

Modular-neck or dual-taper THA femoral stems have recently been reported to have a high failure rate. Molloy et al[15] conducted a retrospective analysis of 15 patients who underwent THA with a modular-neck hip system with ceramic-on-ceramic (COC) bearings. Patients were implanted with an ABG II dual modular hip system (Stryker) that consisted of a titanium-alloy stem (Ti-12Mo-6Zr-2Fe) and an exchangeable CoCr neck. At a mean follow-up of 42.3 months, cobalt ion levels were elevated in all patients, but chromium ion levels were within the normal range. Medial femoral calcar erosion was present in almost 50% of the patients. All patients who had radiographic grade-2 or grade-3 calcar erosion had MRI findings consistent with an ALTR. Staining and necrosis of the tissue, bone necrosis, and pseudotumor formation were observed in the seven patients who underwent revision surgery. A histological analysis of the samples collected from the patients who underwent revision surgery confirmed MOM synovitis similar to that seen with MOM bearings. Because the ABG II dual modular hip system was associated with a high rate of early failure as a result of fretting and corrosion at the femoral neck-stem taper, the component was recalled. Cooper et al[16] also reported ALTRs as a result of corrosion at the femoral neck-body junction in a dual-taper titanium femoral stem (titanium-molybdenum-zirconium-iron alloy) and a CoCr-alloy modular neck. The authors performed a retrospective study of 12 hips in 11 patients (a multicenter, multisurgeon series) who underwent revision surgery for failed THA as a result of ALTRs. The authors reported that serum levels had a higher elevation of cobalt ions (mean, 6.0 ng/mL) than chromium (mean, 0.6 ng/mL) or titanium ions (mean, 3.4 ng/mL). Eight of nine patients demonstrated evidence of ALTRs on metal artifact reduction sequence MRIs. Intraoperatively, all hips had large soft-tissue masses, tissue damage, and noticeable corrosion at the modular femoral neck-body junction.

In 7 of 10 patients, histology demonstrated large areas of tissue necrosis, and the viable capsular tissue demonstrated a dense lymphocyte infiltrate. Stereolight and scanning electron microscopic analyses were consistent with modular neck-body interface fretting and crevice corrosion. The authors concluded that corrosion at the modular neck-body junction in dual-tapered stems may lead to the release of metal ions and debris, which may result in local tissue destruction. As early as 1994, Urban et al[17] identified chromium orthophosphate as a potent osteolytic moiety and a by-product of dual-tapered stems.

Clinical Outcomes

The long-term effects of alternative bearings, such as MOM and modularity, in THA on revision surgery rates are not encouraging. Mihalko et al[18] performed a systematic review of clinical studies (level IV or higher) that were performed between 1998 and 2013 and that had a minimum follow-up of 5 years. The authors also included registry data studies that had a minimum follow-up of 7 years; however, retrieval studies and case reports were excluded. Thirty-two studies on MOM, 19 studies on COC, 20 studies on modular stem designs, and 11 registry reports met the inclusion criteria. The authors reported no evidence in the clinical studies that either MOM or COC bearings in THA have decreased revision surgery rates compared with conventional bearing couples; however, the registry data showed that large-head MOM implants had lower 7- to 10-year survivorship compared with polyethylene bearings. Both the registry data and the clinical studies showed that modular exchangeable femoral neck implants had a lower 10-year survival rate compared with combined registry primary THA implant survivorship. This systematic review showed that, in reality, both large-head MOM THA and added modularity have lowered the survival rate of hip prostheses.

Conclusions

The authors of this chapter, based on their experiences with modular femoral neck corrosion and other taper-related problems, share the opinion expressed by Padgett and Wright[19] with regard to the ineffectiveness of the 510(k) pathway, in which established implant systems are used to reference substantial equivalence to new designs. The available evidence shows that fretting corrosion and ALTRs are prevalent in MOM implants. MOM bearings and added modularity have not improved the survivorship of THAs. In MOM bearings, edge-loading is the most important factor responsible for the variation in wear rates; however, multiple factors apart from the acetabular cup inclination angle are involved in the process. There is a relationship between titanium taper corrosion and CoCr bearing wear in large-head MOM THAs, and the simultaneous existence of both processes cannot be excluded. Implant design changes, such as larger femoral heads, smaller trunnions, and dual-tapered stems, are implicated as causes of taper material deterioration. Undoubtedly, innovations are necessary to improve quality and achieve better clinical outcomes; however, there is a need for more rigorous premarket clinical research before substantial innovations are introduced and broadly adopted by the orthopaedic community.

Update on Ceramics

The clinical use of alumina ceramic as a hard-on-hard bearing dates back to the early 1970s, with the Mittelmeier Autophor COC cup (Smith & Nephew) being cleared for use in the United States for THA in 1982[20] (**Figure 2**). However, early failures, which were attributed to poor implant design, component positioning, acetabular component loosening, and low-quality ceramics that resulted in fractures and debris generation, dampened enthusiasm for their use.[21-23] Subsequently, alumina and zirconia ceramic femoral head components were introduced as low-friction metallic substitutes to reduce ultra-high–molecular-weight polyethylene (UHMWPE) wear debris in THA. These materials are highly biocompatible and substantially smoother, harder, and more scratch resistant than their metallic counterparts, with superior wear, lubrication, and friction properties.[24]

The quality of alumina ceramic currently in use is much improved and has minimized impurities, which are potential stress risers. Furthermore, the reduction of grain boundaries has substantially increased material strength and toughness, and better quality control through proof-testing has substantially reduced the prevalence of component fracture. Laboratory studies continually document dramatic reductions in wear volume for these alumina ceramic couples (**Figure 3**), which offer increased in vivo longevity and a decreased potential for osteolytic response.[25-29]

Although alumina is a superior bearing surface compared with other ceramic materials, efforts are continual to make it stronger and more fracture resistant. Newer alumina composite ceramics made with other additives, such as zirconia, strontium, and chromium, have been developed. These new

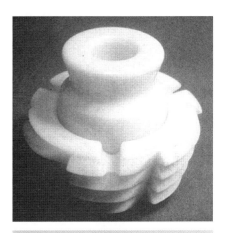

Figure 2   Clinical photograph of an early Mittelmeier Autophor ceramic-on-ceramic cup (Smith & Nephew). (Reproduced with permission from Greenwald AS, Garino JP; American Academy of Orthopaedic Surgeons Committee on Biomedical Engineering; American Academy of Orthopaedic Surgeons Committee on Hip and Knee Arthritis: Alternative bearing surfaces: The good, the bad, and the ugly. *J Bone Joint Surg Am* 2001; 83[suppl 2 pt 2]:68-72.)

composites are nearly twice as fracture resistant as the already safe and reliable alumina ceramic that has been used worldwide for the previous two decades[30-32] (**Figure 4**).

As hip replacement in younger, more active patient populations increases, there will be a need for bearing solutions with increased longevity that promise satisfactory patient outcomes[33,34] (**Figure 5**). Ceramics certainly offer this prospect, both as an articulation against enhanced polyethylenes and as a hard-on-hard solution.[14] Although most medical device manufacturers have a specific COC acetabular cup design, several contemporary modular systems facilitate the use of both polymer and ceramic liners as well as provide durable metal shell-bone fixation. The armamentarium of the hip replacement surgeon has expanded; however, COC

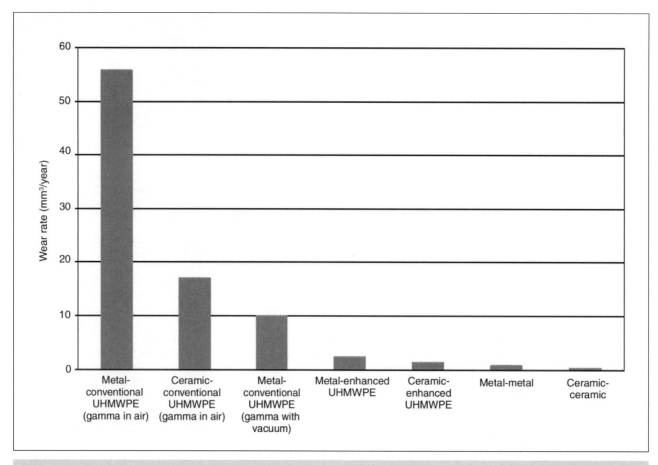

Figure 3 Bar graph demonstrates the wear rates for various types of hip bearing couples. UHMWPE = ultra-high–molecular-weight polyethylene.

bearing couples are technically more demanding because the components need to be optimally placed to avoid impingement of the neck against the rim, and because the tapers need to be clean, perfectly dry, and undamaged to ensure an optimal outcome.[35]

The contemporary appreciation of ceramic bearings, beyond their dramatic reduction in the generation of wear particulate compared with their alternatives, includes their allowance for larger diameter femoral heads that help address hip instability in both primary and revision surgery situations.[36] With the recent recalls of MOM articulations for both hip resurfacing and THA applications, ceramics provide a bioinert alternative that allows for

biomechanical restoration in patients who have instability. Studies of relatively small populations have reported that ceramic femoral heads may decrease the potential for fretting corrosion caused by the femoral head-neck taper.[37,38] If longer term studies with increased numbers continue to support this finding, ceramic femoral heads could easily outpace their metallic counterparts in the coming years with respect to primary THA[39] (**Figure 6**).

Ceramic femoral heads, by virtue of their improved structural integrity, low particulate debris burden, and relative absence of adverse soft- and hard-tissue responses, will pave the way for further increased use in both primary and revision THA applications. Although

both enhanced polyethylenes and ceramic liners offer the reconstructive surgeon material alternatives, the type of liner used will be influenced by patient activity and the increased cost associated with each liner. Surgeons must appreciate that, for a successful outcome, hard-on-hard bearings require a technical proficiency that is more demanding compared with conventional techniques.

Modern Polymers in Orthopaedic Surgery
Ultra-High–Molecular-Weight Polyethylene
Since Charnley's application of UHMWPE as a bearing surface in hip replacement, the science of UHMWPE

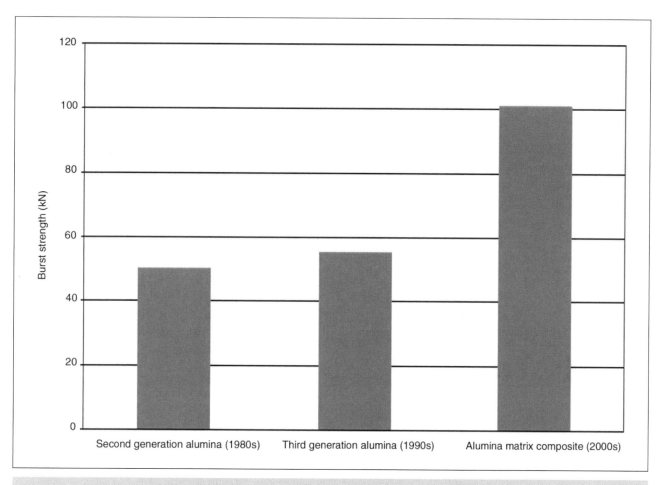

Figure 4   Bar graph demonstrates the burst strength for various types of alumina femoral heads.

as a biomaterial has grown. Polyethylene is composed of carbon and hydrogen atoms. UHMWPE denotes that the polyethylene chain is as long as 200,000 ethylene units, which gives UHMWPE a molecular weight of 3.5 to 7.5 million g/mol.[40] This long chain of ethylene units can rotate and fold about the covalent bonds that connect the carbon atoms and can form amorphous and crystalline regions. Structural variations in the polyethylene chain and the relationship between adjoining UHMWPE molecules can have an important effect on the mechanical properties of the material.

UHMWPE has higher ultimate strength and impact strength than the shorter chain high-density polyethylene.

UHMWPE also is more abrasion resistant and wear resistant than the shorter chain high-density polyethelene. Important insights have led to improvements in UHMWPE's durability as a bearing material. First, the sterilization process affects the material properties of UHMWPE. Before 1995, most UHMWPE implants were sterilized with gamma irradiation in air, which may lead to polyethylene-chain scission and oxidation and a subsequent degradation of the favorable material properties of UHMWPE. For the purposes of this chapter, UHMWPE gamma sterilization in air will be referred to as "historical" UHMWPE. In 1998, gamma sterilization in air was abandoned for alternate methods that

do not accelerate the oxidation process (gamma inert, gas plasma, and ethylene oxide). Irradiation of UHMWPE for sterilization (radiation dose of 35 to 40 kGy) in an inert environment leads to a low level of cross-linking within the polyethylene chain.[41] For the purposes of this chapter, such UHMWPE will be referred to as "conventional" UHMWPE.

The packaging of an UHMWPE implant also affects its performance and wear characteristics. Packaging an irradiated UHMWPE implant in air allows the implant to oxidize on the shelf. After this was understood by manufacturers, the packaging of UHMWPE implants was altered to limit the oxidation of the implant in the package.

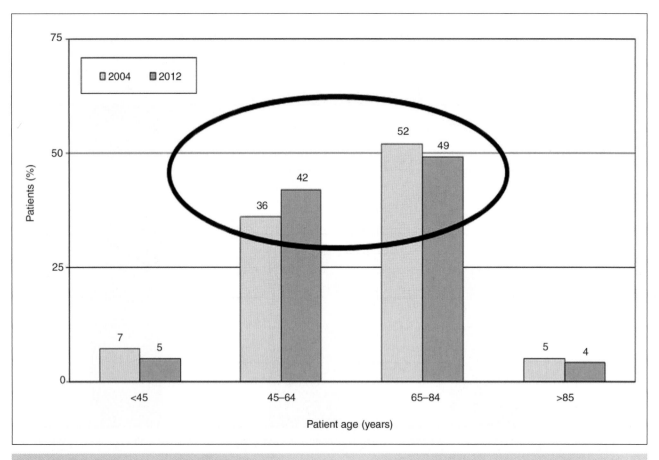

Figure 5 Bar graph demonstrates the age ranges of patients who undergo primary total hip arthroplasty. The black oval highlights the fact that, over time, more patients in younger age groups (specifically, patients aged 45 to 65 years) are undergoing primary total hip arthroplasty.

Particulate wear of the UHMWPE surface is an important contributing factor to osteolysis. In the hip, cross-linking of polyethylene that has been irradiated in an inert environment (highly cross-linked UHMWPE) reduces linear wear rates from approximately 0.1 mm/y to below the osteolysis threshold of 0.05 mm/y.[42] Cross-linking can be achieved with gamma or electron beam irradiation in doses that range from 50 to 100 kGy. After irradiation, free radicals are reduced, and cross-linking is enhanced by either annealing (warming below the melt temperature) or remelting the polyethylene. The reheating process, which is called quenching, reduces the percentage of crystalline polyethylene in the material and allows the polyethylene chains to reconform and establish more cross-links. Quenching reduces not only wear, but also the remaining free radicals in the material, which reduces the polyethylene's potential to oxidize.

Ten-year clinical follow-up studies of highly cross-linked UHMWPE acetabular components have reported virtually unmeasurable rates of linear wear and no clinically significant evidence of osteolysis.[43] Cross-linking and quenching of polyethylene does come with a small mechanical cost, however. Cracks in the material from fatigue propagate more rapidly, and, ultimately, tensile strength, yield strength, and fracture toughness are reduced. This has led to some failures of polyethylene in acetabular locking mechanisms that concentrate stress in small areas, particularly if the acetabular component is poorly positioned. However, given the remarkable success of highly cross-linked UHMWPE in reducing wear, it is now the preferred acetabular bearing for hip replacement.

Second-generation highly cross-linked polyethylene was developed to take advantage of the favorable wear characteristics that are afforded by cross-linking but to avoid the negative material property and fatigue consequences of quenching. It was hoped that second-generation highly

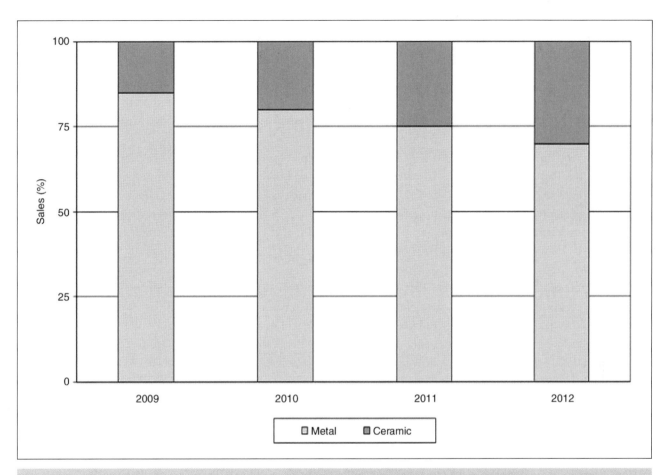

Figure 6   Bar graph demonstrates metal and ceramic femoral head sales in the United States.

cross-linked polyethylene would improve wear in settings other than the hip, such as the knee, without increasing fatigue-associated wear and failure. Vitamin E, a powerful antioxidant, can be diffused into polyethylene (a process called doping) to avoid oxidation of the polyethylene after it is irradiated. This eliminates the need for quenching; however, it does involve some reheating of the material to potentiate the diffusion of vitamin E. The polyethylene retains a higher degree of crystallinity, which improves its material properties. Wear-simulator studies and other mechanical testing studies of highly cross-linked UHMWPE that has been doped with vitamin E have confirmed the retention of improved wear behavior and

favorable material properties.[44-46] In addition, highly cross-linked polyethylene that has been doped with vitamin E should be resistant to in vivo oxidation, which was a potential problem with first generation highly cross-linked polyethylene. Highly cross-linked UHMWPE that has been doped with vitamin E became commercially available in 2007 for hips and in 2008 for knees. Long-term studies on the clinical performance of antioxidant-doped, second-generation highly cross-linked UHMWPE are not yet available.

Application in Total Knee Arthroplasty

The standard bearing surface for the tibial component in total knee

arthroplasty (TKA) is conventional UHMWPE. Given the success of highly cross-linked UHMWPE in THA, there was an interest to apply this same technology in TKA. The conventional UHMWPE wear particles produced in vivo from TKA are substantially different from those from THA.[47] TKA wear particles have a greater variety of shape, size, and texture than wear particles from THA, and fewer knee particles are submicron in size, which indicates a different wear mechanism. Wear-simulator studies have reported that highly cross-linked polyethylene demonstrates approximately 60% to 85% less wear than conventional polyethylene in both cruciate-retaining and posterior-stabilized designs;[48-50]

however, it is unclear whether these studies capture the complexity and variability of in vivo loading and would be predictive of in vivo outcomes. Currently, both conventional, which commonly has some degree of cross-linking as a result of sterilization via irradiation, and highly cross-linked UHMWPE are available for TKA. The degree of cross-linking and quenching as well as the methods of sterilization and packaging for commercially available highly cross-linked UHMWPE vary greatly among manufacturers.

Whether cross-linking of polyethylene is a benefit in vivo for TKA remains controversial. Hinarejos et al[51] performed a randomized prospective trial of conventional versus highly cross-linked polyethylene in 34 TKA patients. At 1-year follow-up, the authors aspirated the knee joints of the patients and reported no difference in the number of polyethylene particles in the synovial fluid samples between the two polyethylene groups. In addition, there was no difference reported in particle size and morphology between the two polyethylene groups. The authors concluded that polyethylene wear in TKA is dependent on many factors, and cross-linking of polyethylene did not influence wear substantially. Kim and Park[52] reported on a series of 308 patients who underwent bilateral posterior-stabilized TKA, in which one knee received a conventional polyethylene bearing and the other knee received a highly cross-linked bearing. The authors found no difference in clinical outcomes, no catastrophic failure of the polyethylene, and no radiographic evidence of osteolysis in either group.

Registry data on the use of highly cross-linked UHMWPE in TKA are just beginning to shed light on this topic. The 2013 Australian Orthopaedic Association National Joint Replacement Registry Annual Report shows that, overall, highly cross-linked polyethylene is beneficial compared with conventional polyethylene for both cruciate-retaining and posterior-stabilized total knee replacements;[53] however, careful evaluation of the data reveals that this benefit appears to be implant specific.

Application in Total Shoulder Arthroplasty

UHMWPE is the standard glenoid bearing surface for total shoulder arthroplasty (TSA). All glenoid components that are currently available for TSA use UHMWPE as a bearing surface. Fixation of the glenoid component with cement is the benchmark, but it has been problematic because radiolucencies at the cement-bone interface are common, even immediately postoperatively. Wear and osteolysis also are of concern. In a recent, large retrospective review of 359 TSAs, Raiss et al[54] reported that 43% of the shoulders had radiographic evidence of proximal humerus osteolysis at a mean follow-up of 8.2 years. The authors reported that radiographic proximal humerus osteolysis was related to lower Constant scores, less shoulder elevation, and less external shoulder rotation; however, none of the humeral components had actually loosened as a result of the osteolysis.

In a wear-simulator study that compared conventional polyethylene with highly cross-linked polyethylene for TSA, Wirth et al[55] reported a substantial reduction in wear for the highly cross-linked polyethylene group; however, the relevance of a simulator study such as this to the in vivo condition has yet to be determined. Retrieval studies have reported that wear of TSA glenoid components is usually caused by abrasion and fatigue.[56] This is similar to wear in the knee and distinct from the adhesive wear mechanism that predominates in THA. Furthermore, because TSA glenoid components are thin, usually unsupported by metal, and subject to high-contact stresses, there are concerns with respect to fractures of highly cross-linked UHMWPE in this setting. Currently, highly cross-linked polyethylene is being offered by some manufacturers for glenoid components in TSA but at radiation doses that are 50 kGy. Currently, there are no in vivo follow-up studies on these implants in the peer-reviewed literature.

The use of reverse TSA (RTSA) has grown since its introduction in the United States in 2004. Conventional UHMWPE is the current standard bearing surface for RTSA; however, there are concerns with respect to wear and osteolysis. RTSA is more constrained and, thus, has different biomechanics than conventional TSA. Because the biomechanics are theoretically similar to THA, there has been an interest to introduce highly cross-linked UHMWPE as a bearing for RTSA. In a recent wear-simulator study that compared conventional UHMWPE with highly cross-linked UHMWPE, Peers et al[57] reported that volumetric wear was reduced by 54% in the highly cross-linked group. However, small retrieval studies have reported that the predominant wear area for an UHMWPE bearing is on the rim and the inferior quadrant of the implant rather than concentrically in the body of the implant.[58,59] Thus, it is unclear whether the use of highly cross-linked UHMWPE is beneficial in RTSA.

Application in Total Elbow Arthroplasty

The most commonly used primary total elbow arthroplasty is fundamentally different from primary THAs, TKAs, or TSAs because it incorporates a linked, semiconstrained hinge design with UHMWPE bushings. Revision of the bushings is performed if they have worn or failed, and osteolysis is an important failure mode in this type of implant. In a recent study that evaluated the wear debris present in total elbow arthroplasties, Day et al[60] reported that polyethylene, cement, and metal debris were present. The polyethylene particles reported were of a size known to be associated with an osteolytic response. Currently, conventional UHMWPE is the standard for total elbow arthroplasty.

Application in Total Ankle Arthroplasty

Total ankle arthroplasty became generally available in the United States in the late 1990s. UHMWPE has been the standard bearing surface since its introduction. An important failure mode involved wear and osteolysis. Recently, highly cross-linked UHMWPE was introduced as a bearing surface in some implant designs. In a recent wear-simulator study that compared conventional UHMWPE with highly cross-linked UHMWPE, Bischoff et al[61] reported a 74% reduction in volumetric wear in the highly cross-linked UHMWPE group; however, as with other joints, it remains to be seen whether the simulator data are replicated in in vivo loading. Because highly cross-linked UHMWPE for total ankle arthroplasty has just recently been introduced to the market, clinical outcomes have yet to be determined.

Application in the Spine

Total disk arthroplasty implants became available in the United States in 2004; however, there was experience in Europe with these types of implants long before then. The original total disk arthroplasty implants that used historical UHMWPE were reported to develop wear, and there were reported cases of associated osteolysis similar to that seen in THAs and TKAs. Retrieval analyses of contemporary total disk arthroplasty implant designs with conventional UHMWPE reveal improved biomaterial performance. In a recent study that examined the periprosthetic tissues of 12 contemporary lumbar disk replacements that were revised for pain, Veruva et al[62] reported that one-half of the tissue specimens had measurable amounts of polyethylene debris and macrophage infiltration at a mean follow-up of 3.4 years. Compared with historical UHMWPE, this was reported as an improvement; however, more research is necessary to determine whether contemporary designs will have improved longevity and function. Total disk arthroplasty in the cervical spine has surpassed total disk arthroplasty in the lumbar spine, likely because of the decreased forces transmitted in the cervical spine and the relatively more straightforward anterior exposure for implantation. Conventional UHMWPE remains the standard bearing surface for total disk arthroplasty implants, and midterm clinical results have shown promise.

Polyetheretherketone

Polyetheretherketone (PEEK) falls into the category of polyaryletherketones, and is the most common type of polyaryletherketone used in orthopaedic surgery. PEEK has many material properties that make it well suited for orthopaedic use.[63] It is a chemically stable, biocompatible material that is insensitive to chemical and radiation damage and stronger than many metals on a per unit mass basis. PEEK's elastic modulus is comparable to dense cancellous bone, and, if PEEK is prepared as a composite material with carbon fiber, it can have stiffness similar to that of cortical bone and even titanium alloy.

In 1998, PEEK became available in orthopaedic implants, and it is currently used in a variety of settings. One interesting and potentially useful feature of PEEK is that it can be a part of a composite material, with the other component being a bioactive material, such as hydroxyapatite. Such a composite can be engineered to have a range of material properties depending on the intended use. PEEK also can be engineered to have a variety of porosities and surface textures. Because of its versatility as a material, PEEK's use is continually evolving.

Application in the Spine

The use of PEEK in orthopaedics began in the 1990s as a cage material for lumbar interbody fusions. In contrast to titanium cages, a PEEK cage had lower stiffness and, importantly, did not interfere with MRI and CT evaluation of the spine. In addition, PEEK cages could be manufactured in a variety of shapes and sizes to accommodate variations in patient anatomy. The clinical use of various PEEK formulations, with and without carbon-fiber reinforcement, has been successful in both the cervical and lumbar spine. PEEK is now widely used in the spine as a cage material.

There has been interest in augmenting the progression of fusion with the formulation of a composite material that combines PEEK and a bioactive material, such as hydroxyapatite, β-tricalcium phosphate, or growth factors.[63] In addition, Kakinuma et al[64] have investigated the addition of silver to PEEK to prevent infection. These bioactive composite materials for the spine are currently in various stages of development, and clinical reports are not available. PEEK rods also have been developed for posterior spinal fusion. Currently, early clinical reports are available, but the case numbers are too small; whether there are any advantages of PEEK rods over metal rods in the setting of posterior spinal fusion remains unclear.[65]

Application in Trauma

There has been continued interest in the development of PEEK composites as internal fixation devices for fractures. Plates and intramedullary nails that are composed of PEEK have been studied in various animal models, with the hypothesis that the lower elastic modulus of PEEK would promote more rapid bone healing. Although limited clinical data, particularly in relation to distal radius fractures, are just becoming available, PEEK and other polymer materials have yet to demonstrate a substantial effect in fracture fixation.[66]

Application for Soft-Tissue Reconstruction and Repair

PEEK has had success and is commonly used as a biointerference screw for ligament reconstruction. PEEK also is used in suture anchors for the repair of soft tissues to bone. Radiolucency and excellent biocompatibility are the main advantages of PEEK.

Conclusions

UHMWPE and PEEK are two polymers that have become widely used in orthopaedic surgery. Continued research and development have resulted in the refinement of their material properties, which has made them the standard materials for various orthopaedic interventions. Research and development in this area are ongoing. The formulation of new polymers and bioactive composites may expand the applications for these and other polymers in the future.

Additive Manufacturing

The traditional manufacturing process uses subtractive manufacturing, in which material is modified to its desired shape by a controlled removal process. Recently, additive manufacturing has been developed. The additive manufacturing process uses layers to build a three-dimensional (3D) product that is based on a computer model. In the additive manufacturing process, also known as 3D printing, the fine sections of the computer model are printed layer by layer until the product is completed. The layers are bonded with the use of a variety of energy sources, such as ultraviolet (UV), laser, electron beam, microwave, and ultrasound. Initially, material choices were limited; however, many options are currently available for orthopaedic applications, including polymers, ceramics, and metals.

Techniques

Initially, additive manufacturing was used for rapid prototyping with a stereolithographic apparatus. In this process, photopolymers are placed in a container with a build plate. A thin layer of polymer on the build plate is exposed to controlled UV radiation, which causes local polymerization. The build plate is then moved downward, which allows another layer of photopolymer to cover the object; it is then subjected again to UV radiation. This process is repeated until the 3D object is created.

Many newer techniques have allowed for the use of a wide variety of substrates and have changed additive manufacturing from a development tool to a manufacturing process. A substantial advance was the development of 3D printing with the use of laser inkjet technology. Two processes, fused deposition modeling and selective laser sintering, use the sintering technique, which fuses substrates into a solid state without complete mixing and melting. In fused deposition modeling, a thermoplastic substrate is heated to just above the melting point and then extruded onto a layer. During cooling, the substrate polymerizes to the layer below and rapid cooling causes hardening. In selective laser sintering, the powder in each layer is selectively fused via laser energy. Selective laser melting allows more complex models to be manufactured.

Additive manufacturing of metals, such as titanium and CoCr alloys, is of interest to orthopaedic surgeons. Three methods are available for metals: direct laser deposition, shaped metal deposition, and electron beam deposition. In direct laser deposition, fine metal powders or wires are sintered with the use of laser energy. The process is relatively slow, and the mechanical properties are not as good as those of other techniques. Direct laser deposition is limited to porous devices and requires further heat treatment to achieve improved mechanical performance. A modification of direct laser deposition is laser melting, which uses higher levels of energy but induces high internal stresses and requires further treatment to achieve acceptable material properties. Shaped metal deposition is performed with the use of tungsten inert gas welding in an argon atmosphere. Larger pieces of material up to 1 m^3 can be manufactured quickly. Electron beam melting uses high-energy electron beams that are focused on metal powders or wires, which causes them to melt. The electron beam is created by electrons that are released from a heated tungsten wire and are accelerated by a strong potential difference across the electrodes. The beam is focused on the substrate with the use of magnetic fields. This is performed in a vacuum to avoid oxidation problems. The high temperature during printing is maintained, which reduces the formation of internal stresses compared with the other methods. The electron beam melting process has been approved by the FDA for medical devices and is used for hip arthroplasty in Europe. An advantage of 3D printing of metals is that porosity, trabecular size, relative density, and roughness can be optimized for maximum bone ingrowth.

The process of additive manufacturing begins with a 3D computer-aided drawing.[67] For medical applications, this is often based on CT or MRI taken with a minimum of 1- to 2-mm slice thickness. Through a process of segmentation, a region of interest is chosen based on thresholds of physical parameters, such as Hounsfield units. Software then converts the model to a stereolithographic format, which is used in most additive manufacturing equipment. The model is reconstructed in layers and then printed layer by layer.

Clinical Application

Additive manufacturing has many potential clinical applications, including education and training, the development of patient-specific implants and instruments, and the manufacture of medical devices, prosthetics, and tissue-engineering scaffolds. A variety of biocompatible polymers, ceramics, and metals can be manufactured. Additive manufacturing can substantially reduce the amount of time necessary to create a custom implant and, thus, lower costs. Initially, additive manufacturing was used for patients who had cranial and maxillofacial defects.[68,69] Implants for more complex patients, such as those with tracheomalacia, have proven to be lifesaving.[70] Custom implants created with additive manufacturing have been reported to be beneficial in patients who have congenital abnormalities, in patients who have reconstruction after tumor resection, and in patients who sustained trauma.[71-74]

Orthotics and Prosthetics

Additive manufacturing is ideally suited for the rapid production of custom orthotic and prosthetic devices. Standard methods for the creation of custom devices require patients to have a cast made (the generation of a negative form) from which the final device is created. The final device then undergoes modification to improve function and fit. The alternative process—additive manufacturing—can produce custom devices rapidly, at substantially lower costs, and from a wide range of suitable materials.[75,76] One problem is dimensional accuracy, which may be lost because of shrinkage; however, methods to correct this have proven effective. Examples of prosthetic devices that are created with additive manufacturing include ankle-foot orthoses, lower limb prostheses, foot orthotics, upper extremity prostheses, and spinal orthoses for scoliosis.[75,77] An important advantage of additive manufacturing of prosthetic devices is that the process can easily be distributed anywhere. In resource-scarce regions, war, natural disasters, and neglect of trauma and congenital diseases have created large populations that require prosthetic devices. In countries such as Sudan and Haiti, upper and lower extremity prostheses are being manufactured with the use of additive manufacturing.

Surgical Education and Planning

Additive manufacturing can be used to aid in surgical planning and education. Surgical plans that are based on CT or MRI are converted from digital imaging and communications in medical images to a stereolithographic format and printed. The 3D-printed models can then be used for surgical planning and education. The 3D-printed models can be sterilized, which may aid in execution, expand minimally invasive surgery, and reduce surgical time. For complex anatomic areas, such as the acetabulum and the clavicle, 3D-printed models allow osteosynthetic plates to be precontoured, which, in the case of the clavicle, allows fixation with a minimally invasive surgical approach.[78] Custom and disposable instruments can act as guides to aid in safe fixation. 3D-printed pedicle screw drilling blocks created from CT scans were used to safely place screws in a preoperative model and, then, at the time of surgery in 10 patients.[79] In addition, an exact anatomic model that is available during surgery facilitates execution of the surgical plan.

Patient-Specific Implants

Additive manufacturing has made patient-specific joint implants possible. CT scans can help in the design of a patient-specific implant that is

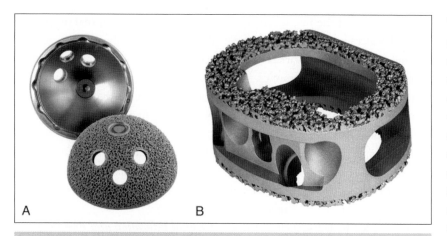

Figure 7 Illustrations show acetabular liners (**A**) and an interbody cage (**B**) that were made with the use of electron beam melting. (Courtesy of Renovis Surgical Technology, Redland, CA.)

manufactured with the use of standard metallurgical methods. Additive manufacturing can then be used to create a custom disposable instrument set for surgery. The proposed advantages include reduced inventory that is stored at the hospital and better approximation of the implant to the patient. The benefits of this approach have not yet been proven.

New Manufacturing Method

The additive manufacturing of metal devices with the use of electron beam melting has been approved, and several joint prosthetic devices have gained FDA approval via the 510(k) clearance process. Devices that contain both titanium and CoCr alloys can be produced. The devices produced for arthroplasty are nonbearing surfaces, such as tibial tray liners and acetabular shells (**Figure 7, A**). Interbody cages are available for the spine (**Figure 7, B**). The material properties of these devices can be designed to be equal or improved compared with traditional manufacturing methods. One potential advantage of electron beam melting is in regard to the porous coating. Instead of sintering,

electron beam melting creates a stronger structure that is less likely to delaminate. In many hip, knee, and spine explants, third-body wear has been reported as a result of delaminated porous coating. Additive manufacturing theoretically reduces such wear. Furthermore, the porous coating structure can easily be optimized to bone biology. The marginal costs of additive manufacturing are substantially reduced while dimensional quality is maintained.

Limitations

Currently, patients have limited access to medical devices that are manufactured with additive processes. Although some techniques of additive manufacturing have FDA approval, medical devices are limited to custom applications in the United States. Regulatory burden for routine use will be high for this technology and most likely will require large randomized clinical trials. Devices that are created with additive technology may have different mechanical properties than devices that are created with traditional manufacturing methods and may undergo changes in unknown ways after implantation.

The dimensional accuracy of additive manufacturing is variable, depending on the manufacturing process used and the resolution of the layering; however, several investigations have reported that the dimensional accuracy of additive manufacturing is sufficient for orthopaedics, including prosthetics, arthroplasty, and spine surgery.[80-82] Sterilization is a concern because microorganisms may be encapsulated during the manufacturing process and released after implantation, which may result in in vivo implant degradation.

Summary

The failure of orthopaedic devices, especially in arthroplasty, is often related to the type of biomaterials used. When selecting an implant, it is important that orthopaedic surgeons have a complete understanding of the material choice, the intended use of the device, how the device will affect specific tissues, and how the device will react to the in vivo environment. New devices that are made with new materials or manufacturing processes require extensive preclinical and clinical testing before they can be used. Surgeons should recognize that laboratory investigations that use today's standards may not predict subsequent in vivo behavior and, thus, should be cautious with the use of new technologies until sufficient long-term clinical results are available.

References

1. Lehil MS, Bozic KJ: Trends in total hip arthroplasty implant utilization in the United States. *J Arthroplasty* 2014;29(10):1915-1918.

2. Corten K, MacDonald SJ: Hip resurfacing data from national joint registries: What do they tell us? What do they not tell us? *Clin Orthop Relat Res* 2010;468(2):351-357.

3. Hug KT, Watters TS, Vail TP, Bolognesi MP: The withdrawn ASR™ THA and hip resurfacing systems: How have our patients fared over 1 to 6 years? *Clin Orthop Relat Res* 2013;471(2):430-438.

4. Griffin WL: Metal ion levels: How can they help us? *J Arthroplasty* 2014;29(4):659-660.

5. Witt F, Bosker BH, Bishop NE, Ettema HB, Verheyen CC, Morlock MM: The relation between titanium taper corrosion and cobalt-chromium bearing wear in large-head metal-on-metal total hip prostheses: A retrieval study. *J Bone Joint Surg Am* 2014;96(18):e157.

6. Daniel J, Ziaee H, Kamali A, Pradhan C, Band T, McMinn DJ: Ten-year results of a double-heat-treated metal-on-metal hip resurfacing. *J Bone Joint Surg Br* 2010;92(1):20-27.

7. Hart AJ, Muirhead-Allwood S, Porter M, et al: Which factors determine the wear rate of large-diameter metal-on-metal hip replacements? Multivariate analysis of two hundred and seventy-six components. *J Bone Joint Surg Am* 2013;95(8):678-685.

8. Jacobs JJ, Wimmer MA: An important contribution to our understanding of the performance of the current generation of metal-on-metal hip replacements. *J Bone Joint Surg Am* 2013;95(8):e53.

9. Esposito CI, Wright TM, Goodman SB, Berry DJ; Clinical, Biological and Bioengineering Study Groups from Carl T. Brighton Workshop: What is the trouble with trunnions? *Clin Orthop Relat Res* 2014;472(12):3652-3658.

10. Porter DA, Urban RM, Jacobs JJ, Gilbert JL, Rodriguez JA, Cooper HJ: Modern trunnions are more flexible: A mechanical analysis of THA taper designs. *Clin Orthop Relat Res* 2014;472(12):3963-3970.

11. Nassif NA, Nawabi DH, Stoner K, Elpers M, Wright T, Padgett DE: Taper design affects failure of large-head metal-on-metal total hip replacements. *Clin Orthop Relat Res* 2014;472(2):564-571.

12. Elkins JM, Callaghan JJ, Brown TD: Stability and trunnion wear potential in large-diameter metal-on-metal total

hips: A finite element analysis. *Clin Orthop Relat Res* 2014;472(2):529-542.

13. Cook RB, Bolland BJ, Wharton JA, Tilley S, Latham JM, Wood RJ: Pseudotumour formation due to tribocorrosion at the taper interface of large diameter metal on polymer modular total hip replacements. *J Arthroplasty* 2013;28(8):1430-1436.

14. Cook SD, Thomas KA, Harding AF, et al: The in vivo performance of 250 internal fixation devices: A follow-up study. *Biomaterials* 1987;8(3):177-184.

15. Molloy DO, Munir S, Jack CM, Cross MB, Walter WL, Walter WK Sr: Fretting and corrosion in modular-neck total hip arthroplasty femoral stems. *J Bone Joint Surg Am* 2014;96(6):488-493.

16. Cooper HJ, Urban RM, Wixson RL, Meneghini RM, Jacobs JJ: Adverse local tissue reaction arising from corrosion at the femoral neck-body junction in a dual-taper stem with a cobalt-chromium modular neck. *J Bone Joint Surg Am* 2013;95(10):865-872.

17. Urban RM, Jacobs JJ, Gilbert JL, Galante JO: Migration of corrosion products from modular hip prostheses: Particle microanalysis and histopathological findings. *J Bone Joint Surg Am* 1994;76(9):1345-1359.

18. Mihalko WM, Wimmer MA, Pacione CA, Laurent MP, Murphy RF, Rider C: How have alternative bearings and modularity affected revision rates in total hip arthroplasty? *Clin Orthop Relat Res* 2014;472(12):3747-3758.

19. Padgett DE, Wright TM: That's why we call it BIOmechanics! Commentary on an article by H. John Cooper, MD, et al.: "Adverse local tissue reaction arising from corrosion at the femoral neck-body junction in a dual-taper stem with a cobalt-chromium modular neck." *J Bone Joint Surg Am* 2013;95(10):e71.

20. Greenwald AS, Garino JP; American Academy of Orthopaedic Surgeons Committee on Biomedical Engineering; American Academy of Orthopaedic Surgeons Committee on Hip and Knee Arthritis: Alternative bearing surfaces: The good, the bad, and the ugly. *J Bone Joint Surg Am* 2001; 83(suppl 2 pt 2):68-72.

21. O'Leary JF, Mallory TH, Kraus TJ, Lombardi AV Jr, Lye CL: Mittelmeier ceramic total hip arthroplasty: A retrospective study. *J Arthroplasty* 1988;3(1):87-96.

22. Mahoney OM, Dimon JH III: Unsatisfactory results with a ceramic total hip prosthesis. *J Bone Joint Surg Am* 1990;72(5):663-671.

23. Huo MH, Martin RP, Zatorski LE, Keggi KJ: Total hip replacements using the ceramic Mittelmeier prosthesis. *Clin Orthop Relat Res* 1996;332:143-150.

24. Schmalzried T, Clarke I, McKellop H: Bearing surfaces, in Callaghan JJ, Rosenberg HE, Rubash HE, eds: *The Adult Hip*. Philadelphia, PA, Lippincott Williams & Wilkins, 1998, pp 247-265.

25. McKellop H, Shen FW, Lu B, Campbell P, Salovey R: Development of an extremely wear-resistant ultra high molecular weight polyethylene for total hip replacements. *J Orthop Res* 1999;17(2):157-167.

26. Clarke IC, Good V, Williams P, et al: Ultra-low wear rates for rigid-on-rigid bearings in total hip replacements. *Proc Inst Mech Eng H* 2000;214(4):331-347.

27. Clarke IC, Gustafson A: Clinical and hip simulator comparisons of ceramic-on-polyethylene and metal-on-polyethylene wear. *Clin Orthop Relat Res* 2000;379:34-40.

28. Heros R, Willmann G: Ceramics in total hip arthroplasty: History, mechanical properties, clinical results, and current manufacturing state of the art. *Seminars in Arthroplasty* 1998;9(2):114-122.

29. Hatton A, Nevelos JE, Matthews JB, Fisher J, Ingham E: Effects of clinically relevant alumina ceramic wear particles on TNF-alpha production by human peripheral blood mononuclear phagocytes. *Biomaterials* 2003;24(7):1193-1204.

30. Toni A, Affatao S, Bordini B: Simulator testing of the wear couple ZTA-on-polyethylene, in Willmann G, Zweymüller K, eds: *Bioceramics in Hip Joint Replacement: Proceedings 5th International CeramTec Symposium, Febr, 18/19, 2000*. Stuttgart, Germany, Thieme, 2000, pp 124-126.

31. Insley G, Turner I, Fisher J, Streicher R: In-vitro testing and validation of zirconia toughened alumina (ZTA), in Zippel H, Dietrich M, eds: *Bioceramics in Joint Arthroplasty 2002: 7th International Biolox Symposium.* Stuttgart, Germany, Thieme, 2002, pp 26-31.

32. Merkert P: Next generation ceramic bearings, in Zippel H, Dietrich M, eds: *Bioceramics in Joint Arthroplasty.* Berlin, Germany, Steinkopff Verlag, 2003, pp 123-125.

33. Agency for Health Care Research and Quality: Healthcare Cost and Utilization Project (HCUP). Rockville, MD, Agency for Healthcare Research and Quality, 2014. Available at: http://www.hcupnet.ahrq.gov. Accessed November 7, 2014.

34. Rajpura A, Kendoff D, Board TN: The current state of bearing surfaces in total hip replacement. *Bone Joint J* 2014;96(2):147-156.

35. Tateiwa T, Clarke IC, Williams PA, et al: Ceramic total hip arthroplasty in the United States: Safety and risk issues revisited. *Am J Orthop (Belle Mead NJ)* 2008;37(2):E26-E31.

36. Banerjee S, Pivec R, Issa K, Kapadia BH, Khanuja HS, Mont MA: Large-diameter femoral heads in total hip arthroplasty: An evidence-based review. *Am J Orthop (Belle Mead NJ)* 2014;43(11):506-512.

37. Kurtz SM, Kocagöz SB, Hanzlik JA, et al: Do ceramic femoral heads reduce taper fretting corrosion in hip arthroplasty? A retrieval study. *Clin Orthop Relat Res* 2013;471(10):3270-3282.

38. Hallab NJ, Messina C, Skipor A, Jacobs JJ: Differences in the fretting corrosion of meta-metal and ceramic-metal modular junctions of total hip replacements. *J Orthop Res* 2004;22(2):250-259.

39. Mendenhall Associates, Inc: 2014 hip and knee implant review. *Orthopedic Network News* July 2014;25(3):1-20.

40. Sobieraj MC, Rimnac CM: Ultra high molecular weight polyethylene: Mechanics, morphology, and clinical behavior. *J Mech Behav Biomed Mater* 2009;2(5):433-443.

41. Berry DJ, Currier BH, Mayor MB, Collier JP: Gamma-irradiation sterilization in an inert environment: A partial solution. *Clin Orthop Relat Res* 2012;470(7):1805-1813.

42. Dumbleton JH, Manley MT, Edidin AA: A literature review of the association between wear rate and osteolysis in total hip arthroplasty. *J Arthroplasty* 2002;17(5):649-661.

43. Glyn-Jones S, Thomas GE, Garfjeld-Roberts P, et al: The John Charnley Award: Highly crosslinked polyethylene in total hip arthroplasty decreases long-term wear. A double-blind randomized trial. *Clin Orthop Relat Res* 2015;473(2):432-438.

44. Shen J, Gao G, Liu X, Fu J: Natural polyphenols enhance stability of crosslinked UHMWPE for joint implants. *Clin Orthop Relat Res* 2015;473(3):760-766.

45. Bladen CL, Teramura S, Russell SL, et al: Analysis of wear, wear particles, and reduced inflammatory potential of vitamin E ultrahigh-molecular-weight polyethylene for use in total joint replacement. *J Biomed Mater Res B Appl Biomater* 2013;101(3):458-466.

46. Affatato S, Bracco P, Costa L, Villa T, Quaglini V, Toni A: In vitro wear performance of standard, cross-linked, and vitamin-E-blended UHMWPE. *J Biomed Mater Res A* 2012;100(3):554-560.

47. Schmalzried TP, Campbell P, Schmitt AK, Brown IC, Amstutz HC: Shapes and dimensional characteristics of polyethylene wear particles generated in vivo by total knee replacements compared to total hip replacements. *J Biomed Mater Res* 1997;38(3):203-210.

48. Wang A, Yau SS, Essner A, Herrera L, Manley M, Dumbleton J: A highly crosslinked UHMWPE for CR and PS total knee arthroplasties. *J Arthroplasty* 2008;23(4):559-566.

49. Stoler AP, Johnson TS, Popoola OO, Humphrey SM, Blanchard CR: Highly crosslinked polyethylene in posterior-stabilized total knee arthroplasty: In vito performance evaluation of wear, delamination, and tibial post durability. *J Arthroplasty* 2011;26(3):483-491.

50. Iwakiri K, Minoda Y, Kobayashi A, et al: In vivo comparison of wear particles between highly crosslinked polyethylene and conventional polyethylene in the same design of total knee arthroplasties. *J Biomed Mater Res B Appl Biomater* 2009;91(2):799-804.

51. Hinarejos P, Piñol I, Torres A, Prats E, Gil-Gómez G, Puig-Verdie L: Highly crosslinked polyethylene does not reduce the wear in total knee arthroplasty: In vivo study of particles in synovial fluid. *J Arthroplasty* 2013;28(8):1333-1337.

52. Kim YH, Park JW: Comparison of highly cross-linked and conventional polyethylene in posterior cruciate-substituting total knee arthroplasty in the same patients. *J Bone Joint Surg Am* 2014;96(21):1807-1813.

53. Australian Orthopaedic Association: Annual Report 2012-2013. Sydney, Australia, September 2013. Available at: http://www.aoa.org.au/about-aoa/resources/annual-reports. Accessed May 14, 2015.

54. Raiss P, Edwards TB, Deutsch A, et al: Radiographic changes around humeral components in shoulder arthroplasty. *J Bone Joint Surg Am* 2014;96(7):e54.

55. Wirth MA, Klotz C, Deffenbaugh DL, McNulty D, Richards L, Tipper JL: Cross-linked glenoid prosthesis: A wear comparison to conventional glenoid prosthesis with wear particulate analysis. *J Shoulder Elbow Surg* 2009;18(1):130-137.

56. Kurtz SM: *UHMWPE Biomaterials Handbook: Ultra-High Molecular Weight Polyethylene in Total Joint Replacement and Medical Devices,* ed 2. Burlington, MA, Academic Press, 2009, pp 117-135.

57. Peers S, Moravek JE Jr, Budge MD, et al: Wear rates of highly cross-linked polyethylene humeral liners subjected to alternating cycles of glenohumeral flexion and abduction. *J Shoulder Elbow Surg* 2015;24(1):143-149.

58. Day JS, MacDonald DW, Olsen M, Getz C, Williams GR, Kurtz SM: Polyethylene wear in retrieved reverse total shoulder components. *J Shoulder Elbow Surg* 2012;21(5):667-674.

59. Nam D, Kepler CK, Nho SJ, Craig EV, Warren RF, Wright TM:

Observations on retrieved humeral polyethylene components from reverse total shoulder arthroplasty. *J Shoulder Elbow Surg* 2010;19(7):1003-1012.

60. Day JS, Baxter RM, Ramsey ML, et al: Characterization of wear debris in total elbow arthroplasty. *J Shoulder Elbow Surg* 2013;22(7):924-931.

61. Bischoff JE, Fryman JC, Parcell J, Orozco Villaseñor DA: Influence of crosslinking on the wear performance of polyethylene within total ankle arthroplasty. *Foot Ankle Int* 2015;36(4):369-376.

62. Veruva SY, Lanman TH, Isaza JE, MacDonald DW, Kurtz SM, Steinbeck MJ: UHMWPE wear debris and tissue reactions are reduced for contemporary designs of lumbar total disc replacements. *Clin Orthop Relat Res* 2015;473(3):987-998.

63. Kurtz SM, Devine JN: PEEK biomaterials in trauma, orthopedic, and spinal implants. *Biomaterials* 2007;28(32):4845-4869.

64. Kakinuma H, Ishii K, Ishihama H, et al: Antibacterial polyetheretherketone implants immobilized with silver ions based on chelate-bonding ability of inositol phosphate: Processing, material characterization, cytotoxicity, and antibacterial properties. *J Biomed Mater Res A* 2015;103(1):57-64.

65. Mavrogenis AF, Vottis C, Triantafyllopoulos G, Papagelopoulos PJ, Pneumaticos SG: PEEK rod systems for the spine. *Eur J Orthop Surg Traumatol* 2014;24(suppl 1):S111-S116.

66. Tarallo L, Mugnai R, Adani R, Zambianchi F, Catani F: A new volar plate made of carbon-fiber-reinforced polyetheretherketon for distal radius fracture: Analysis of 40 cases. *J Orthop Traumatol* 2014;15(4):277-283.

67. Horn TJ, Harrysson OL: Overview of current additive manufacturing

technologies and selected applications. *Sci Prog* 2012;95(pt 3):255-282.

68. Lethaus B, Poort L, Böckmann R, Smeets R, Tolba R, Kessler P: Additive manufacturing for microvascular reconstruction of the mandible in 20 patients. *J Craniomaxillofac Surg* 2012;40(1):43-46.

69. Peltola MJ, Vallittu PK, Vuorinen V, Aho AA, Puntala A, Aitasalo KM: Novel composite implant in craniofacial bone reconstruction. *Eur Arch Otorhinolaryngol* 2012;269(2):623-628.

70. Joseph S: Doctors use a dissolvable 3D-printed tracheal splint to save a baby's life. Smithsonian.com. May 22, 2013. Available at: http://www.smithsonianmag.com/science-nature/doctors-use-a-dissolvable-3d-printed-tracheal-splint-to-save-a-babys-life-77862492/?no-ist. Accessed May 14, 2015.

71. Wu XB, Wang JQ, Zhao CP, et al: Printed three-dimensional anatomic templates for virtual preoperative planning before reconstruction of old pelvic injuries: Initial results. *J Chin Med J (Engl)* 2015;128(4):477-482.

72. Jeong HS, Park KJ, Kil KM, et al: Minimally invasive plate osteosynthesis using 3D printing for shaft fractures of clavicles: Technical note. *Arch Orthop Trauma Surg* 2014;134(11):1551-1555.

73. Gouin F, Paul L, Odri GA, Cartiaux O: Computer-assisted planning and patient-specific instruments for bone tumor resection within the pelvis: A series of 11 patients. *Sarcoma* 2014;2014:842709.

74. Trainor PA, Richtsmeier JT: Facing up to the challenges of advancing craniofacial research. *Am J Med Genet A* 2015;167(7):1451-1454.

75. Creylman V, Muraru L, Pallari J, Vertommen H, Peeraer L: Gait

assessment during the initial fitting of customized selective laser sintering ankle foot orthoses in subjects with drop foot. *Prosthet Orthot Int* 2013;37(2):132-138.

76. Devasconcellos P, Balla VK, Bose S, Fugazzi R, Dernell WS, Bandyopadhyay A: Patient specific implants for amputation prostheses: Design, manufacture and analysis. *Vet Comp Orthop Traumatol* 2012;25(4):286-296.

77. Salles AS, Gyi DE: An evaluation of personalised insoles developed using additive manufacturing. *J Sports Sci* 2013;31(4):442-450.

78. Chung KJ, Hong Y, Kim YT, Yang I, Park YW, Kim HN: Preshaping plates for minimally invasive fixation of calcaneal fractures using a real-size 3D-printed model as a preoperative and intraoperative tool. *Foot Ankle Int* 2014;35(11):1231-1236.

79. Sugawara T, Higashiyama N, Kaneyama S, et al: Multistep pedicle screw insertion procedure with patient-specific lamina fit-and-lock templates for the thoracic spine: Clinical article. *J Neurosurg Spine* 2013;19(2):185-190.

80. Wu AM, Shao ZX, Wang JS, et al: The accuracy of a method for printing three-dimensional spinal models. *PLoS One* 2015;10(4):e0124291.

81. Otawa N, Sumida T, Kitagaki H, et al: Custom-made titanium devices as membranes for bone augmentation in implant treatment: Modeling accuracy of titanium products constructed with selective laser melting. *J Craniomaxillofac Surg* 2015.

82. Salmi M, Paloheimo KS, Tuomi J, Wolff J, Mäkitie A: Accuracy of medical models made by additive manufacturing (rapid manufacturing). *J Craniomaxillofac Surg* 2013;47(7):603-609.

Principles of Antibiotic Prophylaxis in Total Joint Arthroplasty: Current Concepts

Joseph Bosco, MD
Jared Bookman, BA
James Slover, MD, MS
Emmanuel Edusei, BS
Brett Levine, MD, MS

Abstract

Infection is a rare, serious complication after total joint arthroplasty and constitutes a considerable emotional and financial burden for patients, surgeons, and healthcare systems. Prevention of surgical site and periprosthetic joint infections is crucial. This requires knowledge of the microorganisms that commonly cause these infections, including Staphylococcus species. Selection of the appropriate antibiotic regimen to treat infection remains controversial, but cefazolin and cefuroxime are the most commonly recommended antibiotics for prophylaxis. Appropriate timing of administration before surgery, with redosing performed as needed, can help to ensure optimal antibiotic concentration during surgery. Given the increasing evidence that S aureus colonization is a risk factor for periprosthetic joint infection, an exploration of the potential benefits of preoperative S aureus carrier screening and decolonization protocols is warranted. The use of antibiotic-loaded bone cement in primary total joint arthroplasty and antibiotic powder at wound closure are other controversial topics that require additional research.

Instr Course Lect 2016;65:467–476.

Despite numerous advances in arthroplasty, infections continue to occur. Although rare, infection is a devastating complication and a common indication for revision surgery.[1,2] It has been estimated that, by 2030, more than 4 million primary total hip arthroplasty (THA) and total knee arthroplasty (TKA) procedures will be performed annually in the United States.[3,4] Deep infection rates of approximately 1% to 2% within 2 years after TKA and THA have been reported.[5,6] If these rates remain constant, by 2030, the estimated number of deep infections after joint arthroplasty will be 40,000 to 80,000 per year. Infections are associated with serious morbidity, often require several reoperations, and are expensive to manage. Treatment of a single periprosthetic joint infection (PJI) has been reported to cost approximately $50,000; serious infections involving

Dr. Bosco or an immediate family member has received royalties from Genoval; has received research or institutional support from CareFusion and MAKO Surgical; and serves as a board member, owner, officer, or committee member of the Orthopaedic Learning Center. Dr. Slover or an immediate family member has received research or institutional support from Biomet and DJO Global. Dr. Levine or an immediate family member serves as a paid consultant to Link Orthopaedics, OrthoView, and Zimmer; has received research or institutional support from Biomet and Zimmer; and serves as a board member, owner, officer, or committee member of the American Association of Hip and Knee Surgeons and the Council of Orthopaedic Residency Directors. Neither of the following authors nor any immediate family member has received anything of value from or has stock or stock options held in a commercial company or institution related directly or indirectly to the subject of this chapter: Mr. Bookman and Mr. Edusei.

antibiotic-resistant organisms can cost more than $100,000.[7,8] If the conservative cost estimate of $50,000 per infection is used, the annual cost of treating infections will be $2 to $4 billion by 2030.

Various measures are used to prevent this devastating complication in arthroplasty patients, including optimizing medical comorbidities and patient risk factors, managing the operating room environment (eg, laminar flow, body exhaust suits, minimizing operating room traffic), using proper skin preparation, and carefully selecting and effectively using antibiotic prophylaxis.[2,9] Surgeons should be familiar with current concepts of antibiotic prophylaxis in total joint arthroplasty (TJA), including the rationale for antibiotic use and common microorganisms covered; antibiotic selection, timing, and dosing; *Staphylococcus aureus* carrier screening and decolonization; the role of antibiotic-laden bone cement; and local application of antibiotics during wound closure.

Historical and Theoretical Perspective

Studies published in the late 1950s and early 1960s established the effectiveness of prophylactic antibiotics in preventing surgical site infections (SSIs).[10,11] In a 1970 study of spine surgeries, Fogelberg et al[12] described the prophylactic use of penicillin. In the antibiotic group (120 patients) the infection rate was 1.7%, whereas the rate in the control group (112 patients) was 8.9%. However, the authors demonstrated a caveat of prophylactic antibiotic use—the development of antimicrobial resistance. Rates of resistant *S aureus* increased from 20% in the first year of the study to 31% in the second year and 60% in the third year. Therefore, despite the

lower infection rates, it is possible that antibiotic prophylaxis increases the complexity of infection.

Common Microorganisms

The creation of guidelines for antibiotic prophylaxis and appropriate decision making on antibiotic administration rely on the identification of organisms most likely to cause infection. Early infections (within 1 year postoperatively) and infections in patients with continuous pain since the index surgery are commonly thought to be caused by direct inoculation during the perioperative period, whereas late infections are thought to occur via hematogenous seeding of the prosthesis or through compromised local tissues.[13]

Many studies have demonstrated that gram-positive bacteria are most commonly associated with PJIs, particularly *S aureus* (methicillin-sensitive *S aureus* and methicillin-resistant *S aureus* [MRSA]) and coagulase-negative staphylococci, such as *Staphylococcus epidermidis*.[13,14] Other gram-positive organisms, including *Streptococcus* and *Enterococcus* species, also can cause infections. Infections caused by *Staphylococcus*, especially by *S epidermidis*, may be very difficult to treat because of the bacteria's ability to adhere to orthopaedic implants and form a local biofilm, which creates an ideal environment for bacterial replication, accelerates mutation rates, confers a relative resistance to host defenses, and impairs effective penetration of antibiotics.[15] Gram-negative organisms of concern are *Escherichia coli*, *Pseudomonas* species, and *Klebsiella* species. Gram-negative infections are less common and reportedly account for 10% to 20% of infections.[16] Approximately 20% of PJIs are polymicrobial.[17]

Other organisms, such as *Propionibacterium acnes* infection, have been associated with infections of specific joints after shoulder arthroplasty. *P acnes* is a gram-positive, non–spore-forming, anaerobic bacillus that was historically considered nonpathogenic but recently has been regarded as a pathogen in many infections with a late presentation.[18-20] However, its antibiotic susceptibility profile is good, with low rates of resistance, especially to first- and second-generation cephalosporin antibiotics (eg, cefazolin, cefuroxime) commonly used for prophylaxis.[19] All of these microorganisms can be part of normal skin flora. Therefore, direct infection from the patient's skin or airborne contamination from the surgical environment is the most likely route of inoculation.

Antibiotic Selection and Dosage

Systemic antibiotics are effective in reducing the infection rate; however, antibiotic selection remains controversial.[21] The most commonly recommended antibiotics for prophylaxis are cefazolin and cefuroxime.[22,23] Cefazolin is often dosed at 1 g for patients who weigh less than 80 kg or 2 g for patients who weigh more than 80 kg (**Table 1**). In patients who weigh more than 120 kg, a 3-g dose may be considered.[24] Cefuroxime is dosed at 1.5 g. Both of these cephalosporins are safe and have an effective spectrum of action against the most commonly encountered organisms, specifically gram-positive bacteria and 40% of gram-negative bacteria.[25] The most recent information statement on antibiotic prophylaxis from the American Academy of Orthopaedic Surgeons stated that cefazolin and cefuroxime are the preferred antibiotics for use in the absence of a β-lactam allergy.[22] A first- or second-generation cephalosporin should be the treatment of choice for routine prophylaxis.[8]

Clindamycin and vancomycin can be used if cephalosporins are contraindicated because of an allergy or if patients have known risk factors for antibiotic-resistant organisms, including MRSA. A 900-mg dose of clindamycin offers superior effectiveness against the common gram-positive bacteria of concern—*Streptococcus* and *Staphylococcus* species. Although clindamycin is effective against many MRSA species, vancomycin is a bactericidal agent that provides coverage against a greater percentage of MRSA species, which makes it a better choice to cover MRSA.

Patient-specific factors should be considered with respect to vancomycin dosage. One study reported that 69% of patients who receive vancomycin at the standard 1-g dose were being underdosed based on their actual weight.[26] This suggests that, given the high rates of obesity in arthroplasty patients, a weight-based dose of 15 mg/kg should be used. To maintain therapeutic concentration from the time of incision to the time of wound closure, cefazolin should be redosed every 2 to 5 hours during an extended surgical procedure; cefuroxime, clindamycin, and vancomycin should be redosed every 3 to 4 hours, 3 to 6 hours, and 6 to 12 hours, respectively.[27,28]

With regard to the selection and effectiveness of antibiotic prophylaxis, the clinician must consider whether the organism identified on cultures at presentation was within the spectrum of the original prophylaxis administered at the time of the primary surgery. A recent study of 163 patients with PJI

Table 1
Routine Antibiotic Prophylaxis Dosage and Schedule

Antibiotic	Recommended Dose	Redosing Schedule (hr)
Cefazolin	1 g (<80 kg body weight)	2–5
	2 g (60–120 kg body weight)	
	3 g (>120 kg body weight)	
Cefuroxime	1.5 g	3–4
Clindamycin	900 mg	3–6
Vancomycin	15 mg/kg (weight-based)	6–12

demonstrated that, in 63% of patients, the infections were caused by a bacteria that was resistant to the original prophylaxis.[29] MRSA was isolated from 26% of patients with cultures positive for infection.[29] Given the varying levels of antibiotic-resistant organisms present at institutions, it is important to customize antibiotics based on local trends. The use of a local and up-to-date antibiogram and consultation with an infectious disease specialist can help clinicians estimate the prevalence of antibiotic-resistant organisms, which aids in the selection of effective prophylactic agents.

Given the increasing prevalence of MRSA, surgeons must specifically address whether every arthroplasty patient should routinely receive vancomycin, either as a single medication or as a supplemental antibiotic. Current guidelines suggest that vancomycin is a reasonable choice of antibiotic for patients who have a β-lactam allergy, patients known to be colonized with MRSA, and patients in whom the risk of a MRSA infection is high (eg, patients in regions with a high prevalence of MRSA, institutionalized patients, healthcare workers).[22,25] The 2013 Proceedings of the International Consensus on Periprosthetic Joint Infection broadly support the routine

use of vancomycin in patients who are known MRSA carriers, patients with a known anaphylactic allergy to penicillin, or patients in whom the risk of a MRSA infection is high.[23] In addition, the routine use of dual antibiotics is generally not supported.[8]

In a retrospective study, Smith et al[30] analyzed PJI data after an increase in THA and TKA infection rates drove an institution to switch from cefazolin to vancomycin for routine prophylaxis. By comparing two historical cohorts before and after the switch, the authors reported that overall infection rates dropped from 1.0% to 0.5% after the switch to vancomycin. In addition, the infections that did occur were more successfully treated with irrigation and débridement alone after the switch (76.9% versus 22.2%), and the use of two-stage resection arthroplasty was required less frequently.

Sewick et al[31] compared dual prophylaxis with cefazolin and vancomycin versus cefazolin alone. In their retrospective analysis of 1,828 primary THAs and TKAs, the authors reported that the rates of infection with cefazolin and vancomycin versus cefazolin alone did not significantly differ (1.1% and 1.4%, respectively; $P = 0.636$) at 1-year follow-up. The prevalence of MRSA infections was significantly lower in the dual-antibiotic group than in the cefazolin group (0.02% and 0.08%, respectively; $P < 0.05$). However, these infections were very rare in the cohort; therefore, the number needed to treat to prevent one MRSA infection was very high (138). Tyllianakis et al[32] reported that the use of dual antibiotic agents (including vancomycin) was no better than cefuroxime alone in preventing PJIs, even at an institution with a higher than 25% prevalence of MRSA and methicillin-resistant *S epidermidis*.

Currently, the evidence to support the use of vancomycin for routine prophylaxis is mixed. This may represent a failure in terms of the effectiveness of the antibiotic or a failure to use the appropriate dosage (suggested dose, 15 mg/kg). Therefore, vancomycin is generally recommended for patients with β-lactam allergy, patients with a known MRSA colonization, or patients in institutions with a high prevalence of MRSA. In a systematic review of the literature, Cranny et al[33] used an economic model in an attempt to establish the prevalence level of MRSA at which an institutional switch from nonglycopeptide antibiotics (eg, cefazolin, clindamycin) to glycopeptide antibiotics (eg, vancomycin, teicoplanin) would be warranted. The authors found no clear evidence to determine any such threshold prevalence.

Timing and Duration of Action

The goal should be to infuse antibiotics within 1 hour of incision or the use of a tourniquet (whichever comes first); this results in optimal antibiotic concentration at the surgical site when the procedure begins.[25] In a large, multicenter observational study of the relationship between antibiotic timing and

SSI risk in various surgeries (including nonorthopaedic procedures), SSI risk increased incrementally with a longer interval between infusion and incision. Administration of antibiotics within 30 minutes before the incision was associated with a trend toward a lower risk of infection (1.6%) than administration 31 to 60 minutes (2.4%) before incision (odds ratio, 1.74; 95% confidence interval, 0.98 to 3.04).[34] If administered too rapidly, vancomycin can cause a histamine release, which results in hypotension and a skin reaction called red man syndrome; therefore, infusion of vancomycin should take place over a longer period of time than that for other antibiotics—60 to 120 minutes instead of the typical 30 to 60 minutes.[25] In addition, tissue penetration affects the varying infusion times for antibiotics. Cefazolin has a rapid tissue penetration into bone, synovium, and soft tissue.[9] Slower tissue penetration adds to the need to administer vancomycin earlier. The only exception to these guidelines is in the setting of revision arthroplasty if preoperative cultures of aspiration are negative but there is a high index of suspicion for an infection. In these cases, prophylactic antibiotics should not be administered until deep intra-articular cultures are obtained. After these cultures are obtained, then the antibiotics can be administered.

To maintain adequate serum concentrations, antibiotics should be redosed during longer surgeries (eg, 4 hours) and if there is increased blood loss (>2,000 mL) and/or fluid resuscitation (>2,000 mL).[8,22,23,35] Finally, 24 hours is considered the ideal duration for prophylactic antibiotic treatment. Many studies have failed to demonstrate any benefit associated with the use of antibiotics beyond 24 hours in elective, clean

surgical cases.[36-38] In a study of the short-term use of antibiotic prophylaxis in patients who underwent THA and TKA procedures, Heydemann and Nelson[36] reported no difference in infection rates between a 24-hour and a 7-day dose of nafcillin or cefazolin. In a retrospective review of 1,341 THA and TKA procedures, Williams and Gustilo[37] reported no difference in infection rates in patients who were treated with either a 24-hour or a 3-day course of cefazolin. The risks of excessive antimicrobial treatment, including toxicity and development of antibiotic-resistant organisms, have led to the recommendation for a 24-hour course of antibiotics.[22] Limiting unnecessary antibiotic exposure can minimize adverse effects associated with overuse, such as *Clostridium difficile* infection.[39] Hospital-associated *C difficile* infections carry serious morbidity and result in extended hospital stays and increased costs of care.[40]

S aureus Carrier Screening and Decolonization

There is increasing evidence that *S aureus* colonization is a risk factor for PJI. Patients who undergo orthopaedic surgery are colonized with *S aureus* at rates similar to those of the general population and, in patients who undergo TJA, nearly 20% are *S aureus* carriers.[41-43] Nasal carriers have increased rates of skin colonization, which is important to note because the skin is directly exposed to the surgical field at incision. Maoz et al[44] reported that *S aureus* colonization was a risk factor for infection after THA; compared with patients without preoperative colonization, patients colonized with the bacteria had a 2.36 relative risk for infection. In patients with multiple risk factors, *S aureus* colonization can further magnify the risk of infection

(**Table 2**). The authors also reported that patients who were obese (body mass index >30 kg/m^2), were colonized with *S aureus*, and actively used tobacco had a statistically significant relative risk of infection of 12.36 after THA compared with patients who did not have these risk factors (*P* < 0.002). In a study of 4,030 patients who underwent orthopaedic surgery, neurosurgery, or general surgery procedures, patients had a 0.42 relative risk of perioperative infection after treatment with nasal mupirocin.[43] Given the consequences of infection, exploring the potential effects of preoperative decolonization is warranted.

Two authors of this chapter developed a universal program for *S aureus* screening and decolonization before high-risk orthopaedic procedures (eg, TJA, spine fusion).[41] Patients' nares are cultured 7 to 10 days before the procedure. All patients are then given a prescription for nasal mupirocin for decolonization. On the day of surgery, patients are asked if they complied with the protocol. For those who report compliance, the cultures are checked and, if they test positive for MRSA, they receive vancomycin prophylaxis within 30 minutes of the skin incision and the typical preoperative preparation for their surgery. Patients whose cultures are negative receive the typical cephalosporin prophylaxis before the incision. If patients did not comply with the protocol and their cultures are negative or positive for methicillin-sensitive *S aureus* only, they also receive the typical cephalosporin or clindamycin prophylactic antibiotics before the incision. Patients who did not comply and have nasal cultures positive for MRSA receive preoperative vancomycin prophylaxis, are decolonized with mupirocin after surgery, and placed on

isolation precautions after surgery until the decolonization protocol is complete.

After adoption of this universal screening and decolonization protocol, the overall MRSA burden for the hospital was shown to decrease, and the overall deep infection rate associated with TJA was reduced from 1.45% to 1.28%.[41,45] However, this difference was not statistically significant and, to reach adequate power, 57,604 patients would be needed in each group. Despite the reduced rate of postoperative infections associated with a carrier screening protocol, several concerns exist. In a study of patient compliance with the universal protocol, Ramos et al[46] surveyed 100 patients who underwent TJA or spine surgery and reported that more than 80% complied with the protocol, but up to 41% incurred some out-of-pocket expense, with 7% reporting that this expense was substantial (mean cost, $31; range, $2 to $115). Because the protocol requires monitoring of preoperative cultures, it can be an operational challenge to obtain the cultures in a timely fashion so that the next steps of the protocol—antibiotic selection, decolonization, and isolation—can be initiated as needed.

As an alternative to obtaining preoperative cultures, polymerase chain reaction (PCR)-based testing has emerged as an effective tool for detecting MRSA colonization.[42,43,47] The accuracy of PCR-based tests for detection of *S aureus* has been validated in the literature and found to be sensitive, specific, and cost-effective.[48,49] In a systematic review of the accuracy of culture- and PCR-based tests, the PCR test was reported to be the most sensitive and specific for detecting MRSA colonization compared with nine other tests.[48] In addition, the universal carrier screening

Table 2

Patient Factors Associated With a High Risk of Infection

Prior prosthetic joint infection

Morbid obesity

Diabetes mellitus

Corticosteroid use

Inflammatory arthritis

Immunosuppression

and decolonization protocol requires universal treatment of high-risk patients with mupirocin, which raises concerns for overuse and antibiotic resistance. A randomized, controlled open-label trial of mupirocin and nasal povidone-iodine for *S aureus* decolonization was conducted to determine if decolonization could be completed without universal mupirocin treatment.[50] The use of povidone-iodine would have the advantage of being completed on the day of surgery, allowing treatment of culture-positive patients only and avoiding overtreatment and concerns for mupirocin resistance. An intention-to-treat analysis with more than 760 patients in each group demonstrated that povidone-iodine was equally successfully for decolonizing orthopaedic surgery patients.[50] This has led to a screening protocol with increased preoperative use of PCR-based tests to identify colonized patients and the use of nasal povidone-iodine in colonized patients only, rather than universal mupirocin treatment.

There is increasing evidence that *S aureus* carrier screening and decolonization have the ability to decrease perioperative infection rates; these procedures can be highly cost-effective and may improve outcomes.[51] It should be noted that the decolonization is not permanent, and patients who are decolonized have a substantial risk of being recolonized.[52] This means that patients who are decolonized for a procedure will need to be rescreened if they undergo a second procedure or if their surgery is postponed. Additional studies are necessary to determine the ideal screening and decolonization protocol and whether it is the decolonization process itself, administration of vancomycin for MRSA-colonized patients, or a combination of the two that is driving the trend of reduced infection rates.

Antibiotic-loaded Bone Cement

Polymethyl methacrylate (PMMA) bone cement serves as a grout to afford load transfer from the bone to the prosthesis. Initial medical applications of PMMA were in dentistry beginning in 1940 and in orthopaedic surgery with John Charnley's early work on THA in the 1950s and 1960s.[53] Although bone cement does not share many of the advantages of biologic fixation, it is commonly used for fixation of THA and TKA components.

Mixing antibiotics into bone cement allows for direct delivery of antibiotics to the implant and surgical site immediately after surgery. This practice is common and widely accepted in revision arthroplasty either in the creation of a spacer in the first stage of the procedure or as part of the cementing process in the replantation stage.[54] However, the use of antibiotic-loaded bone cement in primary THA and TKA is controversial; questions of efficacy, mechanical strength, and antibiotic resistance have been raised.[55]

Several properties of bone cement are important to consider when creating an antibiotic-cement mixture.[55,56] First, PMMA polymerization is an exothermic reaction; therefore, antibiotics must be heat stable. Second, the antibiotic itself must be water soluble to allow diffusion into the surrounding tissues. It must have a bactericidal effect at the tissue concentration and be released gradually over an extended period of time. Finally, the antibiotic must result in minimal local inflammatory or allergic reaction.

The mechanical and chemical stability of a variety of antibiotic-cement combinations has been studied. Aminoglycoside antibiotics (eg, gentamicin, tobramycin) have favorable properties for this application.[54] Other antibiotics, including vancomycin, erythromycin, and colistin, also have been used.

Historically, concerns about whether antibiotic loading decreases the strength of PMMA cement have been expressed. Lautenschlager et al[57] reported that adding large doses of gentamicin (>4.5 g per 40 g cement) or liquid antibiotics caused a substantial decrease in compressive strength to substandard levels. However, at the lower doses used for prophylaxis (<2 g per 40 g cement), this change in strength is likely negligible.[58,59] In a prospective randomized controlled trial of 25 patients who underwent THA with tobramycin-containing cement, Bohm et al[60] reported no increased motion of femoral stems (measured by radiostereometric analysis) at 2-year follow-up. This suggests that concerns about impaired strength associated with the use of antibiotic-loaded bone cement are largely theoretical. No in vivo clinical evidence has demonstrated an increased risk of mechanical failure associated with the use of antibiotic cement.[2,55]

Outside the United States, the use of antibiotic cement for routine primary THA or TKA has been well studied.

Large studies of data from the Scandinavian registry established the efficacy of antibiotic cement in THA.[61-63] Data on THAs from the Norwegian arthroplasty register (10,905 procedures)[61] and the long-term results of 22,170 procedures[62] showed lower revision rates if antibiotic prophylaxis was given both systemically and in cement versus prophylaxis alone (cement only or systemic only). Similarly, a study[63] of 92,675 THAs from the Swedish database that were performed from 1978 to 1990 showed substantially decreased rates of revision for infection with the use of gentamicin-containing cement. In a recent study of TKAs from the Canadian registry, Bohm et al[64] analyzed a sample of 36,681 TKAs. In 45% of these procedures, antibiotic-loaded cement was used. No significant difference between the groups treated with or without antibiotic-loaded cement was found with regard to 2-year revision rates for infection or any other cause.

In a large, prospective, randomized controlled trial, Hinarejos et al[65] examined the efficacy of antibiotic-loaded cement in reducing the incidence of infection after TKA. The authors randomized 2,948 patients to TKA with standard cement or with erythromycin/colistin-containing cement. The authors reported comparable rates of deep infection in the two groups: a rate of 1.4% in the antibiotic group versus 1.35% in the standard-cement group ($P = 0.96$). Currently no conclusive evidence exists regarding the efficacy of antibiotic-loaded cement in TJA.

Finally, the issue of cost is critical. The average cost of premixed antibiotic in PMMA is approximately $300 per bag.[2] Illingworth et al[2] reported that the cost of premixed antibiotic-loaded bone cement for 100 procedures (two bags per procedure) would be about $60,000. This is similar to the cost of treating one prosthetic infection. Therefore, for routine antibiotic-loaded cement to be cost-effective, it would have to demonstrably prevent one infection for every 100 primary arthroplasty procedures. An absolute decrease in infection rate of 1% would be difficult to achieve in practice, given that the baseline infection rates are already low (1% to 2%). Gutowski et al[66] performed a similar cost analysis for antibiotic-loaded bone cement used in TKA and reported that there is likely a cost benefit with hand-mixed cement, with the average cost per infection prevented ranging from $2,112 to $37,176. This is lower than the cost of a revision procedure. The cost of premixed cement for TKA was $112,606 per infection spared.

Currently, given the mixed results regarding its efficacy, no recommendation can be made with regard to the routine use of antibiotic-loaded cement in primary arthroplasty. One common practice is to use it only in patients with a high risk of infection (eg, patients with diabetes mellitus, morbid obesity, prior history of PJI). The 2013 Proceedings of the International Consensus on Periprostheic Joint Infection echoes this recommendation, with more than 90% agreement on the statement that antibiotic-loaded PMMA should be used in elective arthroplasty in high-risk patients only.[23]

Antibiotic Powder at Wound Closure

The application of topical vancomycin powder to surgical wounds has been used in both pediatric and adult spine surgery, with evidence demonstrating its efficacy and safety.[67-69] The use of intrawound vancomycin is associated with lower rates of SSI, with undetectable systemic absorption of vancomycin.[69,70] However, there are currently no studies demonstrating the efficacy of intrawound vancomycin powder in the setting of TJA. Qadir et al[71] recently created a biomechanical model to simulate wear behavior and reported that the addition of vancomycin powder to the total joint construct had no effect on wear rates of the ultra-high-molecular-weight polyethylene liner. The authors also highlighted one additional benefit of vancomycin powder—cost. Vancomycin powder is relatively inexpensive ($10 to $12 per patient) compared with the cost of antibiotic-loaded cement ($300 to $400 per patient).[71] However, given the lack of data on the efficacy of the powder in arthroplasty, the rates of allergic/adverse reactions, and the development of antibiotic resistance, it is difficult to draw definitive conclusions on the role of topical intrawound application of vancomycin powder at this time.

Summary

Antibiotic prophylaxis plays a critical role in the prevention of infection after TJA. Currently, infection rates are low, which makes careful study of antibiotic efficacy critical in reducing infections to the lowest attainable levels. Different systemic and local antibiotics each have a specific role and must be carefully considered to ensure the most effective prophylaxis regimen is selected for each patient, with the minimum of unintended effects. An ongoing research effort and close collaboration with infectious disease specialists will be required to provide all patients who undergo TJA the best protection against infection.

References

1. Jafari SM, Coyle C, Mortazavi SM, Sharkey PF, Parvizi J: Revision hip arthroplasty: Infection is the most common cause of failure. *Clin Orthop Relat Res* 2010;468(8):2046-2051.

2. Illingworth KD, Mihalko WM, Parvizi J, et al: How to minimize infection and thereby maximize patient outcomes in total joint arthroplasty: A multicenter approach. AAOS exhibit selection. *J Bone Joint Surg Am* 2013;95(8):e50.

3. Kurtz S, Ong K, Lau E, Mowat F, Halpern M: Projections of primary and revision hip and knee arthroplasty in the United States from 2005 to 2030. *J Bone Joint Surg Am* 2007;89(4):780-785.

4. Kurtz SM, Ong KL, Lau E, Bozic KJ: Impact of the economic downturn on total joint replacement demand in the United States: Updated projections to 2021. *J Bone Joint Surg Am* 2014;96(8):624-630.

5. Ong KL, Kurtz SM, Lau E, Bozic KJ, Berry DJ, Parvizi J: Prosthetic joint infection risk after total hip arthroplasty in the Medicare population. *J Arthroplasty* 2009;24(suppl 6):105-109.

6. Kurtz SM, Ong KL, Lau E, Bozic KJ, Berry D, Parvizi J: Prosthetic joint infection risk after TKA in the Medicare population. *Clin Orthop Relat Res* 2010;468(1):52-56.

7. Kurtz SM, Lau E, Watson H, Schmier JK, Parvizi J: Economic burden of periprosthetic joint infection in the United States. *J Arthroplasty* 2012;27(suppl 8):61-65.e1.

8. Parvizi J, Pawasarat IM, Azzam KA, Joshi A, Hansen EN, Bozic KJ: Periprosthetic joint infection: The economic impact of methicillin-resistant infections. *J Arthroplasty* 2010;25(suppl 6):103-107.

9. Prokuski L: Prophylactic antibiotics in orthopaedic surgery. *J Am Acad Orthop Surg* 2008;16(5):283-293.

10. Burke JF: The effective period of preventive antibiotic action in experimental incisions and dermal lesions. *Surgery* 1961;50:161-168.

11. Tachdjian MO, Compere EL: Postoperative wound infections in

orthopedic surgery: Evaluation of prophylactic antibiotics. *J Int Coll Surg* 1957;28(6 pt 1):797-805.

12. Fogelberg EV, Zitzmann EK, Stinchfield FE: Prophylactic penicillin in orthopaedic surgery. *J Bone Joint Surg Am* 1970;52(1):95-98.

13. Aslam S, Darouiche RO: Prosthetic joint infections. *Curr Infect Dis Rep* 2012;14(5):551-557.

14. Pandey R, Berendt AR, Athanasou NA; The OSIRIS Collaborative Study Group, Oxford Skeletal Infection Research and Intervention Service: Histological and microbiological findings in non-infected and infected revision arthroplasty tissues. *Arch Orthop Trauma Surg* 2000;120(10):570-574.

15. Zimmerli W, Moser C: Pathogenesis and treatment concepts of orthopaedic biofilm infections. *FEMS Immunol Med Microbiol* 2012;65(2):158-168.

16. Lamagni T: Epidemiology and burden of prosthetic joint infections. *J Antimicrob Chemother* 2014;69(suppl 1):i5-i10.

17. Del Pozo JL, Patel R: Clinical practice: Infection associated with prosthetic joints. *N Engl J Med* 2009;361(8):787-794.

18. Dodson CC, Craig EV, Cordasco FA, et al: Propionibacterium acnes infection after shoulder arthroplasty: A diagnostic challenge. *J Shoulder Elbow Surg* 2010;19(2):303-307.

19. Crane JK, Hohman DW, Nodzo SR, Duquin TR: Antimicrobial susceptibility of Propionibacterium acnes isolates from shoulder surgery. *Antimicrob Agents Chemother* 2013;57(7):3424-3426.

20. Bjerke-Kroll BT, Christ AB, McLawhorn AS, Sculco PK, Jules-Elysée KM, Sculco TP: Periprosthetic joint infections treated with two-stage revision over 14 years: An evolving microbiology profile. *J Arthroplasty* 2014;29(5):877-882.

21. Hill C, Flamant R, Mazas F, Evrard J: Prophylactic cefazolin versus placebo in total hip replacement: Report of a multicentre double-blind randomised trial. *Lancet* 1981;1(8224):795-796.

22. American Academy of Orthopaedic Surgeons: Information statement: Recommendations for the use of intravenous antibiotic prophylaxis in primary total joint arthroplasty. AAOS information statement 1027. Revised March 2014. Available at: http://www.aaos.org/about/papers/advistmt/1027.asp. Accessed May 18, 2015.

23. Parvizi J, Gehrke T, Chen AF: Proceedings of the International Consensus on Periprosthetic Joint Infection. *Bone Joint J* 2013;95(11):1450-1452.

24. Ho VP, Nicolau DP, Dakin GF, et al: Cefazolin dosing for surgical prophylaxis in morbidly obese patients. *Surg Infect (Larchmt)* 2012;13(1):33-37.

25. Bratzler DW, Dellinger EP, Olsen KM, et al: Clinical practice guidelines for antimicrobial prophylaxis in surgery. *Surg Infect (Larchmt)* 2013;14(1):73-156.

26. Catanzano A, Phillips M, Dubrovskaya Y, Hutzler L, Bosco J III: The standard one gram dose of vancomycin is not adequate prophylaxis for MRSA. *Iowa Orthop J* 2014;34:111-117.

27. Fletcher N, Sofianos D, Berkes MB, Obremskey WT: Prevention of perioperative infection. *J Bone Joint Surg Am* 2007;89(7):1605-1618.

28. Dellinger EP, Gross PA, Barrett TL, et al: Quality standard for antimicrobial prophylaxis in surgical procedures. *Infect Control Hosp Epidemiol* 1994;15(3):182-188.

29. Peel TN, Cheng AC, Buising KL, Choong PF: Microbiological aetiology, epidemiology, and clinical profile of prosthetic joint infections: Are current antibiotic prophylaxis guidelines effective? *Antimicrob Agents Chemother* 2012;56(5):2386-2391.

30. Smith EB, Wynne R, Joshi A, Liu H, Good RP: Is it time to include vancomycin for routine perioperative antibiotic prophylaxis in total joint arthroplasty patients? *J Arthroplasty* 2012;27(suppl 8):55-60.

31. Sewick A, Makani A, Wu C, O'Donnell J, Baldwin KD, Lee GC: Does dual antibiotic prophylaxis better prevent surgical site infections in total joint arthroplasty? *Clin Orthop Relat Res* 2012;470(10):2702-2707.

32. Tyllianakis ME, Karageorgos ACh, Marangos MN, Saridis AG, Lambiris EE: Antibiotic prophylaxis in primary hip and knee arthroplasty: Comparison between cefuroxime and two specific antistaphylococcal agents. *J Arthroplasty* 2010;25(7):1078-1082.

33. Cranny G, Elliott R, Weatherly H, et al: A systematic review and economic model of switching from non-glycopeptide to glycopeptide antibiotic prophylaxis for surgery. *Health Technol Assess* 2008;12(1):iii-iv, xi-xii, 1-147.

34. Steinberg JP, Braun BI, Hellinger WC, et al: Timing of antimicrobial prophylaxis and the risk of surgical site infections: Results from the trial to reduce antimicrobial prophylaxis errors. *Ann Surg* 2009;250(1):10-16.

35. Swoboda SM, Merz C, Kostuik J, Trentler B, Lipsett PA: Does intraoperative blood loss affect antibiotic serum and tissue concentrations? *Arch Surg* 1996;131(11):1165-1171.

36. Heydemann JS, Nelson CL: Short-term preventive antibiotics. *Clin Orthop Relat Res* 1986;205:184-187.

37. Williams DN, Gustilo RB: The use of preventive antibiotics in orthopaedic surgery. *Clin Orthop Relat Res* 1984;190:83-88.

38. Wymenga AB, Hekster YA, Theeuwes A, Muytjens HL, van Horn JR, Slooff TJ: Antibiotic use after cefuroxime prophylaxis in hip and knee joint replacement. *Clin Pharmacol Ther* 1991;50(2):215-220.

39. Tokarski AT, Karam JA, Zmistowski B, Deirmengian CA, Deirmengian GK: Clostridium difficile is common in patients with postoperative diarrhea after hip and knee arthroplasty. *J Arthroplasty* 2014;29(6):1110-1113.

40. Campbell R, Dean B, Nathanson B, Haidar T, Strauss M, Thomas S: Length of stay and hospital costs among high-risk patients with hospital-origin Clostridium difficile-associated diarrhea. *J Med Econ* 2013;16(3):440-448.

41. Hadley S, Immerman I, Hutzler L, Slover J, Bosco J: Staphylococcus aureus decolonization protocol decreases surgical site infections for total joint replacement. *Arthritis* 2010;2010:924518.

42. Kim DH, Spencer M, Davidson SM, et al: Institutional prescreening for detection and eradication of

methicillin-resistant Staphylococcus aureus in patients undergoing elective orthopaedic surgery. *J Bone Joint Surg Am* 2010;92(9):1820-1826.

43. Bode LG, Kluytmans JA, Wertheim HF, et al: Preventing surgical-site infections in nasal carriers of Staphylococcus aureus. *N Engl J Med* 2010;362(1):9-17.

44. Maoz G, Phillips M, Bosco J, et al: The Otto Aufranc Award: Modifiable versus nonmodifiable risk factors for infection after hip arthroplasty. *Clin Orthop Relat Res* 2015;473(2):453-459.

45. Mehta S, Hadley S, Hutzler L, Slover J, Phillips M, Bosco JA III: Impact of preoperative MRSA screening and decolonization on hospital-acquired MRSA burden. *Clin Orthop Relat Res* 2013;471(7):2367-2371.

46. Ramos N, Skeete F, Haas JP, et al: Surgical site infection prevention initiative: Patient attitude and compliance. *Bull NYU Hosp Jt Dis* 2011;69(4):312-315.

47. Hacek DM, Robb WJ, Paule SM, Kudrna JC, Stamos VP, Peterson LR: Staphylococcus aureus nasal decolonization in joint replacement surgery reduces infection. *Clin Orthop Relat Res* 2008;466(6):1349-1355.

48. Luteijn JM, Hubben GA, Pechlivanoglou P, Bonten MJ, Postma MJ: Diagnostic accuracy of culture-based and PCR-based detection tests for methicillin-resistant Staphylococcus aureus: A meta-analysis. *Clin Microbiol Infect* 2011;17(2):146-154.

49. Shrestha NK, Shermock KM, Gordon SM, et al: Predictive value and cost-effectiveness analysis of a rapid polymerase chain reaction for preoperative detection of nasal carriage of Staphylococcus aureus. *Infect Control Hosp Epidemiol* 2003;24(5):327-333.

50. Phillips M, Rosenberg A, Shopsin B, et al: Preventing surgical site infections: A randomized, open-label trial of nasal mupirocin ointment and nasal povidone-iodine solution. *Infect Control Hosp Epidemiol* 2014;35(7):826-832.

51. Slover J, Haas JP, Quirno M, Phillips MS, Bosco JA III: Cost-effectiveness of a Staphylococcus aureus screening and decolonization program for high-risk orthopedic patients. *J Arthroplasty* 2011;26(3):360-365.

52. Immerman I, Ramos NL, Katz GM, Hutzler LH, Phillips MS, Bosco JA III: The persistence of Staphylococcus aureus decolonization after mupirocin and topical chlorhexidine: Implications for patients requiring multiple or delayed procedures. *J Arthroplasty* 2012;27(6):870-876.

53. Charnley J: The bonding of prostheses to bone by cement. *J Bone Joint Surg Br* 1964;46:518-529.

54. Joseph TN, Chen AL, Di Cesare PE: Use of antibiotic-impregnated cement in total joint arthroplasty. *J Am Acad Orthop Surg* 2003;11(1):38-47.

55. Jiranek WA, Hanssen AD, Greenwald AS: Antibiotic-loaded bone cement for infection prophylaxis in total joint replacement. *J Bone Joint Surg Am* 2006;88(11):2487-2500.

56. Arora M, Chan EK, Gupta S, Diwan AD: Polymethylmethacrylate bone cements and additives: A review of the literature. *World J Orthop* 2013;4(2):67-74.

57. Lautenschlager EP, Jacobs JJ, Marshall GW, Meyer PR Jr: Mechanical properties of bone cements containing large doses of antibiotic powders. *J Biomed Mater Res* 1976;10(6):929-938.

58. Bourne RB: Prophylactic use of antibiotic bone cement: An emerging standard. In the affirmative. *J Arthroplasty* 2004;19(4 suppl 1):69-72.

59. Hanssen AD: Prophylactic use of antibiotic bone cement: An emerging standard. In opposition. *J Arthroplasty* 2004;19(4 suppl 1):73-77.

60. Bohm E, Petrak M, Gascoyne T, Turgeon T: The effect of adding tobramycin to Simplex P cement on femoral stem micromotion as measured by radiostereometric analysis: A 2-year randomized controlled trial. *Acta Orthop* 2012;83(2):115-120.

61. Espehaug B, Engesaeter LB, Vollset SE, Havelin LI, Langeland N: Antibiotic prophylaxis in total hip arthroplasty: Review of 10,905 primary cemented total hip replacements reported to the Norwegian arthroplasty register, 1987 to 1995. *J Bone Joint Surg Br* 1997;79(4):590-595.

62. Engesaeter LB, Lie SA, Espehaug B, Furnes O, Vollset SE, Havelin LI: Antibiotic prophylaxis in total hip arthroplasty: Effects of antibiotic prophylaxis systemically and in bone cement on the revision rate of 22,170 primary hip replacements followed 0-14 years in the Norwegian Arthroplasty Register. *Acta Orthop Scand* 2003;74(6):644-651.

63. Malchau H, Herberts P, Ahnfelt L: Prognosis of total hip replacement in Sweden: Follow-up of 92,675 operations performed 1978-1990. *Acta Orthop Scand* 1993;64(5):497-506.

64. Bohm E, Zhu N, Gu J, et al: Does adding antibiotics to cement reduce the need for early revision in total knee arthroplasty? *Clin Orthop Relat Res* 2014;472(1):162-168.

65. Hinarejos P, Guirro P, Leal J, et al: The use of erythromycin and colistin-loaded cement in total knee arthroplasty does not reduce the incidence of infection: A prospective randomized study in 3000 knees. *J Bone Joint Surg Am* 2013;95(9):769-774.

66. Gutowski CJ, Zmistowski BM, Clyde CT, Parvizi J: The economics of using prophylactic antibiotic-loaded bone cement in total knee replacement. *Bone Joint J* 2014;96(1):65-69.

67. O'Neill KR, Smith JG, Abtahi AM, et al: Reduced surgical site infections in patients undergoing posterior spinal stabilization of traumatic injuries using vancomycin powder. *Spine J* 2011;11(7):641-646.

68. Sweet FA, Roh M, Sliva C: Intrawound application of vancomycin for prophylaxis in instrumented thoracolumbar fusions: Efficacy, drug levels, and patient outcomes. *Spine (Phila Pa 1976)* 2011;36(24):2084-2088.

69. Bridwell KH, Anderson PA, Boden SD, Kim HJ, Vaccaro AR, Wang JC: What's new in spine surgery. *J Bone Joint Surg Am* 2014;96(12):1048-1054.

70. Gans I, Dormans JP, Spiegel DA, et al: Adjunctive vancomycin powder in pediatric spine surgery is safe. *Spine (Phila Pa 1976)* 2013;38(19):1703-1707.

71. Qadir R, Ochsner JL, Chimento GF, Meyer MS, Waddell B, Zavatsky JM: Establishing a role for vancomycin powder application for prosthetic joint infection prevention: Results of a wear simulation study. *J Arthroplasty* 2014;29(7):1449-1456.

Cardiovascular Considerations for Joint Replacement Surgery

Jasmine Saleh, MD

Erik Wright, BS

Mouhanad M. El-Othmani, MD

J.M. Lane, MD

William M. Mihalko, MD, PhD

Khaled J. Saleh, BSc, MD, MSc, FRCSC, MHCM

Abstract

Heart disease is the leading cause of death in the United States. Cardiovascular complications are associated with higher morbidity and mortality rates for patients who undergo orthopaedic surgery. Therefore, the clinical importance of a comprehensive preoperative evaluation and medical clearance is crucial and may substantially improve postoperative outcomes. A thorough knowledge of cardiovascular perioperative planning and management can enable healthcare professionals to identify patients who are potentially at risk for cardiovascular complications, and eventually improve both short- and long-term patient outcomes and satisfaction.

Instr Course Lect 2016;65:477–486.

Cardiovascular complications are some of the most common causes of postoperative morbidity and mortality and are expected to increase with the rising number of surgeries performed on patients who have multiple comorbidities. Therefore, it is crucial that orthopaedic surgeons have a comprehensive understanding and knowledge of cardiovascular risk factors and complications. This understanding may help improve preoperative evaluation and perioperative management, which could potentially result in a substantial reduction in the cost of hospitalization, the length of hospitalization, and postoperative morbidity and mortality. It is important for orthopaedic surgeons to understand the most frequently encountered complications in patients who have underlying cardiovascular diseases as well as perioperative management and strategies to improve postoperative outcomes.

Perioperative Cardiovascular Risk Assessment

Orthopaedic procedures are classified as intermediate-risk surgeries.[1] According to the American College of Cardiology (ACC) and the American Heart Association (AHA), an intermediate risk implies a less than or equal to 5% chance of an adverse postoperative cardiovascular complication. To reduce patient risk, orthopaedic surgeons need to employ appropriate perioperative management by identifying and assessing a patient's cardiac risks before surgery. Lee et al[2] identified and included six independent predictors of complications for noncardiac surgery in the Revised Cardiac Risk Index (RCRI). These variables include high-risk surgery (intrathoracic, intra-abdominal, or suprainguinal vascular), a history of ischemic heart disease, a history of congestive heart failure (CHF), a history of cerebrovascular disease, type 1 diabetes mellitus, and a preoperative serum creatinine level higher than 2 mg/dL.

Lee et al[2] reported that the incidence of perioperative cardiac events increases from 0.5% in patients without any risk factors to 9% in patients who have more than three risk factors. Likewise, a prospective cohort study by Ackland et al[3] demonstrated that an RCRI score greater than or equal to 3 is associated with higher postoperative noncardiac morbidity and a prolonged hospital stay after orthopaedic surgery. This implies that the RCRI can contribute to objective risk stratification of postoperative cardiovascular mortality and morbidity, which makes it a potentially useful preoperative assessment tool.

Some studies recommend that advanced patient age also be included in the RCRI.[4-7] Welten et al[7] reported that adding patient age to the RCRI improves its predictive value for adverse cardiovascular events because adverse cardiac events were noted to be higher among patients aged 75 years or older versus patients younger than 75 years (0.76 versus 0.62, respectively). A prospective cohort analysis showed that perioperative complications occurred in 4.3% of patients aged 59 years or younger, 5.7% of patients aged 60 to 69 years, 9.6% of patients aged 70 to 79 years, and 12.5% of patients aged 80 years or older.[6]

Cardiovascular Complications
Myocardial Infarction

Patients who have experienced a recent preoperative myocardial infarction (MI) are at a greater risk for cardiac death, mortality, and other complications after orthopaedic surgery compared with patients who have not had a recent MI.[8] Patients undergoing surgical fixation for femoral neck fractures were determined to have a substantially higher risk of mortality up to 12 days after MI.[9] Furthermore, recent data suggest that patients who have surgery for hip fractures and lower extremity amputations within 30 days of an MI, are at a considerably higher risk for recurrent MI, 30-day mortality, and 1-year mortality.[10] An MI within 6 months of orthopaedic surgery also has been shown to substantially increase a patient's risk for surgical site infections and ventilator dependence, which results in longer hospital stays.[11] For patients who undergo total knee or total hip replacements, a history of MI substantially increases the risk of the development of additional postoperative cardiac complications, including another ischemic event, CHF, and arrhythmia.[12]

Orthopaedic surgeons need to consider the timing of a previous ischemic event in relation to a planned surgical procedure to determine the overall risk of mortality and reinfarction.[13] The ACC and the AHA recommend postponing elective surgery at least 4 to 6 weeks after MI occurs.[14] However, studies have shown that the probability of postoperative infarction is as high as 27% if a patient has had MI up to 3 months before surgery.[15] The risk for reinfarction drops to 5.7% if surgery is postponed 4 to 6 months after MI occurs and to 3.3% if surgery is postponed more than 6 months after MI occurs.[16] Further research is necessary to determine an optimal timeframe for elective orthopaedic surgery in patients who have a recent history of MI.

Patients who have not experienced previous ischemic events are still considered to be at moderate risk for MI after orthopaedic surgery.[16] A study of patients who underwent elective total hip arthroplasty (THA) or total knee arthroplasty (TKA) reported that 6.4% of patients had a postoperative MI.[17] In a study of patients who were treated for femoral neck fractures, 1 in every 5 patients experienced MI within the first 2 days after surgery.[18] For patients who underwent surgery to repair a hip fracture, the risk for developing perioperative MI was reported to be substantially higher up to 7 days after the surgical procedure.[19] MIs have been reported to be the cause of death in 26% of total mortality cases that occur within

Dr. Lane or an immediate family member serves as a paid consultant to or is an employee of Bone Therapeutics, CollPlant, and Graftys; has received research or institutional support from Merck; has stock or stock options held in DFINE and CollPlant; and serves as a board member, owner, officer, or committee member of the American Academy of Orthopaedic Surgeons, the Association of Bone and Joint Surgeons, the American Orthopaedic Association, the American Society for Bone Mineral Research, the Musculoskeletal Tumor Society, and the Orthopaedic Research Society. Dr. Mihalko or an immediate family member has received royalties from Aesculap/B. Braun; is a member of a speakers' bureau or has made paid presentations on behalf of Aesculap/B. Braun; serves as a paid consultant to or is an employee of Aesculap/B. Braun and Medtronic; has received research or institutional support from Aesculap/B. Braun, Smith & Nephew, and Stryker; and serves as a board member, owner, officer, or committee member of the American Board of Orthopaedic Surgery, the American Orthopaedic Association, and ASTM International. Dr. K. Saleh or an immediate family member has received royalties from Aesculap/B. Braun; is a member of a speakers' bureau or has made paid presentations on behalf of Aesculap/B. Braun; serves as a paid consultant to or is an employee of Aesculap/B. Braun, the Memorial Medical Center Co-Management Orthopaedic Board, the Southern Illinois University School of Medicine, and Watermark Research Partners; has received research or institutional support from the NIH/NIAMS, the Orthopaedic Research and Education Foundation, and Smith & Nephew; and serves as a board member, owner, officer, or committee member of the American Academy of Orthopaedic Surgeons, the American Board of Orthopaedic Surgeons, the American Orthopaedic Association, the Board of Specialty Societies, Notify, and the Orthopaedic Research and Education Foundation. None of the following authors nor any immediate family member has received anything of value from or has stock or stock options held in a commercial company or institution related directly or indirectly to the subject of this chapter: Dr. J. Saleh, Mr. Wright, and Dr. El-Othmani.

© 2016 AAOS Instructional Course Lectures, Volume 65

90 days of THA.[20] Moreover, a prospective study of orthopaedic patients in whom a postoperative MI developed revealed that 1-year mortality rates may reach as high as 70%.[21]

Coronary Artery Disease

Coronary artery disease (CAD) is most commonly a result of arterial blood flow obstruction from atherosclerotic plaques.[22,23] This obstruction may compromise myocardial blood flow, which results in inadequate levels of oxygen and nutrient delivery necessary to meet metabolic tissue requirements.[22,23] Because orthopaedic surgery is associated with blood loss and hemodynamic changes, patients with CAD are at a higher risk for the development of perioperative MI.[22,23] Oberweis et al[24] reported that subjects with CAD had an increased risk for both perioperative thrombotic and bleeding complications, with an incidence of myocardial necrosis and major bleeding of up to 5.8% and 5.4%, respectively.

Functional capacity is an important indicator of perioperative outcomes in patients who have CAD.[25-27] Functional capacity is expressed in metabolic equivalents (METs), with 1 MET defined as 3.5 mL of oxygen uptake/kg per minute, which is the resting oxygen uptake of a person in a sitting position.[25,26] It has been reported that poor functional capacity (<4 METs) is associated with increased adverse cardiac events in patients who undergo noncardiac surgery.[26,27] Therefore, the ACC/AHA guidelines recommend that patients with no or intermediate clinical predictors for cardiovascular complications do not need additional cardiac testing unless they are unable to meet a functional capacity of 4 METs during daily activities.[25]

Some studies have reported that patients who undergo noncardiac surgery within 6 weeks after stenting may have an increased risk of perioperative and postoperative complications, including MI, stent thrombosis, bleeding, and death.[25,28,29] It is recommended that surgical intervention be postponed for 6 weeks after coronary stenting to allow patients to complete an antiplatelet prophylaxis regimen, therefore reducing the risk of stent thrombosis and bleeding complications.[28] The risk for perioperative thrombotic events may be caused by premature discontinuation of antiplatelet prophylaxis and the thrombotic state generated by the surgery; however, the continuation of medication in the perioperative period may predispose patients to an increased risk of perioperative bleeding and hemorrhage.[25,29] Nevertheless, it has been reported that patients on continued antiplatelet therapy have lower perioperative morbidity and mortality rates compared with patients who are not on continued antiplatelet therapy.[25,29] The ACC and the AHA recommend that elective noncardiac surgery be postponed 4 to 6 weeks for patients who have nonpharmacologic stents, without discontinuing aspirin at time of surgery.[25,29] Clopidogrel should be discontinued at least 5 days before surgery.[25,29] Surgery should be postponed 1 year for patients who have pharmacologic stents, without discontinuing aspirin at the time of surgery.[25,29]

Congestive Heart Failure

The clinical findings of CHF are characterized by jugular vein distention, the presence of a third heart sound, shortness of breath, weight gain, lower extremity edema, and an elevated serum B-type natriuretic peptide level.[5,25]

Several studies report that patients with CHF are at an increased risk for perioperative complications, including MI, worsening heart failure, and death.[25] Some studies have reported that the rate of perioperative heart failure was 2% among patients with no history of heart failure, 6% among patients with a history of heart failure, and 35% among patients with heart failure.[5,30] Similarly, Hammill et al[31] reported that patients with CHF who undergo surgery have substantially higher risks of hospital readmission and perioperative mortality compared with patients who have not had heart failure. In addition, Healy et al[30] reported that decreased left ventricular ejection fraction (<30%) is associated with a substantially higher risk of adverse perioperative outcomes. In their study of 174 patients who underwent intermediate- or high-risk, noncardiac surgery, 53 patients (30.5%) had at least one adverse perioperative complication, including 14 deaths within 30 days (8.1%), 26 MIs (14.9%), and 44 CHF exacerbations (25.3%).[30] According to ACC/AHA guidelines, it is important not only to diagnose and assess the severity of CHF, but also to identify its cause because different etiologies may lead to different risks and complications.[25]

Hypertension

The ACC and the AHA define stage 1 or stage 2 hypertension as systolic blood pressure below 180 mm/Hg and diastolic blood pressure below 110 mm/Hg.[14] Some studies have reported that mild or moderate hypertension is not an independent risk factor for perioperative cardiovascular morbidity or mortality.[5,14] Therefore, patients who have stage 1 or stage 2 hypertension and no history of substantial cardiovascular comorbidities can proceed with surgery under tight heart rate control.[14] Antihypertensive medications, especially β-blockers and clonidine, should be continued throughout the perioperative period to avoid potential rebound hypertension and its associated sequelae and complications.[14] Patients who have hypertension and are treated with angiotensin-converting enzyme inhibitors and angiotensin receptor blockers may have lower intravascular volume. As a result, they are predisposed to intraoperative hypotension and are at a higher risk for the development of perioperative cardiac and renal complications.[14,32] Therefore, it is recommended that angiotensin-converting enzyme inhibitors and angiotensin receptor blockers are withheld from patients the morning of orthopaedic surgery.[14,32]

Stage 3 hypertension is characterized as systolic blood pressure greater than or equal to 180 mm/Hg and diastolic blood pressure greater than or equal to 110 mm/Hg.[14] It may be beneficial to delay surgical intervention for patients who have stage 3 hypertension until a normotensive state is acheived.[14] Normalizing blood pressure can delay surgery for days or weeks. This may be acceptable for elective surgeries; however, for urgent surgeries, blood pressure can be controlled with rapidly acting intravenous agents.[14] The literature remains inconclusive in defining the benefits associated with a delay in surgical intervention.[14,33] Some studies have observed no statistically significant difference in postoperative complications between patients who underwent noncardiac surgery as planned and patients who had surgery postponed.[14,33] The ACC and the AHA recommend that orthopaedic surgeons weigh the potential risks and benefits of delaying surgery for each patient.[14]

Stroke

Stroke is the fourth leading cause of death in the United States.[34] Undergoing orthopaedic surgery increases the risk for the development of a postoperative stroke, even in patients with no history of stroke.[35,36] Lalmohamed et al[37] reported that during the first 2 weeks after THA, patients had a 4.7 and 4.4 times higher risk for the development of an ischemic or hemorrhagic stroke, respectively, than patients who did not undergo surgery. Postoperative stroke can be catastrophic for patients and physicians because it is associated with higher healthcare costs, a higher incidence of disability, and an eightfold increase in the risk of postoperative mortality.[38,39]

The strongest predictors of postoperative stroke are a history of stroke and hip fracture repair surgery.[36,40] Bateman et al[36] reported that THA is associated with higher postoperative stroke rates in patients who have a history of stroke. Popa et al[40] reported that the risk of postoperative ischemic stroke was 2.71 times greater for patients who underwent hip fracture repair compared with patients underwent THA. Because history of stroke is a substantial predictor of postoperative mortality, it is recommended that surgeons meticulously plan and tailor perioperative management to meet each patient's needs (such as close blood pressure monitoring and adjustment of antihypertensive medication to prevent cerebral hypoperfusion).[35,36,40]

Jørgensen et al[41] reported that patients have a higher risk of mortality if surgery is performed within 9 months of a stroke. Although the risk decreases if surgery is postponed at least 9 months after a stroke, the risk is still higher compared with patients who have no previous history of stroke.[41] Further research is necessary to investigate the risk variation in relation to the duration between a previous stroke and orthopaedic intervention.

Pulmonary Embolism

Pulmonary embolism (PE) is a common surgical complication that substantially increases postoperative morbidity and mortality rates.[42] A patient's age, the type of surgery being performed, and the presence of deep vein thrombosis (DVT), hyperglycemia, and anemia are variables that affect a patient's relative risk for the development of a PE after an orthopaedic procedure.[43,44] Studies have reported that PE develops in 28% of patients who undergo total joint arthroplasty.[45,46] For TKA patients and patients who undergo orthopaedic intervention after pelvic trauma, the PE incidence rate is reported to be 10%.[47,48] The incidence of PE has considerably decreased since the introduction of modern pharmacologic and mechanical prophylactic measures, yet it continues to be a serious complication in orthopaedic surgery.[49] Because surgery is believed to be a cause of acquired hypercoagulable states, the risk for the development of a fatal PE remains high for 3 to 6 weeks postoperatively.[50] PE is one of the most common preventable causes of in-hospital mortality;[51] however, despite the administration of both mechanical and chemical postoperative thromboprophylaxis, which are considered highly protective against PE, the condition may still develop.[52] Because PE may be expressed silently, the diagnosis and treatment of PE require a very high index of suspicion. A recent cohort study reported that the mortality rate for orthopaedic patients in whom a postoperative PE developed was higher than 15%.[52] PE was found to be the second most frequent cause of death in patients who undergo elective lower extremity total joint arthroplasty.[53] In addition to being a higher risk factor for short-term mortality, a primary perioperative PE is a strong risk factor for a recurrent PE, with incidence rates reaching 4.86% at 5 years postoperatively and 5.94% at 8 years postoperatively.[54,55] These recurrent events are associated with a fatality rate higher than 50%.[56]

Deep Vein Thrombosis

The risk for development of postoperative DVT increases with older age, history of DVT, obesity, and the type of the orthopaedic intervention.[56-58] On average, DVT develops in more than one-half of patients who undergo THA and TKA without thromboprophylaxis.[59] It has been reported that even with prophylactic measures in place, DVT still occurs in 46% of patients who undergo orthopaedic surgery.[60,61] More specifically, proximal lower extremity DVT occurs in approximately 10% of those patients.[62] Proximal DVT is more clinically significant than distal DVT because it is more frequently associated with postthrombotic syndrome.[63] Postthrombotic syndrome is a serious concern for orthopaedic surgeons because it is a potentially disabling condition characterized by extreme pain, edema, and severe leg ulcers.[64] The incidence of postthrombotic syndrome among patients in whom DVT develops after THA and TKA can be as high as 16.7% at 18 months postoperatively and 24% at 2 to 4 years postoperatively.[60,65]

The detection and diagnosis of postoperative DVT does not always occur while the patient is in the hospital.[66] In a study of more than 5,000 patients, it was reported that the mean time to DVT diagnosis was 17 days after TKA and 27 days after THA.[67] Subsequent studies have reported that 50% to 75% of DVTs are not diagnosed until after patients are discharged from the hospital.[68] Discharged patients have a higher risk for DVT because their care shifts to an outpatient treatment in which detection and management of DVT is more complicated.[69] Surgeons can help prevent DVT in discharged patients by understanding the risk factors and timeframe for DVT development and by providing appropriate prophylaxis for high-risk patients.[52]

Perioperative Medical Therapy

Aspirin

Because aspirin inhibits platelet aggregation and thrombus formation, it relatively reduces the risk of MI and other major cardiovascular complications by approximately 25%.[70] There is strong evidence that aspirin also prevents venous thromboembolism (VTE) after orthopaedic surgery.[71] In a study that compared hip fracture and elective arthroplasty in patients who received aspirin versus a placebo, Bozic et al[71] reported a 36% reduction in DVT and a 58% reduction in PE among the patients who received aspirin. In comparison with anticoagulants, however, aspirin may be associated with a higher risk of DVT after orthopaedic surgery.[72] In a systematic review that compared the efficacy of VTE prophylaxis agents, the incidence of postoperative VTE was reported to be higher in patients who received aspirin compared with patients who received anticoagulation therapy.[73] The American College of Chest Physicians recommends against the use of aspirin as a sole VTE prophylaxis.[74] With respect to the risk of DVT and PE, Patel et al[75] found no significant difference in the efficacy of aspirin and pneumatic compression devices (PCDs) compared with low-molecular-weight heparin and PCDs. Guidelines from the American College of Chest Physicians and the American Academy of Orthopaedic Surgeons recommend that, for patients who undergo elective TKA or for patients who have a contraindication to pharmacologic prophylaxis and undergo a THA or hip fracture surgery, aspirin combined with PCDs is as effective as VTE prophylaxis.[74]

Although aspirin provides several advantages for orthopaedic patients, it increases the risk of bleeding complications.[76] The Perioperative Ischemic Evaluation 2 trial reported a hazard ratio of 1.23 for major bleeding in patients who received aspirin compared with patients who received a placebo.[76] A higher rate of postoperative transfusions also was reported for patients who received aspirin.[77] However, a meta-analysis reported that after hip fracture repair surgery and arthroplasty, the risk of bleeding was lower with aspirin than with anticoagulants.[72] Similarly, Brown et al[78] reported that the relative surgical site bleeding risks of vitamin K antagonists, low-molecular-weight heparin, and pentasaccharides were all higher than the relative surgical site bleeding risk of aspirin.

Although aspirin is associated with an increased risk for bleeding complications, withdrawing it preoperatively may substantially increase the risk of thromboembolic complications.[79] O'Riordan et al[79] reported that perioperative withdrawal of aspirin is associated with a 10% risk of vascular events. Several studies agree that the increased risk for bleeding with aspirin continuation should not outweigh the risks of thromboembolism, and encourage perioperative management of aspirin based on an optimal risk-benefit ratio that ensures the best possible patient care.[79,80]

Statins

Statins are well recognized for lowering cholesterol and treating hyperlipidemia.[81] They possess anti-inflammatory effects and have the ability to decrease airway hyperreactivity and hypercoagulability.[81] The preoperative use of statins in noncardiac procedures is associated with a decrease in respiratory complications, infectious complications (sepsis and organ space infection), and VTE.[81] Evidence suggests that statins reduce not only major noncardiac complications, but also adverse cardiovascular events, including atrial fibrillation and MI.[82] Some studies have reported that in intermediate-risk, noncardiac surgeries, the 30-day overall mortality rate was reduced fivefold in patients who received statins.[25,82] This finding suggests that perioperative statin use is associated with a reduction in adverse postoperative cardiovascular events, morbidity, and mortality with respect to intermediate-risk, noncardiac surgery.

Although recent data demonstrate that statins can improve perioperative cardiac outcomes by inhibiting inflammatory response, some studies suggest that withdrawing statins after orthopaedic and other noncardiac surgeries may increase inflammation and, thus, increase cardiovascular morbidity and mortality.[83] Le Manach et al[83] reported that withdrawal of statins for 4 days may be an independent predictor of postoperative troponin leak and MI.

Therefore, the ACC and the AHA advocate for the continued use of statins in patients who currently receive them and plan to undergo orthopaedic surgery.[14]

Statins can exert pleiotropic effects, including improved endothelial dysfunction, enhanced angiogenesis, and possible anabolic effects on osteogenesis with neovascularization.[84] Mundy et al[84] reported that statins can have an anabolic effect on bone formation, both in vitro and in vivo, by activating the promoter of the bone morphogenetic protein-2 gene. A study of rabbit models by Oka et al[85] demonstrated the efficacy of low-dose simvastatin for the promotion of tendon-bone healing after ACL reconstruction. Although these studies suggest that statins may enable a new strategy to promote healing after ACL reconstruction and tendon rupture, further investigations in both animal and human models are necessary.

β-Blockers

β-blockers decrease myocardial oxygen demand by slowing heart rate and reducing contractility.[86] β-blockers are reported to reduce the risk of perioperative MI and cardiovascular mortality in intermediate- and high-risk patients (RCRI ≥2).[86] Some studies have reported that the overall 6-month, 1-year, and 2-year mortality rates were significantly lower for surgical patients who received atenolol compared with surgical patients who received a placebo.[87,88] The Dutch Echocardiographic Cardiac Risk Evaluation Applying Stress Echocardiography study reported that the incidence of cardiac deaths and nonfatal MIs was significantly reduced in patients who received bisoprolol.[89] Likewise, the results of a meta-analysis by Devereaux et al[90] revealed that patients who received

perioperative β-blockers had a statistically significant lower relative risk for cardiovascular mortality, nonfatal MI, and nonfatal cardiac arrest.

The benefits associated with perioperative β-blockers in noncardiac surgery remain inconsistent throughout the literature. Although the Perioperative Ischemic Evaluation 2 trial reported fewer major perioperative cardiovascular events among patients who received metoprolol compared with patients who received a placebo, more deaths occurred among the patients who received metoprolol because of a higher incidence of stroke.[86,91] This may be related to the higher incidence of significant hypotension and bradycardia in the metoprolol group.[86,91] Nevertheless, the AHA guidelines state that "the weight of evidence–especially in aggregate– suggests a benefit to perioperative beta blockade during noncardiac surgery in high-risk patients," and recommend the administration of β-blockers to patients who are at risk for perioperative cardiac events.[14]

The initiation of β-blocker therapy a few days before surgery may not be beneficial.[92] In a recent cohort study, Wijeysundera et al[92] reported that patients who received β-blocker therapy less than 8 days before surgery had a higher risk for 30-day mortality compared with patients who received β-blocker therapy 8 to 30 days and more than 31 days before surgery.[92] However, 1 to 7 days of preoperative β-blocker therapy was not significantly associated with higher 1-year mortality rates, 30-day MI, or 30-day ischemic stroke.[92] This implies that perioperative β-blockers should be initiated several days to weeks before orthopaedic surgery.

The ACC/AHA guidelines emphasize the importance of tight heart rate control in reducing perioperative cardiovascular events.[14] The dosage of β-blockers should be titrated to achieve a resting heart rate of 60 beats/min preoperatively and 60 to 65 beats/min intraoperatively and postoperatively.[14,93] Feringa et al[94] reported an increased incidence of MI, troponin T release, and long-term mortality in association with higher heart rates. The authors concluded that tight heart rate control with an absolute mean perioperative heart rate of less than 70 beats/min is associated with reduced perioperative cardiovascular events.[94]

Available evidence strongly suggests that perioperative discontinuation of β-blockers increases the risk of postoperative cardiovascular morbidity and mortality. van Klei et al[95] reported that the discontinuation of β-blockers during the first week after TKA or THA was significantly associated with postoperative MI and mortality. Therefore, the ACC/AHA guidelines advocate against the withdrawal of β-blocker therapy in noncardiac surgical patients, including low-risk patients.[14]

Summary

Patients who have a history of cardiovascular diseases, including CAD, MI, or CHF, are predisposed to a substantially higher risk of postoperative morbidity and mortality. Successful perioperative evaluation and treatment of these patients requires a comprehensive understanding of a variety of cardiovascular conditions as well as the required medical treatment and management. A thorough knowledge of cardiovascular conditions may substantially reduce the cost of hospitalization, the length of hospitalization, and postoperative morbidity and mortality for orthopaedic surgery patients.

References

1. Eagle KA, Berger PB, Calkins H, et al: ACC/AHA guideline update for perioperative cardiovascular evaluation for noncardiac surgery: Executive summary. A report of the American College of Cardiology/American Heart Association Task Force on Practice Guidelines (Committee to Update the 1996 Guidelines on Perioperative Cardiovascular Evaluation for Noncardiac Surgery). *Circulation* 2002;105(10):1257-1267.

2. Lee TH, Marcantonio ER, Mangione CM, et al: Derivation and prospective validation of a simple index for prediction of cardiac risk of major noncardiac surgery. *Circulation* 1999;100(10):1043-1049.

3. Ackland GL, Harris S, Ziabari Y, Grocott M, Mythen M; SOuRCe Investigators: Revised cardiac risk index and postoperative morbidity after elective orthopaedic surgery: A prospective cohort study. *Br J Anaesth* 2010;105(6):744-752.

4. Bhattacharyya T, Iorio R, Healy WL: Rate of and risk factors for acute inpatient mortality after orthopaedic surgery. *J Bone Joint Surg Am* 2002;84(4):562-572.

5. Goldman L, Caldera DL, Nussbaum SR, et al: Multifactorial index of cardiac risk in noncardiac surgical procedures. *N Engl J Med* 1977;297(16):845-850.

6. Polanczyk CA, Marcantonio E, Goldman L, et al: Impact of age on perioperative complications and length of stay in patients undergoing noncardiac surgery. *Ann Intern Med* 2001;134(8):637-643.

7. Welten GM, Schouten O, van Domburg RT, et al: The influence of aging on the prognostic value of the revised cardiac risk index for postoperative cardiac complications in vascular surgery patients. *Eur J Vasc Endovasc Surg* 2007;34(6):632-638.

8. Topkins MJ, Artusio JF Jr: Myocardial infarction and surgery: A five year study. *Anesth Analg* 1964;43:716-720.

9. Thiagarajah S, Fenton A, Sivardeen Z, Stanley D: The management and mortality of patients undergoing hip fracture surgery following recent acute myocardial infarction. *Acta Orthop Belg* 2011;77(5):626-631.

10. Livhits M, Ko CY, Leonardi MJ, Zingmond DS, Gibbons MM, de Virgilio C: Risk of surgery following recent myocardial infarction. *Ann Surg* 2011;253(5):857-864.

11. Lim S, Edelstein AI, Jain U, Puri L, Kim JY: Impact of preoperative myocardial infarction on surgical outcomes in inpatient orthopaedic surgery. *Int Orthop* 2013;37(12):2483-2489.

12. Basilico FC, Sweeney G, Losina E, et al: Risk factors for cardiovascular complications following total joint replacement surgery. *Arthritis Rheum* 2008;58(7):1915-1920.

13. Auerbach A, Goldman L: Assessing and reducing the cardiac risk of noncardiac surgery. *Circulation* 2006;113(10):1361-1376.

14. Fleisher LA, Beckman JA, Brown KA, et al: ACC/AHA 2007 Guidelines on Perioperative Cardiovascular Evaluation and Care for Noncardiac Surgery: Executive summary. A report of the American College of Cardiology/American Heart Association Task Force on Practice Guidelines (Writing Committee to revise the 2002 Guidelines on Perioperative Cardiovascular Evaluation for Noncardiac Surgery): Developed in collaboration with the American Society of Echocardiography, American Society of Nuclear Cardiology, Heart Rhythm Society, Society of Cardiovascular Anesthesiologists, Society for Cardiovascular Angiography and Interventions, Society for Vascular Medicine and Biology, and Society for Vascular Surgery. *Circulation* 2007;116(17):1971-1996.

15. Steen PA, Tinker JH, Tarhan S: Myocardial reinfarction after anesthesia and surgery. *JAMA* 1978;239(24):2566-2570.

16. Shah KB, Kleinman BS, Sami H, Patel J, Rao TL: Reevaluation of perioperative myocardial infarction in patients with prior myocardial infarction undergoing noncardiac operations. *Anesth Analg* 1990;71(3):231-235.

17. Goodman SM, Mackenzie CR: Cardiovascular risk in the rheumatic disease patient undergoing

orthopedic surgery. *Curr Rheumatol Rep* 2013;15(9):354.

18. Urban MK, Jules-Elysee K, Loughlin C, Kelsey W, Flynn E: The one year incidence of postoperative myocardial infarction in an orthopedic population. *HSS J* 2008;4(1):76-80.

19. Aynardi M, Jacovides CL, Huang R, Mortazavi SM, Parvizi J: Risk factors for early mortality following modern total hip arthroplasty. *J Arthroplasty* 2013;28(3):517-520.

20. Hietala P, Strandberg M, Strandberg N, Gullichsen E, Airaksinen KE: Perioperative myocardial infarctions are common and often unrecognized in patients undergoing hip fracture surgery. *J Trauma Acute Care Surg* 2013;74(4):1087-1091.

21. Huddleston JM, Gullerud RE, Smither F, et al: Myocardial infarction after hip fracture repair: A population-based study. *J Am Geriatr Soc* 2012;60(11):2020-2026.

22. Devereaux PJ, Goldman L, Cook DJ, Gilbert K, Leslie K, Guyatt GH: Perioperative cardiac events in patients undergoing noncardiac surgery: A review of the magnitude of the problem, the pathophysiology of the events and methods to estimate and communicate risk. *CMAJ* 2005;173(6):627-634.

23. Chan YC, Cheng SW, Irwin MG: Perioperative use of statins in noncardiac surgery. *Vasc Health Risk Manag* 2008;4(1):75-81.

24. Oberweis BS, Nukala S, Rosenberg A, et al: Thrombotic and bleeding complications after orthopedic surgery. *Am Heart J* 2013;165(3):427-33.e1.

25. Fleisher LA, Fleischmann KE, Auerbach AD, et al: 2014 ACC/AHA Guideline on Perioperative Cardiovascular Evaluation and Management of Patients Undergoing Noncardiac Surgery: A report of the American College of Cardiology/American Heart Association Task Force on Practice Guidelines. *J Am Coll Cardiol* 2014;64(22):e77-e137.

26. Karnath BM: Preoperative cardiac risk assessment. *Am Fam Physician* 2002;66(10):1889-1896.

27. Gerson MC, Hurst JM, Hertzberg VS, et al: Cardiac prognosis in noncardiac geriatric surgery. *Ann Intern Med* 1985;103(6 pt 1):832-837.

28. Kałuza GL, Joseph J, Lee JR, Raizner ME, Raizner AE: Catastrophic outcomes of noncardiac surgery soon after coronary stenting. *J Am Coll Cardiol* 2000;35(5):1288-1294.

29. Ramos GC: Relevant aspects of coronary artery disease in candidates for non-cardiac surgery. *Rev Bras Anestesiol* 2010;60(6):659-665, 366-369.

30. Healy KO, Waksmonski CA, Altman RK, Stetson PD, Reyentovich A, Maurer MS: Perioperative outcome and long-term mortality for heart failure patients undergoing intermediate- and high-risk noncardiac surgery: Impact of left ventricular ejection fraction. *Congest Heart Fail* 2010;16(2):45-49.

31. Hammill BG, Curtis LH, Bennett-Guerrero E, et al: Impact of heart failure on patients undergoing major noncardiac surgery. *Anesthesiology* 2008;108(4):559-567.

32. Brabant SM, Bertrand M, Eyraud D, Darmon PL, Coriat P: The hemodynamic effects of anesthetic induction in vascular surgical patients chronically treated with angiotensin II receptor antagonists. *Anesth Analg* 1999;89(6):1388-1392.

33. Weksler N, Klein M, Szendro G, et al: The dilemma of immediate preoperative hypertension: To treat and operate, or to postpone surgery? *J Clin Anesth* 2003;15(3):179-183.

34. Burke JF, Lisabeth LD, Brown DL, Reeves MJ, Morgenstern LB: Determining stroke's rank as a cause of death using multicause mortality data. *Stroke* 2012;43(8):2207-2211.

35. Sanders RD, Bottle A, Jameson SS, et al: Independent preoperative predictors of outcomes in orthopedic and vascular surgery: The influence of time interval between an acute coronary syndrome or stroke and the operation. *Ann Surg* 2012;255(5):901-907.

36. Bateman BT, Schumacher HC, Wang S, Shaefi S, Berman MF: Perioperative acute ischemic stroke in noncardiac and nonvascular surgery: Incidence,

risk factors, and outcomes. *Anesthesiology* 2009;110(2):231-238.

37. Lalmohamed A, Vestergaard P, Cooper C, et al: Timing of stroke in patients undergoing total hip replacement and matched controls: A nationwide cohort study. *Stroke* 2012;43(12):3225-3229.

38. Mashour GA, Shanks AM, Kheterpal S: Perioperative stroke and associated mortality after noncardiac, nonneurologic surgery. *Anesthesiology* 2011;114(6):1289-1296.

39. Selim M: Perioperative stroke. *N Engl J Med* 2007;356(7):706-713.

40. Popa AS, Rabinstein AA, Huddleston PM, Larson DR, Gullerud RE, Huddleston JM: Predictors of ischemic stroke after hip operation: A population-based study. *J Hosp Med* 2009;4(5):298-303.

41. Jørgensen ME, Torp-Pedersen C, Gislason GH, et al: Time elapsed after ischemic stroke and risk of adverse cardiovascular events and mortality following elective noncardiac surgery. *JAMA* 2014;312(3):269-277.

42. Paiement GD, Mendelsohn C: The risk of venous thromboembolism in the orthopedic patient: Epidemiological and physiological data. *Orthopedics* 1997;20:7-9.

43. Parvizi J, Huang R, Raphael IJ, Arnold WV, Rothman RH: Symptomatic pulmonary embolus after joint arthroplasty: Stratification of risk factors. *Clin Orthop Relat Res* 2014;472(3):903-912.

44. Mraovic B, Hipszer BR, Epstein RH, Pequignot EC, Parvizi J, Joseph JI: Preadmission hyperglycemia is an independent risk factor for in-hospital symptomatic pulmonary embolism after major orthopedic surgery. *J Arthroplasty* 2010;25(1):64-70.

45. Phillips CB, Barrett JA, Losina E, et al: Incidence rates of dislocation, pulmonary embolism, and deep infection during the first six months after elective total hip replacement. *J Bone Joint Surg Am* 2003;85(1):20-26.

46. Mantilla CB, Horlocker TT, Schroeder DR, Berry DJ, Brown DL: Frequency of myocardial infarction, pulmonary embolism, deep venous

thrombosis, and death following primary hip or knee arthroplasty. *Anesthesiology* 2002;96(5):1140-1146.

47. Geerts W, Ray JG, Colwell CW, et al: Prevention of venous thromboembolism. *Chest* 2005;128(5):377S-376S.

48. Montgomery KD, Geerts WH, Potter HG, Helfet DL: Thromboembolic complications in patients with pelvic trauma. *Clin Orthop Relat Res* 1996;329:68-87.

49. Goldhaber SZ, Bounameaux H: Pulmonary embolism and deep vein thrombosis. *Lancet* 2012;379(9828):1835-1846.

50. Schulman S; Duration of Anticoagulation Study Group: The effect of the duration of anticoagulation and other risk factors on the recurrence of venous thromboembolisms. *Wien Med Wochenschr* 1999;149(2-4):66-69.

51. Alikhan R, Peters F, Wilmott R, Cohen AT: Fatal pulmonary embolism in hospitalised patients: A necropsy review. *J Clin Pathol* 2004;57(12):1254-1257.

52. Gudipati S, Fragkakis EM, Ciriello V, et al: A cohort study on the incidence and outcome of pulmonary embolism in trauma and orthopedic patients. *BMC Med* 2014;12:39.

53. Poultsides LA, Gonzalez Della Valle A, Memtsoudis SG, et al: Meta-analysis of cause of death following total joint replacement using different thromboprophylaxis regimens. *J Bone Joint Surg Br* 2012;94(1):113-121.

54. Heit JA, Mohr DN, Silverstein MD, Petterson TM, O'Fallon WM, Melton LJ III: Predictors of recurrence after deep vein thrombosis and pulmonary embolism: A population-based cohort study. *Arch Intern Med* 2000;160(6):761-768.

55. Prandoni P, Villalta S, Bagatella P, et al: The clinical course of deep-vein thrombosis: Prospective long-term follow-up of 528 symptomatic patients. *Haematologica* 1997;82(4):423-428.

56. Warwick D, Rosencher N: The "critical thrombosis period" in major orthopedic surgery: When to start and when to stop prophylaxis. *Clin Appl Thromb Hemost* 2010;16(4):394-405.

57. Samama MM: An epidemiologic study of risk factors for deep vein thrombosis in medical outpatients: The Sirius study. *Arch Intern Med* 2000;160(22):3415-3420.

58. Stringer MD, Steadman CA, Hedges AR, Thomas EM, Morley TR, Kakkar VV: Deep vein thrombosis after elective knee surgery: An incidence study in 312 patients. *J Bone Joint Surg Br* 1989;71(3):492-497.

59. Arcelus JI, Kudrna JC, Caprini JA: Venous thromboembolism following major orthopedic surgery: What is the risk after discharge? *Orthopedics* 2006;29(6):506-516.

60. Schindler OS, Dalziel R: Post-thrombotic syndrome after total hip or knee arthroplasty: Incidence in patients with asymptomatic deep venous thrombosis. *J Orthop Surg (Hong Kong)* 2005;13(2):113-119.

61. Maynard MJ, Sculco TP, Ghelman B: Progression and regression of deep vein thrombosis after total knee arthroplasty. *Clin Orthop Relat Res* 1991;273:125-130.

62. Piovella F, Wang CJ, Lu H, et al: Deep-vein thrombosis rates after major orthopedic surgery in Asia: An epidemiological study based on postoperative screening with centrally adjudicated bilateral venography. *J Thromb Haemost* 2005;3(12):2664-2670.

63. Cordell-Smith JA, Williams SC, Harper WM, Gregg PJ: Lower limb arthroplasty complicated by deep venous thrombosis: Prevalence and subjective outcome. *J Bone Joint Surg Br* 2004;86(1):99-101.

64. Sullivan SD, Kahn SR, Davidson BL, Borris L, Bossuyt P, Raskob G: Measuring the outcomes and pharmacoeconomic consequences of venous thromboembolism prophylaxis in major orthopaedic surgery. *Pharmacoeconomics* 2003;21(7):477-496.

65. Siragusa S, Beltrametti C, Barone M, Piovella F: Clinical course and incidence of post-thrombophlebitic syndrome after profound asymptomatic deep vein thrombosis: Results of a transverse epidemiologic study. *Minerva Cardioangiol* 1997;45(3):57-66.

66. White RH, Romano PS, Zhou H, Rodrigo J, Bargar W: Incidence and time course of thromboembolic outcomes following total hip or knee arthroplasty. *Arch Intern Med* 1998;158(14):1525-1531.

67. Dahl OE, Gudmundsen TE, Haukeland L: Late occurring clinical deep vein thrombosis in joint-operated patients. *Acta Orthop Scand* 2000;71(1):47-50.

68. Scurr JH: How long after surgery does the risk of thromboembolism persist? *Acta Chir Scand Suppl* 1990;556:22-24.

69. Anderson FA Jr, Spencer FA: Risk factors for venous thromboembolism. *Circulation* 2003;107(23 suppl 1):I9-I16.

70. Cannon CP; CAPRIE Investigators: Effectiveness of clopidogrel versus aspirin in preventing acute myocardial infarction in patients with symptomatic atherothrombosis (CAPRIE trial). *Am J Cardiol* 2002;90(7):760-762.

71. Bozic KJ, Vail TP, Pekow PS, Maselli JH, Lindenauer PK, Auerbach AD: Does aspirin have a role in venous thromboembolism prophylaxis in total knee arthroplasty patients? *J Arthroplasty* 2010;25(7):1053-1060.

72. Drescher FS, Sirovich BE, Lee A, Morrison DH, Chiang WH, Larson RJ: Aspirin versus anticoagulation for prevention of venous thromboembolism major lower extremity orthopedic surgery: A systematic review and meta-analysis. *J Hosp Med* 2014;9(9):579-585.

73. Lussana F, Squizzato A, Permunian ET, Cattaneo M: A systematic review on the effect of aspirin in the prevention of post-operative arterial thrombosis in patients undergoing total hip and total knee arthroplasty. *Thromb Res* 2014;134(3):599-603.

74. Stewart DW, Freshour JE: Aspirin for the prophylaxis of venous thromboembolic events in orthopedic surgery patients: A comparison of the AAOS and ACCP guidelines with review of the evidence. *Ann Pharmacother* 2013;47(1):63-74.

75. Patel AR, Crist MK, Nemitz J, Mayerson JL: Aspirin and compression devices versus low-molecular-weight heparin and PCD for VTE prophylaxis in orthopedic

oncology patients. *J Surg Oncol* 2010;102(3):276-281.

76. Devereaux PJ, Mrkobrada M, Sessler DI, et al: Aspirin in patients undergoing noncardiac surgery. *N Engl J Med* 2014;370(16):1494-1503.

77. Anekstein Y, Tamir E, Halperin N, Mirovsky Y: Aspirin therapy and bleeding during proximal femoral fracture surgery. *Clin Orthop Relat Res* 2004;418:205-208.

78. Brown GA: Venous thromboembolism prophylaxis after major orthopaedic surgery: A pooled analysis of randomized controlled trials. *J Arthroplasty* 2009;24(6 suppl):77-83.

79. O'Riordan JM, Margey RJ, Blake G, O'Connell PR: Antiplatelet agents in the perioperative period. *Arch Surg* 2009;144(1):69-76.

80. Gerstein NS, Schulman PM, Gerstein WH, Petersen TR, Tawil I: Should more patients continue aspirin therapy perioperatively? Clinical impact of aspirin withdrawal syndrome. *Ann Surg* 2012;255(5):811-819.

81. Iannuzzi JC, Rickles AS, Kelly KN, et al: Perioperative pleiotropic statin effects in general surgery. *Surgery* 2014;155(3):398-407.

82. Raju MG, Pachika A, Punnam SR, et al: Statin therapy in the reduction of cardiovascular events in patients undergoing intermediate-risk noncardiac, nonvascular surgery. *Clin Cardiol* 2013;36(8):456-461.

83. Le Manach Y, Ibanez Esteves C, Bertrand M, et al: Impact of preoperative statin therapy on adverse postoperative outcomes in patients undergoing vascular surgery. *Anesthesiology* 2011;114(1):98-104.

84. Mundy G, Garrett R, Harris S, et al: Stimulation of bone formation in vitro and in rodents by statins. *Science* 1999;286(5446):1946-1949.

85. Oka S, Matsumoto T, Kubo S, et al: Local administration of low-dose simvastatin-conjugated gelatin hydrogel for tendon-bone healing in anterior cruciate ligament reconstruction. *Tissue Eng Part A* 2013;19(9-10):1233-1243.

86. Flynn BC, Vernick WJ, Ellis JE: β-Blockade in the perioperative management of the patient with cardiac disease undergoing non-cardiac surgery. *Br J Anaesth* 2011;107(suppl 1):i3-i15.

87. Mangano DT, Layug EL, Wallace A, Tateo I; Multicenter Study of Perioperative Ischemia Research Group: Effect of atenolol on mortality and cardiovascular morbidity after noncardiac surgery. *N Engl J Med* 1996;335(23):1713-1720.

88. Ashton JN, Hatton KW, Flynn JD, Smith KM: Perioperative beta-blockade in patients undergoing noncardiac surgery. *Orthopedics* 2010;33(7):488-491.

89. Poldermans D, Schouten O, Bax J, Winkel TA: Reducing cardiac risk in non-cardiac surgery: Evidence from the DECREASE studies. *Eur Heart J Suppl* 2009;11(suppl A):A9-A14.

90. Devereaux PJ, Beattie WS, Choi PT, et al: How strong is the evidence for the use of perioperative beta blockers in non-cardiac surgery? Systematic review and meta-analysis of randomised controlled trials. *BMJ* 2005;331(7512):313-321.

91. POISE Study Group, Devereaux PJ, Yang H, et al: Effects of extended-release metoprolol succinate in patients undergoing non-cardiac surgery (POISE trial): A randomised controlled trial. *Lancet* 2008;371(9627):1839-1847.

92. Wijeysundera DN, Beattie WS, Wijeysundera HC, Yun L, Austin PC, Ko DT: Duration of preoperative β-blockade and outcomes after major elective noncardiac surgery. *Can J Cardiol* 2014;30(2):217-223.

93. Graham L: ACC/AHA Release Guidelines on Perioperative Cardiovascular Evaluation for Noncardiac Surgery. *Am Fam Physician* 2008;77(12):1748-1751.

94. Feringa HH, Bax JJ, Boersma E, et al: High-dose beta-blockers and tight heart rate control reduce myocardial ischemia and troponin T release in vascular surgery patients. *Circulation* 2006;114(1 suppl):I344-I349.

95. van Klei WA, Bryson GL, Yang H, Forster AJ: Effect of beta-blocker prescription on the incidence of postoperative myocardial infarction after hip and knee arthroplasty. *Anesthesiology* 2009;111(4):717-724.

Renal and Gastrointestinal Considerations in Patients Undergoing Elective Orthopaedic Surgery

Peter Pyrko, MD, PhD

Javad Parvizi, MD, FRCS

Abstract

To minimize perioperative complications after elective orthopaedic procedures, patients may undergo preoperative medical optimization, which includes an assessment of their renal function and gastrointestinal system. The gastrointestinal and renal systems are complex, and their proper optimization in the preoperative period can influence the success of any procedure. Several factors, including a thorough evaluation and screening, with particular emphasis on anemia and its renal and gastrointestinal causes; the management of medications that are metabolized by the liver and excreted by the kidneys; and careful attention to the patient's nutritional status, can prevent complications and reduce morbidity, mortality, and the cost of care after elective orthopaedic procedures.

Instr Course Lect 2016;65:487–496.

Elective orthopaedic surgery, such as total joint arthroplasty, alleviates pain and improves the quality of life for patients who have end-stage arthritis.[1] The overall rate of complications after orthopaedic procedures is low, and improvements in quality of life equal or surpass those realized after procedures such as coronary artery bypass graft or renal dialysis.[2] To reduce postoperative complications, patients typically are assessed for the presence of various conditions that could compromise the outcomes of elective procedures. Such assessment has been reported to reduce the rate of perioperative complications during and after elective orthopaedic surgery.[3] Patients are evaluated to identify modifiable risk factors that can be controlled and optimized before the elective procedure. It is important for surgeons to understand that some of the important renal and gastrointestinal (GI) conditions can be optimized before an elective procedure. Patients who have renal and GI conditions share numerous common complications, including anemia, increased perioperative blood loss as a result of platelet dysfunction, increased infection rates,[4,5] wound-related issues,[6] and the potential for fluid imbalance. Other complications are specific to each organ system. It is important to note that some patients who have severe renal and/or GI issues should not be subjected to elective orthopaedic procedures until these issues are resolved completely.

The authors of this chapter believe that all patients who undergo elective inpatient surgery—and those deemed at risk for renal or GI dysfunction who undergo more minor procedures—should be screened for anemia and renal dysfunction. Elderly patients older than 80 years should be screened for

Dr. Parvizi or an immediate family member serves as a paid consultant to CeramTec, ConvaTec, Medtronic, Smith & Nephew, TissueGene, and Zimmer; has stock or stock options held in CD Diagnostics, Hip Innovation Technology, and PRN; has received research or institutional support from 3M, Cempra, CeramTec, DePuy, the National Institutes of Health, the Orthopaedic Research and Education Foundation, Smith & Nephew, StelKast, Stryker, and Zimmer; and serves as a board member, owner, officer, or committee member of the Eastern Orthopaedic Association and the Muller Foundation. Neither Dr. Pyrko nor any immediate family member has received anything of value from or has stock or stock options held in a commercial company or institution related directly or indirectly to the subject of this chapter.

Table 1
Pricing of Common Laboratory Tests at the Institution of the Authors of this Chapter

Test	Price
Complete blood count with differential	$67
Basic metabolic panel	$381
PT/INR	$47
PTT	$76
Serum albumin	$50
Prealbumin	$184
Serum transferrin	$160

PT/INR = prothrombin time/international normalized ratio, PTT = partial thromboplastin time.

Table 2
Common Conditions That Affect Patients Who Have Renal Disease

Anemia resulting from reduced erythropoietin production

Deficiency of active vitamin D, leading to hypocalcemia, secondary hyperparathyroidism, hypophosphatemia, and renal osteodystrophy

Decreased acid and water secretion, leading to hypertension volume overload and edema (acidosis compounded by surgery) and cardiac and pulmonary overload

Hyperkalemia, leading to arrhythmia and other cardiac complications

Reduced renal clearance of some medications

Platelet dysfunction and increased risk of bleeding

Wound-related complications from delayed healing

Increased infection rates and mortality

Malnutrition from proteinuria or reduced production of albumin

Obtunded immunity caused by dysfunction of cell-mediated and humoral immune system

---

malnutrition, as should patients who have a body mass index (BMI) less than 18.5 kg/m^2 and greater than 35 kg/m^2. Understandably, the additional laboratory evaluation adds to cost. The pricing of common laboratory tests at the institution of the authors of this chapter is presented in **Table 1**.

Renal Considerations

Several issues negatively affect the outcomes of patients with renal conditions who undergo orthopaedic procedures. Awareness of these issues may enable optimization of these conditions before elective procedures. Any patient who has a new diagnosis of renal insufficiency or known renal dysfunction with a glomerular filtration rate (GFR) less than 50 should undergo further evaluation before elective orthopaedic surgery. **Table 2** lists common conditions that affect patients who have renal disease.

Renal insufficiency is classified based on the GFR: 60 to 89 is mild, 30 to 59 is moderate, 15 to 29 is severe, and less than 15 represents renal failure. Any level of kidney disease increases surgical risks. The authors of this chapter recommend that any elevation in creatinine and any reduction in GFR encountered during the preoperative laboratory evaluation be followed with additional workup by a specialist.

Anemia

The presence of anemia negatively affects the outcome of any surgical procedure, including orthopaedic procedures. In a recent study of 13,593 patients who underwent total joint arthroplasty, Viola et al[7] reported that patients with anemia had a higher rate of complications compared with patients without anemia (odds ratio, 2.11). The largest single complication was cardiovascular, which occurred in 26.5% of patients who had anemia compared with 11.8% of those without anemia. Genitourinary complications occurred in 3.9% of patients who had anemia compared with 0.9% of those without anemia. Patients with anemia had a fourfold increase in the rate of infection (4.5%) compared with those without anemia (1.12%). In addition, the length of hospital stay was substantially longer for patients who had anemia compared with those without anemia.

Patients with anemia should be assessed and their condition should be optimized before undergoing elective orthopaedic procedures. The increased complication rate in patients who have anemia may be multifactorial. Patients who have anemia are more likely to require allogeneic blood transfusion, with all its adverse consequences.[8] Anemia, as a result of renal disease, is the consequence of the underproduction of erythropoietin, which is the hormone that stimulates erythrocyte production.[9] In a diseased kidney, the underproduction of erythropoietin ensues, which is directly proportional to residual kidney function. Identification and treatment of preoperative anemia can help reduce mortality and associated complications such as infection.[10,11] Therefore, all patients who undergo elective orthopaedic procedures should have a complete blood count performed to detect anemia. Patients who have anemia should be evaluated and treated. The administration of hematinics, such as iron and vitamins, or erythropoietin should be considered, and all efforts should be made to return the hemoglobin level to normal before surgery.[12]

Vitamin D Metabolism

Human marrow stromal cells respond to 1α, 25-dihydroxyvitamin D during their conversion to osteoblasts and actively participate in vitamin D metabolism by converting 25-dihydroxyvitamin D_3 to 1α, $25(OH)_2D_3$. Chronic kidney disease (CKD) is linked to the impaired biosynthesis of 1α, $25(OH)_2D$.[13] The absence of the active form of vitamin D leads to hypocalcemia, secondary hyperparathyroidism, hypophosphatemia, and, as a result, renal osteodystrophy. Patients who have renal osteodystrophy may present with low bone quality as a result of osteomalacia. Although not easily correctable preoperatively, the low quality of bone must be recognized and should prompt a discussion with the patient about the increased risk of iatrogenic fractures and the difficulty in achieving bony fixation. Patients who have osteomalacia may require a modified surgical technique and implant selection to minimize the potential for complications. An increasing number of orthopaedic patients are at risk for vitamin D deficiency. Therefore, it may be reasonable to check vitamin D levels in patients who undergo complex orthopaedic procedures to ensure that vitamin D deficiency, if present, is corrected before surgery. Patients with vitamin D deficiency have a higher risk of fracture, impaired bone healing, and diminished neuromuscular function.[14] It also is crucial to continue vitamin D and calcium repletion in the postoperative period, based on the established guidelines.

Edema and Acidosis

A decrease in water and acid clearance leads to volume overload and edema in patients who have chronic renal disease. Edema in the extremity places patients who have chronic renal disease at risk for wound-healing complications and should be corrected preoperatively with the use of appropriate diuretics and dialysis, if possible.[15] Edema and volume overload also may lead to cardiac and pulmonary complications. A monitored setting may be required in the immediate postoperative period to closely monitor the cardiac and pulmonary statuses of patients who have renal issues. Because metabolic acidosis may be compounded by the insult of surgery, it should be corrected preoperatively by an experienced nephrologist.

Hyperkalemia

The accumulation of potassium occurs in patients who have chronic renal failure. The homeostasis of potassium is achieved via two mechanisms.[16] In the first mechanism, the kidneys are responsible for excreting excess potassium; this is a slow process that takes several hours. In patients who have renal failure, this process is obtunded. In response, the excretion of potassium by the gut is increased, but this increase is insufficient to maintain homeostasis in the presence of renal excretory insufficiency; thus, hyperkalemia ensues. The second mechanism involves an internal system that maintains potassium balance via intracellular shifts of potassium in response to hormonal stimulus; this is a rapid process that occurs in minutes. Of all potassium in the body, 98% is found intracellularly, and the remaining 2% is maintained in the extracellular space. This uneven distribution indicates that small shifts from the

intracellular space to the extracellular space can cause severe hyperkalemia, and that small shifts into the cells can easily correct profound hyperkalemia. The first process causes the increased serum potassium seen in CKD, and the second process is exploited for rapid correction and treatment. The ultimate treatment of hyperkalemia in patients who have chronic renal failure is dialysis and removal of potassium from the blood stream. Maintenance of normal potassium levels is crucial because hyperkalemia, if left untreated, can lead to cardiac complications, including arrhythmias and cardiac arrest.[17]

Renal Dosing of Medications

The kidneys metabolize and excrete several common medications used in orthopaedic surgery, and dosing must be adjusted based on creatinine clearance. Several medications should be avoided in patients who have CKD. The avoidance of anticoagulants that are secreted by the kidney, such as enoxaparin, is particularly important because these drugs may accumulate in the bloodstream and cause substantial postoperative bleeding.[18] Alternative anticoagulation must be used in patients who have CKD. Contrast material is nephrotoxic and should be avoided in patients who have CKD.[19] This may compel the surgeon to use imaging modalities that do not rely on the administration of contrast material. Many of the antibiotics administered intraoperatively and postoperatively also are nephrotoxic and should be avoided.[18] Narcotic medications can accumulate in patients who have CKD; therefore, doses should be adjusted and their effects monitored by an internist to avoid respiratory depression.[20] Common medications used in orthopaedic surgery that

Table 3

Common Medications That Require Renal Dosing Before Orthopaedic Surgery

Medication	Dosage
Enoxaparin	Severe renal disease: Administer different anticoagulant.
	CrCl <30 mL/min: Administer 30 mg q 24 h.
Cefazolin	CrCl 35–54 mL/min: Unchanged.
	CrCl 11–34 mL/min: Administer usual dose x 1, then decrease dose 50%.
	CrCl <10 mL/min: Administer usual dose x 1, then 50% q 18–24 h.
Vancomycin	CrCl 50–90 mL/min: Administer 15 mg/kg x 1, then usual dose q 12–24 h.
	CrCl 10–50 mL/min: Administer 15 mg/kg x 1, then usual dose q 24–96 h.
	CrCl <10 mL/min: Administer 15 mg/kg x 1, then usual dose q 4–7 d.
Morphine	CrCl 10–50 mL/min: Decrease dose 25%.
	CrCl <10 mL/min: Decrease dose 50%, monitor respiratory status.

CrCl = creatine clearance, q = every.

require renal dosing or avoidance are presented in **Table 3**.

Platelet Dysfunction and Increased Risk of Bleeding

Patients who have renal disease in general and those being treated with dialysis in particular are known to have platelet dysfunction. The mechanism of this phenomenon is typically linked to uremia or the damage of platelets during dialysis or may be secondary to the administration of anticoagulation medication during dialysis. A platelet count and the bleeding time may need to be assessed in patients who have CKD, particularly in those who have a prior history of excessive bleeding, before they undergo elective orthopaedic surgery.[21] Evidence has shown that a subpopulation of patients who have renal disease is resistant to the antiplatelet action of aspirin.[22]

Wound-Related Complications From Delayed Healing

The rate of wound complications is increased in patients with CKD who have edema, uremia, skin dryness, and rashes. A high association of CKD with

diabetes mellitus as well as the presence of peripheral vascular disease in conjunction with an increased susceptibility to infection also increase the rate of wound complications in patients who have CKD.[6,23] In addition, patients being treated with dialysis have been reported to have dermal angiopathy, a macrovascular disease that leads to delayed wound healing.[24] It is essential for surgeons to understand this phenomenon and discuss it with patients who have CKD and those being treated with dialysis to minimize wound complications. Preoperative optimization that focuses on reducing systemic edema and careful surgical technique with an emphasis on cautious soft-tissue manipulation and meticulous closure also are critical. The orthopaedic procedure may need to be canceled if these serious issues cannot be addressed.

Increased Infection and Mortality Rates

It is well established that patients with CKD have an increased risk of infection after elective orthopaedic surgery.[4,25-27] The direct cause of this phenomenon is not well understood

but is likely multifactorial. Patients with renal impairment have more associated comorbidities, which increase complications and mortality because of the underlying pathology. Patients being treated with dialysis may be subject to the entry of pathogens into the bloodstream, which can result in a subsequent infection. In addition, some patients who have CKD, especially those who have had a renal transplant, may be on immunosuppressive therapy. Because of these mechanisms and the direct effect of renal impairment, patients with CKD have an increased risk of complications and mortality.[26] Another important fact to consider is that patients being treated with renal dialysis are often carriers of methicillin-resistant *Staphylococcus aureus*;[28,29] therefore, antibiotic prophylaxis should be adjusted for patients being treated with dialysis to include methicillin-resistant *S aureus* coverage.

The presence of impaired renal function also has been correlated with an increased mortality rate.[27,30-32] This correlation is not surprising because cardiac and pulmonary complications develop in patients who have renal impairment and can be fatal. The higher rate of infection in these patients also increases the risk of mortality.

Acute Kidney Injury After Orthopaedic Surgery

Acute kidney injury (AKI) is a serious complication that leads to an increased risk for mortality after orthopaedic surgery. Despite advances in treatment, the mortality rate in patients with acute renal failure from all causes has remained at approximately 50% in the past 50 years.[33] It is critical for surgeons to identify patients who are at risk for AKI in the perioperative period to avoid this potentially fatal complication. In one study, the overall incidence of AKI after elective or emergent orthopaedic procedures was 8.9%.[34] The risk factors for AKI in the study were dehydration, a history of diabetes mellitus, preexisting kidney disease, perioperative shock, and the administration of NSAIDs or nephrotoxic antibiotics. The authors recommended a thorough preoperative evaluation and close postoperative monitoring for patients who have these risk factors. Jafari et al[35] evaluated 17,000 joint arthroplasties that were performed at their institution over a period of 7 years. The authors reported that the rate of AKI or acute renal injury (0.55%) was much smaller than the 8.9% cited earlier. The authors identified a high BMI, an elevated preoperative creatinine level, chronic obstructive pulmonary disease, congestive heart failure, hypertension, and underlying cardiac disease as risk factors for AKI or acute renal injury. In the study, renal impairment was correlated closely with a longer hospital stay as well as increased in-hospital and 1-year all-cause mortality. The authors recommended perioperative optimization for patients who had the risk factors that were established. In addition, patients with kidney and liver transplants have an increased risk of AKI after hip arthroplasty, and solid organ transplantation has been reported to be an independent risk factor for AKI.[36]

GI Considerations

Patients undergoing orthopaedic procedures may have underlying GI conditions that can affect the outcome of the surgical intervention. **Table 4** lists some of the common GI conditions that may affect patients who undergo elective orthopaedic surgery.

Malnutrition

Malnutrition is a serious preoperative risk factor for any patient, regardless of BMI, who undergoes elective orthopaedic surgery. Multiple studies have reported adverse outcomes in malnourished patients who underwent elective orthopaedic surgery.[37-39] A correlation exists between malnutrition, poor wound healing, and subsequent infection. In one study, 35% of patients with drainage who did not respond to irrigation and débridement were reported to be malnourished compared with 5% of patients in the group who responded to irrigation and débridement.[39] In an observational study, Huang et al[37] evaluated for the presence of malnutrition in more than 2,000 patients who underwent total joint arthroplasty. The authors reported that 8.5% of the patients were malnourished. The incidence of all complications, including hematoma formation, infection, and renal and cardiac events, was substantially higher in patients who were malnourished compared with patients who were not malnourished (12% versus 3.9%, respectively). Surprisingly, obesity, which is defined as a BMI greater than 30 kg/m^2, was present in more than 40% of malnourished patients; this underscores the need for nutritional screening in patients who are obese. In fact, some authors define malnutrition as not only the deficiency of nutrients but also an excess of nutrients, which is the case in patients who are obese.[38] Obesity in itself is associated with multiple intraoperative and postoperative complications, including increased surgical times, persistent wound drainage, and infection, which may lead to local wound complications.[40]

Malnutrition is rarely obvious clinically and should be screened for in

Table 4

Gastrointestinal Conditions That Affect Elective Orthopaedic Surgery

Malnutrition

Metabolic syndrome (eg, obesity, hypertension, dyslipidemia, and diabetes mellitus)

Chronic liver disease and cirrhosis

Alcohol consumption

Viral hepatitis

Dose adjustment of medications metabolized by the liver

Inflammatory bowel disease

Ileus

Anemia resulting from poor nutrition or acute gastrointestinal blood loss

at-risk populations, including those older than 80 years and those who have a BMI greater than 35 kg/m^2. The most common screening tests are the serum total lymphocyte count, which is positive for malnutrition if less than 1,500 cells are present per cubic millimeter, and the serum albumin concentration, which is positive for malnutrition if the concentration is less than 3.5 g/dL. Prealbumin and transferrin tests also are used. Anthropomorphic measurements, including body composition measurements such as calf muscle circumference (<31 cm) and arm muscle circumference (<22 mm), can indicate malnutrition; however, these measurements better reflect a patient's long-term nutritional status and underestimate acute nutritional changes. Various nutritional scoring tools, such as the Mini Nutritional Assessment, also have been proposed.[38]

Perioperative Considerations in Patients Who Have Liver Disease

Many patients who have liver disease are asymptomatic; hence, the condition may go undetected. Therefore, vigilant screening of patients via a careful history and physical examination is recommended to detect potential risk factors for liver disease. For patients in whom active liver disease is newly discovered, it is recommended that elective surgery be postponed until the underlying cause of the liver disease can be determined, eliminated, or treated. Cirrhosis of the liver leads to hyperdynamic circulation, with increased cardiac output and decreased peripheral vascular resistance. Pulmonary hypertension, ascites, and bleeding varices often are present. Because of these issues, perioperative morbidity and mortality are greatly increased in patients who have cirrhosis of the liver.[41] Liver cirrhosis also is associated with increased rates of periprosthetic joint infections, prolonged hospital stay, discharge to a nursing facility, readmission, urinary tract infection, renal failure, blood transfusion, intestinal hemorrhage, dislocation, and revision surgery.[42,43] Acute liver failure, active viral hepatitis, alcoholic hepatitis, cardiomyopathy, hypoxemia, and coagulopathy recalcitrant to treatment are considered contraindications to elective surgery.

In patients who have liver disease, coagulopathy is caused by the decreased production of clotting factors secondary to reduced liver synthetic function or depletion of vitamin K stores. Liver disease also causes mild disseminated intravascular coagulation, which may lead to thrombocytopenia. Other causes of thrombocytopenia include the splenic sequestration of platelets and alcohol-induced bone marrow suppression.

To ensure improved outcomes of orthopaedic procedures, patients who have liver disease should be optimized in collaboration with an internist. A risk assessment of patients with liver disease who undergo elective surgery can be performed using established risk assessment tools such as the Model for End-stage Liver Disease and the Child-Pugh score.

Alcohol Consumption

Excessive alcohol consumption (>40 units per week, which is equal to 400 g of pure alcohol) is associated with an increased risk of infectious and noninfectious postoperative complications.[44] Alcohol induces enzymatic liver activity, which may lead to an increased need for anesthetic agents and the decreased efficacy of other medications because of enhanced breakdown. At least 4 weeks of alcohol abstinence has been suggested as necessary to reverse the pathophysiologic changes that increase the risk of postoperative morbidity and mortality in patients with excessive alcohol consumption.[45]

Viral Hepatitis

As discussed earlier, acute viral hepatitis is a contraindication to elective surgery. Chronic hepatitis is associated with an increased risk of perioperative complications.[46,47] To the knowledge of the authors of this chapter, no official medical optimization guidelines are available for patients who have chronic hepatitis. In one study, patients with chronic hepatitis C were reported to have a higher risk of infection and bleeding.[48] In recent years, immunotherapy has gained attention for the treatment of patients who have hepatitis; some agents propose to "cure" the condition. Therefore, it is important that a patient who has hepatitis be referred to a hepatologist for possible treatment and medical optimization prior to any elective orthopaedic procedures.

Medication Dosing in Liver Disease

Liver disease can lead to an increased duration of action for certain drugs because of reduced liver metabolic activity and lower than normal serum levels of albumin. It also can lead to a decreased duration of action secondary to an increased volume of distribution because of ascites. It is important for surgeons to follow each drug's dosing guidelines in patients who have liver disease to avoid overdosing. In particular, care must be taken to minimize the use of benzodiazepines and opioids in patients who have liver disease.

Inflammatory Bowel Disease

Chronic inflammatory bowel disease (CIBD), including Crohn disease and ulcerative colitis, may present a variety of problems in the perioperative period, including increased rates of thromboembolic events.[49] Anemia is common in patients who have CIBD for a variety of reasons, including the increased incidence of intestinal bleeding, the reduced absorption of hematinics and nutrients through the small bowel, and the state of chronic disease. Patients with CIBD have been reported to be more susceptible to infections and poor wound healing,[50] which may be secondary to the autoimmune nature of the disease or to the administration of immunosuppressive medications used for its treatment. Many of the medications used for the treatment of CIBD are the same disease-modifying antirheumatic drugs (DMARDs) used in the management of inflammatory arthropathies.[51] Although the optimal management of patients who are being treated with DMARDs is currently unknown, the association between the increased risk of infection and the severity of infection, if it occurs, led the attendees of the International Consensus Meeting on Periprosthetic Joint Infection to recommend that DMARDs be discontinued before elective arthroplasty[52] (**Table 5**).

Ileus Prevention

Postoperative ileus, which is defined as the cessation of bowel motility, is common after orthopaedic procedures, particularly after spine surgery. Ileus manifests as the delayed passage of flatus and stool as well as increased abdominal distention. Ileus likely results from a sympathetic stress response to surgery, the effect of endogenous and administered opioids on bowel movement, immobility, prolonged recumbent positioning, and bowel manipulation in transabdominal spine surgery. Ileus also may be associated with hypokalemia. Postoperative ileus has been linked to reduced postoperative intake, prolonged hospital stays, patient discomfort, increased pain, pulmonary complications, delayed wound healing, and an increased cost of surgery.[53] Therefore, the focus should be on the prevention of ileus via the early ambulation of patients whenever possible, the administration of medications to increase GI mobility, the minimization of opioid use for pain control, and well-balanced nutrition.

Anemia and GI Bleeding

Anemia that results from GI disorders is of particular importance because it often is correctable and has the potential to make the treatment of other forms of anemia ineffective if not corrected.[53] In addition to the causes previously discussed, anemia can result from insufficient absorption of iron or other nutrients that are important in red

Table 5
Recommended Preoperative Cessation of Chronic Inflammatory Bowel Disease Medications

Medication	Half-Life	Recommended Discontinuation Before Surgery
Methotrexate	0.7–5.8 h	1 wk prior
Azathioprine	7.6 h	Before 1 wk prior
Infliximab	8–10 d	3 wk prior
Adalimumab	12–14 d	1 mo prior
Certolizumab	12–14 d	1 mo prior
Glucocorticoids	12–48 h	Administer stress dose in OR

OR = operating room.

blood cell turnover and regeneration. Malabsorption issues are corrected easily by treating bowel inflammation or with the supplemental administration of iron and folic acid. In addition, it is important for surgeons to recognize iron deficiency anemia in conjunction with other causes of anemia because erythropoietin treatment may be less effective in the presence of an iron deficiency, and coadministration of iron may be required.[54]

GI bleeding is another common cause of anemia, especially in elderly patients. It is important to screen for gastroesophageal reflux disease and inquire about its symptoms in patients who have anemia. The stress of surgery can exacerbate the symptoms of gastroesophageal reflux disease and cause intestinal bleeding. Appropriate preoperative treatment and perioperative prophylaxis are recommended. A stool guaiac test can detect the presence of blood in the stool. This test can be performed easily during preoperative clearance of a patient who has anemia.

Summary

A thorough evaluation and screening—with the objective of identifying and optimizing renal and GI conditions,

such as anemia, malnutrition, and alcohol abuse—are vital to improve the outcomes of patients who undergo elective orthopaedic procedures.

References

1. Charnley J: The long-term results of low-friction arthroplasty of the hip performed as a primary intervention: 1972. *Clin Orthop Relat Res* 1995;319:4-15.

2. Lavernia CJ, Guzman JF, Gachupin-Garcia A: Cost effectiveness and quality of life in knee arthroplasty. *Clin Orthop Relat Res* 1997;345:134-139.

3. Radcliff KE, Orozco FR, Quinones D, Rhoades D, Sidhu GS, Ong AC: Preoperative risk stratification reduces the incidence of perioperative complications after total knee arthroplasty. *J Arthroplasty* 2012;27(8, suppl): 77-80.e8.

4. Poultsides LA, Ma Y, Della Valle AG, Chiu YL, Sculco TP, Memtsoudis SG: In-hospital surgical site infections after primary hip and knee arthroplasty: Incidence and risk factors. *J Arthroplasty* 2013;28(3):385-389.

5. Bozic KJ, Ong K, Lau E, et al: Estimating risk in Medicare patients with THA: An electronic risk calculator for periprosthetic joint infection and mortality. *Clin Orthop Relat Res* 2013;471(2):574-583.

6. Jones RE, Russell RD, Huo MH: Wound healing in total joint replacement. *Bone Joint J* 2013; 95(11, suppl A):144-147.

7. Viola J, Gomez MM, Restrepo C, Maltenfort MG, Parvizi J: Preoperative anemia increases postoperative complications and mortality following total joint arthroplasty. *J Arthroplasty* 2015;30(5):846-848.

8. Augustin ID, Yeoh TY, Sprung J, Berry DJ, Schroeder DR, Weingarten TN: Association between chronic kidney disease and blood transfusions for knee and hip arthroplasty surgery. *J Arthroplasty* 2013;28(6):928-931.

9. McClellan W, Aronoff SL, Bolton WK, et al: The prevalence of anemia in patients with chronic kidney disease. *Curr Med Res Opin* 2004;20(9):1501-1510.

10. Eschbach JW, Egrie JC, Downing MR, Browne JK, Adamson JW: Correction of the anemia of end-stage renal disease with recombinant human erythropoietin: Results of a combined phase I and II clinical trial. *N Engl J Med* 1987;316(2):73-78.

11. Rosencher N, Poisson D, Albi A, Aperce M, Barré J, Samama CM: Two injections of erythropoietin correct moderate anemia in most patients awaiting orthopedic surgery. *Can J Anaesth* 2005;52(2):160-165.

12. Goodnough LT, Maniatis A, Earnshaw P, et al: Detection, evaluation, and management of preoperative anaemia in the elective orthopaedic surgical patient: NATA guidelines. *Br J Anaesth* 2011;106(1):13-22.

13. Zhou S, Leboff MS, Waikar SS, Glowacki J: Vitamin D metabolism and action in human marrow stromal cells: Effects of chronic kidney disease. *J Steroid Biochem Mol Biol* 2013;136:342-344.

14. Patton CM, Powell AP, Patel AA: Vitamin D in orthopaedics. *J Am Acad Orthop Surg* 2012;20(3):123-129.

15. Carrasco LR, Chou JC: Perioperative management of patients with renal disease. *Oral Maxillofac Surg Clin North Am* 2006;18(2):203-212, vi.

16. Allon M: Hyperkalemia in end-stage renal disease: Mechanisms and management. *J Am Soc Nephrol* 1995;6(4):1134-1142.

17. Shingarev R, Allon M: A physiologic-based approach to the treatment of acute hyperkalemia. *Am J Kidney Dis* 2010;56(3):578-584.

18. Hartmann B, Czock D, Keller F: Drug therapy in patients with chronic renal failure. *Dtsch Arztebl Int* 2010;107(37):647-656.

19. Rudnick MR, Berns JS, Cohen RM, Goldfarb S: Contrast media-associated nephrotoxicity. *Semin Nephrol* 1997;17(1):15-26.

20. Kurella M, Bennett WM, Chertow GM: Analgesia in patients with ESRD: A review of available evidence. *Am J Kidney Dis* 2003;42(2):217-228.

21. Dorgalaleh A, Mahmudi M, Tabibian S, et al: Anemia and thrombocytopenia in acute and chronic renal failure. *Int J Hematol Oncol Stem Cell Res* 2013;7(4):34-39.

22. Kilickesmez KO, Kocas C, Abaci O, Okcun B, Gorcin B, Gurmen T: Follow-up of aspirin-resistant patients with end-stage kidney disease. *Int Urol Nephrol* 2013;45(4):1097-1102.

23. Seth AK, De la Garza M, Fang RC, Hong SJ, Galiano RD: Excisional wound healing is delayed in a murine model of chronic kidney disease. *PLoS One* 2013;8(3):e59979.

24. Lundin AP, Fani K, Berlyne GM, Friedman EA: Dermal angiopathy in hemodialysis patients: The effect of time. *Kidney Int* 1995;47(6):1775-1780.

25. Deegan BF, Richard RD, Bowen TR, Perkins RM, Graham JH, Foltzer MA: Impact of chronic kidney disease stage on lower-extremity arthroplasty. *Orthopedics* 2014;37(7):e613-e618.

26. McCleery MA, Leach WJ, Norwood T: Rates of infection and revision in patients with renal disease undergoing total knee replacement in Scotland. *J Bone Joint Surg Br* 2010;92(11):1535-1539.

27. Miric A, Inacio MC, Namba RS: Can total knee arthroplasty be safely performed in patients with chronic renal disease? *Acta Orthop* 2014;85(1):71-78.

28. Schmid H, Romanos A, Schiffl H, Lederer SR: Persistent nasal methicillin-resistant staphylococcus aureus carriage in hemodialysis outpatients: A predictor of worse outcome. *BMC Nephrol* 2013;14:93.

29. Otter JA, French GL: Nosocomial transmission of community-associated methicillin-resistant Staphylococcus aureus: An emerging threat. *Lancet Infect Dis* 2006;6(12):753-755.

30. Miric A, Inacio MC, Namba RS: The effect of chronic kidney disease on total hip arthroplasty. *J Arthroplasty* 2014;29(6):1225-1230.

31. Aynardi M, Jacovides CL, Huang R, Mortazavi SM, Parvizi J: Risk factors for early mortality following modern total hip arthroplasty. *J Arthroplasty* 2013;28(3):517-520.

32. Bozic KJ, Lau E, Kurtz S, et al: Patient-related risk factors for periprosthetic joint infection and postoperative mortality following total hip arthroplasty in Medicare patients. *J Bone Joint Surg Am* 2012;94(9):794-800.

33. Ympa YP, Sakr Y, Reinhart K, Vincent JL: Has mortality from acute renal failure decreased? A systematic review of the literature. *Am J Med* 2005;118(8):827-832.

34. Kateros K, Doulgerakis C, Galanakos SP, Sakellariou VI, Papadakis SA, Macheras GA: Analysis of kidney dysfunction in orthopaedic patients. *BMC Nephrol* 2012;13:101.

35. Jafari SM, Huang R, Joshi A, Parvizi J, Hozack WJ: Renal impairment following total joint arthroplasty: Who is at risk? *J Arthroplasty* 2010; 25(6, suppl):49-53.e2.

36. Choi YJ, Lee EH, Hahm KD, Kwon K, Ro YJ: Transplantation is a risk factor for acute kidney injury in patients undergoing total hip replacement arthroplasty for avascular necrosis: An observational study. *Transplant Proc* 2013;45(6):2220-2225.

37. Huang R, Greenky M, Kerr GJ, Austin MS, Parvizi J: The effect of malnutrition on patients undergoing elective joint arthroplasty. *J Arthroplasty* 2013;28(8, suppl):21-24.

38. Cross MB, Yi PH, Thomas CF, Garcia J, Della Valle CJ: Evaluation of malnutrition in orthopaedic surgery. *J Am Acad Orthop Surg* 2014;22(3):193-199.

39. Jaberi FM, Parvizi J, Haytmanek CT, Joshi A, Purtill J: Procrastination of wound drainage and

malnutrition affect the outcome of joint arthroplasty. *Clin Orthop Relat Res* 2008;466(6):1368-1371.

40. Liabaud B, Patrick DA Jr, Geller JA: Higher body mass index leads to longer operative time in total knee arthroplasty. *J Arthroplasty* 2013;28(4):563-565.

41. Bhangui P, Laurent A, Amathieu R, Azoulay D: Assessment of risk for non-hepatic surgery in cirrhotic patients. *J Hepatol* 2012;57(4):874-884.

42. Tiberi JV III, Hansen V, El-Abbadi N, Bedair H: Increased complication rates after hip and knee arthroplasty in patients with cirrhosis of the liver. *Clin Orthop Relat Res* 2014;472(9):2774-2778.

43. Jiang SL, Schairer WW, Bozic KJ: Increased rates of periprosthetic joint infection in patients with cirrhosis undergoing total joint arthroplasty. *Clin Orthop Relat Res* 2014;472(8):2483-2491.

44. Bradley KA, Rubinsky AD, Sun H, et al: Alcohol screening and risk of postoperative complications in male VA patients undergoing major non-cardiac surgery. *J Gen Intern Med* 2011;26(2):162-169.

45. Tonnesen H, Rosenberg J, Nielsen HJ, et al: Effect of preoperative abstinence on poor postoperative outcome in alcohol misusers: Randomised controlled trial. *BMJ* 1999;318(7194):1311-1316.

46. Orozco F, Post ZD, Baxi O, Miller A, Ong A: Fibrosis in hepatitis C patients predicts complications after elective total joint arthroplasty. *J Arthroplasty* 2014;29(1):7-10.

47. Best MJ, Buller LT, Klika AK, Barsoum WK: Increase in perioperative complications following primary total hip and knee arthroplasty in patients with hepatitis C without cirrhosis. *J Arthroplasty* 2015;30(4):663-668.

48. Pour AE, Matar WY, Jafari SM, Purtill JJ, Austin MS, Parvizi J: Total joint arthroplasty in patients with hepatitis C. *J Bone Joint Surg Am* 2011;93(15):1448-1454.

49. Kumar A, Auron M, Aneja A, Mohr F, Jain A, Shen B: Inflammatory bowel disease: Perioperative pharmacological considerations. *Mayo Clin Proc* 2011;86(8):748-757.

50. Sholter DE, Armstrong PW: Adverse effects of corticosteroids on the cardiovascular system. *Can J Cardiol* 2000;16(4):505-511.

51. Scanzello CR, Figgie MP, Nestor BJ, Goodman SM: Perioperative management of medications used in the treatment of rheumatoid arthritis. *HSS J* 2006;2(2):141-147.

52. Parvizi J, Gehrke T, Chen AF: Proceedings of the International Consensus on Periprosthetic Joint Infection. *Bone Joint J* 2013;95(11):1450-1452.

53. Thompson M, Magnuson B: Management of postoperative ileus. *Orthopedics* 2012;35(3):213-217.

54. Auerbach M, Ballard H, Trout JR, et al: Intravenous iron optimizes the response to recombinant human erythropoietin in cancer patients with chemotherapy-related anemia: A multicenter, open-label, randomized trial. *J Clin Oncol* 2004;22(7):1301-1307.

37

Perioperative Treatment of Patients With Rheumatoid Arthritis

Khaled J. Saleh, BSc, MD, MSc, FRCS(C), MHCM
Alexander Kurdi, BSc
Mouhanad M. El-Othmani, MD
Benjamin Voss, BS
Tony H. Tzeng, BS
Jasmine Saleh, MD
J.M. Lane, MD
William M. Mihalko, MD, PhD

Abstract

Rheumatoid arthritis is an autoimmune disease mediated by a widespread, chronic, and systematic inflammatory process that causes joint deterioration, which leads to pain, disability, and poor quality of life. The increased use of disease-modifying antirheumatic drugs has been shown to markedly slow disease progression, which has translated into a decrease in the need for orthopaedic intervention in this population. However, in a substantial percentage of patients with the disease, optimal pharmacologic treatment fails and surgical intervention is required. A thorough understanding of medical considerations in these patients and improved knowledge of the medical complications caused by the disease process and the pharmacologic therapy used to treat it may lead to improved preoperative planning and medical clearance, which may ultimately improve the overall postoperative outcome.

Instr Course Lect 2016;65:497–508.

Rheumatoid arthritis (RA) is a chronic systemic inflammatory disease characterized by joint deterioration that leads to pain, disability, systemic complications, poor quality of life, and a shortened life span. Improved knowledge of the medical complications caused by the disease and the pharmacologic therapy that these patients receive may result in improved overall surgical outcomes.[1-4] RA is the most common inflammatory arthritis, with an estimated incidence of 20 to 50 cases per 100,000 persons in North America and Northern Europe.[3,5-7] Inflammation primarily affects the synovial membrane of joints, but it also affects other organ systems.[8] The most notable extra-articular features of RA include cardiovascular disease (CVD),[9-11] rheumatoid nodules, interstitial lung disease, and an increased infection rate; all of these features play a major role in increasing the mortality rate (up to threefold) in patients who have RA.[4,8,12] Assessment of medical comorbidities associated with both the disease process and the treatment of RA is an important part of the patient evaluation for medical clearance before orthopaedic surgery.

The introduction of disease-modifying antirheumatic drugs (DMARDs) has drastically improved patient survival and has led to a decreased number of patients who require orthopaedic intervention.[13-15] In addition, the widespread use of other immunosuppressive drugs, such as glucocorticoids and NSAIDs, has played a considerable role in improving the quality of life in patients who have RA.[13-15] However, despite optimal medical treatment, some patients still exhibit progressive destruction of the joints that requires surgical intervention.[16] Although suppressing immune function is essential for the treatment of RA, the increased risk of postoperative complications is considerable in some patients.[17] At the time of total knee arthroplasty (TKA), patients with joint destruction secondary to RA tend to be approximately 10 years younger than other orthopaedic populations, such as those with osteoarthritis (OA).[18,19] The limited life span of the implant is a critical implication and consideration for these patients. Although patients with RA may have lower activity levels, prostheses with longer survivorship are essential because these patients receive the implant at a younger age, have poorer bone quality, and are predisposed to infection because of the immunosuppressive treatment regimen. These factors potentially increase the surgical revision rate secondary to loosening, polyethylene wear, and periprosthetic joint infection.[19] Thus, with the inherent increase in comorbidities and surgical complications, orthopaedic surgeons must consider the medical conditions that accompany RA because they may add serious risk factors that can affect the postoperative outcome. Surgeons should be aware of specific considerations in the perioperative medical management and clearance of patients with RA to optimize surgical outcomes.

Timing, Surgical Sequence, and Intervention

Optimal timing for surgical intervention has been a subject of debate among rheumatologists and orthopaedic surgeons.[20] However, because of the progressive joint erosion and destruction associated with RA, it may be better to introduce orthopaedic intervention earlier in the disease process because later stages of joint damage may limit treatment options.[21] Studies have shown that postoperative functional results are highly correlated with preoperative function in patients with RA who undergo total hip arthroplasty (THA) or TKA.[22] In addition, postponement of surgical intervention increases the patients' risk of complications.[22] This suggests that an earlier orthopaedic consultation or intervention may lead to improved outcomes in patients who have RA.[20,22]

The appropriate sequence of surgical intervention for patients with RA who have multiple joint involvement may be challenging. The primary goal of surgical intervention is to help patients sustain a satisfactory quality of life. This may be better accomplished by performing lower extremity procedures before upper extremity procedures to preserve the patient's ambulatory capacity.[23-25] The upper extremities, when repaired first, may be at risk of damage during the rehabilitation process after lower extremity procedures.[23-25] If the use of a walker or cane is too painful for the patient secondary to joint involvement in the upper extremities, it may be beneficial to proceed with upper extremity procedures, postponing the intervention on the lower extremities until the patient is able to tolerate rehabilitation with these devices.[25]

The sequence of surgical intervention for the lower limb is forefoot, hip, knee, hindfoot, and ankle.[23] Procedures are combined whenever possible to minimize the number of surgeries and hospital stays.[25] Forefoot procedures are typically performed first because they provide symptomatic relief and lower the risk of ulcer and infection without any adverse risk to future total joint arthroplasties.[26] If both THA and TKA are indicated, it is ideal to perform the THA first to ensure proper femoral length and alignment of the knees and to aid postoperative rehabilitation.[23] THA provides increased range

Dr. K. Saleh or an immediate family member has received royalties from and is a member of a speakers' bureau or has made paid presentations on behalf of Aesculap/B. Braun; is an employee of Southern Illinois University School of Medicine; serves as a paid consultant to Aesculap/B. Braun, Memorial Medical Center, and Watermark Research Partners; has received research or institutional support from Smith & Nephew, the Orthopaedic Research and Education Foundation, and the National Institute of Arthritis and Musculoskeletal and Skin Diseases; and serves as a board member, owner, officer, or committee member of the American Academy of Orthopaedic Surgeons, the American Orthopaedic Association, the Orthopaedic Research and Education Foundation, the American Board of Orthopaedic Surgeons, the Board of Specialty Societies, and Notify. Dr. Lane or an immediate family member serves as a paid consultant to Bone Therapeutics, CollPlant, Graftys, Harvest, ISTO Technologies, and BiologicsMD; has stock or stock options held in Dfine and CollPlant; has received research or institutional support from Merck; and serves as a board member, owner, officer, or committee member of the American Academy of Orthopaedic Surgeons, the Orthopaedic Research Society, the Musculoskeletal Tumor Society, the Association of Bone and Joint Surgeons, the American Osteopathic Association, and the American Society for Bone and Mineral Research. Dr. Mihalko or an immediate family member has received royalties from and is a member of a speakers' bureau or has made paid presentations on behalf of Aesculap/B. Braun; serves as a paid consultant to Aesculap/B. Braun, Medtronic, and Panoramic Healthcare Communications; has received research or institutional support from Aesculap/B. Braun, MicroPort, Smith & Nephew, and Stryker; and serves as a board member, owner, officer, or committee member of the American Board of Orthopaedic Surgery, the American Orthopaedic Association, and ASTM International. None of the following authors or any immediate family member has received anything of value from or has stock or stock options held in a commercial company or institution related directly or indirectly to the subject of this chapter: Mr. Kurdi, Dr. El-Othmani, Mr. Voss, Mr. Tzeng, and Dr. J. Saleh.

of motion at the hip joint, allowing optimal knee flexion, which is beneficial for TKA recovery.[23] Performing bilateral TKA or THA, especially in patients with flexion contractures, allows for the straightening of both lower extremities and supports the rehabilitation process.[25]

It may be preferable to perform hindfoot procedures first in some scenarios (eg, cases of fixed varus, valgus, or equinus deformities) if abnormal forces may be placed on a knee arthroplasty.[25] In the setting of a flexible foot deformity, such as a posterior tibial tendon rupture, a TKA may be performed before intervention on the foot.[25] In a valgus knee, there is increased risk of recurrent foot deformity if the hindfoot is repaired first; thus, the procedure at the knee should precede the intervention on the foot.[25,27,28]

Surgical interventions on the hands and wrists also are important treatment options that can substantially improve the quality of life in patients who have RA. Hand procedures (eg, nerve decompression, synovectomy for synovitis or impending tendon rupture, and flexor tendon reconstruction to provide enhanced grip and incentive to use the hand) typically start at the level of the soft tissue to provide short-term functional relief.[23,29-32] This is followed by bone procedures, including fusion of the wrist, interphalangeal joints of the fingers, and the interphalangeal and metacarpophalangeal joints of the thumb.[23,30-32] With the wrist stabilized, attention can shift to the elbow, followed by the shoulder. The rationale behind this sequence can be explained by the increased functionality provided by elbow arthroplasty compared with that provided by shoulder arthroplasty.[30,33,34] The shoulder may be treated

before the elbow in patients who have decreased shoulder rotation, thus minimizing abnormal levels of stress on the elbow joint.[35]

Preoperative Assessment

Patients who have RA present with more comorbidities than does the average patient. Because of the chronic systemic inflammation, these patients are at increased risk of cardiovascular problems, such as venous thromboembolism (VTE),[36] atherosclerosis, myocardial infarction, congestive heart failure, and stroke.[37-39] Research has shown that the risk of mortality associated with CVD in patients with RA is approximately 50% higher than the risk in the general population.[39]

Although cardiovascular conditions receive the most attention, pulmonary concerns are often overlooked. Approximately 10% to 20% of RA-associated deaths are secondary to pulmonary complications.[40-43] The airway, parenchyma, vasculature, and the pleura of the lungs may be affected, leading to interstitial lung disease, a deadly lung condition associated with RA.[43] In patients with these complications, consultation with a pulmonologist is advised for clearance because no consensus guideline exists for perioperative management.[44]

Cervical spine involvement in patients who have RA is common and progressive and may potentially become devastating.[45] In a study of 113 patients with RA who underwent THA or TKA, 69 (61%) had cervical spine instability.[46] Because intubation requires hyperextension of the neck, it is important to perform a preoperative radiographic assessment of the range of motion at the cervical spine for all patients who undergo major surgery.[46-48] In patients

who have cervical spine instability, TKA and THA are best performed under regional anesthesia, but fiberoptic intubation should be used if general anesthesia is required.[25] MRI should be used if abnormalities are found on the screening radiographs or if neurologic impairment is noted.[49] Patients with RA have an elevated risk of subaxial instability and basilar invagination, and 80% of patients have atlantoaxial instability.[24,46] Although surgical intervention on the spine is not commonly required, if instability is present, early and aggressive surgical intervention may be used to prevent further deterioration or neurologic injuries.[45]

Perioperative Pharmacologic Management
Disease-modifying Antirheumatic Drugs
A wide range of immunosuppressive medications are available to manage and treat RA and other chronic inflammatory diseases. DMARDs used to manage RA include methotrexate (MTX), leflunomide, azathioprine, hydroxychloroquine, and biologic response modifiers that inhibit tumor necrosis factor (TNF)-α and interleukin (IL)-1 (eg, etanercept, adalimumab).[15] These drugs are often stopped one drug half-life before surgery to reduce infection, which may result in the added risk of increased perioperative flares that may hinder rehabilitation. Typically, the drugs are restarted after healing has occurred, at approximately 2 weeks postoperatively.[25]

The most commonly used DMARD for first-line treatment of RA is MTX, a cytotoxic drug that is commonly prescribed to improve symptoms and reduce the progression of joint destruction.[50] MTX works through the inhibition of dihydrofolate reductase as well as through other enzymes that inhibit cytokine production, increasing the release of extracellular adenosine, blocking lymphocyte and monocyte proliferation, and promoting cell apoptosis.[51] MTX has been shown to inhibit the expression of receptor activator of nuclear factor ϰ-B ligand, thus preventing osteoclast formation.[52]

Studies have shown that patients with RA who underwent elective orthopaedic surgery showed no short-term increases in infection risk or surgical complications if MTX treatment was continued through the procedure.[53-55] However, inflammatory flare-ups were observed in those who discontinued MTX treatment perioperatively.[53] In a study of long-term results in patients with RA who were being treated with MTX at the time they underwent elective orthopaedic surgery, no long-term complications associated with the perioperative continuation of MTX were reported at a 10-year follow-up.[56] This suggests that, for patients with disease controlled by MTX, treatment should not be discontinued before the surgical procedure.[53,56]

Treatment of RA with MTX should be approached with caution in cases of delayed healing or nonunion of fractures. Although some studies found that MTX caused no suppression of osteoblast function or bone formation,[57,58] others noted a suppression in bone formation when osteoblastic differentiation was inhibited.[59,60] Caution also should be exercised in elderly patients and in patients with comorbidities (eg, renal or hepatic insufficiency) that affect the drug's metabolism because the buildup of metabolites may lead to MTX toxicity.[55] In this population, MTX should be withheld

1 week preoperatively and at least 1 to 2 weeks postoperatively.[48,61,62] Withholding MTX any longer may increase the risk of flare-ups, which are typically seen at approximately 4 weeks without MTX.[53,63]

Leflunomide inhibits pyrimidine synthesis.[64] Compared with patients being treated with MTX, patients being treated with leflunomide monotherapy have a substantially increased risk of surgical wound infection.[65] As a result, discontinuation of leflunomide 1 to 2 days before the procedure is recommended, with cholestyramine used to rapidly reduce blood levels of the active metabolite.[15,65] Leflunomide may be reinstated 1 to 2 weeks postoperatively, after the wound has healed, the patient is stable, minimal narcotic pain medication is required, and antibiotic therapy has been discontinued.[15]

TNF-α, a macrophage-derived cytokine, mediates inflammation and subsequent joint destruction in patients who have RA, making this cytokine an attractive target for pharmacotherapy.[66,67] TNF-α inhibitors, such as infliximab, etanercept, and adalimumab, are effective in controlling the disease,[68,69] reducing the number of patients who reach end-stage joint destruction.[13,70] However, because of the role that TNF-α plays in the immune response through the apoptosis of infected cells and the destruction of intracellular organisms, patients being treated with TNF-α inhibitors have an increased risk of serious, opportunistic infections.[71-76]

Since the introduction of TNF-α inhibitors, there has been an influx in the literature investigating their safety and efficacy in surgical patients. Several studies have reported conflicting results on the risk of infection in patients being treated with TNF-α

inhibitor therapy.[71,73,77-79] In a recent retrospective study of 50,359 orthopaedic patients, including 1,329 patients with RA, 878 patients were being treated with DMARDs or TNF-α inhibitors before they underwent orthopaedic procedures.[80] The authors noted that patients who were being treated with TNF-α inhibitors with or without other conventional DMARDs had a tenfold increase in the rate of infection if the drug was given within one administration interval (ie, 3.5 days for etanercept 25 mg, 7 days for etanercept 50 mg, 14 days for adalimumab 40 mg, 56 days for infliximab 3 to 5 mg/kg of body weight) before the procedure.[80] These findings were consistent with those of a meta-analysis that showed that patients being treated with TNF-α inhibitor therapy had a substantial increase in the rate of serious infection, even after adjusting for other predictive factors, such as disease severity and patient age.[71]

Because of the increased rates of infection and negative outcomes related to the use of TNF-α inhibitors, the Club Rhumatismes et Inflammation presented guidelines that clarify preoperative administration of TNF-α based on pharmacologic properties.[81] The three types of TNF-α inhibitors commonly used in the United States (etanercept, adalimumab, and infliximab) follow different algorithms. The Club Rhumatismes et Inflammation recommends that patients being treated with etanercept discontinue the medication at least 1 week before surgery, and those being treated with adalimumab or infliximab should discontinue the medication at least 4 weeks before surgery.[81] For high-risk surgical procedures, such as total joint arthroplasty or revision, the Club Rhumatismes et Inflammation and Härle et al[17] suggest

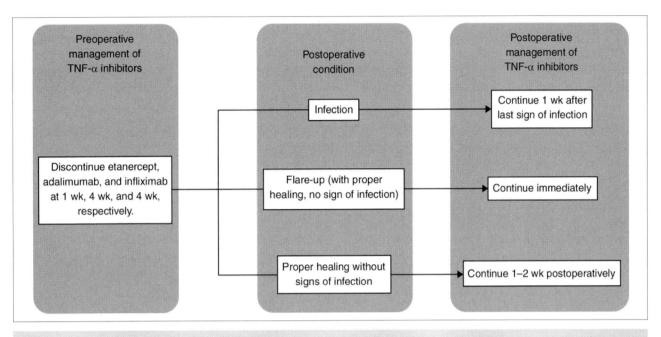

Figure 1   Algorithm shows perioperative management of tumor necrosis factor (TNF)-α inhibitors.

that it is appropriate to wait four to five half-lives for each medication before surgery. Although preoperative discontinuation of TNF-α inhibitors is generally advised, it remains unclear when medication should be restarted postoperatively. Because TNF-α inhibitors are linked to impaired wound healing,[82] some believe treatment should resume only after 2 weeks of healing without any sign of infection.[83] According to the American College of Rheumatology guidelines, these medications may be restarted 1 week after the procedure.[84] However, if RA flare-ups are noted postoperatively and there is no sign of infection, TNF-α inhibitors should be restarted immediately to prevent flare-ups from hindering rehabilitation[17,53,85] (**Figure 1**).

Several reports have shown that more powerful immunosuppression can be elicited by combining immunosuppressive therapies that target different steps of the immune response.[17,86,87] A double-blind, randomized controlled study compared two treatment strategies in DMARD-naïve patients who had early RA.[88] The authors showed that combination therapy with MTX and a TNF-α inhibitor led to a greater reduction in the progression of joint destruction than did MTX and placebo. However, combination therapy with TNF-α and an IL-1 inhibitor was found to provide no additional benefit compared with IL-1 monotherapy.[89] This combination also drastically increased the rates of infection and neutropenia. Given the paucity of data on perioperative management of combination therapy, drugs taken in combination can be managed individually, just as they are managed for monotherapy.

Steroids

For patients who have inflammatory diseases, glucocorticoids are a common treatment option because of their relatively low cost and fast-acting nature compared with other RA treatments.[13,14] Glucocorticoids have a faster onset of action than DMARDs, which results in quicker relief of symptoms.[17,90]

However, prolonged use of glucocorticoids compromises the immune system, decreases bone quality, and impairs wound healing.[15,91-94] Teriparatide is considered a beneficial adjunctive therapy, with steroids used to increase bone mineral density and reduce the risk of fractures.[95,96] In patients with RA who are being treated with a chronic, low-dose oral glucocorticoid, the hypothalamic-pituitary-adrenal axis is suppressed, which implies a decrease in corticotropin-releasing hormone secretion and steroidogenic enzymes of the adrenal glands.[24,94] This inhibits the release of cortisol after a surgical procedure and causes acute perioperative adrenal insufficiency, leading to fatal circulatory shock.[15,94] Administration of a physiologic dose of glucocorticoids followed by a gradual tapering to preoperative doses has proved to be beneficial in preventing the risk of these complications.[94,97] It is crucial that surgeons tailor the administration of glucocorticoids for each patient to create a balance between preventing acute adrenal insufficiency or addisonian crisis and avoiding impaired wound healing and infection.[24,94]

Nonsteroidal Anti-inflammatory Drugs

Traditional NSAIDs used to be the first line of treatment for pain and stiffness in patients with RA.[98] With the advent of DMARDs, the use of NSAIDs became limited to adjunctive therapy with MTX.[48] Aspirin is the most widely used NSAID;[99] it causes irreversible inhibition of cyclooxygenase ([COX], mostly COX-1), thereby inhibiting platelet function and thrombosis.[100] Other NSAIDs (eg, ibuprofen, naproxen) act as reversible competitive inhibitors of COX-1 and COX-2; hence, perioperative management should be based on the respective dosage and the half-life of the drug.[101] Preoperatively, NSAIDs should be withheld for three to five half-lives, or up to 10 days, to prevent an increased risk of perioperative bleeding.[94] Because of its irreversible activity, perioperative doses of aspirin should be based on the turnover rate of COX rather than the drug's half-life.[101] Platelets have a life span of 8 to 10 days and have an estimated turnover rate of 10% per day if aspirin is discontinued, resulting in normal platelet COX-1 activity in approximately 10 days.[94,102] However, the manifestation of normal platelet hemostasis may occur in patients who have only 20% of COX-1 activity,[103,104] with normal platelet function achieved in less than 72 hours.[105] Discontinuing aspirin 72 hours before surgery and restarting it no earlier than 8 to 10 days postoperatively may minimize the risk of perioperative bleeding.[106] Aspirin's effect on the risk of perioperative bleeding and the blood transfusion requirement is unclear. Some research has shown that

aspirin taken perioperatively may substantially increase the risk of bleeding and the need for blood transfusion during orthopaedic surgery.[106-108] Other studies have shown only a relatively moderate increase in intraoperative and postoperative bleeding associated with the use of NSAIDs, with no increase in blood transfusion rates reported.[109]

Although the risk of perioperative bleeding is a possible concern with the use of aspirin, continued use is preferred in some circumstances.[110] A recent study showed no reduction in myocardial infarctions or VTE in patients who were treated with perioperative aspirin versus a placebo;[106] however, it is widely accepted that patients with preexisting CVD should be treated with aspirin without interruption.[111-113] Continuation of aspirin to prevent CVD, coronary artery disease, and peripheral vascular disease is strongly supported for all patients who undergo surgery.[114] Studies also have shown that discontinuation of aspirin may trigger the onset of aspirin withdrawal syndrome characterized by a prothrombotic rebound period that results in an increase in thromboxane production and a decrease in fibrinolysis, thereby increasing the thromboembolic risk[114] (**Table 1**).

Perioperative Prevention of VTE

With regard to prophylaxis and prevention of VTE, patients who have RA may be treated similar to those with OA. The American Academy of Orthopaedic Surgeons (AAOS) Clinical Practice Guidelines on the prevention of VTE were based on a review of high- or medium-quality randomized controlled studies of patients who underwent elective THA or TKA. The guidelines include a moderate recommendation on

the use of pharmacologic agents and/or mechanical compressive devices for patients who undergo elective THA or TKA if they are not at increased risk of VTE or bleeding beyond the risk of the surgery itself.[115] However, no evidence indicated that one specific prophylactic strategy was superior to other strategies.[115] Early acceptance of prophylaxis as the standard of care for patients who undergo elective total joint arthroplasty has made it difficult to compare different prophylactic strategies because of the paucity of placebo-controlled trials.[115]

The AAOS guidelines also recommend discontinuing antiplatelet agents, such as aspirin or clopidogrel, before THA or TKA.[115] In addition to obtaining a thorough patient history, including screening for VTE, patients may be assessed for active liver disease and bleeding disorders, such as hemophilia. For patients who have these conditions, mechanical compressive devices may be used because they pose a low risk of bleeding and are "consistent with current practice."[115] For those who have a history of VTE, the guidelines recommend the use of both pharmacologic prophylaxis and mechanical compression devices.[115] The literature on the efficacy of inferior vena cava filters to prevent VTE remains unclear; therefore, the AAOS guidelines do not recommend for or against the use of these filters in patients who have a history of VTE or a contraindication to chemoprophylaxis.[115] The use of neuraxial anesthesia was suggested to help reduce blood loss. Postoperatively, early mobilization is advised to prevent VTE because it poses minimal risk and is "consistent with current practice."[115] Finally, the AAOS guidelines recommend against routine postoperative

Table 1

Summary of Recommendations for Drugs Used for the Perioperative Management of Rheumatoid Arthritis

Medication	Half-life	Recommendation
NSAIDs	2–17 hr	Therapy should be discontinued within 1 wk before surgery. Aspirin should be discontinued at least 72 hr before surgery.
Methotrexate	0.7–5.8 hr	Continue perioperatively.
Sulfasalazine	5 hr	Discontinue therapy 1 wk before surgery.
Azathioprine	7.6 hr	Discontinue therapy 1 wk before surgery.
Leflunomide	~2 wk	Can be discontinued 1–2 d before surgery, with cholestyramine used to remove active metabolite; may be reinstated 1–2 wk postoperatively.
Hydroxychloroquine	1–2 mo	Therapy can continue up to and including the day of surgery.
Etanercept	4.3 d	Hold for at least 1 wk before surgery. Reinstate 1–2 wk postoperatively.
Infliximab	8–10 d	Hold for 4 wk before surgery; may be reinstated 1–2 wk postoperatively (with no sign of infection).
Golimumab	8–10 d	Hold for 4 wk before surgery; may be reinstated 1–2 wk postoperatively (with no sign of infection).
Tocilizumab	12–14 d	Hold for 1 mo before surgery.
Abatacept	12–14 d	Hold for 1 mo before surgery.
Adalimumab	12–14 d	Hold for 1 mo before surgery.
Certolizumab	12–14 d	Hold for 1 mo before surgery.
Rituximab	21 d	Hold for 2 mo before surgery.

Data from Parvizi J, Gehrke T, eds: *Proceedings of the International Consensus Meeting on Periprosthetic Joint Infection.* Brooklandville, MD, Data Trace Publishing Company, 2013.

duplex ultrasonography screening in patients who are undergoing elective THA or TKA.

Rehabilitation and Patient Outcomes

Patients with active RA have longer hospital stays and demonstrate slower functional improvement than do patients with OA.[24,116] Thus, patients with RA should have minimal bed rest and immediately begin physiotherapy to help prevent immobilization injuries and contractures as well as to improve muscle strength and joint motion.[23] Preoperative physiotherapy also may improve outcomes by providing patient education, preoperative assessments, and therapy to optimize postoperative rehabilitation.[117,118] This is especially helpful for patients with multiple joint involvement and ensures that the appropriate durable medical equipment and modifications are readily available. Although surgical outcomes are better in patients who have OA than in those who have RA secondary to the compromised immune system and healing potential, patients with RA have a lower risk of deep vein thrombosis (DVT).[119,120] Niki et al[120] reported that patients with RA had a lower incidence of postoperative DVT than did those with OA. When patients being treated with NSAIDs and those older than 65 years were excluded from the study, the incidence of DVT was equal in both patient populations.[120] This difference in outcome may be attributed to the younger age of patients with RA and the potential effect of NSAIDs on platelet activity.

A recent meta-analysis and systematic review compared the complication rates after total joint arthroplasty in patients who had RA and those who had OA.[121] The authors found that patients with RA had an increased risk of hip dislocation after THA and an increased risk of infection after TKA. Postoperative hip dislocation in these patients may be attributable to poorer soft-tissue quality[122] and reduced abductor strength.[123] Finally, the study found that there were no differences in the risk of revision surgeries, DVT, or mortality within 90 days of surgery.[121] However, the lack of difference in DVT risk factors between the two populations may be attributed to selection bias and the possibility that healthier patients who have RA are being approved for surgery, reducing the risk of thromboembolism to match that of those who have OA.

Summary

RA is a debilitating disease caused by a chronic inflammatory process. With the introduction of DMARDs, the number of patients with RA who progress to joint deformity and disability has decreased, reducing the need for orthopaedic interventions in this population. However, a considerable number of these patients still require surgery. It is important for orthopaedic surgeons to be familiar with common medical conditions encountered in this population. These comorbidities affect multiple organ systems and can be the direct result of the disease process or an adverse effect of the number of medications that these patients receive. A comprehensive understanding of these comorbidities may lead to appropriate perioperative medical management, which is vital for improving postoperative outcomes and preventing life-threatening complications.

References

1. Aksu K, Donmez A, Keser G: Inflammation-induced thrombosis: Mechanisms, disease associations and management. *Curr Pharm Des* 2012;18(11):1478-1493.

2. Myasoedova E, Davis JM III, Crowson CS, Gabriel SE: Epidemiology of rheumatoid arthritis: Rheumatoid arthritis and mortality. *Curr Rheumatol Rep* 2010;12(5):379-385.

3. Firestein GS: Evolving concepts of rheumatoid arthritis. *Nature* 2003;423(6937):356-361.

4. Gullick NJ, Scott DL: Co-morbidities in established rheumatoid arthritis. *Best Pract Res Clin Rheumatol* 2011;25(4):469-483.

5. Rossini M, Rossi E, Bernardi D, et al: Prevalence and incidence of rheumatoid arthritis in Italy. *Rheumatol Int* 2014;34(5):659-664.

6. Alamanos Y, Voulgari PV, Drosos AA: Incidence and prevalence of rheumatoid arthritis, based on the 1987 American College of Rheumatology criteria: A systematic review. *Semin Arthritis Rheum* 2006;36(3):182-188.

7. Carbonell J, Cobo T, Balsa A, Descalzo MA, Carmona L; SERAP Study Group: The incidence of rheumatoid arthritis in Spain: Results from a nationwide primary care registry. *Rheumatology (Oxford)* 2008;47(7):1088-1092.

8. McInnes IB, Schett G: The pathogenesis of rheumatoid arthritis. *N Engl J Med* 2011;365(23):2205-2219.

9. Masuda H, Miyazaki T, Shimada K, et al: Disease duration and severity impacts on long-term cardiovascular events in Japanese patients with rheumatoid arthritis. *J Cardiol* 2014;64(5):366-370.

10. Ajeganova S, Andersson ML, Frostegård J, Hafström I: Disease factors in early rheumatoid arthritis are associated with differential risks for cardiovascular events and mortality depending on age at onset: A 10-year observational cohort study. *J Rheumatol* 2013;40(12):1958-1966.

11. Avouac J, Meune C, Chenevier-Gobeaux C, et al: Inflammation and disease activity are associated with high circulating cardiac markers in rheumatoid arthritis independently of traditional cardiovascular risk factors. *J Rheumatol* 2014;41(2):248-255.

12. Naz SM, Symmons DP: Mortality in established rheumatoid arthritis. *Best Pract Res Clin Rheumatol* 2007;21(5):871-883.

13. Louie GH, Ward MM: Changes in the rates of joint surgery among patients with rheumatoid arthritis in California, 1983-2007. *Ann Rheum Dis* 2010;69(5):868-871.

14. Carmona L, Cross M, Williams B, Lassere M, March L: Rheumatoid arthritis. *Best Pract Res Clin Rheumatol* 2010;24(6):733-745.

15. Howe CR, Gardner GC, Kadel NJ: Perioperative medication management for the patient with rheumatoid arthritis. *J Am Acad Orthop Surg* 2006;14(9):544-551.

16. Momohara S, Tanaka S, Nakamura H, et al: Recent trends in orthopedic surgery performed in Japan for rheumatoid arthritis. *Mod Rheumatol* 2011;21(4):337-342.

17. Härle P, Straub RH, Fleck M: Perioperative management of immunosuppression in rheumatic diseases: What to do? *Rheumatol Int* 2010;30(8):999-1004.

18. Stundner O, Danninger T, Chiu YL, et al: Rheumatoid arthritis vs osteoarthritis in patients receiving total knee arthroplasty: Perioperative outcomes. *J Arthroplasty* 2014;29(2):308-313.

19. Lee JK, Choi CH: Total knee arthroplasty in rheumatoid arthritis. *Knee Surg Relat Res* 2012;24(1):1-6.

20. Simmen BR, Bogoch ER, Goldhahn J: Surgery insight: Orthopedic treatment options in rheumatoid arthritis. *Nat Clin Pract Rheumatol* 2008;4(5):266-273.

21. Rheumatic diseases: Surgical treatment. A systematic literature review by SBU: The Swedish Council on Technology Assessment in Health Care. *Acta Orthop Scand Suppl* 2000;294:1-88.

22. Nelissen RG: The impact of total joint replacement in rheumatoid arthritis. *Best Pract Res Clin Rheumatol* 2003;17(5):831-846.

23. Wilkinson JM, Stanley D, Getty CJ: Surgical management of the rheumatoid patient. *Curr Orthop* 2004;18(5):357-370.

24. Clement ND, Breusch SJ, Biant LC: Lower limb joint replacement in rheumatoid arthritis. *J Orthop Surg Res* 2012;7:27.

25. Goodman SM, Figgie M: Lower extremity arthroplasty in patients with inflammatory arthritis: Preoperative and perioperative management. *J Am Acad Orthop Surg* 2013;21(6):355-363.

26. Stockley I, Betts RP, Getty CJ, Rowley DI, Duckworth T: A prospective study of forefoot arthroplasty. *Clin Orthop Relat Res* 1989;248:213-218.

27. Meding JB, Keating EM, Ritter MA, Faris PM, Berend ME, Malinzak RA: The planovalgus foot: A harbinger of failure of posterior cruciate-retaining total knee replacement. *J Bone Joint Surg Am* 2005;87(suppl 2):59-62.

28. Keenan MA, Peabody TD, Gronley JK, Perry J: Valgus deformities of the feet and characteristics of gait in patients who have rheumatoid arthritis. *J Bone Joint Surg Am* 1991;73(2):237-247.

29. Papp SR, Athwal GS, Pichora DR: The rheumatoid wrist. *J Am Acad Orthop Surg* 2006;14(2):65-77.

30. Stanley J: The rheumatoid wrist. *Curr Orthop* 2001;15(5):329-337.

31. Connor J, Nalebuff EA: Current recommendations for surgery of the rheumatoid hand and wrist. *Curr Opin Rheumatol* 1995;7(2):120-124.

32. Herren DB, Ishikawa H: Partial arthrodesis for the rheumatoid wrist. *Hand Clin* 2005;21(4):545-552.

33. Ovesen J, Olsen BS, Johannsen HV, Søjbjerg JO: Capitellocondylar total elbow replacement in late-stage rheumatoid arthritis. *J Shoulder Elbow Surg* 2005;14(4):414-420.

34. Ewald FC, Simmons ED Jr, Sullivan JA, et al: Capitellocondylar total elbow replacement in rheumatoid arthritis: Long-term results. *J Bone Joint Surg Am* 1993;75(4):498-507.

35. Neer CS II, Kirby RM: Revision of humeral head and total shoulder arthroplasties. *Clin Orthop Relat Res* 1982;170:189-195.

36. Bacani AK, Gabriel SE, Crowson CS, Heit JA, Matteson EL: Noncardiac vascular disease in rheumatoid arthritis: Increase in venous thromboembolic events? *Arthritis Rheum* 2012;64(1):53-61.

37. Nicola PJ, Maradit-Kremers H, Roger VL, et al: The risk of congestive heart failure in rheumatoid arthritis: A population-based study over 46 years. *Arthritis Rheum* 2005;52(2):412-420.

38. Maradit-Kremers H, Crowson CS, Nicola PJ, et al: Increased unrecognized coronary heart disease and sudden deaths in rheumatoid arthritis: A population-based cohort study. *Arthritis Rheum* 2005;52(2):402-411.

39. Aviña-Zubieta JA, Choi HK, Sadatsafavi M, Etminan M, Esdaile JM, Lacaille D: Risk of cardiovascular mortality in patients with rheumatoid arthritis: A meta-analysis of observational studies. *Arthritis Rheum* 2008;59(12):1690-1697.

40. Minaur NJ, Jacoby RK, Cosh JA, Taylor G, Rasker JJ: Outcome after 40 years with rheumatoid arthritis: A prospective study of function, disease activity, and mortality. *J Rheumatol Suppl* 2004;69:3-8.

41. Sihvonen S, Korpela M, Laippala P, Mustonen J, Pasternack A: Death rates and causes of death in patients with rheumatoid arthritis: A population-based study. *Scand J Rheumatol* 2004;33(4):221-227.

42. Brown KK: Rheumatoid lung disease. *Proc Am Thorac Soc* 2007;4(5):443-448.

43. Bongartz T, Nannini C, Medina-Velasquez YF, et al: Incidence and mortality of interstitial lung disease in rheumatoid arthritis: A population-based study. *Arthritis Rheum* 2010;62(6):1583-1591.

44. Choi SM, Lee J, Park YS, et al: Postoperative pulmonary complications after surgery in patients with interstitial lung disease. *Respiration* 2014;87(4):287-293.

45. da Côrte FC, Neves N: Cervical spine instability in rheumatoid arthritis. *Eur J Orthop Surg Traumatol* 2014;24(suppl 1):S83-S91.

46. Collins DN, Barnes CL, FitzRandolph RL: Cervical spine instability in rheumatoid patients having total hip or knee arthroplasty. *Clin Orthop Relat Res* 1991;272:127-135.

47. Neva MH, Häkkinen A, Mäkinen H, Hannonen P, Kauppi M, Sokka T: High prevalence of asymptomatic cervical spine subluxation in patients with rheumatoid arthritis waiting for orthopaedic surgery. *Ann Rheum Dis* 2006;65(7):884-888.

48. Danoff JR, Moss G, Liabaud B, Geller JA: Total knee arthroplasty considerations in rheumatoid arthritis. *Autoimmune Dis* 2013;2013:185340.

49. Neva MH, Myllykangas-Luosujärvi R, Kautiainen H, Kauppi M: Mortality associated with cervical spine disorders: A population-based study of 1666 patients with rheumatoid arthritis who died in Finland in 1989. *Rheumatology (Oxford)* 2001;40(2):123-127.

50. Weinblatt ME, Maier AL, Fraser PA, Coblyn JS: Long-term prospective study of methotrexate in rheumatoid arthritis: Conclusion after 132 months of therapy. *J Rheumatol* 1998;25(2):238-242.

51. Wessels JA, Huizinga TW, Guchelaar HJ: Recent insights in the pharmacological actions of methotrexate in the treatment of rheumatoid arthritis. *Rheumatology (Oxford)* 2008;47(3):249-255.

52. Revu S, Neregård P, af Klint E, Korotkova M, Catrina AI: Synovial membrane immunohistology in early-untreated rheumatoid arthritis reveals high expression of catabolic bone markers that is modulated by methotrexate. *Arthritis Res Ther* 2013;15(6):R205.

53. Grennan DM, Gray J, Loudon J, Fear S: Methotrexate and early postoperative complications in patients with rheumatoid arthritis undergoing elective orthopaedic surgery. *Ann Rheum Dis* 2001;60(3):214-217.

54. Murata K, Yasuda T, Ito H, Yoshida M, Shimizu M, Nakamura T: Lack of increase in postoperative complications with low-dose methotrexate therapy in patients with rheumatoid arthritis undergoing elective orthopedic surgery. *Mod Rheumatol* 2006;16(1):14-19.

55. Pieringer H, Stuby U, Biesenbach G: The place of methotrexate perioperatively in elective orthopedic surgeries in patients with rheumatoid arthritis. *Clin Rheumatol* 2008;27(10):1217-1220.

56. Sreekumar R, Gray J, Kay P, Grennan DM: Methotrexate and postoperative complications in patients with rheumatoid arthritis undergoing elective orthopaedic surgery: A ten year follow-up. *Acta Orthop Belg* 2011;77(6):823-826.

57. Minaur NJ, Jefferiss C, Bhalla AK, Beresford JN: Methotrexate in the treatment of rheumatoid arthritis: I. In vitro effects on cells of the

osteoblast lineage. *Rheumatology (Oxford)* 2002;41(7):735-740.

58. Minaur NJ, Kounali D, Vedi S, Compston JE, Beresford JN, Bhalla AK: Methotrexate in the treatment of rheumatoid arthritis: II. In vivo effects on bone mineral density. *Rheumatology (Oxford)* 2002;41(7):741-749.

59. Uehara R, Suzuki Y, Ichikawa Y: Methotrexate (MTX) inhibits osteoblastic differentiation in vitro: Possible mechanism of MTX osteopathy. *J Rheumatol* 2001;28(2):251-256.

60. Annussek T, Kleinheinz J, Thomas S, Joos U, Wermker K: Short time administration of antirheumatic drugs: Methotrexate as a strong inhibitor of osteoblast's proliferation in vitro. *Head Face Med* 2012;8:26.

61. Morgacheva O, Furst DE: Use of MTX in the elderly and in patients with compromised renal function. *Clin Exp Rheumatol* 2010; 28(5 suppl 61):S85-S94.

62. Rosandich PA, Kelley JT III, Conn DL: Perioperative management of patients with rheumatoid arthritis in the era of biologic response modifiers. *Curr Opin Rheumatol* 2004;16(3):192-198.

63. Kremer JM, Rynes RI, Bartholomew LE: Severe flare of rheumatoid arthritis after discontinuation of long-term methotrexate therapy: Double-blind study. *Am J Med* 1987;82(4):781-786.

64. Kalden JR, Schattenkirchner M, Sörensen H, et al: The efficacy and safety of leflunomide in patients with active rheumatoid arthritis: A five-year followup study. *Arthritis Rheum* 2003;48(6):1513-1520.

65. Fuerst M, Möhl H, Baumgärtel K, Rüther W: Leflunomide increases the risk of early healing complications in patients with rheumatoid arthritis undergoing elective orthopedic surgery. *Rheumatol Int* 2006;26(12):1138-1142.

66. Choy EH, Panayi GS: Cytokine pathways and joint inflammation in rheumatoid arthritis. *N Engl J Med* 2001;344(12):907-916.

67. Maini RN, Breedveld FC, Kalden JR, et al: Therapeutic efficacy of multiple intravenous infusions of anti-tumor necrosis factor alpha monoclonal antibody combined with low-dose weekly methotrexate in rheumatoid arthritis. *Arthritis Rheum* 1998;41(9):1552-1563.

68. Chen YF, Jobanputra P, Barton P, et al: A systematic review of the effectiveness of adalimumab, etanercept and infliximab for the treatment of rheumatoid arthritis in adults and an economic evaluation of their cost-effectiveness. *Health Technol Assess* 2006;10(42):iii-iv, xi-xiii, 1-229.

69. Furst DE, Keystone EC, So AK, et al: Updated consensus statement on biological agents for the treatment of rheumatic diseases, 2012. *Ann Rheum Dis* 2013;72(suppl 2):ii2-ii34.

70. Finckh A, Choi HK, Wolfe F: Progression of radiographic joint damage in different eras: Trends towards milder disease in rheumatoid arthritis are attributable to improved treatment. *Ann Rheum Dis* 2006;65(9):1192-1197.

71. Bongartz T, Sutton AJ, Sweeting MJ, Buchan I, Matteson EL, Montori V: Anti-TNF antibody therapy in rheumatoid arthritis and the risk of serious infections and malignancies: Systematic review and meta-analysis of rare harmful effects in randomized controlled trials. *JAMA* 2006;295(19):2275-2285.

72. Bernatsky S, Habel Y, Rahme E: Observational studies of infections in rheumatoid arthritis: A meta-analysis of tumor necrosis factor antagonists. *J Rheumatol* 2010;37(5):928-931.

73. Giles JT, Bartlett SJ, Gelber AC, et al: Tumor necrosis factor inhibitor therapy and risk of serious postoperative orthopedic infection in rheumatoid arthritis. *Arthritis Rheum* 2006;55(2):333-337.

74. Tubach F, Salmon D, Ravaud P, et al: Risk of tuberculosis is higher with anti-tumor necrosis factor monoclonal antibody therapy than with soluble tumor necrosis factor receptor therapy: The three-year prospective French Research Axed on Tolerance of Biotherapies registry. *Arthritis Rheum* 2009;60(7):1884-1894.

75. Dixon WG, Hyrich KL, Watson KD, et al: Drug-specific risk of tuberculosis in patients with rheumatoid arthritis treated with anti-TNF therapy: Results from the British Society for Rheumatology Biologics Register (BSRBR). *Ann Rheum Dis* 2010;69(3):522-528.

76. Dao KH, Herbert M, Habal N, Cush JJ: Nonserious infections: Should there be cause for serious concerns? *Rheum Dis Clin North Am* 2012;38(4):707-725.

77. Bibbo C, Goldberg JW: Infectious and healing complications after elective orthopaedic foot and ankle surgery during tumor necrosis factor-alpha inhibition therapy. *Foot Ankle Int* 2004;25(5):331-335.

78. Galloway JB, Hyrich KL, Mercer LK, et al: Anti-TNF therapy is associated with an increased risk of serious infections in patients with rheumatoid arthritis especially in the first 6 months of treatment: Updated results from the British Society for Rheumatology Biologics Register with special emphasis on risks in the elderly. *Rheumatology (Oxford)* 2011;50(1):124-131.

79. Ruyssen-Witrand A, Gossec L, Salliot C, et al: Complication rates of 127 surgical procedures performed in rheumatic patients receiving tumor necrosis factor alpha blockers. *Clin Exp Rheumatol* 2007;25(3):430-436.

80. Scherrer CB, Mannion AF, Kyburz D, Vogt M, Kramers-de Quervain IA: Infection risk after orthopedic surgery in patients with inflammatory rheumatic diseases treated with immunosuppressive drugs. *Arthritis Care Res (Hoboken)* 2013;65(12):2032-2040.

81. Strand V, Smolen JS, van Vollenhoven RF, et al: Certolizumab pegol plus methotrexate provides broad relief from the burden of rheumatoid arthritis: Analysis of patient-reported outcomes from the RAPID 2 trial. *Ann Rheum Dis* 2011;70(6):996-1002.

82. Mooney DP, O'Reilly M, Gamelli RL: Tumor necrosis factor and wound healing. *Ann Surg* 1990;211(2):124-129.

83. Goh L, Jewell T, Laversuch C, Samanta A: Should anti-TNF therapy be discontinued in rheumatoid arthritis patients undergoing elective orthopaedic surgery? A systematic review of the evidence. *Rheumatol Int* 2012;32(1):5-13.

84. Nannini C, Medina-Velasquez YF, Achenbach SJ, et al: Incidence and mortality of obstructive lung disease in rheumatoid arthritis: A population-based study. *Arthritis Care Res (Hoboken)* 2013;65(8):1243-1250.

85. Momohara S, Hashimoto J, Tsuboi H, et al: Analysis of perioperative clinical features and complications after orthopaedic surgery in rheumatoid arthritis patients treated with tocilizumab in a real-world setting: Results from the multicentre TOcilizumab in Perioperative Period (TOPP) study. *Mod Rheumatol* 2013;23(3):440-449.

86. Detert J: Early use of biological agents after first DMARD in rheumatoid arthritis: Yes. *Dtsch Med Wochenschr* 2013;138(37):1850.

87. Edwards CK III, Green JS, Volk HD, et al: Combined anti-tumor necrosis factor-α therapy and DMARD therapy in rheumatoid arthritis patients reduces inflammatory gene expression in whole blood compared to DMARD therapy alone. *Front Immunol* 2012;3:366.

88. Detert J, Bastian H, Listing J, et al: Induction therapy with adalimumab plus methotrexate for 24 weeks followed by methotrexate monotherapy up to week 48 versus methotrexate therapy alone for DMARD-naive patients with early rheumatoid arthritis: HIT HARD. An investigator-initiated study. *Ann Rheum Dis* 2013;72(6):844-850.

89. Genovese MC, Cohen S, Moreland L, et al: Combination therapy with etanercept and anakinra in the treatment of patients with rheumatoid arthritis who have been treated unsuccessfully with methotrexate. *Arthritis Rheum* 2004;50(5):1412-1419.

90. Kirwan JR; The Arthritis and Rheumatism Council Low-Dose Glucocorticoid Study Group: The effect of glucocorticoids on joint destruction in rheumatoid arthritis. *N Engl J Med* 1995;333(3):142-146.

91. Chmell MJ, Scott RD: Total knee arthroplasty in patients with rheumatoid arthritis: An overview. *Clin Orthop Relat Res* 1999;366:54-60.

92. Luessenhop CP, Higgins LD, Brause BD, Ranawat CS: Multiple prosthetic infections after total joint arthroplasty: Risk factor analysis. *J Arthroplasty* 1996;11(7):862-868.

93. Anstead GM: Steroids, retinoids, and wound healing. *Adv Wound Care* 1998;11(6):277-285.

94. Pieringer H, Stuby U, Biesenbach G: Patients with rheumatoid arthritis undergoing surgery: How should we deal with antirheumatic treatment? *Semin Arthritis Rheum* 2007;36(5):278-286.

95. Saag KG, Shane E, Boonen S, et al: Teriparatide or alendronate in glucocorticoid-induced osteoporosis. *N Engl J Med* 2007;357(20):2028-2039.

96. Saag KG, Zanchetta JR, Devogelaer JP, et al: Effects of teriparatide versus alendronate for treating glucocorticoid-induced osteoporosis: Thirty-six-month results of a randomized, double-blind, controlled trial. *Arthritis Rheum* 2009;60(11):3346-3355.

97. Shaw M, Mandell BF: Perioperative management of selected problems in patients with rheumatic diseases. *Rheum Dis Clin North Am* 1999;25(3):623-638, ix.

98. Scott DL, Wolfe F, Huizinga TW: Rheumatoid arthritis. *Lancet* 2010;376(9746):1094-1108.

99. Schairer WW, Vail TP, Bozic KJ: What are the rates and causes of hospital readmission after total knee arthroplasty? *Clin Orthop Relat Res* 2014;472(1):181-187.

100. Campbell CL, Smyth S, Montalescot G, Steinhubl SR: Aspirin dose for the prevention of cardiovascular disease: A systematic review. *JAMA* 2007;297(18):2018-2024.

101. Lack WD, Fredericks D, Petersen E, et al: Effect of aspirin on bone healing in a rabbit ulnar osteotomy model. *J Bone Joint Surg Am* 2013;95(6):488-496.

102. Burch JW, Stanford N, Majerus PW: Inhibition of platelet prostaglandin synthetase by oral aspirin. *J Clin Invest* 1978;61(2):314-319.

103. Patrono C, Ciabattoni G, Patrignani P, et al: Clinical pharmacology of platelet cyclooxygenase inhibition. *Circulation* 1985;72(6):1177-1184.

104. Bradlow BA, Chetty N: Dosage frequency for suppression of platelet function by low dose aspirin therapy. *Thromb Res* 1982;27(1):99-110.

105. Jimenez AH, Stubbs ME, Tofler GH, Winther K, Williams GH, Muller JE: Rapidity and duration of platelet suppression by enteric-coated aspirin in healthy young men. *Am J Cardiol* 1992;69(3):258-262.

106. Devereaux PJ, Mrkobrada M, Sessler DI, et al: Aspirin in patients undergoing noncardiac surgery. *N Engl J Med* 2014;370(16):1494-1503.

107. Manning BJ, O'Brien N, Aravindan S, Cahill RA, McGreal G, Redmond HP: The effect of aspirin on blood loss and transfusion requirements in patients with femoral neck fractures. *Injury* 2004;35(2):121-124.

108. Thrombosis prevention trial: Randomised trial of low-intensity oral anticoagulation with warfarin and low-dose aspirin in the primary prevention of ischaemic heart disease in men at increased risk. The Medical Research Council's General Practice Research Framework. *Lancet* 1998;351(9098):233-241.

109. Samama CM, Bastien O, Forestier F, et al: Antiplatelet agents in the perioperative period: Expert recommendations of the French Society of Anesthesiology and Intensive Care (SFAR) 2001. Summary statement. *Can J Anaesth* 2002;49(6):S26-S35.

110. Keating EM, Meding JB, Faris PM, Ritter MA: Long-term followup of nonmodular total knee replacements. *Clin Orthop Relat Res* 2002;404:34-39.

111. Chassot PG, Marcucci C, Delabays A, Spahn DR: Perioperative antiplatelet therapy. *Am Fam Physician* 2010;82(12):1484-1489.

112. McEntegart A, Capell HA, Creran D, Rumley A, Woodward M, Lowe GD: Cardiovascular risk factors, including thrombotic variables, in a population with rheumatoid arthritis. *Rheumatology (Oxford)* 2001;40(6):640-644.

113. Wållberg-Jonsson S, Dahlén GH, Nilsson TK, Rånby M, Rantapää-Dahlqvist S: Tissue plasminogen activator, plasminogen activator inhibitor-1 and von Willebrand factor in rheumatoid arthritis. *Clin Rheumatol* 1993;12(3):318-324.

114. Gerstein NS, Schulman PM, Gerstein WH, Petersen TR, Tawil I: Should more patients continue aspirin therapy perioperatively? Clinical impact of aspirin withdrawal syndrome. *Ann Surg* 2012;255(5):811-819.

115. Mont MA, Jacobs JJ, Boggio LN, et al: Preventing venous thromboembolic disease in patients undergoing elective hip and knee arthroplasty. *J Am Acad Orthop Surg* 2011;19(12):768-776.

116. Nguyen-Oghalai TU, Ottenbacher KJ, Caban M, Granger CV, Grecula M, Goodwin JS: The impact of rheumatoid arthritis on rehabilitation outcomes after lower extremity arthroplasty. *J Clin Rheumatol* 2007;13(5):247-250.

117. Stross JK, Banwell BF, Wolf FM, Becker MC: Evaluation of an education program on the management of rheumatic diseases for physical therapists. *J Rheumatol* 1986;13(2):374-378.

118. Vukomanović A, Popović Z, Durović A, Krstić L: The effects of short-term preoperative physical therapy and education on early functional recovery of patients younger than 70 undergoing total hip arthroplasty. *Vojnosanit Pregl* 2008;65(4):291-297.

119. van Heereveld HA, Laan RF, van den Hoogen FH, Malefijt MC, Novakova IR, van de Putte LB: Prevention of symptomatic thrombosis with short term (low molecular weight) heparin in patients with rheumatoid arthritis after hip or knee replacement. *Ann Rheum Dis* 2001;60(10):974-976.

120. Niki Y, Matsumoto H, Hakozaki A, Mochizuki T, Momohara S: Rheumatoid arthritis: A risk factor for deep venous thrombosis after total knee arthroplasty? Comparative study with osteoarthritis. *J Orthop Sci* 2010;15(1):57-63.

121. Ravi B, Croxford R, Hollands S, et al: Increased risk of complications following total joint arthroplasty in patients with rheumatoid arthritis. *Arthritis Rheumatol* 2014;66(2):254-263.

122. Jain A, Nanchahal J, Troeberg L, Green P, Brennan F: Production of cytokines, vascular endothelial growth factor, matrix metalloproteinases, and tissue inhibitor of metalloproteinases 1 by tenosynovium demonstrates its potential for tendon destruction in rheumatoid arthritis. *Arthritis Rheum* 2001;44(8):1754-1760.

123. Lakstein D, Backstein DJ, Safir O, Kosashvili Y, Gross AE: Modified trochanteric slide for complex hip arthroplasty: Clinical outcomes and complication rates. *J Arthroplasty* 2010;25(3):363-368.

Effect of Smoking on Joint Replacement Outcomes: Opportunities for Improvement Through Preoperative Smoking Cessation

Erik Wright, BS
Tony H. Tzeng, BS
Michael Ginnetti, BSc
Mouhanad M. El-Othmani, MD
Jamal K. Saleh, BSc
Jasmine Saleh, MD
J.M. Lane, MD
William M. Mihalko, MD, PhD
Khaled J. Saleh, BSc, MD, MSc, FRCSC, MHCM

Abstract

Because orthopaedic surgeons focus on identifying serious potential complications, such as heart attack, stroke, and deep vein thrombosis, during the preoperative assessment, correctable factors, such as smoking, may be overlooked. Chronic exposure to nicotine has been correlated with perioperative complications that lead to worse outcomes, including decreased patient satisfaction, longer hospitalization periods, and an increased rate of hospital readmission. It has been proven that smoking is a negative risk factor for decreased bone mineral density, which leads to increased fracture risk, heightened pain, postoperative wound and bone healing complications, decreased fusion rates, and postoperative tendon and ligament healing complications. Physician-led preoperative smoking cessation programs that include, but are not limited to, pharmacotherapy plans have been shown to improve primary surgical outcomes and smoking cessation rates. Smoking has detrimental effects on specialty-specific physiology; however, there are many effective options for intervention that can improve primary outcomes.

Instr Course Lect 2016;65:509–520.

Smoking releases toxins, such as nicotine and carbon monoxide, and has a negative effect on postoperative outcomes.[1] Since the 1944 publication of Morton's landmark study on smoking and pulmonary complications after surgery,[2] hundreds of other studies have further described the adverse effects of tobacco on the human body. Many studies link smoking not only to chronic health conditions and mortality, but also to perioperative complications, including delayed wound healing, infection, heightened pain, delayed bone healing, and cardiopulmonary complications.[3-5]

Despite the known negative effects of smoking on a person's health and standard of living, smoking remains a substantial health concern that often has deadly consequences. On average, worldwide, 50% of men and 10% of women will become smokers in their lifetime.[6] Furthermore, global statistics have shown that annual smoking-related deaths will rise from approximately 5 million in 2010 to 10 million by 2030.[7] In addition to increased mortality rates, smoking costs the US healthcare industry between $289 billion and $333 billion each year.[8]

As the 42 million adult smokers in the United States continue to age, the implications and importance of understanding the effects and the risk factors of smoking for this patient population are evident.[8,9] It is important for surgeons to understand the effects of tobacco on the musculoskeletal system, tissue healing, bone union, and perioperative pain. In addition, surgeons should understand the use and optimal implementation of preoperative smoking cessation techniques.

Cigarette Smoke

Cigarettes release more than 4,000 known toxins as part of either a particulate phase or a volatile phase.[10] The particulate phase contains 3,500 chemicals, including nicotine, and is most responsible for the carcinogenic effect of cigarette smoke.[11] The volatile phase contains the remaining 500 chemicals, mostly in gaseous form, including carbon monoxide.[12] A smoker inhales roughly 2 to 3 mg of nicotine and 20 to 30 mL of carbon monoxide with the consumption of one cigarette.[12]

Nicotine mediates its effects by binding to sympathetic nicotinic acetylcholine receptors in the central nervous system, which causes an increase in excitatory transmission.[13] Nicotine increases the release of epinephrine, which causes peripheral vasoconstriction and decreases the activity of natural killer cells and neutrophils.[14] These combined effects decrease a patient's ability to rebuild and repair tissue after surgical trauma.[3-5] Nicotine has a half-life of 3 hours and is subsequently metabolized by the liver and excreted into the urine as a detectable metabolite.[3]

Carbon monoxide works by binding to hemoglobin within an erythrocyte and forming carboxyhemoglobin. In this state, carbon monoxide has a half-life of 5 to 6 hours, depending on a person's age, sex, and level of physical activity.[15] Carbon monoxide, because of its interactions within the erythrocyte, binds with hemoglobin at a much higher affinity than oxygen and impairs a person's ability to transport oxygen to the peripheral tissues. Smoking one pack of cigarettes per day, a total ingestion of 400 to 600 mL of carbon monoxide, has been shown to induce a permanent hypoxic state in some peripheral tissues.[15]

Smoking and Wound Complications

Smoking has been identified as a modifiable risk factor for wound healing time and infection rates.[16] During the inflammatory phase of healing, smoking increases leukocyte counts and concomitantly decreases chemotaxis.[17-19] Furthermore, smoking impairs the ability of macrophages to detect bacteria and decreases their production of proinflammatory cytokine interleukin-1.[19] With respect to bacterial destruction, neutrophil and monocyte oxidative burst are reduced in smokers by 58% and 68%, respectively.[14] During the proliferative phase of healing, smoking hinders fibroblast migration, fibroblast function, epithelial cell regeneration, and extracellular matrix production, all of which result in longer healing time and an increased incidence of wound dehiscence.[18,20]

Compared with nonsmokers, smokers have an increased risk for the development of wound complications after surgery.[21] In a meta-analysis that investigated the incidence of perioperative

Mr. Saleh or an immediate family member has received royalties from Aesculap/B. Braun; is a member of a speakers' bureau or has made paid presentations on behalf of CareFusion; serves as a paid consultant to or is an employee of Aesculap/B. Braun and Watermark Research Partners; has received research or institutional support from the National Institutes of Health (NIAMS & NICHD) and Smith & Nephew; and serves as a board member, owner, officer, or committee member of the American Board of Orthopaedic Surgeons, the American Orthopaedic Association, and the Blue Cross Blue Shield Association. Dr. Lane or an immediate family member serves as a paid consultant to or is an employee of Bone Therapeutics, CollPlant, and Graftys; has received research or institutional support from Merck; has stock or stock options held in DFINE and CollPlant; and serves as a board member, owner, officer, or committee member of the American Academy of Orthopaedic Surgeons, the Association of Bone and Joint Surgeons, the American Orthopaedic Association, the American Society for Bone Mineral Research, the Musculoskeletal Tumor Society, and the Orthopaedic Research Society. Dr. Mihalko or an immediate family member has received royalties from Aesculap/B. Braun; is a member of a speakers' bureau or has made paid presentations on behalf of Aesculap/B. Braun; serves as a paid consultant to or is an employee of Aesculap/B. Braun and Medtronic; has received research or institutional support from Aesculap/B. Braun, Smith & Nephew, and Stryker; and serves as a board member, owner, officer, or committee member of the American Board of Orthopaedic Surgery, the American Orthopaedic Association, and ASTM International. Dr. K. Saleh or an immediate family member has received royalties from Aesculap/B. Braun; is a member of a speakers' bureau or has made paid presentations on behalf of Aesculap/B. Braun; serves as a paid consultant to or is an employee of Aesculap/B. Braun, the Memorial Medical Center Co-Management Orthopaedic Board, the Southern Illinois University School of Medicine, and Watermark Research Partners; has received research or institutional support from the NIH/NIAMS, the Orthopaedic Research and Education Foundation, and Smith & Nephew; and serves as a board member, owner, officer, or committee member of the American Academy of Orthopaedic Surgeons, the American Board of Orthopaedic Surgeons, the American Orthopaedic Association, the Board of Specialty Societies, Notify, and the Orthopaedic Research and Education Foundation. None of the following authors nor any immediate family member has received anything of value from or has stock or stock options held in a commercial company or institution related directly or indirectly to the subject of this chapter: Mr. Wright, Mr. Tzeng, Mr. Ginnetti, Dr. J. Saleh, and Dr. El-Othmani.

complications, smokers were found to have a higher risk of surgical site infections and dehiscence.[22] Smokers undergoing breast reduction surgery also have a significantly higher risk of perioperative infection.[23,24] Another set of studies determined that smokers had a significantly increased rate of skin flap necrosis and greater levels of digit replantation failure.[25,26] Smokers who underwent gastrointestinal surgery were found to have an increased risk for surgical site infection as well as a number of pulmonary complications, including pneumonia, failure to wean from a ventilator, and reintubation.[27] Wound complications, mediastinitis, respiratory distress syndrome, and heart attack are more likely to develop in smokers after undergoing cardiac surgery.[28-30]

Furthermore, smoking has anatomic-specific implications on outcomes after orthopaedic surgery, with a substantially increased risk for the development of wound complications. A recent study reported that 21% of patients who underwent total joint arthroplasty and in whom a perioperative infection developed were active smokers.[4] Moreover, smokers undergoing external skeletal fixation are reported to have a significantly higher rate of pin site infection.[31] Smokers have a substantially longer wound healing time after open reduction and internal fixation of calcaneal fractures.[32] Smoking also increases the risk for the development of an infection and the need for subsequent surgical intervention in patients with calcaneal fractures.[33] In addition, a retrospective study of patients undergoing surgery across all orthopaedic specialties reported that surgical site infections are 6.4 times more likely to develop in smokers than nonsmokers.[34]

Smokers also have impaired healing abilities in their tendons, ligaments, and cartilage. Clinical studies on the results of rotator cuff repairs report lower American Shoulder and Elbow Surgeons Subjective Shoulder Scale scores at 6-month follow-up and decreased mean improvement in University of California-Los Angeles Shoulder Rating Scale scores at 1-year follow-up for patients who smoke.[35] Smokers who underwent shoulder arthroscopy had almost twice the risk for the development of complications compared with nonsmokers.[36] It also was reported that smoking increases negative outcomes and subsequent revision surgery for patients who have glenoid labrum tears.[37] Smokers have a 7.5 times higher probability of a complete distal biceps tendon rupture than nonsmokers.[38] Smokers undergoing anterior cruciate ligament reconstruction have greater knee instability and worse functional outcomes compared with nonsmokers.[39] A statistical analysis by Amin et al[40] reported that smokers have a twofold greater risk for excessive cartilage loss at the medial tibiofemoral joint and the patellofemoral joint than nonsmokers. Clinical studies investigating the surgical repair of cartilage defects in the knee have found that smokers have significantly higher negative outcomes for chondrocyte implantation, débridement, and radiofrequency chondroplasty.[41-43]

Smoking and Bone Health

Tobacco use negatively affects multiple protective mechanisms of bone health, which results in decreased bone mineral density (BMD) and an increased risk of fractures.[44] The World Health Organization Fracture Risk Assessment Tool, an internationally validated method for determining the risk of fracture within

a 10-year timeframe, includes current tobacco use as one of only eight clinical risk factors that have an effect on overall fracture risk.[45]

High levels of nicotine, found in those who smoke more than or equal to one pack of cigarettes per day, may decrease osteoblast proliferation and osteocalcin synthesis, which can ultimately cause bone cell death.[46] Smoking decreases the function of aromatase and increases sex hormone-binding globulin levels, which can lead to a reduction in free levels of the bone-protective sex hormone, estrogen.[47] In patients with normal estrogen levels, osteocytes, osteoclasts, and osteoblasts inhibit bone remodeling, decrease bone resorption, and maintain bone density.[48] In addition, studies have determined that smokers have decreased levels of 25-hydroxycholecalciferol, 1,25-dihydroxycholecalciferol, and parathyroid hormone.[49] Low levels of active vitamin D and parathyroid hormone are correlated with decreased BMD, sarcopenia, and an increased fracture risk.[50,51] A substantial increase in the urinary N-telopeptide/creatinine ratio was reported in heavy smokers, which suggests another possible mechanism for the low BMD present in smokers.[52]

Smoking is the most important risk factor for the development of osteomyelitis after nonunion.[53] The risk for the development of osteomyelitis in open tibia fractures is 3.7 times higher in smokers than nonsmokers.[54] In a study of patients who underwent mandibular surgery, the most common cause of osteomyelitis was a current history of smoking.[55] Furthermore, 71% of failed procedures for patients who underwent limb salvage because of chronic osteomyelitis occurred in smokers.[56]

Smoking is significantly correlated with an increased risk for the development of spinal disorders. A retrospective study revealed that the relative risk for the development of lumbar disk disease and cervical disk disease is higher in smokers compared with nonsmokers.[57] In addition, current smokers are at a significantly higher risk for recurrent lumbar disk herniation.[58] Another study determined that the risk for the development of prolapsed disks is 20% higher in cigarette smokers than in nonsmokers.[59] Smokers also are statistically more likely to be hospitalized for surgical fixation of disk disorders than nonsmokers.[60]

Moreover, patients who smoke are at a higher risk for the development numerous negative outcomes after spine surgery. A retrospective case study of patients who underwent spinal fusion surgery found that pseudarthrosis developed in smokers 24 months after surgery at a rate five times higher than nonsmokers.[61] In a study of patients who underwent lumbar spinal fusion for the treatment of lumbar stenosis, compared with nonsmokers, smokers had higher dissatisfaction rates at 2-year follow-up, more regular use of analgesic agents, less improvement in walking ability, and a significantly inferior quality of life when measured with the Oswestry Low Back Pain Disability Questionnaire.[62] Smokers who undergo lumbar spine arthrodesis have higher nonunion rates than nonsmokers and a three times greater risk for nonunion than nonsmokers.[63] Smokers also have significantly higher rates of reoperation after spinal surgery compared with nonsmokers.[64]

The clinical effects of smoking on BMD vary in males and females. Specifically in males, smoking negatively affects BMD at all bone sites, especially the hip.[65] A population-based study of adult males reported that, in comparison with nonsmokers, smokers had a significantly lower BMD of the total body, lumbar spine, femoral neck, and greater trochanter.[66] When compared with age- and sex-matched nonsmokers, young males who smoke are reported to have a significantly impaired ability to generate bone mass, which leads to decreased peak bone mass.[67] In elderly men, a statistically increased risk of fracture is correlated, in a dose-response relationship, with the length of smoking history.[68] Specifically, smoking has been linked to an increased risk for osteoporotic fractures of the humerus, radius, pelvis, hip, and vertebrae.[69] In addition, a current history of smoking is attributed to one-half of all incurred fractures in men older than 65 years.[70]

Female smokers have been shown to have decreased BMD, increased fracture risk, and a higher incidence of osteoporosis.[71,72] A meta-analysis by Hermann et al[73] reported that smoking significantly reduces bone mass in the lumbar spine, femoral neck, and total body of young women. In an investigation of female twins, it was reported that the twin who smoked a pack of cigarettes per day during adulthood had a 5% to 10% lower BMD compared with the respective twin who was a nonsmoker.[74] Research has found that women who smoke reach menopause, on average, 1.74 years earlier than nonsmokers.[75] Furthermore, in a study of postmenopausal women, Bjarnason and Christiansen[76] reported that smokers have a 4% lower BMD than nonsmokers, and that the increase in smokers' serum estradiol levels during hormone replacement therapy is only one-half that of the increased serum estradiol levels of nonsmokers.

Smoking and Bone Union

The chemical composition of smoke negatively affects bone union after orthopaedic surgery.[77] Nicotine and carbon monoxide are believed to negatively affect bone growth because they decrease the level of available oxygen.[78] One study reported a 23.8% and 29% decrease in tissue oxygenation after a smoker inhaled a first cigarette and then a second cigarette, respectively.[25] Furthermore, the hypoxic effects of inhaling a single cigarette are reported to last for 30 to 50 minutes.[79] The amount of carbon monoxide and nicotine ingested by smokers who consume one pack of cigarettes per day induces a permanent hypoxic state in several peripheral tissues.[15] Smoking may also increase platelet aggregation, which can lead to thrombin formation and the further impairment of tissue oxygenation.[80]

The hypoxic effects of smoking negatively affect bone union after open fractures, which causes long-term impairments in functional outcomes.[81] In a retrospective study of patients with diaphyseal fractures of the femur, tibia, or humerus, smoking was reported to be the most significant negative predictor of bone healing.[82] Reoperation and implant failure rates for femur fractures are higher in patients who have a current history of tobacco use.[83,84] Similarly, smoking prolongs the time to achieve bone union and increases nonunion rates for open fractures of the humerus.[85]

In addition, smokers with tibial shaft fractures have an increased median time to clinical union.[86] In a review of patients who had open tibia fractures, Castillo et al[54] determined that smokers were 37% less likely than nonsmokers to achieve union after 24 months. Further investigation by Adams et al[87] suggested that patients with open tibia fractures who smoke are more likely than nonsmokers to require a bone graft to complete union. In addition, in a study of patients who received a composite bone graft to treat a nonunion fracture, Ziran et al[88] reported that only 67% of smokers achieved proper healing compared with 87% of nonsmokers.

Radiographic findings are currently considered the preferred method to diagnose nonunion; however, recent evidence suggests that certain molecules may also serve as predictors for nonunion.[89] A promising new biomarker for fracture healing, transforming growth factor β-1, has been reported to be significantly lower in smokers 4 weeks after open fracture surgery compared with nonsmokers.[90] It also has been reported that low serum osteocalcin levels are correlated with delayed bone healing.[91] Procollagen type I aminoterminal propeptide has been useful in measuring bone turnover and early stages of bone formation,[92] but despite its use as a diagnostic tool for fracture healing in Europe, it is not, at this time, used in the United States except for research purposes.[93]

Smoking and Pain

Recent literature links a current history of smoking with higher self-reported pain scores, both before and after surgery. In a nationally representative survey of 9,282 adults, respondents who reported themselves as current smokers were twice as likely to report having medically unexplained chronic back and neck pain within the past year than nonsmokers.[94] Smokers with spinal cord injuries who are exposed to nicotine have heightened complex neuropathic pain compared with nonsmokers who are exposed to nicotine.[95] In a study

examining the effects of smoking deprivation and pain, Pauli et al[96] reported that 12 hours of smoking cessation did not alter pain thresholds, but that smoking a cigarette during the same timeframe negatively affected pain thresholds. Research investigating patients before and after smoking a cigarette revealed that smoking increases trigeminal nerve pain processing at the supraspinal level.[97] In a study of previous smokers who were undergoing chemotherapy, Ditre et al[98] reported an inverse correlation between pain severity and the number of years smokers had abstained from smoking.

Smoking Cessation

Preoperative smoking cessation reduces perioperative complications.[99] A systematic review by Sørensen[100] determined that smoking cessation restores the tissue microenvironment and the inflammatory response within 4 weeks. A study of perioperative wound complications after head and neck surgery revealed a significant stepwise correlation between smoking cessation time before surgery and improvements in wound healing.[101] Patients who cease smoking more than 4 weeks before surgery have significantly better primary outcomes than patients who cease smoking less than 4 weeks before surgery, with each additional week of cessation reducing the relative risk of negative primary outcomes by 19%.[102] A systematic review by Wong et al[103] reported that the risk of wound complications for smokers who began a cessation intervention program remained constant until 3 to 4 weeks, at which point improvements became substantial. In a randomized trial conducted on patients who underwent surgery (hip or knee prosthesis, hernia repair, or laparoscopic cholecystectomy), an

intention-to-treat analysis revealed that the complication rate for smokers was 41%, whereas patients who started a cessation intervention program 4 weeks before surgery had a complication rate of 21%.[104] Smoking intervention initiated 6 to 8 weeks before knee or hip arthroplasty reduces the overall complication rate from 52% to 18%.[105] In a study investigating postoperative smoking cessation, Glassman et al[106] found that smoking cessation has statistically significant positive effects on primary outcomes for patients undergoing spinal fusion. In addition, when comparing pain scores for smokers to those who quit smoking before the treatment of spinal disorders, patients who quit smoking had significantly greater improvements in reported worst, current, and average weekly pain.[107] Pain also can serve as a barrier for smokers. A study by Zale et al[108] reported that smokers who experienced pain within the past month had more difficulty quitting smoking than smokers who did not experience pain in the past month.

For many patients, a negative aspect of smoking cessation is weight gain. Smoking causes increased energy expenditure in the peripheral tissues, which leads to an overall increased basal metabolic rate.[109] Smokers have been reported to have a 10% greater energy expenditure over a 24-hour period than nonsmokers.[110] For many smokers, the idea of gaining weight after smoking cessation may hinder participation in smoking cessation programs and overall success.[111] Smokers who have a low body mass index (BMI; below 18) have a greater probability of gaining weight after cessation than smokers who have a normal BMI.[112] Low BMI is associated with a poorer immunologic status and, therefore, worse surgical outcomes.[113]

In this specific patient population, however, smoking cessation may likely play a more considerable role in improving surgical outcomes.

Physician Involvement

Physician-led, preoperative smoking cessation intervention programs not only increase smoking cessation rates at the time of surgery, but also increase patient odds for attaining long-term smoking cessation.[114] Physicians may be concerned that confronting patients about their smoking habits and urging them to quit may cause them to seek treatment from another medical provider; however, a study by Rechtine et al[115] reported this to be an unfounded concern. Comparisons of intensive interventions (more than one meeting or phone call over several weeks) with brief interventions (one meeting or phone call or letter) revealed that patients who were involved in the intensive intervention had higher smoking cessation rates 12 months postoperatively.[116] A meta-analysis by Kottke et al[117] examined the differences among 108 intervention programs in relation to smoking cessation rates at 6 months and 12 months after the initiation of the intervention. The authors reported that the highest smoking cessation rates resulted from intervention programs that centered on face-to-face advice from a physician, intervention programs with multiple interactions, and intervention programs with the longest duration of contact.[117] In a study investigating the effectiveness of an intervention program, Ratner et al[118] reported that patients who participated in an intervention program were more likely to quit smoking preoperatively and to achieve higher abstinence rates 6 months postoperatively than patients

who did not participate in an intervention program. Although a greater motivation to quit smoking has been reported if physicians inform patients of the perioperative risks associated with tobacco use,[116,119] some patients report that the thought of smoking cessation is impossible when dealing with the stress of an impending surgery.[120]

In addition to personal intervention methods, physicians may also consider first-line pharmacotherapy to aid patients in preoperative smoking cessation.[119] Nicotine replacement therapy (NRT), most commonly in the form of chewing gum and transdermal nicotine patches, has been extensively used by individuals who attempt to quit smoking.[121] Chewing gum provides a 2-mg dose of nicotine per piece, and transdermal patches are manufactured to deliver 7 to 21 mg of nicotine over a 24-hour period.[122] Dosages of both chewing gum and patches should be based on the number of cigarettes a patient consumed daily, with patients who smoked more than or equal to one pack of cigarettes per day receiving the highest dose.[123] Relatively uncommon side effects of NRT include nausea, dizziness, vomiting, and heart palpitations.[124] Although NRT exposes patients to nicotine, exposure to nicotine alone leads to only moderate impairments in the inflammatory response and, clinically, does not negatively affect postoperative wound or tissue healing.[125]

Sustained-release bupropion (bupropion SR), a norepinephrine-dopamine reuptake inhibitor and nicotinic-acetylcholine receptor antagonist, is another pharmacologic option that can be used to reduce withdrawal symptoms.[126] Bupropion SR, which is safe for long-term treatment, usually takes approximately 1 week to reach maximal

effectiveness; therefore, a smoking cessation date needs to be established before beginning use.[127] The most common side effects of bupropion SR are rash, irritability, insomnia, dry mouth, headache, and tremors.[128] Bupropion SR, because of its availability, has been reported to be abused via nasal inhalation or intravenous injection, with individuals reporting increased energy and libido as well as adverse effects, such as seizures, paranoia, hallucinations, and tachycardia.[129]

Another pharmacologic alternative is varenicline, a drug that acts as a partial agonist to the $\alpha_4\beta_2$ nicotinic-acetylcholine receptors, which is used to decrease smoking satisfaction and reduce withdrawal symptoms.[130] Varenicline should be started 7 days before the determined smoking cessation date and should be administered on a titration schedule, reaching the maximal dose at day 7, to reduce adverse effects.[131] The most common side effects of varenicline are nausea, insomnia, headache, flatulence, and constipation.[132] The FDA has recently released a black-box warning for varenicline as a result of the increased risk for suicidal behavior, aggression, and depression.[133]

In a meta-analysis conducted on the effectiveness of NRT, bupropion SR, and varenicline, Wu et al[134] reported that, compared with placebo controls, all three interventions significantly improved smoking cessation rates at 3-month follow-up and at 1-year follow-up. Varenicline is more effective than bupropion SR in maintaining smoking cessation for the first 4 weeks, 44% versus 29.5%, respectively, and from weeks 9 to 52, 21.9% versus 16.1%, respectively.[135] In a study of long-term cessation rates after an 8-week course of varenicline versus NRT, Hsueh et al[136] reported that varenicline has a substantial advantage over NRT at 36-month follow-up. Varenicline, however, has only a modest advantage over NRT at 24-week follow-up.[137] Of the most popular NRT options, transdermal nicotine patches have higher smoking cessation rates at 6-month follow-up and 1-year follow-up compared with smoking cessation rates of chewing gum.[138] Furthermore, a study by Jorenby et al[139] reported that if NRT and bupropion SR are administered in combination, smoking cessation rates are higher at 7-week follow-up compared with the smoking cessation rates of the therapies individually.

Electronic cigarettes are rapidly gaining worldwide popularity among smokers to assist in smoking cessation.[140] In a Web-based survey administered to current and former cigarette smokers, Giovenco et al[141] reported that almost 50% of the survey respondents reported trying electronic cigarettes at least once. Although electronic cigarettes are not associated with second-hand smoke exposure and the multiple chemicals that are found in traditional cigarettes,[142] electronic cigarettes still increase the smoker's exposure to nicotine, with reports of delivery levels between 2 to 15 mg of inhaled nicotine per cartridge.[143]

Orthopaedic surgeons can help patients overcome the difficulties of smoking cessation and take charge of their own health by increasing patient activation. An activated patient is defined as a patient who has the confidence and knowledge necessary to understand his or her own current health and subsequently takes action to maintain and/or improve his or her condition.[144] In a study of more than 25,000 patients, Greene and Hibbard,[145] using patient activation measures, determined that patient activation is strongly related to improved patient outcomes and a decreased probability of smoking. In addition, patients who are activated are more likely to participate in physical therapy and have higher postoperative physical functional status scores.[146,147] Activated patients also are more likely to adhere to and be compliant with pharmacotherapy treatment plans.[148] Ultimately, activated patients have higher satisfaction with their health care and lower overall healthcare costs.[149]

Future Research

Although the current literature has provided physicians with an understanding of the effect of smoking on surgical outcomes and new interventional methods to improve cessation rates, further research is required to expand on this foundation. Recent studies have found a link between smoking and the risk for the development of perioperative osteomyelitis; however, because the studies lacked size and direct correlation, further exploration is necessary. Indirect intervention methods that can help improve smokers' perioperative outcomes also need to be investigated. For example, research in animal models has shown that hyperbaric oxygen therapy substantially decreases the risk for surgical site infection and improves fracture healing; however, these studies are mostly limited to animal models and need further follow up in human trials.[150,151] Preoperative smoking cessation has been shown to improve primary outcomes; however, the results need to be further investigated and duplicated. Finally, further research is needed to develop effective techniques that surgeons can use to improve patient activation because this is an excellent opportunity for improving primary outcomes.

Summary

The current literature demonstrates a substantial correlation between smoking and negative perioperative consequences involving wound and bone healing; BMD; infection rates; and cartilage, tendon, and ligament healing. Orthopaedic surgeons who guide interventions in smokers with upcoming surgeries, especially elective, need to have a thorough understanding of these negative perioperative consequences and the multiple ways to increase perioperative cessation rates in order to improve surgical outcomes and achieve greater patient satisfaction. Surgeons and other healthcare professionals should use surgery as an opportunity to activate patients in an effort to assist in long-term smoking cessation and reduce perioperative morbidity.

References

1. Sadr Azodi R, Bellocco R, Eriksson K, Adami J: The impact of tobacco use and body mass index on the length of stay in hospital and the risk of post-operative complications among patients undergoing total hip replacement. *J Bone Joint Surg Br* 2006;88(10):1316-1320.

2. Morton HJV: Tobacco smoking and pulmonary complications after operation. *Lancet* 1944;243(6290):368-370.

3. Masquelet AC: The dangers of peri-operative smoking in orthopaedic surgery. *European Instructional Lectures* 2014;14:17-23.

4. Pruzansky JS, Bronson MJ, Grelsamer RP, Strauss E, Moucha CS: Prevalence of modifiable surgical site infection risk factors in hip and knee joint arthroplasty patients at an urban academic hospital. *J Arthroplasty* 2014;29(2):272-276.

5. Truntzer J, Vopat B, Feldstein M, Matityahu A: Smoking cessation and

bone healing: Optimal cessation timing. *Eur J Orthop Surg Traumatol* 2015;25(2):211-215.

6. Jha P, Peto R: Global effects of smoking, of quitting, and of taxing tobacco. *N Engl J Med* 2014;370(1):60-68.

7. Peto R, Lopez AD: The future worldwide health effects of current smoking patterns, in Koop CE, Pearson CE, Schwarz MR, eds: *Critical Issues in Global Health*. San Francisco, CA, Wiley (Jossey-Bass), 2001, pp 154-161.

8. US Department of Health and Human Services: *The Health Consequences of Smoking—50 Years of Progress: A Report of the Surgeon General*. Atlanta, GA, US Department of Health and Human Services, Centers for Disease Control and Prevention, National Center for Chronic Disease Prevention and Heath Promotion, Office on Smoking and Health, 2014, pp 1-944.

9. Schnell S, Friedman SM, Mendelson DA, Bingham KW, Kates SL: The 1-year mortality of patients treated in a hip fracture program for elders. *Geriatr Orthop Surg Rehabil* 2010;1(1):6-14.

10. Whiteford L: Nicotine, CO and HCN: The detrimental effects of smoking on wound healing. *Br J Community Nurs* 2003;8(12):S22-S26.

11. Scolaro JA, Schenker ML, Yannascoli S, Baldwin K, Mehta S, Ahn J: Cigarette smoking increases complications following fracture: A systematic review. *J Bone Joint Surg Am* 2014;96(8):674-681.

12. Hadley MN, Reddy SV: Smoking and the human vertebral column: A review of the impact of cigarette use on vertebral bone metabolism and spinal fusion. *Neurosurgery* 1997;41(1):116-124.

13. McGehee DS, Heath MJ, Gelber S, Devay P, Role LW: Nicotine enhancement of fast excitatory synaptic transmission in CNS by presynaptic receptors. *Science* 1995;269(5231):1692-1696.

14. Sørensen LT, Nielsen HB, Kharazmi A, Gottrup F: Effect of smoking and abstention on oxidative burst and reactivity of neutrophils and monocytes. *Surgery* 2004;136(5):1047-1053.

15. Middleton ET, Morice AH: Breath carbon monoxide as an indication of smoking habit. *Chest* 2000;117(3):758-763.

16. Argintar E, Triantafillou K, Delahay J, Wiesel B: The musculoskeletal effects of perioperative smoking. *J Am Acad Orthop Surg* 2012;20(6):359-363.

17. Noble RC, Penny BB: Comparison of leukocyte count and function in smoking and nonsmoking young men. *Infect Immun* 1975;12(3):550-555.

18. Guo S, Dipietro LA: Factors affecting wound healing. *J Dent Res* 2010;89(3):219-229.

19. Carel RS, Tockman MS, Baser M: Smoking, leukocyte count, and ventilatory lung function in working men. *Chest* 1988;93(6):1137-1143.

20. Wong LS, Martins-Green M: First-hand cigarette smoke alters fibroblast migration and survival: Implications for impaired healing. *Wound Repair Regen* 2004;12(4):471-484.

21. Myles PS, Iacono GA, Hunt JO, et al: Risk of respiratory complications and wound infection in patients undergoing ambulatory surgery: Smokers versus nonsmokers. *Anesthesiology* 2002;97(4):842-847.

22. Sørensen LT: Wound healing and infection in surgery: The clinical impact of smoking and smoking cessation. A systematic review and meta-analysis. *Arch Surg* 2012;147(4):373-383.

23. Bikhchandani J, Varma SK, Henderson HP: Is it justified to refuse breast reduction to smokers? *J Plast Reconstr Aesthet Surg* 2007;60(9):1050-1054.

24. Schumacher HH: Breast reduction and smoking. *Ann Plast Surg* 2005;54(2):117-119.

25. van Adrichem LN, Hovius SE, van Strik R, van der Meulen JC: Acute effects of cigarette smoking on microcirculation of the thumb. *Br J Plast Surg* 1992;45(1):9-11.

26. Chang DW, Reece GP, Wang B, et al: Effect of smoking on complications in patients undergoing free TRAM flap breast reconstruction. *Plast Reconstr Surg* 2000;105(7):2374-2380.

27. Gajdos C, Hawn MT, Campagna EJ, Henderson WG, Singh JA, Houston T: Adverse effects of smoking on postoperative outcomes in cancer patients. *Ann Surg Oncol* 2012;19(5):1430-1438.

28. Christenson JT, Aeberhard JM, Badel P, et al: Adult respiratory distress syndrome after cardiac surgery. *Cardiovasc Surg* 1996;4(1):15-21.

29. Voors AA, van Brussel BL, Plokker HW, et al: Smoking and cardiac events after venous coronary bypass surgery: A 15-year follow-up study. *Circulation* 1996;93(1):42-47.

30. Abboud CS, Wey SB, Baltar VT: Risk factors for mediastinitis after cardiac surgery. *Ann Thorac Surg* 2004;77(2):676-683.

31. Sharma SK, Vati J, Wali I, Sen R: The effect of smoking on pin site infection rate among patients with external skeletal fixation. *Nursing and Midwifery Research Journal* 2008;4(2):68-71.

32. Abidi NA, Dhawan S, Gruen GS, Vogt MT, Conti SF: Wound-healing risk factors after open reduction and internal fixation of calcaneal fractures. *Foot Ankle Int* 1998;19(12):856-861.

33. Folk JW, Starr AJ, Early JS: Early wound complications of operative treatment of calcaneus fractures: Analysis of 190 fractures. *J Orthop Trauma* 1999;13(5):369-372.

34. Jain RK, Shukla R, Singh P, Kumar R: Epidemiology and risk factors for surgical site infections in patients requiring orthopedic surgery. *Eur J Orthop Surg Traumatol* 2015;25(2):251-254.

35. Mallon WJ, Misamore G, Snead DS, Denton P: The impact of preoperative smoking habits on the results of rotator cuff repair. *J Shoulder Elbow Surg* 2004;13(2):129-132.

36. Martin CT, Gao Y, Pugely AJ, Wolf BR: 30-day morbidity and mortality after elective shoulder arthroscopy: A review of 9410 cases. *J Shoulder Elbow Surg* 2013;22(12):1667-1675.e1.

37. Park MJ, Hsu JE, Harper C, Sennett BJ, Huffman GR: Poly-L/D-lactic acid anchors are associated with reoperation and failure of SLAP repairs. *Arthroscopy* 2011;27(10):1335-1340.

38. Safran MR, Graham SM: Distal biceps tendon ruptures: Incidence, demographics, and the effect of smoking. *Clin Orthop Relat Res* 2002;404:275-283.

© 2016 AAOS Instructional Course Lectures, Volume 65

39. Kim SJ, Lee SK, Kim SH, Kim SH, Ryu SW, Jung M: Effect of cigarette smoking on the clinical outcomes of ACL reconstruction. *J Bone Joint Surg Am* 2014;96(12):1007-1013.

40. Amin S, Niu J, Guermazi A, et al: Cigarette smoking and the risk for cartilage loss and knee pain in men with knee osteoarthritis. *Ann Rheum Dis* 2007;66(1):18-22.

41. Jaiswal PK, Macmull S, Bentley G, Carrington RW, Skinner JA, Briggs TW: Does smoking influence outcome after autologous chondrocyte implantation? A case-controlled study. *J Bone Joint Surg Br* 2009;91(12):1575-1578.

42. Spahn G, Kahl E, Mückley T, Hofmann GO, Klinger HM: Arthroscopic knee chondroplasty using a bipolar radiofrequency-based device compared to mechanical shaver: Results of a prospective, randomized, controlled study. *Knee Surg Sports Traumatol Arthrosc* 2008;16(6):565-573.

43. Kanneganti P, Harris JD, Brophy RH, Carey JL, Lattermann C, Flanigan DC: The effect of smoking on ligament and cartilage surgery in the knee: A systematic review. *Am J Sports Med* 2012;40(12):2872-2878.

44. Law MR, Hackshaw AK: A meta-analysis of cigarette smoking, bone mineral density and risk of hip fracture: Recognition of a major effect. *BMJ* 1997;315(7112):841-846.

45. Shuler FD, Conjeski J, Kendall D, Salava J: Understanding the burden of osteoporosis and use of the World Health Organization FRAX. *Orthopedics* 2012;35(9):798-805.

46. Rothem DE, Rothem L, Soudry M, Dahan A, Eliakim R: Nicotine modulates bone metabolism-associated gene expression in osteoblast cells. *J Bone Miner Metab* 2009;27(5):555-561.

47. Yoon V, Maalouf NM, Sakhaee K: The effects of smoking on bone metabolism. *Osteoporos Int* 2012;23(8):2081-2092.

48. Khosla S, Oursler MJ, Monroe DG: Estrogen and the skeleton. *Trends Endocrinol Metab* 2012;23(11):576-581.

49. Brot C, Jorgensen NR, Sorensen OH: The influence of smoking on vitamin D status and calcium metabolism. *Eur J Clin Nutr* 1999;53(12):920-926.

50. Wang TJ, Pencina MJ, Booth SL, et al: Vitamin D deficiency and risk of cardiovascular disease. *Circulation* 2008;117(4):503-511.

51. Visser M, Deeg DJ, Lips P; Longitudinal Aging Study Amsterdam: Low vitamin D and high parathyroid hormone levels as determinants of loss of muscle strength and muscle mass (sarcopenia): The Longitudinal Aging Study Amsterdam. *J Clin Endocrinol Metab* 2003;88(12):5766-5772.

52. Rapuri PB, Gallagher JC, Balhorn KE, Ryschon KL: Smoking and bone metabolism in elderly women. *Bone* 2000;27(3):429-436.

53. Hogan A, Heppert VG, Suda AJ: Osteomyelitis. *Arch Orthop Trauma Surg* 2013;133(9):1183-1196.

54. Castillo RC, Bosse MJ, MacKenzie EJ, Patterson BM; LEAP Study Group: Impact of smoking on fracture healing and risk of complications in limb-threatening open tibia fractures. *J Orthop Trauma* 2005;19(3):151-157.

55. Calhoun KH, Shapiro RD, Stiernberg CM, Calhoun JH, Mader JT: Osteomyelitis of the mandible. *Arch Otolaryngol Head Neck Surg* 1988;114(10):1157-1162.

56. Siegel HJ, Patzakis MJ, Holtom PD, Sherman R, Shepherd L: Limb salvage for chronic tibial osteomyelitis: An outcomes study. *J Trauma* 2000;48(3):484-489.

57. An HS, Silveri CP, Simpson JM, et al: Comparison of smoking habits between patients with surgically confirmed herniated lumbar and cervical disc disease and controls. *J Spinal Disord* 1994;7(5):369-373.

58. Miwa S, Yokogawa A, Kobayashi T, et al: Risk factors of recurrent lumbar disc herniation: A single center study and review of the literature. *J Spinal Disord Tech* 2015;28(5):E265-E269.

59. Kelsey JL, Githens PB, O'Conner T, et al: Acute prolapsed lumbar intervertebral disc: An epidemiologic study with special reference to driving automobiles and cigarette smoking. *Spine (Phila Pa 1976)* 1984;9(6):608-613.

60. Kaila-Kangas L, Leino-Arjas P, Riihimäki H, Luukkonen R, Kirjonen J: Smoking and overweight as predictors of hospitalization for back disorders. *Spine (Phila Pa 1976)* 2003;28(16):1860-1868.

61. Brown CW, Orme TJ, Richardson HD: The rate of pseudoarthrosis (surgical nonunion) in patients who are smokers and patients who are nonsmokers: A comparison study. *Spine (Phila Pa 1976)* 1986;11(9):942-943.

62. Sandén B, Försth P, Michaëlsson K: Smokers show less improvement than nonsmokers two years after surgery for lumbar spinal stenosis: A study of 4555 patients from the Swedish spine register. *Spine (Phila Pa 1976)* 2011;36(13):1059-1064.

63. Stephens BF, Murphy GA, Mihalko WM: The effects of nutritional deficiencies, smoking, and systemic disease on orthopaedic outcomes. *Instr Course Lect* 2014;63:393-399.

64. Mok JM, Cloyd JM, Bradford DS, et al: Reoperation after primary fusion for adult spinal deformity: Rate, reason, and timing. *Spine (Phila Pa 1976)* 2009;34(8):832-839.

65. Ward KD, Klesges RC: A meta-analysis of the effects of cigarette smoking on bone mineral density. *Calcif Tissue Int* 2001;68(5):259-270.

66. Lorentzon M, Mellström D, Haug E, Ohlsson C: Smoking is associated with lower bone mineral density and reduced cortical thickness in young men. *J Clin Endocrinol Metab* 2007;92(2):497-503.

67. Rudäng R, Darelid A, Nilsson M, et al: Smoking is associated with impaired bone mass development in young adult men: A 5-year longitudinal study. *J Bone Miner Res* 2012;27(10):2189-2197.

68. McCloskey E, Johansson H, Oden A, Kanis JA: Fracture risk assessment. *Clin Biochem* 2012;45(12):887-893.

69. Jutberger H, Lorentzon M, Barrett-Connor E, et al: Smoking predicts incident fractures in elderly men: Mr OS Sweden. *J Bone Miner Res* 2010;25(5):1010-1016.

70. Olofsson H, Byberg L, Mohsen R, Melhus H, Lithell H, Michaëlsson K: Smoking and the risk of fracture in older men. *J Bone Miner Res* 2005;20(7):1208-1215.

71. Høidrup S, Prescott E, Sørensen TI, et al: Tobacco smoking and risk of hip fracture in men and women. *Int J Epidemiol* 2000;29(2):253-259.

72. Oncken C, Prestwood K, Kleppinger A, Wang Y, Cooney J, Raisz L: Impact of smoking cessation on bone mineral density in postmenopausal women. *J Womens Health (Larchmt)* 2006;15(10):1141-1150.

73. Hermann AP, Brot C, Gram J, Kolthoff N, Mosekilde L: Premenopausal smoking and bone density in 2015 perimenopausal women. *J Bone Miner Res* 2000;15(4):780-787.

74. Abate M, Vanni D, Pantalone A, Salini V: Cigarette smoking and musculoskeletal disorders. *Muscles Ligaments Tendons J* 2013;3(2):63-69.

75. McKinlay SM, Bifano NL, McKinlay JB: Smoking and age at menopause in women. *Ann Intern Med* 1985;103(3):350-356.

76. Bjarnason NH, Christiansen C: The influence of thinness and smoking on bone loss and response to hormone replacement therapy in early postmenopausal women. *J Clin Endocrinol Metab* 2000;85(2):590-596.

77. Al-Hadithy N, Sewell MD, Bhavikatti M, Gikas PD: The effect of smoking on fracture healing and on various orthopaedic procedures. *Acta Orthop Belg* 2012;78(3):285-290.

78. Santiago-Torres J, Flanigan DC, Butler RB, Bishop JY: The effect of smoking on rotator cuff and glenoid labrum surgery: A systematic review. *Am J Sports Med* 2015;43(3):745-751.

79. Jensen JA, Goodson WH, Hopf HW, Hunt TK: Cigarette smoking decreases tissue oxygen. *Arch Surg* 1991;126(9):1131-1134.

80. Padmavathi P, Reddy VD, Maturu P, Varadacharyulu N: Smoking-induced alterations in platelet membrane fluidity and Na(+)/K(+)-ATPase activity in chronic cigarette smokers. *J Atheroscler Thromb* 2010;17(6):619-627.

81. Moghaddam A, Zimmermann G, Hammer K, Bruckner T, Grützner PA, von Recum J: Cigarette smoking influences the clinical and occupational outcome of patients with tibial shaft fractures. *Injury* 2011;42(12):1435-1442.

82. Hernigou J, Schuind F: Smoking as a predictor of negative outcome in diaphyseal fracture healing. *Int Orthop* 2013;37(5):883-887.

83. Ricci WM, Streubel PN, Morshed S, Collinge CA, Nork SE, Gardner MJ: Risk factors for failure of locked plate fixation of distal femur fractures: An analysis of 335 cases. *J Orthop Trauma* 2014;28(2):83-89.

84. Evanson BJ, Mullis BH, Anglen JO: Nonunion of a pertrochanteric femur fracture due to a low-velocity gunshot. *Am J Orthop (Belle Mead NJ)* 2011;40(1):E5-E9.

85. Murray IR, Amin AK, White TO, Robinson CM: Proximal humeral fractures: Current concepts in classification, treatment and outcomes. *J Bone Joint Surg Br* 2011;93(1):1-11.

86. Schmitz MA, Finnegan M, Natarajan R, Champine J: Effect of smoking on tibial shaft fracture healing. *Clin Orthop Relat Res* 1999;365:184-200.

87. Adams CI, Keating JF, Court-Brown CM: Cigarette smoking and open tibial fractures. *Injury* 2001;32(1):61-65.

88. Ziran BH, Hendi P, Smith WR, Westerheide K, Agudelo JF: Osseous healing with a composite of allograft and demineralized bone matrix: Adverse effects of smoking. *Am J Orthop (Belle Mead NJ)* 2007;36(4):207-209.

89. Pountos I, Georgouli T, Pneumaticos S, Giannoudis PV: Fracture nonunion: Can biomarkers predict outcome? *Injury* 2013;44(12):1725-1732.

90. Moghaddam A, Weiss S, Wölfl CG, et al: Cigarette smoking decreases TGF-b1 serum concentrations after long bone fracture. *Injury* 2010;41(10):1020-1025.

91. Oni OO, Mahabir JP, Iqbal SJ, Gregg PJ: Serum osteocalcin and total alkaline phosphatase levels as prognostic indicators in tibial shaft fractures. *Injury* 1989;20(1):37-38.

92. Ivaska KK, Gerdhem P, Akesson K, Garnero P, Obrant KJ: Effect of fracture on bone turnover markers: A longitudinal study comparing marker levels before and after injury in 113 elderly women. *J Bone Miner Res* 2007;22(8):1155-1164.

93. Coulibaly MO, Sietsema DL, Burgers TA, Mason J, Williams BO, Jones CB: Recent advances in the use of serological bone formation markers to monitor callus development and fracture healing. *Crit Rev Eukaryot Gene Expr* 2010;20(2):105-127.

94. Ditre JW, Brandon TH, Zale EL, Meagher MM: Pain, nicotine, and smoking: Research findings and mechanistic considerations. *Psychol Bull* 2011;137(6):1065-1093.

95. Richardson EJ, Richards JS, Stewart CC, Ness TJ: Effects of nicotine on spinal cord injury pain: A randomized, double-blind, placebo controlled crossover trial. *Top Spinal Cord Inj Rehabil* 2012;18(2):101-105.

96. Pauli P, Rau H, Zhuang P, Brody S, Birbaumer N: Effects of smoking on thermal pain threshold in deprived and minimally-deprived habitual smokers. *Psychopharmacology (Berl)* 1993;111(4):472-476.

97. Holle D, Heber A, Naegel S, Diener HC, Katsarava Z, Obermann M: Influences of smoking and caffeine consumption on trigeminal pain processing. *J Headache Pain* 2014;15(1):39.

98. Ditre JW, Gonzalez BD, Simmons VN, Faul LA, Brandon TH, Jacobsen PB: Associations between pain and current smoking status among cancer patients. *Pain* 2011;152(1):60-65.

99. Cavichio BV, Pompeo DA, Oller GA, Rossi LA: Duration of smoking cessation for the prevention of surgical wound healing complications. *Rev Esc Enferm USP* 2014;48(1):174-180.

100. Sørensen LT: Wound healing and infection in surgery: The pathophysiological impact of smoking, smoking cessation, and nicotine replacement therapy. A systematic review. *Ann Surg* 2012;255(6):1069-1079.

101. Kuri M, Nakagawa M, Tanaka H, Hasuo S, Kishi Y: Determination of the duration of preoperative smoking cessation to improve wound healing after head and neck surgery. *Anesthesiology* 2005;102(5):892-896.

102. Mills E, Eyawo O, Lockhart I, Kelly S, Wu P, Ebbert JO: Smoking cessation reduces postoperative complications: A systematic review and meta-analysis. *Am J Med* 2011;124(2):144-154.e8.

103. Wong J, Lam DP, Abrishami A, Chan MT, Chung F: Short-term preoperative smoking cessation and postoperative complications: A systematic review and meta-analysis. *Can J Anaesth* 2012;59(3):268-279.

104. Lindström D, Sadr Azodi O, Wladis A, et al: Effects of a perioperative smoking cessation intervention on postoperative complications: A randomized trial. *Ann Surg* 2008;248(5):739-745.

105. Møller AM, Villebro N, Pedersen T, Tønnesen H: Effect of preoperative smoking intervention on postoperative complications: A randomised clinical trial. *Lancet* 2002;359(9301):114-117.

106. Glassman SD, Anagnost SC, Parker A, Burke D, Johnson JR, Dimar JR: The effect of cigarette smoking and smoking cessation on spinal fusion. *Spine (Phila Pa 1976)* 2000;25(20):2608-2615.

107. Behrend C, Prasarn M, Coyne E, Horodyski M, Wright J, Rechtine GR: Smoking cessation related to improved patient-reported pain scores following spinal care. *J Bone Joint Surg Am* 2012;94(23):2161-2166.

108. Zale EL, Ditre JW, Dorfman ML, Heckman BW, Brandon TH: Smokers in pain report lower confidence and greater difficulty quitting. *Nicotine Tob Res* 2014;16(9):1272-1276.

109. Audrain-McGovern J, Benowitz NL: Cigarette smoking, nicotine, and body weight. *Clin Pharmacol Ther* 2011;90(1):164-168.

110. Hofstetter A, Schutz Y, Jéquier E, Wahren J: Increased 24-hour energy expenditure in cigarette smokers. *N Engl J Med* 1986;314(2):79-82.

111. Meyers AW, Klesges RC, Winders SE, Ward KD, Peterson BA, Eck LH: Are weight concerns predictive of smoking cessation? A prospective analysis. *J Consult Clin Psychol* 1997;65(3):448-452.

112. Lycett D, Munafò M, Johnstone E, Murphy M, Aveyard P: Weight change over eight years in relation to alcohol consumption in a cohort of continuing smokers and quitters. *Nicotine Tob Res* 2011;13(11):1149-1154.

113. Okamura Y, Maeda A, Matsunaga K, Kanemoto H, Uesaka K: Negative impact of low body mass index on surgical outcomes after hepatectomy for hepatocellular carcinoma. *J Hepatobiliary Pancreat Sci* 2012;19(4):449-457.

114. Møller A, Villebro N: Interventions for preoperative smoking cessation. *Cochrane Database Syst Rev* 2005;3:CD002294.

115. Rechtine GR II, Frawley W, Castellvi A, Gowski A, Chrin AM: Effect of the spine practitioner on patient smoking status. *Spine (Phila Pa 1976)* 2000;25(17):2229-2233.

116. Thomsen T, Tønnesen H, Møller AM: Effect of preoperative smoking cessation interventions on postoperative complications and smoking cessation. *Br J Surg* 2009;96(5):451-461.

117. Kottke TE, Battista RN, DeFriese GH, Brekke ML: Attributes of successful smoking cessation interventions in medical practice: A meta-analysis of 39 controlled trials. *JAMA* 1988;259(19):2883-2889.

118. Ratner PA, Johnson JL, Richardson CG, et al: Efficacy of a smoking-cessation intervention for elective-surgical patients. *Res Nurs Health* 2004;27(3):148-161.

119. Thomsen T, Villebro N, Møller AM: Interventions for preoperative smoking cessation. *Cochrane Database Syst Rev* 2014;3:CD002294.

120. Warner DO, Patten CA, Ames SC, Offord K, Schroeder D: Smoking behavior and perceived stress in cigarette smokers undergoing elective surgery. *Anesthesiology* 2004;100(5):1125-1137.

121. Stead LF, Perera R, Bullen C, Mant D, Lancaster T: Nicotine replacement therapy for smoking cessation. *Cochrane Database Syst Rev* 2008;1:CD000146.

122. Silagy C, Lancaster T, Stead L, Mant D, Fowler G: Nicotine replacement therapy for smoking cessation. *Cochrane Database Syst Rev* 2004;3:CD000146.

123. Herman AI, Sofuoglu M: Comparison of available treatments for tobacco addiction. *Curr Psychiatry Rep* 2010;12(5):433-440.

124. Tonstad S, Gustavsson G, Kruse E, Walmsley JM, Westin Å: Symptoms of nicotine toxicity in subjects achieving high cotinine levels during nicotine replacement therapy. *Nicotine Tob Res* 2014;16(9):1266-1271.

125. Sørensen LT, Jorgensen LN, Zillmer R, Vange J, Hemmingsen U, Gottrup F: Transdermal nicotine patch enhances type I collagen synthesis in abstinent smokers. *Wound Repair Regen* 2006;14(3):247-251.

126. Jorenby DE, Hays JT, Rigotti NA, et al: Efficacy of varenicline, an alpha4beta2 nicotinic acetylcholine receptor partial agonist, vs placebo or sustained-release bupropion for smoking cessation: A randomized controlled trial. *JAMA* 2006;296(1):56-63.

127. Haustein KO: Bupropion: Pharmacological and clinical profile in smoking cessation. *Int J Clin Pharmacol Ther* 2003;41(2):56-66.

128. Woolacott NF, Jones L, Forbes CA, et al: The clinical effectiveness and cost-effectiveness of bupropion and nicotine replacement therapy for smoking cessation: A systematic review and economic evaluation. *Health Technol Assess* 2002;6(16):1-245.

129. Paillet-Loilier M, Cesbron A, Le Boisselier R, Bourgine J, Debruyne D: Emerging drugs of abuse: Current perspectives on substituted cathinones. *Subst Abuse Rehabil* 2014;5:37-52.

130. Garrison GD, Dugan SE: Varenicline: A first-line treatment option for smoking cessation. *Clin Ther* 2009;31(3):463-491.

131. Kaur K, Kaushal S, Chopra SC: Varenicline for smoking cessation: A review of the literature. *Curr Ther Res Clin Exp* 2009;70(1):35-54.

132. Oncken C, Gonzales D, Nides M, et al: Efficacy and safety of the novel selective nicotinic acetylcholine receptor partial agonist, varenicline, for smoking cessation. *Arch Intern Med* 2006;166(15):1571-1577.

133. Moore TJ, Singh S, Furberg CD: The FDA and new safety warnings. *Arch Intern Med* 2012;172(1):78-80.

134. Wu P, Wilson K, Dimoulas P, Mills EJ: Effectiveness of smoking cessation therapies: A systematic review and meta-analysis. *BMC Public Health* 2006;6:300.

135. Gonzales D, Rennard SI, Nides M, et al: Varenicline, an alpha4beta2 nicotinic acetylcholine receptor partial agonist, vs sustained-release bupropion and placebo for smoking cessation: A randomized controlled trial. *JAMA* 2006;296(1):47-55.

136. Hsueh KC, Hsueh SC, Chou MY, et al: Varenicline versus transdermal nicotine patch: A 3-year follow-up in a smoking cessation clinic in Taiwan. *Psychopharmacology (Berl)* 2014;231(14):2819-2823.

137. Cahill K, Stead LF, Lancaster T: Nicotine receptor partial agonists for smoking cessation. *Cochrane Database Syst Rev* 2012;4:CD006103.

138. Eisenberg MJ, Filion KB, Yavin D, et al: Pharmacotherapies for smoking cessation: A meta-analysis of randomized controlled trials. *CMAJ* 2008;179(2):135-144.

139. Jorenby DE, Leischow SJ, Nides MA, et al: A controlled trial of sustained-release bupropion, a nicotine patch, or both for smoking cessation. *N Engl J Med* 1999;340(9):685-691.

140. King BA, Patel R, Nguyen KH, Dube SR: Trends in awareness and use of electronic cigarettes among U.S. adults, 2010-2013. *Nicotine Tob Res* 2015;17(2):219-227.

141. Giovenco DP, Lewis MJ, Delnevo CD: Factors associated with e-cigarette use: A national population survey of current and former smokers. *Am J Prev Med* 2014;47(4):476-480.

142. McAuley TR, Hopke PK, Zhao J, Babaian S: Comparison of the effects of e-cigarette vapor and cigarette smoke on indoor air quality. *Inhal Toxicol* 2012;24(12):850-857.

143. Goniewicz ML, Hajek P, McRobbie H: Nicotine content of electronic cigarettes, its release in vapour and its consistency across batches: Regulatory implications. *Addiction* 2014;109(3):500-507.

144. Hibbard JH, Stockard J, Mahoney ER, Tusler M: Development of the Patient Activation Measure (PAM): Conceptualizing and measuring activation in patients and consumers. *Health Serv Res* 2004;39(4 pt 1):1005-1026.

145. Greene J, Hibbard JH: Why does patient activation matter? An examination of the relationships between patient activation and health-related outcomes. *J Gen Intern Med* 2012;27(5):520-526.

146. Mosen DM, Schmittdiel J, Hibbard J, Sobel D, Remmers C, Bellows J: Is patient activation associated with outcomes of care for adults with chronic conditions? *J Ambul Care Manage* 2007;30(1):21-29.

147. Skolasky RL, Mackenzie EJ, Wegener ST, Riley LH III: Patient activation and adherence to physical therapy in persons undergoing spine surgery. *Spine (Phila Pa 1976)* 2008;33(21):E784-E791.

148. Marshall R, Beach MC, Saha S, et al: Patient activation and improved outcomes in HIV-infected patients. *J Gen Intern Med* 2013;28(5):668-674.

149. Hibbard JH, Greene J: What the evidence shows about patient activation: Better health outcomes and care experiences; fewer data on costs. *Health Aff (Millwood)* 2013;32(2):207-214.

150. Demirtaş A, Azboy I, Bulut M, et al: The effect of hyperbaric oxygen therapy on fracture healing in nicotinized rats. *Ulus Travma Acil Cerrahi Derg* 2014;20(3):161-166.

151. Demirtas A, Azboy I, Bulut M, Ucar BY, Alabalik U, Ilgezdi S: Effect of hyperbaric oxygen therapy on healing in an experimental model of degloving injury in tails of nicotine-treated rats. *J Hand Surg Eur Vol* 2013;38(4):405-411.

Effect of Vitamin D on Joint Replacement Outcomes

Michael Ginnetti, BSc
Mouhanad M. El-Othmani, MD
Erik Wright, BS
Tony H. Tzeng, BS
Jasmine Saleh, MD
J.M. Lane, MD
William M. Mihalko, MD, PhD
Khaled J. Saleh, BSc, MD, MSc, FRCSC, MHCM

Abstract

Vitamin D is a steroid hormone that affects not only bone metabolism and strength but also a variety of musculoskeletal health and surgical outcomes that are relevant to orthopaedic medicine. Risk factors for vitamin D deficiency include sex, age, skin pigmentation, obesity, and preexisting conditions such as nephritic syndrome and malabsorption syndrome. Furthermore, vitamin D deficiency is associated with the development of postoperative complications, such as an increased risk of infection, morbidity, and mortality. The standardization of vitamin D terminology as well as a thorough understanding of the medical considerations associated with vitamin D deficiency can improve preoperative planning and clearance, and, ultimately, patient outcomes and satisfaction.

Instr Course Lect 2016;65:521–530.

Background

Vitamin D is a steroid hormone that is traditionally known to prevent and cure rickets.[1] Recent research suggests that the effects of vitamin D extend to a variety of organ systems and disease processes beyond calcium absorption and bone metabolism.[2,3] Adequate levels of vitamin D are associated with good musculoskeletal health, proper immune system function, and improved surgical outcomes—all of which are important in the field of orthopaedic surgery.[4-6]

Despite their importance, vitamin D levels often are underestimated or not evaluated in surgical patients.[7] Hypovitaminosis D, the accepted term for insufficient or deficient levels of vitamin D, is a prevalent condition that affects an estimated one billion people worldwide.[8,9] In the United States, 30% to 50% of children and adults are vitamin D deficient, with higher rates of vitamin D deficiency occurring in females and minorities.[10-13] Furthermore, a recent study comparing US population trends in vitamin D insufficiency from 1988 to 1994 with those from 2001 to 2004 found that the average vitamin D level per person has decreased, which suggests that hypovitaminosis D is rising.[14]

It is critical for surgeons to have an increased awareness of hypovitaminosis D and its effects on surgical outcomes.[7] Management of hypovitaminosis D has traditionally been confined to the primary care physician; however, in recent years, orthopaedic surgeons have placed a greater emphasis on hypovitaminosis D management.[15] Because of their increased role in the management of vitamin D deficiency, it is essential that orthopaedic surgeons understand the basic concepts related to vitamin D metabolism, the risk factors and prevalence of vitamin D deficiency, and the effects

Table 1

Dietary Sources of Vitamin D

Source	Vitamin D Content (IU)
Cod liver oil, 1 tbsp	1360
Sockeye salmon (raw), 3 oz	375
Bluefin tuna (raw), 3 oz	193
Atlantic sardines (canned in oil), 3 oz	164
Fortified 2% milk, 8 oz	98
Large egg (raw)	41
Shiitake mushrooms (raw), 3 oz	15
Cheddar cheese, 1 oz	7

Data from the United States Department of Agriculture, Agricultural Research Service, Nutrient Data Laboratory: United States Department of Agriculture National Nutrient Database for Standard Reference, Release 27. August 2014. Available at: www.ars.usda.gov/nutrientdata. Accessed August 21, 2015.

of vitamin D levels on orthopaedic surgery outcomes.

Vitamin D Metabolism

The term vitamin D is generally used to describe ergocalciferol (vitamin D_2) and cholecalciferol (vitamin D_3), but it also can be used to refer to 25-hydroxyvitamin D or 1,25-dihydroxyvitamin D, which are the hydroxylated forms of vitamin D_3.[9,16] Vitamin D is primarily obtained from exposure to sunlight, which converts 7-dehydrocholesterol to previtamin D_3 and then isomerizes to vitamin D_3.[3] Vitamin D also can be obtained from dietary sources and oral vitamin D_2 or vitamin D_3 supplements.[16] The primary natural dietary sources of vitamin D include cod liver oil, salmon, tuna, mushrooms, and fortified breakfast cereals and dairy products[13] (**Table 1**).

Vitamin D obtained from exposure to sunlight or dietary sources and supplements is either taken up by adipose tissue for storage or metabolized in the liver into 25-hydroxyvitamin D.[2,17] Metabolically inactive 25-hydroxyvitamin D is the major circulating form of vitamin D and is generally used to determine a patient's vitamin D levels.[18,19] Eighty-five percent to 90% of the circulating 25-hydroxyvitamin D is bound to vitamin D–binding protein, 10% to 15% is bound to albumin, and less than 1% exists in a free unbound form.[20-22] 25-hydroxyvitamin D is converted in the kidney into 1,25-dihydroxyvitamin D—the metabolically active form of vitamin D—by renal 25-hydroxyvitamin D-1α-hydroxylase.[19,23] The activity of renal 25-hydroxyvitamin D-1α-hydroxylase and, thereby, the production of 1,25-dihydroxyvitamin D is regulated by parathyroid hormone, fibroblast growth factor 23, and circulating 1,25-dihydroxyvitamin D.[24]

Activated vitamin D exerts its metabolic effect through a vitamin D receptor (VDR), which is a nuclear receptor protein that contains 427 amino acids.[19] The binding of 1,25-dihydroxyvitamin D to the VDR facilitates the formation of a heterodimer with a retinoic acid receptor.[2] The binding of the VDR-retinoic acid receptor heterodimer to specific DNA sequences—known as vitamin D response elements—upregulates transcription of the target genes through interactions with various transcription factors.[2]

Vitamin D Measurement

Various techniques, such as competitive vitamin D protein binding assay, radioimmunoassay, and high-performance liquid chromatography, can be used to determine a patient's serum 25-hydroxyvitamin D levels.[25] These techniques generally measure total 25-hydroxyvitamin D levels versus free 25-hydroxyvitamin D

Dr. Lane or an immediate family member serves as a paid consultant to or is an employee of Bone Therapeutics, CollPlant, and Graftys; has received research or institutional support from Merck; has stock or stock options held in DFINE and CollPlant; and serves as a board member, owner, officer, or committee member of the American Academy of Orthopaedic Surgeons, the Association of Bone and Joint Surgeons, the American Orthopaedic Association, the American Society for Bone Mineral Research, the Musculoskeletal Tumor Society, and the Orthopaedic Research Society. Dr. Mihalko or an immediate family member has received royalties from Aesculap/B. Braun; is a member of a speakers' bureau or has made paid presentations on behalf of Aesculap/B. Braun; serves as a paid consultant to or is an employee of Aesculap/B. Braun and Medtronic; has received research or institutional support from Aesculap/B. Braun, Smith & Nephew, and Stryker; and serves as a board member, owner, officer, or committee member of the American Board of Orthopaedic Surgery, the American Orthopaedic Association, and ASTM International. Dr. K. Saleh or an immediate family member has received royalties from Aesculap/B. Braun; is a member of a speakers' bureau or has made paid presentations on behalf of Aesculap/B. Braun; serves as a paid consultant to or is an employee of Aesculap/B. Braun, the Memorial Medical Center Co-Management Orthopaedic Board, the Southern Illinois University School of Medicine, and Watermark Research Partners; has received research or institutional support from the National Institutes of Health/National Institute of Arthritis and Musculoskeletal and Skin Diseases, the Orthopaedic Research and Education Foundation, and Smith & Nephew; and serves as a board member, owner, officer, or committee member of the American Academy of Orthopaedic Surgeons, the American Board of Orthopaedic Surgeons, the American Orthopaedic Association, the Board of Specialty Societies, Notify, and the Orthopaedic Research and Education Foundation. None of the following authors nor any immediate family member has received anything of value from or has stock or stock options held in a commercial company or institution related directly or indirectly to the subject of this chapter: Mr. Ginnetti, Dr. El-Othmani, Mr. Wright, Mr. Tzeng, and Dr. J. Saleh.

levels.[26] Because a substantial portion of the circulating 25-hydroxyvitamin D is bound to vitamin D–binding protein, decreased levels of this protein may result in decreased levels of 25-hydroxyvitamin D.[20,22] Lower vitamin D–binding protein levels can be a result of genetic factors, such as polymorphisms in the vitamin D–binding protein gene, which are highly prevalent among African Americans,[26] as well as acquired pathologic conditions, such as liver and renal diseases.[20] Current assays may underestimate the vitamin D levels of these patient populations because their total 25-hydroxyvitamin D levels are decreased, but their free, bioavailable 25-hydroxyvitamin D levels are within normal range.[20,26] In addition, substantial variability exists among the results reported from different assays and laboratories; this lack of standardization for reporting vitamin D measurements should be considered in cases in which the vitamin D levels of patients are being evaluated.[27-29]

Hypovitaminosis D generally refers to insufficient or deficient levels of vitamin D;[9] however, there are conflicting opinions on the thresholds for vitamin D deficiency, insufficiency, and sufficiency. Although it is not uncommon for 10 ng/mL or 15 ng/mL to be the threshold for vitamin D deficiency, most experts define vitamin D deficiency as 25-hydroxyvitamin D levels less than 20 ng/mL.[8,30,31] There is less consensus on what constitutes optimal levels of vitamin D.[8] The Institute of Medicine defines vitamin D sufficiency as 25-hydroxyvitamin D levels greater than 20 ng/mL;[16] however, it has been suggested that this threshold may be low. At levels less than 29.8 ng/mL, 25-hydroxyvitamin D concentration is negatively correlated with serum parathyroid hormone levels.[32] Furthermore, in a study examining intestinal calcium transport, it was reported that women who had 25-hydroxyvitamin D levels of 32 ng/mL had a 65% increase in calcium absorption compared with women who had 25-hydroxyvitamin D levels of 20 ng/mL.[33] These findings, among others, have led experts to suggest that a sufficient level of vitamin D is greater than 30 ng/mL, with levels less than 30 ng/mL qualifying as insufficiency and levels less than 20 ng/mL indicating deficiency.[8,34]

Hypovitaminosis D in Orthopaedics
Epidemiology
A high prevalence of hypovitaminosis D has been established in orthopaedic patients. A study by Bogunovic et al[35] reported that 40% of all patients who underwent orthopaedic surgery were vitamin D deficient. The authors also reported that the trauma service had the highest prevalence rates of hypovitaminosis D, with 61% of patients who were vitamin D deficient.[35] In patients undergoing total hip arthroplasty, the prevalence rates for hypovitaminosis D were reported to range from 46.6% to 65%.[6,36] Another study reported that 24% of patients who underwent total hip arthroplasty had vitamin D levels less than 15 ng/mL.[37] Hypovitaminosis D also is highly prevalent in patients who experience back pain. A study by Al Faraj and Al Mutairi[38] reported that 83% of patients with chronic back pain had 25-hydroxyvitamin D levels less than 9 ng/mL. Similarly, preoperative testing of patients who underwent spinal fusion surgery identified that 57% of patients were vitamin D insufficient.[39] A study by Davies et al[40] reported that 32% of pediatric orthopaedic patients were vitamin D deficient, thereby confirming that hypovitaminosis D is not confined to the adult patient population.

Risk Factors
Inadequate exposure to sunlight is a common cause of vitamin D deficiency. People who live in the circles of latitude above the 37th parallel in the northern hemisphere or below the 37th parallel in the southern hemisphere produce little, if any, vitamin D during the winter because of decreased levels of ultraviolet B radiation, which puts them at a particularly high risk for vitamin D deficiency.[18] Another risk factor for vitamin D deficiency is darker skin pigmentation.[18] Melanin, which absorbs ultraviolet B radiation, is responsible for decreased synthesis and lower circulating levels of vitamin D in darker-skinned individuals.[18,41] Elderly adults who are exposed to ultraviolet B radiation produce three times less vitamin D than young adults who are exposed to ultraviolet B radiation, which suggests that increasing age is a substantial risk factor for vitamin D deficiency.[42] Obesity also is associated with vitamin D deficiency, possibly because vitamin D is sequestrated in adipose tissue or is volumetrically diluted within the increased mass.[43,44] In addition, pregnancy and lactation are considered risk factors for vitamin D deficiency.[45] A study by Lee et al[46] reported that 73% of pregnant women and 80% of their infants were vitamin D deficient despite the women taking a prenatal dose of 400 IU of vitamin D per day. Malabsorption syndrome, nephritic syndrome, chronic kidney disease, and primary or tertiary hyperparathyroidism also are risk factors for vitamin D deficiency.[13]

Vitamin D and Musculoskeletal Health

The presence of the VDR in human muscle tissue and an observation of muscle weakness and pain as symptoms of osteomalacia suggest that vitamin D plays a role in muscle function.[5,47,48] Histologic examinations of skeletal muscle fibers have further associated vitamin D with muscle function. Biopsies of skeletal muscle from patients who have vitamin D deficiency have shown type II muscle fiber atrophy.[49,50] In addition, decreased vitamin D levels are associated with increased fat infiltration in muscle.[51] In a study of patients who had torn rotator cuffs, Oh et al[52] reported vitamin D levels to be negatively correlated with fatty degeneration of torn cuff muscles; however, this degeneration may be reversible. In a randomized controlled trial of elderly women, Sato et al[53] reported that supplementation of 1,000 IU of vitamin D_2 per day increased the relative number and size of type II muscle fibers.

The effect of vitamin D supplementation on muscle performance has been controversial. Observational studies have shown a positive association between vitamin D concentration and lower extremity function, grip strength, and overall physical performance.[54-56] Conversely, in a systematic review and meta-analysis of 17 randomized controlled trials, Stockton et al[57] reported that vitamin D supplementation had no significant effect on muscle strength except in patients who had severe vitamin D deficiency (25-hydroxyvitamin D levels <10 ng/mL). In contrast, a more recent meta-analysis by Muir and Montero-Odasso[58] reported that a supplemental dose of 800 to 1,000 IU of vitamin D per day consistently demonstrated beneficial effects on strength and balance. Some studies have suggested that improvements in muscle strength and balance may explain the well-established association between adequate vitamin D levels and reduced fall risk.[58-61]

Vitamin D supplementation can help reduce the risk of both hip and nonvertebral fractures. In a meta-analysis of 12 randomized controlled trials, Bischoff-Ferrari et al[62] reported that an oral dose of 700 to 800 IU of vitamin D per day reduced the risk of nonvertebral fractures and hip fractures by 23% and 26%, respectively. Studies suggest that the benefits of vitamin D on hip fracture risk not only are limited to its effects on calcium absorption and bone density but also extend to its nonskeletal effects, such as improved muscle strength and balance, thereby reducing the risk of a fall.[5,63] However, the effects of vitamin D on fracture healing are unclear. In a recent systemic review, Gorter et al[64] reported that data investigating the effects of vitamin D deficiency or vitamin D supplementation on fracture healing were inconclusive.

Similarities between the symptoms of osteomalacia and chronic low back pain have led researchers to examine the association between low back pain and vitamin D levels.[65,66] In addition to finding that hypovitaminosis D is highly prevalent in patients who have chronic low back pain, researchers also noted that low back pain symptoms improved with vitamin D supplementation.[38,65,67]

Vitamin D levels affect arthroplasty outcomes and significantly positively correlate with both preoperative and postoperative Harris hip scores.[37] In a study of patients who underwent primary total hip arthroplasty, Lavernia et al[6] reported that patients who had 25-hydroxyvitamin D levels less than 30 ng/mL had a lower mean preoperative Harris hip score (43) and a lower mean postoperative Harris hip score (83) compared with patients who had sufficient levels of vitamin D (53 and 92, respectively). However, inadequate levels of vitamin D appear to have no effect on the attainment of in-hospital functional milestones (eg, the ability to transfer, walking distance, and the ability to climb stairs).[36]

Vitamin D and Infection

Vitamin D plays an important role in modulating both the innate and adaptive immune systems.[4] By binding to the VDR, 1,25-dihydroxyvitamin D stimulates the transcription of antimicrobial peptides, such as cathelicidin and defensin β2.[68] Cathelicidin, which protects against bacteria, viruses, and fungi, is maximally expressed at 25-hydroxyvitamin D levels between 30 ng/mL and 35 ng/mL.[69-71] In addition, vitamin D suppresses B cell and T cell proliferation, which results in decreased production of inflammatory cytokines (interleukin-17 and interleukin-21).[72] These findings suggest that vitamin D has both antimicrobial and anti-inflammatory properties; thus, an adequate level of vitamin D may help prevent infection.

Infections that occur after orthopaedic surgery are serious complications. Common examples of postoperative infections include pneumonia, urinary tract infection (UTI), surgical site infection, sepsis, and severe sepsis—all of which can lead to both increased mortality rates and procedure costs.[73] Deficient levels of vitamin D (<20 ng/mL) are associated with increased infection rates in surgical intensive care unit patients.[74,75] In a study of gastric bypass patients, Quraishi et al[76] reported that patients who had 25-hydroxyvitamin D levels less than 30 ng/mL had a fourfold increase in surgical site infections compared with vitamin D–sufficient patients. Another study found that patients who underwent revision surgery for a periprosthetic joint infection had a significant decrease in vitamin D levels compared with patients undergoing revision arthroplasty for aseptic loosening.[77] However, the specific association between vitamin D levels and surgical site and periprosthetic joint infections with respect to orthopaedic patients requires further examination.

Several underpowered studies suggest an association between inadequate levels of vitamin D and sepsis.[78,79] In a study of 3,386 intensive care unit patients, Moromizato et al[80] found the risk of sepsis to be 1.21-fold higher in patients who had 25-hydroxyvitamin D levels between 15 ng/mL and 30 ng/mL and 1.6-fold higher in patients who had 25-hydroxyvitamin D levels less than or equal to 15 ng/mL compared with patients who had adequate 25-hydroxyvitamin D levels. The same study also found that patients with sepsis and hypovitaminosis D had an increased risk of 30-day mortality compared with vitamin D–sufficient patients.[80]

Because UTI is the most common in-hospital infection that occurs after total joint arthroplasty (occurring at a rate of 3.26%), vitamin D supplementation has recently been suggested as a potential measure for prevention.[73] However, vitamin D supplementation increases the expression of cathelicidin in bladders that are infected with uropathogenic *Escherichia coli*, the primary causative agent of UTIs.[81,82] In addition, recurrent UTIs in postmenopausal women are associated with vitamin D deficiency.[83]

Vitamin D and Mortality

Inadequate levels of vitamin D are associated with increased all-cause mortality;[84,85] however, vitamin D supplementation can reduce mortality risk.[85-87] In an examination specifically of critically ill surgical patients, two studies reported that 25-hydroxyvitamin D levels were inversely related to mortality risk.[88,89] In a study of hip fracture patients, Nurmi-Lüthje et al[90] reported that calcium plus vitamin D supplementation was associated with a 36% and 43% reduction in deaths in females and males, respectively, at 36-month follow-up. Similarly, home-discharged hip fracture patients who purchased vitamin D supplements or calcium plus vitamin D supplements had a decreased 1-year mortality risk compared with hip fracture patients who did not purchase the supplements.[91]

The discovery of the VDR in cardiomyocytes, vascular smooth muscle cells, and endothelial cells has led to an increase in research on the relationship between vitamin D and cardiovascular disease.[92-94] The Framingham Offspring study found that individuals who had 25-hydroxyvitamin D levels less than 15 ng/mL had an increased risk for cardiovascular events.[95] Cardiovascular disease is commonly cited as a significant risk factor for mortality after arthroplasty, with myocardial infarction (MI) being the most common cause of death after total joint arthroplasty.[96-101]

In a prospective study of men who did not have a diagnosed cardiovascular disease, Giovannucci et al[102] found that during the 10 years of follow-up, MI was twice as likely to develop in patients who had 25-hydroxyvitamin D levels less than 15 ng/mL than in patients who had sufficient levels of 25-hydroxyvitamin D. The association between perioperative MI and vitamin D has not been extensively studied in orthopaedic patients; however, inadequate 25-hydroxyvitamin D levels have been found to increase the risk of major adverse cardiac and cerebrovascular events, including in-hospital death, stroke, MI, and low output syndrome, after cardiac surgery.[103] Interestingly, in a study of hip fracture patients, Fisher et al[104] reported that perioperative myocardial injury and in-hospital all-cause mortality were associated with elevated parathyroid hormone levels but were independent of 25-hydroxyvitamin D levels.

Vitamin D Supplementation

The supply of vitamin D that the body obtains from exposure to sunlight decreases during the winter season, which leaves dietary sources as the primary means to satisfy the body's vitamin D requirements. Because most foods do not contain sufficient levels of vitamin D, supplementation is the only way to meet the body's vitamin D requirements.[13] Supplemental vitamin D is available as vitamin D_2 or vitamin D_3. Although there has been some controversy with regard to the efficacy of vitamin D_2 compared with vitamin D_3, most studies indicate that vitamin D_3 is more effective than vitamin D_2 at increasing 25-hydroxyvitamin D levels.[105-107] Vitamin D supplementation can be administered orally or intramuscularly, and both means are relatively safe and effective.[108]

Currently, there is no consensus on the appropriate recommended daily allowance of vitamin D. The Institute of Medicine recommends 400 IU of vitamin D per day for infants younger than 1 year, 600 IU per day for persons aged 1 to 70 years, and 800 IU per day for persons older than 70 years.[16] Both the International Osteoporosis Foundation and the National Osteoporosis Foundation recommend higher daily allowances of up to 1,000 IU of vitamin D per day for persons older than 50 years.[109,110] Because these daily allowances may be too low to achieve adequate serum 25-hydroxyvitamin D concentration, higher recommendations should potentially be used.[13]

An adult who is exposed to a single, minimal erythemal dose of ultraviolet radiation will produce an estimated 10,000 IU of vitamin D, which is enough to satisfy the body's daily requirements.[111] In adults, every 100 IU of vitamin D ingested increases the serum 25-hydroxyvitamin D concentration by 1 ng/mL.[111,112] Without exposure to sunlight, a supplemental dose of 1,500 to 2,000 IU of vitamin D per day and vitamin D–fortified foods may be necessary to reach vitamin D sufficiency.[13]

Higher doses of vitamin D supplementation are required in patients with hypovitaminosis D to correct 25-hydroxyvitamin D levels. A common treatment strategy for patients with vitamin D deficiency consists of administering 50,000 IU of vitamin D_2 per week for 8 to 12 weeks, which helps the patient achieve sufficient vitamin D levels; this is followed by the administration of a maintenance dose of 2,000 IU of vitamin D per day, which helps prevent the recurrence of vitamin D deficiency.[9,13,113] This treatment strategy may help correct vitamin D levels without reaching levels of vitamin D toxicity. Supplementation of more than 600,000 IU of vitamin D during the

course of 60 days has been shown to correct vitamin D deficiency without causing vitamin D toxicity.[114]

Vitamin D toxicity is observed at 25-hydroxyvitamin D levels greater than 150 ng/mL.[8] To reduce the risk of vitamin D toxicity, the Institute of Medicine has established 4,000 IU of vitamin D per day as the tolerable upper intake level for adults;[16] however, because there is little evidence that supports the toxicity of moderate doses of vitamin D, most of the literature suggests that these limits are more conservative than necessary.[13,115] Certain experts recommend 10,000 IU of vitamin D per day as the safe upper limit of vitamin D supplementation for the adult patient population.[13,116,117]

Summary

Vitamin D deficiency is a highly prevalent condition that affects 40% of orthopaedic patients. Vitamin D plays a role in not only bone metabolism but also musculoskeletal health, immune system function, cardiovascular events, and even mortality. It is crucial for orthopaedic surgeons to have a comprehensive understanding of the postoperative complications associated with vitamin D deficiency as well as the necessary perioperative medical management to avoid them.

Although many studies suggest that vitamin D is an important component of health, very few of these studies include orthopaedic patients. The inconsistency in the definitions of vitamin D deficiency, insufficiency, and sufficiency, as well as discrepancies in the recommended daily allowance of vitamin D must be addressed. Standardization of these terms and values will lead not only to consistency within the literature but also to a unified approach for the

treatment of hypovitaminosis D and clear recommendations for vitamin D supplementation.

References

1. Holick MF: Resurrection of vitamin D deficiency and rickets. *J Clin Invest* 2006;116(8):2062-2072.

2. Jones G, Strugnell SA, DeLuca HF: Current understanding of the molecular actions of vitamin D. *Physiol Rev* 1998;78(4):1193-1231.

3. Holick MF: Vitamin D: Importance in the prevention of cancers, type 1 diabetes, heart disease, and osteoporosis. *Am J Clin Nutr* 2004;79(3):362-371.

4. Chun RF, Liu PT, Modlin RL, Adams JS, Hewison M: Impact of vitamin D on immune function: Lessons learned from genome-wide analysis. *Front Physiol* 2014;5:151.

5. Bischoff-Ferrari HA: Relevance of vitamin D in muscle health. *Rev Endocr Metab Disord* 2012;13(1):71-77.

6. Lavernia CJ, Villa JM, Iacobelli DA, Rossi MD: Vitamin D insufficiency in patients with THA: Prevalence and effects on outcome. *Clin Orthop Relat Res* 2014;472(2):681-686.

7. Dipaola CP, Bible JE, Biswas D, Dipaola M, Grauer JN, Rechtine GR: Survey of spine surgeons on attitudes regarding osteoporosis and osteomalacia screening and treatment for fractures, fusion surgery, and pseudo-arthrosis. *Spine J* 2009;9(7):537-544.

8. Holick MF: Vitamin D deficiency. *N Engl J Med* 2007;357(3):266-281.

9. Patton CM, Powell AP, Patel AA: Vitamin D in orthopaedics. *J Am Acad Orthop Surg* 2012;20(3):123-129.

10. Sullivan SS, Rosen CJ, Halteman WA, Chen TC, Holick MF: Adolescent girls in Maine are at risk for vitamin D insufficiency. *J Am Diet Assoc* 2005;105(6):971-974.

11. Zadshir A, Tareen N, Pan D, Norris K, Martins D: The prevalence of hypovitaminosis D among US adults: Data from the NHANES III. *Ethn Dis* 2005;15(4, suppl 5):S5-97-S5-101.

12. Tangpricha V, Pearce EN, Chen TC, Holick MF: Vitamin D insufficiency

among free-living healthy young adults. *Am J Med* 2002;112(8):659-662.

13. Holick MF: Vitamin D and health: Evolution, biologic functions, and recommended dietary intakes for vitamin D. *Clin Rev Bone Miner Metab* 2009;7(1):2-19.

14. Ginde AA, Liu MC, Camargo CA Jr: Demographic differences and trends of vitamin D insufficiency in the US population, 1988-2004. *Arch Intern Med* 2009;169(6):626-632.

15. Tosi LL, Gliklich R, Kannan K, Koval KJ: The American Orthopaedic Association's "own the bone" initiative to prevent secondary fractures. *J Bone Joint Surg Am* 2008;90(1):163-173.

16. Ross AC, Taylor CL, Yaktine AL, Del Valle HB; Institute of Medicine (IOM): *Dietary Reference Intakes for Calcium and Vitamin D*. Washington, DC, The National Academies Press, 2011.

17. Blunt JW, DeLuca HF, Schnoes HK: 25-hydroxycholecalciferol: A biologically active metabolite of vitamin D3. *Biochemistry* 1968;7(10):3317-3322.

18. Holick MF: Sunlight and vitamin D for bone health and prevention of autoimmune diseases, cancers, and cardiovascular disease. *Am J Clin Nutr* 2004;80(6 suppl):1678S-1688S.

19. DeLuca HF: Overview of general physiologic features and functions of vitamin D. *Am J Clin Nutr* 2004; 80(6 suppl):1689S-1696S.

20. Yousefzadeh P, Shapses SA, Wang X: Vitamin D binding protein impact on 25-hydroxyvitamin D levels under different physiologic and pathologic conditions. *Int J Endocrinol* 2014;2014:981581.

21. Chun RF, Peercy BE, Orwoll ES, Nielson CM, Adams JS, Hewison M: Vitamin D and DBP: The free hormone hypothesis revisited. *J Steroid Biochem Mol Biol* 2014; 144(pt A):132-137.

22. Bikle DD, Gee E, Halloran B, Kowalski MA, Ryzen E, Haddad JG: Assessment of the free fraction of 25-hydroxyvitamin D in serum and its regulation by albumin and the vitamin D-binding protein. *J Clin Endocrinol Metab* 1986;63(4):954-959.

23. Holick MF, Schnoes HK, DeLuca HF, Suda T, Cousins RJ: Isolation and identification of 1,25-dihydroxycholecalciferol: A metabolite of vitamin D active in intestine. *Biochemistry* 1971;10(14):2799-2804.

24. Henry HL: Regulation of vitamin D metabolism. *Best Pract Res Clin Endocrinol Metab* 2011;25(4):531-541.

25. Su Z, Narla SN, Zhu Y: 25-hydroxyvitamin D: Analysis and clinical application. *Clin Chim Acta* 2014;433:200-205.

26. Powe CE, Evans MK, Wenger J, et al: Vitamin D-binding protein and vitamin D status of black Americans and white Americans. *N Engl J Med* 2013;369(21):1991-2000.

27. Lai JK, Lucas RM, Clements MS, Harrison SL, Banks E: Assessing vitamin D status: Pitfalls for the unwary. *Mol Nutr Food Res* 2010;54(8):1062-1071.

28. Binkley N, Krueger DC, Morgan S, Wiebe D: Current status of clinical 25-hydroxyvitamin D measurement: An assessment of between-laboratory agreement. *Clin Chim Acta* 2010;411(23-24):1976-1982.

29. Moon HW, Cho JH, Hur M, et al: Comparison of four current 25-hydroxyvitamin D assays. *Clin Biochem* 2012;45(4-5):326-330.

30. Lips P: Relative value of 25(OH) D and 1,25(OH)2D measurements. *J Bone Miner Res* 2007;22(11):1668-1671.

31. Thomas MK, Lloyd-Jones DM, Thadhani RI, et al: Hypovitaminosis D in medical inpatients. *N Engl J Med* 1998;338(12):777-783.

32. Holick MF, Siris ES, Binkley N, et al: Prevalence of Vitamin D inadequacy among postmenopausal North American women receiving osteoporosis therapy. *J Clin Endocrinol Metab* 2005;90(6):3215-3224.

33. Heaney RP, Dowell MS, Hale CA, Bendich A: Calcium absorption varies within the reference range for serum 25-hydroxyvitamin D. *J An Coll Nutr* 2003;22(2):142-146.

34. Stein EM, Shane E: Vitamin D in organ transplantation. *Osteoporos Int* 2011;22(7):2107-2118.

35. Bogunovic L, Kim AD, Beamer BS, Nguyen J, Lane JM: Hypovitaminosis D in patients scheduled to undergo orthopaedic surgery: A single-center analysis. *J Bone Joint Surg Am* 2010;92(13):2300-2304.

36. Unnanuntana A, Rebolledo BJ, Gladnick BP, et al: Does vitamin D status affect the attainment of in-hospital functional milestones after total hip arthroplasty? *J Arthroplasty* 2012;27(3):482-489.

37. Nawabi DH, Chin KF, Keen RW, Haddad FS: Vitamin D deficiency in patients with osteoarthritis undergoing total hip replacement: A cause for concern? *J Bone Joint Surg Br* 2010;92(4):496-499.

38. Al Faraj S, Al Mutairi K: Vitamin D deficiency and chronic low back pain in Saudi Arabia. *Spine (Phila Pa 1976)* 2003;28(2):177-179.

39. Stoker GE, Buchowski JM, Bridwell KH, Lenke LG, Riew KD, Zebala LP: Preoperative vitamin D status of adults undergoing surgical spinal fusion. *Spine (Phila Pa 1976)* 2013;38(6):507-515.

40. Davies JH, Reed JM, Blake E, Priesemann M, Jackson AA, Clarke NM: Epidemiology of vitamin D deficiency in children presenting to a pediatric orthopaedic service in the UK. *J Pediatr Orthop* 2011;31(7):798-802.

41. Clemens TL, Adams JS, Henderson SL, Holick MF: Increased skin pigment reduces the capacity of skin to synthesise vitamin D3. *Lancet* 1982;1(8263):74-76.

42. Holick MF, Matsuoka LY, Wortsman J: Age, vitamin D, and solar ultraviolet. *Lancet* 1989;2(8671):1104-1105.

43. Drincic AT, Armas LA, Van Diest EE, Heaney RP: Volumetric dilution, rather than sequestration best explains the low vitamin D status of obesity. *Obesity (Silver Spring)* 2012;20(7):1444-1448.

44. Vanlint S: Vitamin D and obesity. *Nutrients* 2013;5(3):949-956.

45. Hollis BW, Wagner CL: Assessment of dietary vitamin D requirements during pregnancy and lactation. *Am J Clin Nutr* 2004;79(5):717-726.

46. Lee JM, Smith JR, Philipp BL, Chen TC, Mathieu J, Holick MF: Vitamin D deficiency in a healthy group of mothers and newborn infants. *Clin Pediatr (Phila)* 2007;46(1):42-44.

47. Bischoff-Ferrari HA, Borchers M, Gudat F, Dürmüller U, Stähelin HB, Dick W: Vitamin D receptor expression in human muscle tissue decreases with age. *J Bone Miner Res* 2004;19(2):265-269.

48. Francis RM, Selby PL: Osteomalacia. *Baillieres Clin Endocrinol Metab* 1997;11(1):145-163.

49. Ceglia L: Vitamin D and its role in skeletal muscle. *Curr Opin Clin Nutr Metab Care* 2009;12(6):628-633.

50. Yoshikawa S, Nakamura T, Tanabe H, Imamura T: Osteomalacic myopathy. *Endocrinol Jpn* 1979;26(suppl):65-72.

51. Gilsanz V, Kremer A, Mo AO, Wren TA, Kremer R: Vitamin D status and its relation to muscle mass and muscle fat in young women. *J Clin Endocrinol Metab* 2010;95(4):1595-1601.

52. Oh JH, Kim SH, Kim JH, Shin YH, Yoon JP, Oh CH: The level of vitamin D in the serum correlates with fatty degeneration of the muscles of the rotator cuff. *J Bone Joint Surg Br* 2009;91(12):1587-1593.

53. Sato Y, Iwamoto J, Kanoko T, Satoh K: Low-dose vitamin D prevents muscular atrophy and reduces falls and hip fractures in women after stroke: A randomized controlled trial. *Cerebrovasc Dis* 2005;20(3):187-192.

54. Bischoff-Ferrari HA, Dietrich T, Orav EJ, et al: Higher 25-hydroxyvitamin D concentrations are associated with better lower-extremity function in both active and inactive persons aged > or =60 y. *Am J Clin Nutr* 2004;80(3):752-758.

55. Visser M, Deeg DJ, Lips P; Longitudinal Aging Study Amsterdam: Low vitamin D and high parathyroid hormone levels as determinants of loss of muscle strength and muscle mass (sarcopenia): The Longitudinal Aging Study Amsterdam. *J Clin Endocrinol Metab* 2003;88(12):5766-5772.

56. Wicherts IS, van Schoor NM, Boeke AJ, et al: Vitamin D status predicts physical performance and its decline in older persons. *J Clin Endocrinol Metab* 2007;92(6):2058-2065.

57. Stockton KA, Mengersen K, Paratz JD, Kandiah D, Bennell KL: Effect of vitamin D supplementation on muscle strength: A systematic review and meta-analysis. *Osteoporos Int* 2011;22(3):859-871.

58. Muir SW, Montero-Odasso M: Effect of vitamin D supplementation on muscle strength, gait and balance in older adults: A systematic review and meta-analysis. *J Am Geriatr Soc* 2011;59(12):2291-2300.

59. Bischoff-Ferrari HA, Dawson-Hughes B, Willett WC, et al: Effect of Vitamin D on falls: A meta-analysis. *JAMA* 2004;291(16):1999-2006.

60. Kalyani RR, Stein B, Valiyil R, Manno R, Maynard JW, Crews DC: Vitamin D treatment for the prevention of falls in older adults: Systematic review and meta-analysis. *J Am Geriatr Soc* 2010;58(7):1299-1310.

61. Jackson C, Gaugris S, Sen SS, Hosking D: The effect of cholecalciferol (vitamin D3) on the risk of fall and fracture: A meta-analysis. *QJM* 2007;100(4):185-192.

62. Bischoff-Ferrari HA, Willett WC, Wong JB, Giovannucci E, Dietrich T, Dawson-Hughes B: Fracture prevention with vitamin D supplementation: A meta-analysis of randomized controlled trials. *JAMA* 2005;293(18):2257-2264.

63. Parkkari J, Kannus P, Palvanen M, et al: Majority of hip fractures occur as a result of a fall and impact on the greater trochanter of the femur: A prospective controlled hip fracture study with 206 consecutive patients. *Calcif Tissue Int* 1999;65(3):183-187.

64. Gorter EA, Hamdy NA, Appelman-Dijkstra NM, Schipper IB: The role of vitamin D in human fracture healing: A systematic review of the literature. *Bone* 2014;64:288-297.

65. Lotfi A, Abdel-Nasser AM, Hamdy A, Omran AA, El-Rehany MA: Hypovitaminosis D in female patients with chronic low back pain. *Clin Rheumatol* 2007;26(11):1895-1901.

66. Gifre L, Peris P, Monegal A, Martinez de Osaba MJ, Alvarez L, Guañabens N: Osteomalacia revisited: A report on 28 cases. *Clin Rheumatol* 2011;30(5):639-645.

67. Waikakul S: Serum 25-hydroxy-calciferol level and failed back surgery syndrome. *J Orthop Surg (Hong Kong)* 2012;20(1):18-22.

68. Wang TT, Nestel FP, Bourdeau V, et al: Cutting edge: 1,25-dihydroxyvitamin D3 is a direct inducer of antimicrobial peptide gene expression. *J Immunol* 2004;173(5):2909-2912.

69. Dürr UH, Sudheendra US, Ramamoorthy A: LL-37, the only human member of the cathelicidin family of antimicrobial peptides. *Biochim Biophys Acta* 2006;1758(9):1408-1425.

70. Bhan I, Camargo CA Jr, Wenger J, et al: Circulating levels of 25-hydroxyvitamin D and human cathelicidin in healthy adults. *J Allergy Clin Immunol* 2011;127(5):1302-1304.e1.

71. Quraishi SA, Litonjua AA, Moromizato T, et al: Association between prehospital vitamin D status and hospital-acquired bloodstream infections. *Am J Clin Nutr* 2013;98(4):952-959.

72. Aranow C: Vitamin D and the immune system. *J Investig Med* 2011;59(6):881-886.

73. Rasouli MR, Maltenfort MG, Purtill JJ, Hozack WJ, Parvizi J: Has the rate of in-hospital infections after total joint arthroplasty decreased? *Clin Orthop Relat Res* 2013;471(10):3102-3111.

74. Flynn L, Zimmerman LH, McNorton K, et al: Effects of vitamin D deficiency in critically ill surgical patients. *Am J Surg* 2012;203(3):379-382.

75. Youssef DA, Ranasinghe T, Grant WB, Peiris AN: Vitamin D's potential to reduce the risk of hospital-acquired infections. *Dermatoendocrinol* 2012;4(2):167-175.

76. Quraishi SA, Bittner EA, Blum L, Hutter MM, Camargo CA Jr: Association between preoperative 25-hydroxyvitamin D level and hospital-acquired infections following Roux-en-Y gastric bypass surgery. *JAMA Surg* 2014;149(2):112-118.

77. Maier GS, Horas K, Seeger JB, Roth KE, Kurth AA, Maus U: Is there an

association between periprosthetic joint infection and low vitamin D levels? *Int Orthop* 2014;38(7):1499-1504.

78. Cecchi A, Bonizzoli M, Douar S: Vitamin D deficiency in septic patients at ICU admission is not a mortality predictor. *Minerva Anestesiol* 2011;77(12):1184-1189.

79. Ginde AA, Camargo CA Jr, Shapiro NI: Vitamin D insufficiency and sepsis severity in emergency department patients with suspected infection. *Acad Emerg Med* 2011;18(5):551-554.

80. Moromizato T, Litonjua AA, Braun AB, Gibbons FK, Giovannucci E, Christopher KB: Association of low serum 25-hydroxyvitamin D levels and sepsis in the critically ill. *Crit Care Med* 2014;42(1):97-107.

81. Hertting O, Holm Å, Lüthje P, et al: Vitamin D induction of the human antimicrobial peptide cathelicidin in the urinary bladder. *PLoS One* 2010;5(12):e15580.

82. Svanborg C, Godaly G: Bacterial virulence in urinary tract infection. *Infect Dis Clin North Am* 1997;11(3):513-529.

83. Nseir W, Taha M, Nemarny H, Mograbi J: The association between serum levels of vitamin D and recurrent urinary tract infections in premenopausal women. *Int J Infect Dis* 2013;17(12):e1121-e1124.

84. Schöttker B, Jorde R, Peasey A, et al: Vitamin D and mortality: Meta-analysis of individual participant data from a large consortium of cohort studies from Europe and the United States. *BMJ* 2014;348:g3656.

85. Zittermann A, Iodice S, Pilz S, Grant WB, Bagnardi V, Gandini S: Vitamin D deficiency and mortality risk in the general population: A meta-analysis of prospective cohort studies. *Am J Clin Nutr* 2012;95(1):91-100.

86. Autier P, Gandini S: Vitamin D supplementation and total mortality: A meta-analysis of randomized controlled trials. *Arch Intern Med* 2007;167(16):1730-1737.

87. Bjelakovic G, Gluud LL, Nikolova D, et al: Vitamin D supplementation for prevention of mortality in adults. *Cochrane Database Syst Rev* 2014;1:CD007470.

88. Matthews LR, Ahmed Y, Wilson KL, Griggs DD, Danner OK: Worsening severity of vitamin D deficiency is associated with increased length of stay, surgical intensive care unit cost, and mortality rate in surgical intensive care unit patients. *Am J Surg* 2012;204(1):37-43.

89. Quraishi SA, Bittner EA, Blum L, McCarthy CM, Bhan I, Camargo CA Jr: Prospective study of vitamin D status at initiation of care in critically ill surgical patients and risk of 90-day mortality. *Crit Care Med* 2014;42(6):1365-1371.

90. Nurmi-Lüthje I, Lüthje P, Kaukonen JP, et al: Post-fracture prescribed calcium and vitamin D supplements alone or, in females, with concomitant anti-osteoporotic drugs is associated with lower mortality in elderly hip fracture patients: A prospective analysis. *Drugs Aging* 2009;26(5):409-421.

91. Nurmi-Lüthje I, Sund R, Juntunen M, Lüthje P: Post-hip fracture use of prescribed calcium plus vitamin D or vitamin D supplements and antiosteoporotic drugs is associated with lower mortality: A nationwide study in Finland. *J Bone Miner Res* 2011;26(8):1845-1853.

92. Chen S, Glenn DJ, Ni W, et al: Expression of the vitamin D receptor is increased in the hypertrophic heart. *Hypertension* 2008;52(6):1106-1112.

93. Wu-Wong JR, Nakane M, Ma J, Ruan X, Kroeger PE: Effects of vitamin D analogs on gene expression profiling in human coronary artery smooth muscle cells. *Atherosclerosis* 2006;186(1):20-28.

94. Merke J, Milde P, Lewicka S, et al: Identification and regulation of 1,25-dihydroxyvitamin D3 receptor activity and biosynthesis of 1,25-dihydroxyvitamin D3: Studies in cultured bovine aortic endothelial cells and human dermal capillaries. *J Clin Invest* 1989;83(6):1903-1915.

95. Wang TJ, Pencina MJ, Booth SL, et al: Vitamin D deficiency and risk of cardiovascular disease. *Circulation* 2008;117(4):503-511.

96. Aynardi M, Jacovides CL, Huang R, Mortazavi SM, Parvizi J: Risk factors for early mortality following modern

total hip arthroplasty. *J Arthroplasty* 2013;28(3):517-520.

97. Tarity TD, Herz AL, Parvizi J, Rothman RH: Ninety-day mortality after hip arthroplasty: A comparison between unilateral and simultaneous bilateral procedures. *J Arthroplasty* 2006;21(6, suppl 2):60-64.

98. Cusick LA, Beverland DE: The incidence of fatal pulmonary embolism after primary hip and knee replacement in a consecutive series of 4253 patients. *J Bone Joint Surg Br* 2009;91(5):645-648.

99. Singh JA, Lewallen DG: Ninety-day mortality in patients undergoing elective total hip or total knee arthroplasty. *J Arthroplasty* 2012;27(8):1417-1422.e1.

100. Parvizi J, Sullivan TA, Trousdale RT, Lewallen DG: Thirty-day mortality after total knee arthroplasty. *J Bone Joint Surg Am* 2001;83(8):1157-1161.

101. Smith EJ, Maru M, Siegmeth A: Thirty-day mortality after elective hip and knee arthroplasty. *Surgeon* 2015;13(1):5-8.

102. Giovannucci E, Liu Y, Hollis BW, Rimm EB: 25-hydroxyvitamin D and risk of myocardial infarction in men: A prospective study. *Arch Intern Med* 2008;168(11):1174-1180.

103. Zittermann A, Kuhn J, Dreier J, Knabbe C, Gummert JF, Börgermann J: Vitamin D status and the risk of major adverse cardiac and cerebrovascular events in cardiac surgery. *Eur Heart J* 2013;34(18):1358-1364.

104. Fisher AA, Southcott EK, Srikusalanukul W, et al: Relationships between myocardial injury, all-cause mortality, vitamin D, PTH, and biochemical bone turnover markers in older patients with hip fractures. *Ann Clin Lab Sci* 2007;37(3):222-232.

105. Logan VF, Gray AR, Peddie MC, Harper MJ, Houghton LA: Long-term vitamin D3 supplementation is more effective than vitamin D2 in maintaining serum 25-hydroxyvitamin D status over the winter months. *Br J Nutr* 2013;109(6):1082-1088.

106. Heaney RP, Recker RR, Grote J, Horst RL, Armas LA: Vitamin D(3) is more potent than vitamin D(2)

in humans. *J Clin Endocrinol Metab* 2011;96(3):E447-E452.

107. Tripkovic L, Lambert H, Hart K, et al: Comparison of vitamin D2 and vitamin D3 supplementation in raising serum 25-hydroxyvitamin D status: A systematic review and meta-analysis. *Am J Clin Nutr* 2012;95(6):1357-1364.

108. Tellioglu A, Basaran S, Guzel R, Seydaoglu G: Efficacy and safety of high dose intramuscular or oral cholecalciferol in vitamin D deficient/insufficient elderly. *Maturitas* 2012;72(4):332-338.

109. Dawson-Hughes B, Mithal A, Bonjour JP, et al: IOF position statement: Vitamin D recommendations for older adults. Position Paper. New York, NY, National AIDS Treatment Advocacy Project (NATAP), July 2010. Available at: www.natap.org/2010/HIV/072310_01.htm. Accessed June 25, 2014.

110. National Osteoporosis Foundation: Calcium and vitamin D: What you need to know. Washington, DC, National Osteoporosis Foundation. Available at: www.nof.org/aboutosteoporosis/prevention/vitamind. Accessed June 25, 2014.

111. Heaney RP, Davies KM, Chen TC, Holick MF, Barger-Lux MJ: Human serum 25-hydroxycholecalciferol response to extended oral dosing with cholecalciferol. *Am J Clin Nutr* 2003;77(1):204-210.

112. Holick MF, Biancuzzo RM, Chen TC, et al: Vitamin D2 is as effective as vitamin D3 in maintaining circulating concentrations of 25-hydroxyvitamin D. *J Clin Endocrinol Metab* 2008;93(3):677-681.

113. Kennel KA, Drake MT, Hurley DL: Vitamin D deficiency in adults: When to test and how to treat. *Mayo Clin Proc* 2010;85(8):752-758.

114. Pepper KJ, Judd SE, Nanes MS, Tangpricha V: Evaluation of vitamin D repletion regimens to correct vitamin D status in adults. *Endocr Pract* 2009;15(2):95-103.

115. Vieth R: Vitamin D supplementation, 25-hydroxyvitamin D concentrations, and safety. *Am J Clin Nutr* 1999;69(5):842-856.

116. Vieth R: Vitamin D toxicity, policy, and science. *J Bone Miner Res* 2007;22(suppl 2):V64-V68.

117. Rizzoli R, Boonen S, Brandi ML, Burlet N, Delmas P, Reginster JY: The role of calcium and vitamin D in the management of osteoporosis. *Bone* 2008;42(2):246-249.

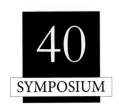

40
SYMPOSIUM

Outpatient Arthroplasty is Here Now

Adolph V. Lombardi, Jr, MD, FACS
John W. Barrington, MD
Keith R. Berend, MD
Michael E. Berend, MD
Lawrence D. Dorr, MD
William Hamilton, MD
Jason M. Hurst, MD
Michael J. Morris, MD
Giles R. Scuderi, MD

Abstract

Substantial advances have been made in arthroplasty to minimize surgical trauma and maximize perioperative pain control, which has enabled patients to regain mobility within hours of surgical intervention and be safely discharged to home the same day. Surgeons should understand the indications and contraindications for the safe performance of outpatient arthroplasty in a hospital and ambulatory surgical center setting as well as know how to optimize, medically manage, prepare, and rehabilitate patients. To undertake outpatient arthroplasty, surgeons must be knowledgeable in multimodal anesthesia techniques, effective venous thromboembolism prophylaxis, blood management, and wound management. In addition, surgeons must learn the subtle nuances of specialized surgical techniques that lend themselves to outpatient arthroplasty, including partial knee, muscle-sparing total hip, less invasive total knee, and total shoulder techniques.

Instr Course Lect 2016;65:531–546.

The concept of minimally invasive joint arthroplasty was introduced to the orthopaedic community and its patients approximately 10 years ago. The expectation of a more rapid return of function secondary to diminished surgical trauma as a result of smaller surgical incisions was very attractive to patients. Fortunately, the concept of a rapid recovery program, which incorporated perioperative planning, pain control, and rehabilitation, was introduced coincident with the introduction of minimally invasive surgery.[1-3]

At the time that one of the authors of this chapter (A.V.L.) started his practice in 1987, patients were hospitalized for 7 to 10 days after joint arthroplasty.

Immediately after surgery, patients were taken to a mini-intensive care unit and kept on bed rest for at least 24 hours. The lengths of incisions were not regarded as important. Knees were immobilized and wrapped in bulky, multilayered, compressive Robert Jones dressings with splints, and hips were closed with Charnley compression buttons. Patients were allowed to dangle the legs at the bedside the first day after surgery and stand and walk the second or third day after surgery. Several years later, after the introduction of skilled nursing facilities within acute care hospitals, patients were hospitalized in the acute portion of the facility for the first 3 days after surgery and then transferred to the skilled nursing facility for the next 4 to 10 days. The mobilization of patients followed a similar protocol. In the ensuing few years, patients were mobilized on the first day after surgery

Table 1

Ten Steps for Successful Execution of Outpatient Arthroplasty

1. Orthopaedic assessment
2. Preoperative medical clearance
3. Preoperative education
4. Preoperative physical therapy and rehabilitation
5. Preoperative analgesic agents
6. Perioperative anesthetic agents
7. Efficient performance of the surgical procedure
8. Wound healing adjuncts
9. Establishment of clinical pathways
10. Explicit postdischarge instructions

and transferred to outside skilled facilities on the third day after surgery.

Twelve years ago, one of the authors of this chapter (A.V.L.) was instrumental in establishing a specialty hospital for orthopaedics. The creation of this specialty hospital coincided with the development of minimally invasive surgical techniques and rapid recovery protocols.[1-3] In the specialty hospital, patients were mobilized the day of surgery, and discharge planning was instituted for either late on the first or second postoperative day. As time passed, increasing numbers of patients were discharged on the first day after surgery, with the mean hospital length of stay decreasing to 1.5 days. More recently, the authors of this chapter began to question whether patients even had to stay in the hospital. Certainly, a large number of patients could be discharged to home on the day of surgery. This concept was tested first at the specialty hospital, and then, ultimately, an outpatient surgical facility was created to address this new need. Surgeons who wish to pursue outpatient arthroplasty must surround themselves with individuals of a similar mindset. Office personnel, medical assistants, physician assistants, perioperative nurses, physical therapists, and each individual who has contact with the patient must echo the benefits and the reality of outpatient surgery.

Preparing for Outpatient Arthroplasty

The successful execution of outpatient arthroplasty requires 10 steps (**Table 1**). The first step is the orthopaedic assessment. As the orthopaedic surgeon evaluates the patient, he or she must determine the need for surgical intervention and if the patient comprehends the surgical procedure that is being prescribed. Will the patient be able to follow the recommendations? Does the patient have home support? Four of the authors of this chapter (A.V.L., K.R.B., J.M.H., and M.J.M.) have found that patients generally do not wish to stay in the hospital and are happy to learn that arthroplasty can be an outpatient procedure; consequently, patients are more excited to undergo the surgical intervention. Thus, the orthopaedic surgeon plants a seed in a patient's mind that motivates the patient to proceed; however, ultimately, it is the patient's decision whether to proceed with surgery.

The second step involves preoperative medical clearance. The role of the medical consultant is to identify any problems, correct those that are correctable, and then point out those that are uncorrectable. This begins with a comprehensive history and physical examination followed by appropriate laboratory studies and other tests and, if indicated, referral to an appropriate

Dr. Lombardi or an immediate family member has received royalties from Biomet, Innomed, and OrthoSensor; serves as a paid consultant to or is an employee of Biomet, OrthoSensor, and Pacira Pharmaceuticals; has received research or institutional support from Biomet, Kinamed, and Pacira Pharmaceuticals; and serves as a board member, owner, officer, or committee member of the Hip Society, the Knee Society, the Mount Carmel Education Center at New Albany, and Operation Walk USA. Dr. Barrington or an immediate family member has received royalties from Biomet; serves as a paid consultant to or is an employee of Biomet, OrthoSensor, Pacira Pharmaceuticals, and Smith & Nephew; has stock or stock options held in Iconacy Orthopedic Implants; has received research or institutional support from Biomet; and has received nonincome support (such as equipment or services), commercially derived honoraria, or other non-research–related funding (such as paid travel) from Tier 1 Group Healthcare Education and Research. Dr. K.R. Berend or an immediate family member has received royalties from Biomet; serves as a paid consultant to or is an employee of Biomet; has received research or institutional support from Biomet, Kinamed, and Pacira Pharmaceuticals; and serves as a board member, owner, officer, or committee member of the American Academy of Orthopaedic Surgeons Board of Specialty Societies and the American Association of Hip and Knee Surgeons. Dr. M.E. Berend or an immediate family member has received royalties from Biomet; serves as a paid consultant to or is an employee of Biomet; has stock or stock options held in OrthAlign; has received research or institutional support from Biomet, Stryker, and Johnson & Johnson; and serves as a board member, owner, officer, or committee member of Piedmont Orthopaedic Associates, the American Association of Hip and Knee Surgeons, and the Joint Replacement Surgeons of Indiana Research Foundation. Dr. Dorr or an immediate family member has received royalties from DJ Orthopaedics; serves as a paid consultant to or is an employee of Encore Medical Technologies; serves as an unpaid consultant to Total Joint Orthopedics; has stock or stock options held in Joint Research and Development; and serves as a board member, owner, officer, or committee member of Operation Walk USA. Dr. Hamilton or an immediate family member is a member of a speakers' bureau or has made paid presentations on behalf of DePuy; serves as a paid consultant to or is an employee of DePuy; and has received research or institutional support from DePuy, Inova, and Biomet. Dr. Hurst or an immediate family member serves as a paid consultant to or is an employee of Biomet, and has received research or institutional support from Biomet, Kinamed, and Pacira Pharmaceuticals. Dr. Morris or an immediate family member serves as a paid consultant to or is an employee of Biomet, and has received research or institutional support from Biomet, Kinamed, and Pacira Pharmaceuticals. Dr. Scuderi or an immediate family member has received royalties from Zimmer; is a member of a speakers' bureau or has made paid presentations on behalf of Pacira Pharmaceuticals, Zimmer, Medtronic, and ConvaTec; serves as a paid consultant to or is an employee of Merz Pharmaceuticals, Pacira Pharmaceuticals, Zimmer, Medtronic, and ConvaTec; has received research or institutional support from Pacira Pharmaceuticals; and serves as a board member, owner, officer, or committee member of the International Congress for Joint Reconstruction and Operation Walk USA.

© 2016 AAOS Instructional Course Lectures, Volume 65

medical specialist. Medical consultants perform medication reconciliation and provide appropriate instructions on which medications should be stopped preoperatively and which should be dosed on the day of surgery. Medical consultants also offer advice on the appropriate venue for the surgical procedure; that is, should it be performed at an outpatient surgical center with 23-hour observation, an orthopaedic specialty hospital, or a full-service hospital?

Previous or ongoing comorbidities that may contraindicate surgery in an outpatient setting include (1) cardiac issues, such as prior revascularization, congestive heart failure, or valve disease; (2) pulmonary issues, including chronic obstructive pulmonary disease, home use of supplemental oxygen, untreated sleep apnea, or a body mass index greater than 50 kg/m2; (3) renal disease, such as hemodialysis or a severely elevated serum creatinine level; (4) gastrointestinal issues, such as a history of postoperative ileus or chronic hepatic disease; (5) genitourinary issues, including a history of urinary tract infection or severe benign prostatic hyperplasia; (6) hematologic issues, including chronic warfarin use, coagulopathy, anemia with a hemoglobin level less than 13.0 g/dL, or thrombophilia; (7) neurologic issues, including a history of cerebrovascular accident, delirium, or dementia; and (8) solid organ transplant. Four of the authors of this chapter (A.V.L., K.R.B., J.M.H., and M.J.M.) have used a consistent group of physicians to perform preoperative medical clearance throughout their entire practice. Meding et al[4] reported that, as a result of a preoperative medical clearance evaluation, a remarkable number of new diagnoses were established, and 2.5% of patients were deemed unacceptable as surgical candidates.

The third step in the process is preoperative education. The educators are the surgeon, office staff, and perioperative nurses. Comprehensive educational materials will answer the most commonly asked questions and offer patients sound advice on what to do before surgery, what to do on the day of surgery, and what to expect after surgery.

The fourth step is preoperative physical therapy and rehabilitation. It has been reported that if patients are aware of their immediate postoperative functional expectations, then there is a considerable decrease in the level of fear and anxiety preoperatively.[1-3] It is the role of the physical therapist to outline in a stepwise process how a patient will address activities of daily living. The physical therapist relates to the patient timeline for convalescence after the surgical intervention; however, patients can best learn the exercises they will need for recovery before rather than after the surgical intervention.

The fifth step is preoperative analgesia. A multimodal program should be developed with both internists and anesthesiologists.[5-7] Preoperative medications to control postoperative pain, such as celecoxib, acetaminophen, corticosteroids, pregabalin or gabapentin; and prophylactic antiemetics, including dexamethasone, ondansetron, and a scopolamine transdermal patch, should be administered. The control of pain before the onset of noxious stimuli improves pain control postoperatively.[5-7]

The sixth step is perioperative anesthetic agents. Surgeons should align themselves with a competent and involved anesthesiologist. The first function of the anesthesiologist is to calm the patient. Anesthesiologists should provide not only the anesthetic agent for the surgical intervention but also the much-needed postoperative analgesic agents, which include neuraxial and regional anesthesia as well as appropriate medications.

The seventh step relies entirely on the surgeon. Surgery should be performed as efficiently as possible; however, efficiency does not mean speed. Efficiency means to perform the surgery in a timely fashion with as much precision as humanly possible.

The eighth step is wound-healing adjuncts. Currently, the most commonly used wound-healing adjunct is intravenous or topical tranexamic acid,[8-10] which has been reported in several studies to produce substantial hemostasis. Blood is a noxious stimulant; therefore, a decrease in postoperative hematoma will lead to a decrease in pain and suffering.

The ninth step involves the establishment of clinical pathways. The preoperative and postanesthesia care unit nurses will develop and institute several targets that the patient will need to attain. Patients generally move from the acute postanesthesia care unit to a step-down center and then are discharged to home.

The final step occurs after discharge. The discharge instructions must be very explicit. All medications should be reviewed, and specific instructions on physiotherapy must be provided. At the institution of four of the authors of this chapter (A.V.L., K.R.B., J.M.H., and M.J.M.), physical therapists evaluate the patient before discharge and discuss specific instructions for various maneuvering techniques. Patients are contacted by the outpatient surgical facility 24 hours after discharge to review any questions or concerns.

To date, four of the authors of this chapter (A.V.L., K.R.B., J.M.H., and M.J.M.) and their partners have performed nearly 2,000 outpatient total joint procedures with 98% satisfaction. Outpatient total joint arthroplasty (TJA) certainly is here and now. The requisites for the development of an outpatient TJA program begin with the physician champion. Orthopaedic surgeons must establish and embrace a team of associates who will execute the delivery of outpatient TJA care in a methodical fashion.

Anesthesia Protocols

Outpatient arthroplasty of the large joints has gained popularity in recent years because it has been reported to be safe and efficacious with reduced cost of care.[11-26] Multiple centers have implemented clinical pathways coupled with multimodal pain management protocols to accelerate the early recovery of patients and reduce their hospital length of stay.[1-3,18,19,27-30] Mitigating the risks and side effects of surgical intervention by combining efficient surgery with an effective anesthetic program that minimizes pain, nausea, sedation, and motor loss enables rapid mobilization of patients and safe discharge to home in a timely manner.

An enhanced understanding of pain management through a multimodal approach has been paramount in the advancement of the rapid recovery movement. The anesthesia staff members are key elements of the care team. To reduce patient anxiety, the anesthesiologist should visit the patient in the preoperative holding area and provide a detailed explanation on the management of postoperative pain. At the facility of one of the authors of this chapter (M.J.M.), most patients who undergo outpatient joint arthroplasty are treated with either a single-shot, short-acting spinal anesthetic agent (50 to 60 mg of lidocaine; hip patients), a combination adductor canal block (15 mL of 0.5% ropivacaine) and sciatic nerve block (15 mL of 0.1% ropivacaine; knee patients), or an interscalene block (shoulder patients). The avoidance of narcotics in the intrathecal space helps minimize potential postoperative sedation, nausea, and pruritus, which can slow down early recovery. Preoperatively, patients receive a combination of 400 mg of celecoxib, 300 to 600 mg of gabapentin, and 1,000 mg of acetaminophen orally as well as 10 mg of both dexamethasone and metoclopramide intravenously. Hydration is usually instituted with 1,000 mL of crystalloid before the surgical procedure. Scopolamine transdermal patches are considered to further combat perioperative nausea, unless contraindicated. In addition to the perioperative antibiotic, patients receive 1 g of tranexamic acid and 4 mg of ondansetron intravenously as well as aggressive hydration during the surgical intervention. Narcotics are minimized, and short-acting anesthetic agents are used during the actual procedure. Furthermore, periarticular injections are used to deliver analgesic agents directly into the soft tissue of the joint. The intra-articular injection currently administered by four of the authors of this chapter (A.V.L., K.R.B., J.M.H., and M.J.M.) consists of 60 mL of 0.5% ropivacaine and 0.5 mL of 1:1,000 epinephrine. For patients who have normal renal function, 30 mg of ketorolac are added. The intra-articular injection is administered throughout all soft tissues in and around the joint.

Postoperatively, the acetaminophen and tranexamic acid doses are repeated. Patients are given intravenous narcotics (hydromorphone) as needed in the immediate postanesthesia care unit and transitioned to oral narcotics in the form of oxycodone as quickly as possible. The oxycodone, coupled with celecoxib and acetaminophen, is continued for the first few days postoperatively. Patients are encouraged to transition to hydrocodone and acetaminophen as soon as they feel comfortable. Patients who have known benign prostatic hypertrophy and male patients who received spinal anesthesia are provided 20 mg of bethanechol postoperatively to minimize the risk of urinary retention. These anesthesia protocols enabled four of the authors of this chapter (A.V.L., K.R.B., J.M.H., and M.J.M.) to perform outpatient arthroplasty on more than 1,300 patients during 2014. Of those patients, only 8% required an overnight bed, with most patients staying overnight because they lived more than 2 hours away or their procedures were completed in the late afternoon or early evening.

Liposomal Bupivacaine Infiltration

Despite the success of TJA, pain after surgery can be severe and difficult to manage.[31] Many complications after TJA may be associated with pain management strategies. Opioid analgesic agents, including patient-controlled intravenous and oral analgesic agents, have been a standard modality for postoperative pain management but are associated with a risk of nausea, pruritus, vomiting, respiratory depression, prolonged ileus, and cognitive dysfunction.[32-34] Regional pain control techniques, such as femoral nerve blockade, may limit exposure to opioid-related adverse events but may cause quadriceps weakness, neuropathy, and postoperative falls.[35,36] Periarticular injections (PAIs) have been reported to decrease pain, increase function, and reduce opioid-related adverse events after TJA.[37-39] In addition, PAIs are cheaper and easier to perform than other regional modalities, such as femoral nerve blocks.[31]

Recently, a single-dose local analgesic agent that uses bupivacaine in combination with a liposomal time-released product delivery platform has been introduced. To date, few clinical data exist to understand the effect of the time-released mechanism on patient-reported pain among differing PAI modalities. One of the authors of this chapter (J.W.B.) conducted a study that compared a large sample of patients in whom novel extended-release liposomal bupivacaine was used during PAI with a control group of patients in whom PAI was performed without liposomal bupivacaine (John W. Barrington, Plano, TX, unpublished data, 2015). Pain control was used as the primary outcome measure. Because of the time-released mechanism that was incorporated in the liposomal bupivacaine, the author hypothesized that the liposomal bupivacaine group would have demonstrably lower visual analog scale (VAS) pain scores in the immediate postoperative period compared with the control group.

The study included 2,248 consecutive hip and knee arthroplasties that were performed by one of four surgeons in a dedicated arthroplasty practice. The first half of these patients (the "pre" group) was treated with well-established multimodal analgesia, including PAIs with bupivacaine, ketorolac, and morphine and therapy protocols. A matching number of 1,124 consecutive hip and knee arthroplasties were performed with similar therapy protocols, but the established PAIs were substituted with an FDA-approved liposomal bupivacaine surgical site soft-tissue PAI technique (the "post" group). The primary outcome measures were the mean VAS pain score and the percentage of VAS pain scores that were 0 during hospitalization, which was a result of a patient having no pain (John W. Barrington, Plano, TX, unpublished data, 2015).

VAS pain scores were significantly lower for patients in the post group compared with the VAS scores for those in the pre group for hip arthroplasty (1.67 versus 2.30, P < 0.0001), knee arthroplasty (2.21 versus 2.52, P < 0.0001), and both procedures combined (1.98 versus 2.43, P < 0.0001). The percentage of patients who reported having no pain was significantly higher in the post group compared with the pre group for both hip (57.3% versus 43.4%, P < 0.0001) and knee (47.2% versus 42.1%, P < 0.0001) arthroplasty. Regression analysis also demonstrated that the post group had significantly lower VAS pain scores by 0.39 (P < 0.0001) compared with the pre group, after controlling for available demographic and surgical factors. Regression analysis also demonstrated that the post group had higher pain scores by 0.15 on the day of surgery compared with the pre group but had lower pain scores on days 1 to 4, ranging from 0.62 to 0.96 points lower (P < 0.0001) compared with the pre group (John W. Barrington, Plano, TX, unpublished data, 2015).

One of the authors of this chapter (J.W.B.) reported a substantial improvement in pain relief in a large series of TJA patients at his surgical center after the introduction of liposomal bupivacaine as part of an already well-established multimodal protocol. The author reported improved pain relief for both hip and knee procedures, as measured by both mean VAS pain scores and the percentage of patients who reported no pain (John W. Barrington, Plano, TX, unpublished data, 2015). Pain control plays a critical role in patient prognosis after large joint arthroplasty because it encourages earlier ambulation and the initiation of physiotherapy.[40] Aggressive pain control improves patient compliance with rehabilitation immediately after surgery.[35] Conversely, poorly controlled pain can lead to delayed or diminished ambulation, anxiety, delays in the recovery of normal function and lifestyle, poor sleep, urinary retention, and reduced quality of life,[41] as well as an increased cost of care.[42-44]

Other than slower rehabilitation, adverse outcomes associated with poorly controlled pain include delayed wound healing, an increased risk of pulmonary morbidity (including pneumonia) and thrombosis, an increased risk of mortality, and hypertension.[41] The elimination of analgesic gaps,[45-47] preemptive procedure or site-specific analgesia, and cognitive, age, and cultural barriers[48-50] may be the mechanisms by which many patients in the study experienced improved pain control.

The primary difference in the post group was the administration of liposomal bupivacaine as part of the analgesic protocol. Liposomal bupivacaine is a 72-hour local anesthetic formulation that was FDA approved in 2013 for surgical site soft-tissue injection. This formulation uses a novel delivery system to combine the well-established benefits of bupivacaine with time-released delivery and the prolonged duration of effect. The efficacy and safety of liposomal bupivacaine have been established in more than 21 clinical trials, including 10 double-blind, randomized controlled trials that collectively involved 823 patients who underwent a range of surgical procedures, including total knee arthroplasty (TKA).[37,51-59]

It is important to note that the study discussed in this section describes a surgical soft-tissue injection, not an intra-articular infusion.[60] Regional techniques, such as liposomal bupivacaine, act as a substitute for traditional methods of pain control, primarily patient-controlled morphine or other opioids. By reducing narcotic consumption, there is a great potential to reduce nausea and vomiting, reduce the hospital length of stay, improve patient satisfaction, and increase physical therapy participation.[35]

Blood Management

The optimization of blood management and the reduction or elimination of postoperative blood transfusions is a critical component of outpatient TJA. Blood transfusions may not be available at some outpatient centers, and it may not be feasible from a time or workflow standpoint to transfuse patients after surgery if same-day discharge is planned. It is possible to reduce the transfusion rate enough to make outpatient TJA safe and feasible. There are several techniques to reduce perioperative blood loss and the subsequent transfusion rate; the use of all of them synergistically can almost eliminate the need for postoperative transfusions.

The preoperative identification of patients who have a high risk for requiring a transfusion can help reduce the transfusion rate. One of the biggest predictors of postoperative hemoglobin levels is the preoperative hemoglobin level,[61] and after a certain preoperative hemoglobin threshold is reached (13 g/dL), the transfusion rate drops close to zero.[62] The identification of patients who have preoperative anemia will allow the surgeon to either perform the procedures for these patients in an inpatient setting or increase their hemoglobin level preoperatively. Patients who have lower overall blood volumes at baseline are more likely to experience a clinically substantial hemoglobin drop for the same volume of blood loss. Overall, females have less blood volume than males; therefore, compared with males, females are more likely to have a larger drop in hemoglobin levels for the same volume of blood loss. Small statured patients, especially females, have a higher risk of a large hemoglobin drop. Certain procedures, including revision surgery, bilateral surgery, and total hip arthroplasty (THA), have higher blood losses compared with TKAs or unicondylar arthroplasties.[63]

Several steps can be taken to reduce blood loss during surgery. An efficient surgery with shorter surgical time and careful attention to hemostasis can reduce intraoperative blood loss. Surgeons should be wary of performing new procedures or new surgical approaches in the outpatient setting. Several studies have reported a learning curve for surgeons who perform the anterior approach to the hip, with higher early blood loss.[63,64] Comfort and consistency should be achieved with any procedure to reduce the chance for complications and possible transfusion. Regional anesthesia has been reported to reduce overall blood loss and transfusion rates,[65,66] either from the effects of the anesthesia on the vascular system or the hypotension that frequently accompanies regional anesthesia. Hypotension with mean arterial pressures at or below 60 mm Hg can reduce intraoperative bleeding.[67,68]

The most important tool to reduce blood loss and subsequent transfusion rates is tranexamic acid. Tranexamic acid is an antifibrinolytic agent that reduces the rate of clot breakdown without increasing the rate of clot formation.[69] Multiple studies have reported that mean calculated perioperative blood loss can be substantially reduced with the use of tranexamic acid. Tranexamic acid can be dosed either intravenously or topically, with similar effectiveness via either route.[10,70,71] Intravenous dosing can be administered via either a weight-based or a standard dosing regimen and can be given both preoperatively and postoperatively. The surgical center of one of the authors of this chapter (W.H.) currently administers 1 g of tranexamic acid intravenously before incision and a second 1-g dose intravenously in the recovery room. Topical dosing is usually administered toward the end of the procedure by mixing 2 to 3 g of topical tranexamic acid in 50 to 100 mL of saline and allowing the mixture to soak in the wound during closure. If a drain is used postoperatively, it has been recommended that the drain be clamped for 30 to 60 minutes to allow the mixture to soak into the wound. Regardless of the technique, studies consistently report that tranexamic acid reduces blood loss and lowers transfusion rates without increasing the rate of thrombotic events.[8-10,70,71]

The final tool to reduce perioperative transfusion rates is to modify classic transfusion triggers. Historic practices have set numerical thresholds for the administration of blood transfusions (ie, hemoglobin level of 10 g/dL); however, evidence does not support this practice. Rather, patients should be evaluated clinically to determine if symptoms of anemia, such as orthostatic hypotension or tachycardia, are present. Substantially lower hemoglobin levels can be tolerated, especially by younger, healthier patients. The surgical center of one of the authors of this chapter (W.H.) currently follows the algorithm described by Pierson et al.[72] Transfusion is considered only if the patient's hemoglobin level is less than 7 g/dL or if the patient's hemoglobin level is less than 8 g/dL and the patient shows symptoms of anemia and does not respond to volume resuscitation. Most patients who demonstrate dizziness, fatigue, or nausea are symptomatic from hypovolemia, not anemia. This combination of tools can systematically help reduce blood loss and acceptably lower the rate of blood transfusion. Preoperative patient screening, intraoperative hypotension, regional anesthesia, efficient and facile surgical technique, tranexamic acid, and modified blood transfusion triggers should lower blood transfusion rates for primary THAs and primary TKAs to less than 3% and 1%, respectively.

Outpatient Partial Knee Arthroplasty

Outpatient arthroplasty procedures represent the next wave of arthroplasty surgery. This trend has already occurred for procedures that were formerly regarded as inpatient procedures, such as upper extremity surgery, arthroscopy, anterior cruciate ligament reconstruction, foot and ankle procedures, and rotator cuff repair. The refinement of surgical techniques, anesthesia protocols, and patient selection has facilitated this transformation. The outpatient arthroplasty program at the surgical center of one of the authors of this chapter (M.E.B.) is based on collective evidence from more than 50,000 joint arthroplasties and hundreds of peer-reviewed publications on arthroplasty outcomes. The program was initiated with a focus on a mobile-bearing partial knee arthroplasty (PKA) system for the treatment of medial compartment knee disease, a fixed-bearing partial knee for the treatment of lateral disease, and patellofemoral replacement for the treatment of patellofemoral disease. The surgical center of the author of this chapter (M.E.B.) has expanded the program to include THA and TKA.

Outpatient PKA can be highly beneficial for patients, surgeons, anesthesiologists, ambulatory surgery centers, and payers because arthroplasty procedures shift to the outpatient space. It is the belief of one of the authors of this chapter (M.E.B.) that it will always cost more to perform arthroplasty procedures in a hospital. A less efficiently run inpatient hospital setting demands overtreatment of each patient to fit him or her into the mold of inpatient surgery. A study of the Medicare database indicates that 7% of unicompartmental knee arthroplasties are already performed as outpatient procedures.[73] Patient satisfaction is very high in the outpatient setting.[19,21,23] Patients can recover in their own homes, with reduced inpatient services and use of outpatient services for nursing and physical therapy. The surgeon efficiently controls the local environment, and, thus, overall patient experience and satisfaction are improved for procedures performed in the outpatient setting.

The surgeon's role changes from that of a commoditized technician in the hospital setting to that of a coordinator of the entire care experience, including preoperative care, imaging, anesthesia, perioperative care mapping, postoperative care, and enhanced coordination with therapy providers, in the outpatient setting.

In general, any patient who has met the indications for a PKA, THA, or TKA may potentially receive care as an outpatient. At the surgical center of one of the authors of this chapter (M.E.B.), same-day discharge has been safe and very likely if patients are younger than 60 to 63 years, have no substantial cardiovascular history, and live within 1 to 2 hours of the center. In facilities that have overnight (23-hour) capability, these indications may expand to include older patients and those who live further from the center and do not want to drive home late in the evening. Because 23-hour stays are possible at many ambulatory surgery centers in most states, most PKA, TKA, and THA patients (50% to 75%) may qualify for outpatient or 23-hour (overnight) stay possibilities.

Partial knee replacement represents more than 50% of the care for the treatment of an arthritic knee; in 2012, 53% of primary knee arthroplasties performed by one of the authors of this chapter (M.E.B.) were PKAs. This rate has steadily increased in the past 10 years, with proven data and expanded indication criteria. A better understanding of these expanded indications, which are supported in the literature,[27] will give the orthopaedic surgeon the confidence necessary to perform PKA as an outpatient procedure.

Medical optimization is critical to the safety and the success of outpatient PKA arthroplasty. Surgeons and outpatient centers are strongly encouraged to adopt a standardized format for preadmission testing.[4] Input from the anesthesiologist and local medical doctors in the creation of customized preadmission testing templates is highly beneficial. Preoperative education is essential to prepare the patient for same-day discharge. At the surgical center of one of the authors of this chapter (M.E.B.), the patient is provided with a CD that contains an educational PowerPoint presentation and/or website-based patient education on outpatient surgery. Preoperatively, the patient may tour the surgery center to become familiar and more comfortable with the setting. The patient also has a preoperative session with a physical therapist for gait training and home exercise training. One to 2 weeks after surgery, the patient is seen for follow-up at the surgeon's office for a wound check, which is performed by a physician assistant. The patient then returns at 6 to 8 weeks postoperatively for clinical and radiographic assessment.

Perioperatively, the patient is given 400 mg of celecoxib, 300 mg of gabapentin, 1 g of acetaminophen intravenously, and 80 mg of dexamethasone.[74] Intraoperatively, a laryngeal mask airway for light general sedation and an ultrasound-guided adductor canal block are used for knee patients. The surgical center of one of the authors of this chapter (M.E.B.) uses a periarticular capsular injection that includes 20 mL of liposomal bupivacaine as an injectable suspension, 25 mL of 0.5% bupivacaine with epinephrine, 0.5 mL of 1:1,000 epinephrine, and, in patients who have sufficient renal function, 30 mg of ketorolac. Postoperative management includes three medications that are administered intravenously

for 4 to 6 hours (1 g of acetaminophen, 15 or 30 mg of ketorolac, and an antibiotic), with four additional oral doses after discharge; oral narcotics of choice, such as oxycodone, without acetaminophen for 12 to 24 hours; ketorolac tromethamine spray every 6 hours for 3 days; and a motorized cryotherapy unit for comfort. Aspirin and a portable, battery-powered intermittent pneumatic compression ambulatory calf-pump device are used for venous thromboembolism prophylaxis.

The outpatient PKA program focuses on patient, surgeon, and center satisfaction and success. Close, caring follow-up is critical. Outpatient PKA requires slightly more attention from the center and its staff than inpatient PKA. Routine phone calls on the day after surgery and at 1 week postoperatively are encouraged. Patients can call the surgeon or the center with any questions, and routine follow-up is at the discretion of the surgeon.

Outpatient THA and TKA

In the past 15 years, the mean hospital length of stay for THA and TKA patients has gradually decreased from several days to overnight. The most logical and safest next step is outpatient THA and TKA. In the era of minimally invasive surgery, the most intriguing advancements were not related to the surgery itself but instead to the areas of rapid recovery techniques and perioperative protocols. Rapid recovery techniques and perioperative protocols have been refined to allow for same-day discharge with improved outcomes.[1-3]

The initial critical step in planning outpatient THA or TKA involves the clinic visit. Traditionally, the purpose of the office visit was to determine candidacy for THA or TKA via a thorough

history and physical examination. In the era of outpatient arthroplasty, the office visit also must involve education for the patient and the family, as well as a discussion that joint arthroplasties do not need to be performed at a hospital with a lengthy inpatient stay. The focus of this education involves presenting the patient with evidence that he or she does not need a hospital. By addressing patient and family fears, mitigating perioperative risk, and reducing or eliminating the side effects of treatment, orthopaedic surgeons can safely allow patients to be discharged to home the same day of either THA or TKA.

By providing the patient with education and preoperative physical therapy, fear, which is caused by the belief that something is dangerous, likely to cause pain, or a threat, can be eliminated or reduced. A standardized medical prescreening examination evaluates patients for known risk factors, including obstructive sleep apnea, diabetes, and ischemic heart disease.[4] Together with the anesthesiologist, the medical team and the orthopaedic team establish a list of patient factors and comorbidities that are acceptable, concerning, or unacceptable for outpatient THA and TKA. The team of providers uses this list to determine the appropriateness of outpatient joint arthroplasty for each individual patient.

As previously mentioned, the single most important advancement from the minimally invasive surgery era was the multimodal approach to pain management for patients who underwent arthroplasty. In addition to blood loss management with the use of tranexamic acid and hypotensive anesthetic techniques, a multimodal program is the most important variable in reducing or avoiding side effects. Side effects that need to be addressed in any arthroplasty procedure include the negative effects of narcotics and blood loss. Anesthetic techniques that use local nerve blocks, such as the adductor canal block and sciatic blocks for knees and short-acting spinal blocks for hips, augment intraoperative anesthesia and provide postoperative pain relief and quicker mobilization. In addition, pericapsular injection that contains local anesthetic may help with pain relief and recovery as well as reduce the amount of oral narcotics used in the early postoperative period.

Multimodal perioperative protocols can help avoid narcotics and the side effects of nausea. In addition, four of the authors of this chapter (K.R.B., A.V.L., J.M.H., and M.J.M.) use an aggressive prophylactic antiemetic program that consists of dexamethasone, ondansetron, and a scopolamine patch. Patients who do not have any substantial cardiovascular history are given celecoxib preoperatively, which is continued for approximately 2 weeks postoperatively. Acetaminophen and additional dexamethasone are administered intravenously immediately after the procedure.

This multimodal program was used between June 2013 and October 2014 at the outpatient arthroplasty center of four of the authors of this chapter (K.R.B., A.V.L., J.M.H., and M.J.M.) to perform 1,441 outpatient arthroplasties, 482 of which were THAs, 460 of which were TKAs, and 461 of which were PKAs. Seven percent of the patients who underwent outpatient arthroplasties stayed overnight, with approximately one-half staying overnight for convenience and one-half staying overnight for medical or anesthetic reasons (Keith R. Berend, MD, New Albany, OH, unpublished data,

2015). The multimodal protocols that address fear, risk, and side effects will increase patient eligibility for outpatient surgery and decrease the need for overnight hospitalization. By focusing on the patient and avoiding overtreatment, outpatient arthroplasty will become the standard of care for THA and TKA in the same way other hospital inpatient procedures have transitioned to ambulatory procedures.

Outpatient Total Shoulder Arthroplasty

As lower extremity arthroplasty procedures move to the outpatient setting, the progression of total shoulder arthroplasty (TSA) to the outpatient setting also has occurred.[75-78] Because most TSA patients can ambulate almost immediately after the procedure, the transition to the outpatient setting is typically a smooth one. The basic principles of outpatient TSA are similar to those for lower extremity arthroplasty, but some unique concerns must be considered.

As with TKA and THA, outpatient TSA begins with adequate patient selection and preoperative clearance. Although it is always imperative to obtain preoperative medical clearance for TSA patients, it is just as important for the clearing medical physician to be aware that TSA will be performed in an outpatient setting. In addition, it is useful for the surgeon, the clearing physician, and the outpatient center's anesthesiologists to develop a strict contraindications list. Contraindications for outpatient TSA include, but are not limited to, substantial cardiac disease, renal dysfunction, coagulopathy, severe urinary retention, cerebrovascular disease, liver cirrhosis, and substantial pulmonary disease.

Pulmonary disease is a particular concern for TSA patients. Because the anesthetic procedure of choice for TSA is the interscalene block and there is always an inherent risk of inadvertent phrenic nerve blockade, it is important for TSA patients to have a robust pulmonary system without chronic obstructive pulmonary disease or other pulmonary conditions. Obstructive sleep apnea is currently a common condition; however, if the sleep apnea is severe, uncontrolled, or newly diagnosed, it is prudent to observe such patients for at least 23 hours after the procedure. Because patients who have sleep apnea usually require full intubation if placed in the beach-chair or raised position, it is even more important that their pulmonary status be stout enough to rebound from surgery in a reasonable time period for same-day discharge.

Most TSA procedures currently are performed under nerve blockade with or without indwelling perineural catheters. The use of indwelling perineural catheters is safe and effective in outpatient TSA;[75,76] however, the use of indwelling perineural catheters is at the discretion of the surgeon and not imperative in the development of a successful program for outpatient TSA. Although indwelling perineural catheters provide excellent pain relief for multiple days after the procedure, there are substantial costs and catheter-management issues related to their use. Some surgeons prefer a single-shot blockade for early neurologic evaluation, early active-assisted shoulder motion, and the elimination of indwelling perineural catheters. As with all outpatient arthroplasty procedures, it is very important that a good strategy exists to adequately control nausea and pain after the nerve blockade has stopped. Patient education is the key to help patients control their pain, and there should always be an easy way for patients to obtain advice on pain management in the first few days after the surgery.

Indwelling perineural catheters are not used at the surgical center of one of the authors of this chapter (J.M.H.); instead, only a single-shot interscalene block with ropivacaine is used for all outpatient TSA procedures. Narcotics are used sparingly, and nausea is controlled aggressively with adequate hydration, the preoperative intravenous administration of dexamethasone, ondansetron, and topical scopolamine patches for patients who have a history of anesthesia-associated nausea. Oral hydration and bland foods are started within 2 hours after surgery to ensure that patients can tolerate liquids and food before discharge. All patients are screened by a licensed physical therapist before discharge to ensure that they can safely ambulate and use the sling. Patients are encouraged to attend outpatient physical therapy on the first postoperative day. One of the authors of this chapter (J.M.H.) typically prescribes oxycodone, celecoxib, and acetaminophen as the primary regimen for oral pain control after discharge, with low-dose hydromorphone prescribed for a pain crisis. The literature on outpatient TSA is limited, and few studies focus on the feasibility and safety of TSA with the use of perineural catheters;[75-78] however, most high-volume TSA surgeons would agree that the outpatient setting is reasonable and attractive to many healthy patients who do not have the medical contraindications previously identified or poor pulmonary status. As the interest and trust in outpatient TSA grows, the substantial void in outpatient TSA literature will likely be filled.

Outpatient Venous Thromboembolism Prophylaxis

One of the authors of this chapter (L.D.D.) is now in his 10th year of experience with outpatient THA, and his proposed recommendations for outpatient THA are supported by his extensive clinical experience.[22,79-81] First, outpatient arthroplasty is a wonderful option, particularly for patients who are still in their productive years or those who have busy family obligations. Because time is a valuable commodity to these patients and they fear the surgical recovery will severely affect their necessary functions, many hesitate to have a needed THA. The concept of same-day discharge greatly boosts a patient's confidence, and nothing creates a better recovery than exceeding a patient's expectations.[79] Same-day discharge for outpatient THA patients can boost a surgeon's practice.

The outpatient protocols of one of the authors of this chapter (L.D.D.) initially mimicked those of Richard A. Berger, MD, who is credited with the initiation of outpatient THAs and TKAs.[13-21] The author (L.D.D.) deviates from Berger's pain management and recovery program in two ways: (1) One unit of blood is transfused for blood doping of the patient; this reduces dizziness and lethargy as well as promotes the patient's confidence to be discharged to home. (2) Aspirin is used for venous thromboprophylaxis, which has been the author's (L.D.D.) routine since the 1980s. The author's (L.D.D.) multimodal program with the use of chemical anticoagulant prophylaxis only for patients who are at high risk is very safe and as effective as any published treatment.[80] An aspirin suppository of 650 mg is given to the patient in the recovery room, and subsequently one adult 325-mg dose of aspirin is given orally twice a day. Other surgeons give patients 81 mg, but if the patient tolerates an adult dose, it has the secondary effect of an anti-inflammatory agent for pain relief. Aspirin prevents heterotopic ossification, a complication that does not exist in the author's (L.D.D.) patient population. Aspirin provides protection against arterial complications, such as myocardial infarction and stroke. Aspirin is administered twice a day to neutralize all circulating platelets. The spleen continuously makes platelets, and an aspirin taken in the morning neutralizes every circulating platelet in the blood for approximately 20 minutes; however, new platelets made during the day are not affected. A second dose administered in the evening neutralizes the new platelets.

Outpatient arthroplasty patients use calf compression in the hospital before their discharge, which is the equivalent of 6 hours of treatment. Patients are discharged to home with calf-high antithromboembolic stockings, which are worn until the patient can walk 1 mile or for 20 minutes. Most patients remove the antithromboembolic stockings within 1 week. In high-risk patients who are being treated with warfarin transiently for venous thromboprophylaxis and patients who are being treated with warfarin permanently, such as for atrial fibrillation, 81 mg of aspirin should be administered once a day for 2 to 4 weeks to prevent heterotopic ossification. The warfarin dosage may be adjusted if it is affected by the 81 mg of aspirin.

The efficacy of this treatment protocol is validated by patient outcomes. In 10 years, not one incidence of pulmonary embolus or clinically diagnosed deep vein thrombosis has been reported at the facility of one of the authors of this chapter (L.D.D.). There have been no readmissions for any reason. The first 150 patients returned 7 to 10 days postoperatively for an ultrasound, and not a single clot was identified, including calf clots (Lawrence D. Dorr, MD, Los Angeles, CA, unpublished data, 2015). These results can be attributed more to the activity level of patients who were not in a hospital than to just the use of aspirin. One of the authors of this chapter (L.D.D.) believes that the rapid mobilization of these patients and the physical therapy of a daily walk outdoors was the most effective prevention against clots. Data published previously by Dorr et al[22] on outpatient THA document the recovery patterns for the author's (L.D.D.) patients; however, it must be noted that the patients in this study underwent a posterior mini-incision approach, which refutes the notion of an advantage with an anterior incision approach for outpatient THA.[81] The results of Dorr et al[22] can be summarized as follows: One week postoperatively, 42% of patients who worked had returned to work, 75% of patients could walk 1 mile or 30 minutes per day, and 48% of patients were independent for activities of daily living. Three weeks postoperatively, 69% of patients who worked had returned to work, 84% of patients were able to drive, 98% of patients could walk 1 mile or 30 minutes per day, and 73% of patients were independent for activities of daily living.

The Contrarian: Neither My Patients nor I Will Consider Outpatient Arthroplasty

The increases in both TKA and THA volume have been driven by both the aging baby boomer generation, which has become aware that TJA is a successful procedure with the potential for resumption of an active lifestyle; and an aging population, which is encumbered by their arthritic hips and knees but have been under successful medical management despite being viable surgical candidates. As the demand for TJA increases, hospitals and surgeons will seek to optimize the efficiency by which they deliver these procedures because of an associated increase in costs. Possible options to reduce the related expenses include reducing the hospital length of stay and minimizing perioperative complications.[82] Recent advances in minimally invasive surgical techniques, perioperative multimodal analgesia, regional anesthesia, and postoperative clinical pathways have led to rapid recovery programs, which have shortened the hospital length of stay and the subsequent length of recovery for TJA patients. The trend of decreasing the hospital length of stay has further shifted some TJA procedures to the outpatient surgery setting; however, this strategy relies on risk stratification, in which younger, healthy patients who have lower Charlson comorbidity scores undergo outpatient TJA, some even in ambulatory surgery centers, and older patients who have associated comorbidities undergo inpatient TJA at hospitals with varying hospital lengths of stay.

Although advocates for outpatient TJA have been able to perform the TJA in an ambulatory setting, patient safety takes precedence. Most patients who undergo TJA have multiple medical comorbidities. In a review of 516,745 elective TKAs that were performed in patients aged 40 to 95 years, Pugely et al[83] reported that only 12.7% of patients had no comorbidities, whereas 32.6% of patients had three or more comorbidities, with the most common comorbidities being hypertension (67.8%), diabetes mellitus (20.0%), and obesity (19.8%). Patients who had multiple comorbidities required increased hospital resources and had an increased hospital length of stay, which placed a financial burden on many of the hospitals and healthcare systems that performed the procedures. As already mentioned, minimizing perioperative and postoperative complications is an important strategy to reduce costs associated with TJA.[25]

Medical comorbidities are not the sole contributors to postoperative complications. Psychological comorbidities, such as anxiety and depression, are risk factors for moderate to severe postoperative pain.[84] Many times, there is an incongruence between patient- and physician-reported comorbidities; therefore, due diligence is necessary in the preoperative patient interview to accurately assess comorbidities, especially psychological comorbidities.[85] Strategies that focus on the optimization of medical and psychological comorbidities may help improve outcomes and reduce postoperative complications.[86]

The inherent trade-off between shorter hospital lengths of stay and outpatient joint arthroplasties includes a greater need for stringent preoperative evaluation to identify and manage comorbidities, a greater need for a structured program for postoperative acute care, and higher readmission rates. Although some site-specific studies have reported that a shorter hospital length of stay or outpatient surgery via a defined clinical pathway does not increase short-term complications,[24,87,88] this observation may not be universally applied to all hospitals. In a study of a cohort of patients who underwent outpatient TJA, Berger et al[19] reported a 3.6% readmission rate within the first week postoperatively and concluded that the patients would have been better treated in an inpatient setting. Vegari et al[89] also reported a higher readmission rate (10.2%) within 30 days postoperatively for patients who underwent outpatient TJA. If emergency department visits are included as part of the readmission number for unplanned care episodes, 12.4% of outpatients required either hospital readmission or an unplanned further episode of care. These reports support appropriate patient selection to minimize perioperative and postoperative complications. Specific exclusion criteria for outpatient TJA includes patients older than 70 years, myocardial infarction within 1 year, prior pulmonary embolus or deep vein thrombosis, sleep apnea, a body mass index greater than 40 kg/m2, and three or more medical comorbidities.[19]

Pain management is a critical component of a rapid recovery program. Preemptive analgesia, neuraxial anesthesia, periarticular injections, and a pharmacopeia of medications are integral components of a multimodal pain management program. This multimodal approach allows for earlier participation in postoperative rehabilitation, faster attainment of functional milestones, and reduced hospital length of stay. Pain control with this multimodal approach is better if the surgery is performed early in the day because it allows for medication adjustment; however, this may pose a scheduling challenge. Although it may be preferable to

perform the outpatient cases early in the day, the same argument could be made for patients with multiple comorbidities who will need closer monitoring during their hospitalization.

Reduced hospital length of stay may lead to reduced vigilance in monitoring for early signs of superficial wound infections and complications, such as deep vein thrombosis, in the early postoperative period, which could potentially result in readmission for more serious complications. All patients who undergo TJA should receive preoperative patient education, have a mechanism for communication with postoperative care providers, and arrange appropriate follow-up care.

The widespread practice of reducing the hospital length of stay to less than 3 days may be associated with some negative consequences if not managed properly.[25] In the past decade, there has been a marked decline in Medicare patient hospital lengths of stay from 7.9 days (1991 to 1994) to 3.5 days (2007 to 2010), which reflects improvements in the clinical pathway.[90] However, this also has generated more scrutiny on outcomes and transparency with the reporting of infection rates, complications, and readmissions, all of which affect the hospital length of stay. Therefore, it is important to improve clinical outcomes with the implementation of a risk reduction program, appropriate coding of all preoperative comorbidities, and the evaluation and treatment of all complications. There is concern that a decrease in hospital lengths of stay is accompanied by an increase in hospital readmission rates. Under the Patient Protection and Affordable Care Act and the Medicare Hospital Readmission Reduction Program, hospitals that have excess readmissions within

30 days of discharge are penalized with fines from the US Centers for Medicare & Medicaid Services (CMS). Since the implementation of this law in 2012, the CMS began evaluating the readmissions for THAs and TKAs. The number of hospitals that have been fined has increased, and the fine can be 1% to 3% of a hospital's Medicare payments. It is imperative that a great deal of scrutiny is used in planning patient discharge and that readmission is minimized with meticulous perioperative surveillance.

Although a reduction in the hospital length of stay will affect TJA costs, the CMS is taking into account the procedure time, the hospital length of stay, and accelerated recovery programs in their calculation of the work relative value units related to THA and TKA. In 2014, the work relative value units were decreased by 5% for THA and by 11% for TKA. Furthermore, beginning in 2017, the CMS is reducing the global procedure to "0 days" because it appears that the current global payments are too high and include more postoperative services than are actually provided.

An orthopaedic surgeon's focus should be on a gradual transition to reduced hospital length of stay so that all patients can be safely optimized for discharge and the implementation of protocols that are beyond the current capabilities of hospital systems can be avoided. This includes the preoperative optimization of each patient with appropriate identification and management of comorbidities; preoperative patient education with engagement of family caregivers; preoperative discharge planning, preferably to the home; surgical efficiencies; and postoperative clinical pathways that follow a team approach and employ current evidence-based clinical guidelines. Patient selection, hospital specialization, and an appropriate follow-up protocol will facilitate a rapid recovery program and further safely reduce the hospital length of stay.

Summary

Currently, THA, TKA, and TSA can be safely performed as outpatient procedures if surgical and anesthetic protocol refinements are implemented. Outpatient TJA is one step further in the rapid recovery protocols for TJA. Rapid recovery TJA changed the entire paradigm of how health care is delivered. Understanding and safely addressing the reasons that surgeons and patients believe they need a hospital admission for arthroplasty procedures is the cornerstone of outpatient arthroplasty. The avoidance of a hospital stay negates the possibility of hospital-acquired infections. The promotion of early mobilization and early same-day discharge to home may decrease the incidence of postoperative pneumonia, atelectasis, ileus, and venous thromboembolism. The risk of surgical interventions can be mitigated by controlling and minimizing pain, nausea, somnolence, and bleeding, which allows patients to recover faster and enables large joint arthroplasty to be performed safely in an outpatient setting with high patient satisfaction. The singular focus on the patient and the avoidance of overtreatment will become the standard of care for TJA in much the same way it did for other procedures that were once deemed inpatient surgeries. In properly selected patients, the risk-benefit ratio favors the benefits to patients.

References

1. Berend KR, Lombardi AV Jr, Mallory TH: Rapid recovery protocol for peri-operative care of total hip and total knee arthroplasty patients. *Surg Technol Int* 2004;13:239-247.

2. Lombardi AV Jr, Viacava AJ, Berend KR: Rapid recovery protocols and minimally invasive surgery help achieve high knee flexion. *Clin Orthop Relat Res* 2006;452:117-122.

3. Lombardi AV, Berend KR, Adams JB: A rapid recovery program: Early home and pain free. *Orthopedics* 2010;33(9):656.

4. Meding JB, Klay M, Healy A, Ritter MA, Keating EM, Berend ME: The prescreening history and physical in elective total joint arthroplasty. *J Arthroplasty* 2007;22(6 suppl 2):21-23.

5. Mallory TH, Lombardi AV Jr, Fada RA, Dodds KL: Anesthesia options: Choices and caveats. *Orthopedics* 2000;23(9):919-920.

6. Mallory TH, Lombardi AV Jr, Fada RA, Dodds KL, Adams JB: Pain management for joint arthroplasty: Preemptive analgesia. *J Arthroplasty* 2002;17(4 suppl 1):129-133.

7. Lombardi AV Jr, Berend KR, Mallory TH, Dodds KL, Adams JB: Soft tissue and intra-articular injection of bupivacaine, epinephrine, and morphine has a beneficial effect after total knee arthroplasty. *Clin Orthop Relat Res* 2004;428:125-130.

8. Chimento GF, Huff T, Ochsner JL Jr, Meyer M, Brandner L, Babin S: An evaluation of the use of topical tranexamic acid in total knee arthroplasty. *J Arthroplasty* 2013;28(8 suppl):74-77.

9. Gandhi R, Evans HM, Mahomed SR, Mahomed NN: Tranexamic acid and the reduction of blood loss in total knee and hip arthroplasty: A meta-analysis. *BMC Res Notes* 2013;6:184.

10. Gilbody J, Dhotar HS, Perruccio AV, Davey JR: Topical tranexamic acid reduces transfusion rates in total hip and knee arthroplasty. *J Arthroplasty* 2014;29(4):681-684.

11. Aynardi M, Post Z, Ong A, Orozco F, Sukin DC: Outpatient surgery as a means of cost reduction in total hip arthroplasty: A case-control study. *HSS J* 2014;10(3):252-255.

12. Bertin KC: Minimally invasive outpatient total hip arthroplasty: A financial analysis. *Clin Orthop Relat Res* 2005;435:154-163.

13. Berger RA: Total hip arthroplasty using the minimally invasive two-incision approach. *Clin Orthop Relat Res* 2003;417:232-241.

14. Berger RA, Jacobs JJ, Meneghini RM, Della Valle C, Paprosky W, Rosenberg AG: Rapid rehabilitation and recovery with minimally invasive total hip arthroplasty. *Clin Orthop Relat Res* 2004;429:239-247.

15. Berger RA, Sanders S, Gerlinger T, Della Valle C, Jacobs JJ, Rosenberg AG: Outpatient total knee arthroplasty with a minimally invasive technique. *J Arthroplasty* 2005; 20(7 suppl 3):33-38.

16. Berger RA: A comprehensive approach to outpatient total hip arthroplasty. *Am J Orthop (Belle Mead NJ)* 2007;36(9 suppl):4-5.

17. Berger RA, Sanders S, D'Ambrogio E, et al: Minimally invasive quadriceps-sparing TKA: Results of a comprehensive pathway for outpatient TKA. *J Knee Surg* 2006;19(2):145-148.

18. Berger RA, Sanders SA, Thill ES, Sporer SM, Della Valle C: Newer anesthesia and rehabilitation protocols enable outpatient hip replacement in selected patients. *Clin Orthop Relat Res* 2009;467(6):1424-1430.

19. Berger RA, Kusuma SK, Sanders SA, Thill ES, Sporer SM: The feasibility and perioperative complications of outpatient knee arthroplasty. *Clin Orthop Relat Res* 2009;467(6):1443-1449.

20. Chen D, Berger RA: Outpatient minimally invasive total hip arthroplasty via a modified Watson-Jones approach: Technique and results. *Instr Course Lect* 2013;62:229-236.

21. Cross MB, Berger R: Feasibility and safety of performing outpatient unicompartmental knee arthroplasty. *Int Orthop* 2014;38(2):443-447.

22. Dorr LD, Thomas DJ, Zhu J, Dastane M, Chao L, Long WT: Outpatient total hip arthroplasty. *J Arthroplasty* 2010;25(4):501-506.

23. Gondusky JS, Choi L, Khalaf N, Patel J, Barnett S, Gorab R: Day of surgery discharge after unicompartmental knee arthroplasty: An effective perioperative pathway. *J Arthroplasty* 2014;29(3):516-519.

24. Kolisek FR, McGrath MS, Jessup NM, Monesmith EA, Mont MA: Comparison of outpatient versus inpatient total knee arthroplasty. *Clin Orthop Relat Res* 2009;467(6):1438-1442.

25. Lovald ST, Ong KL, Malkani AL, et al: Complications, mortality, and costs for outpatient and short-stay total knee arthroplasty patients in comparison to standard-stay patients. *J Arthroplasty* 2014;29(3):510-515.

26. Lovald S, Ong K, Lau E, Joshi G, Kurtz S, Malkani A: Patient selection in outpatient and short-stay total knee arthroplasty. *J Surg Orthop Adv* 2014;23(1):2-8.

27. Berend KR, Lombardi AV Jr: Liberal indications for minimally invasive Oxford unicondylar arthroplasty provide rapid functional recovery and pain relief. *Surg Technol Int* 2007;16:193-197.

28. Carmichael NM, Katz J, Clarke H, et al: An intensive perioperative regimen of pregabalin and celecoxib reduces pain and improves physical function scores six weeks after total hip arthroplasty: A prospective randomized controlled trial. *Pain Res Manag* 2013;18(3):127-132.

29. Mears DC, Mears SC, Chelly JE, Dai F, Vulakovich KL: THA with a minimally invasive technique, multi-modal anesthesia, and home rehabilitation: Factors associated with early discharge? *Clin Orthop Relat Res* 2009;467(6):1412-1417.

30. Sculco PK, Pagnano MW: Perioperative solutions for rapid recovery joint arthroplasty: Get ahead and stay ahead. *J Arthroplasty* 2015;30(4):518-520.

31. Affas F, Nygårds EB, Stiller CO, Wretenberg P, Olofsson C: Pain control after total knee arthroplasty: A randomized trial comparing local infiltration anesthesia and continuous femoral block. *Acta Orthop* 2011;82(4):441-447.

32. Wheeler M, Oderda GM, Ashburn MA, Lipman AG: Adverse events associated with postoperative opioid analgesia: A systematic review. *J Pain* 2002;3(3):159-180.

33. Oderda GM, Said Q, Evans RS, et al: Opioid-related adverse drug events in surgical hospitalizations: Impact on costs and length of stay. *Ann Pharmacother* 2007;41(3):400-406.

34. Cepeda MS, Farrar JT, Baumgarten M, Boston R, Carr DB, Strom BL: Side effects of opioids during short-term administration: Effect of age, gender, and race. *Clin Pharmacol Ther* 2003;74(2):102-112.

35. Sharma S, Iorio R, Specht LM, Davies-Lepie S, Healy WL: Complications of femoral nerve block for total knee arthroplasty. *Clin Orthop Relat Res* 2010;468(1):135-140.

36. Beaupre LA, Johnston DB, Dieleman S, Tsui B: Impact of a preemptive multimodal analgesia plus femoral nerve blockade protocol on rehabilitation, hospital length of stay, and postoperative analgesia after primary total knee arthroplasty: A controlled clinical pilot study. *ScientificWorldJournal* 2012;2012:273821.

37. Kerr DR, Kohan L: Local infiltration analgesia: A technique for the control of acute postoperative pain following knee and hip surgery. A case study of 325 patients. *Acta Orthop* 2008;79(2):174-183.

38. Parvataneni HK, Shah VP, Howard H, Cole N, Ranawat AS, Ranawat CS: Controlling pain after total hip and knee arthroplasty using a multimodal protocol with local periarticular injections: A prospective randomized study. *J Arthroplasty* 2007;22(6 suppl 2):33-38.

39. Busch CA, Shore BJ, Bhandari R, et al: Efficacy of periarticular multimodal drug injection in total knee arthroplasty: A randomized trial. *J Bone Joint Surg Am* 2006;88(5):959-963.

40. Paul JE, Arya A, Hurlburt L, et al: Femoral nerve block improves analgesia outcomes after total knee arthroplasty: A meta-analysis of randomized controlled trials. *Anesthesiology* 2010;113(5):1144-1162.

41. American Society of Anesthesiologists Task Force on Acute Pain Management: Practice guidelines for acute pain management in the perioperative setting: An updated report by the American Society of Anesthesiologists Task Force on Acute Pain Management. *Anesthesiology* 2012;116(2):248-273.

42. Kehlet H: Surgical stress: The role of pain and analgesia. *Br J Anaesth* 1989;63(2):189-195.

43. Pavlin DJ, Chen C, Penaloza DA, Buckley FP: A survey of pain and other symptoms that affect the recovery process after discharge from an ambulatory surgery unit. *J Clin Anesth* 2004;16(3):200-206.

44. Wu CL, Naqibuddin M, Rowlingson AJ, Lietman SA, Jermyn RM, Fleisher LA: The effect of pain on health-related quality of life in the immediate postoperative period. *Anesth Analg* 2003;97(4):1078-1085.

45. Carr DB, Reines HD, Schaffer J, Polomano RC, Lande S: The impact of technology on the analgesic gap and quality of acute pain management. *Reg Anesth Pain Med* 2005;30(3):286-291.

46. Ng A, Hall F, Atkinson A, Kong KL, Hahn A: Bridging the analgesic gap. *Acute Pain* 2000;3(4):194-199.

47. Chen PP, Chui PT, Ma M, Gin T: A prospective survey of patients after cessation of patient-controlled analgesia. *Anesth Analg* 2001;92(1):224-227.

48. Green CR, Anderson KO, Baker TA, et al: The unequal burden of pain: Confronting racial and ethnic disparities in pain. *Pain Med* 2003;4(3):277-294.

49. Atherton MJ, Feeg VD, el-Adham AF: Race, ethnicity, and insurance as determinants of epidural use: Analysis of a national sample survey. *Nurs Econ* 2004;22(1):6-13, 3.

50. Joshi GP, Kehlet H: Procedure-specific pain management: The road to improve postsurgical pain management? *Anesthesiology* 2013;118(4):780-782.

51. Davidson EM, Barenholz Y, Cohen R, Haroutiunian S, Kagan L, Ginosar Y: High-dose bupivacaine remotely loaded into multivesicular liposomes demonstrates slow drug release without systemic toxic plasma concentrations after subcutaneous

administration in humans. *Anesth Analg* 2010;110(4):1018-1023.

52. Bergese SD, Ramamoorthy S, Patou G, Bramlett K, Gorfine SR, Candiotti KA: Efficacy profile of liposome bupivacaine, a novel formulation of bupivacaine for postsurgical analgesia. *J Pain Res* 2012;5:107-116.

53. Dasta J, Ramamoorthy S, Patou G, Sinatra R: Bupivacaine liposome injectable suspension compared with bupivacaine HCl for the reduction of opioid burden in the postsurgical setting. *Curr Med Res Opin* 2012;28(10):1609-1615.

54. Golf M, Daniels SE, Onel E: A phase 3, randomized, placebo-controlled trial of DepoFoam® bupivacaine (extended-release bupivacaine local analgesic) in bunionectomy. *Adv Ther* 2011;28(9):776-788.

55. Cohen SM: Extended pain relief trial utilizing infiltration of Exparel(®), a long-acting multivesicular liposome formulation of bupivacaine: A Phase IV health economic trial in adult patients undergoing open colectomy. *J Pain Res* 2012;5:567-572.

56. Marcet JE, Nfonsam VN, Larach S: An extended pain relief trial utilizing the infiltration of a long-acting multivesicular liposome formulation of bupivacaine, EXPAREL (IMPROVE): A Phase IV health economic trial in adult patients undergoing ileostomy reversal. *J Pain Res* 2013;6:549-555.

57. Vogel JD: Liposome bupivacaine (EXPAREL®) for extended pain relief in patients undergoing ileostomy reversal at a single institution with a fast-track discharge protocol: An IMPROVE Phase IV health economics trial. *J Pain Res* 2013;6:605-610.

58. Haas E, Onel E, Miller H, Ragupathi M, White PF: A double-blind, randomized, active-controlled study for post-hemorrhoidectomy pain management with liposome bupivacaine, a novel local analgesic formulation. *Am Surg* 2012;78(5):574-581. Medline

59. Bergese SD, Onel E, Morren M, Morganroth J: Bupivacaine extended-release liposome injection exhibits a favorable cardiac safety profile. *Reg Anesth Pain Med* 2012;37(2):145-151.

60. Syed HM, Green L, Bianski B, Jobe CM, Wongworawat MD: Bupivacaine and triamcinolone may be toxic to human chondrocytes: A pilot study. *Clin Orthop Relat Res* 2011;469(10):2941-2947.

61. Rosencher N, Kerkkamp HE, Macheras G, et al: Orthopedic Surgery Transfusion Hemoglobin European Overview (OSTHEO) study: Blood management in elective knee and hip arthroplasty in Europe. *Transfusion* 2003;43(4):459-469.

62. Hatzidakis AM, Mendlick RM, McKillip T, Reddy RL, Garvin KL: Preoperative autologous donation for total joint arthroplasty: An analysis of risk factors for allogenic transfusion. *J Bone Joint Surg Am* 2000;82(1):89-100.

63. Woolson ST, Pouliot MA, Huddleston JI: Primary total hip arthroplasty using an anterior approach and a fracture table: Short-term results from a community hospital. *J Arthroplasty* 2009;24(7):999-1005.

64. Seng BE, Berend KR, Ajluni AF, Lombardi AV Jr: Anterior-supine minimally invasive total hip arthroplasty: Defining the learning curve. *Orthop Clin North Am* 2009;40(3):343-350.

65. Park JH, Rasouli MR, Mortazavi SM, Tokarski AT, Maltenfort MG, Parvizi J: Predictors of perioperative blood loss in total joint arthroplasty. *J Bone Joint Surg Am* 2013;95(19):1777-1783.

66. Juelsgaard P, Larsen UT, Sørensen JV, Madsen F, Søballe K: Hypotensive epidural anesthesia in total knee replacement without tourniquet: Reduced blood loss and transfusion. *Reg Anesth Pain Med* 2001;26(2):105-110.

67. Sharrock NE, Salvati EA: Hypotensive epidural anesthesia for total hip arthroplasty: A review. *Acta Orthop Scand* 1996;67(1):91-107.

68. Eroglu A, Uzunlar H, Erciyes N: Comparison of hypotensive epidural anesthesia and hypotensive total intravenous anesthesia on intraoperative blood loss during total hip replacement. *J Clin Anesth* 2005;17(6):420-425.

69. Duncan CM, Gillette BP, Jacob AK, Sierra RJ, Sanchez-Sotelo J, Smith HM: Venous thromboembolism and mortality associated with

tranexamic acid use during total hip and knee arthroplasty. *J Arthroplasty* 2015;30(2):272-276.

70. Wind TC, Barfield WR, Moskal JT: The effect of tranexamic acid on transfusion rate in primary total hip arthroplasty. *J Arthroplasty* 2014;29(2):387-389.

71. Konig G, Hamlin BR, Waters JH: Topical tranexamic acid reduces blood loss and transfusion rates in total hip and total knee arthroplasty. *J Arthroplasty* 2013;28(9):1473-1476.

72. Pierson JL, Hannon TJ, Earles DR: A blood-conservation algorithm to reduce blood transfusions after total hip and knee arthroplasty. *J Bone Joint Surg Am* 2004;86(7):1512-1518.

73. Bolognesi MP, Greiner MA, Attarian DE, et al: Unicompartmental knee arthroplasty and total knee arthroplasty among Medicare beneficiaries, 2000 to 2009. *J Bone Joint Surg Am* 2013;95(22):e174.

74. Berend ME, Berend KR, Lombardi AV Jr: Advances in pain management: Game changers in knee arthroplasty. *Bone Joint J* 2014;96(11 suppl A):7-9.

75. Ilfeld BM, Wright TW, Enneking FK, et al: Total shoulder arthroplasty as an outpatient procedure using ambulatory perineural local anesthetic infusion: A pilot feasibility study. *Anesth Analg* 2005;101(5):1319-1322.

76. Ilfeld BM, Vandenborne K, Duncan PW, et al: Ambulatory continuous interscalene nerve blocks decrease the time to discharge readiness after total shoulder arthroplasty: A randomized, triple-masked, placebo-controlled study. *Anesthesiology* 2006;105(5):999-1007.

77. Gallay SH, Lobo JJ, Baker J, Smith K, Patel K: Development of a regional model of care for ambulatory total shoulder arthroplasty: A pilot study. *Clin Orthop Relat Res* 2008;466(3):563-572.

78. Shah A, Nielsen KC, Braga L, Pietrobon R, Klein SM, Steele SM: Interscalene brachial plexus block for outpatient shoulder arthroplasty: Postoperative analgesia, patient satisfaction and complications. *Indian J Orthop* 2007;41(3):230-236.

79. Dorr LD, Thomas D, Long WT, Polatin PB, Sirianni LE: Psychologic reasons for patients preferring minimally invasive total hip arthroplasty. *Clin Orthop Relat Res* 2007;458:94-100.

80. Dorr LD, Gendelman V, Maheshwari AV, Boutary M, Wan Z, Long WT: Multimodal thromboprophylaxis for total hip and knee arthroplasty based on risk assessment. *J Bone Joint Surg Am* 2007;89(12):2648-2657.

81. Dorr LD, Maheshwari AV, Long WT, Wan Z, Sirianni LE: Early pain relief and function after posterior minimally invasive and conventional total hip arthroplasty: A prospective, randomized, blinded study. *J Bone Joint Surg Am* 2007;89(6):1153-1160.

82. Larsen K, Hansen TB, Thomsen PB, Christiansen T, Søballe K: Cost-effectiveness of accelerated perioperative care and rehabilitation after total hip and knee arthroplasty. *J Bone Joint Surg Am* 2009;91(4):761-772.

83. Pugely AJ, Martin CT, Gao Y, Belatti DA, Callaghan JJ: Comorbidities in patients undergoing total knee arthroplasty: Do they influence hospital costs and length of stay? *Clin Orthop Relat Res* 2014;472(12):3943-3950.

84. Singh JA, Lewallen DG: Medical and psychological comorbidity predicts poor pain outcomes after total knee arthroplasty. *Rheumatology (Oxford)* 2013;52(5):916-923.

85. Gad BV, Higuera CA, Klika AK, Elsharkawy KA, Barsoum WK: Validity of patient-reported comorbidities before total knee and hip arthroplasty in patients older than 65 years. *J Arthroplasty* 2012;27(10):1750-1756.e1.

86. Singh JA, Lewallen DG: Depression in primary TKA and higher medical comorbidities in revision TKA are associated with suboptimal subjective improvement in knee function. *BMC Musculoskelet Disord* 2014;15:127.

87. Teeny SM, York SC, Benson C, Perdue ST: Does shortened length of hospital stay affect total knee arthroplasty rehabilitation outcomes? *J Arthroplasty* 2005;20(7 suppl 3):39-45.

88. Isaac D, Falode T, Liu P, I'Anson H, Dillow K, Gill P: Accelerated rehabilitation after total knee replacement. *Knee* 2005;12(5):346-350.

89. Vegari DN, Mokris JG, Odum SM, Springer BD: Paper No. 367. Implications of outpatient vs inpatient total joint arthroplasty on hospital readmission rates. *AAOS 2014 Annual Meeting Proceedings*. Rosemont, IL, American Academy of Orthopaedic Surgeons, 2014.

90. Cram P, Lu X, Kates SL, Singh JA, Li Y, Wolf BR: Total knee arthroplasty volume, utilization, and outcomes among Medicare beneficiaries, 1991-2010. *JAMA* 2012;308(12):1227-1236.

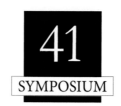
Outpatient Hip and Knee Replacement: The Experience From the First 15 Years

Richard A. Berger, MD
Michael B. Cross, MD
Sheila Sanders, RN, BSN, DNC

Abstract

Rapid recovery and early discharge after total joint arthroplasty are becoming more common. To develop a successful, safe, outpatient arthroplasty practice, surgeons must have the support of a multidisciplinary team, which includes an orthopaedic surgeon, an anesthesiologist, nurses, physical therapists, and a discharge planner. The authors of this chapter recommend surgeons start with healthier, motivated patients and focus on total hip replacements and unicompartmental knee replacements in the learning curve phase of the transition to outpatient total joint arthroplasty. It is important for orthopaedic surgeons to establish an outpatient joint arthroplasty protocol as well as ways to avoid complications and delays in discharge.

Instr Course Lect 2016;65:547–552.

DThe Inception of Outpatient Hip and Knee Replacement

In 1999, the senior author of this chapter (R.A.B.) began to develop a minimally invasive total hip replacement procedure that would accelerate patient recovery, and soon after, he began to develop a minimally invasive knee replacement procedure. To ensure patient safety, the senior author of this chapter performed more than 40 minimally invasive hip replacement surgeries on cadaver models before the first tissue-sparing minimally invasive total hip replacement was performed on a patient in 2000.[1] After a similar cadaver model learning curve for minimally invasive knee replacement surgeries, the senior author of this chapter began performing minimally invasive total knee replacements with a quadriceps-sparing approach on patients in 2002.[2]

Because of these tissue-sparing surgical innovations, patients began to recover faster, and it became clear that the entire perioperative recovery process needed to be restructured to keep pace with the rapid recovery that was resulting from the improved surgical techniques. Outpatient arthroplasty, which would allow patients to be discharged to home a few hours after surgery, was the natural culmination of the synergy between the refinement of rapid recovery protocols and the improvement of minimally invasive surgical techniques.

The first outpatient, same day, total hip replacement was performed in 2001 at Rush University Medical Center by the senior author of this chapter. Many articles have since been published on the surgical techniques and rapid recovery protocols that were used for outpatient total hip replacements.[1,3-5] Shortly after routine outpatient total hip replacements were successfully accomplished, the total hip protocols at

Dr. Berger or an immediate family member has received royalties from Zimmer, and serves as a paid consultant to or is an employee of MicroPort. Dr. Cross or an immediate family member has received royalties from Smith & Nephew, and serves as a paid consultant to or is an employee of Acelity, Exactech, Intellijoint, LinkBio, and Smith & Nephew. Neither Ms. Sanders nor any immediate family member has received anything of value from or has stock or stock options held in a commercial company or institution related directly or indirectly to the subject of this chapter.

Table 1

Length of Hospital Stay for Patients Who Underwent Hip or Knee Replacement Surgery at Rush University Medical Center With Richard A. Berger, MD

Year	Outpatient (n)	1 day (n)	>1 day (n)
2004	200	88	296
2005	281	189	252
2006	341	253	95
2007	596	281	44
2008	591	301	36
2009	616	306	43
2010	639	381	43
2011	636	382	46
2012	676	405	45
2013	797	380	22
Total	**5,373**	**2,966**	**922**

Rush University Medical Center were modified and combined with minimally invasive, quadriceps-sparing, knee arthroplasty techniques. The knowledge acquired from the outpatient hip replacement procedures was applied to knees and resulted in the first outpatient unicompartmental knee replacement and the first outpatient total knee replacement in 2002 and 2003, respectively.[2,6-9]

Since the development of these outpatient hip and knee replacement procedures at Rush University Medical Center, the senior author of this chapter has continually increased the number of patients who have outpatient hip and knee replacement procedures[9,10] (**Table 1**). In 2013, the senior author of this chapter successfully discharged 797 patients from the hospital the same day of surgery and 380 patients from the hospital the day after surgery. These numbers represent 98% of all arthroplasties being performed as either outpatient procedures or next-day discharge procedures by the senior author of this chapter.

The senior author of this chapter performed 5,373 outpatient hip and knee replacements from 2004 to 2013. During the same time, the senior author of this chapter performed 2,966 hip and knee replacement procedures in patients who were discharged the day after surgery. Since 2007, 62% of the senior author's primary hip and knee replacements were successfully discharged the same day as surgery, 34% of the senior author's primary hip and knee replacements stayed in the hospital overnight, and only 4% of the senior author's primary hip and knee replacements stayed in the hospital more than one night. These data represent every primary hip and knee replacement performed by the senior author of this chapter. The hip and knee replacement procedures the senior author of this chapter performed in 2013 include 241 total hip replacements, 479 total knee replacements, and 87 unicompartmental knee replacements in patients who were discharged the same day as surgery. **Table 1** shows the length of hospital stay for patients who underwent hip and knee replacement surgery with the senior author of this chapter in the past decade.

Current Interest in Outpatient Hip and Knee Replacement

The current healthcare industry is attempting to reduce costs while maintaining the same level of care. Most healthcare entities, from orthopaedic surgeons to hospital administrators and insurance companies, are attempting to safely decrease the length of hospital stay to lower costs while concurrently diminishing the risks of hospital-acquired infections and complications.[11-15] With respect to cost savings, Bertin[16] reported that the mean hospital bill for outpatient total hip arthroplasty was $4,000 less than the mean hospital bill for inpatient total hip arthroplasty. Rapid recovery rehabilitation protocols have been increasingly implemented in many practices to take advantage of these cost savings. The synergy from the combination of a less invasive surgical approach, a multimodal anesthesia protocol, a multimodal postoperative pain regimen, and rapid recovery physical therapy allows for a more rapid recovery and allows for outpatient total hip and knee arthroplasty to be safely performed.[3,9,14] However, a multidisciplinary team, which includes an orthopaedic surgeon, an anesthesiologist, nurses, physical therapists, and a discharge planner, is necessary to ensure that patients who are candidates for outpatient hip and knee replacement are discharged home safely and early.[3-10]

Preoperative Management

A patient's main concerns with being discharged after total hip arthroplasty are the fear of uncontrollable pain and dependency on others.[3] Preoperative patient education is essential to allay these concerns and helps build patient confidence and trust in the patient-care team. Preoperative patient education also will set a patient's expectations of early discharge to home and assure him or her that it is safe.[17] All patients should attend a preoperative joint arthroplasty education class that is taught by a clinical nurse; the postoperative primary caregiver is encouraged to attend with the patient. In the preoperative joint arthroplasty education class, the nurse will explain the procedure, postoperative pain regimen (which includes a multimodal anesthesia approach), and the degree of dependency required as well as allow time to answer all of the patients' questions. This process takes place over the course of 2 hours. When Rush University Medical Center began preoperative joint arthroplasty education classes more than a decade ago, patients also attended a physical therapy session at which they learned how to ambulate with the use of various ambulatory assistive devices, such as walkers, crutches, and canes. For more than a decade, Rush University Medical Center has discharged patients from the hospital who have ambulated without any assistive device just a few hours after surgery. Because patients did not require much physical therapy before discharge and because they routinely received only a cane and rarely used it, Rush University Medical Center has discontinued preoperative physical therapy.

Rush University Medical Center's preoperative protocol requires that patients also see an internal medicine attending physician to obtain clearance for elective joint arthroplasty. Similarly, all patients have a discharge planner contact them and their caregiver preoperatively to arrange all postoperative services, including transportation home, home care nursing services, and home physical therapy. These crucial steps are required to facilitate rapid discharge and minimize patients' fears of dependency. The initiation of preoperative pain management decreases early postoperative pain and fear of pain; therefore, patients who will be treated with postoperative narcotics are treated with 10 mg of controlled-release oxycodone hydrochloride the morning of surgery. In addition, a scopolamine patch is placed in the holding area and is applied before surgery to decrease the incidence of severe nausea that may be caused by the narcotics used preoperatively, intraoperatively, and postoperatively. A scopolamine patch should be avoided in older men, patients who have a history of urinary retention, and patients who have glaucoma issues.

Anesthesia

Multimodal anesthesia uses different classes of analgesic agents and different sites of analgesic agent administration to provide superior dynamic pain relief with reduced analgesic-related side effects. Regional anesthesia facilitates a rapid recovery program by decreasing the amount of narcotics required immediately after and during surgery, which decreases the number of patients in whom postoperative nausea or hypotension develops. All patients who participate in Rush University Medical Center's rapid recovery protocol receive epidural anesthesia. Patients are treated with a dose of midazolam before the epidural is placed, which further alleviates and allays the preconceived fears of the use of epidurals. The epidural is dosed as follows: fentanyl 10 μg/mL plus 0.1% bupivacaine at 6 mL of continuous infusion, 1 mL every 15 minutes with a 40-mL 4-hour lockout. In addition to the epidural, a titrated dose of propofol is administered intraoperatively.

The Surgery

Currently, a minimally invasive modified Watson-Jones approach is used for total hip replacements.[10] Similarly, a quadriceps-sparing, minimally invasive approach is used for total knee replacements and unicompartmental knee replacements.[6-9] By using these minimally invasive approaches, soft-tissue trauma is minimized, which decreases postoperative pain and allows for less use of perioperative medications (eg, narcotics). Less perioperative medications lead to less perioperative side effects and medication-related complications. The use of only epidural anesthesia that includes minimal propofol does not provide the soft-tissue laxity that general anesthesia provides. Although epidural anesthesia makes the surgical approach and visualization challenging for the surgeon, patients benefit greatly.

Intraoperative and Postoperative Care

In addition to minimal sedation, all patients are given intravenous acetaminophen, appropriate intravenous fluids, and a unit of autologous blood. After the procedure is complete and before closure, the periarticular soft tissues of all patients are treated with 60 mg of 0.5% bupivacaine. The authors of this chapter have learned that complex cocktails for injection are not necessary if surgery is performed with great care so as not to injure the surrounding soft tissues. In all patients, the placement of a Foley catheter helps decrease the risk of postoperative urinary retention from the epidural. The catheter is removed immediately after surgery. In the recovery room, patients are given 4 mg of ondansetron. The scopolamine patch, which was placed preoperatively, is maintained for 72 hours. The epidural is discontinued immediately after surgery. Physical therapy is initiated 2 to 4 hours after surgery. Although postoperative care is provided predominantly by the recovery room nursing staff, a clinical nurse who works directly with the surgeon oversees the recovery process to ensure the protocol is effective as well as that all patients are well cared for and have all their questions answered efficiently. The protocols at Rush University Medical Center require that each patient, whether an outpatient or an overnight stay patient, independently transfer from the bed to a standing position, ambulate 100 feet, ascend and descend one flight of stairs, demonstrate stable vital signs, have adequate pain control, tolerate a regular diet, and be willing to be discharged home before they are discharged.

At the time of discharge, most patients are given 325 mg of enteric-coated aspirin, which should be taken every 12 hours for 3 weeks for pharmacologic thromboprophylaxis. Currently, approximately 94% of the patients at Rush University Medical Center are given 325 mg of enteric-coated aspirin. Patients receive 1 to 2 weeks of home physical therapy, after which they progress to outpatient physical therapy for an additional 2 to 6 weeks, depending on their progress.

Postoperative Pain Regimen

Every attempt should be made to avoid intravenous narcotic pain medication postoperatively. Depending on age, tolerance, and history of narcotic use,

patients either should not be treated with controlled-release oxycodone hydrochloride or should be treated with 10 mg or 20 mg of controlled-release oxycodone hydrochloride twice daily, which should be tapered over 5 days after surgery. In addition, depending on age, tolerance, and history of narcotic use, patients should be treated either with acetaminophen, tramadol, or 10 mg/325 mg of hydrocodone/acetaminophen every 4 to 6 hours as needed for breakthrough pain in the first 6 weeks. In addition, Rush University Medical Center treats all their patients with 75 mg of diclofenac every 12 hours for 3 months and 40 mg of pantoprazole every day for 3 months for gastrointestinal prophylaxis. Patients are treated with a 50-mg dose of pregabalin every 12 hours for the first 2 weeks. Pregabalin is added to the multimodal postoperative pain regimen to minimize the risk of sciatic flare-ups, which may be caused by the transition to a more normalized gait pattern. If patients have tight muscles, baclofen also may be added to the multimodal postoperative pain regimen.

Patients are monitored with a phone call 1 day after surgery and 1 week after surgery as well as physically seen in the office 2 to 3 weeks after surgery for clinical and radiographic evaluation. Patients are encouraged to contact the primary surgeon or one of the clinical nurses directly with any questions or concerns. The patient is given very specific discharge instructions, including a tailored medication graph and emergency contact information. The emergency contact information includes the primary surgeon's home telephone number and the clinic nurses' cell phone numbers, which are answered 24 hours a day, 7 days a week.

Summary

Outpatient hip and knee replacements have been successfully performed at Rush University Medical Center for almost 15 years. Same-day arthroplasty represents more than 60% of the senior author's practice for hip and knee replacements. Outpatient arthroplasty can be safely performed with the support of a multidisciplinary team, which includes an orthopaedic surgeon, an anesthesiologist, nurses, physical therapists, and a discharge planner. After 15 years of experience, a few lessons have been learned. If surgeons are attempting to adopt an outpatient total joint arthroplasty program, patients should first be selected as candidates. In the learning curve phase of the transition to outpatient total joint arthroplasties, the authors of this chapter recommend surgeons begin with relatively healthy, motivated patients and focus on outpatient total hip replacements and outpatient unicompartmental knee replacements. After the protocol and follow-up program improves, surgeons may then perform outpatient total knee replacements and outpatient total joint arthroplasty on any patient. To successfully implement an outpatient total joint arthroplasty program, the multidisciplinary team must work together to avoid and manage problems that may potentially prevent day-of-surgery discharge, including postoperative nausea, poor pain control, urinary retention, oversedation, hypotension, and the patient's and patient's family's fears. Preoperative patient education that outlines the surgical procedure and sets patients' expectations for early or outpatient discharge is necessary. The surgical team and the anesthesia team must work together to limit the use of multimodal anesthesia that includes epidural and intravenous narcotics; this will prevent any side effects from narcotics that may delay early discharge. The authors of this chapter have learned that if multimodal anesthesia is used appropriately, most patients can be safely discharged to home the same day as surgery.

References

1. Berger RA: Total hip arthroplasty using the minimally invasive two-incision approach. *Clin Orthop Relat Res* 2003;417:232-241.

2. Berger RA, Deirmengian CA, Della Valle CJ, Paprosky WG, Jacobs JJ, Rosenberg AG: A technique for minimally invasive, quadriceps-sparing total knee arthroplasty. *J Knee Surg* 2006;19(1):63-70.

3. Berger RA, Sanders SA, Thill ES, Sporer SM, Della Valle C: Newer anesthesia and rehabilitation protocols enable outpatient hip replacement in selected patients. *Clin Orthop Relat Res* 2009;467(6):1424-1430.

4. Berger RA, Jacobs JJ, Meneghini RM, Della Valle C, Paprosky W, Rosenberg AG: Rapid rehabilitation and recovery with minimally invasive total hip arthroplasty. *Clin Orthop Relat Res* 2004;429:239-247.

5. Berger RA: A comprehensive approach to outpatient total hip arthroplasty. *Am J Orthop (Belle Mead NJ)* 2007;36(9, suppl):4-5.

6. Berger RA, Kusuma SK, Sanders SA, Thill ES, Sporer SM: The feasibility and perioperative complications of outpatient knee arthroplasty. *Clin Orthop Relat Res* 2009;467(6):1443-1449.

7. Berger RA, Sanders S, D'Ambrogio E, et al: Minimally invasive quadriceps-sparing TKA: Results of a comprehensive pathway for outpatient TKA. *J Knee Surg* 2006;19(2):145-148.

8. Berger RA, Sanders S, Gerlinger T, Della Valle C, Jacobs JJ, Rosenberg AG: Outpatient total knee arthroplasty with a minimally invasive technique. *J Arthroplasty* 2005; 20(7, suppl 3):33-38.

9. Cross MB, Berger R: Feasibility and safety of performing outpatient unicompartmental knee arthroplasty. *Int Orthop* 2014;38(2):443-447.

10. Chen D, Berger RA: Outpatient minimally invasive total hip arthroplasty via a modified Watson-Jones approach: Technique and results. *Instr Course Lect* 2013;62:229-236.

11. Mason JB: The new demands by patients in the modern era of total joint arthroplasty: A point of view. *Clin Orthop Relat Res* 2008;466(1):146-152.

12. Booth RE Jr: Truth in advertising: The ethical limits of direct-to-consumer marketing. *Orthopedics* 2006;29(9):780-781.

13. Bozic KJ, Smith AR, Hariri S, et al: The 2007 ABJS Marshall Urist Award: The impact of direct-to-consumer advertising in orthopaedics. *Clin Orthop Relat Res* 2007;458:202-219.

14. Healy WL, Iorio R, Ko J, Appleby D, Lemos DW: Impact of cost reduction programs on short-term patient outcome and hospital cost of total knee arthroplasty. *J Bone Joint Surg Am* 2002;84(3):348-353.

15. Hayes JH, Cleary R, Gillespie WJ, Pinder IM, Sher JL: Are clinical and patient assessed outcomes affected by reducing length of hospital stay for total hip arthroplasty? *J Arthroplasty* 2000;15(4):448-452.

16. Bertin KC: Minimally invasive outpatient total hip arthroplasty: A financial analysis. *Clin Orthop Relat Res* 2005;435:154-163.

17. Kearney M, Jennrich MK, Lyons S, Robinson R, Berger B: Effects of preoperative education on patient outcomes after joint replacement surgery. *Orthop Nurs* 2011;30(6):391-396.

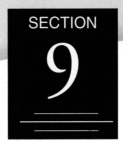

The Practice of Orthopaedics

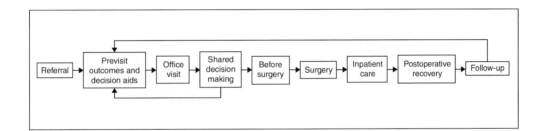

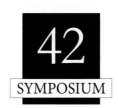

Implementation of Bundled Payment Initiatives for Total Joint Arthroplasty: Decreasing Cost and Increasing Quality

James P. Doran, MD
Alan H. Beyer, MD
Joseph Bosco, MD
Peggy L. Naas, MD, MBA
Brian S. Parsley, MD
James Slover, MD, MS
Stephen J. Zabinski, MD
Joseph D. Zuckerman, MD
Richard Iorio, MD

Abstract

Although the Bundled Payments for Care Improvement (BPCI) Initiative began generating data in January 2013, it may be years before the data can determine if the BPCI Initiative enhances value without decreasing quality. Private insurers have implemented other bundled payment arrangements for the delivery of total joint arthroplasty in a variety of practice settings. It is important for surgeons to review the early results of the BPCI Initiative and other bundled payment arrangements to understand the challenges and benefits of healthcare delivery systems with respect to total joint arthroplasty. In addition, surgeons should understand methods of cost control and quality improvement to determine the effect of the BPCI Initiative on the value-quality equation with respect to total joint arthroplasty.

Instr Course Lect 2016;65:555–566.

History and Overview of Bundled Payment Models

Total joint arthroplasty (TJA) procedures currently account for one of the largest portions of healthcare payments made to US hospitals by the Centers for Medicare & Medicaid Services (CMS).[1,2] The demand for TJA is expected to increase substantially over the next 15 years.[3] The predicted increase in procedure volume in combination with the current unsustainable rate of healthcare spending will place a massive economic burden on the US healthcare system. As a result, various stakeholders, such as the CMS, government policy makers, hospitals, industry thought leaders, payers, and physician groups, have begun to examine the utility of alternative healthcare delivery and payment strategies.

Transition from fee-for-service (FFS) models, which traditionally have incentivized healthcare providers based on the volume rather than the value of care delivered and, thus, led to the excessive utilization of services and increased healthcare expenditures, is taking place. One alternative to FFS models is global capitation, which delivers cost-containing incentives by giving physicians and healthcare decision makers a fixed budget for all the care their enrollees may require. This model has been explored with accountable care organizations (ACOs); however, the ACO system has been criticized because it does not work well for independent practitioners who are not highly integrated with a healthcare system and, therefore, lack the necessary means to coordinate episodes of care.

Value-based models, such as episode of care or bundled payment models, can be considered a middle ground between the FFS model and global capitation. Bundled payment models are designed to incentivize providers who use a vertically integrated, multidisciplinary healthcare approach with the goals of enhanced quality and efficiency of care, improved patient satisfaction, and controlled cost. In this model, physicians are financially accountable for the cost of care that is in excess of the established target payment for the episode of care. Physicians and hospitals are financially aligned through gainsharing, and only those physicians who provide high-quality care at a cost below the established target payment benefit from shared cost savings. Potential savings in an episode-based bundled payment model result from a decrease in the use of fixed cost services or items, a decrease in the cost of implants through reference pricing, a reduction in the hospital length of stay (LOS), control of inpatient and postdischarge expenses, and a reduction in complications and readmissions.

Several studies have demonstrated the effectiveness of bundled payments in reducing healthcare costs.[4,5] Some of the early bundled payment models adopted pilot programs, such as ProvenCare (Geisinger) and Provider Payment Reform for Outcomes, Margins, Evidence, Transparency, Hassle-reduction, Excellence, Understandability and Sustainability (PROMETHEUS; Health Care Incentives Improvement Institute). These programs demonstrated early success, but also highlighted the difficulties providers encountered as they implemented the models.[6,7] The CMS also have developed bundled payment programs. In 2009, the CMS introduced the Acute Care Episode Demonstration program, which included bundles for various cardiac and orthopaedic procedures.[8] This program eventually evolved into the BPCI Initiative, which began patient enrollment in 2013.[9] The BPCI Initiative is a 3-year program that is composed of four innovative models, which cover 48 orthopaedic and nonorthopaedic diagnosis-related groups (DRGs).[9,10] Although it may be years before data can determine if the BPCI Initiative enhances value without decreasing quality, early results of the BPCI Initiative are available for a variety of clinical settings.

Bundled Payment Participation From the Health System Perspective
Advantages
There are many incentives for health systems that participate in a bundled payment initiative (BPI). First and foremost, BPIs provide a direct advantage to patients. Patients have the potential to benefit from higher quality of care, experience more coordinated care from multiple healthcare professionals, receive a personalized standardization of treatment, suffer fewer complications, receive more comprehensible billing, and have more predictable costs in cases of self-pay. There are many advantages for the health system as well. Luft et al[11] reported that hospitals increase their volume of patients by providing higher quality care at a decreased cost. BPIs help hospitals gain an understanding of the total cost of care and better appreciate the consequences (financial and clinical) of complications and readmissions. In addition, BPIs help foster a collaborative relationship between physicians and care providers in the service line or across the continuum. BPIs provide many benefits, including insight on how to leverage and prioritize process improvement efforts, allocate scarce resources, and eliminate waste in the most effective and key areas; additional financial incentives within alignment models (comanagement, professional service agreements, clinical integration networks); and opportunities to leverage work across multiple payers

Dr. Bosco or an immediate family member has received royalties from Genoval; has received research or institutional support from CareFusion and MAKO Surgical; and serves as a board member, owner, officer, or committee member of the Orthopaedic Learning Center. Dr. Naas or an immediate family member serves as a board member, owner, officer, or committee member of the American Academy of Orthopaedic Surgeons. Dr. Parsley or an immediate family member has received royalties from ConforMIS; is a member of a speakers' bureau or has made paid presentations on behalf of ConforMIS and Nimbic Systems; serves as a paid consultant to or is an employee of Nimbic Systems; has stock or stock options held in Nimbic Systems; has received research or institutional support from ConforMIS; and serves as a board member, owner, officer, or committee member of the American Association of Hip and Knee Surgeons. Dr. Slover or an immediate family member has received research or institutional support from Biomet and DJO Global. Dr. Zuckerman or an immediate family member has received royalties from Exactech; serves as a paid consultant to the Musculoskeletal Transplant Foundation; serves as an unpaid consultant to the Arnold P. Gold Foundation and J3Personica/Residency Select; has stock or stock options held in AposTherapy and Hip Innovation Technology; and serves as a board member, owner, officer, or committee member of the American Orthopaedic Association. Dr. Iorio or an immediate family member serves as a paid consultant to Kyocera/International Material Data System; has received research or institutional support from Pacira Pharmaceuticals; and serves as a board member, owner, officer, or committee member of the American Association of Hip and Knee Surgeons, The Hip Society, and The Knee Society. None of the following authors nor any immediate family member has received anything of value from or has stock or stock options held in a commercial company or institution related directly or indirectly to the subject of this chapter: Dr. Doran, Dr. Beyer, and Dr. Zabinksi.

with the use of common contracting strategies. Current BPIs have the potential to act as dress rehearsals for more sweeping and inclusive future Medicare and Medicaid government (federal and state) payment models and alternative commercial payment models. Finally, BPIs may offer methodologies that can be applied to manage and predict a stakeholder's own employee and dependent covered lives for which they are self-insured. Orthopaedic surgeons also benefit from the same advantages gained by the patients and the health system, with the additional benefit of increased selected per-case revenue through gainsharing.

Disadvantages

Despite the potential advantages for a health system to pursue a bundled payment program, there are many reasons that dissuade participation. Reasons for health systems to not participate in a bundled payment program include overall satisfaction with the current payment model; solid, secure, and continuing financial success with FFS models; no interest in the local or germane market for bundled payments; and physician groups may have already aggressively become bundled payment owners, such that the current rules of precedence preclude gain for the health system within those bundles. Access to the proper patient population also plays an important role. For example, health systems may not participate in bundled payment programs if their payer mix has a small percentage of Medicare or Medicaid exposure, if they have no or only minimally offered services within specific bundles, or if their minimal volume is such that small variation can have a large consequence for risk exposure.

From a data-gathering perspective, some health systems may already have a solid foundation of preexisting knowledge on the total cost of delivery for specific services and bundles of services across the continuum, and it may appear that there is not much to gain by switching models. In addition, if a health system already has current population knowledge on the financial and clinical consequences of outliers, there is not much to gain from the additional data offered by bundled payments. A strong infrastructure and physician-hospital alignment also is required. It may not be feasible for a health system to participate in a BPI model if leadership and management have a perception of physician resistance, physician reluctance, or a lack of skill sets for potential participating physicians; if there is a perception or reality of a lack of intellectual capital or skills within the health system leadership with which to be successful with bundles; or if there is a lack of financial capital with which to create and deploy necessary infrastructure for BPI success. Last, if the health system misses the enrollment or participation deadlines, then it will not be able to use the federal bundled payment model.

Bundled Payments at a Large, Urban, Academic Medical Center
Overview

There are three fundamental questions an academic medical center should answer if a bundled payment program for TJA patients is being considered. These questions should be addressed in order because if the answers to all three questions are not "yes," then a bundled payment program should not be pursued.

Question one: "Is there sufficient initial interest to investigate the possibility of the BPCI Initiative program?" This question requires input from three different perspectives. First, from an administrative standpoint, is there an understanding of the program? Second, from a financial standpoint, are data available? And third, from a clinical standpoint, is there physician leadership in place?

Question two: "Based on an in-depth analysis of the BPCI Initiative models and clinical programs, is there a bundled model that best fits with the institution?" The four bundled payment models that are available include a retrospective model for acute care hospital stays only, a retrospective model for acute care hospital stays plus postacute care (30, 60, or 90 days), a retrospective model for postacute care only, and a prospective model for acute care hospital stays only. It also is essential for an academic medical center to know and research the DRGs that qualify for the models under consideration. Sixteen of the 48 DRGs that qualify for the BPCI Initiative models are musculoskeletal related; they include amputation; back and neck except spinal fusion; cervical spinal fusion; combined anterior posterior spinal fusion; complex noncervical spinal fusion; double joint replacement of the lower extremity; fractures femur and hip/pelvis; hip and femur procedures except major joint; lower extremity and humerus procedures except hip, foot, femur; major joint replacement of the lower extremity; major joint replacement of the upper extremity; medical noninfectious orthopaedic; other knee procedures; removal of orthopaedic devices; revision of the hip or knee; and spinal fusion (noncervical).[9] After consideration of the available bundled models and qualifying DRGs, the academic medical center should decide which model and which DRGs are the most appropriate for their institution or should at least have narrowed the options substantially.

Question three: "Does the institution have the resources (clinical, personnel, infrastructure, and administrative) to design and implement the BPCI Initiative program?" First, the model and clinical parameters need to be assessed. For the model parameters, the decision should be based on where the greatest opportunity exists, where the most substantial effects can be made, and which model provides the most opportunity to effectively control and monitor care. For the clinical parameters, the decision should take into account if there is sufficient patient volume and physician expertise, if the surgeons are amenable to a standardized clinical pathway, if there are cost-savings opportunities, if there is strong leadership, and if there is potential for physician-institution alignment. The second part of the decision-making process involves proceeding with the chosen model and selecting the DRGs that are eligible for participation.

Implementation for Medicare TJA

The Department of Orthopaedic Surgery at New York University Langone Medical Center (NYULMC) proceeded with bundled Model 2, which is a retrospective model in which an episode of care covered within the bundle is defined as the services provided 72 hours before hospital admission, the inpatient stay, and 90 days postdischarge. NYULMC selected the following DRGs for inclusion within bundled Model 2: major joint replacement of the

lower extremity (DRG 469: with major complication or comorbidity, and DRG 470: without major complication or comorbidity) and spinal fusion (noncervical; DRG 459: with major complication or comorbidity, and DRG 460: without major complication or comorbidity). To make the BPCI Initiative effort successful, NYULMC made a commitment to provide administrative, information technology, and care management resources. Without the support of the institution, accurate data, and adequate care management, it would be difficult to successfully implement the BPCI Initiative program. Therefore, departmental leadership was essential to align the surgeons from the institution and to deliver cost-effective, high-quality care. NYULMC's goals were to improve efficiency, enhance the coordination of care, and increase value for patients. Model 2 of the BPCI Initiative provides health systems with the opportunity to align the incentives of hospitals, surgeons, and postacute care providers, while quality is maintained or improved.

Total hip arthroplasty (THA) and total knee arthroplasty (TKA) are, predictably, clinically successful interventions that represent some of the highest CMS expenditures under the DRG payment system.[1,12] All Medicare beneficiaries admitted to NYULMC under DRGs 469 and 470 were included in Model 2 of the BPCI Initiative program and were not eligible to receive financial incentives. An episode of care was defined as all Medicare Part A and Part B services provided by an entity wholly owned or operated by the admitting hospital in the 72 hours before admission, the hospital facility services provided during the hospital stay, and services provided

during the 90-day postdischarge period at any location. Claims to Medicare by the physicians and hospital and payments to the physicians and hospital by the CMS were made in the standard fashion. All admitting physicians were required to participate. Retrospectively, claims were reconciled against the target price. If reconciled claim sums were lower than the target price, then the hospital received a check for the difference. If reconciled claim sums were higher than the target price, then the awardee repaid the difference to the CMS. The hospital received Medicare funds for cost savings that exceeded an agreed-upon discount; however, they also incurred risk for expenditures made above the agreed-upon discount. Physician reimbursement above the standard Medicare rates was determined by a gainsharing formula that was agreed upon with the hospital. Physician gainsharing was capped at 50% above the standard Medicare reimbursement rates.

Implementation Strategy

The formula for the successful implementation of a cost-effective episode of care for primary TJA patients initially involved a three-pronged approach: improved care coordination and preoperative patient education to set expectations and maximize communication; implementation of clinical pathways and standardization of care with the use of evidence-based medicine standards that all clinical providers were comfortable with; and minimal use of postacute care inpatient facilities, if unnecessary, and utilization of the clinical care coordination infrastructure to manage postacute care in a cost-effective manner. These pathways and protocols were instituted through the cooperative effort of the division chief, adult reconstruction attending physicians, the Joint Pathway Implementation Committee, the BPCI Initiative Committee, and the NYU Department of Population Management.

Care coordination ensures that best practices are followed, improves communication between providers and patients, ensures follow-up after care transitions, and optimizes patient expectations and outcomes. These goals can be achieved through the standardization of clinical pathways, workflows, and order sets, which increase efficiency, improve the provider's ability to monitor and study individual patient factors, and improve team communication. Studies have reported that the implementation of clinical pathways decreases hospital LOS, improves clinical outcomes, reduces costs, and increases patient satisfaction.[13-18]

To maximize efficiency and quality, NYULMC sought to create a standard clinical pathway for patients that included preoperative, inpatient, and postacute care components. NYULMC's goal was to have a minimum of 80% of patients follow the pathway, with exceptions based on evidence-based criteria rather than individual preference. For organizational purposes, this task was divided into three teams: the preoperative committee, the inpatient committee, and the postacute committee. As pathway components were developed, implementation teams were required to educate staff about the pathway. It was essential for all providers across each of the disciplines to understand the pathway, the progression of milestones and their role in that progression within their discipline, and the documentation required for success.

The preoperative pathway concentrated on patient education, management of patient and family expectations, and improvements in efficiency. Patient expectations and preparations for TJA were met through the creation of a standardized surgical booking and equipment ordering platform, a new patient assessment tool that helped identify important patient health factors and determine the required preoperative evaluations, a TJA patient education guide, and preoperative care management assessment tools to identify barriers for discharge and required support measures.

The inpatient pathways and protocols coordinated the roles of clinical care coordinators, nurse practitioners, physical therapists, nurses, care managers, social workers, residents, fellows, and attending physicians to achieve a median 3-day hospital LOS. A dashboard located in the electronic medical records was used as a basis for daily interdisciplinary rounds to discuss patient progress toward discharge, facilitate communication among caregivers, and document patient progress along the care pathway. Each member of the healthcare team had access to patient progress on the dashboard. Real-time communication via email was used to keep the healthcare team informed about patient progress along the pathway. If a patient deviated from the pathway, then an email that described the issue and potential solutions was triggered. The implementation of evidence-based protocols, which involved anesthesia, blood management, radiology, pathology, catheterization, and laboratory testing, affected operating room efficiency and perioperative medical treatment along the pathway (**Table 1**). In addition, the use of hospitalists to manage

routine medical issues was encouraged, and routine inpatient use of consultants was discouraged, unless medical complexity required such expertise.

The postacute pathways formalized communication with postacute providers. The appropriate use of postacute inpatient facilities was emphasized while maximizing the rate of home discharge with services. Postacute inpatient facilities were a major cost driver for the episode of care. Improved communication of postacute protocols at the time of transfer and the electronic exchange of information with postacute partners were critical. For patients without complications, routine follow-up appointments were limited to two in the first 90 days after surgical intervention. Although the role of the clinical care coordinators was to manage the entire 90-day episode of care, they played a prominent role in this stage of the pathway. The clinical care coordinators preoperatively counseled patients with respect to discharge needs and expectations that were based on a validated risk stratification tool. In addition, readmission risks were evaluated during year two of the BPCI contract with the use of an internal evaluation tool that was based on modifiable patient-derived risk factors. To ensure coordination of care throughout the 90-day episode, the clinical care coordinators followed BPCI Initiative patients postoperatively if they were discharged to home with services or to inpatient facilities. The clinical care coordinators also ensured delivery of essential services and maintenance of communication between all caregivers to minimize the need for unnecessary office visits, emergency department visits, and readmissions.

Table 1

Elements, Interventions, and Intended Results of Evidence-Based Clinical Pathways

Element	Interventions	Intended Results
Anesthesia	Regional anesthesia and peripheral blocks	Early ambulation
	Multimodal analgesia protocols and periarticular intraoperative anesthesia injections	Pain control
		Decrease venous thromboembolic disease
Blood management	Discontinuation of routine autologous blood donation or preoperative pharmacologic optimization (erythropoietin, etc.) without medical necessity	Patient safety
	Transfusion only to patients in true need, as determined by symptoms	Cost-effectiveness
	Tranexamic acid administration protocol (1 g before incision and 1 g during closure)	Minimize blood loss
	Discontinuation of radiofrequency bipolar sealer	Decrease infections
	Discontinuation of reinfusion drains	
Radiology	Discontinuation of routine postoperative primary total knee arthroplasty radiographs	Patient safety
		Cost-effectiveness
		Decrease surgical time
Pathology	Pathology specimen evaluation only performed for primary total joint arthroplasty if a diagnosis is needed	Cost-effectiveness
Catheterization	No routine urinary catheterization	Decrease infections
	Bladder scanning to evaluate urinary retention	Improve efficiency
	If catheterization is required, intermittent catheterization performed in lieu of an indwelling catheter	Early mobilization
Laboratory testing	Preoperative urinalysis avoided unless patient is symptomatic	Patient safety
	Routine prothrombin time/partial thromboplastin time and international normalized ratio not required unless patient is currently being treated with anticoagulants or has a preexisting blood and/or liver disorder	Cost-effectiveness

Readmissions

During the first year of the BPCI Initiative implementation, NYULMC found that it was difficult to control readmissions with the care coordination methodology alone. As a result, NYULMC discovered that several patients who required readmission had modifiable risk factors, which could be optimized before surgery. A risk-factor stratification and modification program was implemented to delay surgery in high-risk patients who were most likely to have complications (**Table 2**). Physician quality and performance metrics for BPCI Initiative patients were circulated biweekly to monitor results and are now available

in real time on the dashboard. Hospital LOS, discharge disposition, readmissions, and ranking against division averages and expectations were reported. Preliminary results demonstrated that readmission rates decreased from 14% at 90 days in 2012 to 2013 to 8% at 90 days in late 2014. Mean hospital LOS decreased from 4.5 days to 3.1 days. Discharge to inpatient postacute facilities decreased from 70% to 30%. The cost of each episode of care decreased approximately $7,000 as a result of the BPCI Initiative program (New York University Langone Medical Center, Department of Orthopaedic Surgery, New York, NY, unpublished data, 2013).

Bundled Payments at a Physician-Owned Private Hospital

Hoag Orthopedic Institute, a physician-owned private hospital that is a 51% to 49% joint venture between a community not-for-profit hospital and 44 physician shareholders, most of whom are orthopaedic surgeons, participates in a commercial bundled payment program for TJA. Hoag Orthopedic Institute is composed of 70 beds, an inpatient facility with 9 operating rooms, and 2 ambulatory surgery centers. The institute is managed by physician leaders and chosen administrative staff, not by the hospital itself. The physician shareholders, in conjunction with the hospital

Table 2

Perioperative Interventions to Optimize At-Risk Total Joint Arthroplasty Patients

Intervention Classification	Patient Risk Factors	Interventions
Medical	Coronary artery disease/ myocardial infarction	Perioperative cardiovascular optimization and stroke prevention (PT, high-dose statins, and ACE inhibitors)
	Cerebrovascular disease/stroke	
	Uncontrolled diabetes mellitus	Diabetes mellitus control and nutritional interventions (hard stop for blood glucose >180)
	Poor nutrition	
	History of or risk factors for VTED	Coagulation profile screening for high-risk VTED patients
	Morbid obesity	Aggressive weight control (hard stop for BMI >40)
Infection	*Staphylococcus* colonization	MRSA screening and decolonization
	High risk for infection	Weight-based antibiotic dosing and use of vancomycin and gentamicin
Social	Active smoker	Smoking cessation (hard stop)
	Drug and alcohol abuse	Illicit drug and alcohol interventions
Patient education	Physical deconditioning	PT and fall prevention education
Other	Pain catastrophizing	Catastrophizing avoidance and counseling

ACE = angiotensin-converting enzyme, BMI = body mass index, MRSA = methicillin-resistant *Staphylococcus aureus*, PT = physical therapy, VTED = venous thromboembolic disease.

and several payers, defined patients who would qualify for the commercial bundled payment program as those who were insured by one of the payers participating in the program; were aged 18 to 64 years; had an anesthesia risk rating of 2 or less; had a body mass index less than 38 kg/m^2; did not have active cancer, end-stage renal disease, or active HIV/AIDS; and fell within the complications and comorbidities for the DRG codes that were initially selected. All services associated with inpatient charges, such as implants; in-hospital testing; inpatient pharmacy; all inpatient professional fees, including those of the surgeon and assistant; radiology; consultations; and hospitalist treatment, were included in the bundled payment model. Outpatient rehabilitation also was included. All services associated with readmission related to the DRGs, such as venous thromboembolic diseases and surgical site infections, and all services associated with the inpatient

skilled rehabilitation setting were included in the bundled payment model. Services associated with subacute skilled nursing facilities or nursing facilities that provide care beyond rehabilitation, home health care nursing charges, nurse visits to the home, durable medical equipment, and outpatient pharmacy were excluded from the bundled payment model. To develop the bundled payment model price, professional fees for the physicians were established based on the highest preferred provider organization contracts currently held in the state. Facility fees were equal to the direct cost of care or the episode cost with a built-in margin. The cost of stop-loss coverage for readmissions, a small fee for administration costs, and a margin to cover readmission deductibles were included.

Reconciliation of the bundles is performed yearly, and, after payments are made to both the facility and the participating physicians, the remaining risk

pool is split among the surgeons based on a formula that takes into account the surgeons' surgical volume. Surgeons' outcomes are compared with the institute's standardized report cards, and surgeons who provide a higher quality of care based on these outcomes are rewarded at a higher level per case. Examples of quality metrics include LOS; readmission percentage; the use of postacute care facilities; and various quality parameters, such as the use of venous thromboembolic prophylaxis, infection rates, the use of implants, and so on. The hospital does not participate in this split. The margin for the hospital also is built into the bundled payment model.

Advantages

There are many advantages for a physician-owned private hospital to participate in a bundled payment model. A bundled payment model grants a private hospital access to previously inaccessible patients. Payers are more likely to direct patients to health systems that use bundled payment models and demonstrate high-quality outcomes. Bundled payment models provide payers with a more predictable cost of care and a warranty for certain readmissions because surgeons will be accountable for these costs. Bundled payment models also provide surgeons with the opportunity to critically evaluate cost-of-care factors that may have been previously overlooked. Surgeons who provide high-quality, efficient care can strengthen the physician-hospital relationship. Coordination of care and services within the health system is essential to maximize the benefit of the bundled payment.

The key to a successful bundled payment model in a physician-owned hospital is similar to that in other clinical settings: alignment on multiple levels. Alignment is required from orthopaedic surgeon to orthopaedic surgeon because the physicians have to determine and agree on clinical pathways, implant selection, and discharge dispositions. The hospital and the orthopaedic surgeons have to agree on implant selection, which has substantial effects on cost. Specific issues that need to be discussed include vendor negotiations, especially in terms of whether to use single- or dual-source vendors or to set a price point at which companies meet; revision implants; and the management of wasted implants. The physicians and the hospital must work together to reconcile the bundle.

Results

Overall, the bundled payment model at Hoag Orthopedic Institute resulted in many improvements compared with the years prior to participation in the program. The current surgical site infection rate is 0.44%, which is down from the approximately 1% rate it was 4 years ago. The overall readmission rate is 3.4%, and the readmission rate for TJA patients is 1.4%. Currently, approximately 84% of patients are being discharged home compared with approximately 60% in previous years. In addition, Hospital Consumer Assessment of Healthcare Providers and Systems survey scores have remained in the high 90s (New York University Langone Medical Center, Department of Orthopaedic Surgery, New York, NY, unpublished data, 2013).

Bundled Payments for Medicare and Non-Medicare TJA at a Community Hospital
History

In late 2010, the director of Shore Orthopaedic University Associates, a private practice group of eight orthopaedic surgeons, was approached by Horizon Blue Cross Blue Shield of New Jersey and invited to participate in a TJA episode of care program as a physician advisory board member. This program was the first of its kind to be built and implemented by a commercial payer in the state of New Jersey.[19] Quarterly meetings commenced in January 2011, and four other orthopaedic groups were represented on the initial advisory board.

In phase 1 of the project, which lasted until January 2012, all parties developed and agreed on the parameters of an episode-based BPI. The parties defined the episode of care duration (30 days preoperatively to 90 days postoperatively), quality measures, inclusion criteria, grouper technology, best practices, standards of care, patient outcome and satisfaction measurement tools, and never events. Patient episode of care data, outcomes, and cost collection began in January 2012. All primary, elective, unilateral TJA patients who were older than 18 years and had Horizon Blue Cross Blue Shield of New Jersey insurance coverage were enrolled in the BPI. Episode of care budgets were based on individual patient severity and determined with the use of the five orthopaedic groups' historical claims data averages from the 24 months before the program was initiated. The patient-severity adjusted budget for each episode of care was determined with the use of PROMETHEUS grouper technology.[20] In each quarter of 2012, a retrospective, shared-savings report and payment based on the patient episodes of care and actual spending relative to the budget were delivered to each orthopaedic group. During this timeframe, there was no risk for the participating orthopaedic groups, and all negative (over budget) episodes of care were eliminated.

Phase 2 of the project began in January 2013. In this phase, all episodes of care above and below the target cost were used to generate the shared savings payments; however, a downside limitation for severely over-budget episodes of care was put into effect, and substantially over-budget outlier episodes of care were protected at a maximum of 115% of the severity adjusted budget. Currently, the program is converting orthopaedic practices that are enrolled in the program to a more easily adopted historical practice-based budget, which does not adjust each individual patient episode of care relative to severity. Because of regulatory and reimbursement hurdles, the final phase of the project, in which a prospective, global bundled payment is dispensed to the participating orthopaedic groups at the onset of the episode of care, has yet to be achieved.

The BPCI Initiative for Medicare TJA

In 2012, two of the primary health systems that Shore Orthopaedic University Associates used to perform TJAs decided not to participate in the CMS bundled payment programs. The reasons the health systems provided for rejection of the CMS bundled payment programs involved the notion that the health systems' programs were already tightly managed; therefore, the CMS bundled payment programs posed too much risk for too little gain. In addition, the health systems believed that the large amount of data and analysis required would offer minimal benefit. In contrast, a third participating health system in the area, which benefits from more aligned systems, has a history of substantially higher episode of care costs, has an active ACO program, and has a history of self-insurance, did elect to participate in the prospective CMS bundled payment program. The health system is currently in the early stages of data analysis.

Practice Goals and Initiatives

Shore Orthopaedic University Associates entered the bundled payment program with three goals: decrease the overall cost of a TJA episode of care by decreasing complications, improving postoperative patient function (decrease hospital LOS and increase discharge to home), and making both system and practice improvements; improve the quality of care and patient satisfaction while reducing cost; and increase surgeon and practice reimbursement for TJA via shared savings payments and increased patient volume from referrals.

Practice Modifications

To achieve these goals, Shore Orthopaedic University Associates instituted new evidence-based protocols for their preoperative, perioperative, and postoperative practices. Preoperative protocols emphasized patient education, preoperative physical therapy and exercise, medical comorbidity optimization with standardized clearance protocols, and hospital-based TJA nurse navigation. Perioperative protocols emphasized standardized implant choices with options for demand matching; improved pain control; full compliance with postoperative day zero ambulation; diminished transfusion rate; reduced urinary, hemodynamic, and gastrointestinal complications; and the elimination of unnecessary medical device use. Some surgeons also altered their surgical approaches and techniques. Postoperative protocols emphasized discharge disposition, the reduction in unnecessary readmissions, and the earlier transition of patients from formal physical therapy to home exercise programs if medically appropriate. To facilitate the adoption of these protocols, a comanagement agreement was established between the orthopaedic surgeons and the health system. This agreement established metrics for quality and efficiency and empowered the orthopaedic surgeons, in conjunction with the health system, to participate in vendor negotiations and system alterations, with the ultimate goals of decreasing cost and improving both quality and patient satisfaction.

Results

Horizon Blue Cross Blue Shield of New Jersey provided patient episode of care data to Shore Orthopaedic University Associates on a quarterly basis. The

episode of care was divided into four stages: stage one included the 30-day preoperative period; stage two included the acute hospital stay and related surgical costs; stage three included the first 30 postoperative days; and stage four included postoperative days 31 to 90.

For TKA, 78.6% of the spending occurred in stage two, and 17.1% of the spending occurred in stage three. For THA, 85.2% of the spending occurred in stage two, and 7.3% of the spending occurred in stage three. Only a small portion of the total episode of care cost occurred in the preoperative (stage one) and late postoperative (stage four) time periods (Horizon Blue Cross Blue Shield of New Jersey, Newark, NJ, and Shore Orthopaedic University Associates, Galloway, NJ, unpublished data, 2013 through 2014).

The mean hospital LOS decreased substantially for both TKA and THA. The hospital LOS for TKA decreased from 3.3 days to 1.9 days, and the hospital LOS for THA decreased from 2.9 days to 1.8 days. The transfusion rate decreased from 23.2% to 4.45%. Discharge to inpatient rehabilitation also substantially decreased. In 2011, approximately 66.3% of patients were discharged to inpatient rehabilitation compared with 33.17% of patients in 2013 and 2014. Thirty-day readmission rates decreased from 3.2% to 2.7%. Deep infection and major wound complication rates remained low at 0.9%. The mean device cost per patient decreased from $6,301 to $4,972, with a mean device cost per patient of $4,585 in the final 6 months of 2014 (Horizon Blue Cross Blue Shield of New Jersey, Newark, NJ, and Shore Orthopaedic University Associates, Galloway, NJ, unpublished data, 2013 through 2014).

There was a substantial difference between the site of service costs for the health systems in Shore Orthopaedic University Associates' catchment area. Average inpatient spending that occurred in stage two was $10,800 for the primary health system compared with more than $25,000 for the health system in the northern portion of the catchment area. The average episode of care budget was $25,365 for TKA and $23,580 for THA. For Horizon Blue Cross Blue Shield of New Jersey patients who were enrolled from January 2012 to December 2013, Shore Orthopaedic University Associates was under budget for 65 of 78 TKA episodes of care and 27 of 38 THA episodes of care. The total savings relative to the budget for all Horizon Blue Cross Blue Shield of New Jersey patients over the course of this 2-year period exceeded $524,000, which resulted in a savings-based payment of $262,445 (an average of $2,262 per patient) to Shore Orthopaedic University Associates for the 2-year timeframe (Horizon Blue Cross Blue Shield of New Jersey, Newark, NJ, and Shore Orthopaedic University Associates, Galloway, NJ, unpublished data, 2013 through 2014).

Creating Value in TJA

To assess the efficacy of strategies for creating value in TJA, it is first important to define value. Value can be defined as outcomes/cost. Given this definition, a 10% decrease in positive outcomes with a 50% decrease in cost could theoretically create value. Because the ethics of medicine preclude any increase in value as a result of a decrease in quality, the numerator can never decrease in the value equation. Several scenarios for creating value exist, depending on how outcomes and cost

are altered. Strategies that improve outcomes and increase cost are good strategies for creating value. Better strategies for creating value are those that result in no change in outcomes with a concomitant decrease in cost. The best strategies for creating value improve outcomes while decreasing cost.

Increasing Cost and Improving Outcomes

The use of new technology is a common strategy for creating value in TJA. Historically, technologic advancements in medicine tend to increase the cost of care;[21] therefore, most new technologies that improve outcomes can create value if the cost is reasonable. New technologies that result in any decrease in positive outcomes are unacceptable, even if value is created, and thus, rejected. If a new technology does improve outcomes, then it is important to determine if the potential benefit is cost effective. The incremental cost-effectiveness ratio may be used to analyze the cost-benefit of new technologies. For example, the incremental cost-effectiveness ratio can be used to analyze a new implant with improved bearing surfaces that demonstrates a decrease in polyethylene wear in vitro but is more expensive compared with currently used implants. Furthermore, quality-adjusted life-years should also be used to assess the cost-benefit of new technologies. An implant that has improved bearing surfaces and wear properties may not result in an increase in quality-adjusted life years for a 70-year-old patient. To determine if improved outcomes justify increased cost, institutions should have new product committees and a formalized mechanism that qualitatively, if not quantitatively, determines the incremental cost-effectiveness ratio.

Decreasing Cost Without Affecting Outcomes

There are many strategies a health system can implement to reduce the cost of a TJA episode of care. The elimination of certain interventions, such as routine blood work and the use of autotransfusion devices and cell savers, may help health systems decrease cost without affecting outcomes. In addition, the elimination of implant waste and the control of implant price both decrease cost without affecting quality. Several years ago, NYULMC implemented a reference pricing program that established ceiling prices for commonly used implants. Through physician-hospital alignment, the program resulted in a 25% reduction in implant costs without affecting implant market share or demand matching.[22]

The elimination of implant waste may also help health systems decrease cost without affecting outcomes. The NYULMC Orthopaedic Surgery Department recorded implant waste by division, surgeon, and procedure to create physician awareness, with the ultimate goal of decreasing implant waste. In 1 year, the reduction of implant waste resulted in a cost savings of 50% of the total amount spent on wasted implants from the previous year.

Decreasing Cost and Improving Outcomes

The best strategies for creating value in TJA are those that improve outcomes and decrease the cost of the episode of care simultaneously. Because of the wide variation in cost between discharge scenarios, discharge dispositions are one way value can be created in TJA. Inpatient rehabilitation may cost $15,000, whereas discharge to home with home physical therapy may cost $2,000.

NYULMC analyzed the discharge dispositions of patients who underwent primary THA and TKA to determine if improved outcomes justified the cost differential and created value. Results showed that THA patients who were discharged to an inpatient rehabilitation facility were more likely to be readmitted compared with THA patients who were discharged to home with health services (P = 0.027).[23] Discharge patterns after TJA varied widely between physicians at NYULMC. Patients who were discharged home did not have a longer hospital LOS or a higher rate of readmission than patients who were discharged to a rehabilitation center or skilled nursing facility. The large interphysician variance in discharge cost did not correlate with a difference in the quality of care, as measured by the hospital LOS and readmission rates; therefore, the results indicate that discharge disposition provides surgeons with an opportunity to create value by reducing cost and increasing quality.[24]

Blood management practices, specifically the use of tranexamic acid (TXA), also were studied for the potential to create value in a TJA episode of care. A control group of 1,827 TJA patients from 2012 who did not receive TXA was compared with a treatment group of 2,016 TJA patients from 2013 who received TXA. Transfusion rates were 20.8% for the control group and 9.1% for the TXA treatment group (P < 0.003). The cost associated with blood products decreased by 35% for the TXA treatment group. The mean per-patient cost for blood transfusions was $198.82 for the control group and $128.45 for the TXA treatment group (after accounting for the additional cost of TXA administration). The cost of 1 g/10 mL of TXA was $25.98, and the cost of 1 unit of packed red blood cells was $414.43. These data show that TXA decreased costs and improved outcomes, which created value (New York University Langone Medical Center, Department of Orthopaedic Surgery, New York, NY, unpublished data, 2012 through 2014).

Physician-specific metrics are used at NYULMC to monitor value. To determine the quality of care, ratios of observed versus expected venous thromboembolic events, readmissions, and surgical site infection events were analyzed. In addition, physician resource use and quality of care for the 2012 and 2013 fiscal years were plotted on a 2 × 2 analysis matrix. Physicians who were a part of the Division of Adult Reconstruction had their performance from both years plotted separately into one of four quadrants: low quality/high cost, low quality/low cost, high quality/high cost, and high quality/low cost. Although many strategies exist for creating value in TJA, as a rule, only the interventions that create value without negatively affecting patient outcomes are acceptable for implementation.

Summary

The ability to create value by initiating stakeholder alignment, standardized care, evidence-based medicine protocols, minimal use of resources, communication among stakeholders, care coordination, and patient education is essential to the success of BPIs. Early results from the CMS BPCI Initiative at NYULMC demonstrate decreased hospital LOS, decreased discharge to inpatient facilities, decreased episode of care costs, improvements in all quality metrics, and a positive result for hospital reimbursement and surgeon gainsharing, without accounting for the administrative expenses associated with the program; however, NYULMC did not substantially alter the readmission rates of BPCI Initiative patients until the institution focused on the preoperative optimization of patients who had a high risk for readmission. Changes in care coordination, clinical care pathways, and evidence-based protocols are the keys to improve the quality metrics and cost-effectiveness of the BPCI Initiative at a large, urban, academic center and, thus, increase value in TJA.

The key components to the success of a bundled payment program at a physician-owned private hospital are: (1) coordinated care across the health system, (2) a well-defined patient population, (3) established best practices and pathways (access to bundled payment patients is only given to physicians who follow the pathways), (4) near real-time quality matrix reporting, (5) a highly developed cost-accounting system, (6) a stop-loss coverage reserve fund for catastrophic patient complications, (7) a payer that is motivated, and (8) collaboration between the hospital and physicians to control the flow of funds.

Shore Orthopaedic University Associates' implementation of a private practice-based commercial BPI at a community hospital successfully decreased the orthopaedic group's cost of a TJA episode of care compared with their average cost of a TJA episode of care before 2011. This cost reduction has primarily resulted from a decrease in the length of inpatient stay, an increase in discharge to home, a reduction in implant costs, improvements in the readmission rate, and the migration of patients to lower cost sites of service. Participation in the bundled payment program has resulted in higher practice reimbursement via shared savings payments.

References

1. United States Department of Health & Human Services, Agency for Healthcare Research and Quality: Healthcare Cost and Utilization Project (HCUP): Nationwide Inpatient Sample (NIS). Available at: http://hcupnet.ahrq.gov. Accessed March 5, 2015.

2. Centers for Medicare & Medicaid Services: Medicare & Medical Statistical Supplement: 2013 Edition. Chapter 5: Medicare Short Stay Hospitals. Table 5.7: Discharges, Total Days of Care, Total Charges and Program Payments for Medicare Beneficiaries Discharged from Short-Stay Hospitals, by Leading Diagnosis-Related Groups (DRGs). Calendar Year 2012. 2014. Available at: http://www.cms.gov/Research-Statistics-Data-and-Systems/Statistics-Trends-and-Reports/MedicareMedicaidStatSupp/2013.html. Accessed March 5, 2015.

3. Kurtz S, Ong K, Lau E, Mowat F, Halpern M: Projections of primary and revision hip and knee arthroplasty in the United States from 2005 to 2030. *J Bone Joint Surg Am* 2007;89(4):780-785.

4. Luft HS: Economic incentives to promote innovation in healthcare delivery. *Clin Orthop Relat Res* 2009;467(10):2497-2505.

5. Cutler DM, Ghosh K: The potential for cost savings through bundled episode payments. *N Engl J Med* 2012;366(12):1075-1077.

6. Satin DJ, Miles J: Performance-based bundled payments: Potential benefits and burdens. *Minn Med* 2009;92(10):33-35.

7. Hussey PS, Ridgely MS, Rosenthal MB: The PROMETHEUS bundled payment experiment: Slow start shows problems in implementing new payment models. *Health Aff (Millwood)* 2011;30(11):2116-2124.

8. Centers for Medicare & Medicaid Services: Medicare Acute Care Episode (ACE) Demonstration. Available at: http://innovation.cms.gov/initiatives/ACE. Accessed January 5, 2015.

9. Centers for Medicare & Medicaid Services: Bundled Payments for Care Improvement (BPCI) Initiative: General Information. Available at: http://innovation.cms.gov/initiatives/bundled-payments/index.html. Accessed October 20, 2014.

10. Froimson MI, Rana A, White RE Jr, et al: Bundled payments for care improvement initiative: The next evolution of payment formulations. AAHKS Bundled Payment Task Force. *J Arthroplasty* 2013;28(8, Suppl):157-165.

11. Luft HS, Hunt SS, Maerki SC: The volume-outcome relationship: Practice-makes-perfect or selective-referral patterns? *Health Serv Res* 1987;22(2):157-182.

12. Paxton EW, Namba RS, Maletis GB, et al: A prospective study of 80,000 total joint and 5000 anterior cruciate ligament reconstruction procedures in a community-based registry in the United States. *J Bone Joint Surg Am* 2010;92(suppl 2):117-132.

13. Duncan CM, Moeschler SM, Horlocker TT, Hanssen AD, Hebl JR: A self-paired comparison of perioperative outcomes before and after implementation of a clinical pathway in patients undergoing total knee arthroplasty. *Reg Anesth Pain Med* 2013;38(6):533-538.

14. Ibrahim MS, Khan MA, Nizam I, Haddad FS: Peri-operative interventions producing better functional outcomes and enhanced recovery following total hip and knee arthroplasty: An evidence-based review. *BMC Med* 2013;11:37.

15. Barbieri A, Vanhaecht K, Van Herck P, et al: Effects of clinical pathways in the joint replacement: A meta-analysis. *BMC Med* 2009;7:32.

16. Ibrahim MS, Alazzawi S, Nizam I, Haddad FS: An evidence-based review of enhanced recovery interventions in knee replacement surgery. *Ann R Coll Surg Engl* 2013;95(6):386-389.

17. Gooch K, Marshall DA, Faris PD, et al: Comparative effectiveness of alternative clinical pathways for primary hip and knee joint replacement patients: A pragmatic randomized, controlled trial. *Osteoarthritis Cartilage* 2012;20(10):1086-1094.

18. Healy WL, Iorio R, Ko J, Appleby D, Lemos DW: Impact of cost reduction programs on short-term patient outcome and hospital cost of total knee arthroplasty. *J Bone Joint Surg Am* 2002;84(3):348-353.

19. Horizon Blue Cross Blue Shield of New Jersey: Horizon Healthcare Innovations. 2014. Available at: http://www.horizonblue.com/providers/products-programs/horizon-healthcare-innovations. Accessed October 20, 2014.

20. Healthcare Incentives Improvement Institute. Available at: http://www.hci3.org. Accessed October 20, 2014.

21. Skinner JS: The costly paradox of health-care technology. MIT Technology Review. Cambridge, MA, Massachusetts Institute of Technology, September 5, 2013. Available at: http://www.technologyreview.com/news/518876/the-costly-paradox-of-health-care-technology. Accessed March 5, 2015.

22. Bosco JA, Alvarado CM, Slover JD, Iorio R, Hutzler LH: Decreasing total joint implant costs and physician specific cost variation through negotiation. *J Arthroplasty* 2014;29(4):678-680.

23. Ramos NL, Karia RJ, Hutzler LH, Brandt AM, Slover JD, Bosco JA: The effect of discharge disposition on 30-day readmission rates after total joint arthroplasty. *J Arthroplasty* 2014;29(4):674-677.

24. Ramos NL, Wang EL, Karia RJ, Hutzler LH, Lajam CM, Bosco JA: Correlation between physician specific discharge costs, LOS, and 30-day readmission rates: An analysis of 1,831 cases. *J Arthroplasty* 2014;29(9):1717-1722.

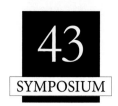

Evidence, Quality, Costs, and Reimbursement: Connecting the Dots

David S. Jevsevar, MD, MBA
John W. Karl, MD, MPH
Mohit Bhandari, MD, PhD, FRCSC
Kevin J. Bozic, MD, MBA
Mark A. Piasio, MD, MBA
Stuart L. Weinstein, MD

Abstract

Healthcare costs in the United States continue to rise, and substantial variations in the type, quality, and location of that care persist. It is critically important for all healthcare stakeholders to address and define value in orthopaedic care delivery. Evidence-based orthopaedic care delivery, reliable quality and performance measurement, and the delivery of the best care at the lowest cost are the key strategies to improve the value of musculoskeletal care. A failure to implement these strategies could negatively affect the reimbursement of all healthcare providers—at both the private and government payer levels.

Instr Course Lect 2016;65:567–576.

Healthcare costs in the United States continue to rise as a result of many factors, including inefficient care, technologic advances, administrative costs, and the practice of defensive medicine because of a fear of litigation.[1] In 2012, the United States spent $8,745 per person on health care, which is 42% more than the spending per person in Norway, the second highest spender.[2] In the same year, the United States spent 16.9% of its gross domestic product on health care, which is almost 1.5 times higher than the 12.1% of gross domestic

product the next highest country, the Netherlands, spent on health care.[3] It has not always been this way. In 1970, the United States was in line with other developed countries, with healthcare spending at 6.7% of the gross domestic product. After 1980, spending rose steadily, which brought the United States to its current level of spending. Far from being abstract economic indicators, increased healthcare costs are felt by average Americans. From 2008 to 2011, health insurance premiums increased by 10% or more each year, so

that the current annual cost per family is nearly $17,000.[4] Despite spending more per capita on health care, the United States consistently ranks lower on health outcomes and measures, such as access, efficiency, and quality, compared with other high-income countries.[5]

Within the United States, variation exists in spending, which may be a result of either increased healthcare consumption or higher costs for the same care. Fisher et al[6] reported that patients who live in higher spending regions of the country received 60% more care than those who live in lower spending regions. Patients who live in the higher spending regions had more of everything: physician visits, inpatient visits, diagnostic testing, minor procedures, and specialty care. The escalation of costs, coupled with substantial variations in the quality and effectiveness of health care, have affected reimbursement for all healthcare providers. It is important for orthopaedic surgeons to understand how evidence-based medicine (EBM), reliable quality and performance measurement, and the delivery of the best care at the lowest cost affect reimbursement costs in both the private and public sectors.

EBM in Health Care

EBM has been defined as the integration of the best research evidence with clinical expertise and patient values.[7] EBM generally refers to the conscientious use of the current best evidence from clinical care research to make healthcare decisions; however, clinical decision making still requires a physician's clinical experience and expertise as well as each patient's unique values and social and life circumstances.

A level-of-evidence hierarchy was developed to ascribe rank to the clinical research that is used to make clinical decisions.[8] Randomized controlled trials (RCTs) minimize the effects of bias (which may cause the observed effect to be unrepresentative of the true or accurate effect) and confounding (which may lead to the conclusion that a spurious relationship exists between the independent and dependent variables). Although RCTs remain the preferred method to determine the efficacy of a diagnostic test or treatment, many issues surround the use of RCTs in surgery.

Underpowered surgical clinical trials are an example of the difficulties encountered. Surgical RCTs are generally underpowered by a factor of 10, which limits the conclusions that can be drawn.[9] One way in which underpowered studies are limited involves the concept of fragility.[10] The Fragility Index measures the minimum number of patients whose status would need to change from a nonevent to an event to turn a statistically significant result to a nonsignificant result. In orthopaedics, examples of fragility can be found in several studies that address the use of bone morphogenetic protein-2 for the treatment of tibial nonunions.[11,12] Changes in outcomes of only three patients in the control group would lead to a different conclusion on the efficacy of bone morphogenetic protein-2 for the treatment of tibial nonunions.[12]

To attain stronger conclusions from clinical research, much larger studies are needed. Multicenter, international studies provide surgeons with the opportunity to obtain large enough patient sample sizes to support the conclusions that can be drawn from clinical research. Big data, with the help of administrative databases, registries, payer databases, electronic medical records, and external patient sources, present exciting opportunities that address the need for large sample sizes; however, care must be taken to ensure

that accurate conclusions are made from these sources. The mere presence of correlation does not necessarily indicate causation. EBM remains the foundation for clinical decision making that can improve outcomes and reduce variation.

The Move Toward Emphasizing Value in Health Care

To address the rising and unsustainable growth in healthcare spending and to improve health outcomes, the Institute of Medicine issued a call to improve the quality of care. Several strategies have been implemented to improve the quality of care, including clinical practice guidelines (CPGs), which describe best practices to manage a disease or condition and are developed by a systematic review of all published studies. New payment models, such as bundled payments and pay-for-performance, that incentivize value-based care instead of the volume of care have the potential to improve outcomes (and not just slow the growth of spending) by driving improvements in care coordination; however, to determine if any of these initiatives truly improve quality, stakeholders must agree on what constitutes quality care and how it is measured. Numerous stakeholders, including payers, policymakers, providers, and patients, have varying perspectives on the definition of quality, which adds to the complexity of implementing a system of quality measurement and reporting.[13]

The Importance of Measurement

Although it may be difficult to attain consensus among multiple stakeholders on what constitutes quality health care, it is imperative for stakeholders to

Dr. Bhandari or an immediate family member serves as a paid consultant to or is an employee of Amgen, Eli Lilly, Stryker, Smith & Nephew, Zimmer, Moximed, and Bioventus, and has received research or institutional support from Smith & Nephew, DePuy, Eli Lilly, and Bioventus. Dr. Bozic or an immediate family member serves as a paid consultant to or is an employee of the Institute for Healthcare Improvement, and serves as a board member, owner, officer, or committee member of the American Academy of Orthopaedic Surgeons, the American Association of Hip and Knee Surgeons, and the Orthopaedic Research and Education Foundation. Dr. Piasio or an immediate family member has stock or stock options held in Bristol-Myers Squibb, Eli Lilly, GE Healthcare, GlaxoSmithKline, Johnson & Johnson, Merck, Pfizer, and Procter & Gamble. None of the following authors nor any immediate family member has received anything of value from or has stock or stock options held in a commercial company or institution related directly or indirectly to the subject of this chapter: Dr. Jevsevar, Dr. Karl, and Dr. Weinstein.

© 2016 AAOS Instructional Course Lectures, Volume 65

find a way to stretch healthcare dollars by improving value (defined as health outcomes achieved per dollar amount spent). Performance improvement can be measured with the use of collected data, and healthcare quality can be evaluated in terms of appropriateness, prevention, population health, patient engagement, safety, and care coordination. The results of these evaluations may lead to the implementation of changes and, then, reevaluation.

The Performance Measures Committee of the American Academy of Orthopaedic Surgeons (AAOS) is tasked with the development, validation, implementation, and testing of orthopaedic performance measures. The committee used a performance measures development process (roadmap) that includes the steps shown in **Figure 1**. If new performance measures are being evaluated, selected, and prioritized, the committee considers existing performance measures, the ability for the performance measures to be harmonized, the clinical and economic burden of the condition for which the new performance measures are being proposed, the feasibility of performance measurement, and how the performance measures would ultimately be used. Other considerations include the following: (1) Does the new performance measure provide improved relevance for clinical decision making or reduce practice variation compared with existing performance measures? (2) Is there sufficient evidence on which to base the new performance measure? (3) Is the topic a national health priority, or does it have potential for a large effect (eg, based on the number of people affected, high cost)? (4) Is there potential for improvement (is there substantial variation in diagnosis

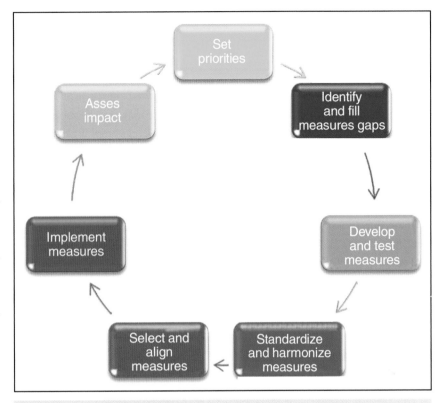

Figure 1   Illustration shows the performance measures development process roadmap developed by the Performance Measures Committee of the American Academy of Orthopaedic Surgeons.

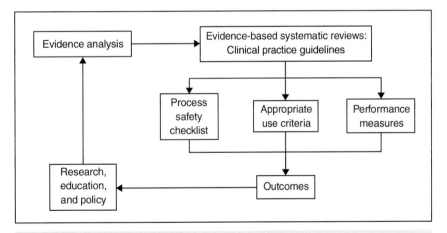

Figure 2   Algorithm shows the cycle of quality developed by the American Academy of Orthopaedic Surgeons.

or treatment)? (5) Do data sources exist for measurement and implementation? (6) What are the planned uses for the performance measure? Evidence from systematic reviews and CPGs is used to inform the development of performance measures. Outcomes based on these performance measures are then incorporated into research and evidence analysis, which leads to revised CPGs. This process is known as the cycle of quality (**Figure 2**).

Performance Measures and Assessment

Performance measures can be classified as structural measures, process measures, patient-experience measures, efficiency measures, and outcomes measures. Structural measures, such as the adoption of electronic medical records and nursing ratios, may be easy to define but are difficult for providers to implement. Process measures, such as the administration of prophylactic antibiotics, may be easy to measure and actionable but are difficult to correlate with clinical outcomes.[1] Patient-experience measures are important because they are patient centered, but they may be affected by patient expectations and cultural norms. An example of a patient-experience measure is the Hospital Consumer Assessment of Healthcare Providers and Systems survey. Efficiency measures, which include the utilization of care and the costs of care, are objective but may vary based on perspective and the time frame.[1] Outcomes measures, such as infection rates or functional status, are the most direct assessment of the quality of care; however, they need to be risk adjusted because other factors, such as patient comorbidities, can affect outcomes. Outcomes also may be difficult to measure, and a substantial time lag may exist between care delivery and the outcome.

Performance measures should be selective, focused, measurable, and actionable. They are tools for quality measurement and should be based on evidence from systematic reviews and CPGs that demonstrate a correlation between a specific healthcare process and outcome (for structural and process measures) or that a specific outcome can be modified by a provider intervention (for outcomes measures). For performance measurement and data collection, orthopaedic organizations and physicians must move from simply measuring what they can to thinking about what is important to measure and how it can be measured. Both the clinical relevance of the measures and the feasibility of measurement should be considered. Performance measurement and data collection methods should be accurate and replicable as well as accompanied by appropriate risk adjustment and efficient yet feasible reporting mechanisms.[14]

The Relationship Between Cost and Quality

Although some may argue that the United States spends more on health care than its peers, the higher level of care that American patients expect and receive justifies the higher cost. Yet, despite spending twice as much on health care, life expectancy in the United States is 3 years less than the average life expectancy in comparable countries.[2] Similarly, regions of the United States with increased spending do not necessarily have better quality of care, functional status, or patient satisfaction than regions of the United States with less spending; in fact, regions of the United States with increased spending have been associated with an increased risk of death.[6,15] Even among individual hospitals in different cities, a wide variation exists in quality of care and spending, with no substantial relationship between spending and quality of care.[16]

In contrast to current research, research from 1984 to 1998 showed that the benefits of new medical technology outweighed the costs, which suggested that during this period, more spending had led to better care.[17] Skinner et al[18] reconciled this apparent contradiction with the use of an expanded database that contained information from 1986 to 2003. The authors reported that outcomes in all regions of the United States improved initially as spending increased but then trailed off in the late 1990s as costs continued to rise. The authors also reported that regions in the United States with higher spending did not improve outcomes as much as regions in the United States with lower spending.[18]

If different hospitals and healthcare systems provide different amounts of quality health care with the same resource inputs, then economists would describe them as being on different production functions. Production functions are curves that describe the health quality of care outputs that can be produced by a healthcare system at different levels of monetary inputs. These curves have diminishing marginal returns, which means that each additional dollar spent yields slightly less than the last. This indicates that earlier studies, which reported improved outcomes with increased spending, were analyzing the earlier, steeper part of the different production curves, and that later studies were analyzing the flatter portion of the different production curves.

Furthermore, Skinner et al[18] suggested that differences in efficiency of production between different hospitals and regions in the United States describe different production curves, not different points along the same curve. This theory has been empirically supported by studies that showed that hospitals that readily adopted high-efficacy, low-cost treatments for myocardial infarction, such as aspirin, β-blockers, and early percutaneous coronary

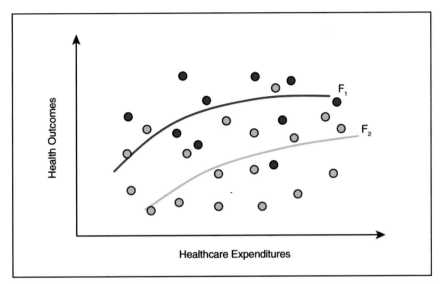

Figure 3   Scatter plot shows the relationship between expenditures and outcomes among various providers (circles) in managing a hypothetical condition. The blue circles represent providers who use a comparatively cost-effective mix of interventions for the hypothetical condition, albeit at different levels of intensity (expenditure). The green circles represent providers who use a less cost-effective mix of services. The curves F_1 and F_2 show the associations between expenditures among providers who practice more (F_1) and less (F_2) cost-effective medicine. (Reproduced with permission from Weinstein MC, Skinner JA: Comparative effectiveness and health care spending—Implications for reform. *N Engl J Med* 2010;362[5]:460-465.)

interventions, had better rates of patient survival at no additional cost and, thus, had defined a more efficient production function[19,20] (**Figure 3**).

The development of these differing production curves can be rational and describe a model based on productivity spillovers, in which physicians in high-intensity regions become better at delivering high-intensity care by working with other physicians who are more skilled in rendering high-intensity care. As a result, physicians achieve better outcomes from delivering high-intensity care compared with low-intensity care in the same region. At the same time, physicians in low-intensity regions become better at delivering low-intensity care and achieve better outcomes from delivering low-intensity care compared with high-intensity care in the same region.[21] Both strategies are rational and

deliver comparable results but at very different price points. In essence, higher intensity regions are on a less efficient production curve. In this situation, the reduction of healthcare spending or reimbursement alone will not work without changing the production functions on which providers operate; it only will move a system down its current curve. To shift to a higher production curve, on which better outcomes are produced at the same or lower cost, the orthopaedic profession needs to improve the efficiency of its processes (**Figure 4**).

Although the idea of changing a production function may seem daunting and abstract, there are many simple, concrete examples of how providers can achieve this goal. The standardization of either implants/devices or care, attention to logistics and supply-chain negotiation strategies, and tying physician

preference to outcomes are a few examples of pragmatic processes that can affect production functions.

Transparency and Accountability in Pay for Value

As representatives of the payer community, orthopaedic physicians face a new world order of better informed consumers who, armed with quality and cost data from multiple credible sources, are introducing a new wave of transparency and accountability that the orthopaedic profession and industry has never previously experienced. It is clear that attempts to ignore this trend as another futile attempt to question physician sovereignty will result in mutual peril. Consumerism is alive and well and represents one of the greatest threats, or opportunities, that the medical industry (and specifically orthopaedics) has ever faced.

The Affordable Care Act, value programming from the Centers for Medicare and Medicare Services (CMS), Medicaid expansion and state responses, benefit changes, silver plans and high deductibles, and self-insured entities are now the rule, not the exception. Accountable care organizations, transparent pricing, tiered networks, and patient steering are now commonplace in all markets, and the effects will be even more dramatic going forward. These ideas are not fads. Well-respected media sources are fully aware of the Dartmouth Atlas of Health Care, and many credible research studies are raising serious questions about the value of what orthopaedic physicians do. This comes as no surprise to Consumer Reports or the National Business Group on Health. Medical tourism is no longer an import; it is interstate

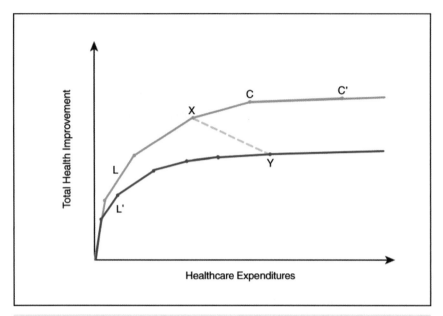

Figure 4 Line graph shows the relationship between expenditures and health gains (as measured in quality-adjusted life-years) in two hypothetical healthcare delivery systems. The purple curve represents an allocation of expenditures to health interventions that maximizes health improvements for any level of expenditure. The blue curve represents an allocation that is inefficient in the sense that it falls short of the maximum attainable health gain for any level of expenditure. The line segments that make up both of the curves represent incremental additions of health interventions or substitutions of more beneficial but more expensive interventions for less expensive but less beneficial alternatives. For example, line segments L and L' both represent a hypothetical intervention that is very cost-effective relative to the other interventions to the right; however, in the inefficient allocation (blue curve), this highly cost-effective intervention is underutilized, which is represented by the shorter length of L' compared with L. The line segments become progressively less steep from left to right, which reflects diminishing health value as expenditures increase. The points on the curves represent possible allocations of health expenditures. For example, point X on the purple curve represents an allocation that achieves more health gain at a lower cost than the allocation represented by point Y on the blue curve. The shallow slope of the line segment connecting points C and C' reflects the fact that the intervention it represents is a relatively cost-ineffective one, although it is still beneficial. (Reproduced with permission from Weinstein MC, Skinner JA: Comparative effectiveness and health care spending—Implications for reform. *N Engl J Med* 2010;362[5]:460-465.)

commerce driven by large multinational and American corporations that seek better value for their enormous, unprecedented healthcare costs. The numerous CMS initiatives—including the Medicare Shared Savings Program, accountable care organizations, hierarchical condition categories, value-based purchasing, quality rating systems for qualified health plans, physician quality reporting systems, and star ratings systems—hopefully have now received full attention. The National Quality Foundation is creating new quality measures, with little input from orthopaedic physicians and groups. Why can orthopaedics professionals not be trusted to put patients first? Without honest action to bring real value to patients and whoever pays for their care, orthopaedic surgeons simply will be excluded from the process of creating new quality measures.

As major payers, with integrated finance and delivery systems, orthopaedic surgeons currently have several strategies, or levers of opportunity, that can drive out volume and waste and bring value to spending (**Table 1**). Reference-based pricing is currently being used in California for total joint surgery and in many areas of the United States for colonoscopies. Essentially, reference-based pricing is the commoditization of a procedure; if there is unexplained cost variation, then ceiling limits are placed on total spending. The patient covers the excess, not the deductible. This tactic is currently highly effective but only against true outliers, and the future return is limited. Tiered networks and the steerage of patients to high-value providers are well known, except that these tactics have had little effect with prior benefit design. Patient-centered medical home programs, high deductibles, and narrow networks, all of which are now commonplace, will only enhance the effect.

Reimbursement redesign that rewards value, not volume, holds great promise. The dearth of reliable quality metrics and their ease of capture retard the development of reimbursement design. The cost or efficiency components are well understood and easily and reliably gleaned from administrative datasets. Orthopaedic surgeons can create quality and efficiency scores for fee schedule modifications or bonus payments with the use of medical grouper software. Episodic payments, or bundles, also hold great promise and have been very successful in other high-cost, frequent interventions, such as cardiothoracic surgery and oncology. Much work will occur in the episodic/bundled payment arena, especially for joint arthroplasty, spinal surgery, and, possibly, discretionary sports medicine surgery. Gain share, risk share, and accountable care organizations are more of a challenge if specialty models are being created, but some form of participation is expected in select markets. A practicing physician will need to understand how gain share, risk share, and accountable care organizations work and where the opportunities exist. Physicians know all too well about utilization management, which is here to stay. The effectiveness of transparency and profiling tools that are entering the marketplace is currently being studied.

Grouper software will be used to collect services into procedure or diagnostic groups that can be measured for comparative costs, quality, and efficiency. Many software programs are available in the marketplace, each with nuances but all very robust and accurate. These programs will allow a payer to measure a surgeon's performance for quality and complication against comparative costs and market adjustments. Utilization rates as well as unit costs will be compared and quality and risk adjusted with performance scores. These software programs are accurate and reliable. The only current weakness is the lack of evidence-based metrics and appropriate use criteria in the methodology. Now is the opportunity to get these remaining details right. Administrative data sets will be required. Such data initially will be used to profile the format for quality improvement, but physician groups should expect the profiles to be released to other physicians for steering and, eventually, to the public for transparency and tiering.

The payer community is requesting cooperation, honest research, and true evidence-based guidelines and appropriate use criteria, which are necessary to create value payment models for the orthopaedic specialist. Physicians must ensure that their literature is free of commercial or self-serving bias, they fully support the efforts of their peers to make hard decisions in the interest of their patients, and society pays for patient care. Physicians must pursue scalable reliable metrics that can be coded and administratively collected. The United States has a robust longitudinal dataset on all patients and their healthcare claims. Such data are rich, comprehensive, and only now being explored to their fullest potential. Robust longitudinal data are the best registry data and can easily accommodate outcome data by means of G (Therapy Functional Reporting), V (Supplementary Classification of Factors Influencing Health Status and Contact With Health Services), and CPT (Current Procedural Terminology) Category II coding. The current quality registry sets measure complications but not cost, efficiency, utilization, regional effects, or appropriate use, and they are not transparent nor easily populated.

The National Quality Forum is currently the nation's steward for quality metrics in health care, and orthopaedic physicians should fully participate in its robust process of creating national standards for quality health care. Reduce, refine, and relate should be the core principles in metric development. Measures must have manageable reporting requirements, be aligned by reporting entities, and focus on clinical outcomes, not processes, to provide utility to the consumer. Orthopaedic professionals must pursue endorsement

Table 1
Levers of Opportunity for Orthopaedic Pay-for-Value Programs

Benefit redesign
  Reference-based pricing
  Steering
  Tiered networks

Reimbursement redesign
  Fee-for-service schedule enhancements/value modifier
  Bundled payments per episode
  Prospective
  Retrospective
  Gain share and risk share

Medical management
  Prior authorization and utilization review

Transparency
  Profiling and steering

by the National Quality Forum, ease of data collection, cross-cutting measures across multiple conditions for both overutilization and underutilization, and a parsimonious measure set. They must strive to create outcomes measures so that a prudent physician will succeed. Physicians cannot let malpractice be the standard and must lead, seize the moral high ground, and establish a mutually profitable collaborative to ensure high-quality, cost-effective care that patients deserve.

Orthopaedic Quality Advocacy Efforts for the Public Sector

Congress views these issues in the context of the three main issues plaguing US health care: high and unsustainable costs, variable quality, and substantial numbers of Americans who lack adequate healthcare coverage. Congress is particularly concerned about the growth in Medicare spending in the past decade, which is secondary to the growth in volume and the intensity of physician services. Congress is concerned about the 212% increase in insurance premiums in the past 15 years because earnings increased by only 54%. Congressional members recognize that companies in their districts that have employer-based insurance systems are facing ever-increasing healthcare costs for their employees, which affects company profitability and business expansion. Congress also is aware that healthcare spending is the largest factor that contributes to the federal debt.

Congress also is asking important questions about US healthcare. Why do cost differences exist depending on the site of service? Why should a colonoscopy cost 118% more if performed in a hospital versus a doctor's office? Why should a spinal fusion cost $62,000 in the United States but $9,000 in Singapore? Why does so much variability exist in US healthcare spending without better outcomes for such expenditures? Congress understands that most Americans will spend one-third of their lives on Medicare and that, without healthcare reform, they will not be able to afford it.

Orthopaedic surgeons are squarely in the congressional and CMS cross hairs. Almost one-fourth of the CPT codes are related to the musculoskeletal system. The number one diagnosis-related group in Medicare is for joint arthroplasty, and as the population ages in the next 15 years, the need for joint arthroplasty, particularly total knee replacements, will increase exponentially.

The sustainable growth rate formula emerged in 1997 in the Balanced Budget Act as an attempt to stem rising healthcare costs. By 2002, it was clear that the formula was flawed and needed to be repealed and replaced. Thirteen years

of advocacy finally led to the passage of the Medicare Access and Children's Health Insurance Program Reauthorization Act of 2015 (HR 2). All stakeholders were included in the planning of the bill during the 3 years that led up to its passage. The bill had overwhelming support from both Democrats and Republicans in both the House and the Senate. HR 2 has been euphemistically called the "Doc Fix" because it stabilized physician reimbursement under Medicare. The bill ensures that patients have access to care and changes the way physicians will be paid in the future. The ultimate goal of the bill is to replace payment for volume with payment for value. The federal government and all payers want to align the incentives for payment to reward quality care—outcomes achieved per dollar spent. In drafting the legislation, Congress gave physicians the right to determine what quality care means for patients. Physicians cannot abrogate this responsibility. If physicians do not rise to the challenge and take advantage of this opportunity, the identification of what quality care means for patients will be determined by individuals external to the medical community.

Although the AAOS and other organizations have been working on quality metrics for some time, the passage of HR 2 put these organizations on the clock. They have a 5-year window in which to put forth a substantial effort to define metrics for quality. As an expert-based discipline, orthopaedics will never have a strong evidence base for guidelines but orthopaedic surgeons must nevertheless continue to develop them. However, there is a strong base for the development of important appropriate use criteria and performance measures, which must be generated

with the most rigorous of development processes. The AAOS cannot do this alone; it will take a coordinated effort by the AAOS, specialty societies, and others. If appropriate use criteria or performance measures have been developed by a collaborative, a healthcare system, or other source with the use of rigorous methodology, orthopaedic organizations must adopt them rather than starting from scratch. Every specialty and subspecialty society must make this priority number one.

To be effective advocates for issues in Washington, DC, orthopaedic organizations need to be both players and contributors. After fighting for 13 years to get the sustainable growth rate repealed and replaced, orthopaedic organizations, for the first time, are at the table for every iteration of the replacement process. Orthopaedic organizations need to be part of the solution rather than be viewed by members of Congress as part of the problem. At every visit to Capitol Hill that is related to an orthopaedic issue, be it medical liability reform, the preservation of in-office ancillary services, or a discussion of the implementation of the 10th revision of the International Statistical Classification of Diseases and Related Health Problems, orthopaedic organizations must be able to show members of Congress what they are doing in the quality arena. Orthopaedic organizations need to thank Congress for their support of HR 2 and show them how the profession has taken advantage of Congress's faith in their ability to determine what quality care means for patients.

Summary

The United States is spending more money on health care than it can afford, and the outcomes being achieved are not commensurate with that spending. Outcomes are not determined by how much money is spent but by how the money is spent. There are huge inefficiencies in physician systems, some of which can be controlled. Providers must work to eliminate these inefficiencies and tie together quality and cost; without solid evidence on quality, payers will choose based on cost only, to the detriment of both patients and providers.

References

1. Saleh KJ, Bozic KJ, Graham DB, et al: Quality in orthopaedic surgery—an international perspective: AOA critical issues. *J Bone Joint Surg Am* 2013;95(1):e3.

2. The Henry J. Kaiser Family Foundation: *Health Costs.* Available at: http://kff.org/health-costs. Accessed June 30, 2015.

3. Organisation for Economic and Co-operation and Development (OECD): *OECD Health Statistics 2014 – Frequently Requested Data.* Available at: http://www.oecd.org/els/health-systems/oecd-health-statistics-2014-frequently-requested-data.htm. Accessed February 4, 2015.

4. Gruber J: Growth and variability in health plan premiums in the individual insurance market before the Affordable Care Act. *Issue Brief (Commonw Fund)* 2014;11:1-12.

5. Davis K, Stremikis K, Squires D, Schoen C: *Mirror, mirror on the wall, 2014 update: How the U.S. health care system compares internationally.* New York, NY, The Commonwealth Fund, 2014. Available at: www.commonwealthfund.org/publications/fund-reports/2014/jun/mirror-mirror. Accessed June 30, 2015.

6. Fisher ES, Wennberg DE, Stukel TA, Gottlieb DJ, Lucas FL, Pinder EL: The implications of regional variations in Medicare spending: Part 1. The content, quality, and accessibility of care. *Ann Intern Med* 2003;138(4):273-287.

7. Sackett DL, Rosenberg WM, Gray JA, Haynes RB, Richardson WS: Evidence based medicine: What it is and what it isn't. *BMJ* 1996;312(7023):71-72.

8. Wright JG, Swiontkowski MF, Heckman JD: Introducing levels of evidence to the journal. *J Bone Joint Surg Am* 2003;85(1):1-3.

9. Maggard MA, O'Connell JB, Liu JH, Etzioni DA, Ko CY: Sample size calculations in surgery: Are they done correctly? *Surgery* 2003;134(2):275-279.

10. Walsh M, Srinathan SK, McAuley DF, et al: The statistical significance of randomized controlled trial results is frequently fragile: A case for a Fragility Index. *J Clin Epidemiol* 2014;67(6):622-628.

11. Aro HT, Govender S, Patel AD, et al: Recombinant human bone morphogenetic protein-2: A randomized trial in open tibial fractures treated with reamed nail fixation. *J Bone Joint Surg Am* 2011;93(9):801-808.

12. Govender S, Csimma C, Genant HK, et al: Recombinant human bone morphogenetic protein-2 for treatment of open tibial fractures: A prospective, controlled, randomized study of four hundred and fifty patients. *J Bone Joint Surg Am* 2002;84(12):2123-2134.

13. Bumpass DB, Samora JB, Butler CA, Jevsevar DS, Moffatt-Bruce SD, Bozic KJ: Orthopaedic quality reporting: A comprehensive review of the current landscape and a roadmap for progress. *JBJS Rev* 2014;2(8):e5.

14. Marjoua Y, Bozic KJ: Brief history of quality movement in US healthcare. *Curr Rev Musculoskelet Med* 2012;5(4):265-273.

15. Fisher ES, Wennberg DE, Stukel TA, Gottlieb DJ, Lucas FL, Pinder EL: The implications of regional variations in Medicare spending: Part 2. Health outcomes and satisfaction with care. *Ann Intern Med* 2003;138(4):288-298.

16. Yasaitis L, Fisher ES, Skinner JS, Chandra A: Hospital quality and intensity of spending: Is there an association? *Health Aff (Millwood)* 2009;28(4):w566-w572.

17. Cutler DM, McClellan M: Is technological change in medicine worth it? *Health Aff (Millwood)* 2001;20(5):11-29.

18. Skinner JS, Staiger DO, Fisher ES: Is technological change in medicine always worth it? The case of acute myocardial infarction. *Health Aff (Millwood)* 2006;25(2):w34-w47.

19. Weinstein MC, Skinner JA: Comparative effectiveness and health care spending—implications for reform. *N Engl J Med* 2010;362(5):460-465.

20. Skinner J, Staiger D: Technology diffusion and productivity growth in health care: NBER Working Paper No. 14865. Cambridge, MA, National Bureau of Economic Research, April 2009. Available at: http://www.nber.org/papers/w14865. Accessed June 30, 2015.

21. Chandra A, Staiger DO: Productivity spillovers in healthcare: Evidence from the treatment of heart attacks. *J Polit Econ* 2007;115:103-140.

Outcome Measure Development

Nicholas G. Mohtadi, MD, MSc, FRCSC

Abstract

Measuring patient-reported outcomes is the current method for conducting clinical research. Creating a new outcome measure is an exhaustive process that should be carefully monitored and concentrated on only important and common conditions. The evaluation of an existing outcome measure should involve assessing its internal consistency, reliability, floor and ceiling effects, validity, and ability to measure clinically meaningful change. The most important characteristic of a patient-reported outcome is that it is developed with direct input from its target patient population. Item generation and reduction is the most critical step in the development process because it "guarantees" that patients have communicated what is important to them and represents content validity. Outcome measures should not change; rather, they should demonstrate responsiveness by being reproducible and reliable if a patient's clinical condition is stable or reflect differences if a patient's clinical condition varies. Validation is an iterative process and requires patients from different settings and circumstances.

Instr Course Lect 2016;65:577–582.

Outcome measures can be called instruments, tools, scales, scores, indices, measures, outcomes, or questionnaires; these terms are used interchangeably throughout this chapter. Outcome measures can be classified in many ways. The purpose of an outcome measure can be classified as either disease specific (eg, to assess osteoarthritis),[1] joint specific (eg, to assess the outcome of a particular joint or region, such as the shoulder, hip, or knee),[2-5] or generic (eg, the Medical Outcomes Study 36-Item Short Form [SF-36] and the Medical Outcomes Study 12-Item Short Form).[6,7] Outcome measures also can be classified according to the person who completes the assessment. Traditionally, outcomes have been assessed by clinicians and have included objective measures, such as radiographic assessments. In addition, the clinician would ask the patient about pain or other subjective symptoms. These clinician-based or clinician-administered tools may introduce bias because of the way they are administered; more importantly, however, they may not capture a patient's perceived outcomes. Because of these drawbacks, patient-based and patient-administered tools have been created.[3,4,8-14] These patient-reported outcome (PRO) measures are typically self-administered, which eliminates clinician bias, and give patients the opportunity to provide their clinicians with important information about their condition in a neutral setting. PROs are considered standard references for reporting the results of clinical trials.[15-17] A PRO measure can range from a simple visual analog scale (VAS) for pain to a complex multidomain questionnaire. Despite being called a PRO, the content of the questions may be clinician and/or patient derived; therefore, it is necessary and critical to ensure that the target patient population of a PRO has direct input into the content of the PRO.

Developing a New PRO Measure

The question to ask before developing a new outcome measure is whether the condition, disease, or patient population

Dr. Mohtadi or an immediate family member serves as a board member, owner, officer, or committee member of the Arthroscopy Association of Canada.

is common and important enough to evaluate. An exhaustive search of the literature should then be performed to determine if an existing instrument is available. For example, the Harris hip score was revised as the Modified Harris hip score (mHHS) by eliminating the elements of "deformity...and range of motion."[18] Eliminating these two elements, which required a physical examination, essentially changed a clinician-determined and clinician-administered outcome measure into one that can be patient reported. Modifying an existing outcome measure, however, will inevitably change its characteristics and can potentially invalidate the measurement properties of the new outcome measure.

According to Guyatt et al,[19] two different strategic models can be used to develop a new outcome measure: the Rolls-Royce model and the Volkswagen model. Patient input is critically emphasized in the Rolls-Royce model. Item selection and generation is the single most important phase in outcome measure development. It is an exhaustive process of identifying every possible item of concern from 50 to 100 patients who have the disease in question; in other words, it surveys to the point of redundancy.[20] Without this process of obtaining patient input, it is possible or even likely that important items may be missed.

For example, not many male surgeons are comfortable asking a female patient about the effect of their hip problem on sexual activity. However, the question, "How much trouble do you have with sexual activity because of your hip?" was included in the International Hip Outcome Tool (iHOT-33) and the short version of the International Hip Outcome Tool (iHOT-12)

because patients recognized it as an important issue or item of concern.[3] Examples of item generation also can be observed in the Anterior Cruciate Ligament Quality of Life (ACL-QOL) questionnaire, which started with 167 items, and the iHOT-33, which initially generated 146 separate items.[4,14]

After the items have been generated, the next step is item reduction. Item reduction involves requesting another group of patients (eg, the iHOT-33 used 150 patients) to rate each selected item on a scale from 0 to 5, where 0 means that the patient does not experience the particular issue, and 5 means that the patient believes the issue is extremely important. This process allows the developer of the outcome measure to create a "frequency-importance" product for each item and rank the items accordingly. Patient input is a critical element in this step because it has been found that asking surgeons to rate the items on the same scale frequently generates a completely different ranking.[21]

The next step is to determine the preferred questionnaire format and response scale (eg, Likert scale, VAS, nominal yes/no scale). A VAS is typically used because it is easy to calculate the score for each patient and because the responses can be analyzed using parametric statistics, which makes analyses easier to understand. Specific questions are written, and the response scale is attached. If some redundancy is identified during the question-writing process, the questionnaire must be pretested in one-on-one interviews with another group of patients (20 patients are typically required).[19] This ensures that each question is understood, is written in an unambiguous manner, and has the appropriate context.

The most common method for defining the scoring scale is to have a higher score represent a better outcome, measured on a scale from 1 to 100. However, one of the original PROs, the VAS for pain, has a higher score representative of more pain for the patient.[22] Some differences do exist between outcome measures; for example, the Western Ontario and McMaster Universities Osteoarthritis Index uses both a Likert scale and a VAS format, with a higher score representative of a poorer outcome.[1,23-27] Conversely, the Rotator Cuff Quality of Life (RC-QOL) questionnaire, the ACL-QOL questionnaire, and the iHOT-33 all use a VAS format with a higher score representative of a better quality of life or outcome.[4,9,14]

After these initial stages of development, the outcome measure is complete, and it must undergo the essential steps of validation. These steps include assessing the outcome measure's reliability and reproducibility, floor and ceiling effects, responsiveness, ability to determine minimal clinically important differences (MCIDs), and construct validity.

What is a Reliable or Reproducible Outcome Measure?

One component of reliability relates to the internal consistency of an outcome measure and the notion that patients should score approximately the same on questions that test similar attributes. A highly internally consistent questionnaire will have some redundancy. Internal consistency can be statistically measured by using the Cronbach alpha test, which gives a score between 0 and 1. A questionnaire that receives a Cronbach alpha score higher than 0.7 is considered to be internally consistent.[28]

A reliable or reproducible questionnaire must be more than just internally consistent. If a patient's quality of life, function, or pain has not changed since his or her original assessment, then the outcome assessment should render the same result if it is repeated. Retest reliability can be determined by using the intraclass correlation coefficient, which is more appropriate than a simple correlation coefficient because it acknowledges systematic differences.[28] To determine the correlation between responses, a group of patients is given the questionnaire on one occasion and then again, typically 2 weeks later. The assumptions are that patients' clinical circumstances are unlikely to change in 2 weeks, and patients will not remember their responses from the first time the questionnaire was administered. Each separate question and the entire questionnaire or separate domains within the questionnaire are evaluated for reliability. Unreliable questions are removed from the questionnaire at this stage.

What is a Floor or Ceiling Effect?

Questions also should be evaluated to determine if they have a floor or ceiling effect. A ceiling effect or, conversely, a floor effect arises if a high percentage of patients score at the upper or lower levels of the spectrum for a question or the questionnaire. The best example to illustrate a ceiling effect involves using the mHHS to determine the outcome of a professional athlete undergoing hip arthroscopy for femoroacetabular impingement.[29] The mHHS assesses a patient with respect to pain (44 points), gait (33 points), and functional activities (14 points). A professional hockey player who may have problems only with

heavy weight training and sprinting in the offseason or when playing back-to-back games in the midseason would likely score very high on the mHHS. The professional hockey player's gait and functional activities, as defined in the mHHS, may not be compromised, and pain might be reported at a relatively low level, which results in a score of 85 out of 100. Whether this is a low enough score to consider surgery is influenced by the goals of the professional athlete, which are likely to be different from those of a typical patient. The mHHS, therefore, may not be as applicable for professional athletes, and different outcome measures, such as sport-specific performance measures, may be required. In addition, the mHHS may not have a large-enough scale to determine if the measurable improvement in a patient's score is both clinically important and statistically significant.

The same argument can be made for the floor effect. For example, if a patient has a permanent limp because of a limb-length discrepancy and a painful arthritic hip, total hip arthroplasty may substantially improve the patient's overall quality of life but may not necessarily change his or her gait. The gait component of the mHHS will remain low before and after treatment, demonstrating a floor effect. Questions that have obvious floor or ceiling effects should be removed at this stage of validation.

What is a Responsive Outcome Measure?

The psychometric property of responsiveness is an essential element of a credible outcome measure.[19,30-33] Responsiveness can be determined in many ways, but it can be an elusive property unless it is measured in the same

patient population for which outcomes are being compared. As a result, some authors have questioned the concept of responsiveness; however, it remains an intuitively important element of an outcome measure.[34] Responsiveness is the measure of an instrument's ability to detect change and is directly related to the magnitude of difference between scores from patients who have improved or deteriorated and scores from patients who have not changed at all. A responsive questionnaire will demonstrate little variability in stable patients (noise) and a substantial change in patients who have improved or deteriorated (signal).[19,31,32] A high signal-to-noise ratio reflects greater responsiveness.

What is an MCID?

Jaeschke et al[35] originally defined an MCID as "the smallest difference in score in the domain of interest which patients perceive as beneficial and which would mandate, in the absence of troublesome side effects and excessive cost, a change in the patient's management." Since then, several definitions have been offered, all of which describe an MCID as an instrument's ability to measure the "lower boundary of change."[36] MCIDs can be defined statistically, using a distributional approach; by an external standard, such as expert opinion; or by what a patient considers a detectable change in score.[37] Irrespective of how MCIDs are determined or defined, it must take into account what is measurable, it must be more than the inherent error of the instrument, and it must be clinically meaningful.

What is a Valid Outcome Measure?

Validity, in the simplest sense, refers to an outcome measuring what it intends to measure. Validity can be described in several ways, the simplest of which, is face validity. Face validity refers to a PRO that appears to measure the appropriate patient-related characteristics. Ideally, an outcome measure should be compared with a benchmark; if it compares well, then it is likely the outcome is valid. Many clinical outcome measures, particularly PRO measures, do not have benchmarks for comparison; therefore, the concepts of content and construct validity need to be addressed during validation. Using the Rolls-Royce and Volkswagen models for outcome measure development previously described, an outcome measure based on the Volkswagen model would rely on face validity alone. An outcome measure based on the Rolls-Royce model, however, would require excellent content validity and the evaluation of several constructs.

Content validity is the most important measurement property of a PRO questionnaire.[28] Content validity is a measure of a questionnaire's comprehensiveness and how well questions represent all relevant patient concerns. It is critical that patients are involved in shaping the content of questionnaires; otherwise, the content will reflect only the clinician's perspective.[21] A PRO questionnaire should clearly describe its target population and be developed through item generation and reduction methods that involve patients and clinicians.[28] In a truly patient-derived PRO, content validity is most closely linked to and, therefore, ensured through the process of surveying patients to redundancy.[20]

Construct validity can be determined by comparing the new outcome measure with similar existing outcome measures. It is important to recognize that the new outcome measure is not being compared with a benchmark (ie, criterion validity).[19,20] Construct validity also can be demonstrated by establishing reasonable hypotheses and testing them with the new outcome measure. For example, it is reasonable to expect a patient's quality of life to improve after surgical treatment and continue to improve over time. If a patient's outcome scores do not improve and every other indicator suggests that the patient is improving, then the suggested hypothesis would be disproven, and the outcome measure would be considered invalid. If all other measures, such as range of motion, strength, and return to activity or work have improved and the new outcome correlates with these improvements, then the hypothesis would be proven, and the outcome measure would be considered valid.

When is a PRO Measure Completely Validated?

An outcome measure is considered valid after all the steps previously described have been completed and all the questions have been answered. It is imperative, however, to critically assess the manner in which each step was performed, if there was sufficient patient input, and, most importantly, if the correct patient population was used for the validation process. For example, the SF-36 is considered a validated, general health-related PRO; it has been used throughout the world and was developed in accordance with all the principles previously described.[7,38-44] However, if the SF-36 is used as the primary outcome measure to compare two surgical methods of ACL reconstruction, it is unlikely that it would be able to demonstrate that one procedure is better than the other. Even if a randomized clinical trial with several hundred patients was performed and reported a statistically significant difference between the two surgical techniques, the difference would be somewhat meaningless. This is because the SF-36 was intended measure general health outcomes; it was not developed using the young and active individuals that are typical of the ACL-injured or ACL-deficient population. The questions in the SF-36 are not similar to the questions in the disease-specific ACL-QOL questionnaire.[14] Likewise, comparisons between the SF-36 and the RC-QOL questionnaire have shown that the SF-36 is unable to discriminate between patients with large rotator cuff tears (RCTs) and patients with massive RCTs.[9] The hypothesis that the outcome of surgical treatment for a large RCT would be better than the outcome of surgical treatment for a massive RCT is proven with the disease-specific RC-QOL questionnaire, not the SF-36.[9]

Summary

Developing a well-validated PRO is an extensive process that potentially involves several hundred patients and a substantial amount of time and resources. Generic and disease-specific outcome measures are available for most of the common orthopaedic conditions. Clinicians should understand the development process for outcome measures and recognize that the most important element of the process is patient involvement. Many practitioners use simple and short outcome measures to avoid burdening patients; however, most investigators have found that if patients are asked relevant and important questions, they are more than happy to answer them. With their continued use, surgeons will become more reliant on the critically important information that validated outcome measures provide.

References

1. Bellamy N, Buchanan WW, Goldsmith CH, Campbell J, Stitt LW: Validation study of WOMAC: A health status instrument for measuring clinically important patient relevant outcomes to antirheumatic drug therapy in patients with osteoarthritis of the hip or knee. *J Rheumatol* 1988;15(12):1833-1840.

2. Constant CR, Murley AH: A clinical method of functional assessment of the shoulder. *Clin Orthop Relat Res* 1987;214:160-164.

3. Griffin DR, Parsons N, Mohtadi NG, Safran MR; Multicenter Arthroscopy of the Hip Outcomes Research Network: A short version of the International Hip Outcome Tool (iHOT-12) for use in routine clinical practice. *Arthroscopy* 2012;28(5):611-618.

4. Mohtadi NG, Griffin DR, Pedersen ME, et al: The development and validation of a self-administered quality-of-life outcome measure for young, active patients with symptomatic hip disease: The International Hip Outcome Tool (iHOT-33). *Arthroscopy* 2012;28(5):595-605, quiz 606-610.e1.

5. Marx RG, Stump TJ, Jones EC, Wickiewicz TL, Warren RF: Development and evaluation of an activity rating scale for disorders of the knee. *Am J Sports Med* 2001;29(2):213-218.

6. Ware J Jr, Kosinski M, Keller SD: A 12-Item Short-Form Health Survey: Construction of scales and preliminary tests of reliability and validity. *Med Care* 1996;34(3):220-233.

7. Ware JE Jr, Sherbourne CD: The MOS 36-item short-form health survey (SF-36): I. Conceptual framework and item selection. *Med Care* 1992;30(6):473-483.

8. Dawson J, Fitzpatrick R, Carr A: Questionnaire on the perceptions of patients about shoulder surgery. *J Bone Joint Surg Br* 1996;78(4):593-600.

9. Hollinshead RM, Mohtadi NG, Vande Guchte RA, Wadey VM: Two 6-year follow-up studies of large and massive rotator cuff tears: Comparison of outcome measures. *J Shoulder Elbow Surg* 2000;9(5):373-381.

10. Hudak PL, Amadio PC, Bombardier C; The Upper Extremity Collaborative Group (UECG): Development of an upper extremity outcome measure: The DASH (disabilities Disabilities of the Arm, Shoulder, and Hand) [corrected]. *Am J Ind Med* 1996;29(6):602-608.

11. Kirkley A, Alvarez C, Griffin S: The development and evaluation of a disease-specific quality-of-life questionnaire for disorders of the rotator cuff: The Western Ontario Rotator Cuff Index. *Clin J Sport Med* 2003;13(2):84-92.

12. Kirkley A, Griffin S, McLintock H, Ng L: The development and evaluation of a disease-specific quality of life measurement tool for shoulder instability: The Western Ontario Shoulder Instability Index (WOSI). *Am J Sports Med* 1998;26(6):764-772.

13. Lo IK, Griffin S, Kirkley A: The development of a disease-specific quality of life measurement tool for osteoarthritis of the shoulder: The Western Ontario Osteoarthritis of the Shoulder (WOOS) index. *Osteoarthritis Cartilage* 2001;9(8):771-778.

14. Mohtadi N: Development and validation of the quality of life outcome measure (questionnaire) for chronic anterior cruciate ligament deficiency. *Am J Sports Med* 1998;26(3):350-359.

15. Rothman ML, Beltran P, Cappelleri JC, Lipscomb J, Teschendorf B; Mayo/FDA Patient-Reported Outcomes Consensus Meeting Group: Patient-reported outcomes: Conceptual issues. *Value Health* 2007;10(10 suppl 2):S66-S75.

16. Schipper H, Clinch J, Olweny C: Quality of life studies: Definitions and conceptual issues, in Spilker B, ed: *Quality of Life and Pharmacoeconomics in Clinical Trials*, ed 2. Philadelphia, PA, Lippincott-Raven, 1996, pp 11-23.

17. Scoggins JF, Patrick DL: The use of patient-reported outcomes instruments in registered clinical trials: Evidence from ClinicalTrials.gov. *Contemp Clin Trials* 2009;30(4):289-292.

18. Byrd JW, Jones KS: Hip arthroscopy in the presence of dysplasia. *Arthroscopy* 2003;19(10):1055-1060.

19. Guyatt GH, Bombardier C, Tugwell PX: Measuring disease-specific quality of life in clinical trials. *CMAJ* 1986;134(8):889-895.

20. Burns KE, Duffett M, Kho ME, et al: A guide for the design and conduct of self-administered surveys of clinicians. *CMAJ* 2008;179(3):245-252.

21. Martin RL, Mohtadi NG, Safran MR, et al: Differences in physician and patient ratings of items used to assess hip disorders. *Am J Sports Med* 2009;37(8):1508-1512.

22. Huskisson EC: Measurement of pain. *Lancet* 1974;2(7889):1127-1131.

23. Bellamy N: Pain assessment in osteoarthritis: Experience with the WOMAC osteoarthritis index. *Semin Arthritis Rheum* 1989;18(4 suppl 2):14-17.

24. Bellamy N, Goldsmith CH, Buchanan WW, Campbell J, Duku E: Prior score availability: Observations using the WOMAC osteoarthritis index. *Br J Rheumatol* 1991;30(2):150-151.

25. Bellamy N, Patel B, Davis T, Dennison S: Electronic data capture using the Womac NRS 3.1 Index (m-Womac): A pilot study of repeated independent remote data capture in OA. *Inflammopharmacology* 2010;18(3):107-111.

26. Bellamy N, Wilson C, Hendrikz J: Population-based normative values for the Western Ontario and McMaster (WOMAC) osteoarthritis index and the Australian/Canadian (AUSCAN) hand osteoarthritis index functional subscales. *Inflammopharmacology* 2010;18(1):1-8.

27. Bellamy N, Wilson C, Hendrikz J, et al; EDC Study Group: Osteoarthritis Index delivered by mobile phone (m-WOMAC) is valid, reliable, and responsive. *J Clin Epidemiol* 2011;64(2):182-190.

28. Terwee CB, Bot SD, de Boer MR, et al: Quality criteria were proposed for measurement properties of health status questionnaires. *J Clin Epidemiol* 2007;60(1):34-42.

29. Byrd JW, Jones KS: Prospective analysis of hip arthroscopy with 2-year follow-up. *Arthroscopy* 2000;16(6):578-587.

30. Guyatt G, Walter S, Norman G: Measuring change over time: Assessing the usefulness of evaluative instruments. *J Chronic Dis* 1987;40(2):171-178.

31. Guyatt GH, Feeny DH, Patrick DL: Measuring health-related quality of life. *Ann Intern Med* 1993;118(8):622-629.

32. Guyatt GH, Kirshner B, Jaeschke R: Measuring health status: What are the necessary measurement properties? *J Clin Epidemiol* 1992;45(12):1341-1345.

33. Wright JG, Young NL: A comparison of different indices of responsiveness. *J Clin Epidemiol* 1997;50(3):239-246.

34. Terwee CB, Dekker FW, Wiersinga WM, Prummel MF, Bossuyt PM: On assessing responsiveness of health-related quality of life instruments: Guidelines for instrument evaluation. *Qual Life Res* 2003;12(4):349-362.

35. Jaeschke R, Singer J, Guyatt GH: Measurement of health status: Ascertaining the minimal clinically important difference. *Control Clin Trials* 1989;10(4):407-415.

36. Beaton DE, Boers M, Wells GA: Many faces of the minimal clinically important difference (MCID): A literature review and directions for future research. *Curr Opin Rheumatol* 2002;14(2):109-114.

37. de Vet HC, Ostelo RW, Terwee CB, et al: Minimally important change determined by a visual method integrating an anchor-based and a distribution-based approach. *Qual Life Res* 2007;16(1):131-142.

38. Ware JE Jr: SF-36 health survey update. *Spine (Phila Pa 1976)* 2000;25(24):3130-3139.

39. Ware JE Jr, Gandek B: Overview of the SF-36 Health Survey and the International Quality of Life Assessment (IQOLA) Project. *J Clin Epidemiol* 1998;51(11):903-912.

40. Ware JE Jr, Gandek B, Kosinski M, et al: The equivalence of SF-36 summary health scores estimated using standard and country-specific algorithms in 10 countries: Results from the IQOLA Project. International Quality of Life Assessment. *J Clin Epidemiol* 1998;51(11):1167-1170.

41. Ware JE Jr, Keller SD, Hatoum HT, Kong SX: The SF-36 Arthritis-Specific Health Index (ASHI): I. Development and cross-validation of scoring algorithms. *Med Care* 1999;37(5 suppl):MS40-MS50.

42. Ware JE, Kosinski M: Interpreting SF-36 summary health measures: A response. *Qual Life Res* 2001;10(5):405-413, discussion 415-420.

43. Ware JE Jr, Kosinski M, Bayliss MS, McHorney CA, Rogers WH, Raczek A: Comparison of methods for the scoring and statistical analysis of SF-36 health profile and summary measures: Summary of results from the Medical Outcomes Study. *Med Care* 1995;33(4 suppl):AS264-AS279.

44. Ware JE Jr, Kosinski M, Gandek B, et al: The factor structure of the SF-36 Health Survey in 10 countries: Results from the IQOLA Project. International Quality of Life Assessment. *J Clin Epidemiol* 1998;51(11):1159-1165.

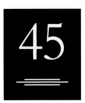

Why Measure Outcomes?

John E. Kuhn, MD

Abstract

The concept of measuring the outcomes of treatment in health care was promoted by Ernest Amory Codman in the early 1900s, but, until recently, his ideas were generally ignored. The forces that have advanced outcome measurement to the forefront of health care include the shift in payers for health care from the patient to large insurance companies or government agencies, the movement toward assessing the care of populations not individuals, and the effort to find value (or cost-effective treatments) amid rising healthcare costs. No ideal method exists to measure outcomes, and the information gathered depends on the reason the outcome information is required. Outcome measures used in research are best able to answer research questions. The methods for assessing physician and hospital performance include process measures, patient-experience measures, structure measures, and measures used to assess the outcomes of treatment. The methods used to assess performance should be validated, be reliable, and reflect a patient's perception of the treatment results. The healthcare industry must measure outcomes to identify which treatments are most effective and provide the most benefit to patients.

Instr Course Lect 2016;65:583–586.

History of Outcomes Assessment

Ernest Amory Codman is largely credited with the development of outcomes research because he was an early proponent of following patient outcomes after treatment. In 1900, he became interested in what he called the "end result idea," which he described as "the common-sense notion that every hospital should follow every patient it treats, long enough to determine whether or not the treatment has been successful, and then to inquire 'if not, why not'?"[1] Although this idea seems reasonable currently, Codman faced a great deal of resistance from the medical community, which was detrimental to his professional career. The notion of following patient outcomes remained dormant until it was resurrected in the latter part of the 20th century as a result of political and economic forces.

Changes in the 20th Century

The relationship between a physician and a patient has traditionally been close and personal without external influences. A physician would provide a service to an individual patient, and the patient would pay the physician for that service. This relationship changed in the 20th century as patients began to organize into payment groups (insurance or government) and as payment for services was routed through these groups or third-party payers. These payers manage a large number of patients and, like any other business, attempt to minimize costs. One way for payers to minimize costs is by demanding cost-effective treatments from physicians.

Simultaneously, political influences in the latter part of the 20th century led to population-based health care. Examples of population-based health care include the vaccination of populations and oversight into the research of populations, both of which are in the interests of patient protection and the use of limited funding. The change to

Dr. Kuhn or an immediate family member serves as a board member, owner, officer, or committee member of the American Orthopaedic Society for Sports Medicine and the American Shoulder and Elbow Surgeons.

population-based health care is reflected in the literature with the publication of fewer case studies and more hypothesis-driven, large-scale population studies. The move toward population-based health care requires outcome measurement, something Codman could not persuade hospitals or physicians to do in the early part of the 20th century.

The Importance of Perspective in Measuring Outcomes

The general understanding of outcomes has dramatically changed in the past few decades. Early attempts to develop scales to measure outcomes were physician derived, meaning that a physician scaled an outcome based on what he or she believed was important. Methods to quantify outcomes after treatment (eg, measuring knee laxity with a KT-1000 arthrometer after anterior cruciate ligament surgery or measuring shoulder range of motion) were developed and believed to be critically important for outcome measurement.[2] Physician-oriented outcome measures, however, can be very different from patient-oriented outcome measures. In the 1990s, orthopaedic medicine transitioned toward patient-oriented outcome measures, in which scales for measuring outcomes were developed with patient input and began to include features such as pain, function, and satisfaction.[3]

Recently, costs for treating patients have risen rapidly, and payers are rightly interested in the value of the care that is being provided. With respect to health care, the value of a service is defined as the outcome relative to its cost. Methods for comparing different types of healthcare interventions have evolved. The quality-adjusted life-year measures how a treatment improves not only the

lifespan of a patient but also the quality of a patient's life. This measure is often used to determine how healthcare dollars should be spent if rationing is required. Fortunately, most orthopaedic treatments substantially improve a patient's quality of life and, therefore, score well with this measure.[4]

Measuring Outcomes for Research

It is relatively easy to determine which outcome measures to use in conducting research. Research is driven by a question from which a testable hypothesis is derived; therefore, the best outcome measure available to answer the research question should be chosen. For example, a researcher who is testing a new technique to improve the healing of rotator cuff tears should choose an outcome measure that is able to assess healing (eg, MRI); patient-reported scores would not be the best outcome measure in this circumstance. Conversely, a researcher who is comparing surgery with physical therapy for the treatment of rotator cuff tears should choose a validated, patient-oriented, disease-specific outcome measure (eg, the Western Ontario Rotator Cuff Index).[5]

Measuring Outcomes to Assess Performance

Historically, physicians have been paid under a fee-for-service model in which there is no accounting for outcomes, experience, or cost. This model of payment is unusual in a service-oriented marketplace in which reimbursement is generally predicated on a successful outcome. In a 2013 report, the National Commission on Physician Payment Reform recognized that the fee-for-service payment system provides incentives to

physicians who perform more procedures and more (possibly unnecessary) care and stated that "our nation cannot control runaway medical spending without fundamentally changing how physicians are paid."[6] Consequently, the commission recommended that physician payment should be based on the value of the services provided (ie, the best possible outcomes for the least possible cost).

In 2000, the Institute of Medicine reported that 44,000 to 98,000 preventable deaths occur each year as a result of healthcare errors and recommended that incentives be given to providers as a reward for and to encourage quality care.[7] In 2001, the Institute of Medicine recommended increased payment for providers of quality care.[8] In 2006, the Institute of Medicine recommended a national system for performance measurement and urged purchasers and insurers to redesign payment models toward this goal.[9] The Medicare Payment Advisory Commission recommends paying providers at different rates based on the quality of care they provide.[10]

The era of value-based health care has arrived. Physicians must continue to be good stewards of the physician-patient relationship while addressing the challenges of measuring performance and quality of care. Medicine is not like other service industries because a deep, personal relationship is formed between physicians and patients as they delve into very personal decisions about life and health. Because the physician-patient relationship is so personal, standard methods for measuring the quality of a service (eg, a survey evaluating the service a waiter provided) may not be adequate. Therefore, multiple methods that provide different perspectives are required to measure the performance and quality of physician care. The four methods currently used to measure performance are process measures, patient-experience measures, structure measures, and outcome measures.

Process Measures

Process measures assess the effectiveness of activities that contribute to better health outcomes for patients (eg, counseling a patient to cease tobacco consumption). Process measures are relatively easy to implement, and most hospitals are already using them to measure the effectiveness of hand washing and perioperative antibiotics. Although process measures are important, they do not necessarily reflect quality in the field of orthopaedics.[11]

Patient-Experience Measures

Payers also are interested in collecting data on patients' perceptions of the quality of care they received and patients' satisfaction with their experience. Examples of patient-experience measures include questions such as the following: "What was the patient's perceived quality of communication with doctors and nurses?", "Was it easy to make an appointment?", and "Were the rooms clean and quiet?"

Structure Measures

Structure measures are used to assess the features and the capabilities of facilities, personnel, and equipment. These system-based measures are often mandated, such as with electronic medical records, which are used to not only store patients' health records but also ultimately collect performance data.

Outcome Measures

Outcome measures are designed to assess the effectiveness of a physician's

treatment on a patient. Outcome measures can be controversial because outcomes may be affected by social and clinical factors unrelated to the treatment, many of which are beyond a physician's control. When measuring outcomes, it is important to include a clear definition of the disease state. The International Classification of Diseases, Ninth Revision, had substantial problems in clearly defining disease states. As a result, the International Classification of Diseases, Tenth Revision, was far more complex and detailed than the previous edition. It also is important to determine how long and how often data should be collected for a given disease state or cycle of care. Some disorders are cured (eg, a fracture), and there is a discrete timeframe in which outcomes can be collected. Other disorders are managed (eg, diabetes mellitus), and it may be important to collect data during a patient's entire lifespan. Finally, it is important to define the tools best able to measure outcomes; they should represent a patient's needs and be valid, responsive, and reliable.

Summary

It has been nearly 100 years since Codman presented his end-result idea. Although Codman's idea was correct, contemporary concerns about malpractice exposure and pride prevented its acceptance by physicians. The globalization of medicine has led to financial and political forces that are now advancing Codman's ideas. The healthcare industry should measure the outcomes of treatments to determine their efficacy, and patients should have access to that information so that they can make decisions about their care. The difficult question of how this can be accomplished has yet to be answered.

References

1. Codman EA: *The Shoulder.* Malabar, FL, Robert E. Krieger Publishing Company, 1934.

2. Zarins B: Are validated questionnaires valid? *J Bone Joint Surg Am* 2005;87(8):1671-1672.

3. Kirkley A, Griffin S: Development of disease-specific quality of life measurement tools. *Arthroscopy* 2003;19(10):1121-1128.

4. Dougherty CP, Howard T: Cost-effectiveness in orthopedics: Providing essential information to both physicians and health care policy makers for appropriate allocation of medical resources. *Sports Med Arthrosc* 2013;21(3):166-168.

5. Kirkley A, Alvarez C, Griffin S: The development and evaluation of a disease-specific quality-of-life questionnaire for disorders of the rotator cuff: The Western Ontario Rotator Cuff Index. *Clin J Sport Med* 2003;13(2):84-92.

6. The National Commission on Physician Payment Reform: Report of the National Commission on Physician Payment Reform. March 2013. Available at: http://physicianpaymentcommission.org/wp-content/uploads/2013/03/physician_payment_report.pdf. Accessed August 17, 2015.

7. Kohn LT, Corrigan JM, Donaldson MS, Committee on Quality Health Care in America, the Institute of Medicine: To Err is Human: Building a Safer Health Care System. Washington, DC, the National Academies Press, 2000. Available at: http://www.nap.edu/catalog.php?record_id=9728. Accessed August 17, 2015.

8. Committee on Quality of Health Care in America, Institute of Medicine: Crossing the Quality Chasm: A New Health System for the 21st Century. Washington, DC, the National Academies Press, 2001. Available at: http://www.nap.edu/catalog.php?record_id=10027. Accessed August 17, 2015.

9. Committee on Redesigning Health Insurance Performance Measures, Payment, and Performance Improvement Programs, Board on Health Care Services, Institute of Medicine

of the National Academies: Performance Measurement: Accelerating Improvement (Pathways to Quality Health Care Series). Washington, DC, the National Academies Press, 2006. Available at: http://www.nap.edu/catalog.php?record_id=11517. Accessed August 17, 2015.

10. Medicare Payment Advisory Commission (MedPAC): Chapter 7: Using incentives to improve the quality of care in Medicare, in Report to the Congress: Variation and Innovation in Medicare. Washington, DC, Medicare Payment Advisory Commission (MedPAC), June 2003. Available at: http://www.medpac.gov/documents/ reports/June03_Entire_Report.pdf?sfvrsn=0. Accessed August 17, 2015.

11. Bhattacharyya T, Freiberg AA, Mehta P, Katz JN, Ferris T: Measuring the report card: The validity of pay-for-performance metrics in orthopedic surgery. *Health Aff (Millwood)* 2009;28(2):526-532.

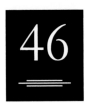

Recommendations for Evaluating and Selecting Appropriately Valued Outcome Measures

Richard J. Hawkins, MD

Abstract

The changing healthcare environment has essentially mandated that outcome scores play an increasing role in orthopaedic research and clinical care. Value is defined as the best outcome at the lowest cost. The reasoning behind the collection of outcome scores can be examined from several perspectives. The process of selecting an appropriate outcome measure involves analyzing its psychometrics in addition to other aspects, such as responsiveness, reliability, validity, and the ability to detect change in a reasonable manner. A minimal clinically important difference measures clinical change, and a minimal detectable change measures statistical change. Orthopaedic surgeons are most interested in minimal clinically important differences because they indicate meaningful clinical changes. Guidelines for selecting appropriately valued outcome measures include the consideration of patient-reported outcomes, proper psychometrics, validated scores, and cost effectiveness.

Instr Course Lect 2016;65:587–592.

Shoulder and elbow outcome scores are being brought to the forefront because of a recent charge from the American Shoulder and Elbow Surgeons (ASES) outcomes subcommittee to develop recommendations for the selection of appropriately valued shoulder and elbow outcome measures. The ASES Value-Based Shoulder Care Committee includes an outcomes subcommittee that was charged with the task of developing appropriately valued outcome measures that could be used universally. The ASES value committee also has subcommittees on cost and registries.

The outcomes subcommittee divided outcome measures into two programs: a basic package for most orthopaedic surgeons and a more robust package for those who conduct research.

The outcomes subcommittee also was tasked with addressing value, which was defined as the best outcome at the lowest cost. Cost remains the primary healthcare driver and probably will continue to be in the foreseeable future. Harvard economists Michael Porter[1] and Robert Kaplan, among others, suggest that in the future, surgical success will be defined by quality measures; the ASES subcommittee determined these quality measures to be patient-reported outcomes (PROs). This paradigm shift may make the fee-for-service model obsolete.

The question of why it is necessary to collect outcome scores has many answers. In the future, physicians may be judged on their quality of care. Outcome scores can help improve patient treatments. Payers and agencies may demand outcome scores. If physicians do not collect outcome scores, others may do so for them. The measures by which physicians are now graded do not truly measure patient outcomes. By defining and shaping outcome measures, physicians can ensure true and appropriately valued outcomes that are central to patient care.

Dr. Hawkins or an immediate family member has received royalties from Össur; serves as a paid consultant to DJ Orthopaedics; and serves as a board member, owner, officer, or committee member of the American Shoulder and Elbow Surgeons.

Table 1

Guidelines for Outcomes Measure Selection

Patient-reported outcomes

Appropriate psychometrics

Validated scores

Ease of use for the patient (ie, simple versus brief [basic package])

Ease of scoring and comprehension for physician

Standardized use nationally and/or internationally

Cost considerations

ASES Outcomes Subcommittee Review Process

The ASES outcomes subcommittee reviewed several papers, reports, and publications that focused on assessing the psychometrics of shoulder and elbow scoring systems. The subcommittee evaluated the responsiveness, reliability, and validity of the scoring systems plus their ability to detect minimal clinically important differences (MCIDs). A minimal detectable change (MDC) measures statistical change, which is less clinically relevant; however, it is important to understand MDCs because if they are accepted as the only outcome measure, they could be misleading.

Currently, physicians are graded by many agencies in what can be described as a pay-for-performance model. For example, in the Greenville Health System Orthopaedic Department, the Hospital Consumer Assessment of Healthcare Providers and Systems survey and the Clinician and Group Consumer Assessment of Healthcare Providers and Systems survey are used to reveal consumers' perception of hospital and doctor's office care. In addition, nonscientific and anonymous grading websites, such as healthgrades.

com, RateMDs.com, and yelp.com, are used to grade hospitals, doctors, and their treatment of patients.

In the hospital setting, external measurement systems include the Surgical Care Improvement Project measures. These measures are important because of the financial implications—essentially a 2% at-risk cost in terms of dollars—that are tied to them as mandated by the Centers for Medicare and Medicaid Services (CMS). The CMS also implemented the Patient Quality Reporting System, which carries financial implications related to Medicare Part B. The FORCE-Total Joint Registry provides a financial bonus from the CMS for physicians who submit data to the registry.

To establish acceptable shoulder and elbow outcome measures, the outcomes subcommittee reviewed multiple papers, reports, and publications.[2,3] A study by Kocher et al[4] reported on how the ASES Subjective Shoulder Scale was validated. A study by Angst et al[5] discussed the psychometrics of multiple shoulder and elbow scoring systems. In addition, a study by Schmidt et al[6] examined the usefulness of PROs. The subcommittee also reviewed a study by van Kampen et al.[7] Based on a review of these studies, the subcommittee established the guidelines listed in **Table 1** for outcome measure selection. The discussion included many aspects, but to arrive at the best scores based on the guidelines for selection, the outcome measures were divided into generic quality of life (QOL) scores, joint- or region-specific scores, and disease-specific scores. The subcommittee agreed that there should be a basic package that would be applicable to most orthopaedic surgeons and a more robust package for researchers at

a university center or for investigators who wish to more closely follow a specific problem (such as rotator cuff tears).

Generic QOL Scores

Generic QOL scores have been used for many years. The rationale for their use is that they allow for comparisons across different diseases (eg, knee arthritis and arthroplasty compared with cancer treatment). The subcommittee analyzed and weighed the various aspects of several QOL scoring systems, such as the Medical Outcomes Study 36-Item Short Form, the Medical Outcomes Study 12-Item Short Form (SF-12), the Medical Outcomes Study 6-Item Short Form, the European Quality of Life-5 Dimensions Questionnaire, the Veterans RAND 36-Item Health Survey, and the Veterans RAND 12-Item Health Survey (VR-12). These scoring systems encompass the domains of physical, mental, and social well-being.

The European Quality of Life-5 Dimensions Questionnaire is extensively used in Europe and consists of five simple questions, each of which can receive a score of 0, 1, or 2; however, because it was currently undergoing revision and the 0, 1, or 2 scoring was difficult to interpret, the subcommittee eliminated this scoring system from the study. Ideally, scoring systems with scores based on a 100-point scale, with 100 being the best, are the simplest to interpret. The Medical Outcomes Study 36-Item Short Form, the standard quality outcome measure used throughout the world, has 36 questions and is a comparatively long questionnaire for patients and doctors. The SF-12 is briefer, standardized, and well accepted, particularly in North America. Unfortunately, all of the short form scores are available only commercially.

The available public domain scoring systems are the Veterans RAND 36-Item Health Survey and the VR-12, both of which were developed by the RAND Corporation. The VR-12 is similar to the SF-12 but with slight wording differences. It involves 14 questions, is scored on a 100-point scale, and is a Likert-type questionnaire (divides the questions into categories of "unable to do," "can do with difficulty," "perform normally," etc.). The advantages of the VR-12 are its appropriate psychometrics, validated status, and availability in the public domain at no cost, which made it very attractive because it achieved the same goals as the SF-12. Therefore, the VR-12 was selected as the generic QOL scoring system for the shoulder and elbow.

Joint-Specific Scores

Next, the outcomes subcommittee analyzed joint-specific scoring systems. Multiple joint-specific scoring systems exist for the shoulder, including the University of California–Los Angeles Shoulder Rating Scale, the Hospital for Special Surgery Shoulder Score, and the Constant assessment score. After applying the selection criteria and analyzing each system's psychometrics, the subcommittee narrowed down the joint-specific scoring systems to the ASES Subjective Shoulder Scale and the Oxford Shoulder Score (OSS); there was almost no disagreement in selecting these systems. The OSS consists of 12 questions with a total score of 60 (higher is better). It has great psychometrics and is extensively used in Europe, often supplementing the commonly used Constant assessment score.

The ASES Subjective Shoulder Scale is used more extensively in North America and is a validated scoring system with excellent psychometrics. It consists of 10 questions, with 50 points for function and 50 points for pain (higher is better). However, it has only one question for evaluating pain: "What is your pain today?" The outcomes subcommittee was concerned that this pain measure may not represent the pain aspect many orthopaedic patients experience (such as night pain or worse pain). This pain measure, with the failure of conservative care, often drives patients and surgeons to consider surgical treatment. Therefore, the committee added a visual analog scale (VAS) for pain ranging from 1 to 100 with the question, "What is your pain at its worst?" A score of 1 to 10 could then be converted to a percentage.

After applying the selection criteria and analyzing the psychometrics, the subcommittee recommended that the ASES Subjective Shoulder Scale should be the primary joint-specific shoulder outcome measure in North America. The OSS was deemed an acceptable joint-specific shoulder outcome measure for those in Europe.

Region-Specific Scores

The outcomes subcommittee also discussed region-specific scoring systems, such as the Disabilities of the Arm, Shoulder and Hand (DASH) questionnaire and the QuickDASH questionnaire, but thought that these systems did not lend themselves well to the shoulder. Because the DASH and the QuickDASH questionnaires are generic scoring systems that are used to measure general upper extremity disability, they were thought to be more applicable to the entire upper limb, not primarily the shoulder or elbow.

The outcomes subcommittee also reviewed the Single Assessment Numeric Evaluation (SANE) method, which asks the following question: "What percentage of normal is your shoulder or elbow?" Because the SANE method is simple, is brief, and closely correlates with the ASES Subjective Shoulder Scale and the International Knee Documentation Committee Subjective Knee Evaluation Form, it was selected as another joint-specific outcome measure.

The Global Rating of Change (GROC) scale also was discussed. This is a seven-point scale (0 to 7) that asks the following questions: "Are you better, worse, or the same? If better (hopefully), how much better?" The original GROC scale had several descriptive phrases, such as "very, very good," "very good," and "good." To make the GROC scale simpler for both patients and doctors, the outcomes subcommittee converted the seven-point scale to a 100-point scale based on percentages and included the following question: "Are you 25%, 50%, 75%, 90%, or 100% better?" The GROC scale may be an effective scoring system, but it has not been validated, and its psychometrics have not been analyzed. Therefore, the subcommittee chose the SANE method because it has the ability to reflect changes in patient condition.

After a final analysis, the outcomes subcommittee recommended the following outcome measures to the ASES for a basic outcomes package: the VR-12 for the generic QOL score; the ASES Subjective Shoulder Scale for the joint-specific score; the SANE method; and the VAS for pain, with "What is your pain at its worst?" as a separate question.

Disease-Specific Scores

For researchers or individuals who wish to more closely analyze a specific problem, the basic outcomes package can be supplemented with disease-specific scoring systems, such as the Western Ontario Rotator Cuff Index, the Western Ontario Shoulder Instability Index, and the Western Ontario Osteoarthritis of the Shoulder Index. Each of these disease-specific scoring systems consist of approximately 20 questions, are very robust with great psychometrics, and are especially helpful for researchers and individuals who wish to critically analyze a problem. Developed at the University of Western Ontario under the leadership of the late Dr. Sandy Kirkley, these scoring systems have a 100-point scale, with higher scores indicating a worse condition. The scoring systems were established by asking patients questions about their concerns regarding their condition; this resulted in a large number of questions, which were tested and retested through a process known as item selection/generation and item reduction. This was done to reduce the number of questions to a manageable amount, approximately 20.

Another supplemental scoring system that impressed the outcomes subcommittee was the PENN Shoulder Score. The PENN Shoulder Score is a joint-specific scoring system for the shoulder that consists of 20 functional questions for 60 points, 4 pain questions for 30 points, and 1 satisfaction question for 10 points. This system most likely has the best psychometrics of all the joint-specific shoulder scoring systems, but the subcommittee did not include the PENN Shoulder Score in the basic outcomes package because it is long; it was suggested for incorporation in the more robust outcomes package.

After a final analysis, the outcomes subcommittee recommended the following outcome measures to the ASES for a more robust outcomes package: the basic outcomes package; and, depending on diagnosis, the Western Ontario Rotator Cuff Index, the Western Ontario Instability Index, or the Western Ontario Osteoarthritis of the Shoulder Index as the disease-specific scoring systems and the PENN Shoulder Score.

Elbow and Other Subspecialty Scores

In using the same process for the elbow, the outcomes subcommittee suggested that the basic outcomes package for the elbow should include the VR-12 for the generic QOL score; the Mayo Elbow Performance Score (MEPS) for the joint-specific score; and the SANE method, with "What percentage of normal is your elbow?" as a separate question.

After much debate, the outcomes subcommittee determined that the MEPS is the standard in North America (and perhaps worldwide), and it has undergone validation.[8] Based on the selection criteria guidelines, the only questionable shortcoming of the MEPS was physician involvement. Individuals who have experience with the MEPS suggest that it can be performed without physician involvement (ie, a PRO), which is how the MEPS validation study was conducted. There are 100 total points: 45 points for pain, 20 points for range of motion, 10 points for stability, and 25 points for function; the highest score is the best. The subcommittee did not include a separate VAS pain question for the elbow. The elbow does not have disease-specific scoring systems to incorporate into a more robust outcomes package.

Having completed this process for both the shoulder and the elbow, the outcomes subcommittee believes that appropriately valued outcome measures for other joints could be developed using a similar methodology. The Greenville Health System Orthopaedic Department has established outcome measures for other joints; however, the subcommittee recommends using a formal selection process to choose the outcome measures most appropriate to each subspecialty area.

In addition to the shoulder and elbow outcomes scores recommended by the ASES outcomes subcommittee, the Steadman Hawkins Clinic of the Carolinas, along with the Greenville Health System, has established outcomes measures for other joints. The following sports knee outcome measures have been established for patients younger than 50 years: the VR-12 for the generic QOL score; the International Knee Documentation Committee Subjective Knee Evaluation Form for the joint-specific score; the Tegner activity score; the SANE method, with "What percentage of normal is your knee?" as a separate question; and the Marx Activity Rating Scale. The only disease-specific scoring system for the sports knee is the Western Ontario Meniscal Evaluation Tool, which deals with meniscal pathology. The following sports knee outcome measures have been established for patients older than 50 years: the VR-12 for the generic QOL score, the SANE method, the Western Ontario and McMaster Universities Osteoarthritis Index, and the Knee Society Score. The Steadman Hawkins Clinic of the Carolinas and the Greenville Health System are currently establishing outcome measures for the foot and ankle, the hip, the hand,

and the spine that will follow a format similar to that established by the ASES outcomes subcommittee.

The outcomes subcommittee was not involved with implementation, methods of collection, retrieval, or studies for applying these scores to patient treatment. However, implementation may include paper, scanning, computer-based or web-based platforms, and software programs, such as the Standardized Orthopaedic Clinical Research and Treatment Evaluation Software Orthopaedic Outcomes Platform (Ortholink Pty), the Outcomes Based Electronic Research Database (Oberd-Universal Research Solutions), the Research Electronic Data Capture (Vanderbilt University), and the Surgical Outcome System (Arthrex). It is important that clinicians choose a software program based on the needs of their practices and cost of the software. After outcome scores are collected, a repository for storage will be required. One of the main challenges is deciding which software program is the best option to collect, store, and retrieve these outcome scores.

The Patient-Reported Outcomes Measurement Information System

It is important to mention that in the future, the Patient-Reported Outcomes Measurement Information System (PROMIS), which is funded by the National Institutes of Health, may become applicable to orthopaedics. To obtain a QOL score, the system uses the PROMIS Global Health 10-Item Short Form, in which each item is rated on a scale from 1 to 10. PROMIS has not yet been extremely applicable for orthopaedics because the system must identify the appropriate questions for shoulder, knee, elbow, or hip problems. PROMIS has computerized adaptive testing that can narrow down the questions, but its application for orthopaedics is probably still a few years in the future. Nevertheless, it is critical that the American Academy of Orthopaedic Surgeons and orthopaedic subspecialty societies track PROMIS' evolving process.

Summary

The ASES evaluation and selection process that was used to identify appropriately valued outcome measures for shoulder and elbow surgery stresses the importance and benefits of outcome scores for the entire field of orthopaedics. By taking an active role in the selection and implementation of these outcome measures and by engaging key stakeholders throughout the process, it is hoped that appropriate patient-centered measures will be able to accurately reflect patient outcomes and will be used in the future of healthcare policy.

References

1. Porter ME: What is value in health care? *N Engl J Med* 2010;363(26):2477-2481.

2. Richards RR, An KN, Bigliani LU, et al: A standardized method for the assessment of shoulder function. *J Shoulder Elbow Surg* 1994;3(6):347-352.

3. Wright RW, Baumgarten KM: Shoulder outcomes measures. *J Am Acad Orthop Surg* 2010;18(7):436-444.

4. Kocher MS, Horan MP, Briggs KK, Richardson TR, O'Holleran J, Hawkins RJ: Reliability, validity, and responsiveness of the American Shoulder and Elbow Surgeons subjective shoulder scale in patients with shoulder instability, rotator cuff disease, and glenohumeral arthritis. *J Bone Joint Surg Am* 2005;87(9):2006-2011.

5. Angst F, Schwyzer H, Aeschlimann A, Simmen B, Goldhahn J: Measures of adult shoulder function: Disabilities of the Arm, Shoulder, and Hand Questionnaire (DASH) and its short version (QuickDASH), Shoulder Pain and Disability Index (SPADI), American Shoulder and Elbow Surgeons (ASES) Society standardized shoulder assessment form, Constant (Murley) Score (CS), Simple Shoulder Test (SST), Oxford Shoulder Score (OSS), Shoulder Disability Questionnaire (SDQ), and Western Ontario Shoulder Instability Index (WOSI). *Arthritis Care Res (Hoboken)* 2011; 63(11 suppl):S174-S188.

6. Schmidt S, Ferrer M, González M, et al: Evaluation of shoulder-specific patient-reported outcome measures: A systematic and standardized comparison of available evidence. *J Shoulder Elbow Surg* 2014;23(3):434-444.

7. van Kampen DA, Willems WJ, van Beers LW, Castelein RM, Scholtes VA, Terwee CB: Determination and comparison of the smallest detectable change (SDC) and the minimal important change (MIC) of four-shoulder patient-reported outcome measures (PROMs). *J Orthop Surg Res* 2013;8(40).

8. Cusick MC, Bonnaig NS, Azar FM, Mauck BM, Smith RA, Throckmorton TW: Accuracy and reliability of the Mayo Elbow Performance Score. *J Hand Surg Am* 2014;39(6):1146-1150.

Implementation of a Comprehensive Orthopaedic Registry System

John M. Tokish, MD

Thomas C. Alexander Jr, MD

Abstract

Advances in information technology have allowed for improvements in the collection and analysis of large-scale outcomes data. These data can be used in the practice of orthopaedics for benchmarking, value analysis, and comparative effectiveness research. The implementation of registries within a busy surgical practice can be challenging, costly, and inefficient. Content, platform, and characteristics are the key elements required to successfully implement a patient-based orthopaedic outcomes data registry. Specific barriers to implementing registries are discussed, and solutions are proposed, to provide an example for optimal integration within clinical practices that may have varying goals.

Instr Course Lect 2016;65:593–600.

The systematic collection of pertinent outcomes into a comprehensive registry is a powerful tool that can be used to benchmark standards of care, compare regional variation, enable comparative effectiveness research, and, ultimately, improve patient-centered care. Information technology (IT) has been the catalyst for enabling registry creation because it allows large-scale data to be stored, extracted, and analyzed with relative ease. The features of an ideal orthopaedic registry (**Table 1**) would combine patient-reported outcomes (PROs); pertinent objective data from a patient's history, physical examination, and imaging assessments; and treatment details and cost. The ideal platform would be web- or cloud-based, Heath Insurance Portability and Accountability Act-compliant, and allow patients to directly enter pertinent demographic and outcomes-related information. Additional key features would include the ability to export data to statistical software for analysis and the ability to export data into a standardized data dictionary to allow for the combination of data from various sources.

Outcomes measurement in medicine is not a new idea. Almost a century ago, Codman pioneered the concept of the "end result idea" as an early approach to outcome studies. He stressed the importance of critical evaluation and honest reporting of both positive and negative results after surgery. His ideas were met with resentment and criticism during his lifetime, and only recently have his contributions to the "end result idea" and the modern outcomes movement gained the respect they deserve.[1]

The Challenges of Outcomes Implementation

PROs, although not currently in the form of registry systems, have already infiltrated medicine in the United States. Payers and patients are increasingly demanding patient outcomes for healthcare decisions regarding reimbursement and physician choice. Government health agencies and payers collect standardized patient outcomes

Dr. Tokish or an immediate family member serves as a paid consultant to Arthrex, DePuy, and Mitek, and serves as a board member, owner, officer, or committee member of the Arthroscopy Association of North America. Neither Dr. Alexander nor any immediate family member has received anything of value from or has stock or stock options held in a commercial company or institution related directly or indirectly to the subject of this chapter.

Table 1

Features of an Ideal Orthopaedic Registry

Content	Platform	Characteristics
PROs	**Demographics/PROs**	Standardized "data-dictionary" ensures data from multiple sources are mapped consistently in database
Generalized health score (VR-12, SANE)	Patient self-enrolled, self-entered	
Anatomic-specific PROs (ASES score, MEPI, etc.)	Data entry via e-mail or "kiosk" portal	
Disease-specific PROs (eg, WOSI Index for shoulder instability)		
Critical objective findings	**Objective data linked to EMR**	Maximize discrete data fields, minimize free text
Origin of chief complaint (eg, traumatic versus atraumatic)	Allows autopopulation of data from chart	
Range of motion/strength of affected joint	Critical objective findings	
	Imaging data	
	Insurance data	
	Surgical detail capture	
Imaging findings	**Automatic follow up**	Data exportable to standard statistical software packages
Radiography	Enrolled patients automatically contacted via e-mail at predetermined time periods	
MRI		
CT	Outcomes staff notified of noncompliance to allow direct patient contact for follow-up	
Ultrasonography		
Treatment details		Modifiable centrally to allow change as new outcomes measures become available
Rehabilitation prescription		
Surgical details of procedures performed, pathology encountered, etc.		
Cost of care		
Return to work		
Return to activity		

ASES = American Shoulder and Elbow Surgeons, EMR = electronic medical record, MEPI = Mayo Elbow Performance Index, PRO = patient-reported outcome, SANE = single assessment numeric evaluation, VR-12 = Veterans RAND 12-Item Health Survey, WOSI = Western Ontario Shoulder Instability.

through the Hospital Consumer Assessment of Healthcare Providers and Systems survey and the Clinician and Group Consumer Assessment of Healthcare Providers and Systems survey. The Internet is replete with multiple web-based physician rating systems that allow unregulated and nonvalidated patient-reported outcomes and opinions of physician services. Unfortunately, such systems of "quality" assessment may say more about the quality of a patient's experience rather than the proper diagnosis and treatment of his or her condition. Orthopaedic surgeons, and physicians in general, have the opportunity and responsibility to ensure that what is defined as "quality

outcomes" represents patient-reported measures that are valid and valuable to patients, providers, and payers.

The collection of meaningful outcomes has traditionally been a labor-intensive and costly endeavor for orthopaedic physicians and practices. Many individuals perceive that the IT revolution and the development of electronic medical records (EMRs) have made the collection and storage of outcomes measures into medical records automatic. Unfortunately, the interface between data collection, storage, and analysis and the logistics of accurate data input by clinicians have failed to live up to expectations of many individuals on both sides of an emerging clinician/IT

schism.[2] There are numerous barriers to the implementation of health IT, in addition to outcomes measurement, into a medical practice, including high initial physician financial and time costs, challenges with technology adaptability and support, data exchange, and physician cultural expectations.[3-5] Studies on the financial implications of EMRs report start-up costs ranging from $16,000 to $36,000 per physician and additional maintenance costs estimated between $8,000 and $17,000 per year.[3-5] The implementation of EMRs causes temporary loss of office productivity secondary to the interruption of normal office workflow. Another barrier to the successful adoption of EMRs is that the level of required physician computer skills[6] and the importance of adequate IT support is often underestimated.[7] As many as two-thirds of physicians polled in studies have identified these user-satisfaction factors as barriers to the implementation of EMRs.[6,7] Although the implementation of EMRs into medical practices is difficult, the integration of outcomes data into an electronic platform that is compatible with EMRs creates further complications. Because of these difficulties, much outcomes research remains outside of the EMR system and is either collected manually or input into a separate system; this can require substantial resources and can be inefficient, therefore making the widespread acceptance of outcomes collection challenging.

The field of orthopaedic surgery has particular challenges in registry creation because meaningful orthopaedic outcomes may differ from outcomes routinely collected in a medical record. For example, a cardiovascular surgeon might designate survival rate, revision surgery, or ejection fraction as an outcome, all of which are routinely searchable in a medical record or Medicare database without any necessary input from a surgeon or staff. Meaningful outcomes in many aspects of orthopaedics, however, include questions about return to sport, functional activities, and patient questionnaires, all of which are outcomes not yet included in searchable EMR platforms. Orthopaedists have access to many validated PRO measures, ranging from generic quality-of-life scores, such as the Medical Outcomes Study 12-Item Short Form, to joint-specific scores, such as the American Shoulder and Elbow Surgeons score for the shoulder, to disease-specific scores, such as

Western Ontario Shoulder Instability index for shoulder instability, all of which are not included in searchable EMR platforms.[8]

Solutions in Outcomes Collection and the Creation of Registries

The implementation of a comprehensive orthopaedic outcomes registry can be discussed on three fronts: content, platform, and characteristics (**Table 1**). The first question to be considered is the purpose of the registry itself. Different platforms and depth may be required depending on the purpose of the registry. For example, physicians who wish to satisfy meaningful use or simple practice benchmarking may choose an abbreviated platform, unlike those who wish to perform comparative effectiveness research. The overall purpose of the data collection will determine the depth of each of the critical aspects of outcomes acquisition.

Content

The foundation for comprehensive data includes PROs, minimally essential objective data from the patient history and physical examination, pertinent findings on imaging examinations, and treatment details. There is no consensus in the United States as to which PROs should be collected. The American Shoulder and Elbow Surgeons has recently established a task force and has formulated a dual set of recommendations for the shoulder and elbow, depending on the goals of the physician, which have been adopted by the Arthroscopy Association of North America. This process can be expanded to all anatomic regions and could form the recommended PROs, as vetted by the subspecialty stakeholders involved.

Defining the critical objective data to be documented in a registry is more difficult because it is diagnostically specific. For example, if a patient receives a diagnosis of shoulder instability, any reasonable objective dataset should include the results of an apprehension test. If a patient receives a diagnosis of anterior cruciate ligament (ACL) injury, the objective dataset should include the results of a Lachman test. Furthermore, treatments that include surgical intervention are dependent on diagnosis, and, thus, should be organized in a registry as such. Fortunately, there is a minimum critical dataset that could satisfy most of the objective details for both standard and robust tracks of data captured for patient history, physical examination, imaging, surgical treatment, and postoperative protocol. An example of the objective data that should be captured for shoulder instability is listed in **Tables 2** and **3**.

Platform and Characteristics

The power of a registry comes from its ability to manage large sets of data. Therefore, it is not surprising that the rise in the importance of registries has corresponded with the development of IT. Electronic platforms that maximize discrete data fields (drop-down choices) are preferred more than free-text data because they can be searched, combined, and analyzed across populations. Given the time and resource costs previously discussed, the system should be as efficient as possible (**Figure 1**). The patient should be able to enter PROs and demographic information data directly into the system. This can be enabled by an e-mail-associated, web-based system, and, if patient e-mail addresses and diagnoses are not known, a kiosk-based system in which patients

Table 2
Discrete Fields for Objective Surgical Findings of Shoulder Instability

Field Name	Field Input
Exam under anesthesia	Symmetric/asymmetric to contralateral
	Stable/anterior instability/posterior instability/MDI
Glenoid bone loss	As percentage in 5% increments
Humeral bone loss	Measured as millimeters from medial edge of defect to cuff insertions
Labral pathology	Amount of clock face involved with labrum
Number of anchors	
Type of anchors	Metal/polyetheretherketone/biocomposite/biocompatible/all suture
Associated procedures	Drop-down box with CPT shoulder codes

CPT = Current Procedural Terminology, MDI = multidirectional shoulder instability.

Table 3
Discrete Fields for Objective Clinical Findings of Shoulder Instability

Field Name	Field Input
ROM (drop down box in 5° increments)	Forward flexion
	External rotation
	Internal rotation
Apprehension test	+/−
Inferior sulcus test	+/−
Posterior push-pull test	+/−
Jerk test	+/−
Load and shift test	Anterior: Normal/to glenoid rim/over glenoid rim
	Posterior: Normal/to glenoid rim/over glenoid rim
Radiographs	Glenoid bone loss: +/−
	Humeral bone loss: +/−
MRI	Labral pathology: none/superior/anterior/posterior/combined
	Bone loss glenoid: +/−
	Humeral bone loss: +/−
	Associated pathology: humeral avulsion of the glenohumeral ligament, anterior labral periosteal sleeve avulsion, rotator cuff tear, coracoid fracture, etc.

ROM = range of motion.

can self-register in the office at initial presentation can be used.

The registry platform should use a minimum critical dataset that can describe objective data in as many discrete fields as possible. Data that only the clinician can enter must be efficiently collected in a comprehensive

manner. The data collected by the clinician (eg, body mass index, pain levels) ideally should be linked to the EMR and automatically extracted into the registry.

Cost effectiveness is becoming increasingly important to all stakeholders in health care, and cost data are critically important to a comprehensive registry. Cost data are another element that can be linked to more modern EMRs, and the combination of these data with outcomes can provide the first truly comprehensive evaluation of value in health care.

After patients are enrolled in the system, follow-up e-mails should be automated. Predetermined time points can be established to generate follow-up e-mails with links to the registry to solicit patients to complete PRO questionnaires. For example, a patient undergoing treatment for shoulder instability may fill out PROs preoperatively, at 6 weeks, 3 months, 6 months, 1 year, and annually thereafter. The registry platform should have a schedule created to send the patient an e-mail to complete the follow-up questionnaires at the designated time points. Patients who do not complete the questionnaires should be flagged and the registry data custodian should be automatically alerted to contact these patients directly.

One of the most critical functions of an outcomes registry is its ability to organize, export, and analyze the data it contains. Although this is not difficult from an IT standpoint, it is critical for data to be stored in standardized formats that allow them to be imported into statistical software packages. Furthermore, it is critical that a standardized data dictionary be used for large datasets that are being entered by multiple sources. The data dictionary is the

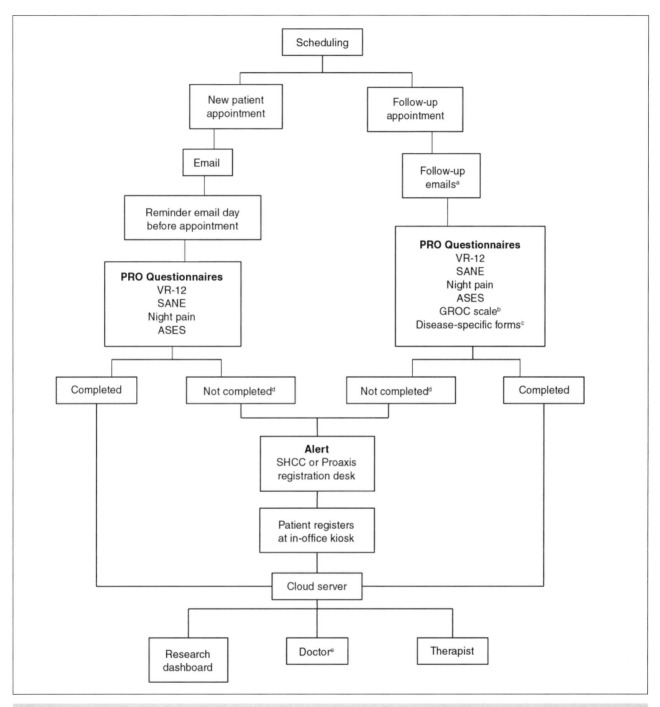

Figure 1 Algorithm demonstrates an example of process flow for efficient registry implementation. ASES = American Shoulder and Elbow Surgeons, GROC = Global Rating of Change, PRO = patient-reported outcome, Proaxis = Proaxis Therapy, SANE = single assessment numeric evaluation, SHCC = Steadman Hawkins Clinic of the Carolinas, VR-12 = Veterans RAND 12-Item Health Survey, WOOS = Western Ontario Osteoarthritis of the Shoulder, WORC = Western Ontario Rotator Cuff, WOSI = Western Ontario Shoulder Instability.
[a]3m (± 3wk), 6m (± 5wk), 12m (± 2m), 24m (± 3m).
[b]Every follow-up.
[c]For example, WOOS Index for shoulder arthritis, WOSI Index for shoulder instability, and WORC Index for rotator cuff disease.
[d]No response to e-mail and visit within defined collection.
[e]Determines disease-specific forms necessary for follow-up PRO questionnaires.

governing document that determines how the data are organized within the registry. For example, it is important that all patients entering their data for a pain score enter it into the same cell in the registry. This becomes critically important to keep the dataset consistent and valid if registries are combined.

Another critical aspect to the registry platform is adaptability. The data considered important may change over time. For example, the importance of bone loss to the outcomes of arthroscopic treatment has only been recognized for approximately 15 years. Undoubtedly, new discoveries will have an effect on outcomes measures as science advances; therefore, registries must be sufficiently adaptable and modifiable to keep up with these changes.

Current Examples and the Senior Author's Experience

Several national registries have substantially contributed to the field of orthopaedics over the past 20 years. For example, use of the Australian Orthopaedic Association National Joint Replacement Registry allowed for the recognition of early failure and complications associated with certain metal-on-metal hip prostheses.[9] National registries have acknowledged their limitations with respect to data from PROs. Most national registries either do not collect or collect only minimal PROs with short-term follow-up.[10] Recognizing this deficiency, governments have mandated that national joint registries point out the obstacles of agreeing on which outcomes to collect, selection bias, and incomplete and missing data.[11]

The Scandinavian ACL Registry may be the most progressive national registry with respect to collecting and incorporating PROs. Founded in 2004,

this registry combines the individual registries of Norway, Denmark, and Sweden, includes nearly 20,000 patients, and attempts to collect a Knee Injury and Osteoarthritis Outcome Score for every patient who has undergone ACL reconstruction. A recently published study comparing PROs in primary versus revision ACL reconstruction reported worse PROs in the revision setting with respect to quality of life, pain, and sports participation.[12] In addition to producing paradigm-shifting work, these registries also provide insight into the challenges of completeness and compliance with PROs that are integrated into a national registry system. Denmark's ACL registry, despite being government mandated by law, reported a 27% patient compliance rate initially and a 33% patient compliance rate at 1-year follow-up.[13]

The experience of the senior author (J.M.T) of this chapter has allowed for a critical evaluation of the strengths and challenges of implementing an orthopaedic registry. In January 2013, the Society of Military Orthopaedic Surgeons Quality Assurance Outcomes Registry was established at the Tripler Army Medical Center. More than 5,000 military members are currently enrolled in the registry, and the goal is to track patient outcomes and military readiness.[14] The process and success rate of obtaining initial PROs and the effectiveness of an electronic registry system was documented.[14] Surgical schedulers entered patient information into the Standardized Orthopaedic Clinical Research and Treatment Evaluation Software (SOCRATES) Orthopaedic Outcomes Platform (Ortholink Pty), including name, date of birth, date of surgery, diagnosis, planned surgical procedure, outcomes protocol, and e-mail

address. The SOCRATES Orthopaedic Outcomes Platform then automatically sent each patient a welcome e-mail with all assigned questionnaires. The automatic compliance rate, defined as patients who completed all of the initial questionnaires from the welcome e-mail without any further intervention by office staff, was 42%.[14] When arriving for the preoperative appointment, all patients were audited for completion. Patients who remained noncompliant were then re-invited to enter their data at the office kiosks. The additional compliance of this group increased the total compliance to 75%. The surgeon entered the objective, imaging, and surgical data in a discrete field system, requiring several additional minutes of time per surgery.

The senior author (J.M.T.) of this chapter studied the results of the study and analyzed variables that affected patient participation by modifying factors such as paper- versus electronic-based platforms and the length of PRO forms. Patient compliance improved from 59% to 67% with the use of an electronic-based platform. Patient compliance improved from 70% to 89% with the use of short PRO forms.[14] In addition, physician involvement improved compliance, as patients were more likely to complete the forms if the physician encouraged participation.

Summary

All registries, even if they are ideal, have strengths and weaknesses. Not all relevant data can be captured, and registries cannot replace prospective studies or randomized controlled trials. However, registries are an efficient way to track outcomes, benchmark results, and achieve population sizes that can answer many of the most meaningful questions in patient care. The future of orthopaedics and medicine points toward an increasing demand for PROs from patients, government, and payers. Orthopaedists have the opportunity to help guide this process by ensuring that valid and meaningful outcomes are collected.[1] Thoughtful implementation of patient-reported registry systems that are able to overcome substantial logistical challenges have the immense potential to advance standards of care through the analysis and identification of meaningful outcomes from large-scale data.

References

1. Mallon WJ: E. Amory Codman, surgeon of the 1990s. *J Shoulder Elbow Surg* 1998;7(5):529-536.

2. Saleh KJ, Novicoff W, Shaha JS, et al: Symposium. Why can't we all get along: Solving a growing gap in EMR satisfaction between clinicians and IT professionals. *AAOS 2015 Annual Meeting Proceedings*. Rosemont, IL, American Academy of Orthopaedic Surgeons, 2015.

3. Fleming NS, Culler SD, McCorkle R, Becker ER, Ballard DJ: The financial and nonfinancial costs of implementing electronic health records in primary care practices. *Health Aff (Millwood)* 2011;30(3):481-489.

4. Miller RH, West C, Brown TM, Sim I, Ganchoff C: The value of electronic health records in solo or small group practices. *Health Aff (Millwood)* 2005;24(5):1127-1137.

5. Wang SJ, Middleton B, Prosser LA, et al: A cost-benefit analysis of electronic medical records in primary care. *Am J Med* 2003;114(5):397-403.

6. Boonstra A, Broekhuis M: Barriers to the acceptance of electronic medical records by physicians from systematic review to taxonomy and interventions. *BMC Health Serv Res* 2010;10:231.

7. Loomis GA, Ries JS, Saywell RM Jr, Thakker NR: If electronic medical records are so great, why aren't family physicians using them? *J Fam Pract* 2002;51(7):636-641.

8. Wright RW, Baumgarten KM: Shoulder outcomes measures. *J Am Acad Orthop Surg* 2010;18(7):436-444.

9. de Steiger RN, Hang JR, Miller LN, Graves SE, Davidson DC: Five-year results of the ASR XL Acetabular System and the ASR Hip Resurfacing System: An analysis from the Australian Orthopaedic Association National Joint Replacement Registry. *J Bone Joint Surg Am* 2011;93(24):2287-2293.

10. Phillips JR, Hopwood B, Arthur C, Stroud R, Toms AD: The natural history of pain and neuropathic pain after knee replacement: A prospective cohort study of the point prevalence of pain and neuropathic pain to a minimum three-year follow-up. *Bone Joint J* 2014;96(9):1227-1233.

11. Franklin PD, Harrold L, Ayers DC: Incorporating patient-reported outcomes in total joint arthroplasty registries: Challenges and opportunities. *Clin Orthop Relat Res* 2013;471(11):3482-3488.

12. Lind M, Menhert F, Pedersen AB: Incidence and outcome after revision anterior cruciate ligament reconstruction: Results from the Danish registry for knee ligament reconstructions. *Am J Sports Med* 2012;40(7):1551-1557.

13. Rahr-Wagner L, Thillemann TM, Lind MC, Pedersen AB: Validation of 14,500 operated knees registered in the Danish Knee Ligament Reconstruction Register: Registration completeness and validity of key variables. *Clin Epidemiol* 2013;5:219-228.

14. Tokish J, Manansala J, Nguyen G, et al: Poster No. 283. Implementation of an electronic patient based orthopaedic outcomes system: How "automatic" can the system be? *AAOS 2014 Annual Meeting Proceedings*. Rosemont, IL, American Academy of Orthopaedic Surgeons, 2014.

Practical Quality Improvement Implementation in Orthopaedic Clinical Practice

David S. Jevsevar, MD, MBA

Kevin G. Shea, MD

Alexandra Styhl, BA

Karl Koenig, MD, MS

Abstract

The passage of the Medicare Access and Children's Health Insurance Program Reauthorization Act of 2015 (HR 2) helps ensure patient access to care and stable physician reimbursement for the near future. HR 2's underlying theme is the improvement of value to address the unsustainable rise in national healthcare spending. Quality improvement and performance improvement, which affect outcomes and costs as well as address variation, are the keys to improve the value of orthopaedic healthcare delivery. Orthopaedic surgeons should examine quality and performance strategies as well as several examples before they begin to implement these processes to improve quality and performance in their practices.

Instr Course Lect 2016;65:601–608.

On April 16, 2015, President Obama signed the Medicare Access and Children's Health Insurance Program Reauthorization Act of 2015 (HR 2), which stabilized physician reimbursement under Medicare.[1] The bill strives to replace payment for volume with payment for value. Value, with respect to health care, is the outcomes achieved with the dollars spent for care of a patient or a patient episode. HR 2 explicitly calls

for professional medical organizations, such as the American Academy of Orthopaedic Surgeons (AAOS) and affiliated specialty societies, to define quality, performance, and value for patient care. Orthopaedic surgeons should follow a pragmatic approach for the implementation of quality and performance improvements within their practices and use resources, such as electronic medical records (EMRs), to aid in these

improvements. Orthopaedic surgeons also should review real case-based examples before they begin to implement measures to improve quality and performance in their practices.

Quality Improvement and Process Improvement

Evidence-based medicine is defined as the integration of the best research evidence with clinical expertise and patient values.[2] High-quality research is required to establish best available care strategies for patient diagnosis and treatment; however, surgical research presents several specific challenges. Surgical studies are generally

Dr. Shea or an immediate family member serves as an unpaid consultant to Clinical Data Solutions and Source Trust, and serves as a board member, owner, officer, or committee member of the American Academy of Orthopaedic Surgeons, the American Orthopaedic Society for Sports Medicine, the North Pacific Orthopaedic Society, and the Pediatric Orthopaedic Society of North America. None of the following authors nor any immediate family member has received anything of value from or has stock or stock options held in a commercial company or institution related directly or indirectly to the subject of this chapter: Dr. Jevsevar, Ms. Styhl, and Dr. Koenig.

underpowered, and blind studies are impossible in surgical research. If no clinical research exists on a particular subject, consensus-based care (ie, care based on physician expertise and experience) is acceptable. Unfortunately, even if the best care or evidence of efficacy is present, the routine achievement of that care is lacking.[3]

The US Agency for Healthcare Research and Quality defines quality health care as "doing the right thing, at the right time, in the right way, for the right person—and having the best possible results."[4] Walter Shewhart[5] and Edward Deming[6] studied industrial quality improvement (QI) and defined it as a series of discrete processes. Shewhart[5] identified customer needs, the reduction of variations in processes, and the minimization of quality control inspections as critically important for industry success, whereas Deming[6] recognized quality as the essential driver for industry success and subsequently introduced process improvement (PI) methodology to Japanese engineers and executives. The Japanese automobile industry used Shewhart's and Deming's ideas to produce better-quality products, which led to considerable growth and subsequent worldwide recognition of quality. PI is defined as the "systematic approach to closing of process or system performance gaps through streamlining and cycle time reduction, and identification and elimination of causes of below-specifications quality, process variation, and non-value-adding activities."[7] A process is a series of linked steps, which may or may not occur sequentially, that lead to a value-added outcome. In health care, patient care can be thought of as a set of processes that lead to improved patient health or outcomes.

The application of QI and PI methodology in patient care is directed toward the improved efficiency of processes (streamlining), the reduction of errors and adverse events (safety), decreased variation in the choice and use of processes (utilization and standardization), improved communication within the healthcare team (checklists), improved systematization of processes (care pathways), maximal health improvement (outcomes), an enhanced patient experience of care (satisfaction), and the elimination of waste associated with processes (logistics). The elimination of waste in health care is critically important. In just "6 categories of waste—overtreatment, failures of care coordination, failures in execution of care processes, administrative complexity, pricing failures, and fraud and abuse—the sum of the lowest available estimates exceeds 20% of total health care expenditures."[8] The routine application of QI and PI leads to continuous QI.[9] Examples of common QI and PI methodologies used in health care are plan-do-study-act cycle, Lean, and Six Sigma strategies. A broad cross-sectional representation of all stakeholders, including staff, is very important because clinicians are not always aware of administrative, logistic, financial, or workflow effects on proposed change strategies.

QI and PI methodologies require the measurement of variation in the care processes that are affected by the proposed changes. Systematic quality measurement demonstrates whether improvement efforts lead to change in the primary end point in the desired direction, contribute to unintended results in different parts of the system, and require additional efforts to bring a process back into acceptable ranges.[10]

Statistical process control uses data that are collected as part of the care process, including outcomes, to continuously improve the process and provide early detection of problems. If measured outcomes are used as the numerator and total opportunities are used as the denominator, then the care process can be graphed on a control chart that evaluates long-term performance. Variation from perfection occurs in two ways. Assignable or specific cause variation is nonrandom and frequently the cause of sentinel events in health care. Although sometimes seen as "black swan" or "aligned Swiss cheese" events, assignable cause events require an expeditious and detailed analysis to prevent recurrence. Random or common cause variation is variation that is expected within any process. The overriding purpose of QI and PI methodologies is to decrease variation and, occasionally, reset expected baselines (perfection).

The plan-do-study-act cycle strategy is commonly used in healthcare settings, perhaps because of its straightforward approach to improvement. This method involves a trial-and-learning approach in which a suggested process change for improvement is made, and clinical testing is performed on a small scale before any changes are made to the larger system.[11] In the plan phase, suggestions for improvement are collated, goals are established, and task assignments are delegated. The plan phase also includes the description of appropriate measures of improvement (success). The implementation of the proposed changes occurs in the do phase. In healthcare settings, deviations are referred to as variations, and some variations may actually reflect improvements rather than detriments of care. Variations are analyzed in the study phase, with particular emphasis on what went right, what went wrong, what improvement was realized (if any), and what change should be made for the next cycle. The act phase applies the results and lessons learned to patient care. The process is iterative; each rapid cycle may produce only a small incremental improvement in care. The plan-do-study-act cycle strategy, as with all QI and PI strategies, is not meant to be a "one-and-done" strategy to improve health outcomes.

Toyota Motor Corporation developed the Toyota Production System, also known as "Lean production," to address inefficiency and waste in its automotive manufacturing process.[12,13] The Lean strategy eliminates any action or process that does not enhance the value of the product or service. Seven types of waste have been identified in the Lean strategy, including overproduction or underproduction, inventory, rework or rejects (ie, assembly mistakes), motion (ie, poor work area ergonomics), waiting (ie, patients waiting to be seen for appointments), processing (ie, outdated policies and procedures), and transport or handling (ie, transporting patients unnecessarily).[10,14] The Lean PI strategy for health care, which was adapted from "Lean production," uses a series of tools to evaluate and address change in the process.

Developed by Motorola in the mid-1980s, Six Sigma is a rigorous statistical measurement methodology that is designed to reduce cost, decrease process variation, and eliminate errors and defects.[15] Six Sigma refers to a statistical unit that reflects the number of standard deviations a given process is from perfection (ie, no process variation). To achieve the level of Six Sigma, a process must be within 3 SD above or below perfection, which represents approximately 3.4 defects (variations) per million opportunities and is virtually error free (99.9996%). Six Sigma is achieved through a series of five steps: define, measure, analyze, improve, and control.

The specific QI and PI methodology chosen is not as important as a commitment to the process of continuous QI in practice. Setting a goal (often with an "aims" statement), studying the process, implementing change, and purposefully sharing successes with all stakeholders are critical to establish a culture of quality.

Leveraging QI Efforts

Orthopaedic surgeons live and practice in a constantly changing healthcare environment. If orthopaedic surgeons practice in the United States, chances are good that some portion of patient care is provided in conjunction with an EMR. EMR systems vary in scope, from simple data entry and medication recording tools for an office practice to comprehensive systems that include all healthcare information, orders, imaging, and procedures for an entire patient population. With the implementation of meaningful use measures as part of the Affordable Care Act, most healthcare systems have moved toward some form of a comprehensive EMR system. Although EMRs have created a multitude of issues for daily practice, including training, hardware, and implementation problems, they also have provided healthcare systems with an opportunity to align QI efforts.

GreenCare

Since the mid-2000s, many healthcare systems have moved their treatment focus from volume to value. This often requires substantial changes in personnel, process flow, resource allocation, and institutional culture. GreenCare, which was developed at the institution of the authors of this chapter, is one example of the shift from volume to value. The process began with a focus on improving the quality of total knee arthroplasty while increasing efficiency to make total knee arthroplasty sustainable in an environment of declining Medicare reimbursement rates. The authors began by standardizing the clinical care pathway and incorporating robust data collection processes to drive continuous innovation. GreenCare is "a process of care that incorporates the available evidence base and consensus-driven best practices for the treatment of a particular medical condition while collecting prospective clinical data for monitoring patient outcomes as well as driving quality and efficiency improvement efforts" (Sohail K. Mirza, MD, MPH; Karl Koenig, MD, MS; Ivan M. Tomek, MD, Lebanon, NH, unpublished data, 2012).

Although the implementation of a quality-focused change effort was a complex process, it was dramatically enhanced by the well-timed introduction of a new EMR system in the hospital system. The generalized environment of change was ripe for the creation of tools and processes that could simultaneously incorporate the new clinical workflow with an evidence-based standardized treatment pathway. The team was able to create tools that helped them achieve their QI goals in conjunction with EMR training for staff.

Process

The GreenCare story began at the drawing board. A multidisciplinary team of surgeons, physician assistants, nurses, clinical staff, QI experts,

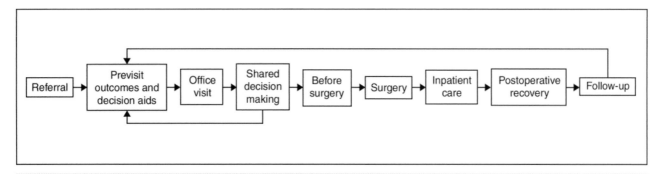

Figure 1 Algorithm shows an episode of care model with preliminary phases of care.

administrators, and patient representatives worked together to carefully map out the current process for an entire episode of care (**Figure 1**). Then, specific phases of care and each patient interaction were defined. The team prepared detailed cost studies to map out which processes were most time and resource intensive. After the current process was defined, the team determined which evidence and best practices were desired for total knee arthroplasty patients. The team used the AAOS Clinical Practice Guidelines and the RAND/UCLA modified-Delphi expert panel method to identify 68 best practices, which were incorporated in the pathway.[16] The institution's arthroplasty surgeons met on multiple occasions to standardize the preoperative and postoperative care pathways, including radiographs, perioperative antibiotics, anticoagulation, mobilization schedules, catheter management, physical therapy protocols, and follow-up schedules. If evidence was good, then it was incorporated. If evidence was lacking, then a consensus was reached among the surgeons with the understanding that further measurement was the goal.

The team then defined 213 data points to collect for each patient throughout an episode of care, which would be used for the evaluation of outcomes and feedback for continuous improvement. Each patient representative believed that a shared decision-making tool for knee osteoarthritis was an integral part of education and treatment. This process of standardization, according to the best available evidence, was long and arduous but absolutely necessary to ensure the success of the next steps.

EMR Incorporation

The institution of the authors of this chapter had the opportunity to embrace a new, comprehensive EMR system at the same time the standardized pathway was being implemented. The EMR system had the capability to build electronic order sets for preoperative and postoperative patient care, which ensured that the standardized pathway could be made easily available for surgeon use. The EMR system has multiple ways to record patient data, depending on the preference of the provider. EMR workflows were established for many of the institution's 213 data elements, and designated team members were assigned to record them. Some data elements, such as limb alignment, did not exist in the record previously, so tools were built to allow them to be recorded in the clinician's note. The key factor was to identify the same elements

for all patients and make it easy for the provider to record them. Field-defined data elements with appropriate discrete responses were necessary to populate the database. Instead of having research assistants or nurses perform chart reviews, the team built a process to record these data prospectively as part of routine clinical care. Because the team defined and standardized the key data up front, they could then build a process to collect it.

The importance of a team care model cannot be overemphasized. None of the data sought were really new to clinical care; however, to ensure that data were captured on every patient at the appropriate time, the work was shared among the team members. For example, a clinical secretary is responsible for six data elements when an appointment is booked. The flow staff record height, weight, medications, and allergies as well as ensure that the patient has completed his or her patient-reported outcomes questionnaires. The questionnaires allow the patient to directly provide substantial information about their symptoms, level of function, and previously used treatments. Nurses participate in the preoperative and postoperative visits with each patient and gather information about their support systems, home environment, discharge

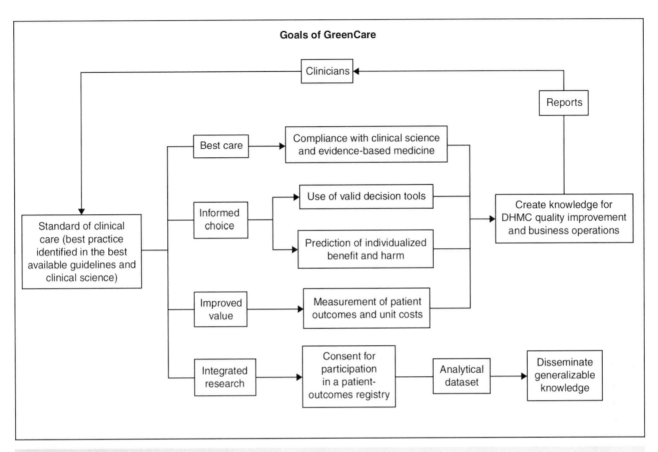

Figure 2   Algorithm shows the GreenCare pathway feedback loop. DHMC = Dartmouth-Hitchcock Medical Center.

expectations, and history of bleeding or clotting issues. The physician or physician assistant then records information about previous knee surgery, physical examination findings, and the radiographic severity of disease. If the patient opts for surgery, then the surgeon also will record information on the surgical approach, the technique, and the intraoperative range of motion. The follow-up appointments have a similar process. Although a discussion with this level of detail may seem unnecessary, planning and the division of labor are necessary for a clinical pathway to succeed. Each role in the clinical pathway has specific instructions on the proper techniques to obtain clinical data and the appropriate location in the EMR in which to record it. The advantage of incorporating the standardized pathway and EMR simultaneously is the ability to train all team members in the same way at the same time, which increases data yield, accuracy, and satisfaction with the process. Feedback reports are crucial at all levels to assist team members with personal improvement in their roles. Each team member wants to know how the team is doing and how to improve. **Figure 2** is a schematic of the feedback loops that were established to address the team's three major goals.

Lessons Learned

The institutional experience of the authors of this chapter in this endeavor has yielded substantial knowledge about shortcomings and strengths. Until a serious inventory of both strengths and shortcomings is taken, it is difficult to move forward; however, after an objective analysis is performed, the leverage of strengths and the improvement of weaknesses become the backbone of the QI process. The key components of a successful clinical pathway include the following: (1) A strong clinical champion to give the process credence and develop interest in the changes that are being made. (2) The creation of data collection tools that are easy to use and make the provider's job easier. A more efficient process does not have to be sold to anyone; it will sell itself. (3) Timely feedback reporting, which will allow the team to thrive on its successes and work hard to improve its weaknesses. Greater team involvement in the clinical pathway process creates substantially greater team engagement. (4) A team effort, in which all stakeholders are included up front and all members of the clinical team feel as if they have input into the process. The engagement of all stakeholders at the first step in the clinical pathway process will yield benefits at every subsequent step.

Physician Engagement in Performance and Quality Improvement Programs

According to the National Healthcare Safety Network, surgical site infections (SSIs) represent 23% of hospital-acquired infections and are one of the leading causes of death.[17-20] Recent reports show that the SSI incidence rate for knee and hip replacements range from 0.58% to 1.6% and 0.67 to 2.4%, respectively,[21] and that up to 35,000 orthopaedic SSIs may occur annually in the United States.[22] SSIs have a negative effect on patients and also add substantial costs and hospital admission days.[23] Methicillin-resistant *Staphylococcus aureus* and other complex multidrug resistant organisms may be very difficult to treat and impossible to eradicate.

Project Zero

In May 2011, St. Luke's Health System in Boise, Idaho, implemented a program to reduce SSIs. Project Zero was implemented in the orthopaedic and neurosurgical departments to reduce SSIs in total joint and spine procedures. The initial goals of the Project Zero team included the following: (1) create a multidisciplinary approach that includes surgeons, infectious disease/infection control staff, administration, surgical and inpatient nursing staff, central instrument processing staff, anesthesiologists, environmental services staff,

engineering (heating, ventilation, air conditioning) staff, and others as needed; (2) create a culture that is focused on patient safety and infection prevention, with improved communication to surgical and nursing staff about SSI prevention; (3) reduce operating room variation, if appropriate; and (4) reduce the SSI rate within the orthopaedic and neurosurgical service lines by 50% in the first 18 months.

Outside Data Sources

The Project Zero team reviewed several resources for guidance on how SSIs could be reduced, including level I and II published literature; practices and recommendations from top-performing organizations; lower level evidence and recommendations from the Association of Perioperative Registered Nurses, the AAOS, the Centers for Disease Control and Prevention, the Infectious Disease Society of America, and the Association for Professionals in Infection Control and Epidemiology; and clean room practices and technology, such as sterile techniques, tissue handling, and air-quality practices, performed at an allograft harvest facility and a computer chip manufacturing facility.

Patient, Procedure, and Environmental Risk Factors

The risk factors for a SSI are multifactorial and may be related to medical comorbidities, operating room practices, and the type of procedure that is performed. Numerous factors have been identified that substantially increase the risk of a SSI, including increased age, obesity, diabetes, tobacco use, malnutrition, and a high American Society of Anesthesiologists Physical Status Classification System score.[24] Nasal

colonization with *S aureus* also increases the risk of a SSI.[25] Procedural factors, such as increased blood loss, drainage, operating room time,[26] the use of implants, and inadequate skin preparation, are associated with an increased risk of a SSI. Regular communication among surgeons on the department's performance and individual surgeon performance is critical to address SSIs. Environmental aspects, including the maintenance of sterile equipment, clean air management, and the monitoring of staff traffic in and out of rooms, all of which are practiced by top-performing organizations and allograft harvest facilities, have been associated with lower infection rates.[27-29] The maintenance of adequate airflow and the minimization of foot traffic may help reduce the risk of SSIs. Environmental factors, including the sterile practices of the staff, operating room staffing patterns, and preoperative planning for procedures and associated instruments, require substantial attention.

Changes Implemented

To address the patient risk factors, a preoperative clinic staffed by primary care providers was implemented. The preoperative clinic created care pathways for patients who had medical comorbidities that increase SSI risk, such as diabetes, nasal colonization with methicillin-sensitive *S aureus* or methicillin-resistant *S aureus*, obesity, poor dentition, malnutrition, and the use of immunosuppressive medications. This allowed the surgeon and the medical staff to ensure that their patients were in the best possible health before surgery. A screening and decolonization program for methicillin-resistant *S aureus* and methicillin-sensitive *S aureus* was introduced. Although there was an associated cost with the preoperative clinic and *S aureus* screening, Urban[30] reported that it may be more financially sound to treat high-risk patients before surgery than to treat SSIs. Protocols for management of environmental and procedural factors also were recommended. Designated surgical uniforms, hand hygiene, surgical instrument sterilization processes, skin preparation processes, postoperative wound care, operating room traffic, and room cleaning processes were standardized and monitored. These changes were paired with educational programs for both operating room personnel and surgeons.

Improved communication between surgeons, the scheduling staff, and the operating room staff also was an area of focus. These groups concentrated on the improvement of case schedule protocols to ensure that all equipment was ready 12 to 24 hours before the procedure and to reduce unnecessary variation in case preparation and management. Case preference cards, which contain items that are normally used in a surgical procedure, were reviewed and revised to ensure that the correct items were available for the procedure. These practices minimized operating room traffic, prevented surgical case delays, reduced turnover times, and likely improved surgeon satisfaction.

Results

During Project Zero's first 18 months, 19 fewer SSIs than expected were reported, based on historical infection rates and case volume. The goal to reduce the SSI rate by half was met by the end of 2012, with the rate reduced from 1.2% to 0.54%. The rates varied throughout 2014 and 2015, but orthopaedic SSI rates have remained close to or below 0.5% (Kevin G. Shea, MD, Boise, ID, unpublished data, 2013).

Lessons Learned

It is critical that input from staff in the operating room, including nurses, surgical technicians, and surgeons, be encouraged. These staff members have valuable ideas and first-hand knowledge of how the process works and may be improved. Communication with all staff, including regular updates about the mission, goals, research, successes, and failures of the project, is important. It is essential that good information on complications, SSI rates, and medical comorbidities is provided to the medical/surgical staff members who will make decisions to improve medical care.

Physician leadership, both medical and surgical, is critically important. Involvement of internal medicine, including inpatient and outpatient medical staff, is crucial. Surgeons are the leaders in the operating room; having them on board with the change process greatly influences the rest of the operating room staff. Regular discussions with key members of the medical staff, including the surgical department chairman and other surgical leaders, are vital to gain buy-in from all surgical departments. Individual surgeon input is crucial to success. Input from infectious disease and epidemiology staff also is critical. These individuals have access to data on SSI rates, infection profiles, antibiotic resistance, and other pertinent issues. Their ability to provide data in a timely manner is critical to success. Access to these data allows for meetings with groups of surgeons to work on the reduction of SSIs. Transformation takes time; patience and flexibility are important for individuals who lead change.

Obstacles may stall the process, and resistance is inevitable. The willingness to work around problems and remain patient with both staff and the institution is important for success.

Future Endeavors

Increasingly, the Project Zero team is working to identify high-risk patient categories before surgery and, if possible, mitigate these risks. A current area of focus includes diabetes and immunosuppression. Future operating room designs and remodeling projects will consider architectural changes that may reduce SSI, such as the development of ultraclean operating room regions that care for high-risk SSI patients during high-risk procedures. There are many challenges going forward. Antibiotic resistance emergence will continue to threaten progress. Obesity remains a substantial risk factor for SSI and will be a challenge to address. Project Zero plans to continue to look to top-performing institutions for guidance and push toward better clean-room standards, which will aid in their overall goal of zero infections.

Summary

Both QI and PI will continue to be emphasized in the attempt to define the value of orthopaedic care delivery in the United States. Although the AAOS and several other organizations work to further the quality mandate on a national level, the most important QI will occur at local and regional levels. Orthopaedic surgeons need to embrace the challenges of QI and find better and more meaningful ways to share this information. Involvement and leadership at the individual orthopaedic surgeon level is the critical first step toward improved orthopaedic healthcare delivery.

References

1. Pub L No. 114-10, 129 Stat 87. Medicare Access and CHIP Reauthorization Act of 2015. 2015.

2. Sackett DL, Rosenberg WM, Gray JA, Haynes RB, Richardson WS: Evidence based medicine: What it is and what it isn't. *BMJ* 1996;312(7023):71-72.

3. McGlynn EA, Asch SM, Adams J, et al: The quality of health care delivered to adults in the United States. *N Engl J Med* 2003;348(26):2635-2645.

4. US Department of Health and Human Services, Agency for Healthcare Research and Quality: Your guide to choosing quality healthcare: A quick look at quality. 2007. Available at: http://archive.ahrq.gov/consumer/qnt/qntqlook.htm. Accessed February 4, 2015.

5. Shewhart WA: *Economic Control of Quality of Manufactured Product.* New York, NY, D. Van Nostrand Company, 1931.

6. Deming WE: *Out of the Crisis.* Cambridge, MA, MIT Press, 1986.

7. BusinessDictionary.com: Process improvement. Available at: http://www.businessdictionary.com/definition/process-improvement.html. Accessed May 15, 2015.

8. Berwick DM, Hackbarth AD: Eliminating waste in US health care. *JAMA* 2012;307(14):1513-1516.

9. Berwick DM: Continuous improvement as an ideal in health care. *N Engl J Med* 1989;320(1):53-56.

10. Varkey P, Reller MK, Resar RK: Basics of quality improvement in health care. *Mayo Clin Proc* 2007;82(6):735-739.

11. Langley GJ, Moen RD, Nolan KM, Nolan TW, Norman CL, Provost LP: *The Improvement Guide: A Practical Approach to Enhancing Organizational Performance,* ed 2. San Francisco, CA, Jossey-Bass, 2009.

12. Holweg M: The genealogy of lean production. *Journal of Operations Management* 2007;25(2):420-437.

13. Young D: Pittsburgh hospitals band together to reduce medication errors. *Am J Health Syst Pharm* 2002;59(11):1014, 1016, 1026.

14. Endsley S, Magill MK, Godfrey MM: Creating a lean practice. *Fam Pract Manag* 2006;13(4):34-38.

15. Chassin MR: Is health care ready for Six Sigma quality? *Milbank Q* 1998;76(4):565-591, 510.

16. SooHoo NF, Lieberman JR, Farng E, Park S, Jain S, Ko CY: Development of quality of care indicators for patients undergoing total hip or total knee replacement. *BMJ Qual Saf* 2011;20(2):153-157.

17. Sievert DM, Ricks P, Edwards JR, et al: Antimicrobial-resistant pathogens associated with healthcare-associated infections: Summary of data reported to the National Healthcare Safety Network at the Centers for Disease Control and Prevention, 2009-2010. *Infect Control Hosp Epidemiol* 2013;34(1):1-14.

18. de Lissovoy G, Fraeman K, Hutchins V, Murphy D, Song D, Vaughn BB: Surgical site infection: Incidence and impact on hospital utilization and treatment costs. *Am J Infect Control* 2009;37(5):387-397.

19. Klevens RM, Edwards JR, Richards CL Jr, et al: Estimating health care-associated infections and deaths in U.S. hospitals, 2002. *Public Health Rep* 2007;122(2):160-166.

20. Evans RP; American Academy of Orthopaedic Surgeons Patient Safety Committee: Surgical site infection prevention and control: An emerging paradigm. *J Bone Joint Surg Am* 2009;91(suppl 6):2-9.

21. Edwards JR, Peterson KD, Mu Y, et al: National Healthcare Safety Network (NHSN) report: Data summary for 2006 through 2008, issued December 2009. *Am J Infect Control* 2009;37(10):783-805.

22. Greene LR: Guide to the elimination of orthopedic surgery surgical site infections: An executive summary of the Association for Professionals in Infection Control and Epidemiology elimination guide. *Am J Infect Control* 2012;40(4):384-386.

23. Whitehouse JD, Friedman ND, Kirkland KB, Richardson WJ, Sexton DJ: The impact of surgical-site infections following orthopedic surgery at a community hospital and a university hospital: Adverse quality of life, excess length of stay, and extra cost. *Infect Control Hosp Epidemiol* 2002;23(4):183-189.

24. Schuster JM, Rechtine G, Norvell DC, Dettori JR: The influence of perioperative risk factors and therapeutic interventions on infection rates after spine surgery: A systematic review. *Spine (Phila Pa 1976)* 2010;35(9 suppl):S125-S137.

25. Kim DH, Spencer M, Davidson SM, et al: Institutional prescreening for detection and eradication of methicillin-resistant Staphylococcus aureus in patients undergoing elective orthopaedic surgery. *J Bone Joint Surg Am* 2010;92(9):1820-1826.

26. Ercole FF, Franco LM, Macieira TG, Wenceslau LC, de Resende HI, Chianca TC: Risk of surgical site infection in patients undergoing orthopedic surgery. *Rev Lat Am Enfermagem* 2011;19(6):1362-1368.

27. Anderson DJ, Kaye KS, Classen D, et al: Strategies to prevent surgical site infections in acute care hospitals. *Infect Control Hosp Epidemiol* 2008;29(suppl 1):S51-S61.

28. Mangram AJ, Horan TC, Pearson ML, Silver LC, Jarvis WR; Centers for Disease Control and Prevention (CDC) Hospital Infection Control Practices Advisory Committee: Guideline for Prevention of Surgical Site Infection, 1999. *Am J Infect Control* 1999;27(2):97-134, discussion 96.

29. Ayliffe GA: Role of the environment of the operating suite in surgical wound infection. *Rev Infect Dis* 1991;13(suppl 10):S800-S804.

30. Urban JA: Cost analysis of surgical site infections. *Surg Infect (Larchmt)* 2006;7(suppl 1):S19-S22.

Getting Ready for ICD-10 and Meaningful Use Stage 2

Jack M. Bert, MD

William R. Beach, MD

Louis F. McIntyre, MD

Ranjan Sachdev, MD, MBA, CMC

Abstract

For the past 24 years, most developed countries have used the International Classification of Diseases, Tenth Revision (ICD-10) to report physician services. In the United States, physicians have continued to use the American Medical Association Current Procedural Terminology, Fourth Edition and the Healthcare Common Procedure Coding System. The ICD-10-Clinical Modification (CM) has approximately 4.9 times more codes than the International Classification of Diseases, Ninth Revision. ICD-10-CM allows for more specific descriptors of a procedure and is broken down by category, etiology, anatomic site, severity, and extension. ICD-10-CM is scheduled to be implemented by Medicare and commercial payers on October 1, 2015. In addition to ICD-10 implementation, physicians have to meet the requirements of the Meaningful Use Electronic Health Record Incentive Program. The Meaningful Use program is designed to promote the use of certified electronic health technology by providing eligible professionals with incentive payments if they meet the defined core and menu objectives of each stage of the program. All core measures must be met; however, providers can choose to meet a preset number of menu measures. Meaningful Use Stage 1 required eligible professionals to meet core and menu objectives that focused on data capture and sharing. Meaningful Use Stage 2 requires eligible professionals to meet core and menu objects that focus on advanced clinical processes for a full year in 2015. Stage 3 has been delayed until 2017, and core and menu measures that will focus on improving outcomes have not yet been defined. It is important for orthopaedic surgeons to understand the history of and techniques for the use of ICD-10-CM in clinical practice. Orthopaedic surgeons also should understand the requirements for Meaningful Use Stages 1 and 2, including the core objectives that must be met to achieve satisfactory attestation.

Instr Course Lect 2016;65:609–622.

The original disease classification system, known as the "Bertillon Classification of Causes of Death," was developed by Dr. Jacques Bertillon and presented at the 1893 World Statistics Congress of the International Statistical Institute. In 1949, the World Health Organization assumed responsibility for the coding system, and the name was changed to the International Classification of Diseases (ICD). The ninth revision of the ICD (ICD-9) became available in 1977 and is the system currently used in the United States. The 10th revision of the ICD (ICD-10) became available in 1994 and is currently used by most developed countries. There are two components to the ICD-10 coding system, one that is used by physicians to report diagnoses, signs, and symptoms (ICD-10-Clinical Modification [CM]), and one that is used by facilities, primarily hospitals, to report hospital inpatient procedural services (ICD-10-Procedural Coding System). Physicians in the United States do not use the ICD-10-Procedural Coding System to report their services, but instead use the American Medical Association (AMA) Current Procedural

Why Convert From ICD-9 to ICD-10?

The conversion to ICD-10 is taking place because, frankly, ICD-9 is out of numbers! The five-digit, all-numeric system of ICD-9 can no longer accommodate new diagnoses. The medical community has reached a critical mass of diagnoses that require a more detailed coding system. Although the addition of a sixth digit to ICD-9 would have sufficed, it would not have answered all the questions that payers ask or achieved the granularity that researchers desire. ICD-10 requires a logical listing of disease states. The desire for a more detailed, granular system has led to the creation of ICD-10. In addition, communication between providers within electronic health records (EHRs) is clearer in ICD-10 irrespective of payment and research considerations.

A new and better ICD would ask and answer the following questions with respect to orthopaedics: Is the condition chronic/degenerative ("M" chapter) or acute/traumatic ("S" chapter)? Does the condition affect the right side of the body or the left side of the body (routinely the sixth digit but occasionally the fifth digit if the primary code has only four characters. For example, the code for osteoarthritis of the hip is M16. The code for unilateral primary osteoarthritis of the hip is M16.1; the code

Terminology, Fourth Edition and the Healthcare Common Procedure Coding System.

for the right hip is M16.11, and the code for the left hip is M16.12. The laterality of the code is in the second to last character, with the letter A, D, or S in the last position for nonfracture codes.)? What is the natural history of the condition (seventh digit)? The creators of ICD-10 were logical in the creation of the coding system, at least with respect to orthopaedics. For example, chronic and degenerative conditions are found in chapter 13 ("M"). Acute and traumatic conditions are found in chapter 19 ("S"). Therefore, the first character of an orthopaedic ICD-10 code usually is the letter M or S.

Routinely, the next four digits depend on the particular diagnosis and, thus, describe the specific condition. For example, a traumatic rotator cuff tear is coded S46.01. The sixth digit of a code describes which side of the body the condition affects; S46.011 is the code for a traumatic right rotator cuff tear, and S46.012 is the code for a traumatic left rotator cuff tear.

The seventh and final digit of a code describes the natural history of the condition. The seventh digit of a code for nonfractures is either an A (initial visit/evaluation of a condition), D (subsequent [follow-up] visit for the same condition), or S (sequelae of that condition). The seventh and final digit of a code for fractures is based on the Gustilo classification and is either an A (initial encounter for a closed fracture), B (initial encounter for an open grade I or II fracture), C (initial encounter for and

open grade III [A, B, or C] fracture), D (subsequent encounter for a closed fracture with routine healing), E (subsequent encounter for an open grade I or II fracture with routine healing), F (subsequent encounter for an open grade III [A, B, or C] fracture with routine healing), G (subsequent encounter for a closed fracture with delayed healing), H (subsequent encounter for an open grade I or II fracture with delayed healing), J (subsequent encounter for an open grade III [A, B, or C] fracture with delayed healing), K (subsequent encounter for a closed fracture with a nonunion), M (subsequent encounter for an open grade I or II fracture with a nonunion), N (subsequent encounter for an open grade III [A, B, or C] fracture with a nonunion), P (subsequent encounter for a closed fracture with a malunion), Q (subsequent encounter for an open grade I or II fracture with a malunion), R (subsequent encounter for an open grade III [A, B, or C] fracture with a malunion), or S (sequelae). The seventh digit can be grouped by fracture type: closed fractures, which include codes for the initial encounter (A), subsequent encounter with routine healing (D), subsequent encounter with delayed healing (G), subsequent encounter with nonunion (K), and subsequent encounter with malunion (P); open grade I or II fractures, which include codes for the initial encounter (B), subsequent encounter with routine healing (E), subsequent encounter with delayed healing (H), subsequent encounter with

Dr. Bert or an immediate family member serves as a paid consultant to or is an employee of Sanofi-Aventis, Smith & Nephew, Exactech, Exscribe Orthopaedic Healthcare Solutions, Luminus Devices, Orthopaedic Practice Management, and Wright Medical Technology, and serves as a board member, owner, officer, or committee member of the Arthroscopy Association of North America. Dr. Beach or an immediate family member serves as a paid consultant to or is an employee of Arthrex, CONMED Linvatec, Mitek, and Smith & Nephew, and serves as a board member, owner, officer, or committee member of the American Academy of Orthopaedic Surgeons and the Arthroscopy Association of North America. Dr. McIntyre or an immediate family member is a member of a speakers' bureau or has made paid presentations on behalf of Quintiles; has stock or stock options held in Tornier; has received research or institutional support from DePuy; and serves as a board member, owner, officer, or committee member of the American Academy of Orthopaedic Surgeons, Advocacy for Improvement in Mobility, the Arthroscopy Association of North America, the Medical Society of the State of New York, the Westchester County Medical Society, and Orthopedic Practice Management. Dr. Sachdev or an immediate family member has stock or stock options held in Exscribe Orthopaedic Healthcare Solutions, Procter & Gamble, and Stryker.

nonunion (M), and subsequent encounter with malunion (Q); and open grade III (A, B, or C) fractures, which include codes for the initial encounter (C), subsequent encounter with routine healing (F), subsequent encounter with delayed healing (J), subsequent encounter with nonunion (N), and subsequent encounter with malunion (R). For fractures, this creates the three times five plus one rule ($3 \times 5 + 1 = 16$). Three types of fractures (closed, open grade I and II, and open grade III), in which only five scenarios can occur (initial encounter, routine healing, delayed healing, nonunion, and malunion), plus the possibility for sequelae.

The process to determine the correct ICD-10 code for a right knee, posterior horn, medial meniscal tear would be as follows. If the condition is degenerative, a physician who is using the AMA 2013 ICD-10 manual would first go to the alphabetical list and find "derangement," or more specifically, "derangement, knee, meniscus, medial = M23.20 (due to old tear or injury)." After the listing is found in the alphabetical list, the physician would then go to the tabular list, which makes up most of the ICD-10 manual. M23.20 is listed as "derangement of unspecified meniscus due to old tear or injury." There are nine sublistings under the listing for unspecified meniscus, and the physician can continue to refine the listing by noting "M23.203, derangement of unspecified medial meniscus due to old tear or injury, right knee." If patient information suggests there is a posterior horn tear, then the physician can be more specific by noting "M23.222, derangement of posterior horn of medial meniscus due to old tear or injury, right knee." The seventh digit is dependent on whether the

encounter is a new or subsequent visit or sequelae of the condition. If this were a new patient encounter, then the final ICD-10 code would be M23.222A. If the condition is acute, a physician who is using the AMA 2013 ICD-10 manual would find the alphabetical listing for "tear, torn—meniscus (S83.209);" there are several sublistings, including bucket-handle, lateral, medial, and old (which refers the reader to the derangement listing). "Medial" includes bucket-handle (S83.21-), complex (S83.23-), peripheral (S83.22), and specified (NEC S83.24) types. These choices direct the physician to the tabular list, which allows the physician to select the most appropriate category (there is no listing for a traumatic posterior horn tear). The code for a peripheral tear of the medial meniscus, current injury, right knee is S83.221. If this were an initial visit, the seventh digit would be an A, and the final ICD-10 code would be S83.221A.

How does a physician learn all this? There are two answers, depending on the desired depth of education. For physicians who have no desire to learn the ICD-10 system, some EHR systems may have cheat sheets with drop-down menus that lead the physician through the coding process. Physicians also can develop their own lists of most commonly used codes. For example, knee, meniscus, tear, acute, right, initial encounter = S83.221A. Alternatively, physicians can learn the fundamentals of the ICD-10 system and refer to the ICD-10 manual for each use. Physicians should begin by reading the conventions section and then review the alphabetical list followed by the tabular list. Physicians should take approximately 2 hours to leaf through the ICD-10 manual and/or CD-ROM; this may be

all that is necessary to understand and employ the new ICD-10.

ICD-10 is here and not likely to be delayed again. Physicians should be prepared, both as physicians and as businesspersons because ICD-10 will change both areas of medical practices. On October 1, 2015, ICD-10 will become the code set required to report medical services and to receive professional reimbursement.

The Structure of ICD-10

ICD-10 is organized as an index and a tabular list. The index alphabetically lists the various medical symptoms and diagnoses and references the categories in the tabular list in which specific conditions can be found. The tabular list is arranged by chapter, and each chapter refers to a specific organ system. The ICD-10 coding system, which has approximately 68,000 codes, is much more specific compared with the ICD-9 coding system, which has approximately 14,000 codes. Nineteen chapters of the 21 in ICD-10 describe diseases, conditions, signs, symptoms, and findings of different organs and systems[1] (**Table 1**).

The ICD-10 code set is arranged as a seven-character alphanumeric display. The first three characters of each code denote the category of disease and are always led by a letter, which indicates the chapter in the ICD-10 manual that corresponds to the disease state or organ system. The category of disease is set off by a decimal point and followed by three additional characters, which correspond to the etiology, anatomic site, and severity of the disease. These characters can be numbers or letters, depending on the given etiology of the disease. The seventh character, or extension, denotes the timeframe

Table 1

Chapters in the International Classification of Diseases, Tenth Revision, Clinical Modification

Chapter No.	Description[a]	Code Category
1	Certain infectious and parasitic diseases	A00-B99
2	**Neoplasms**	C00-D49
3	Diseases of the blood and blood-forming organs and certain disorders involving the immune mechanism	D50-D89
4	Endocrine, nutritional and metabolic diseases	E00-E89
5	Mental, behavioral and neurodevelopmental disorders	F01-F99
6	**Diseases of the nervous system**	G00-G99
7	Diseases of the eye and adnexa	H00-H59
8	Diseases of the ear and mastoid process	H60-H95
9	Diseases of the circulatory system	I00-I99
10	Diseases of the respiratory system	J00-J99
11	Diseases of the digestive system	K00-K94
12	**Diseases of the skin and subcutaneous tissue**	L00-L99
13	**Diseases of the musculoskeletal system and connective tissue**	M00-M99
14	Diseases of the genitourinary system	N00-N99
15	Pregnancy, childbirth and the puerperium	O00-O99
16	Certain conditions originating in the perinatal period	P00-P96
17	**Congenital malformations, deformations and chromosomal abnormalities**	Q00-Q99
18	Symptoms, signs and abnormal clinical and laboratory findings, not elsewhere classified	R00-R99
19	**Injury, poisoning and certain other consequences of external causes**	S00-T88
20	**External causes of morbidity**	V01-Y98
21	Factors influencing health status and contact with health services	Z00-Z99

[a]Descriptions in bold are of interest to orthopaedic surgeons.

Reproduced with permission from Henley MB: ICD 10: What orthopedic surgeons should know, how it will affect them and the cost of implementation? *Sports Med Arthrosc* 2013;21(3):142-147.

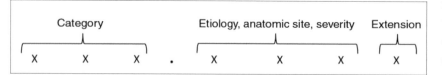

Figure 1   Diagram shows the code structure for the International Classification of Diseases, Tenth Revision, Clinical Modification.

of treatment as initial, subsequent, or sequela, depending on the clinical situation. The seventh character also is used to describe the various clinical scenarios that may arise in the treatment of fractures, including routine healing, delayed healing, nonunion, and malunion (**Figure 1**).

Some six- and seven-character codes use the letter "X" as a placeholder. The "X" is placed in the fifth position for six-character codes and is used to fill in the empty characters if a seventh character extension is required. A seventh character is required for some codes in chapter 13, "Diseases of the musculoskeletal system and connective tissue" (the "M" chapter), and for most codes in chapter 19, "Injury, poisoning and certain other consequences of external cause" (the "S" and "T" chapters). Many of the codes for chronic and degenerative musculoskeletal conditions are listed in chapter 13. The codes for acute conditions, such as fractures, dislocations, sprains, and strains, are listed in chapter 19. Some conditions are found in both chapters based on the etiology of the disease process. For example, degenerative medial meniscal tears are listed as M23 under "derangement," whereas acute meniscal tears are

Table 2
Estimated Costs of Transition to International Classification of Diseases, Tenth Revision in 2008

Aspect of Business Operations	Costs for a Typical Small Practice[a]	Costs for a Typical Medium Practice[b]	Costs for a Typical Large Practice[c]
Staff education and training	$2,405	$4,745	$46,280
Business process analysis of contracts	$6,900	$12,000	$48,000
Changes to superbills	$2,985	$9,950	$99,500
Information technology system changes	$7,500	$15,000	$100,000
Increased documentation costs	$44,000	$178,500	$1,785,000
Cash-flow disruption	$19,500	$65,000	$650,000
Total	**$83,290**	**$285,195**	**$2,728,780**

[a]Assumptions: Three providers and two administrative staff.

[b]Assumptions: Ten providers, one coder, and six administrative staff.

[c]Assumptions: One hundred providers, ten coders, and fifty-four administrative staff.

Adapted with permission from Nachimson Advisors: The impact of implementing ICD-10 on physician practices and clinical laboratories: A report to the ICD-10 coalition. Nachimson Advisors, October 8, 2008, p 6. Available at: http://www.nachimsonadvisors.com/Documents/ICD-10%20Impacts%20 on%20Providers.pdf. Accessed August 10, 2015.

listed as S83. The "M" and "S" chapters contain most of the orthopaedic conditions. Chapter 19, the "S" chapter, is the largest of all the ICD-10 chapters, and both the "M" and "S" chapters require documentation of laterality. The increased specificity of both chapters in addition to the requirement for documentation of laterality and fracture healing characteristics indicate that orthopaedics will be substantially affected by the adoption of ICD-10.

Why Convert to ICD-10?

There are many reasons for physicians to convert to ICD-10. ICD-9-CM is outdated and not consistent with current medical terminology and concepts. ICD-9 is neither flexible nor exact enough to capture aspects of diagnosis and treatment. Many ICD-9 categories are currently filled and no new codes may be entered into them, which limits the system's specificity and usefulness. ICD-10-CM improves the description of diagnoses and services and has updated

terminology, which reflects a modern approach to medical documentation. The specificity of ICD-10 may improve substantiation of medical necessity and enhance accurate payment for services, both of which may decrease supporting documentation requirements. Many individuals hope that ICD-10 will result in fewer denials of claims and aid in tracking health outcomes data.

Effect and Cost of the Transition

ICD-10 will affect all aspects of the practice of medicine and will require changes in orthopaedic office workflow to accommodate the new demands of the code set. Data intake in the reception area and examination rooms will require increased specificity and documentation. Because billing will be completely different, coders will require more time to search for the correct documentation for the more specific coding system, which will decrease their productivity. Because of the increased

specificity of ICD-10, fracture coding will be especially challenging. All of these changes will lead to increased overhead costs and deceased productivity, especially in the transition phase, which begins in October 2015.

Nachimson Advisors[2] were commissioned by medical specialty societies to estimate the costs of the transition to ICD-10 in 2008. The report estimated the cost effect of ICD-10 on three different sizes of provider practices in six different aspects of business operations[2] (**Table 2**). The mean cost per physician for the transition to ICD-10 was approximately $27,000 in 2008. This study was completed before the Health Information Technology for Economic and Clinical Health Act of 2009 was passed and implemented. This act mandated the use of EHRs, which substantially increased the information technology cost burden on practices of all sizes. Nachimson Advisors were commissioned by the AMA to repeat their 2008 study in 2014. Compared with the costs

Table 3

Estimated Costs of Transition to International Classification of Diseases, Tenth Revision in 2014

Aspect of Business Operations	Typical Small Practice	Typical Medium Practice	Typical Large Practice
Training	$2,700–$3,000	$4,800–$7,900	$75,100
Assessment	$4,300–$7,000	$6,535–$9,600	$19,320
Vendor/software upgrades	$0–$60,000	$0–$200,000	$0–$2,000,000
Process remediation	$3,312–$6,701	$6,211–$12,990	$14,874–$31,821
Testing	$15,248–$28,805	$47,906–$93,098	$428,740–$880,660
Productivity loss	$8,500–$20,250	$72,649–$166,649	$726,487–$1,666,487
Payment disruption	$22,579–$100,349	$75,263–$334,498	$752,630–$3,344,976
Total	**$56,639–$226,105**	**$213,364–$824,735**	**$2,017,151–$8,018,364**

Reproduced with permission from American Medical Association: ICD-10 cost estimates increased for most physicians. February 12, 2014. Available at: http://www.ama-assn.org/ama/pub/news/news/2014/2014-02-12-icd10-cost-estimates-increased-for-most-physicians.page. Accessed August 10, 2015.

for business operations in 2008, Nachimson Advisors reported substantially higher costs in all aspects of business operations in 2014[3] (**Table 3**).

Most other first- and second-world countries have already transitioned to ICD-10. The United States will be different in that it will be the only country to use ICD-10 for reimbursement purposes. Because of this, the experience of other countries as a benchmark may not fully reflect the effect that ICD-10 will have on American medicine.

The increased specificity of ICD-10 codes will require orthopaedic surgeons to adjust their history taking and documentation to capture information necessary to arrive at appropriate codes. Orthopaedic surgeons will have to gather and document information on disease acuity, laterality, fracture location, fracture type, and the description of the course of healing. In addition, practicing physicians will need to know specific aspects of ICD-10, such as ICD-10 nomenclature (derangement instead of degeneration) and the degree of specificity of various diagnostic categories.

Implementing ICD-10: How to Minimize the Trauma

The implementation of ICD-10 will require a concerted effort between physicians and their staff to mitigate the potential disruptive effects of the transition, especially with respect to cash flow. Several resources are available from the Centers for Medicare & Medicaid Services,[4] the Centers for Disease Control and Prevention,[5] and the American Academy of Orthopaedic Surgeons[6] to help physicians in their transition to ICD-10. Because physicians will need a working knowledge of the ICD-10 code set, it would be helpful to purchase the ICD-10 Complete Code Set from the AMA. Physicians who spend a few hours looking up common diagnoses in the index and then the tabular list will become familiar with the structure of the code set, nomenclature used, granularity of various diagnostic categories, and conditions in which a seventh character is necessary.

The American Academy of Orthopaedic Surgeons has imbedded ICD-10 search functions in their Orthopaedic Code-X program. These search functions, which prompt surgeons to enter the essential necessary data, help surgeons perform quick searches for and arrive at the appropriate ICD-10 codes. The Orthopaedic Code-X program is currently available for fractures and will be available in the future for other areas of orthopaedics. Orthopaedic surgeons can run reports for their most commonly reported diagnoses to create cheat sheets that list ICD-10 codes, which may then be posted at dictation stations for easy reference (**Figure 2**).

It is essential that orthopaedic surgeons contact vendors involved in the billing and coding cycle to ensure a smooth transition to ICD-10. The insurance carriers a practice accepts need to be contacted to determine their readiness for the ICD-10 transition as well as coding and documentation requirements for timely reimbursement. Orthopaedic surgeons should ask insurance carriers if they will be running ICD-9 codes in parallel with ICD-10 codes, what codes will be required for reimbursement, if they will accept unspecified codes, what should be done for workers compensation and no-fault insurance carriers, and if they will even be using ICD-10. All information technology vendors need to be assessed to determine their readiness for the ICD-10 transition and the tools they have available to search for ICD-10 codes; the easiest way for physicians to search for ICD-10 codes will be as a function of their practice's EHR system, if available and functional. Clearinghouses will need to be contacted with regard to ICD-10 issues for claims transmission. Surgeons should contact all parties who are involved in the billing and coding cycle to determine the resources and support tools available for the conversion to ICD-10.

Surgeons should develop a plan to test the submission of ICD-10 codes through their clearinghouse and to insurance carriers in the third quarter of 2015. Surgeons should expect the productivity of coders to drop by 50% and should add more coders accordingly.[7] Practice surgeons can be enlisted to document and code their own ICD-10 codes to improve efficiency and cost savings. Alternatively, scribes can be trained and enlisted to document for and code ICD-10. It may be prudent for surgeons to establish a line of credit or establish cash reserves to cover potential payment disruptions during the ICD-10 transition process.

The Meaningful Use Program

The Meaningful Use Program was designed to promote the meaningful use of certified EHR technology for the storage of patient information, e-prescribing, the electronic exchange of information to improve the quality of health care, and the reporting of clinical quality measures in a form and manner that is consistent with certain objectives

Red codes require a seventh character (A, D, or S)					
Gold codes are quick codes					
Shoulder				Right	Left
Rotator cuff tear					
	Traumatic			S46.011	S46.012
	Atraumatic				
		Unspecified		M75.101	M75.102
		Incomplete		M75.111	M75.112
		Complete		M75.121	M75.122
Biceps tendon					
	Unspecified			S46.101	S46.102
	Tendinitis			M75.21	M75.22
	Tear			S46.111	S46.112
Instability					
	Acute				
		Unspecified			
			Subluxation	S43.001	S43.002
			Dislocation	S43.004	S43.005
		Anterior			
			Subluxation	S43.011	S43.012
			Dislocation	S43.014	S43.015
		Posterior			
			Subluxation	S43.021	S43.022
			Dislocation	S43.024	S43.025
		Inferior			
			Subluxation	S43.031	S43.032
			Dislocation	S43.034	S43.035
		Other (MDI)			
			Subluxation	S43.081	S43.082
			Dislocation	S43.084	S43.085
	Chronic				
		Recurrent dislocation		M24.411	M24.412
SLAP				S43.431	S43.432
Bursitis				M75.51	M75.52
Impingement				M75.41	M75.42
Adhesive capsulitis				M75.01	M75.02
Calcifying tendinitis				M75.31	M75.32
AC joint					
	Sprain			S43.51x	S43.52x
	Instability				
		Unspecified			
			Subluxation	S43.111	S43.112
			Dislocation	S43.101	S43.102
		100–200% displacement		S43.121	S43.122
		>200% displacement		S43.131	S43.132
SC joint					
		Unspecified			
			Subluxation	S43.201	S43.202
			Dislocation	S43.204	S43.205
		Anterior			
			Subluxation	S43.211	S43.212
			Dislocation	S43.214	S43.215
		Posterior			
			Subluxation	S43.221	S43.222
			Dislocation	S43.224	S43.225
Suprascapular nerve				G56.91	G56.92
Arthritis					
	Osteoarthritis			M19.011	M19.012
	Posttraumatic			M12.511	M12.512
Loose body				M24.011	M24.012

Figure 2   Example of a Shoulder Cheat Sheet for the International Classification of Diseases, Tenth Revision Codes. AC = acromioclavicular, MDI = multidirectional instability, SC = sternoclavicular, SLAP = superior labrum anterior to posterior. (Courtesy of Louis F. McIntyre, MD.)

Table 4

Maximum Incentive Payments Based on the First Calendar Year in Which an Eligible Professional Demonstrates Meaningful Use[a]

Calendar Year	2011	2012	2013	2014
2011	$18,000			
2012	$12,000	$18,000		
2013	$7,840 Reduction ($160)	$11,760 Reduction ($240)	$14,700 Reduction ($80)	
2014	$3,920 Reduction ($80)	$7,840 Reduction ($160)	$11,760 Reduction ($240)	$11,760 Reduction ($240)
2015	$1,960 Reduction ($40)	$3,920 Reduction ($80)	$7,840 Reduction ($160)	$7,840 Reduction ($160)
2016		$1,960 Reduction ($40)	$3,920 Reduction ($80)	$3,920 Reduction ($80)
Total	$43,720	$43,480	$38,220	$23,520

[a]A 2% reduction is applied to any Medicare electronic health record incentive payment for a reporting period that ends on or after April 1, 2013.

Adapted with permission from Centers for Medicare & Medicaid Services: Medicare and Eligible Professional's Guide to Stage 2 of the EHR Incentive Programs. February 2014. Available at: https://www.cms.gov/eHealth/downloads/eHealthU_EPsGuideStage2EHR.pdf. Accessed October 19, 2015.

and measures. It is not enough for physicians just to own a certified EHR system. Eligible professionals (EPs) have to demonstrate to the Centers for Medicare & Medicaid Services that they are using their EHRs in ways that positively affect the care of their patients. The EHR Incentive Program consists of three stages of Meaningful Use, each of which has a distinct focus: stage 1 focuses on data capture and sharing; stage 2 focuses on advanced clinical processes; and stage 3 focuses on improved outcomes.

The Meaningful Use Program began in 2011 and was designed to be implemented in three stages. Stage 1 began in 2011. Stage 2 was originally scheduled to begin in 2013 but was delayed until 2014. The Flexibility Rule allows physicians to optionally delay Stage 2 until 2015; however, a full year of attestation will be required in 2015. Stage 3 was originally scheduled to begin in 2016 but has been delayed until 2017. Interestingly, the criteria for stage 3 have yet to be finalized. The Medicare Access and Children's Health Insurance Program Act of 2015 consolidated and expanded pay-for-performance incentives within the fee-for-service system, which created the new Merit-based Incentive Payment System. Under the Merit-based Incentive Payment System, the Meaningful Use Physician Quality Reporting System, EHR Incentive Program, and Physician Value-based Payment Modifier become part of a single payment adjustment to physician payments beginning in 2019. The Meaningful Use Program offers EPs the opportunity to receive incentive payments (**Table 4**).

Stage 1 Meaningful Use Requirements

In stage 1, which took place from 2011 to 2013, EPs had to meet 20 Meaningful Use objectives in total, 15 of which were core set objectives and 5 of which were menu set objectives. EPs had to report on all core measures and only 5 of the 10 menu measures. EPs also had to report on clinical quality measures, which included three core measures or three alternate core measures, plus three additional measures from a set of 38. EPs could exclude a specific Meaningful Use objective if it was outside the scope of their practice, and the excluded objective would count the same as if it were met. For example, if 3 of the 10 menu set measures did not apply to an EP, then the EP had to meet only 2 out of the 7 that did apply.

In 2014, Meaningful Use EPs were required to attest to a total of 18 objectives, 13 of which were core objectives that all EPs were required to meet and attest to and 5 of which were menu objectives. EPs were required to meet at least five of the nine core measures and were able to defer up to four menu measures. In addition, all EPs were required to meet at least nine clinical quality measures that covered at least three National Quality Strategy domains, which include patient and family engagement, patient safety, care coordination, population and public health, efficient use of healthcare resources, and clinical processes/effectiveness.

In response to feedback from providers, the Centers for Medicare & Medicaid Services changed the 2014 stage 1 requirements. For the core objectives, the Centers for Medicare & Medicaid Services removed the requirement to provide patients with an electronic copy; removed the objective measure to report ambulatory clinical quality measures (still a requirement but no longer an objective measure); removed the requirement for the capability to exchange key clinical information electronically; added the requirement to provide patients with the ability to view, download, and transmit; and increased the age requirement for vitals to 3 years. For the menu objectives, the Centers for Medicare & Medicaid Services removed the requirement to provide patients with timely electronic access.

Stage 2 Meaningful Use Requirements

The final regulations for Meaningful Use stage 2 were published on September 4, 2014. Similar to stage 1 Meaningful Use measures, stage 2 Meaningful Use measures are split into core and menu objectives. EPs must report on all core measures but can choose the menu measures that pertain to their practice. The final rule requires EPs to attest to 17 core measures and 3 of the 6 menu measures. **Table 5** provides a description, details, and exclusions for the 17 required core objectives for Stage 2 Meaningful Use requirements. Under the final regulations, which were published in September 2014, EPs will be required to meet and attest to a full year of these measures in 2015 instead of just 90 days. The six menu objectives

from which EPs are required to meet and attest to three are listed in **Table 6**. **Table 7** lists orthopaedic-relevant clinical quality measures along with their numerator and denominator values.

Choosing Meaningful Use Measures

Physicians can only submit Meaningful Use stage 2 measures that their EHR system is certified to submit. If an EHR system is not certified to submit a specific measure, submission of that measure will not count toward Meaningful Use requirements. Some measures appear simple but may require a great deal of work. For example, the documentation of current medications in the EHR system appears simple; however, a careful analysis of wording reveals that this is not the case. The measure reads "eligible professional attests to documenting a list of current medications to the best of his/her knowledge and ability. This list must include ALL prescriptions, over-the-counter, herbals and vitamin/mineral/dietary (nutritional) supplements AND must contain the medications' name, dosages, frequency and route of administration for all visits occurring during the reporting period." In contrast, functional status assessments for total knee and hip replacements require only two assessments, one preoperative and one postoperative, for a select group of patients.

Audit Risks and Compliance Issues

There are substantial risks for those who provide inaccurate attestation. If an auditor determines that a provider did not meet the attestation requirements, the provider will receive a letter directing him or her to return the overpayment to the government within

30 days to avoid also having to pay interest. The Affordable Care Act clearly states that overpayments must be returned within 60 days of being identified; providers who fail to do so are in violation of the False Claims Act. Physicians also can be fined and penalized under the False Claims Act if false data are submitted. Regulations state that if a provider knowingly fails to meet all of the Meaningful Use requirements but attests that all requirements have been met, all Medicare and Medicaid claims paid during the period of Meaningful Use compliance are deemed a violation of the False Claims Act. It is critical that practices are compliant and accurate in EHR implementation and Meaningful Use attestation.

Summary

ICD-10 will have a profound effect after it is mandated on October 1, 2015. The expansion from 14,000 codes to more than 68,000 codes will challenge even the most organized clinicians. Concerns with regard to the transition from ICD-9 to ICD-10 include coding accuracy; a lack of efficiency for coding experts; the readiness of payers/vendors to accept ICD-10 claims; and the expense of training all healthcare providers, including coders, precerters, physicians, and administrators. In their preparation for the transition, the authors of this chapter identified several codes that do not follow the seven-character convention, most notably the osteoarthritis codes (M19). A physician's need for continual learning must now include ICD-10. The transition also challenges the creators of ICD to standardize every code to seven characters, using X placeholders in cases in which they are necessary. Although the authors of this chapter expect a substantial initial level

Table 5
Eligible Professional (EP) Meaningful Use Core Objectives

Objective No.	Description	Details	Exclusions
1	Use CPOE for medication, laboratory, and radiology orders	Use the EHR's CPOE module to enter at least 60% of medication orders, 30% of laboratory orders, and 30% of radiology orders	EPs who write <100 medication, radiology, or laboratory orders during the reporting period
2	Generate and transmit permissible prescriptions electronically	>50% of all prescriptions have to be compared with at least one drug formulary and sent electronically using a certified EHR—not by phone or fax.	EPs who write <100 prescriptions during the reporting period; or EPs who have no pharmacy that can accept electronic prescriptions within 10 miles of practice location
3	Record demographic information	Record preferred language, sex, race, ethnicity, and date of birth in the EHR for 80% of patients	There are no exclusions.
4	Record and chart changes in vital signs	Record blood pressure in the certified EHR for >80% of patients 3 years and older	EP believes vital signs are not relevant to scope of practice
		Record height and weight in the certified EHR for >80% of patients of any age	EP believes recording blood pressure is not relevant to scope of practice
			EP does not see patients 3 years or older
5	Record smoking status for patients 13 years or older	Record the smoking status for >80% of all patients who are 13 years or older	EP does not see any patients 13 years or older
6	Use clinical decision support to improve performance for high-priority health conditions	Requires certified EHRs with the ability to program clinical decision supports that can trigger alerts or clinical information with certain diagnoses or treatments. EPs must implement 5 clinical decision support rules in EHRs, if possible related to 4 or more of the clinical quality measures EPs report on, at a point in the workflow in which it can have a positive effect on patient care.	There is no exclusion for the first objective. EPs who write <100 medication orders during the reporting period are excluded from the second objective.
		Certified EHR with the ability to automatically check for potentially adverse drug-drug or drug-allergy interactions; EPs must turn this functionality on and keep it on.	
7	Provide patients with the ability to view, download, and transmit their health information	Provide >50% of patients with online access to their health information within 4 business days after the information is available to the EP	EPs who have a practice in an area with low broadband availability
		>5% of all unique patients view, download, or transmit their health information to a third party	
		EPs have to ensure that >5% their patients actually access the online health information made available.	
8	Provide clinical summaries for patients for each office visit	Provide clinical summaries to patients within 1 business day for >50% of office visits	EPs who do not conduct any office visits
9	Protect electronic health information created or maintained by certified EHR technology	Conduct or review a security risk analysis in accordance with the requirements under 45 CFR 164308(a)(1), which includes addressing the encryption/security of data at rest, implementing security updates as necessary, and correcting identified security deficiencies as part of its risk management process	There are no exclusions.

© 2016 AAOS Instructional Course Lectures, Volume 65

Table 5 *(continued)*

Objective No.	Description	Details	Exclusions
10	Incorporate clinical laboratory test results into certified EHR technology	Incorporate >55% of all clinical laboratory tests ordered by the EP during the EHR reporting period whose results are either in a positive/negative or numerical format into certified EHR technology as structured data	EPs who do not order any laboratory tests during the reporting period or no results from the tests come back as a number or as a positive/negative response
11	Generate lists of patients by specific conditions to use for quality improvement, reduction of disparities, research, or outreach	Generate at least one report listing of patients who have specific conditions that are clinically relevant or useful to the EP's practice	There are no exclusions.
12	Use clinically relevant information to identify patients who should receive reminders for preventive/follow-up care	Send a reminder, per patient preference method, to >10% of all unique patients with 2 or more office visits within the 24 months before the beginning of the EHR reporting period	EPs who have no office visits in the 24 months before the reporting period
13	Use certified EHR technology to identify patient-specific education resources	Provide >10% of all unique patients who have office visits with patient-specific education resources	EPs who have no office visits during the reporting period
14	Perform medication reconciliation	Perform medication reconciliation for >50% of transitions of care in which a patient is transitioned into the care of the EP	EPs who did not see any patients after they received care from another provider
15	Provide a summary of care record for each transition of care or referral	EPs must provide a summary of care record for >50% of transitions of care and referrals. EPs must send >10% of summary of care documents electronically, either directly to a recipient or using the eHealth exchange standards. At least one of the summary of care documents that are sent electronically must be sent to someone who is using a completely different EHR vendor or to the CMS-designated test EHR.	EPs who transfer a patient to another setting or refer a patient to another provider <100 times during the reporting period are excluded from all 3 measures.
16	Submit electronic data to immunization registries	Successful ongoing submission of electronic immunization data from a certified EHR technology to an immunization registry or immunization information system for the entire EHR reporting period	EPs who do not administer immunizations EPs who operate in a jurisdiction in which no immunization registry is capable of accepting data, provides timely information on capability to receive immunization data, or is capable of accepting data but cannot enroll any additional EPs
17	Use secure electronic messaging to communicate relevant health information with patients	>5% of patients send a secure message	EPs who have no office visits during the reporting period; or EPs who have a practice in an area with low broadband availability

CFR = Code of Federal Regulations, CMS = Centers for Medicare & Medicaid Services, CPOE = computerized provider order entry, EHR = electronic health record.

Adapted with permission from Centers for Medicare & Medicaid Services: Medicare and Eligible Professional's Guide to Stage 2 of the EHR Incentive Programs. February 2014. Available at: https://www.cms.gov/eHealth/downloads/eHealthU_EPsGuideStage2EHR.pdf. Accessed October 19, 2015.

Table 6
Eligible Professional (EP) Meaningful Use Menu Objectives

Objective No.	Description	Details	Exclusions
1	Capability to submit electronic syndrome surveillance data to public health agencies and actual submission	Successful ongoing submission of electronic surveillance data from certified EHR to public health agency for entire reporting period	EPs who do not collect ambulatory syndrome surveillance information EPs who practice in a jurisdiction in which no registry is capable of accepting data, provides timely information on capability to receive data, or is capable of accepting data but cannot enroll any additional EPs
2	Record electronic notes in patient records	At least one electronic progress note is created, edited, and signed by an EP for >30% of unique patients who have at least one office visit during the EHR reporting period. Electronic progress notes must be text-searchable; non-searchable notes do not qualify.	There are no exclusions.
3	Imaging results are accessible through EHRs	Test results must be accessible through the EHR for >10% of all tests that yield an image, either by storing the image(s) in the EHR or by making a direct link in the EHR that takes the viewer to the image(s) test result.	EPs who order <100 tests that yield an image during the reporting period; or EPs who do not have access to electronic imaging results at the start of the reporting period
4	Record patient family health history as structured data	EPs must record a structured data entry for one or more first-degree relatives for >20% of all unique patients during the EHR reporting period.	EPs who have no office visits during the reporting period
5	Capability to identify and report cancer cases to state cancer registry	Successful ongoing submission of cancer case information from certified EHR technology to a public health central cancer registry for the entire EHR reporting period	EPs who do not diagnose or directly treat cancer EPs who practice in a jurisdiction in which no cancer registry is capable of accepting data, provides timely information on capability to receive data, or is capable of accepting data but cannot enroll any additional EPs
6	Capability to identify and report specific cases to a specialized registry other than cancer registry	Successful ongoing submission of specific case information from certified EHR technology to a specialized registry for the entire EHR reporting period The specialized registry is usually associated with a specific disease and is sponsored or maintained by a national specialty society and/or a public health agency.	EPs who do not diagnose or directly treat any disease associated with a specialized registry EPs who practice in a jurisdiction in which no specialized registry is capable of accepting data, provides timely information on capability to receive data, or is capable of accepting data but cannot enroll any additional EPs

EHR = electronic health record.

Adapted with permission from Centers for Medicare & Medicaid Services: Medicare and Eligible Professional's Guide to Stage 2 of the EHR Incentive Programs. February 2014. Available at: https://www.cms.gov/eHealth/downloads/eHealthU_EPsGuideStage2EHR.pdf. Accessed October 19, 2015.

of frustration by ICD-10 users, they believe that, with some time and energy, end users can prevail.

Meaningful Use regulations were incorporated as part of the EHR Incentive Program to promote the use of certified EHR technology, with the specific goals of improving quality, safety, and efficiency; reducing health disparities; engaging patients and families; improving care coordination; and promoting public health, all while maintaining privacy and security of patient health information. To encourage adoption, financial incentives were provided

© 2016 AAOS Instructional Course Lectures, Volume 65

Table 7
Clinical Quality Measures Relevant to Orthopaedics

CMS eMeasure ID Number	NQF # (Domain)	Measure Title	Numerator	Denominator
CMS138v2	0028 (Population/public health)	Preventive Care and Screening: Tobacco Use: Screening and Cessation Intervention	Patients who were screened for tobacco use at least once within 24 months AND who received tobacco cessation counseling intervention	All patients aged 18 years and older
CMS166v3	0052 (Efficient use of healthcare resources)	Use of Imaging Studies for Low Back Pain	Patients without an imaging study conducted on the date of the outpatient or emergency department visit or in the 28 days after the outpatient or emergency department visit	Patients aged 18 to 50 years who have a diagnosis of low back pain during an outpatient or emergency department visit
CMS123v2	0056 (Clinical process/effectiveness)	Diabetes: Foot Exam	Patients who received a foot examination (visual inspection with a sensory examination and pulse examination) during the measurement period	Patients aged 18 to 75 years who have diabetes mellitus at a visit during the measurement period
CMS68v3	0419 (Patient safety)	Documentation of Current Medications in the Medical Record	EP attests to documenting a list of current medications to the best of his/her knowledge and ability. This list must include ALL prescriptions, over-the-counter medications, herbal and vitamin/mineral/dietary (nutritional) supplements AND must contain the medications' names, dosages, frequency, and route of administration.	All visits occurring during the 12 month reporting period for patients aged 18 years and older before the start of the measurement period
CMS69v2	0421 (Population/public health)	Preventive Care and Screening: BMI Screening and Follow-Up	Patients who have a documented calculated BMI during the encounter or during the previous 6 months, AND, if the BMI is outside of normal parameters, follow-up is documented during the encounter or during the previous 6 months of the encounter with the BMI outside of normal parameters	Initial patient population 1: All patients aged 65 years and older before the beginning of the measurement period with at least 1 eligible encounter during the measurement period. Patient population 2: All patients aged 18 through 64 years before the beginning of the measurement period with at least 1 eligible encounter during the measurement period
CMS139v2	0101 (Patient safety)	Falls: Screening for Future Fall Risk	Patients who were screened for future fall risk at least once within the measurement period	Patients aged 65 years and older who had a visit during the measurement period
CMS50v2	NA (Care coordination)	Closing the referral loop: Receipt of specialist report	Number of patients with a referral, for which the referring provider received a report from the provider to whom the patient was referred	Number of patients, regardless of age, who were referred by one provider to another provider and who had a visit during the measurement period
CMS66v2	NA (Patient and family engagement)	Functional status assessment for knee replacement	Patients who have patient-reported functional status assessment results not >180 days before the primary TKA procedure and at least 60 days and not >180 days after the TKA procedure	Adults, aged 18 years and older, who have a primary TKA and who had an outpatient encounter not >180 days before the procedure and at least 60 days and not >180 days after the TKA procedure

Table 7 (*continued*)
Clinical Quality Measures Relevant to Orthopaedics

CMS eMeasure ID Number	NQF # (Domain)	Measure Title	Numerator	Denominator
CMS56v2	NA (Patient and family engagement)	Functional status assessment for hip replacement	Patients who have patient-reported functional status assessment results not >180 days before the primary THA procedure and at least 60 days and not >180 days after the THA procedure	Adults, aged 18 and older, who have a primary THA and who had an outpatient encounter not >180 days before the procedure and at least 60 days and not >180 days after the THA procedure

BMI = body mass index, CMS = Centers for Medicare & Medicaid Services, EP = eligible professional, NA = not applicable, NQF = National Quality Forum, THA = total hip arthroplasty, TKA = total knee arthroplasty.

to EPs. EPs had to meet certain objectives, which were divided into three stages, to qualify. Stage 1 focused on data sharing and capture, whereas stage 2, which most providers are meeting in 2015, focuses on clinical processes. Stage 3 regulations, which have yet to be finalized, will focus on improving outcomes. Although incentives have increased provider adoption of EHR systems, some of the stated goals have not been met because of a lack of interoperability between software systems. In addition, many systems do not have streamlined workflows or data entry and are considered burdensome by providers. EHRs will truly become a meaningful tool that can be used to improve patient care and health outcomes only after their software usability and interoperability is improved to allow for efficient information sharing.

References

1. Henley MB: ICD 10: What orthopedic surgeons should know, how it will affect them and the cost of implementation? *Sports Med Arthrosc* 2013;21(3):142-147.

2. Nachimson Advisors: The impact of implementing ICD-10 on physician practices and clinical laboratories: A report to the ICD-10 coalition. Nachimson Advisors, October 8, 2008, p 6. Available at: http://www.nachimsonadvisors.com/Documents/ICD-10%20Impacts%20on%20Providers.pdf. Accessed August 10, 2015.

3. American Medical Association: ICD-10 cost estimates increased for most physicians. February 12, 2014. Available at: http://www.ama-assn.org/ama/pub/news/news/2014/2014-02-12-icd10-cost-estimates-increased-for-most-physicians.page. Accessed August 10, 2015.

4. Centers for Medicare & Medicaid Services: ICD-10. July 27, 2015. Available at: http://www.cms.hhs.gov/ICD10. Accessed October 14, 2015.

5. Centers for Disease Control and Prevention: ICD-10-CM Official Guidelines for Coding and Reporting: 2011. Available at: http://www.cdc.gov/nchs/data/icd/10cmguidelines2011_FINAL.pdf. Accessed October 14, 2015.

6. American Academy of Orthopaedic Surgeons: Practice Management Center. Available at: http://www.aaos.org/pracman. Accessed August 10, 2015.

7. Johnson K: Implementation of ICD-10: Experiences and lessons learned from a Canadian hospital. Chicago, IL, American Health Information Management Association, 2004. Available at: http://library.ahima.org/xpedio/groups/public/documents/ahima/bok3_005558.hcsp?dDocName=bok3_005558. Accessed September 3, 2015.

Understanding and Taking Control of Surgical Learning Curves

Wade T. Gofton, BScH, MD, MEd, FRCSC
Steven R. Papp, MD, MSc, FRCSC
Tyson Gofton, PhD
Paul E. Beaulé, MD, FRCSC

Abstract

As surgical techniques continue to evolve, surgeons will have to integrate new skills into their practice. A learning curve is associated with the integration of any new procedure; therefore, it is important for surgeons who are incorporating a new technique into their practice to understand what the reported learning curve might mean for them and their patients. A learning curve should not be perceived as negative because it can indicate progress; however, surgeons need to understand how to optimize the learning curve to ensure progress with minimal patient risk. It is essential for surgeons who are implementing new procedures or skills to define potential learning curves, examine how a reported learning curve may relate to an individual surgeon's in-practice learning and performance, and suggest methods in which an individual surgeon can modify his or her specific learning curve in order to optimize surgical outcomes and patient safety. A defined personal learning contract may be a practical method for surgeons to proactively manage their individual learning curve and provide evidence of their efforts to safely improve surgical practice.

Instr Course Lect 2016;65:623–632.

The field of orthopaedic surgery has dramatically changed over the past decade and continues to evolve at an ever-increasing rate as new techniques and implants are introduced. Based on the rate of medical advances, it is not unreasonable to presume that a surgeon may need to learn a completely new set of skills and procedures 10 years after graduation from a residency training program. As new procedures and less invasive techniques become popular, surgeons who want to offer these options to their patients must acquire new skillsets and technical concepts and integrate them into their practice.

Although new procedures are associated with a learning curve, the number of complications is reduced and outcomes and surgical efficiency improve as the number of procedures

Dr. W.T. Gofton or an immediate family member is a member of a speakers' bureau or has made paid presentations on behalf of Bayer; serves as a paid consultant to or is an employee of MicroPort and Zimmer; and has received nonincome support (such as equipment or services), commercially derived honoraria, or other non–research–related funding (such as paid travel) from Synthes. Dr. Papp or an immediate family member is a member of a speakers' bureau or has made paid presentations on behalf of Stryker, and has received research or institutional support from Synthes. Dr. Beaulé or an immediate family member has received royalties from Corin USA and MicroPort; is a member of a speakers' bureau or has made paid presentations on behalf of Medacta International and Smith & Nephew; serves as a paid consultant to or is an employee of Corin USA, DePuy, Medacta International, and Smith & Nephew; and has received research or institutional support from Corin USA and DePuy. Neither Dr. T. Gofton nor any immediate family member has received anything of value from or has stock or stock options held in a commercial company or institution related directly or indirectly to the subject of this chapter.

performed increases.[1-4] The importance of the surgical learning curve is highlighted in a study by Lekawa et al[5] that described the authors' transition from open to laparoscopic cholecystectomy procedures. The authors found that complication rates were higher with the new laparoscopic technique until surgeons became more proficient. The field of orthopaedic surgery witnessed a similar experience on a smaller scale with the shift to minimally invasive procedures.[6-8]

Although the orthopaedic literature often focuses on the outcomes of a particular procedure, studies are increasingly reporting on the learning curve for a particular procedure. A review of PubMed citations reveals a steady increase in the number of orthopaedic surgery articles published during the past 10 years that directly refer to the learning curve. These articles review the early complication rates and the decrease in surgical efficiency that are associated with a new technique.[9-16] Recent literature reports that even small changes in practices, such as the use of a new implant, can be associated with model-specific learning curves and a higher risk for revision surgery.[17,18]

The authors of this chapter believe that learning curves should not be viewed as uniformly negative because learning is required for surgical techniques to progress. However, it is important for surgeons who are considering incorporating a particular technique into their practice to understand what the reported learning curve might mean and how it may affect patient outcomes. Surgeons who understand learning curves will be able to find the most effective strategies to advantageously manage them, thereby optimizing surgical outcomes and patient safety.

Defining a Surgical Learning Curve

A learning curve is based on the notion that "if one had the means, there would be quantitative measure of 'skill' which if displayed on a chart would show a continuous and elegant geometric curve describing the learning process."[19] There is a fairly clear consensus that a positive correlation exists between the number of surgical procedures a surgeon performs and patient outcomes.[2-4] It also is recognized that many complex new procedures are associated with a learning curve, and that as surgeon experience increases, surgical time decreases,[20-24] the complication rate is lowered,[14,20,22-25] and there are fewer conversions to the standard procedure.[20,23,24] Defining a learning curve for a specific procedure, however, remains a difficult task.

A surgical learning curve represents the association between a surgeon's proficiency with a procedure and the number of times he or she has performed that procedure. The point at which the curve begins to plateau represents the number of procedures that a surgeon needs to perform in order to be proficient enough to independently complete the procedure with a reasonable outcome. The concept of applying learning curves to surgical practice gained popularity as the surgical community attempted to develop threshold numbers that indicated acceptable levels of competence.

Wakefield[26] describes the learning process as "a relatively permanent change in behavior based on an individual's interactional experience with its environment." Although theorists often disagree about what the learning process is, they agree that its effects are cumulative and, therefore, able to be plotted as a curve. A surgical learning curve is a graphic representation of the relationship between a surgeon's experience with a procedure and an outcome variable, which usually is a performance characteristic of clinical interest, such as surgical time.[27] One axis usually represents the number of procedures performed, and the other axis usually represents the number of complications or operating room time. Operating room time is the most commonly used proxy for surgical efficiency. A key element of learning is that it produces a permanent change in an individual's capacity to perform an action (cognitive or psychomotor). Because learning involves the assimilation and retention of knowledge and skills, a curve that only tracks performance against several procedures, but not performance over time, may not sufficiently demonstrate learning.

Orthopaedic studies that review learning curves for a particular procedure generally report improvement in an individual surgeon's performance over time, which demonstrates a degree of skill permanence, and can, therefore, be interpreted as surgical learning curves. The general shape of surgical learning curves is similar to the performance curve described in general motor skills literature[27-29] (**Figure 1**). There are three main features of a learning curve: the starting point, which identifies the initial performance level of a surgeon; the rate of learning, which measures how quickly a surgeon's proficiency improves; and the asymptote or expert level, which is the point at which a surgeon's performance plateaus[30,31] (**Figure 2**). Whether the curve resembles an uphill climb or a downhill slide depends on which variables are mapped to the x and y axes.

Regardless of the axis selected, the shape of a learning curve has several common features (**Figure 2**). The beginning of the curve is relatively flat (phase 1) until an understanding of the concepts and information is acquired. The curve then rises rapidly with early experience (phase 2)[32,33] and plateaus after information is understood and performance is optimized (phase 3). Surgical learning curves tend to have a relatively short phase 1, which may be because experienced surgeons have a background of transferable knowledge and experience, or because surgeons have been trained in or exposed to the procedure in a setting outside of the operating room.

Complex or problematic procedures are often described as having a steep learning curve; however, a learning curve with a steep slope implies a rapid gain in proficiency with a small number of cases or over a short period of time. A procedure with a steep learning curve, therefore, is ideal because only a small number of patients may be exposed to the risks associated with phases 1 and 2. A procedure with a flatter learning curve implies that more cases are required before a surgeon achieves proficiency and is of greater concern for patient safety. This confusion likely developed as the definition of a learning curve has been modified to indicate the amount of effort required for an individual to achieve an appropriate knowledge level within a specific period of time. In discussing learning curves, the colloquial usage of the term "steep" often conveys an assessment of how much effort may be required to achieve surgical expertise.

Because surgical learning curves cannot be precisely measured, they rely on a variety of proxies for learning, such

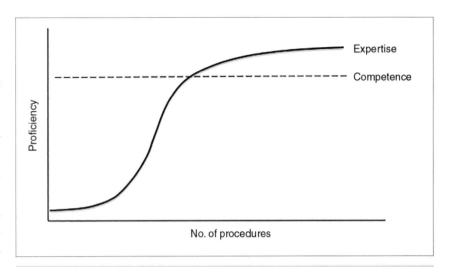

Figure 1 Illustration of a performance curve shows that proficiency improves as the number of procedures (experience) increases and that as experience increases, competence and expertise can be achieved.

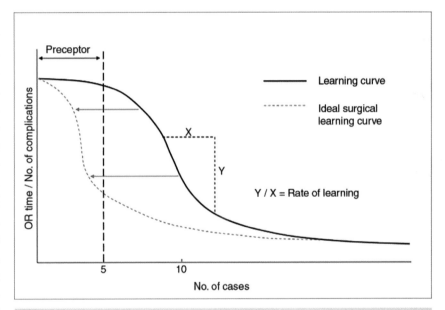

Figure 2 Illustration of a learning curve shows that operating room (OR) time and the number of complications per case generally decrease as the number of cases (experience) increases. The learning curve can be optimized through the presence of a preceptor, who, by providing technical tips, protects the patient from complications that can occur during the early learning phase. (Reproduced from Murnaghan JJ, Hutchison C, Moreau G, Gofton W: Themes: The learning curve and the practicing surgeon. Integrating a new skill/procedure into your practice. *COA Bulletin* Fall 2012;98.)

as surgical time, blood loss, or complication rates; however, learning curves may not be comparable in the absence of a unified measure of surgical proficiency. Because it is expected that a

surgeon's performance will improve as he or she learns, operating room time is often used as a proxy for successful case completion (**Figure 2**). Although operating room time may appear too

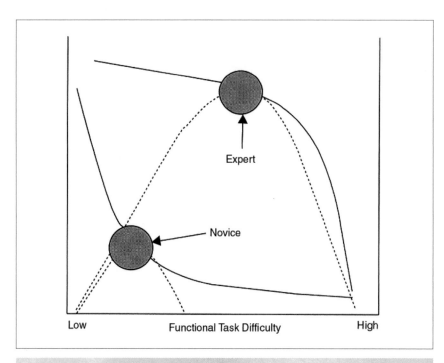

Expert

Novice

Low   Functional Task Difficulty   High

Figure 3 Illustration depicts the relationship between the learning curves (dashed lines), the performance curves (solid lines), and the optimal challenge points (shaded circles) for two performers who have different skill levels as functional task difficulty increases. (Adapted with permission from Guadagnoli MA, Lee TD: Challenge point: A framework for conceptualizing the effects of various practice conditions in motor learning. *J Mot Behav* 2004;36[2]: 212-224.)

blunt a tool to serve as a reliable marker of learning, surgical learning curves for declining surgical time and complication rates are similar.[34] This suggests that increased familiarity with a task increases a surgeon's competency and, therefore, increases speed and decreases errors.[27] Sammon et al[35] have reported that total procedure time may be a relatively reliable indicator of an individual surgeon's location on the learning curve.

Generalizing a Surgical Learning Curve

The surgical literature frequently defines a surgical learning curve as a statistically significant improvement in an individual surgeon's operating room time or a decrease in an individual surgeon's complication rate with procedure volume.[36,37] Unfortunately, it is difficult to translate an individual surgeon's experience to the expected learning outcomes for other surgeons. Performance and learning curves are specific to an individual because the overall shape of an individual surgeon's learning curve may depend on his or her experience, motivation, equipment, team available, or other factors. An individual surgeon's learning curve can provide a heuristic for other surgeons but not a prediction of a generalized learning curve.

Some evidence in the literature suggests that the shape of a learning curve varies for each individual learner and task,[22,24,32,38] a phenomenon that has been recognized in psychology literature with respect to motor skills learning.[28,32] In a study of the effects of task (procedure) difficulty and performer (surgeon) skill level on motor learning, Guadagnoli and Lee[39] introduced the concept of the "challenge point framework." The authors suggest that any specific task carries a nominal level of task difficulty, and that functional task difficulty refers to how challenging a task is relative to the skill level of the performer and to the conditions under which the task is being performed.[39] Surgical performance will decrease with more difficult procedures; however, because of the higher functional task difficulty, this decrease is more substantial for less skilled and less experienced surgeons (**Figure 3**). Learning curves, therefore, should be expected to vary with respect to both functional task difficulty and the level of each surgeon's skills and experience.

In addition, Guadagnoli and Lee[39] suggest that "learning is directly related to the information available and interpretable in a performance instance, which in turn, is tied to the functional difficulty of the task." In other words, although a new procedure represents a certain amount of new information that must be assimilated, the amount learned is dependent on the surgeon and his or her previous experience. For example, a surgeon who has experience with the posterior approach for total hip arthroplasty (THA) is familiar with the principles of arthroplasty and, perhaps the approach itself, thereby making the aspects of a new technique (eg, anterior approach for THA) more easily interpretable and, thus, easier to assimilate. A surgeon who has substantial experience in procedures related to the anterior approach for THA is likely to learn a great deal in the first case or two, after which the slope of the learning curve will decrease because he or she is learning less with each successive case. A new procedure (eg, anterior approach for THA) represents a high level of functional task difficulty for a surgeon who is less familiar with hip arthroplasty; therefore, much of the information available to be learned may not be initially understood. Because less interpretable information is available to the relatively inexperienced surgeon, less information can be assimilated in a single procedure. Accordingly, the learning curve is flatter and more attempts are required to reach the same final level of proficiency. As a result, surgeons who have different backgrounds and skillsets will likely demonstrate substantially different learning curves for the same procedure.

Although it is difficult to interpret and generalize learning curves, it may be useful to evaluate the growing body of learning curve studies before integrating a new surgical procedure. The experience of another surgeon may provide an informal guideline for the number of cases required to reliably perform a procedure with minimal complications. Surgeons reviewing the literature, however, must be aware that a reported learning curve for a particular technique may substantially differ from their own learning curve.

To be able to more accurately extrapolate how their own learning curve may differ from a learning curve reported in a study, surgeons need to be able to make a baseline comparison between their own skills and experience and those of the reported surgeon. It would be valuable for authors who report surgical learning curves to provide an indication of their experience with similar procedures; this would give the reader a preliminary tool with which he or she could calibrate their own expected

learning curve. For example, an author who is reporting on his or her learning curve for a minimally invasive posterior approach for THA would afford value to the reader by providing the approximate number of hip arthroplasties he or she performs per year and his or her experience (surgical time, blood loss, complication rate, etc.) with a classic posterior approach for THA. Functional task difficulty would be anticipated to be substantially reduced for an experienced surgeon who moves from the classic posterior approach to a minimally invasive posterior approach as opposed to a surgeon who is experienced with the anterior or lateral approaches, with limited expertise in the posterior approach, and moves to a minimally invasive posterior approach. By providing comparative benchmarks for similar or related procedures, reported surgical learning curves can be more readily extrapolated to individual learning curves. Comparative benchmarks may also make it easier to anticipate the functional task difficulty relative to other procedures.

With respect to functional task difficulty, it is important for surgeons to determine if a particular surgical learning curve represents a consecutive series of patients or a carefully selected group of patients who were considered ideal for the procedure and how this may relate to their own patient population. Surgeons also should consider how frequently they will perform a new surgical procedure. Although it is not clear what the ideal practice or performance frequency would be for an experienced surgeon, too long of a period between procedures is suboptimal for maximizing the slope of the learning curve. A surgeon also must consider his or her resources relative to those of

the surgeon or surgeons whose results are presented in a published study. The availability of a dedicated assistant, a nursing team, or equipment required for the procedure may all have substantial effects on individual learning curves and outcomes.[14,40] Studies that present an aggregated learning curve from several surgeons at different institutions will better reflect the range of surgical learning curves associated with a particular procedure.

Modifying a Surgical Learning Curve

Every surgeon attempts to minimize potential complications for his or her patients. The Department of Health's response to a public inquiry of the pediatric surgical unit at the Bristol Royal Infirmary was that in these patients, surgery should not be performed by surgeons during the early phase of their learning curves.[41] This ideal presents a challenge for the practicing physician who wants to update or improve his or her skills in order to provide optimal patient care while maintaining an active surgical practice.

Surgeons must continually assess the advantages and disadvantages of new surgical approaches or procedures and the value of these advances to patients. Although a procedure may be beneficial to patients overall, several first patients will inevitably be included in phases 1 and 2 of the learning curve. Because of the risks involved in phases 1 and 2 of the learning curve, "it is the duty of the surgeons embracing a new technique not only to disclose the issue of learning curve to their patients, but also to take concrete steps to reduce the risk to patients."[42]

Fortunately, there are many ways for surgeons to manage the learning curve. Training courses led by surgical experts can help improve the technical understanding of a new procedure and minimize the number of cases in phase 1 of the learning curve. Courses that include manual training are able to enhance learning because they provide surgeons with more information to evaluate, understand, and assimilate. Although bench-top simulation and high-fidelity virtual simulation with haptic feedback are improving and have demonstrated good transfer of learned skills to the operating room for some specialties,[43-46] they have only been available for arthroscopic procedures and remain in the early stages of validation for the field of orthopaedic surgery.[47] Some orthopaedic courses use cadaver model studies to provide a more realistic haptic simulation, but because this form of simulation is expensive, the number of learning opportunities for each surgeon is limited. Ultimately, there is no substitute for the operating room, and there will always be a first live patient for any new procedure or technique.

Some surgical experts are willing to provide interested surgeons a site visit and mini-preceptorship for certain procedures, but because of hospital certification and insurance concerns, there often is little opportunity for manual training. Nevertheless, the learning surgeon is able to observe the expert's tips and tricks for safely and efficiently completing the procedure. Some surgical experts may be willing to visit a learning surgeon's institution to assist in the first few cases that take place during the crucial phase 1 of the learning curve. According to classic learning theory, a performer in the early stages of learning a processing system is too inefficient to manage multiple new information points.[48] The surgical preceptor is able to modify the learning curve in favor of both the patient and the learning surgeon by providing a form of cognitive apprenticeship, which is the combined process of simultaneously teaching a craft and strategic thinking[49-53] (**Figure 2**).

Surgeons who modify their surgical routine to obtain more intraoperative information are able to check their work in real time and can ensure an ideal outcome for a new procedure. For example, an aid, such as intraoperative fluoroscopy, can be a useful adjunct for establishing surgical familiarity with a new minimally invasive technique in which visualization may be decreased. Taking an intraoperative radiograph during a total hip replacement (if a surgeon does not routinely take an intraoperative radiograph during a total hip replacement) is another example of a useful double check.

A practicing surgeon can proactively manage his or her individual learning curve by developing a personal learning contract. Personal learning contracts allow surgeons to consider their options for learning new techniques, educating their team on the techniques, and safely integrating the techniques into practice. To develop a learning contract, a surgeon must consider his or her learning needs for the new procedure. The surgeon must then determine the available learning resources or strategies to address the defined learning needs, and, ideally, establish a timeline to complete his or her goals.[54,55] The surgeon should then focus on completing his or her specified objectives (eg, attend a course, perform a cadaver model study, or observe an expert). Because evaluation is a key element of a learning contract, the surgeon should assess his or her progress.[55] This can be done by reviewing the learning contract and progress with an expert, who functions as a learning mentor. It also can be accomplished by defining outcomes and other metrics that can be collected to demonstrate learning and the safe implementation of the new procedure into practice.[55] A learning contract is valuable because it demonstrates a well-thought-out process for safely learning a new procedure and provides benchmarks and evidence of attained learning objectives in the absence of a formal certification process.

Developing standards and best practices to manage the learning curves of practicing surgeons is an ongoing process. To be successful, standards must not place a burden on surgeons who only want to ensure the best care for their patients. Surgeons must work to improve knowledge transfer among one another, especially in the early phase of the learning curve. Professions that emphasize managing the learning curve, the aviation industry in particular, are subject to substantial regulation and oversight by the government, industry, and professional bodies. Although a degree of regulation is important to ensure that a technique or technology is safe for use and able to be safely used by more than just the designing surgeon, regulation and oversight of individual practicing surgeons may not be appropriate.[56] Accordingly, it is important for the profession to develop and disseminate standards, tools, and best practices for managing learning curves.

To make resources more readily available and to decrease risk in the early phases of the learning curve, surgeons may be encouraged to seek support from associated industry partners (ie, implant manufacturers). Surgeons who are identified as appropriate instructors can help develop cognitive apprenticeship or preceptorship programs. In addition, hospitals must be encouraged to allow visiting learning surgeons or preceptors to maximize real-world learning opportunities in the operating room.

Summary

Orthopaedic surgeons must not simply accept poor outcomes as part of a surgical learning curve.[19,57] Because learning is necessary for surgical advancements, which ultimately benefit patients, a learning curve for a new procedure should not be seen as negative. Instead, surgeons need to understand and manage learning curves to be able to optimize surgical outcomes and minimize complications.

The literature that outlines the learning curves associated with newly introduced orthopaedic techniques provides important insight for surgeons who are considering integrating these new techniques into their practices. Surgeons, however, must understand that learning curves may differ dramatically for each individual surgeon. Therefore, a surgeon must take into account his or her experience, patient population, and available resources that may be relative to the author of a study. Authors can facilitate this process by providing an outline of their experience (performance of similar techniques, approaches, or approximate case volume).

Surgeons who want to introduce a new technique in their practice should consider using peer resources at courses or in organized preceptorships as strategies to optimize the learning curve in their favor. A learning contract can help surgeons outline a safe approach to a new procedure while maximizing learning and patient safety. A learning contract also can be used to demonstrate a safe and complete training program for a new procedure.

Acknowledgments

The authors of this chapter wish to thank Dr. Carol Hutchinson, Dr. John J. Murnaghan, and Dr. Guy Moreau for their contributions to the 2012 Canadian Orthopaedic Association Annual Meeting symposium on the learning curve in orthopaedic surgery.

References

1. Bridgewater B, Grayson AD, Au J, et al: Improving mortality of coronary surgery over first four years of independent practice: Retrospective examination of prospectively collected data from 15 surgeons. *BMJ* 2004;329(7463):421.

2. Cowan JA Jr, Dimick JB, Leveque JC, Thompson BG, Upchurch GR Jr, Hoff JT: The impact of provider volume on mortality after intracranial tumor resection. *Neurosurgery* 2003;52(1):48-54.

3. Hammond JW, Queale WS, Kim TK, McFarland EG: Surgeon experience and clinical and economic outcomes for shoulder arthroplasty. *J Bone Joint Surg Am* 2003;85(12):2318-2324.

4. Katz JN, Losina E, Barrett J, et al: Association between hospital and surgeon procedure volume and outcomes of total hip replacement in the United States Medicare population. *J Bone Joint Surg Am* 2001;83(11):1622-1629.

5. Lekawa M, Shapiro SJ, Gordon LA, Rothbart J, Hiatt JR: The laparoscopic learning curve. *Surg Laparosc Endosc* 1995;5(6):455-458.

6. Bal BS, Haltom D, Aleto T, Barrett M: Early complications of primary total hip replacement performed with a two-incision minimally invasive technique. *J Bone Joint Surg Am* 2005;87(11):2432-2438.

7. Woolson ST, Mow CS, Syquia JF, Lannin JV, Schurman DJ: Comparison of primary total hip replacements performed with a standard incision or a mini-incision. *J Bone Joint Surg Am* 2004;86(7):1353-1358.

8. Archibeck MJ, White RE Jr: Learning curve for the two-incision total hip replacement. *Clin Orthop Relat Res* 2004;429:232-238.

9. Berry DJ: "Minimally invasive" total hip arthroplasty. *J Bone Joint Surg Am* 2005;87(4):699-700.

10. Berry DJ, Berger RA, Callaghan JJ, et al: Minimally invasive total hip arthroplasty: Development, early results, and a critical analysis. Presented at the Annual Meeting of the American Orthopaedic Association, Charleston, South Carolina, USA, June 14, 2003. *J Bone Joint Surg Am* 2003;85(11):2235-2246.

11. Laffosse JM, Chiron P, Accadbled F, Molinier F, Tricoire JL, Puget J: Learning curve for a modified Watson-Jones minimally invasive approach in primary total hip replacement: Analysis of complications and early results versus the standard-incision posterior approach. *Acta Orthop Belg* 2006;72(6):693-701.

12. Bjorgul K, Novicoff WM, Saleh KJ: Learning curves in hip fracture surgery. *Int Orthop* 2011;35(1):113-119.

13. Kempton LB, Ankerson E, Wiater JM: A complication-based learning curve from 200 reverse shoulder arthroplasties. *Clin Orthop Relat Res* 2011;469(9):2496-2504.

14. Nunley RM, Zhu J, Brooks PJ, et al: The learning curve for adopting hip resurfacing among hip specialists. *Clin Orthop Relat Res* 2010;468(2):382-391.

15. Benoit B, Gofton W, Beaulé PE: Hueter anterior approach for hip resurfacing: Assessment of the learning curve. *Orthop Clin North Am* 2009;40(3):357-363.

16. Hoppe DJ, de Sa D, Simunovic N, et al: The learning curve for hip arthroscopy: A systematic review. *Arthroscopy* 2014;30(3):389-397.

17. Peltola M, Malmivaara A, Paavola M: Learning curve for new technology? A nationwide register-based study of 46,363 total knee arthroplasties. *J Bone Joint Surg Am* 2013;95(23):2097-2103.

18. Peltola M, Malmivaara A, Paavola M: Hip prosthesis introduction and early revision risk: A nationwide population-based study covering 39,125 operations. *Acta Orthop* 2013;84(1):25-31.

19. Gallivan S: Paper No. 572: Report to the British Royal Infirmary Inquiry. Learning curves in relation to surgery: A discussion paper. London, United Kingdom, University College London, 2000.

20. Meehan JJ, Georgeson KE: The learning curve associated with laparoscopic antireflux surgery in infants and children. *J Pediatr Surg* 1997;32(3):426-429.

21. Poulin EC, Mamazza J: Laparoscopic splenectomy: Lessons from the learning curve. *Can J Surg* 1998;41(1):28-36.

22. Watson DI, Baigrie RJ, Jamieson GG: A learning curve for laparoscopic fundoplication: Definable, avoidable, or a waste of time? *Ann Surg* 1996;224(2):198-203.

23. Cagir B, Rangraj M, Maffuci L, Herz BL: The learning curve for laparoscopic cholecystectomy. *J Laparoendosc Surg* 1994;4(6):419-427.

24. Soot SJ, Eshraghi N, Farahmand M, Sheppard BC, Deveney CW: Transition from open to laparoscopic fundoplication: The learning curve. *Arch Surg* 1999;134(3):278-282.

25. Kreder HJ, Deyo RA, Koepsell T, Swiontkowski MF, Kreuter W: Relationship between the volume of total hip replacements performed by providers and the rates of postoperative complications in the state of Washington. *J Bone Joint Surg Am* 1997;79(4):485-494.

26. Wakefield JF: *Educational Psychology: Learning to be a Problem Solver.* Boston, MA, Houghton Mifflin, 1996.

27. Rogers DA, Elstein AS, Bordage G: Improving continuing medical education for surgical techniques: Applying the lessons learned in the first decade of minimal access surgery. *Ann Surg* 2001;233(2):159-166.

28. Magill R: *Motor Learning: Concepts and Applications.* Dubuque, IA, WC Brown, 1993.

29. Schmidt RA: *Motor Learning and Performance: From Principles to Practice.* Champaign, IL, Human Kinetics, 1991.

30. Cook JA, Ramsay CR, Fayers P: Statistical evaluation of learning curve effects in surgical trials. *Clin Trials* 2004;1(5):421-427.

31. Raja RJ: The impact of the learning curve in laparoscopic surgery. *World Journal of Laparoscopic Surgery* 2008;1(1):56-59.

32. Lane NE: *Skill Acquisition Rates and Patterns: Issues and Training Implications.* New York, NY, Springer-Verlag, 1987.

33. Ohlsson S: Learning from performance errors. *Psychol Rev* 1996;103(2):241-262.

34. Davis JW, Kreaden US, Gabbert J, Thomas R: Learning curve assessment of robot-assisted radical prostatectomy compared with open-surgery controls from the premier perspective database. *J Endourol* 2014;28(2):560-566.

35. Sammon J, Perry A, Beaule L, Kinkead T, Clark D, Hansen M: Robot-assisted radical prostatectomy: Learning rate analysis as an objective measure of the acquisition of surgical skill. *BJU Int* 2010;106(6):855-860.

36. Hopper AN, Jamison MH, Lewis WG: Learning curves in surgical practice. *Postgrad Med J* 2007;83(986):777-779.

37. Ramsay CR, Wallace SA, Garthwaite PH, Monk AF, Russell IT, Grant AM: Assessing the learning curve effect in health technologies: Lessons from the nonclinical literature. *Int J Technol Assess Health Care* 2002;18(1):1-10.

38. Meinke AK, Kossuth T: What is the learning curve for laparoscopic appendectomy? *Surg Endosc* 1994;8(5):371-376.

39. Guadagnoli MA, Lee TD: Challenge point: A framework for conceptualizing the effects of various practice conditions in motor learning. *J Mot Behav* 2004;36(2):212-224.

40. Cobb JP, Kannan V, Brust K, Thevendran G: Navigation reduces the learning curve in resurfacing total hip arthroplasty. *Clin Orthop Relat Res* 2007;463:90-97.

41. Department of Health: Learning from Bristol: The Department of Health's response to the report of the Public Inquiry into children's heart surgery at the Bristol Royal Infirmary 1984-1995. London, United Kingdom, The Stationary Office, January 2002.

42. Duwelius PJ, Parvizi J, Matsen Ko L: New technology: Safety, efficacy, and learning curves. *Clin Orthop Relat Res* 2014;472(4):1080-1085.

43. Anastakis DJ, Regehr G, Reznick RK, et al: Assessment of technical skills transfer from the bench training model to the human model. *Am J Surg* 1999;177(2):167-170.

44. Sturm LP, Windsor JA, Cosman PH, Cregan P, Hewett PJ, Maddern GJ: A systematic review of skills transfer after surgical simulation training. *Ann Surg* 2008;248(2):166-179.

45. Seymour NE: VR to OR: A review of the evidence that virtual reality simulation improves operating room performance. *World J Surg* 2008;32(2):182-188.

46. Stelzer MK, Abdel MP, Sloan MP, Gould JC: Dry lab practice leads to improved laparoscopic performance in the operating room. *J Surg Res* 2009;154(1):163-166.

47. Pedowitz RA, Esch J, Snyder S: Evaluation of a virtual reality simulator for arthroscopy skills development. *Arthroscopy* 2002;18(6):E29.

48. Sweller J: Cognitive load during problem solving: Effects on learning. *Cognitive Science* 1988;12(2):257-285.

49. Coleman MG, Hanna GB, Kennedy R; National Training Programme Lapco: The National Training Programme for Laparoscopic Colorectal Surgery in England: A new training paradigm. *Colorectal Dis* 2011;13(6):614-616.

50. Adams JA: A closed-loop theory of motor learning. *J Mot Behav* 1971;3(2):111-149.

51. Fitts PM, Posner MI: *Human Performance.* Belmont, CA, Brooks-Cole, 1967.

52. Miller GA: The magical number seven plus or minus two: Some limits on our capacity for processing information. *Psychol Rev* 1956;63(2):81-97.

53. Miskovic D, Wyles SM, Ni M, Darzi AW, Hanna GB: Systematic review

on mentoring and simulation in laparoscopic colorectal surgery. *Ann Surg* 2010;252(6):943-951.

54. Knowles MS: *Using Learning Contracts.* San Francisco, CA, Jossey-Bass, 1986.

55. Hesketh EA, Laidlaw JM: Learning contracts. Edinburgh, Scotland, NHS Education for Scotland, 2007.

56. McCulloch P, Altman DG, Campbell WB, et al: No surgical innovation without evaluation: The IDEAL recommendations. *Lancet* 2009;374(9695):1105-1112.

57. Treasure T: The learning curve. *BMJ* 2004;329(7463):424.

What Do Reported Learning Curves Mean for Orthopaedic Surgeons?

Wade T. Gofton, BScH, MD, MEd, FRCSC
Michael Solomon, MBChB, FRACS (Orth)
Tyson Gofton, PhD
Alex Pagé, MD, FRCSC
Paul R. Kim, MD, FRCSC
Caleb Netting, MD
Mohit Bhandari, MD, PhD, FRCSC
Paul E. Beaulé, MD, FRCSC

Abstract

Practicing orthopaedic surgeons must assess the effects of the learning curve on patient safety and surgical outcomes if a new implant, technique, or approach is being considered; however, it remains unclear how learning curves reported in the literature should be interpreted and to what extent their results can be generalized. Learning curve reports from other surgical specialties and from orthopaedic surgery can be analyzed to identify the strengths and weaknesses of learning curve reporting. Single-surgeon series and registry data can be analyzed to understand learning challenges and to develop a personalized learning plan. Learning curve reports from single-surgeon series have several limitations that result from the limited dataset reported and inconsistencies in the way data are reported. Conversely, learning curve reports from registry data are likely to have greater generalizability, but are largely beneficial retrospectively, after data from a sufficient number of surgeons are assessed. There is a pressing need for surgeons to develop improved and consistent standards for learning curve reporting. Although registry data may provide better prospective measures in the future, the implementation of such registries faces several challenges. Despite substantial limitations, single-surgeon series remain the most effective way for practicing surgeons to assess their learning challenge and develop an appropriate learning plan.

Instr Course Lect 2016;65:633–644.

As new surgical procedures emerge, practicing orthopaedic surgeons must carefully assess the challenges of learning a new technique, approach, or implant. Although innovations are implemented to improve patient care, the increased surgical time and compromised surgical outcomes that may occur during the early phases of the learning curve can be hazardous for patients. The learning curve presents a dilemma for the practicing surgeon: the failure to adopt new techniques denies patients the benefit of meaningful surgical advances; however, the perils of the learning curve are inescapable.[1]

Surgeons and physicians have a professional duty to understand the implications of the learning curve with respect to the health and safety of patients and to minimize its effect on patient care, especially during the early phases of learning. Surgeons should examine learning curve reports to determine when and how surgical innovations should be integrated into their practice. Learning curve reports from other surgical specialties and from orthopaedic surgery can be analyzed to understand the substantial features and complicating factors of learning curves. Single-surgeon series and registry data also can be analyzed to understand learning challenges and to develop a personalized learning plan. Although both single-surgeon series and registry data may be useful tools to decide whether to integrate a new technique, approach, or implant into surgical practice, improved and standardized methods for collecting, reporting, and assessing surgical learning curves need to be developed.

Learning Curves in Other Surgical Specialties

For general surgery, the introduction of laparoscopic cholecystectomy resulted in an unprecedented complication rate.[2,3] The substantial rise in complications led general surgeons to focus on surgical education, especially continuing medical education. The authors of this chapter conducted a nonsystematic PubMed review and identified 928 surgical articles with a focus on the surgical learning curve that were published in the past 15 years, with 127 articles that

were published in the past year alone. What can orthopaedic surgeons learn from the experience of other surgical specialties?

Surgical learning curves typically have a flat "S" shape, regardless whether they are rising or falling. An initial plateau (phase 1) represents the early phase of learning in which learning cues are not well understood and skills develop more slowly. A steeper section (phase 2) represents the phase in which learning cues are better understood and skills are rapidly acquired. Finally, a second plateau (phase 3) represents the phase in which the technique has been well-learned and learning has become incremental. Many surgeons use the term "steep" to describe the learning curve of a challenging procedure; however, a steep curve implies a rapid gain in proficiency and suggests that more information is learned per case. A steep curve is ideal because only a small number of patients are exposed to the increased risk of complications that are associated with the early stages (phases 1 and 2) of learning.[4]

Although many people may assume that individual surgeons and techniques would have substantially different learning curves, there appears to be a certain amount of generalizability in the number of cases required for surgeons

to attain proficiency. For practicing surgeons, the minimum threshold number for essential competence has been suggested to be 40 cases.[5-8] In a study on the learning curve of laparoscopic-assisted distal gastrectomy in patients who had gastric cancer, Hu et al[5] reported that there was a significant decrease in surgical time after the first 40 cases. In a study on the learning curve of endoscopic surgery in patients who had pituitary adenomas, Chi et al[6] reported that the effectiveness of the procedure increased and both the surgical time and postoperative hospital stay decreased after the first 40 cases. Similarly, Silva et al[7] reported that 40 cases were required before surgeons attained proficiency in less invasive approaches for transforaminal lumbar interbody fusion. Similar minimum threshold numbers have been reported for hip arthroplasty (Kevin James Rasuli, MD; Cai Wadden, MD, FRCSC; Richard Lee, BHSc; Jonathan Peck, MD; Tyson Gofton, PhD; Wade Gofton, MD, MEd, FRCSC, Ottawa, Canada, unpublished data, 2014).[8]

The introduction of robotic-assisted surgery has led to more research on learning curves. Although the surgical procedure or approach for robotic-assisted surgery is generally unchanged, the robotic assist presents the learning challenge. In a study on the learning curve of robotic-assisted gastric bypass surgery, Bindal et al[9] reported that after 100 robotic-assisted procedures, surgical time decreased from 216 minutes to 120.9 minutes. Other specialties that have integrated robotic-assisted surgery, such as urology and obstetrics-gynecology, have reported that the number of cases required for surgeons to attain proficiency may be less than 40.[10] In a study on the learning curve

Dr. W.T. Gofton or an immediate family member is a member of a speakers' bureau or has made paid presentations on behalf of Bayer; serves as a paid consultant to or is an employee of MicroPort and Zimmer; and has received nonincome support (such as equipment or services), commercially derived honoraria, or other non-research–related funding (such as paid travel) from Synthes. Dr. Solomon or an immediate family member serves as a paid consultant to or is an employee of Corin USA, Medacta International, and Smith & Nephew. Dr. Kim or an immediate family member serves as a paid consultant to or is an employee of Stryker. Dr. Bhandari or an immediate family member serves as a paid consultant to or is an employee of Amgen, Eli Lilly, Stryker, Smith & Nephew, Zimmer, Moximed, and Bioventus; and has received research or institutional support from Smith & Nephew, DePuy, Eli Lilly, and Bioventus. Dr. Beaulé or an immediate family member has received royalties from Corin USA and MicroPort; is a member of a speakers' bureau or has made paid presentations on behalf of Medacta International and Smith & Nephew; serves as a paid consultant to or is an employee of Corin USA, DePuy, Medacta International, and Smith & Nephew; and has received research or institutional support from Corin USA and DePuy. None of the following authors nor any immediate family member has received anything of value from or has stock or stock options held in a commercial company or institution related directly or indirectly to the subject of this chapter: Dr. T. Gofton, Dr. Pagé, and Dr. Netting.

of robotic-assisted radical prostatectomy, Sammon et al[11] reported that only 25 cases were required for surgeons to attain proficiency. Sammon et al[11] is one of the few studies that assessed more than one surgeon and demonstrated that the learning curves were similar for all three surgeons in the group. Single-surgical site studies may reflect the role of the surgical team in the learning curve; however, further assessment on the importance of surgical teams with respect to learning curves is required.

Although it is not yet clear to what extent surgical learning curves are generalizable, several substantial questions have been raised. In a systemic review of the surgical literature, Ramsay et al[12] reported that surgical time was the most commonly used proxy for surgeon progression in 272 articles that focused on learning curves. Although Darzi et al[13] found surgical time as a proxy for surgeon progression as crude, de Leval et al[14] found it to be at least as good as other measures, such as hand-motion efficiency or the assessment of near misses. Ramsay et al[12] reported that most of the articles reviewed (60%) attempted to demonstrate learning by splitting consecutive series into groups. The authors found that there often was little rationale for the cut points made between the groups, which raised a potential bias for retrospective data-dependent splitting. Moreover, unless the splits were small enough, the groupings may have failed to define an underlying learning curve. Ramsay et al[12] also reported that some articles attempted to demonstrate learning with a univariate test for trend using learning curve fitting procedures. The authors found that these articles often failed to define the rationale for the approach selected, yet frequently defined the curve

as linear, which was likely a reflection of inadequate sampling. The authors reported that a few articles used a cumulative sum analysis, which has been advocated as a method for monitoring surgical performance.[12] Although a systematic study of the recent literature is required to confirm the findings of Ramsay et al,[12] a nonsystematic review of the current literature clearly shows that there are still no consistent standards for learning curve reporting.

Most learning curve reports focus on a single surgeon's experience (case series) and assess the complication profile or the improvement in surgical time with respect to the number of cases.[12] This type of learning curve report has three inherent weaknesses. First, it is difficult to determine the point at which the surgeon is located on the learning curve because there is no comparison with other surgeons. Second, it may be difficult to determine a relationship between surgeon experience and patient complications if complications are infrequent.[12] Moreover, the actual learning challenge may be underestimated if a surgeon carefully selects lower-risk patients in the early parts of the learning curve (phase 1). Third, this type of learning curve report typically relies on retrospective data, which may introduce a reporting bias.[12] Concerns with regard to single-surgeon series are magnified by the fact that most surgeons who report learning curve results are subspecialists with extensive training or focused high-volume practices. The literature clearly demonstrates that increased surgical case volume and increased years of practice are associated with improved performance,[15] which suggests that reported learning curves may underrepresent the learning challenge for other surgeons. Learning

curves may also be confounded to some extent by the skills of the residents or fellows in training if the series takes place at a training center.

Standard measures, such as surgical time, blood loss, and complication rate, may not be effective predictors of favorable clinical outcomes. In a study on the learning curve for conversion from open to robotic-assisted laparoscopic surgery, Thompson et al[16] used a variety of quality-of-life scores and surgical margins in addition to surgical time as a proxy for surgical learning. The authors reported that the initial robotic-assisted surgery results were inferior to the initial open surgery results, with reduced quality of life scores and reduced negative surgical margins.[16] Although robotic-assisted surgery results were superior to open surgery results after a plateau was achieved, the learning curve was long (>300 cases) for this high-volume surgeon. Although many individuals assume that a learning plateau is achieved within 100 cases or within a few years, a recent systematic review by Maruthappu et al[15] suggests that substantial variation exists between individual surgeons with respect to the time it takes to master a procedure. The authors suggest that, depending on the type of procedure performed and the type of evaluation outcomes used, it may take 1 to 15 years or 25 to 750 cases to master a procedure. These findings are not surgeon or technique specific.[15] Because of the wide variation that exists between procedures and outcomes, it may be preferable to assess learning with a surgeon's risk-adjusted patient outcome rather than other proxies, such as the number of cases or surgical time.[15] Maruthappu et al[15] clearly demonstrate that not only surgical time, but also patient outcomes, may be compromised by the learning curve. The authors' findings highlight the need for the prospective monitoring of learning curves and the development of approaches to minimize the effects of the learning curve on patient outcomes.

Vickers[17] noted that the variations within a surgeon's cases and between surgeons' cases may exceed any effects that surgeons might reasonably expect from a novel drug. It has been asked whether it is appropriate for surgeons to take on the challenges of a new procedure if their traditional outcomes are acceptable.[16] Nevertheless, some surgical advances can substantially improve patient outcomes. The careful management of learning curves, including the development of interventions to help surgeons in the early phases of the learning curve or if persistent errors in technique or judgment arise,[17] is required to maintain a balance between patient safety and advances in surgical practice. To empower individual surgeons to optimize patient outcomes, improved and standardized methods for the collection and assessment of surgical outcomes in learning curve reporting must be developed.

Learning Curves in Orthopaedic Surgery

The increased interest in learning curves also is apparent in orthopaedics, with 58 articles with a focus on learning curves published in the past 15 years, 14 of which were published in 2014. Most orthopaedic subspecialties are represented to varying degrees in this literature. Similar to other surgical specialties, reported learning curves in orthopaedic surgery face several systemic limitations.

In a systematic review of the learning curve for minimally invasive spine surgery, Sclafani and Kim[18] reported a postoperative complication rate of 11% and suggested that the learning curve associated with most techniques was overcome for surgical time and complications after 20 to 30 consecutive cases. In a prospective review of the first 100 hip arthroscopies performed by a single surgeon, Konan et al[19] divided patients into three groups based on the order in which they were treated by the surgeon and recorded surgical times and patient satisfaction. The authors proposed a learning curve of 30 cases, with a 40% decrease in surgical time after the first 30 cases. The authors reported that the complication rates were similar to the 1% complication rate generally reported for hip arthroscopy. In a systematic review of the literature for hip arthroscopy, Hoppe et al[20] identified six articles that reported learning curves; only one article reported a bona fide learning curve, and the remainder reported dichotomous split-group comparisons. Hoppe et al[20] reported that only one article[21] used patient-important outcomes, such as patient satisfaction and validated functional scores. This study, by Lee et al,[21] reported improvement in all outcomes and identified 30 cases as the minimum threshold number; however, the systematic review by Hoppe et al[20] did not find sufficient evidence to quantify the learning curve or validate 30 cases as the minimum threshold number for hip arthroscopy. In a study of 73 patients who underwent periacetabular osteotomies, Peters et al[22] reported that nine of the ten major complications occurred in the first 30 cases.

There is marked variability in the learning curves for total joint arthroplasty. In a multicenter study of 1,152 patients who had total hip arthroplasty with the anterior approach, Sprague et al[23] reported that surgeons who performed more than 100 hip procedures per year had lower overall complication rates, which is consistent with the learning curves reported for conventional total hip arthroplasty. Seng et al[24] defined 40 cases as a potential minimum threshold number for high-volume joint surgeons. In the experience of the authors of this chapter, 40 cases also appears to be an important minimum threshold number, at least with respect to measures of surgical time and complications. In a more recent study, Lee et al[25] used cumulative sum analysis to assess if a learning curve exists for optimal acetabular cup orientation. The authors reported that the learning curve for two separate surgeons was less than 50 cases. Similar to general surgery studies, orthopaedic studies also have indicated that surgeon experience and case volume are clearly linked to lower complication rates and decreased surgical time.[26-28] The functional task difficulty is lower for an experienced, high-volume surgeon, which results in a shorter learning curve.[29] Zhang et al[27] reported that surgeons who perform fewer than 15 to 50 Oxford unicompartmental knee arthroplasties per year have a higher complication rate and lower implant survivorship, which suggests that the learning plateau is unlikely to be consistently maintained for surgeons who do not have a sufficient case volume.

Peltola et al[30,31] recently reported that learning curves are not just associated with new techniques, but also with new implants. The authors used the Finnish Arthroplasty Register to examine the survival of various implants after their implementation. The authors reported that simply switching the type of implant used may be associated with a longer learning curve. By comparing the risk of revision for the first 15 cases (phase 1) with the risk of revision after 100 cases (phase 3), the authors were able to assess the hazard ratio of new implants. The authors reported that hazard ratios appear to be implant specific.

Single-Surgeon Series

A single-surgeon series is the method most frequently used to report surgical learning curves. The authors of this chapter carefully monitored the learning curves of three surgeons who incorporated new skills into their practice.

Surgeon A, who learned the anterior Hueter approach for total hip arthroplasty in 2006, was planning to implement the anterior Hueter approach for hip resurfacing. This surgeon had a focused hip practice, had primarily used the lateral or posterior approach for total hip arthroplasty, and had used trochanteric slide osteotomy for more than 200 hip resurfacings. Before Surgeon A began using the anterior Hueter approach for hip resurfacing, a surgeon who was experienced with the approach was invited to lead a cadaver model training experience for 1 week and to assist Surgeon A in the operating room with the first few cases. After initiating the approach, Surgeon A visited, at two different times, two different surgical experts who had experience with the anterior Hueter approach. The authors of this chapter compared Surgeon A's early outcomes for hip resurfacing via the anterior Hueter approach with the outcomes for 50 matched trochanteric slide cases.[8] Surgeon A had a substantial

decrease in surgical time during the first 50 cases via the anterior approach, and a plateau was achieved after 40 cases. The only substantial difference between the two groups was that the proportion of acetabular components with an abduction angle between 45° and 55° was 38% in the anterior Hueter approach group and 16% in the trochanteric slide group.

The authors of this chapter also examined the learning curves of the direct anterior approach for total hip arthroplasty for Surgeon A and another surgeon (Surgeon B). A review of the first 200 cases demonstrated that more complications were apparent early in the learning curve. Some complications, such as two femoral canal perforations and five early infections that were likely related to longer surgical times or less effective soft-tissue preservation, were clearly related to the new technique. Other complications were more likely associated with the implants (two stem loosenings and five failures with a monoblock metal-on-metal total hip) or random events (one deep vein thrombosis and one iliac wing fracture after a fall). In total, there were 22 complications (11%): six (3%) were intraoperative, seven (3.5%) occurred in the 8-week postoperative period and did not need revision surgery, and nine (4.5%) required revision surgery for complications that occurred at a later date. The authors of this chapter attributed some of the cases that required revision surgery to implant design rather than to the surgical approach used. It was difficult for the authors of this chapter to define a surgical learning curve based on the complication rates for these first 200 cases; however, after the authors of this chapter differentiated the complications that were likely associated with

the surgical technique from those that were not, it was clear that complications most commonly occurred in the early learning phase. This may have been more evident if component alignment, specifically, stem alignment and canal fit/fill, was examined. The authors of this chapter note that this case series represents results from an academic center, which is apparent in a review of the learning curves for both surgeons. Both learning curves show a degree of improvement in surgical time relative to the first case; however, later cases in the series often took longer than early cases. The authors of this chapter attributed this change to an increased role of trainees in the procedure.

Another surgeon's (Surgeon C) learning curve was monitored during the transition from a direct lateral approach for total hip arthroplasty to a tissue-sparing posterior approach for total hip arthroplasty. As anticipated, initial surgical times for the tissue-sparing posterior approach were longer than those for the direct lateral approach. Surgical times for the tissue-sparing posterior approach decreased with respect to the case number and became equivalent between cases 40 to 45. Although there was a decrease in surgical time over the first 10 cases, there was an increase in surgical time after Surgeon C made a site visit with a surgical expert on the tissue-sparing posterior approach. The site visit was considered an intervention that altered Surgeon C's understanding of cues, which increased the information available to be learned.

Surgeon C subsequently converted to supercapsular percutaneously-assisted total hip arthroplasty, a tissue-sparing posterior approach that uses a more superior interval. Surgeon C anticipated a relatively short learning curve given that the new approach presented a comparatively minor change in approach. Despite only a small change in approach and the use of intraoperative radiographs, the authors of this chapter noted that the acetabular cups were more anteverted in Surgeon C's first 25 cases. This issue was corrected after it was identified, and Surgeon C's next 25 cases demonstrated more normal acetabular alignment. Surgeon C's correction of the anteverted acetabular cups demonstrates the value of the early review of outcomes, even if a new approach has a low estimated learning challenge. Although the surgical times for supercapsular percutaneously-assisted total hip arthroplasty were shorter than those for the tissue-sparing posterior approach for total hip arthroplasty, the authors of this chapter found that the surgical times for supercapsular percutaneously-assisted total hip arthroplasty were still decreasing after case 50, which suggests that Surgeon C had not yet reached a plateau in the learning curve. Although a shorter learning curve was anticipated for supercapsular percutaneously-assisted total hip arthroplasty, the actual learning curve was longer based on surgical time, which suggests that supercapsular percutaneously-assisted total hip arthroplasty may have subtle cues that are more challenging to understand and learn than those for the tissue-sparing posterior approach for total hip arthroplasty. The complication profile for both approaches was favorable compared with the complication profile for a previous series of 50 consecutive cases performed by Surgeon C with the use of a Hardinge approach for total hip arthroplasty and 50 concurrent cases performed by another surgeon, who worked in the same surgical unit as Surgeon C, with the use of a Hardinge

approach for total hip arthroplasty (Kevin James Rasuli, MD; Cai Wadden, MD, FRCSC; Richard Lee, BHSc; Jonathan Peck, MD; Tyson Gofton, PhD; Wade Gofton, MD, MEd, FRCSC, Ottawa, Canada, unpublished data, 2014).

Surgeons A, B, and C used a variety of tools to improve their individual learning curves. Surgeon A used a site visit, introduced intraoperative radiographs into the procedure, and brought a surgical expert into the operating room to assist with the first four cases to control the early learning curve. The presence of a surgical expert on site makes surgical cues or case-specific nuances more identifiable and understandable, which allows more information to be learned and exposes fewer patients to the risks associated with the early stages of learning. Surgeon C used site visits, practiced with hands-on cadaver models in the local skills laboratory, and introduced routine intraoperative radiographs into the procedure to control the early learning curve.

The authors of this chapter believe their findings are similar to those reported in the literature. Surgical time increased with the introduction of a new technique and decreased with experience. Although a general plateau was observed between 40 and 50 cases, this was not a consistent threshold, even for a single surgeon (Surgeon C). The experience of the authors of this chapter with single-surgeon series demonstrates how a variety of factors can substantially affect standard measures of surgical outcomes, such as surgical time, complication rate, and component placement. For example, strategies to minimize patient risk during the early phases of the learning curve (assistance of an expert or increased intraoperative imaging) may negatively affect surgical

time, but may also limit complications and optimize the number of cases to proficiency. The results of the authors of this chapter illustrate the challenge of accurately reporting the learning curve of a new procedure.

The results of the authors of this chapter for the Hueter, the tissue-sparing posterior, and the supercapsular percutaneously assisted approaches were all single-surgeon series reviews, which limits the generalizability of the learning curves. Although reporting on an individual surgeon's experience with a new procedure, including longer than expected surgical times, changes in surgical times after a surgical expert site visit, and the introduction of intraoperative imaging or changes in component placement, may not be generalizable, it may make reported learning curves more helpful. Surgeons who are contemplating a new approach may be better able to assess their individual learning challenge and make an appropriate learning plan to minimize patient risk during the early stages of the learning curve after they review a report on another surgeon's experience with the same procedure.

Similar to most of the literature on learning curves, the authors of this chapter acknowledge that their data could be improved by including patient-important outcomes, which may better represent improvements in surgical proficiency rather than decreases in surgical time or complication rates. The use of prospective data collection, patient-important outcomes or survivorship, and multisurgeon data could provide surgeons with more robust, generalizable data to assess the safety and challenges associated with a new procedure and strategies to potentially minimize patient risk during the early learning phase.

Table 1

Cumulative Percent Revision of Primary Total Conventional Hip Replacement by Surgeon Experience (Primary Diagnosis: Osteoarthritis)

Surgeon Experience (Years)	N Revised	N Total	1 Year (95% CI)	3 Years (95% CI)	5 Years (95% CI)	7 Years (95% CI)
<3	121	4,306	1.8 (1.4-2.2)	2.7 (2.2-3.3)	4.4 (3.5-5.5)	5.3 (4.1-6.9)
3–7	565	17,243	1.6 (1.4-1.8)	3.2 (2.9-3.5)	5.0 (4.5-5.5)	6.5 (5.9-7.2)
≥8	2,821	93,936	1.4 (1.3-1.5)	2.6 (2.5-2.8)	4.0 (3.9-4.2)	5.4 (5.2-5.7)
Total	3,507	115,485				

CI = confidence interval.

Adapted with permission from the Australian Orthopaedic Association National Joint Replacement Registry: Annual Report: Hip and Knee Arthroplasty. September 1999 to December 2012. Adelaide, Australia, Australian Orthopaedic Association, 2013.

Learning Curves and Registry Data

Increasingly robust national registries are being used to provide more generalizable and accessible information about the outcomes of implants, and, more recently, the effectiveness of surgical techniques.[32] Registry data also have the potential to provide insight into learning curves for new techniques.[30,31] Peltola et al demonstrated how registry data can be used to examine learning curves for total hip[30] and knee[31] implants. Some individuals question if registry data are more informative or more useful than single-surgeon series. Some surgeons have resisted the use of registry data because they fear that it may be used to establish normative outcome reporting for surgeons, which unfairly targets those surgeons in the lower part of the distribution; however, the identification of positive deviance from median outcomes may provide surgeons with valuable clues to improve learning curves and should not be neglected.

The Australian Orthopaedic Association (AOA) dedicated a chapter in their 2013 annual report to the effects of surgeon experience on the revision rate for hip and knee replacement surgery. The AOA recognized the need to establish a National Joint Replacement Registry (NJRR) in 1993 and began collecting data in 1999. The purpose of the AOA NJRR is to define, improve, and maintain the quality of care for individuals who have joint replacement surgery. The AOA believes this can be achieved through the collection of a defined minimum dataset that enables outcomes to be determined based on patient characteristics, prosthesis type and features, method of prosthesis fixation, and surgical technique used. The principal outcome measure that the AOA NJRR uses is time to first revision surgery. Studies of the AOA NJRR data have shown that surgeons who averaged more than 70 procedures per year had the lowest rate of revision surgery for both primary total hip and knee replacement procedures.[33] This finding is consistent with the literature from nonregistry sources, which demonstrates a lower revision rate for higher volume surgeons.[26,28,34] The AOA NJRR reported that the effects of surgical volume varied depending on

the type of prosthesis used. The AOA NJRR also reported variation between individual surgeons who averaged the same number of procedures per year, which was attributed to the type of prosthesis selected; however, another undeniable factor is that different surgeons will have different outcomes.

Studies of registry data have demonstrated that hip revision rates also are related to surgeon experience. Surgeons who have less than 3 years of training also have the highest revision rate, particularly in their first 12 months of practice, which suggests a substantial learning curve; however, the effects of surgeon experience are less evident if the whole 3-year period is evaluated. The AOA NJRR 2013 Annual Report noted that revision rates for surgeons who had less than 3 years of experience were approximately equivalent to revision rates for surgeons who had 3 to 7 years of experience (**Table 1**);[33] however, both groups had higher revision rates than surgeons who had more than 8 years of experience (**Figure 1**).[33] Similar findings were noted for total knee arthroplasty: surgeons with more than 8 years of experience had the lowest

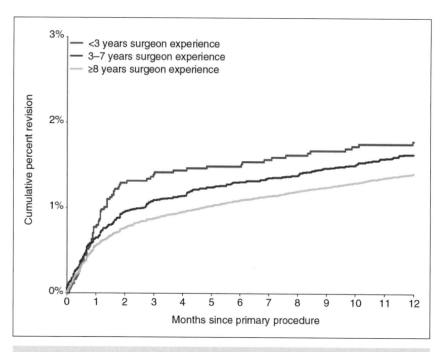

Figure 1 Graph illustrates 1-year cumulative percent revision of primary total conventional hip replacement by surgeon experience (primary diagnosis osteoarthritis). Hazard ratio (HR) is adjusted for age and sex. <3 years surgeon experience vs ≥8 years surgeon experience—0 to 2 weeks: HR = 0.99 (95% confidence interval [CI], 0.54-1.82), P = 0.984; 2 weeks to 3 months: HR = 1.81 (95% CI, 1.35-2.43), P < 0.001; more than 3 months: HR = 0.81 (95% CI, 0.63-1.04), P = 0.104. 3 to 7 years surgeon experience vs ≥8 years surgeon experience—0 to 2 weeks: HR = 1.25 (95% CI, 0.94-1.68), P = 0.126; 2 weeks to 1 month: HR = 1.07 (95% CI, 0.81-1.43), P = 0.625; more than 1 month: HR = 1.20 (95% CI, 1.09-1.33), P < 0.001. <3 years surgeon experience vs 3 to 7 years surgeon experience—0 to 2 weeks: HR = 0.79 (95% CI, 0.42-1.51), P = 0.481; 2 weeks to 3 months: HR = 1.59 (95% CI, 1.16-2.17), P = 0.003; more than 3 months: HR = 0.67 (95% CI, 0.52-0.88), P = 0.003. (Adapted with permission from the Australian Orthopaedic Association National Joint Replacement Registry: Annual Report: Hip and Knee Arthroplasty. September 1999 to December 2012. Adelaide, Australia, Australian Orthopaedic Association, 2013.)

revision rates, followed by surgeons with 3 to 7 years of experience, and surgeons with less than 3 years of experience had the highest revision rate.[33]

The AOA NJRR has not collected data on surgical approaches used for hip replacement surgery, but will in the future. However, a unique opportunity arose for one of the authors of this chapter (M.S.) to review the results of the Quadra-H/Versafit hip implant combination (Medacta International). Because 95% of all Quadra/Versafit hip implant combinations from Medacta

International are inserted with the use of the direct anterior approach, (Michael Solomon, MBChB, FRACS (Orth), Sydney, New South Wales, Australia, unpublished company data from formal letter, 2015) the results of the Quadra-H/Versafit hip implant combination would allow the author (M.S.) to study the effects of the direct anterior approach for hip arthroplasty on revision rates. The direct anterior approach for hip arthroplasty became popular after Medacta International introduced the leg holder technique in

2007. The author (M.S.) submitted a formal request to the AOA NJRR that asked them to extrapolate the results of the Quadra-H/Versafit hip implant combination. The AOA NJRR provided the author (M.S.) with a detailed analysis of the Quadra-H/Versafit hip implant combination's revision rate since its introduction in Australia. The analysis included total conventional hip procedures performed from June 2007 up to and including December 31, 2013; the Quadra-H/Versafit hip implant combination was used for patients who had a primary diagnosis of osteoarthritis. Sixty-eight surgeons used the Quadra-H/Versafit hip implant combination, which suggests that the procedures were done via a direct anterior approach (Medacta International, Castel San Pietro, Switzerland, unpublished company data, 2014). Fifteen surgeons used the Quadra-H/Versafit hip implant combination only once, 50% of the surgeons performed 14 surgeries or less with the Quadra-H/Versafit hip implant combination, 27 surgeons performed at least 50 procedures with the Quadra-H/Versafit hip implant combination, and 13 surgeons performed at least 100 procedures with the Quadra-H/Versafit hip implant combination. The yearly cumulative revision rate confirmed that surgeons who performed more than 50 procedures per year with the Quadra-H/Versafit hip implant combination had a lower revision rate compared with surgeons who performed less than 50 procedures per year with the Quadra-H/Versafit hip implant combination. Moreover, lower case volume correlated with higher revision rates (**Table 2**).

Surgeons who started using the direct anterior approach between 2007 and 2010 had a lower revision rate

Table 2

Yearly Cumulative Percent Revision of Quadra-H/Versafit Total Conventional Hip Replacement by Operation Group[a]

No. of Operations	1 Year (95% CI)	2 Years (95% CI)	3 Years (95% CI)	4 Years (95% CI)	5 Years (95% CI)
1–15	3.4 (2.2-5.1)	3.9 (2.7-5.8)	5.9 (4.2-8.4)	5.9 (4.2-8.4)	5.9 (4.2-8.4)
16–30	2.8 (1.6-4.7)	2.8 (1.6-4.7)	3.2 (1.9- 5.4)	3.2 (1.9-5.4)	3.2 (1.9-5.4)
31–50	2.6 (1.5-4.3)	3.7 (2.3-6.0)	4.7 (3.0-7.5)	4.7 (3.0-7.5)	NA
51–100	1.6 (1.0-2.7)	1.8 (1.1-3.0)	2.5 (1.5-4.2)	3.1 (1.8-5.5)	NA
>100	0.9 (0.6-1.4)	1.3 (0.9-2.0)	1.8 (1.2-2.7)	1.8 (1.2-2.7)	NA

CI = confidence interval, NA = not available.

[a]Unpublished data from Medacta International, Castel San Pietro, Switzerland, 2014 and Michael Solomon, MBChB, FRACS (Orth), Sydney, New South Wales, Australia, 2014.

compared with surgeons who started using the direct anterior approach between 2011 and 2014 (Medacta International, Castel San Pietro, Switzerland, unpublished company data, 2014 and Michael Solomon, MBChB, FRACS (Orth), Sydney, New South Wales, Australia, unpublished data, 2014). The detailed analysis showed that between 2007 and 2010, 22.5% of surgeons using the direct anterior approach had less than 5 years of experience, and 65% of surgeons using the direct anterior approach had more than 10 years of experience. Between 2011 and 2014, 48% of surgeons using the direct anterior approach had less than 5 years of experience, and 38% of surgeons using the direct anterior approach had more than 10 years of experience. It can be concluded that the introduction of a new technique creates a learning curve effect that reflects both the experience of the surgeon (measured in years since qualifying) and the number of procedures performed.

Learning curve reports that are based on registry data are more generalizable and may be more fair comparisons for less subspecialized surgeons to either gauge their outcomes against or predict what their learning curve may look like. Registries have the potential to provide more fine-grained details, which would allow surgeons to compare their learning against an average. Prospective data from many surgeons and institutions could be a valuable resource for the assessment of learning curves and surgical outcomes for new approaches and techniques. Concerns have been raised with respect to who can access registry data and how the data will be used. Even if data in registries are anonymized, individual surgeons and patients may be readily identified, which raises issues related to patient privacy and surgeon liability. The creation and maintenance of registries also is a substantial logistical and financial challenge.[12] To preserve the integrity of registry databases and

the willingness of surgeons to participate in data collection, access to and the reporting of registry data remains limited. Changes in legislation and innovations in technology may mitigate some of these concerns and lead to the wider use of registry data.

Summary

Reports of surgical outcomes, despite their substantial generalizability, are subject to a variety of limitations that may not be explicitly accounted for in any given study. Reported surgical times and other measures of surgical effectiveness, such as blood loss, incision length, or complication rate, may vary between individual surgeons and procedures and may be affected by the presence and participation of trainees or by component implant variation. Reported surgical times and other measures of surgical effectiveness also are subject to variations between sequential case series and case series in which the patient pool has been carefully selected.

Moreover, if compared with patient-important measures, many learning curves may underreport the number of cases that are required to meet or exceed the outcomes achieved with a previous procedure.

The aims of single-surgeon series and registry data are complementary. Single-surgeon series provide a fine-grained sense of the learning process for a new technique, approach, or implant, but sacrifice some of the generalizability of the reported learning curve. Registry data, which draw on the results from a variety of surgeons in a variety of surgical settings, may provide more generalizable results, but are limited by the type of data collected by the registry. Single-surgeon series can be reported either by the developers of the technique, approach, or implant or by other early adopters. Registry data can only provide generality after substantial uptake has occurred.

Reports of single-surgeon series are most useful if they provide fine-grained details on the reporting surgeon's training, surgical experience, learning program, and surgical setting. Single-surgeon series may be thought of as guidelines for estimating the learning challenge and formulating an effective learning plan for a new technique, approach, or implant if little other data are available. Single-surgeon series may be most useful for subspecialists at academic centers and other early adopters, but may be less suited to providing accurate predictions of patient risks in a broader context.

Registry data are most useful if they report on the widest variety of surgeons in the widest variety of surgical settings. Registry data may help provide accurate and generalizable assessments of the relative merits of different techniques,

approaches, and implants and may even provide more fine-grained data on which techniques, approaches, and implants are suited to what types of patients. Although registry data have substantial promise, conclusions drawn from registry data are dependent on the wide uptake of both reporting and the reported data. Registry studies may be best suited for retrospective reporting on comparative benefits after sufficient data have been collected. Concerns with respect to the access and use of registry data will need to be addressed before studies of registry data become commonplace.

Currently, single-surgeon series provide the most practical tool for assessing the learning curves of new procedures. Although the generalizability of such studies may be questioned, these concerns can be mitigated to some extent by multicenter studies[23] or reports from independent surgeons that validate initial results.[26] In all cases, a carefully considered learning plan that includes site visits or expert preceptorships is essential for the ongoing effort to reduce the effects of the surgical learning curve on patient safety and surgical outcomes.

Acknowledgments

Michael Solomon would like to acknowledge the AOA NJRR for their outstanding service to orthopaedics and for providing him with additional data to present on the learning curve effect, especially with respect to the direct anterior approach for hip arthroplasty.

References

1. Gawande A: *Complications: A Surgeon's Notes on an Imperfect Science.* New York, NY, Picador, 2003.

2. Lekawa M, Shapiro SJ, Gordon LA, Rothbart J, Hiatt JR: The laparoscopic learning curve. *Surg Laparosc Endosc* 1995;5(6):455-458.

3. Cuschieri A: Whither minimal access surgery: Tribulations and expectations. *Am J Surg* 1995;169(1):9-19.

4. Gofton WT, Papp SR, Gofton T, Beaulé PE: Understanding and taking control of surgical learning curves. *Instr Course Lect* 2016;65:623-631.

5. Hu WG, Ma JJ, Zang L, et al: Learning curve and long-term outcomes of laparoscopy-assisted distal gastrectomy for gastric cancer. *J Laparoendosc Adv Surg Tech A* 2014;24(7):487-492.

6. Chi F, Wang Y, Lin Y, Ge J, Qiu Y, Guo L: A learning curve of endoscopic transsphenoidal surgery for pituitary adenoma. *J Craniofac Surg* 2013;24(6):2064-2067.

7. Silva PS, Pereira P, Monteiro P, Silva PA, Vaz R: Learning curve and complications of minimally invasive transforaminal lumbar interbody fusion. *Neurosurg Focus* 2013;35(2):E7.

8. Benoit B, Gofton W, Beaulé PE: Hueter anterior approach for hip resurfacing: Assessment of the learning curve. *Orthop Clin North Am* 2009;40(3):357-363.

9. Bindal V, Gonzalez-Heredia R, Masrur M, Elli EF: Technique evolution, learning curve, and outcomes of 200 robot-assisted gastric bypass procedures: A 5-year experience. *Obes Surg* 2015;25(6):997-1002.

10. Paek J, Kim SW, Lee SH, et al: Learning curve and surgical outcome for single-port access total laparoscopic hysterectomy in 100 consecutive cases. *Gynecol Obstet Invest* 2011;72(4):227-233.

11. Sammon J, Perry A, Beaule L, Kinkead T, Clark D, Hansen M: Robot-assisted radical prostatectomy: Learning rate analysis as an objective measure of the acquisition of surgical skill. *BJU Int* 2010;106(6):855-860.

12. Ramsay CR, Wallace SA, Garthwaite PH, Monk AF, Russell IT, Grant AM: Assessing the learning curve effect in health technologies: Lessons from the nonclinical literature. *Int J Technol Assess Health Care* 2002;18(1):1-10.

© 2016 AAOS Instructional Course Lectures, Volume 65

13. Darzi A, Smith S, Taffinder N: Assessing operative skill: Needs to become more objective. *BMJ* 1999;318(7188):887-888.

14. de Leval MR, François K, Bull C, Brawn W, Spiegelhalter D: Analysis of a cluster of surgical failures: Application to a series of neonatal arterial switch operations. *J Thorac Cardiovasc Surg* 1994;107(3):914-924.

15. Maruthappu M, Gilbert BJ, El-Harasis MA, et al: The influence of volume and experience on individual surgical performance: A systematic review. *Ann Surg* 2015;261(4):642-647.

16. Thompson JE, Egger S, Böhm M, et al: Superior quality of life and improved surgical margins are achievable with robotic radical prostatectomy after a long learning curve: A prospective single-surgeon study of 1552 consecutive cases. *Eur Urol* 2014;65(3):521-531.

17. Vickers AJ: What are the implications of the surgical learning curve? *Eur Urol* 2014;65(3):532-533.

18. Sclafani JA, Kim CW: Complications associated with the initial learning curve of minimally invasive spine surgery: A systematic review. *Clin Orthop Relat Res* 2014;472(6):1711-1717.

19. Konan S, Rhee SJ, Haddad FS: Hip arthroscopy: Analysis of a single surgeon's learning experience. *J Bone Joint Surg Am* 2011;93(suppl 2):52-56.

20. Hoppe DJ, de Sa D, Simunovic N, et al: The learning curve for hip arthroscopy: A systematic review. *Arthroscopy* 2014;30(3):389-397.

21. Lee YK, Ha YC, Hwang DS, Koo KH: Learning curve of basic hip arthroscopy technique: CUSUM analysis. *Knee Surg Sports Traumatol Arthrosc* 2013;21(8):1940-1944.

22. Peters CL, Erickson JA, Hines JL: Early results of the Bernese periacetabular osteotomy: The learning curve at an academic medical center. *J Bone Joint Surg Am* 2006;88(9):1920-1926.

23. Sprague S, Matta JM, Bhandari M, et al: Multicenter collaboration in observational research: Improving generalizability and efficiency. *J Bone Joint Surg Am* 2009;91(suppl 3):80-86.

24. Seng BE, Berend KR, Ajluni AF, Lombardi AV Jr: Anterior-supine minimally invasive total hip arthroplasty: Defining the learning curve. *Orthop Clin North Am* 2009;40(3):343-350.

25. Lee YK, Biau DJ, Yoon BH, Kim TY, Ha YC, Koo KH: Learning curve of acetabular cup positioning in total hip arthroplasty using a cumulative summation test for learning curve (LC-CUSUM). *J Arthroplasty* 2014;29(3):586-589.

26. Manley M, Ong K, Lau E, Kurtz SM: Effect of volume on total hip arthroplasty revision rates in the United States Medicare population. *J Bone Joint Surg Am* 2008;90(11):2446-2451.

27. Zhang Q, Zhang Q, Guo W, et al: The learning curve for minimally invasive Oxford phase 3 unicompartmental knee arthroplasty: Cumulative summation test for learning curve (LC-CUSUM). *J Orthop Surg Res* 2014;9:81.

28. Shervin M, Rubash HE, Katz JN: Orthopaedic procedure volume and patient outcomes: A systematic literature review. *Clin Orthop Relat Res* 2007;457:35-41.

29. Guadagnoli MA, Lee TD: Challenge point: A framework for conceptualizing the effects of various practice conditions in motor learning. *J Mot Behav* 2004;36(2):212-224.

30. Peltola M, Malmivaara A, Paavola M: Hip prosthesis introduction and early revision risk: A nationwide population-based study covering 39,125 operations. *Acta Orthop* 2013;84(1):25-31.

31. Peltola M, Malmivaara A, Paavola M: Learning curve for new technology? A nationwide register-based study of 46,363 total knee arthroplasties. *J Bone Joint Surg Am* 2013;95(23):2097-2103.

32. Herberts P, Malchau H: Long-term registration has improved the quality of hip replacement: A review of the Swedish THR Register comparing 160,000 cases. *Acta Orthop Scand* 2000;71(2):111-121.

33. Australian Orthopaedic Association National Joint Replacement Registry: Annual Report: Hip and Knee Arthroplasty. September 1999 to December 2012. Adelaide, Australia, Australian Orthopaedic Association, 2013. Available at: aoanjrr.dmac.adelaide.edu.au/en/annual-reports-2013. Accessed August 17, 2015.

34. Katz JN, Losina E, Barrett J, et al: Association between hospital and surgeon procedure volume and outcomes of total hip replacement in the United States Medicare population. *J Bone Joint Surg Am* 2001;83(11):1622-1629.

Social Media and Orthopaedics: Opportunities and Challenges

Tanishq Suryavanshi
C. David Geier Jr, MD
J. Martin Leland III, MD
Lance Silverman, MD
Naven Duggal, MD

Abstract

Social media presents unique opportunities and challenges for practicing orthopaedic surgeons. Social media, such as blogging, Facebook, and Twitter, provides orthopaedic surgeons with a new and innovative way to communicate with patients and colleagues. Social media may be a way for orthopaedic surgeons to enhance communication with patients and healthcare populations; however, orthopaedic surgeons must recognize the limitations of social media and the pitfalls of increased connectedness in patient care.

Instr Course Lect 2016;65:645–654.

The first implementation of the Internet, which is referred to as Web 1.0, was an industry-produced unidirectional passage of information from the Internet to the consumer.[1] Internet-based healthcare services used this same principle, with their primary purpose being to provide information to patients. This unidirectional passage of information is currently being challenged by Web 2.0, which is a network of information predicated on the concepts of user interaction and participation. Web 2.0 principles are now the foundation for many new healthcare initiatives that aim to create interactive experiences for patients via a multidimensional, user-centric approach to information sharing.

Advances in social media have been made alongside these developments in Internet and healthcare technologies. Originally, social media was a way for individuals to network with one another; however, the recent progression to Web 2.0 has molded social media into a tool that businesses and organizations can use to interact with the public. Currently, social media offers many benefits for organizations that want to interact with the world around them. Social media technologies come in many forms, including video-sharing websites, such as YouTube, and social networking websites, such as Facebook, Twitter, and LinkedIn.[2] Overall, these social media technologies may have tremendous influence on the public (**Figure 1**). In the United States, approximately 61% of

Dr. Geier or an immediate family member serves as a board member, owner, officer, or committee member of the American Academy of Orthopaedic Surgeons, the American Orthopaedic Society for Sports Medicine, and the South Carolina Medical Association. Dr. Leland or an immediate family member serves as a paid consultant to or is an employee of CONMED Linvatec and Stryker; has received research or institutional support from Stryker; and serves as a board member, owner, officer, or committee member of the American Orthopaedic Society for Sports Medicine and the Arthroscopy Association of North America. Dr. Silverman or an immediate family member is a member of a speakers' bureau or has made paid presentations on behalf of Integra. Dr. Duggal or an immediate family member serves as a board member, owner, officer, or committee member of the American Orthopaedic Foot and Ankle Society. Neither Mr. Suryavanshi nor any immediate family member has received anything of value from or has stock or stock options held in a commercial company or institution related directly or indirectly to the subject of this chapter.

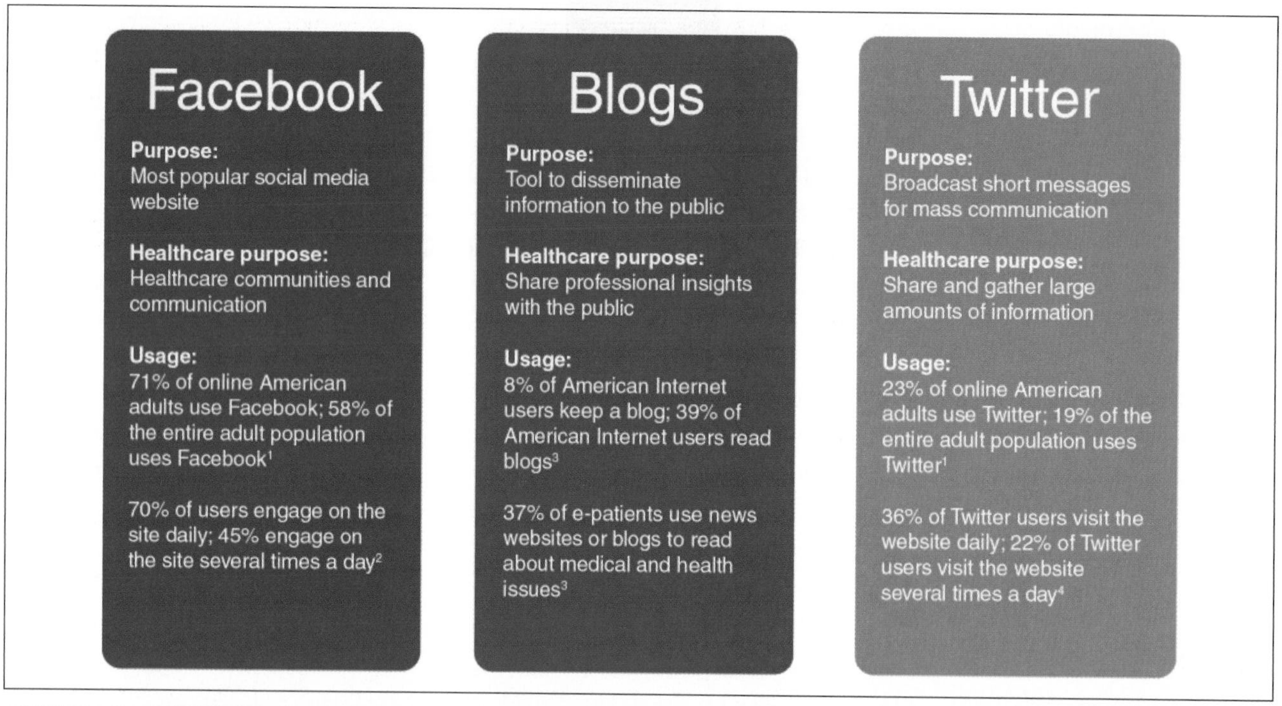

Facebook

Purpose:
Most popular social media website

Healthcare purpose:
Healthcare communities and communication

Usage:
71% of online American adults use Facebook; 58% of the entire adult population uses Facebook[1]

70% of users engage on the site daily; 45% engage on the site several times a day[2]

Blogs

Purpose:
Tool to disseminate information to the public

Healthcare purpose:
Share professional insights with the public

Usage:
8% of American Internet users keep a blog; 39% of American Internet users read blogs[3]

37% of e-patients use news websites or blogs to read about medical and health issues[3]

Twitter

Purpose:
Broadcast short messages for mass communication

Healthcare purpose:
Share and gather large amounts of information

Usage:
23% of online American adults use Twitter; 19% of the entire adult population uses Twitter[1]

36% of Twitter users visit the website daily; 22% of Twitter users visit the website several times a day[4]

Figure 1   Infographic presents an overview of three types of social media, information on their purposes in a normal and healthcare context, as well as their usage statistics.
[1]Duggan M, Ellison NB, Lampe C, Lenhart A, Madden M: Social media update 2014: Demographics of key social networking platforms. Pew Research Center, January 2015. Available at: http://www.pewinternet.org/2015/01/09/demographics-of-key-social-networking-platforms-2. Accessed August 4, 2015.
[2]Duggan M, Ellison NB, Lampe C, Lenhart A, Madden M: Social media update 2014. Pew Research Center, January 2015. Available at: http://www.pewinternet.org/2015/01/09/social-media-update-2014. Accessed August 4, 2015.
[3]Fox S, Purcell K: Chronic disease and the internet: Social media and health. Pew Research Center, March 2010. Available at: http://www.pewinternet.org/2010/03/24/social-media-and-health. Accessed August 4, 2015.
[4]Duggan M, Ellison NB, Lampe C, Lenhart A, Madden M: Social media update 2014: Frequency of social media use. Pew Research Center, January 2015. Available at: http://www.pewinternet.org/2015/01/09/frequency-of-social-media-use-2. Accessed August 4, 2015.

adults report searching online for health information and 39% of adults report using social media, such as Facebook, to search for health information.[3,4] It is clear that social media and Web 2.0 are highly relevant for healthcare patients in current society; however, the value of social media in healthcare from a physician's perspective is a developing topic of research. Thus far, the results have indicated that social media provides substantial value to physicians.

Social Media in Orthopaedics
Opportunities
The benefits of social media technologies in orthopaedics and clinical practice are plentiful. These benefits can be grouped into the broad categories of patient communication and access to healthcare populations.

Patient Communication
Perhaps one of the most obvious and prominent benefits of social media in clinical practice is the potential it has to improve patient communication. Improved patient communication can occur if physicians use social media to disseminate health information to the public or to improve their presence in their community. Blogging, and other social networking services, can be used by physicians to disseminate healthcare information to the public[5] and has the potential to address an unmet need for high-quality healthcare information. Eysenbach and Kohler[6] estimated that approximately 6.5 million health-related search queries occur per day on the Internet. Physician bloggers can satisfy this need for healthcare information by posting their recommendations and thoughts on a blog. Social media allows physicians to suggest approaches and general lifestyle changes for patients who have specific conditions and disease states.[5,7] The patient communication benefits of social media in clinical practice are furthered by the versatility of social media. Social media allows for

    © 2016 AAOS Instructional Course Lectures, Volume 65

the presentation of information in many forms outside of simply text, which has the potential to not only enhance individual patient education but also increase the population size that is able to access the information.

Another important benefit of social media, which emerges from improved patient communication, is the potential for physicians to enhance their physician reputation. Lagu et al[8] identified 33 websites that were dedicated to the user-based rating of physicians, which exemplifies the presence of such websites on the Internet. It is clear that patients often share their opinions of their physicians on social media outlets; physicians who are adept with social media are able to share knowledge, reflect, and debate with patients.[5] Physicians who are aware of online patient opinions now have an opportunity to address and protect their online reputation by providing content that may mitigate any negative information.

Access to Healthcare Populations

The use of social media in clinical practice provides physicians with the ability to access specific healthcare populations. Social media is a vast network that is used by approximately 74% of Internet users,[9] which provides both physicians and clinical researchers with the opportunity to access specific healthcare populations. A multitude of groups and communities exist on the Internet, many of which are relevant to physicians. For example, websites such as www.patientslikeme.com allow patients who have similar illnesses to share their experiences with each other; in addition, many groups have been created via blogs and other social networking websites for individuals with specific illnesses to communicate.[3,10,11] These

groups allow physicians to access specific healthcare populations. For example, treatments or breakthroughs that are relevant to a certain disease are able to be shared by physicians with groups of individuals who have that disease, which allows for the easy dissemination of relevant information.[11] Furthermore, physicians who are specialists are able to reach out to relevant populations, which allows physicians to provide higher quality care where it is needed. This is beneficial for not only the patients who are receiving relevant information, but also the physicians who are able to access healthcare populations that are relevant to their expertise.

In addition to providing benefits in clinical practice, social media also has the potential to enhance the field of clinical research. Social media outlets provide a strong sense of community and interconnectedness.[3,10,11] The formation of communities organizes individuals by specific demographics, which can be used by researchers who are trying to recruit specific individuals for research. For example, a project known as TrialX was launched in 2008 and was designed to connect patients with nearby clinical trial investigators. By making use of social media outlets, namely Twitter, TrialX was able to connect patients with clinical researchers and help the medical research process, which is a key component of the healthcare system.[12]

The Internet is a huge source of data and, likewise, contains large volumes of health-related data. The use of social media in clinical practice allows for the creation of other sources of data that may be useful, such as data from physician rating websites.[8] The data from physician rating websites can be used to improve various aspects of health

care, including physician performance, methods of public medical education, and various public health affairs.[3]

It is clear that there are benefits and incentives for physicians who incorporate social media into their practice; however, the medical community still lags behind in the adoption of these new technologies.[2,13,14] This resistance may be attributed to a variety of concerns that physicians who are skeptical of social media may have because of the confidential nature of their profession. These concerns include the implications of social media on the medical field, the Health Insurance Portability and Accountability Act (HIPAA), and other privacy regulations as well as how social media affects professionalism. These concerns, in combination with physician resistance to social media in health care, likely stem from a lack of time, ignorance of information related to technologies, and worries about privacy issues.

Challenges

There are limitations in and potential problems with incorporating social media into clinical practice. There are several principles that can be used to reduce the barriers and problems associated with social media and clinical practice, such as the concerns with regard to privacy and professionalism as well as the perceived inefficiency of social media in health care.[15]

Privacy and Confidentiality

The first concern that arises if social media is mentioned in clinical practice is the HIPAA and violation of privacy laws.[15] The HIPAA deals with protected health information and outlines limitations for the use of health information.[16] Naturally, the rules of the HIPAA still apply for physicians if social media is incorporated into clinical practice. Fortunately, there are ways to incorporate social media into clinical practice without violating ethical or legal rules. One example, which involves the sharing of photographs by physicians, is called the safe harbor method. This method requires physicians to remove anything that may identify a patient, such as tattoos, birthmarks, or types of personal information, if they are sharing photographs. A variety of factors must be considered to properly deidentify a patient in a photograph.

Professionalism

Professionalism is another relevant concern with regard to social media. Standards of medical professionalism involve putting the interests of the patient above those of the physician.[17] Unfortunately, it may be difficult to determine what this means with respect to the Internet and social media. For example, there are problems that may arise if a physician's social life is merged with his or her professional life, especially if many patients are able to view content that is posted on a physician's personal social media pages. There is much debate on appropriate and inappropriate conduct online because the line between the two is quite difficult to distinguish. Physicians must acknowledge that they are representing their profession when using social media; therefore, social media activities should be conducted in accordance with professional principles.[18]

Blogging

From finding a babysitter to deciding what movie to see, the Internet provides users with hordes of information at the click of a button. Medical information is no different. The old physician reference textbooks now collect dust on a shelf and have been replaced by digital copies that contain ever-changing ideas on best practices, innovative techniques, and scientifically proven data. Sometimes these ideas are shared via medical studies and journals; however, a growing number of medical professionals are turning to less formal options, such as blogs, to disseminate their ideas. The ability of physicians to share professional insights with the use of a more personalized, informal mode of communication is improving the physician-patient relationship. Doctors can always work with patients via more conventional means, such as an office visit or over the phone; however, the ability of physicians to share professional insights through informal methods, such as a blog or in a comments section, is beginning to grow and expand the physician-patient relationship. Blog comments are stated in a more generalized manner because they are not true medical advice; however, they are a means to provide patient education and to help patients make more informed medical decisions. Patients no longer need to take time off of work or pull their child out of school and visit a doctor to obtain more information about a condition. Patients and physicians are connecting via these more informal modes of communication, which helps patients better understand a condition and allows physicians to reach a new clientele who would not have otherwise visited their clinic. Clinic visits after such informal interactions begin with greater levels of trust and knowledge, which allows for a more thorough discussion on the risks and benefits of treatment.

With so many individuals turning to the Internet for answers, it is essential for physicians to pair their physical practice with a digital presence. In addition, because 53% of patients who make online diagnoses talk with a physician about what they found online, it is clear that individuals who are looking for answers also are showing up in the waiting rooms of physicians.[19] Although physicians can provide a great deal of useful information on their website, no forum offers the freedom, spontaneity, or mutualistic benefits quite like a blog.

The unregulated flow of information on the Internet makes it hard for individuals who are seeking information to distinguish more credible sources from less credible sources.[20] In addition, as personal relevance increases or if the knowledge of source credibility is limited, individuals are more motivated to process issue-relevant content.[21] In essence, patients are seeking credible information about relevant health issues because they lack the understanding of a medical professional. Eastin[22] reported that if individuals have little knowledge of online content, then they will perceive information that is attributed to a source with a high level of expertise as more credible than information from a source with less expertise. A blog allows a physician to share credible, trustworthy, and relevant information to the advice-driven public.

It is essential for physicians to provide credible and trustworthy information; however, physicians need to consider the legal and ethical ramifications of the firsthand knowledge they share. The sharing of personal or confidential information online may lead to severe HIPAA violations and revocation of a physician's medical license. The same conventions and limitations that exist in nonelectronic communications should be followed in social media communications.[2] It is essential that every practice develops and adheres to a strict social media policy. Adherence to a social media policy, similar to the adherence to any other employer policy, should be a condition of employment;[23] however, even if attempts are made to follow all the confidentiality obligations, issues can arise if practices are not careful. Sharing a story on social media about a specific procedure that was performed may lead to patient identification through public records. The American Academy of Orthopaedic Surgeons suggests that if blogging medical information, the best practice is to write about composite and/or fictionalized patients or simply obtain patient consent.[23] Ignorance or negligence will not prevent sanctions; therefore, physicians need to be mindful of everything they share on blogs and social media.

A blog also allows physicians the unique ability to collect information from a variety of sources to which they may typically not have access. Blogs are a combination of a website, bulletin board, and e-mail and, thus, are usually one-way and two-ways forms of communication.[24] The amount of participation may vary from session to session and blog to blog, but is determined by the user, not the technology.[25] In a study on the role of Internet-based health information in physician-patient relationships, Ahmad et al[25] reported that physicians often thought that they had to defend their diagnosis or treatment plans if patients came to them with health information they found on the Internet.

There are several best practices to starting and fostering a successful blog. (1) Know the audience of the blog. Write what is relevant to the audience and provide them with consistent developments and insightful content. (2) Respond if someone asks a question, if someone comments on a blog post, or even if someone leaves negative feedback. (3) Collaborate by having former patients or colleagues who are in related industries write a blog post or by contributing a blog post to a former patient's or colleague's website. This will help bring a new audience to the blog and expose knowledge to other readers who may not have otherwise discovered the blog. (4) Be different, and do not just regurgitate what everyone else is saying about the topic. Add personal insights or answer the questions everyone else is avoiding. (5) Follow the rules by not disclosing patient information or writing anything that could be considered a HIPAA violation. If there is uncertainty on whether a particular topic is a violation, it should not be published. (6) Respect others. (7) Separate personal and professional social media accounts. It is wise for solo physicians to create a separate social media account for their practice instead of linking it to a personal social media account.

Health blogging is a great way for physicians to connect with current and prospective patients; however, it is not for everyone. If physicians do not believe they will be able to follow the aforementioned best practices or be able to devote enough time to a blog on a regular basis, then it may not be wise to start a blog. A subpar blog may actually hurt a physician's credibility and steer potential patients away from a practice. Health-orientated blogs from credible sources help improve patient outcomes and the physician-patient relationship. The increased availability of the Internet means that more individuals will have Internet access in the coming years and that these information-driven individuals will continue to discover personal and professional blogs. Physicians should be there to greet them.

Facebook

Founded in 2004, Facebook has grown into one of the biggest and most interactive websites in the world. As of December 31, 2014, Facebook had 1.39 billion people who were monthly active users and 890 million people who were daily active users of Facebook.[26] Although physicians have generally been slow to accept and use social media, they largely maintain a presence in some fashion on Facebook. In a survey on the social media practices of Australian physicians, Brown et al[27] reported that almost three physicians of five (59.9%) used Facebook, which the authors reported to be the social media platform most commonly used by the physicians surveyed. In a survey on the social media practices of 4,033 physicians, Modahl et al[28] reported that 61% of the physicians used Facebook for their personal use, whereas only 15% of the physicians used Facebook for professional purposes.

Although personal uses of Facebook, such as sharing photos and interacting with family and friends, are fairly common for physicians, the use of Facebook for healthcare purposes is growing as more physicians incorporate social media into their daily activities. Physicians who have traditionally been limited to publishing opinions on various topics via academic journals and presentations at medical conferences now have an opportunity to publish on social media platforms such as Facebook.[29-31] There are many benefits for physicians who share information on Facebook. For example, orthopaedic surgeons who specialize in sports medicine can discuss anterior cruciate ligament (ACL) injury prevention programs; joint arthroplasty specialists can weigh in on the pros and cons of different types of exercises after total knee arthroplasty; and orthopaedic surgeons can educate the public on musculoskeletal conditions by sharing information on injuries and treatments in easy-to-understand language. Facebook, like other forms of social media, also allows physicians to interact with other physicians by building professional networks or discussing challenging cases. Physicians can discuss and promote efforts to empower the profession or advocate for change by providing a voice for driving healthcare reforms.[30,31]

Although there are numerous benefits for orthopaedic surgeons who use Facebook, most medical society position statements and journal articles that discuss social media focus on the potential risks. Social media and the increasing role it plays in the lives of people across the world rapidly changes; therefore, it is important for orthopaedic surgeons to understand some basic concerns that currently exist with respect to Facebook (as well as all types of social media) and the concerns that will continue to exist going forward. If orthopaedic surgeons want to discuss a patient's case to obtain advice from other surgeons or to comment on its unusual nature, then they must be careful not to violate patient confidentiality, even unintentionally. Although they do not mention Facebook specifically, both the American Medical Association and the Federation of State Medical Boards recommend that physicians consider separating their social media content into personal efforts and professional efforts.[32,33] The concern that a patient may be able to access information orthopaedic surgeons post on their

personal profiles boils down to professionalism. It is essential and cannot be overemphasized that physicians should demonstrate the same professionalism on Facebook that they exhibit offline.

Increasingly, physicians are faced with patients who send them Facebook friend requests. A survey conducted by Modahl et al[28] found that approximately one-third of physicians reported receiving a friend request from a patient. In addition to concerns on what a patient may see about a physician on his or her personal profile, the Facebook friendship poses a possible conflict for the physician because information in the physician's personal profile may influence future physician-patient interactions.[32]

As social media becomes an integral part of life, it is not surprising that the public is turning to it more often for health-related information. Fox and Duggan[19] reported that approximately one of three American adults uses the Internet as a diagnostic tool. Most individuals who make online diagnoses use search engines, such as Google, to find health information rather than Facebook; however, physicians should be aware of the potential for requests for medical advice from both patients and nonpatients via Facebook.[29] A physician should refrain from discussing the medical care of a patient online, similar to the way in which they would refrain from discussing it in a public setting offline. For example, if a patient asks about his or her weightbearing status on a physician's Facebook page, then the physician should advise the patient to discuss the topic in a proper medical environment, such as the clinic, and document the interaction in the patient's medical record accordingly. Facebook, as well as other social

networking platforms, is not the place to offer specific medical advice.

Twitter

Originally defined as "a short burst of inconsequential information," Twitter has rapidly become one of the world's premier social media platforms and has approximately 300 million monthly users.[34,35] Although physicians have been somewhat slow in their adoption of Twitter, studies have shown a rapid incline in the number of patients who turn to social media for healthcare information. A 2011 poll showed that only 7% of the physicians surveyed had a Twitter account.[36]

Twitter's niche is its emphasis on brevity. Messages posted on Twitter (tweets) are limited to a maximum of 140 characters, which eliminates the paragraphs of information that are sometimes found on other types of social media and forces users to get to the point. Because it may be difficult to get an entire point across in only 140 characters (including spaces), many Twitter users add links to other content on the Internet and embed pictures in their tweets. Similar to the way in which an individual may scan the headlines in a newspaper and read articles that are of interest to them, Twitter users scan tweets and then click on any included links they find appealing.

After a Twitter user opens an account, he or she is immediately directed to his or her main Twitter page and will see a scrolling, reverse chronological list that is populated with the tweets from any individual the user has chosen to follow.[37] Following someone means the account owner is interested in and wants to see what an individual or a group is writing on Twitter. If the user becomes disinterested or no longer wants to see

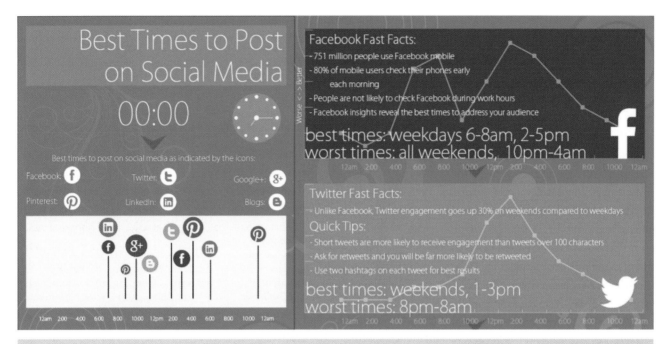

Figure 2   Infographic shows the best times to post on various types of social media. (Reproduced with permission from Bennett S: The best times to post on Facebook, Twitter, Google+, LinkedIn, and Pinterest [Infographic]. *Social Times.* September, 20, 2013. Available at: http://www.adweek.com/socialtimes/social-best-times-post/491030. Accessed July 31, 2015.)

what an individual or a group is tweeting, the user can unfollow the individual or group and will no longer see those tweets on his or her main Twitter page.

There are two types of tweets: original content tweets and re-tweets. Original content tweets may be any text the user wants to tweet, including pictures and links to other webpages. All links and images are condensed down to 20 characters, even if the included link has an extremely long website address. After a user posts a tweet, it appears on his or her main Twitter page and the main Twitter page of any individual who follows that user. In addition, if a user searches for an individual via the "Search Twitter" bar, all of the tweets that individual has posted will be visible. By default, tweets are publicly viewable; however, users can restrict the viewing of their tweets to only those who follow them. Re-tweeting occurs if a user enjoys a tweet by someone else

and decides to tweet it for his or her followers. In this case, the followers of the re-tweeter will see the tweet in its original form on their main page, even if they do not follow the original author.

Another mainstay of Twitter is the hashtag. A hashtag, or "#", is a way to highlight a specific word in a tweet and makes it easier to find in a search. For example, the tweet "Remember to practice #InjuryPrevention drills to decrease the risk of #ACL tears!" would show up in the results if an individual searched Twitter for "#InjuryPrevention" or "#ACL."

Twitter is an extremely effective mode of communication because tweets are disseminated in real time. Even major news networks have teams that monitor Twitter and other social media platforms to look for stories that will appear long before they arrive at the news network via traditional methods.[38] Twitter is frequently used by both large

and small corporations as a marketing tool to publicize information and new research. In medicine, Twitter can be used to make the public aware of newly published research as well as to inform the public of a community health fair or an informational video that has been posted to YouTube by a local physician. The more appealing a tweet, the more likely it is to be re-tweeted and disseminated to a broader audience. Tips to increase the distribution of a tweet include discussing content that is of particular interest to a user's followers and timing the tweet so that it is sent during peak viewing hours (**Figure 2**). Twitter analytics allow users to learn information, such as the geographic distribution, interests, and sex, about their followers. Tweet activity shows users the popularity of their tweets, including how many people viewed each tweet and the engagement rate between a tweet and the individuals who viewed it.

Summary

The use of social media, such as blogging, Facebook, and Twitter, represents new and exciting ways in which the orthopaedic community can communicate with patients and colleagues. It is important for physicians to realize that social media, regardless of the platform, will require engagement and time. Physicians also must be aware of potential pitfalls that are associated with new and evolving forms of patient communication and interaction. The maintenance of professional conduct is just as important in the digital space as it is in the clinical space. The inadvertent disclosure of protected health information and the preservation of patient confidentiality remain important challenges that orthopaedic surgeons must carefully manage.

References

1. Wigand FDL: Adoption of Web 2.0 by Canadian and US governments, in Reddick CG, ed: *Comparative E-Government*. New York, NY, Springer, 2010, p 161-181.

2. Fisher L: Physician participation in social media, in Soyer A, ed: *Social Media in Healthcare: A Primer for Orthopaedic Surgeons*. Rosemont, IL, American Academy of Orthopaedic Surgeons, February 2012, pp 7-9. Available at: http://www3.aaos.org/member/prac_manag/Social_Media_Healthcare_Primer.pdf. Accessed July 30, 2015.

3. Moorhead SA, Hazlett DE, Harrison L, Carroll JK, Irwin A, Hoving C: A new dimension of health care: Systematic review of the uses, benefits, and limitations of social media for health communication. *J Med Internet Res* 2013;15(4):e85.

4. Fox S: The Social Life of Health Information, 2011. Washington, DC, Pew Research Center, May 12, 2011. Available at: http://www.pewinternet.org/2011/05/12/the-social-life-of-health-information-2011. Accessed February 5, 2015.

5. Boulos MN, Maramba I, Wheeler S: Wikis, blogs and podcasts: A new generation of Web-based tools for virtual collaborative clinical practice and education. *BMC Med Educ* 2006;6:41.

6. Eysenbach G, Kohler Ch: What is the prevalence of health-related searches on the World Wide Web? Qualitative and quantitative analysis of search engine queries on the internet. *AMIA Annu Symp Proc* 2003:225-229.

7. Cohen ML: Family medicine meets the blogosphere. *Fam Pract Manag* 2007;14(5):38-40.

8. Lagu T, Hannon NS, Rothberg MB, Lindenauer PK: Patients' evaluations of health care providers in the era of social networking: An analysis of physician-rating websites. *J Gen Intern Med* 2010;25(9):942-946.

9. Pew Research Center: Social networking fact sheet: Highlights of the Pew Internet Project's research related to social networking. Washington, DC, Pew Research Center. Available at: http://www.pewinternet.org/fact-sheets/social-networking-fact-sheet. Accessed March 15, 2015.

10. Sanford AA: "I can air my feelings instead of eating them": Blogging as social support for the morbidly obese. *Communication Studies* 2010;61(5):567-584.

11. Vance K, Howe W, Dellavalle RP: Social internet sites as a source of public health information. *Dermatol Clin* 2009;27(2):133-136, vi.

12. Terry M: Twittering healthcare: Social media and medicine. *Telemed J E Health* 2009;15(6):507-510.

13. Hyman JL, Luks HJ, Sechrest R: Online professional networks for physicians: Risk management. *Clin Orthop Relat Res* 2012;470(5):1386-1392.

14. Spallek H, O'Donnell J, Clayton M, Anderson P, Krueger A: Paradigm shift or annoying distraction: Emerging implications of web 2.0 for clinical practice. *Appl Clin Inform* 2010;1(2):96-115.

15. Antheunis ML, Tates K, Nieboer TE: Patients' and health professionals' use of social media in health care: Motives, barriers and expectations. *Patient Educ Couns* 2013;92(3):426-431.

16. Lifchez SD, McKee DM, Raven RB III, Shafritz AB, Tueting JL: Guidelines for ethical and professional use of social media in a hand surgery practice. *J Hand Surg Am* 2012;37(12):2636-2641.

17. Chretien KC, Kind T: Social media and clinical care: Ethical, professional, and social implications. *Circulation* 2013;127(13):1413-1421.

18. Hawn C: Take two aspirin and tweet me in the morning: How Twitter, Facebook, and other social media are reshaping health care. *Health Aff (Millwood)* 2009;28(2):361-368.

19. Fox S, Duggan M: Health Online 2013. Washington, DC, Pew Research Center. January 15, 2013. Available at: http://www.pewinternet.org/2013/01/15/health-online-2013. Accessed July 30, 2015.

20. Tucher A: Why web warriors might worry. *Columbia Journalism Review* 1997;36(2):35-39.

21. Eagly AH, Chaiken S: *The Psychology of Attitudes*. Fort Worth, TX, Harcourt Brace Jovanovich College Publishers, 1993.

22. Eastin MS: Credibility assessments of online health information: The effects of source expertise and knowledge of content. *Journal of Computer-Mediated Communication* 2001;6(4).

23. Harlow D: Healthcare social media–How to engage online without getting into trouble, in Soyer A, ed: *Social Media in Healthcare: A Primer for Orthopaedic Surgeons*. Rosemont, IL, American Academy of Orthopaedic Surgeons, February 2012, pp 24-27. Available at: http://www3.aaos.org/member/prac_manag/Social_Media_Healthcare_Primer.pdf. Accessed July 30, 2015.

24. Kaye BK: Blog use motivations: An exploratory study, in Tremayne M, ed: *Blogging Citizenship, and the Future of the Media*. New York, NY, Routledge, 2007, pp 127-148.

25. Ahmad F, Hudak PL, Bercovitz K, Hollenberg E, Levinson W: Are physicians ready for patients with Internet-based health information? *J Med Internet Res* 2006;8(3):e22.

26. Facebook.com: Facebook Newsroom: Company Info. http://newsroom. fb.com/company-info. Accessed January 29, 2015.

27. Brown J, Ryan C, Harris A: How doctors view and use social media: A national survey. *J Med Internet Res* 2014;16(12):e267.

28. Modahl M, Tompsett L, Moorhead T: Doctors, Patients & Social Media. QuantiaMD, September 2011. http://www.quantiamd.com/q-qcp/ DoctorsPatientSocialMedia.pdf.

29. George DR, Rovniak LS, Kraschnewski JL: Dangers and opportunities for social media in medicine. *Clin Obstet Gynecol* 2013;56(3):453-462.

30. Vartabedian B: Physicians, risk and opportunity in the digital age. 33 charts, December 12, 2011. Available at: http://33charts.com/2011/12/physicians-risk-opportunity-social-media. html. Accessed February 6, 2015.

31. Vartabedian B: *The Public Physician: Practical Wisdom for Life in a Connected, Always-On World.* Bryan Vartabedian, May 25, 2015.

32. American Medical Association Council on Ethical and Judicial Affairs: Professionalism in the Use of Social Media. November 2010. Available at: https://download.ama-assn.org/ resources/doc/code-medical-ethics/x-pub/9124a.pdf. Accessed February 6, 2015.

33. Federation of State Medical Boards: Model Policy Guidelines for the Appropriate Use of Social Media and Social Networking in Medical Practice. Federation of State Medical Boards of the United States. http:// www.fsmb.org/Media/Default/PDF/ FSMB/Advocacy/pub-social-media-guidelines.pdf. Accessed February 6, 2015.

34. Sarno D: Twitter creator Jack Dorsey illuminates the site's founding document: Part I. Los Angeles Times Blog, February 18, 2009. Available at: http://latimesblogs.latimes.com/ technology/2009/02/twitter-creator. html. Accessed July 30, 2015.

35. Keach S: Instagram now has more users than Twitter. TrustedReviews. com, December 12, 2014. Available at: http://www.trustedreviews.com/ news/instagram-now-has-more-users-than-twitter. Accessed July 30, 2015.

36. McGowan BS, Wasko M, Vartabedian BS, Miller RS, Freiherr DD, Abdolrasulnia M: Understanding the factors that influence the adoption and meaningful use of social media by physicians to share medical information. *J Med Internet Res* 2012;14(5):e117.

37. Johnson S: How Twitter will change the way we live. Time, June 5, 2009. Available at: http:// content.time.com/time/magazine/ article/0,9171,1902818,00.html. Accessed July 30, 2015.

38. Mills A, Chen R, Lee J, Rao RH: Web 2.0 emergency applications: How useful can Twitter be for emergency response? *Journal of Information Privacy and Security* 2009;5(3):3-26.

Index

Page numbers with *f* indicate figures
Page numbers with *t* indicate tables

A

© 2016 AAOS Instructional Course Lectures, Volume 65

© 2016 AAOS Instructional Course Lectures, Volume 65

© 2016 AAOS Instructional Course Lectures, Volume 65

fracture-specific implants, 173–174
glenoid baseplate fixation, 131–132
hemiarthroplasty versus, 161–162, 172, 174
humeral fixation, 130–131
humeral stem retention in, 136*f*
implant design, 159–160
indications, 172–173
emerging, 160
historical, 157–158
modularity of, 136–137
procedure, 161*f*, 165*f*, 171–177
range of motion, 135–136
stem removal, 137*f*
surgical approaches, 174–175
trauma and, 171–179
Reverse total shoulder arthroplasty (RTSA), 104, 116–121, 145
complications, 117–121, 118*t*
acromial fractures, 120, 121*f*
implant disassembly, 120–121
incidence of, 117–118, 118*t*
instability, 119–120
scapular notching, 118–119, 118*f*, 119*t*, 147–156, 148*t*
Grammont-style, 145–146
hemiarthroplasty versus, 104–105
imaging, 116
implant survival, 147–149
indications, 116
periprosthetic infections, 121–123
preoperative evaluation, 116
surgical technique, 116–117
UHMWPE in, 458
Revised Cardiac Risk Index (RCRI), 477, 478
Rheumatoid arthritis (RA)
DVT incidence and, 503
perioperative management of, 497–508, 503*t*
preoperative assessment, 499
rehabilitation, 503–504
reverse shoulder arthroplasty and, 164–165
surgical sequence, 498–499
timing of intervention, 498–499
total shoulder arthroplasty for, 165
Rip-stop effect/construct, 95, 96*f*
Risk factors
modifiable, 202–208
stratifying patients, 208
Robinson classification, 188, 188*f*
Robotic-assisted surgery, learning curves and, 634–635
Rockwood classification, 189–190
Ropivacaine
outpatient arthroplasty, 534, 540
pain management using, 213
Rotator cuff
arthropathy
biomechanical aspects, 128–130
imbalance, 138
severe, 158*f*
shoulder arthroplasty and, 157–158

repair
arthroscopic, 83–92
augmentation in, 95, 102
muscle transfers, 102–103
scaffold devices, 96–97
tendon transfers, 102
tears
arthroplasty for, 103–105
patient characteristics, 103–104
physical examination, 104
resurfacing/hemiarthroplasty, 104
arthroscopic repair, 83–92
débridement, 89
economic effects of, 83–84
full-thickness, 87–89
imaging, 85–86
massive
treatment of, 93–108
tricks in repair of, 93–95
without arthropathy, 162, 163*f*
massive irreparable, 89
partial-thickness, 86–87, 87*f*
patient evaluation, 84
physical examination, 84
postoperative rehabilitation, 89–90
severe, 139*f*
size of, 86–89
symptoms of, 84
tests for, 84–85
transtendinous, 87
Rotator Cuff Quality of Life (RC-QOL) Questionnaire, 578, 580

S

Sagittal balance, 275, 276*f*
Salter-Harris fractures, 346, 382
Scaffold devices
evaluation of, 96–97
in rotator cuff repair, 96–97, 98*t*–101*t*
Scandinavian ACL Registry, 598
Scaphoid fractures, pediatric, 350*f*
Scapular
neck, osseous defect, 146
notching, 118–119, 118*f*, 119*t*, 147–156, 148*t*, 159
avoidance of, 149–150
classification of, 118–119, 118*f*, 146, 147*f*
etiology, 146
implant survival and, 147–149
incidence of, 119*t*, 146, 159
predictors of, 149–150
rate of, 146, 148*t*
Sirveaux grades, 118*f*, 146, 147*f*
winging, 427*f*
Scar formation, outcomes and, 367
Sciatic nerve neurapraxia, 442–443
Selective laser sintering, 460–461
Sentinel events, 272, 602
Sepsis, postoperative, 524, 525
Sex
ankle distraction outcomes and, 314–317

© 2016 AAOS Instructional Course Lectures, Volume 65